Non-Neoplastic Hematopathology and Infections

NON-NEOPLASTIC HEMATOPATHOLOGY AND INFECTIONS

Hernani D. Cualing, MD

Associate Professor, Department of Pathology and Cell Biology
University of South Florida, College of Medicine
Medical Director, IHCFLOW, Inc., Lutz, FL

Parul Bhargava, MD

Assistant Professor of Pathology, Harvard Medical School
Medical Director, Hematology, Coagulation & Flow Cytometry
Beth Israel Deaconess Medical Center, Boston, MA

Ramon L. Sandin, MD

Professor, Oncological Sciences & Pathology, University of South Florida
Medical Director, Clinical Microbiology & Virology
Moffitt Cancer Center and Research Institute, Tampa, FL

⟨JW⟩WILEY-BLACKWELL

A John Wiley & Sons, Inc., Publication

Published by John Wiley & Sons, Inc., Hoboken, New Jersey
Published simultaneously in Canada

For general information on our other products and services or for technical support, please contact our Customer Care Department within the United States at (800) 762-2974, outside the United States at (317) 572-3993 or fax (317) 572-4002.

Wiley also publishes its books in a variety of electronic formats. Some content that appears in print may not be available in electronic formats. For more information about Wiley products, visit our web site at www.wiley.com.

Library of Congress Cataloging-in-Publication Data:

ISBN: 9780470646007

Printed in Singapore

10 9 8 7 6 5 4 3 2 1

I dedicate this book to my beloved family: Rawia, Kareem, Phillip, and Andrew; to my teachers and students; and to my native and adopted country, the Philippines and USA.

HERNANI D. CUALING, MD

To my hematology gurus Dr A Bagg, Dr M Kadin, Dr T Singh and my students for the inspiration and to my husband Pankaj, my daughters Kaveri & Kimya for their unyielding support through the perspiration.

PARUL BHARGAVA, MD

To Mayra, my wife, and Beatriz, my daughter, who constitute the pillars of inspiration and strength in my life!

RAMON L. SANDIN, MD

CONTENTS

CHAPTER **SEVENTEEN**

Mixed Lymph Node Patterns: Stromal and Histiocytic Reactions, NonInfectious   **375**

Hernani D. Cualing

CHAPTER TWENTY

**Mixed Patterns: Emergent/Tropical
Infections with Characterized
Lymphadenopathy**   **447**

Hernani D. Cualing

CONTRIBUTORS

Stephen D. Allen, MD
James Warren Smith Professor of Clinical
  Microbiology
Professor, Department of Pathology and Laboratory
  Medicine
Indiana University School of Medicine
Indiana University Health
Indianapolis, IN

Ernesto Ayala, MD
Assistant Professor
Bone Marrow Transplant Division, Department of
  Oncologic Science
Moffitt Cancer Center and Research Institute
Tampa, FL

Parul Bhargava, MD
Medical Director, Hematology Laboratory at Beth
  Israel Deaconess Medical Center
Assistant Professor
Beth Israel Deaconess Medical Center—Needham
  Campus
Member of Harvard Medical Faculty Physicians
  (HMFP)
Boston, MA

Jeremy W. Bowers, MD
Hematopathology Fellow
Department of Hematopathology and Laboratory
  Medicine
Moffitt Cancer Center and Research Institute
Department of Pathology and Cell Biology
University of South Florida, College of Medicine
Tampa, FL

Sheldon Campbell, MD, PhD, FCAP
Department of Laboratory Medicine
Yale University School of Medicine
Pathology and Laboratory Medicine
VA Connecticut, West Haven, CT

Hernani D. Cualing, MD
Joint Associate Professor, Department of Pathology
  and Cell Biology
University of South Florida, College of Medicine
Medical Director, IHCFLOW, Inc.
Consultant Hematopathologist, Specialty:
  Hematopathology, Cutaneous Lymphomas, and
  Imaging Science
Post-Director of Hematopathology
  Fellowship-Moffitt Cancer Center and Research
  Institute

Shohreh Iravani Dickinson, MD
Assistant Professor, Moffitt Cancer Center and
  Research Institute, Department of Pathology and
  Cell Biology, University of South Florida, COM
Anatomic Pathologist and Hematopathologist

Jason C. Ford, MD, FRCP(C)
Head, Division of Hematopathology, Children's
  and Women's Health Centre of BC
Associate Professor, Faculty of Medicine
University of British Columbia
BC, Canada

Lynne Garcia, MS, MT, FAAM
Clinical Microbiologist
Director, LSG & Associates, Santa Monica, CA

Gary Hellermann, PhD
Assistant Professor
Division of Allergy and Immunology
Department of Internal Medicine
University of South Florida College of Medicine
Tampa, FL

Vandita Johari, MD
Department of Pathology
Division of Clinical Pathology
Director, Hematology Laboratory and Flow
  Cytometry
Assistant Professor of Pathology
Tufts University School of Medicine

Lija Joseph, MD
Staff Hematopathologist
Lowell General Hospital
Adjunct Associate Professor
Boston University School of Medicine
Boston, MA

Loveleen C. Kang, MD
Associate Professor
Department of Pathology
University of South Florida
College of Medicine
Staff Pathologist
James A. Haley VAMC
Tampa, FL

Walid E. Khalbuss, MD, PhD, FIAC
Associate Professor
Director of Cytopathology-UPMC Shadyside
  Hospital
Department of Pathology
University of Pittsburgh Medical Center (UPMC)
UPMC-Shadyside, Pittsburgh, PA, USA

Rebecca Levy, MD
Department of Pathology
Baystate Medical Center
Springfield, MA, USA

Jun Mo, MD
Associate Professor
Pediatric Hematopathology
Division of Pathology
Cincinnati Children's Hospital Medical Center
Cincinnati, OH, USA

Sara E. Monaco, MD
Assistant Professor
Director of Fine Needle Aspiration Biopsy
  Service-UPMC Children's Hospital
  of Pittsburgh
Department of Pathology
University of Pittsburgh Medical Center (UPMC)
UPMC-Shadyside, Pittsburgh, PA, USA

Taiga Nishihori, MD
Assistant Member
Department of Blood and Marrow Transplantation
Moffitt Cancer Center, Tampa, FL

Tal Oren, MD, PhD
Department of Pathology
Stamford Hospital
Suffern, NY, USA

Liron Pantanowitz, MD
Associate Professor
Director of Fine Needle Aspiration Clinic-UPMC
  Shadyside Hospital
Department of Pathology
University of Pittsburgh Medical Center (UPMC)
UPMC-Shadyside, Pittsburgh, PA, USA

Deniz Peker, MD
Clinical Fellow, Hematopathology Fellowship
  Program
Moffitt Cancer Center and Research Institute
Department of Pathology and Cell Biology
University of South Florida College of Medicine

Ramon L. Sandin, MD, MS, FCAP, ABP–MM
Clinical Pathologist
Medical Director, Clinical Microbiology and
  Virology
Senior Member and Professor Department of
  Hematopathology and Laboratory Medicine,
  and Blood and Marrow Transplant Program
Moffitt Cancer Center

Betram Schnitzer, MD
Professor Department of Pathology
University of Michigan Ann Arbor
Ann Arbor, MI

James W. Smith, MD
Nordschow Professor Emeritus
of Tropical Medicine
Van Nuys Medical Science
Former Chair Dept. of Pathology & Laboratory
Medicine
Indiana Univ. School of Medicine
Indianapolis, Indiana

Raul E. Villanueva, MD
Clinical Pathologist
Puget Sound Institute of Pathology
Seattle, WA

Dr. Reza Setoodeh, MD
Department of Pathology and Cell
Biology

University of South Florida College
of Medicine

Ling Zhang, MD
Assistant Professor
Hematopathologist
Department of Hematopathology and Laboratory
Medicine
Moffitt Cancer Center and Research Institute
Department of Pathology and Cell Biology,
USF

Xiaohui Zhang, MD, PhD
Resident-Fellow, Hematopathology Fellowship
Moffitt Cancer Center and Department of Pathology
and Cell Biology
University of South Florida College of Medicine

FOREWORD

Many years ago, when I began my residency in pathology, there seemed to be few, if any, textbooks dealing exclusively with the topic of hematopathology. The general pathology texts then available usually contained only short, cursory chapters on lymph node and bone marrow findings in such diseases as lymphomas and leukemias. However, only multiple rudimentary classifications of these two neoplastic disease entities were described. Ever since the AFIP fascicle on *Classification of Lymphomas* by Dr. Henry Rappaport appeared in 1966, however, numerous books on the subject of hematopathology have been published.

With the exception of the now out-of-date multiple-volume set by William St. Clair Symmers, there are, to my knowledge, no other textbooks combining the fields of hematopathology and Western or tropical infectious diseases. Now, in this book, Dr. Cualing and his fellow contributors have successfully combined these two areas of expertise.

The current volume is especially timely in this era of globalization when people from all over the world travel into our midst, bringing with them diseases that we are unfamiliar with. In other instances, pathologists from other countries send slides for consultation from patients who have a variety of disorders. Thus, more than ever, there is a pressing need for the development of a closer interaction between hematopathology and microbiology in the investigation of infectious and benign reactive diseases particularly those involving lymph nodes, blood, and bone marrow. This book has as its mission the integration of these two disciplines leading to further collaboration and understanding between hematopathologists and microbiologists.

Bertram Schnitzer, MD

PREFACE

This book explores new material at the nexus of hemic-lymphatic manifestations of Western and tropical infectious diseases. It attempts to expand on the classic descriptions of the reactive and inflammatory manifestations of infectious diseases in blood and other related organs. Because many agents seek entry and circulate in blood and lymphatic system, the book begins with the basics of hematology and follows with blood-borne infections. It adds in a survey of patterns of reactions in blood and lymph nodes and ends with hematopathology of bone marrow transplantation. Many of the agents of infections diseases, in addition to human to human transmission, are zoonotic, use a number of vectors, and hence epidemiologic and geographic aspects are included. Upon entry, a number of these agents commandeer blood elements including lymphocytes and macrophages as mobile shuttles. Both blood and lymphatic disorders are therefore elaborated since direct effect by these agents cause red cell, platelets, leucocytes, and tissue immunologic disorders. All these disorders are illustrated with pictures, tables, descriptive and text; illustrated as well are the range of non-neoplastic hematologic disorders, and reactive patterns of noninfectious and infectious agents, and the blood and lymphatic manifestations of familiar infections and the more common infections in the tropics. The epidemiology, pathobiology, and clinical and pathologic manifestations in blood and lymphatic organs as well as the approach to diagnosis, treatment, and prognosis are described. For uniformity of terminology, the book includes WHO-endorsed diagnostic codes based on the International Classification of Disease (ICD-10). Since many infectious agents are also of tropical origin, and since the vast majority of these agents infect a large segment of the world, including transient travelers and immigrants, this book incorporates diseases found in both Western and Eastern Hemispheres. Additionally the microscopic criteria as well as the molecular and laboratory tests provided in this code should prove useful information even for laboratories practicing in resource limited settings besides those with access to modern diagnostic modalities.

We divided the book into four parts. Part I provides an overview of non-neoplastic hematology, Part II addresses blood-borne infections, Part III covers patterns seen in noninfectious and infectious lymphadenopathies, including those commonly seen in tropical countries as well as cytomorphologic findings of reactive adenopathies, and Part IV deals with hematopathologic issues of bone marrow transplantation associated with common and rare infections. We begin the book with a section on the basics of hematology and diagnosis based on peripheral blood findings, then go on to infections related to hematopathology, followed by tissue and pattern-based diagnosis, and finally cover the basics of bone marrow transplantation. In tissue, we proffer an approach using low-power recognition of the histology patterns and proceed from there. The basics of hematology written by practicing experts in the field is completely and succintly covered in Part I, detailing issues on leucocytes, platelets, and red cells disorders including thalassemias. Part II covers blood-borne infections written by well-known practicing microbiologists and includes apicomplexas, flagellates, protobacterias, and fungal infections. In Part III, practicing hematopathologists discuss the issue of reactive lymphadenopathy and present a table detailing the entities under the classic four patterns: follicular, diffuse, sinus, and mixed patterns. The premise for this approach is that knowledge of the salient morphologic findings, the constellation of clinical presentation, the geographic or epidemiological background of the patient, and the key laboratory and the morphologic manifestations will help in arriving at a correct diagnosis. In other words, we begin at the beginning: approach a disease from what we all see under the microscope.

The difficulty in diagnosing reactive lymphadenopathy rivals, if not exceeds, that of the lymphomas. The case of recognizing a reactive lymph node belies its complexity, and contributes to the generally nonchalant attention it receives compared to its malignant cousin. Just as in the case of lymphomas, there is an approach that makes sense of these numerous complexities as well as a framework to formulate diagnoses. Historically the many ways to classify lymphadenopathies has been hindered by the artifice of easy understanding and simple diagnosis. Partly to blame is the notion that "it is just benign, who cares what kind" until the lymphoma is mistaken for a benign diagnosis, or a treatable infection, or one that is highly contagious is missed. Often the lack of clinical history compounds the limited microscopic window that a pathologist initially sees. Hence we use the approach of hematopathologists: we widen the microscopic window to observe what are the pitfalls, the clinical milieu, and the subtle histologic features that differentiate rival entities.

Non-neoplastic hematopathology is a difficult diagnosis not only because of the reactive lymph node's mimicry of lymphomas but also because the field has received less studious attention than its neoplastic counterpart. Inherently, reactive lymph nodes are also difficult to diagnose because lymph nodes, upon stimulation, display a dynamic variability that depends on the patient's age, immune status, phase or duration of reaction, and whether the etiology is infectious or noninfectious. About 30 to 40% of reactive lymph nodes have specific histologic features leading to a definite diagnosis: features in histology suggest a pattern that requires ancillary serology, phenotypic, or serologic tests that may lead to a specific diagnosis. The rest of lymph nodes seen in pathology practice may show a nonspecific histology, but its pattern needs to be stated to initiate a pattern-based differential diagnosis. Even for a nonspecific reactive hyperplasia, such as a mixed follicular and paracortical reaction, diagnosis is important because of the implicit concern for a lymphoma is considered and not favored. A specific reactive lymphadenopathy diagnosis, when suggested by a constellation of clues, needs to be given so that confirmatory tests can be performed. A diagnosis of infection would impel a therapy to commence, surveillance made for endemic and communicable disease, and malignancy ruled out.

We also take a lesson from a *Family Circus* cartoon by Bil Keane: kids looking over an adult reading a book say *"Grown-up books are harder to read … they make you think up your own pictures!!!"* by incorporating many color pictures. We try to fill in with more guideposts a map of non-neoplastic hematopathology that is already dotted with classic landmarks. We are indebted to hematopathology pioneers who described reactive lymphadenopathy and its classic patterns. Bertram Schnitzer (1992) and Lawrence Weiss (2008). As we extend their work into the realm of the infectious diseases, we are indeed navigating a wondrous *terra incognita* as the fictional sailors of Lewis Carroll: We hope the readers will be as excited to fill in the blanks.

He had brought a large map representing the sea,
Without the least vestige of land:
And the crew were much pleased when they found it to be
A map they could all understand.
 … "Other maps are such shapes, with their islands and
  capes!
But we've got our brave Captain to thank"
(So the crew would protest) "that he's brought us the
  best —
A perfect and absolute blank!"
L. Carroll, *Fit the Second, the Hunting of the Snark*

Hernani D. Cualing
Parul Bhargava
Ramon L. Sandin

ACKNOWLEDGMENTS

We, at the onset, would like to express our gratitude to the staff of Wiley-Blackwell Publishers, and especially to our ever gracious medical editor, Thom Moore. We also thank Ian Collins, Editorial Assistant, Dean Gonzalez, Illustration Manager, and Danielle Lacourciere, Senior Production Editor, Maude Akagi and James Hastings of Wiley, as well as Gowri Vasanthkumar of Laserwords, India for their labor and patience in converting our texts to a book as flawless as possible. Since we may not be able to thank all the staff who made this book possible, we ask leave for not including everyone. I would also like to thank my former mentors who started me on the path to hematopathology: Dr. Jen Lin of New York and Drs. Dick Neiman and Atillio Orazi, formerly of Indianapolis, where I had my hematopathology fellowship. Since that time, I collected microscopic slides intending to use them and during my stint as faculty of University of Cincinnati, under Dr. Roger Smith and Dr. Fenoglio-Preiser, for teaching: my first cases of lymph node dirofilariasis and leishmaniasis of bone marrow came from that fellowship and were augmented with pearls to many slide boxes of reactive lymphadenopathies over the years. For the book, additionally would like to thank the following persons and are indebted for their contributions of images, comments, and suggestions.

We are indebted to Dr. Betram Schnitzer for his support and for his endorsement of the book. Much of our tropical infectious digital images were provided by Dr. Wun-Ju Shieh, of the Infectious Diseases Pathology Branch, Division of High-Consequence Pathogens and Pathology, National Center for Emerging and Zoonotic Infectious Diseases, Centers for Disease Control and Prevention at Atlanta, and we could not thank him and his colleagues enough. Dr. Elmer Koneman, a foremost microbiologist, provided us with rare images of infections in tissues, and we also appreciate his comments on materials to include at the front of the book. We thank Dr. Rito Zerpa Larrauri of Servicio de Microbiología, Instituto Nacional de Salud del Niño, Lima, Peru for blood and tissue images of leprosy, bartonellosis, and mycobacteria. We would also like to thank Karen Goraleski, Executive Director of the American Society of Tropical Medicine and Hygiene for allowing us to use digital images of tropical diseases from Dr. Herman Zaiman collections. We are encouraged by the vision and thrust of the ASTMH and support their mission to educate and publish on tropical medicine of widespread emergent or neglected tropical infections. We thank Dr. Fabio Fachetti of the Department of Pathology Spedali Civili-University of Brescia, Italy, for the image of CD123 and for personal communication on plasmacytoid monocytes and lymphadenopathies. We additionally are indebted to Dr. James Smith of Indiana University Medical Center, to Dr. Rodney C. Arcenas of Holywood, Florida, for reviewing most of the manuscript, to Dr. Ronald Jaffe of Pittsburgh Children's Hospital, to Kathy White of Boston Medical Center, and to Dr. J. Ford of Children's Hospital, Vancouver, Canada. We thank Rodney C. Arcenas PhD, Ardeshir Hakam MD of Mofffitt Cancer Center, Antonio Hernandez MD of Quest Dx/Ameripath Center for Advanced Diagnostics, and Dr. Steve Shaw of NIH/NCI for providing scholarly materials discussing the paracortical cords. We also thank Dr. Steve Swerdlow, chief hematopathologist at the University of Pittsburg, for sharing digital images of CML lymphadenitis. We thank Dr. Gary Hellerman for facilitation of email communications at the beginning of the project and for editing parts of the manuscript and also Gary Bentley for helping with line art figures as well as to Dr. Peter Banks for his images on Herpes simplex Lymphadenitis. We are indebted to Ms. Malou Domingo of Manila, the Philippines, for research in tropical pathology and to Dr. Sharon Villanueva of Kyushu University Fukuoka, Japan, for articles on leptospirosis and to Philip Yassin-Cualing, for research and editing work.

Hernani D. Cualing
Lutz, Florida

INTRODUCTION

ROLE OF THE HEMATOPATHOLOGIST

The hematopathologist has a vital role in the laboratory. The hematopathologist functions as both a consultant and diagnostician in anatomic and laboratory medicine evaluations of a clinical pathology nature. In the evaluation of specimen that come to the clinical laboratory medicine, including tissue, blood, and fluids, the hematopathologists act as both a teacher and consultant to residents, clinician practitioners, medical students, and other community practitioners. Often it is the hematopathologist who is charged with arriving at a hematopathology related diagnosis.

In anatomic pathology a thorough hematopathology assessment includes evaluations of lymph node, skin, spleen, thymus, and extranodal flare-ups suggesting lymphoma or leukemia. A classic description of both noninfectious and infectious pattern of lymphadenopathy is included as groundwork for formulating a diagnosis. "Wet" hematology consists of evaluations of peripheral blood smears, body fluids, and the bone marrow, and knowledge of non-neoplastic disorders is a crucial step in further evaluating infectious disorders that target the blood and blood vessels. Hematologic manifestations of infectious agents as well as blood-borne diseases are a critical consideration in the formulation of a diagnosis. This book addresses the need to have the work of the hematopathologist closely integrated with that of the microbiologists and infectious disease practitioners, in evaluating infections from tissue and blood specimens.

When tissue is procured for diagnosis, the clinician, the anatomic pathologist, the cytopathologist, the microbiologist, and the hematopathologist should act as a team to ensure correct handling and processing of the specimen. Along with the need for ancillary tests like flow cytometry, clonality, or molecular cytogenetic studies, specimen portions for culture or direct smears should be processed when they are still fresh and uncontaminated in order to optimize handling and lead to a correct diagnosis. More and more evident is that hematopathologic diseases are related to immune and infectious etiology. In pediatric hospitals, disease patterns suggest congenital and immune reactions. In centers where chemotherapy and organ transplantations are performed, patients are at high risk of contracting infections and hematologic manifestations of infections.

The global economy and the global information superhighway have made people of distant lands neighbors. Hence more and more of the specimens that the hematopathologists see come from across the seas. The differential diagnosis widens to include exotic infectious diseases beyond the typical diseases found in the Western Hemisphere.

This book addresses the confluence of hematopathology and infectious diseases. To the clinicians as well as to medical personnel seeing patients from abroad, the role of hematopathologists extend beyond regional or locally based diagnosis. Today's perplexing disorders include lymphadenopathy, splenomegaly, hemorrhagic fever, unexplained cytopenias, petechiae, and skin rashes associated with common and rare infections. Knowledge of the salient morphologic findings, the constellation of clinical presentation, the geographic or epidemiological background of the patient, and the key laboratory and the morphologic manifestations can help in arriving at a correct diagnosis.

ORGANIZATION OF THE TEXT

The text is divided into four parts. Part I provides an overview of non-neoplastic hematology, Part II addresses blood-borne infections, Part III covers patterns seen in noninfectious and infectious lymphadenopathies, including those commonly seen in tropical countries as well as cytomorphologic findings of reactive adenopathies, and Part IV deals with hematopathologic issues of bone marrow transplantation. In almost all chapters, we included ICD-10 codes (International Classification of Diseases) to advance use of common terminologies.

AIMS AND SCOPE

Our objective is to present new material on hemic-lymphatic diseases, with a view toward their infectious manifestations. The studies in this book expand on the classic descriptions of reactive and inflammatory expressions of infectious diseases in blood and lymph nodes. The many infectious diseases that enter and circulate in blood and the lymphatic system produce patterns of reactions. We attempt to elucidate these patterns, and additionally epidemiologic and geographic factors where the agents of disease are zoonotic and can use a number of vectors. Upon entry some more pernicious agents commandeer lymphocytes and macrophages as mobile shuttles and cause blood and lymphatic disorders. Their direct effects on red cells, platelets, leucocytes, immunologic disorders are elaborated with pictures and tables, and likewise are treated herein the reactive patterns of agents of common infectious and noninfectious diseases. The various diseases' epidemiology, pathobiology, and clinical and pathologic expressions in blood and lymphatic organs are described as well as approaches to diagnoses, treatments, and prognoses. Because many infectious agents are from tropical regions that infect many peoples worldwide, via transient travelers and immigrants, we also cover diseases found at these latitudes of the Eastern and Western Hemispheres.

PART I

NON-NEOPLASTIC HEMATOLOGY

CHAPTER ONE

NON-NEOPLASTIC DISORDERS OF WHITE BLOOD CELLS

Rebecca A. Levy, Vandita P. Johari, and Liron Pantanowitz

OVERVIEW OF WBC PRODUCTION AND FUNCTION

Frequently the first test that suggests an imbalance or disturbance in hematopoiesis is the complete blood count (CBC). The CBC is a simple blood test that is ordered frequently. It may pick up incidental abnormalities or may yield a diagnosis of suspected abnormalities. The CBC is a count of multiple blood components and qualities, and can include a differential of the white blood cells (WBCs). The CBC can suggest infection, inflammatory processes, and malignant processes. Typically a peripheral blood smear and rarely a buffy coat (concentrated white blood cells) are analyzed to help determine a diagnosis (Efrati, 1960). A differential WBC assigns leukocytes to their specific categories as a percentage or absolute count. Manual differential counts tend to be accurate but imprecise, whereas automated counts are fairly precise but sometimes inaccurate (Bain, 2002). It may occasionally be necessary to evaluate both the bone marrow and blood smear to evaluate the quality and quantity of the blood lineages. WBC disorders are classified into quantitative and qualitative conditions, reflecting changes in their number and function, respectively (Stiene-Martin, 1998). This chapter discusses both nonneoplastic quantitative and qualitative disorders of WBCs.

Leukocytes

Hematopoeisis

Hematopoiesis occurs in different parts of the body, depending on the age of the embryo, child, or adult. Initially blood cell formation of the embryo occurs within the yolk sac, in blood cell aggregates called blood islands. As development progresses, the hematopoiesis location changes, and the spleen and liver become the primary sites. As bone marrow develops, it usurps the task of blood cell formation and becomes the site for trilineage hematopoiesis. The bone marrow contains pluripotent stem cells, which can develop into any of the blood cells, including granulocytes, monocytes, and lymphocytes, in response to specific stimulating factors (Andrews, 1994). Several white blood cells (leukocytes) are depicted in Figure 1.1. Maturation, activation, and some proliferation of lymphoid cells occur in secondary lymphoid organs, including the spleen, liver, and lymph nodes. Extramedullary hematopoiesis can take place in the liver, thymus, and spleen and may lead to organomegaly. There is a common myeloid progenitor cell called the CFU-GEMM (Colony-Forming Unit-Granulocyte–Erythroid-Macrophage-Megakaryocyte) that leads to the development of granulocytic, monocytic, eosinophilic, basophilic, erythrocytic, and megakaryocytic precursors.

Non-Neoplastic Hematopathology and Infections, First Edition. Edited by Hernani D. Cualing, Parul Bhargava, and Ramon L. Sandin.
© 2012 Wiley-Blackwell. Published 2012 by John Wiley & Sons, Inc.

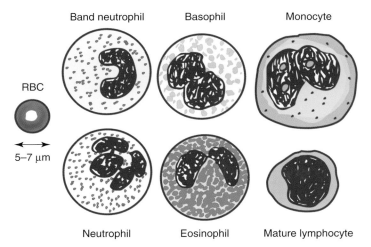

FIGURE 1.1 **Schematic drawings of different white blood cells shown in relation to an erythrocyte**. The band neutrophil (10–18 μm) is characterized by a deeply indented nucleus and secondary granules. The segmented neutrophil (10–15 μm) has 2 to 5 nuclear lobes (4 depicted) connected by thin filaments and contains several cytoplasmic secondary (specific) granules. The basophil (10–15 μm) contains a segmented nucleus and many coarse, dense granules of varying size (that may obscure the nucleus). The eosinophil (10–15 μm) has a bilobed nucleus and cytoplasm filled with coarse, uniform granules. The monocyte (12–20 μm) has an indented nucleus and abundant gray cytoplasm with sparse granules. The presence of nucleoli indicates that this is an immature monocyte (promonocyte). The mature lymphocyte (7–15 μm) has a high nuclear:cytoplasmic ratio (4:1), slightly notched nucleus with dense clumpy chromatin and no nucleolus, and only moderate agranular cytoplasm.

Leukocytosis

Leukocytosis is defined as a total WBC count that is greater than two standard deviations above the mean, or a value >11,000/μL in adults. While leukocytosis is mainly due to a neutrophilia, it may reflect an increase in any of the other leukocytes. Patients with hyperleukocytosis, which is defined as a white cell count (WCC) >100,000/μL, may manifest with hyperviscosity (or so-called symptomatic hyperleukocytosis). The development of symptoms of hyperviscosity syndrome are often correlated with the underlying cause (e.g., hyperproteinemia, erythocytosis, hyperleukocytosis, and thrombocytosis) and is a medical emergency mainly seen with leukemia in blast crisis. The severity of hyperleukocytosis is related to the underlying disorder; hyperviscosity is typically evident in AML with a WCC of >100,100/μL, in ALL with a WCC of >250,000/μL, and in CLL with a WCC of 500,000/μL (Adams, 2009; Rampling, 2003). Spurious leukocytosis can occur because of platelet clumping, increased nucleated erythrocytes, or in cryoglobulinemia (Savage, 1984; Patel, 1987).

Leukemoid Reaction

Leukemoid reaction is used to describe leukocytosis above 50,000/μL. This is usually characterized by a significant increase in early neutrophil precursors including band forms (Figure 1.2). Infants with Down

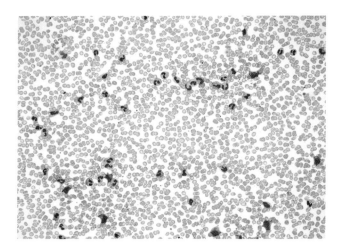

FIGURE 1.2 **Leukemoid reaction observed in a peripheral blood smear**. Notice the significant increase in early neutrophil precursors and band forms in addition to segmented neutrophils.

syndrome may have transient leukemoid reactions (Brodeur, 1980).

Granulocytes

Granulocytes have a single progenitor cell, the myeloblast, that can differentiate into neutrophils, eosinophils, and basophils (Lawrence, 1998). The differentiation process is based on the presence of certain stimulating factors. Neutrophils are the first responders to infection or inflammation, and they respond to cytokines such as interleukin-8 (IL-8), interferon gamma (IFN-gamma), and C5a (Witko-Sarsat, 2000). These chemicals direct the neutrophils migration to areas of need.

Maturation Process

Neutrophils undergo a maturation process as they shift from myeloblasts, to promyelocytes, to myelocytes, to bands; eventually they finish the maturation process as neutrophils which is depicted in Figure 1.3. Only bands and mature neutrophils are normally present in the peripheral blood smear. Other immature cells are very rarely detected in small numbers in the blood of healthy individuals (Oertel, 1998). Band neutrophils constitute about 10 to 15% of the nucleated cells in the bone marrow and around 5 to 10% of the nucleated cells in the peripheral blood (Glassy, 1998). The nucleus of a band is indented to greater than 50% of the diameter of the nucleus (i.e., horseshoe shaped). Eosinophils have the same maturation process; however, the cells are distinctively eosinophilic, with coarse eosinophilic cytoplasmic granules. In this case the myeloblast becomes an eosinophilic myelocyte that matures into an eosinophilic metamyelocyte, then an eosinophilic band, and ultimately an eosinophil. Basophils have a shorter transition from a myeloblast to a basophilic myelocyte and eventually a basophil.

Left Shift

An increase (>20%) in the number of band cells (so-called bandemia) in relation to normal neutrophils is known as a left shift (Figure 1.4) (Nguyen, 2000). With a left shift the band count is usually >700/µL. When a left shift occurs, more immature granulocytes (blasts, promyelocytes, metamyelocytes, myelocytes) are typically released in the peripheral blood. Unless a patient is receiving G-CSF therapy, circulating blasts are not normally seen in reactive conditions. In reactive neutrophilia the left shift contains mainly bands. A left shift may be physiological (e.g., pregnancy) or in response to infection, inflammation, shock, hypoxia, or other marrow stimulation. Newborn infants may

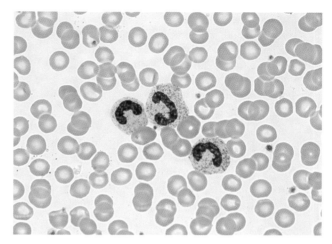

FIGURE 1.4 **Blood smear from a patient with infection showing a bandemia and a left shift.** These band neutrophils all have nuclei that are indented to greater than half the distance from the farthest nuclear margin. Their cytoplasm also contains many toxic granules.

normally show leukocytosis and a leftward shift (Christensen, 1979). Although the diagnostic value of a left shift as an indicator for infection is limited (Seebach, 1997; Gombos, 1998), when the WBC is low, bands may be the only clue of an infection. Occasionally band cell counts are requested to detect infection (e.g., in the neonate) (Bain, 2002). The presence of a left shift and circulating nucleated red blood cells is referred to as a leukoerthyroblastic reaction (or leukoerythroblastosis). There is often also associated erythrocyte anisopoikilocytosis (e.g., teardrop cells or dacrocytes) with anemia and megakaryocyte fragments in a leukoerythrobalstic pattern, indicative of a space-occupying lesion within the marrow (i.e., myelophthisic process).

Monocytes

Monocytes stem from monoblasts and undergo a maturation process as they progress from monoblasts to promonocytes. Monocytes reside in the peripheral blood. They may differentiate further and become macrophages (sometimes referred to as histiocytes) in the tissue.

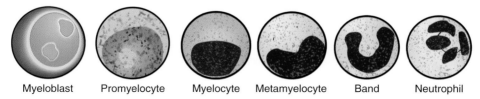

Myeloblast   Promyelocyte   Myelocyte   Metamyelocyte   Band   Neutrophil

FIGURE 1.3 **Neutrophil maturation process.** Neutrophils undergo a maturation process as they shift from myeloblasts, to promyelocytes, to myelocytes, to bands, and eventually to neutrophils.

Lymphocytes

Lymphocytes differentiate from a precursor cell known as a common lymphoid progenitor cell. They can become a precursor T cell/natural killer (NK) cell or a precursor B cell. These cells then become committed to their designation as they develop into Pro-T cells, Pro-NK cells, and Pro-B cells. Further maturation is required as the cells proceed in their development and exhibit morphologically recognizable precursors as Pre-T cells and Pre-B cells. The cells undergo their maturation in distinct locations: B lymphocytes in the bone marrow and T lymphocytes in the thymus. Following this detailed maturation process (Figures 1.5 and 1.6), lymphocytes enter the blood circulation and reside in secondary lymphoid organs, including the spleen and lymph nodes.

QUANTITATIVE DISORDERS OF WBCS

Disorders of Neutrophils

Normal Neutrophil Physiology

In normal adults the bone marrow is the usual site of differentiation, proliferation, and terminal maturation of hematopoietic stem cells into neutrophil progenitors. Maturation of myeloblasts into segmented neutrophils usually occurs in five phases: blast, promyelocyte, myelocyte, metamyelocyte, and mature neutrophil. Division occurs only during the first three stages (i.e., neutrophil blast, promyelocyte, and myelocyte). After the myelocyte stage, the cells are no longer capable of mitosis and enter a large marrow storage pool. After 5 days the cells are released into the blood, where they circulate for a few hours before entering tissues (Nathan, 2006). The physiology of neutrophil function is covered in greater detail in the qualitative disorders of neutrophils section. A neutrophil is also referred to as a polymorphonuclear neutrophil (PMN). The qualitative and quantitative changes of neutrophils noted in response to infection include neutrophilia, left shift, toxic granulation, Döhle bodies, and vacuolization (see below).

Normal Neutrophil Morphology

The nucleus of the circulating neutrophil is segmented, usually with two to four interconnected lobes. The purpose of nuclear segmentation is unknown. In rare situations (mainly with hematological malignancy, but also following G-CSF therapy) neutrophils may have unusual nuclear shapes such as ring/donut or botryoid nuclei or

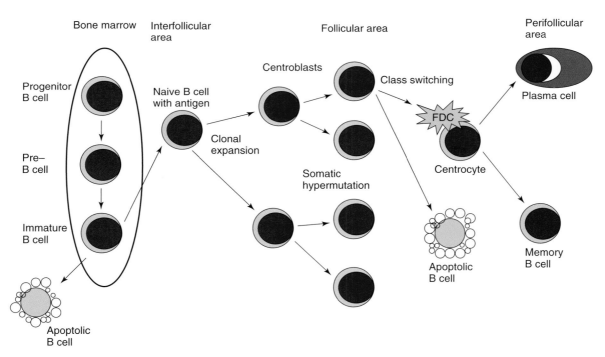

FIGURE 1.5 **Differentiation of B cells**. Precursor B cells may develop into naïve B cells, or may undergo apoptosis. Antigen stimulation of a naïve B cell starts a cascade of events including clonal expansion, somatic hypermutation and class switching of centroblasts. Centroblasts then develop into centrocytes within the follicle center and with the follicle dentritic cell (FDC) or undergo apoptosis. The perifollicular area contains either plasma cells or memory B cells.

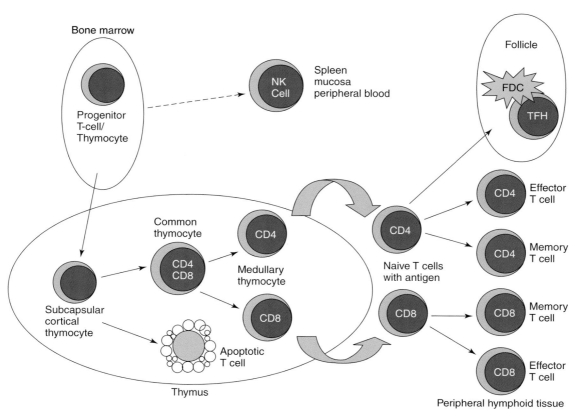

FIGURE 1.6 **Differentiation of T cells**. Progenitor T cells may develop into NK cells in the periphery, or they may enter the thymus where they develop into supcapsular cortical thymocytes and continue on to common thymocytes or apoptotic cells. Common thymocytes are CD4+ and CD8+, which then develop into medullary thymocytes and naïve T cells, either as CD4+ or CD8+. The naïve T cells are stimulated by antigens and transform into effector and memory T cells. T helper cells (TFH) develop from CD4+ naïve T cells within the follicle with the follicle dendritic cell (FDC).

show detached nuclear fragments (Hernandez, 1980; Bain, 2002). Some mature neutrophils in women have a drumstick- or club-shaped nuclear appendage attached to the nuclear lobe by a single fine chromatin strand containing the inactivated X chromosome (Barr body). Females typically have six or more drumsticks per 500 PMNs (Davidson, 1954). In males with Klinefelter syndrome (XXY), drumsticks occur but are fewer in number (Bain, 2002).

The myeloblast is an immature cell with a large oval nucleus, sizable nucleoli, and few or no granules. The promyelocyte stage contains primary (azurophilic or nonspecific) large peroxidase-positive granules that stain metachromatically (reddish-purple) with a polychromatic stain such as the Wright stain. During the myelocyte stage of maturation, secondary (specific) granules are formed that are peroxidase negative. After the myelocyte stage, the primary granules lose their intense staining properties and are no longer evident by light microscopy (DeSantis, 1997). Mature segmented

neutrophils contain primary (peroxidase-positive) granules and specific (peroxidase-negative) granules in a 1:2 ratio. The granules cannot be distinguished individually but are responsible for the pink background color of the neutrophil cytoplasm seen during and after the myelocyte stage. Primary granules contain lysozyme, myeloperoxidase, acid phosphatase, elastase, defensins, and cathepsin G. Secondary granules contain lysozyme, collagenase, lactoferin, B_{12}-binding protein, NADPH oxidase, and cytochrome b. A third type (tertiary) granule identified by electron microscopy has been documented.

When evaluating the granularity of neutrophils, it is important to be aware of possible artifacts such as may arise from prolonged storage and suboptimal staining. Toxic granulation (increased granulation) refers to activated neutrophils that contain large purple or dark blue primary granules (Figure 1.7 and Figure 1.8). With toxic granulation the cytoplasmic

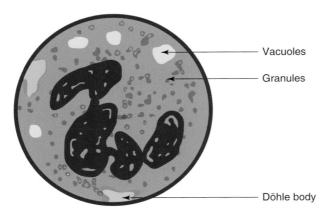

FIGURE 1.7 **Schematic diagram of a toxic segmented neutrophil**. The key features are prominent cytoplasmic granules, clear vacuoles, and Döhle bodies located peripherally adjacent to the cell membrane.

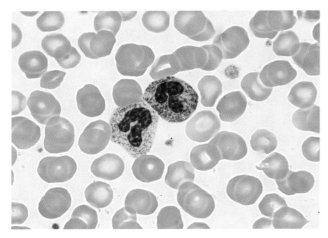

FIGURE 1.8 **Neutrophils with toxic granulation seen in a patient with known infection.**

granules enlarge and stain darker than normal granules (Schofield, 1983). Neutrophils with toxic granules may resemble eosinophils (which have larger granules), basophils, monocytes, or the inclusions of Alder–Reilly anomaly (see later). Activated neutrophils may in addition contain multiple round, empty cytoplasmic vacuoles and Döhle bodies. Blood stored for prolonged periods can artifactually cause vacuoles. Cytoplasmic vacuolation can also be caused by autophagocytosis (e.g., following chloroquine or sulfonamide therapy). Döhle bodies are blue-gray inclusions seen in the cytoplasm that represent areas of rough endoplasmic reticulum. They may be single or multiple and of varying size. Döhle-like bodies can also be found in patients with May–Hegglin anomaly, burns, myelodysplasia, and in pregnancy (see later). In May–Hegglin anomaly these bodies correspond to

amorphous cytoplasmic areas devoid of organelles. Increased granulation is also a characteristic of G-CSF therapy (Schmitz, 1994). Compared to toxic granulation, however, hypergranulation induced by G-CSF therapy has a higher density of granules, which stain more red and often obscure the nucleus (Nguyen, 2000). Other changes that may be encountered in patients receiving growth factor therapy include a neutrophilia with a prominent left shift, Döhle bodies, nuclear segmentation abnormalities (hyposegmentation, hypersegmentation, ring nuclei), leukoerythroblastosis, and rarely a monocytosis, transient lymphocytosis, and eosinophilia. Alder–Reilly anomaly (see later), when present in granulocytes, can also mimic toxic granulation. Alder–Reilly bodies, however, tend to be larger than normal granules. Finally, nuclear projections and cytoplasmic pseudopodia may be observed as rare alterations in toxic neutrophils.

Table 1.1 lists several of the alterations and abnormalities that may be seen in neutrophils. Apoptotic neutrophils may be seen in association with infection, diabetes (Figure 1.9), glucocorticoid administration, and neoplastic diseases (Sudo, 2007; Shidham 2000), but may also occur if blood is left at room temperature for a long time. These are important to recognize as they may mimic nucleated RBCs on low-power examination. Neutrophils may also contain a variety of phagocytosed material such as bacteria, fungi, cryoglobulin, and malarial pigment. (Figure 1.10).

Normal Neutrophil Cytochemistry

The most reliable method for identifying azurophilic granules on blood films is staining the cells for peroxidase with a myeloperoxidase stain. Production of this enzyme by leukemic cells has been the hallmark for distinguishing lymphoblastic from myeloid leukemia. Chloroacetate esterases appear early in maturation and can be used to detect the origin of immature cells.

Reference Range

The normal range for neutrophils is 2.5–7.5 × 10^9/L. However, the normal range can vary. People of African and Middle Eastern descent may have lower counts, which are still normal. At birth, the mean neutrophil count rises rapidly to a peak at 12 hours of age, but then drops by 72 hours of age. Thereafter the neutrophil count slowly decreases so that the lymphocyte becomes the predominant cell at two to three weeks of age (DeSantis, 1997). Several perinatal factors may significantly alter neutrophil dynamics including bacterial disease, maternal hypertension, maternal fever

TABLE 1.1 **Alterations of Neutrophil Morphology**

Abnormality	Condition
Neutrophil nuclei	
Left shift	Pregnancy, infection, shock, hypoxia
Hypersegmentation	Megaloblastic conditions, iron deficiency, uremia, infection, hereditary neutrophil hypersegementation, myelokathexis
Hyposegmentaion	Pelger–Huet anomaly, lactoferin deficiency, MDS, AML
Botryoid (grape-like) nucleus	Heatstroke, hyperthermia, burns
Neutrophil cytoplasm	
Hypogranulation	Lactoferin deficiency, MDS
Hypergranulation	Toxic granulation, pregnancy, infection, inflammation, G-CSF therapy, aplastic anemia, hypereosinophilic syndrome, Alder–Reilly anomaly, chronic neutrophilic leukemia, MDS
Abnormal granules	Chediak-Higashi syndrome, Alder–Reilly anomaly, MDS, AML
Vacuolation	Infection, G-CSF therapy, acute alcohol poisoning, Jordan's anomaly, carinitine deficiency, kwashiorkor, myelokathexis
Döhle bodies/inclusions	Infection, inflammation, burns, pregnancy, G-CSF therapy, May–Hegglin anomaly, Fechtner syndrome, kwashiorkor, MDS, AML

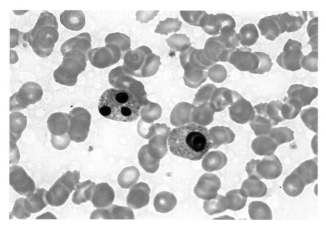

FIGURE 1.9 **Neutrophil apoptosis in the peripheral blood of a patient with diabetes mellitus.** Apoptotic cells have round, dense pyknotic nuclei.

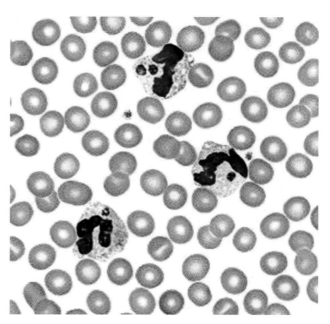

FIGURE 1.10 **Peripheral blood smear from a patient with Ehrlichiosis (human granulocytic anaplasmosis due to infection with the HGA agent *E. phagocytophila*).** The neutrophils contain characteristic intraleukocytic morulae. These may resemble Döhle bodies. Such intracytoplasmic inclusions may be seen in the cytoplasm of neutrophils in many (20–80%) patients with human granulocytic ehrlichiosis and in mononuclear cells in a minority (1–20%) of patients with human monocytic ehrlichiosis.

prior to delivery, hemolytic disease, and periventricular hemorrhage (Manroe, 1979). A diurnal variation of neutrophil counts has been observed in adults, but not infants. Both neutrophilia and neutropenia are defined using the absolute neutrophil count (ANC). The ANC is equal to the product of the WBC count and the percentage of polymorphonuclear cells (PMNs) and band forms noted on the differential analysis:

$$\text{ANC} = \text{WBC (cells/microL)}$$
$$\times \%(\text{PMNs} + \text{bands}) \div 100$$

The ANC is reported to be as sensitive but more specific than the WBC count as an indicator of occult bacteremia (Gombos, 1998).

Neutrophilia

Definition. Neutrophilia is the presence of more than $20.0 \times 10^3/\text{mm}^3$ neutrophils in the circulating blood. In infants with neutrophilia the ANC is

$>10.0 \times 10^3/\text{mm}^3$, in children it is $>8.0 \times 10^3/\text{mm}^3$, and in adults it is $>7.0 \times 10^3/\text{mm}^3$. The term *granulocytosis* has sometimes been used interchangeably with neutrophilia. In strict terms, granulocytes include neutrophils, eosinophils, and basophils. Total granulocyte count (TGC) is the product of the WBC count and the percentage of PMNs, bands, metamyelocytes, myelocytes, and promyelocytes.

ICD-10 Code D72.8

Pathophysiology. Neutrophilia can be due to a reactive or neoplastic process (Table 1.2). Significant causes of neutrophilia in the neonate can be due to maternal factors (smoking, fever, prolonged oxytocin, and dexamethasone administration) and/or fetal factors (stressful delivery, hypoxia, crying, physiotherapy, pain, hypoglycemia, seizures, infection, hemolysis, intraventricular hemorrhage, meconium aspiration, and hyaline membrane disease).

Clinical Approach. Reactive causes of neutrophilia are usually part of an inflammatory or infectious course, or can be drug induced. Pharmaceuticals that are commonly associated with neutrophilia are glucocorticoids, growth factors, and psychiatric medications. The reactive causes can have an associated left shift, meaning that the granulocytes in question have more immature forms circulating in the peripheral blood. However, the presence of immature granulocytes can also suggest a neoplastic process. Therefore a substantial history is required to help differentiate the possible source of neutrophilia.

Morphologic features that characterize a reactive neutrophilia with or without a left shift are toxic granulation, cytoplasmic vacuolation, and Dohle bodies. The absence of these changes and associated basophilia raises the possibility of neoplasia, particularly myeloproliferative neoplasms. A leukocyte alkaline phosphatase (LAP) score can be used that is high in infection (as well as polycythemia vera) but low in CML and PNH. The LAP score, however, may be normal in polycythemia vera and (juvenile) CML.

Differential Diagnosis. Chronic neutrophilic leukemia, essential thrombocythemia and polycythemia vera are usually associated with an absolute neutrophilia without a left shift. Primary myelofibrosis and chronic myeloid leukemia are usually associated with an absolute neutrophilia and left shift. Performing molecular genetic studies on blood for the bcr/abl and JAK2V617F mutation can help differentiate between myeloid neoplasms and a reactive cause of mature neutrophilia. The differentiation from an acute myeloid leukemia depends on both the cell proliferation and maturity of the cell population. If blasts constitute greater than 20% of the differential or abnormal promyelocytes are identified, further workup for acute leukemia should be pursued.

Neutropenia

Definition. Neutropenia is defined as an ANC below $2.5 \times 10^3/\text{mm}^3$ in infants an ANC below $1.5 \times 10^3/\text{mm}^3$ in adults. However, it is important to be aware that neutrophil counts can be naturally lower

TABLE 1.2 Major Causes of Neutrophilia

Acute Neutrophilia	
Physical or emotional stress	Cold, heat, convulsions, pain, labor, panic, depression, infarction, exercise, postoperative period, following seizures, frequent blood transfusion, acute hemorrhage
Infections	Localized and system bacterial, rickettsial and spirochetal infections
Inflammation or tissue necrosis	Burns, electric shock, trauma, vasculitis, antigen-antibody reaction, complement activation
Drugs, hormones, and toxins	Smoking, glucocorticoids, epinephrine, venoms, colony-stimulating factors
Chronic neutrophilia	
Infections	Persistence of infections that cause acute neutrophilia
Inflammation	Acute inflammation involving any organ or systemic such as colitis, nephritis, gout, Sweet's syndrome
Tumors	Carcinoma, lymphoma, brain tumors, melanoma, multiple myeloma, paraneoplastic reaction
Drugs	Continued exposure to drugs that cause acute neutrophilia, lithium, rarely drug reaction
Metabolic and endocrine disorders	Eclampsia, thyroid storm, Cushing's disease, gout, diabetic ketoacidosis
Benign hematologic disorders	Sickle cell disease, hemorrhage, recovery from agranulocytosis, asplenia
Hematologic neoplasms	Myeloproliferative neoplasms
Hereditary and congenital	Down syndrome

TABLE 1.3 **Major Causes of Neutropenia**

Acquired	
Infection	Any overwhelming infection
Autoimmune disease	Felty syndrome, systemic lupus erythematosus
Complement activation	Hemodialysis, filtration leukapheresis acute respiratory distress syndrome
Drug-induced neutropenia	Clozapine, thionamides, sulfasalazine, Chemotherapeutic agents
Toxins	Alcohol, benzene
Non-neoplastic hematologic disorders	Aplastic anemia, marrow replacement, megaloblastic anemia
Hematologic neoplasms	Myelodysplastic syndrome, primary idiopathic myelofibrosis, acute leukemia, T-large granular lymphocytic leukemia, lymphomas with bone marrow involvement
Congenital	
Constitutional	Shwachman–Diamond–Oski syndrome, cyclic neutropenia, Chediak–Higashi syndrome, Kostman syndrome, Fanconi anemia, dyskeratosis

in some ethnic groups such as Africans, African Americans, and Yemenite Jews (Tefferi, 2005). An ANC below $0.5 \times 10^3/mm^3$ is considered to represent severe neutropenia.

ICD-10 Code D70

Pathophysiology. Neutropenia can be caused by decreased production, increased destruction, hereditary disorders, medications, or infections (Table 1.3). The susceptibility to infection in neutropenic patients is related to the ANC. Neutropenia can be classified as follows:

- **Acquired neutropenia:** Postinfection, drug-induced (e.g., penicillin, chloramphenicol, ibuprofen, phenytoin, propylthiouracil, procainamide, chlorpropamide, phenothiazine), autoimmune (e.g., Felty syndrome, lupus erythematosus), isoimmune (e.g., alloimmune neonatal neutropenia), chronic splenomegaly, benign familial neutropenia, benign neutropenia of childhood, chronic idiopathic neutropenia, and nutritional deficiency.
- **Intrinsic defects:** Cyclic neutropenia, Kostmann syndrome (severe infantile agranulocytosis), myelokathexis (neutropenia with tetraploid or cloverleaf nuclei), Schwachman–Diamond–Oski syndrome, Chédiak–Higashi syndrome, reticular dysgenesis, and dyskeratosis congenita.

Neutropenia is often seen accompanying qualitative neutrophil disorders. Neutropenia is also common in several primary immunodeficiency diseases such as CD40L deficiency, WHIM syndrome (warts, hypogammaglobulinemia, immunodeficiency and myelokathexis), X-linked hyper-IgM, X-linked agammaglobulinemia and Chediak-Higashi syndrome (Rezaei, 2009). Congenital neutropenia includes nonsyndromic variants (caused by mutations in ELA2, HAX1, GFI1, or WAS) and syndromic variants (due to mutations in genes controlling glucose metabolism, e.g., SLC37A4 and G6PC3, or lysosomal function, e.g., LYST, RAB27A, ROBLD3/p14, AP3B1, VPS13B) (Klein, 2009). Defects in genes encoding ribosomal proteins (SBDS, RMRP) and mitochondrial proteins (AK2, TAZ) are also associated with some congenital neutropenia syndromes.

Clinical Approach. In some cases there may be telltale signs that will help you make a diagnosis. For example, vitamin B_{12} or folate deficiency results in atypical neutrophils that are hypersegmented, whereas aplastic anemia displays a decrease in bone marrow hematopoiesis. However, the underlying diagnosis resulting in neutropenia will typically require a complete history with additional lab testing. Cyclic neutropenia has a very characteristic history of recurrent episodes of fever and neutropenia in a young child. Neutrophils can also have dysfunctional problems, as are discussed later. A bone marrow evaluation can help determine the cellularity of the bone marrow, presence of malignant cells, chromosomal abnormalities suggesting malignant clones, and myeloid nuclear abnormalities. Also, because certain acquired neutropenias may be associated with the presence of antineutrophil antibodies (directed against neutrophil-specific antigens, e.g., NA1, NA2, NB1, ND1, and NE1 and non–neutrophil-specific HLA antigens), their detection (e.g., by immunofluorescence or agglutination assay) may be helpful. Overall, neutropenia is a worrisome occurrence because patients become susceptible to infections when they do not have adequate numbers of neutrophils to respond to an inflammatory and/or infectious assault.

Disorders of Lymphocytes

Normal Lymphocyte Physiology

Lymphocytes differentiate from lymphoblasts into two major types of lymphocytes:

- **T lymphocytes (T cells)**: These cells identify foreign substances in your body and begin an immune response;
- **B lymphocytes (B cells)**: These cells produce antibodies to foreign substances.

Lymphocytes differentiate further after exposure to an antigen. Upon exposure, lymphocytes become effector or memory lymphocytes (Cianci, 2010). The effector B cells release antibodies and effector T cells release cytotoxic granules or send a signal for helper cells (Malaspina, 2007). The memory cells remain in the peripheral blood and retain the ability to respond to the same antigen in the future.

Normal Lymphocyte Morphology

One cannot reliably distinguish functional and immunological lymphocyte subsets by morphology alone. While normal circulating lymphocytes vary in size and shape, they can arbitrarily be divided into small ("mature") and large ("granular") lymphocytes (Nguyen, 2000). Mimics of reactive lymphocytes include lymphoma cells, lymphoblasts, monocytes, plasma cells, and nucleated red blood cells.

Mature (Small) Lymphocytes. Mature lymphocytes are approximately the same size as red blood cells (i.e., 7 microns in diameter). They have a prominent nucleus with regular nuclear contours and dense chromatin, and only have a small rim of cytoplasm. Nuclear clefts in small lymphocytes may normally be seen in children. Benign binucleated lymphocytes have been documented in some individuals (Troussard, 1997) and also in association with radiation (Bain, 2002). Rare childhood storage disorders can manifest with prominent cytoplasmic vacuoles in lymphocytes. Inclusions within lymphocytes can be seen in Chédiak–Higashi syndrome, Alder–Reilly anomaly, and Tay–Sachs disease (Bain, 2002). Lymphocyte vacuolation can occur in I-cell disease, the mucopolysaccharidoses, Jordan's anomaly, Niemann–Pick disease, Wolman's disease, Pompe's disease, Tay–Sachs disease, Batten–Speilmeyer–Vogt disease, type II sialidosis, and galactosemia (Bain, 2002).

Reactive Lymphocytes. The term *reactive* is used to describe transformed benign lymphocytes, and should not be used interchangeably with *atypical* which should be used to describe malignant-appearing cells (Marty, 1997). Several reactive lymphocyte forms have been described (e.g., Downey classification) (Glassy, 1998). Reactive lymphocytes tend to be larger (9–30 μm) than mature (8–12 μm) lymphocytes. They may also have more abundant basophilic, slightly foamy, or vacuolated cytoplasm. Reactive cells often have an indented surface, which appears scalloped at the edges (Figure 1.11). The nucleus ranges in shape from round to reniform in appearance. Unlike resting small lymphocytes, reactive lymphocytes may have nucleoli. Their nuclear chromatin is typically finer than normal small lymphocytes. Plasmacytoid reactive lymphocytes (sometimes called "plymphs" or Turk cells) resemble plasma cells (Figure 1.12). Plymphs often have a large eccentric nucleus with prominent chromatin clumping, and occasionally a perinuclear hoff may be seen. Reactive lymphocytes that have a plasma cell-like appearance are usually seen as part of a heterogeneous mix of reactive lymphoid cells. They likely represent intermediate B lymphocytes differentiating into plasma cells. Reactive lymphocytes enlarge due to antigen stimulation. More recent studies suggest that reactive lymphocytes are activated T lymphocytes produced in response to infected B lymphocytes (Thomas, 2008). They act as normal lymphocytes in sites of local

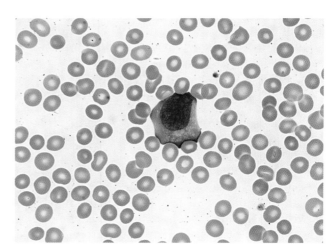

FIGURE 1.11 **Reactive lymphocyte in a patient with infectious mononucleosis (monospot test positive).** The large reactive lymphocyte shown corresponds to a so-called Downey type II cell. These cells have an abundant pale gray-blue amoeboid cytoplasm that partially surrounds adjacent erythrocytes. The curled edges against the RBCs and radiating cytoplasm are slightly darker staining.

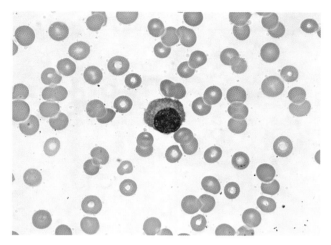

FIGURE 1.12 **Plasmacytoid appearing reactive lymphocyte with coarse chromatin and an eccentric nucleus.**

inflammation, playing a role in the primary cellular immune or helper T-cell response (Simon, 1997).

Large Granular Lymphocytes (LGLs). LGLs are large (T-cell phenotype) lymphocytes with azurophilic granules that contain proteins involved in cell lysis, such as perforin and granzyme B. LGLs normally comprise 10 to 20% of the total lymphocyte population (Nguyen, 2000). Monocytes by comparison contain smaller granules and have a ground-glass cytoplasm.

Natural Killer (NK) Cells. NK cells are a third type of lymphocyte; they are similar to cytotoxic T cells and LGLs, which cause cell lysis of tumor cells and virus-infected cells by releasing granzyme B. NK cells were named as such because they do not require antigen priming to destroy abnormal self-cells. Therefore the cytoxic affect occurs naturally (Morice, 2007). These cells have a large granular lymphocyte appearance; however, NK cells do not display T-cell receptors or pan-T markers (CD3).

Normal Lymphocyte Immunophenotype

In general, T lymphocytes are CD3 positive and individually display CD4 or CD8 staining. Few lymphocytes display both CD4 and CD8 positivity. T-cell LGLs exhibit CD8 and variable CD11b, CD56, and CD 57 positivity. Granzyme B can also be used for T-cell LGL identification (Table 1.4). B lymphocytes display CD20 and CD79a, and are also positive for CD19 on flow cytometry. Plasma cells do not express many surface antigens and are negative for the B cell markers CD19 and CD20 (Table 1.5). They are identified by CD38 and CD138 staining. Natural killer cells display CD16 (FcγRIII), CD56, CD57, CD2, and granzyme B.

Lymphocytosis

Definition. Lymphocytosis is defined as the presence of more than $4 \times 10^3/\text{mm}^3$ lymphocytes in the circulating blood in adults, more than $7 \times 10^3/\text{mm}^3$ in children, and more than $9 \times 10^3/\text{mm}^3$ in infants.

ICD-10 Code D72.8

TABLE 1.4 **T-Cell Phenotype During Stages of Maturation**

	CD7	CD1a	CD2/CD5	CD3	CD4/CD8	TdT
Prothymocyte	+	−	−	−	−	+
Subcapsular thymocyte	+	−	+	Cytoplasmic +	Double +	+
Cortical thymocyte	+	+	+	Surface +	CD4+ or CD8+	+
Medullary thymocyte	+	−	+	Surface +	CD4+ or CD8+	−
Peripheral T cell	+	−	+	Surface +	CD4+ or CD8+	−

TABLE 1.5 **B-Cell Phenotype During Stages of Maturation**

	Antigen	TdT	CD79a	PAX5	CD20
Pro-B	Independent	+	−	−	−
Pre-B	Independent	+	+	+	−
Immature B	Independent	+	+	+	+
Mature naïve B	Independent	−	+	+	+
Germinal center B	Dependent	−	+	+	+
Memory B	Dependent	−	+	+	+
Plasma cell	Dependent	−	+	−	−

TABLE 1.6 **Major Causes of Lymphocytosis**

Reactive causes of lymphocytosis	
Acute viral infections	Infectious mononucleosis (Epstein Barr virus), cytomegalovirus, HIV, hepatitis, adenovirus, chickenpox, herpes simplex and zoster, influenza, mumps, measles
Acute bacterial infections	Pertussis (whooping cough), brucellosis, tuberculosis, typhoid fever, paratyphoid fever
Protozoan infections	Toxoplasmosis, Chaga's disease
Chronic bacterial infections	Tuberculosis, brucellosis, syphilis
Autoimmune disease	Rheumatoid arthritis, idiopathic thrombocytopenic purpura, systemic lupus erythematosus, autoimmune hemolytic anemia
Drug and toxic reactions	Dilantin, dapsone, lead, organic arsenics
Endocrine causes	Stress, Addison's disease, glucocorticoid deficiency, thyrotoxicosis
Miscellaneous	During recovery from acute infections (especially in children), allergic reactions, malnutrition, rickets
Neoplastic causes of lymphocytosis	
Acute lymphoblastic leukemia	
Non-Hodgkin lymphoma	
T-cell large granular lymphocytic leukemia (T-LGL)	

Pathophysiology. Lymphocytosis can be divided into reactive and neoplastic etiologies. Table 1.6 lists some common causes of lymphocytosis. Reactive lymphocytosis is most commonly associated with acute viral illnesses such as infectious mononucleosis due to Epstein Barr virus (EBV) (Nkrumah, 1973; Marty, 1997; Peterson, 1993). Lymphocytosis can also occur with other infections like whooping cough (Kubic, 1990). Reactive lymphocytosis secondary to stress (e.g., myocardial infarction, sickle cell crisis, and trauma) may be more transient (Groom, 1990; Karandikar, 2002).

Clinical Approach

Lymphocytosis is particularly common in children with infection. In viral-induced lymphocytosis there is typically a mixed population of reactive cells, including small lymphocytes, plasmacytoid cells, and few larger lymphocytes. The minimal morphologic criteria for the diagnosis of infectious mononucleosis are (1) 50% or more mononuclear cells (lymphocytes and monocytes) in a blood smear, (2) at least 10 reactive lymphocytes per 100 leukocytes, and (3) marked lymphocyte heterogeneity (Peterson, 2006). Increased numbers of apoptotic lymphocytes are often seen with viral infections. In the elderly population, lymphocytosis is more concerning to be secondary to a neoplastic or lymphoproliferative disorder such as leukemia or lymphoma. Large granular lymphocytes will occur in increased number in large granular lymphocytic leukemia (T-LGL), which can mimic a reactive process and is thus frequently underdiagnosed. T-LGL is known to be associated with several autoimmune and hematologic conditions including myelodysplastic syndromes. Therefore it is important to keep T-LGL in the differential diagnosis of a reactive lymphocytosis. Lymphocytosis after splenectomy is usually mild, and will be accompanied by the presence of Howell–Jolly bodies (Juneja, 1995). Morphological criteria alone may be insufficient to distinguish reactive from malignant lymphocytes. In such cases immunophenotyping (e.g., flow cytometry) and molecular studies (e.g., PCR for IgH gene rearrangement) may be needed.

Lymphocytopenia
Definition. Lymphocytopenia is defined as the presence of less than $1.0 \times 10^3/\text{mm}^3$ lymphocytes in the circulating blood in adults. Children have higher normal levels of lymphocytes, and lymphocytopenia is defined as less than $2.0 \times 10^3/\text{mm}^3$.

ICD-10 Code D72.8

Pathophysiology. Lymphocytopenia can be secondary to congenital immunodeficiency disorders or a reactive process to underlying disease (Table 1.7).

Clinical Approach. Lymphocytopenia is more commonly a reactive etiology that is associated with infectious disease (e.g., AIDS), autoimmune disorders (e.g., rheumatoid arthritis, SLE, myasthenia gravis), nutritional deficiencies (e.g., zinc), systemic diseases (e.g., sarcoidosis, protein-losing enteropathy, renal insufficiency, Hodgkin lymphoma, carcinoma), congenital immunodeficiency disorders, iatrogenic causes (e.g., chemotherapeutic agents, radiation therapy), and idiopathic (idiopathic CD4+ T lymphocytopenia) (Laurence, 1993; Schoentag, 1993, Buckley,

TABLE 1.7 Major Causes of Lymphopenia

Reactive causes of lymphocytopenia	
Infectious diseases	HIV, influenza, hepatitis, tuberculosis, babesiosis, pneumonia, sepsis
Autoimmune disorders	Rheumatoid arthritis, myasthenia gravis, systemic lupus erythematosus
Nutritional disorders	Zinc deficiency, protein malnutrition
Systemic diseases	Renal insufficiency, sarcoidosis, carcinoma, Hodgkin lymphoma
Iatrogenic causes	Radiation therapy, burns
Medications	Chemotherapy, glucocorticoid therapy
Congenital immunodeficiency disordes	
Wiskott–Aldrich syndrome	
Severe combined immunodeficiency disease	
Congenital thymic aplasia (DiGeorge syndrome)	

2000; Datta, 2009). Congenital disorders have classic presentations and dysfunctions. These disorders include severe combine immunodeficiency disease (SCID), DiGeorge syndrome and Wiskott–Aldrich syndrome.

Severe combined immunodeficiency disease (SCID) is also known as Bubble Boy syndrome, alymphocytosis, and Glanzmann–Riniker syndrome. Most cases of SCID are secondary to mutations of the common gamma chain (γ_c). The common gamma chain is a protein of the interleukin receptors, including IL-2, IL-4, IL-7, IL-9, IL-15, and IL-21. A nonfunctional common gamma chain leads to defects of interleukin signaling, development of and differentiation of T and B cells. Consequently this disease is characterized by a dysfunctional immune system with markedly decreased or absent T cells and NK cells and nonfunctional B cells. Patients are commonly affected by recurrent opportunistic infections, ear infections, chronic diarrhea, and oral candidiasis. SCID is severe, and newborns can die within a year if they are not diagnosed and treated early on in the disease process (Gaspar, 2001).

DiGeorge syndrome (congenital thymic aplasia) is characterized by lymphocytopenia and aplasia of the thymus (Figure 1.13) and parathyroid glands. This syndrome is likely secondary to a defect of the third and fourth pharyngeal pouches. These patients have a deletion at q11.2 on chromosome 22 (Hay, 2007; Kobrynski, 2007). They have multiple birth defects, which include congenital heart disease, palate neuromuscular problems (velo-pharyngeal insufficiency), learning disabilities, atypical facial features, and hypocalcemia secondary to parathyroid aplasia. DiGeorge syndrome results in recurrent infections due to the immune system's inability to mediate a T-cell response due to thymic aplasia.

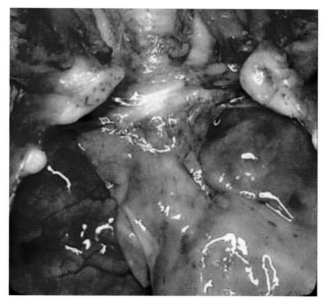

FIGURE 1.13 **Gross image of an opened chest after removal of the breast plate in a patient with complete DiGeorge syndrome**. Note the total absence of any thymic elements, exposing the innominate vein. (Image courtesy of Dr. Ronald Jaffe, Pittsburgh Children's Hospital).

Wiskott–Aldrich syndrome is an X-linked recessive disorder that is characterized by eczema, thrombocytopenia, lymphocytopenia, recurrent infections, and bloody diarrhea. A mutation of the Wiskott–Aldrich syndrome protein (WASP) gene leads to WAS protein dysfunction on the X chromosome (Ochs, 2006). This leads to decreased antibody production and IgM levels are reduced, IgA and IgE levels are elevated, and IgG levels can be reduced or elevated. Initially the patient has relatively normal lymphocyte function, which decreases with time. Eventually the patient has an impaired immune system and hence is subject to recurrent infections.

Disorders of Plasma Cells

Normal Plasma Cell Physiology

While in the spleen or lymph node, T lymphocytes can stimulate B lymphocytes in the germinal centers to differentiate into more specialized cells: plasma cells or memory B lymphocytes. Plasma cells stem form plasmablasts, which divide rapidly and preserve the B-lymphocyte capability of presenting antigens to T cells. A plasmablast will progress to form a differentiated plasma cell. Plasma cells have an indeterminate life span. They can live for days to months after the process of affinity maturation in germinal centers. Plasma cells secrete large amounts of antibodies, but they can only produce a single class of immunoglobin. Each plasma cell can create hundreds to thousands of antibodies per second, which is more than plasmablasts. Plasma cells play a key role in the humoral immune response, even though they cannot switch antibody class or act as antigen-presenting cells like their precursors.

Normal Plasma Cell Morphology

Plasma cells differ morphologically from lymphocytes and granulocytes and are easily recognized. Plasma cells are oval in shape and range in size from 5 to 30 μm. They have basophilic cytoplasm and an eccentrically placed nucleus, which has a characteristic cartwheel or clock-face appearance. Their nuclear structure is due to heterochromatin arrangement. Nucleoli are absent. They also have a characteristic paranuclear hoff, which is a cytoplasmic clearing that contains the golgi apparatus. The remaining cytoplasm contains an abundant rough endoplasmic reticulum. The cytoplasmic constituents make plasma cells well suited for secreting large amounts of immunoglobulins. Plasma cells may contain crystals. Cells with globular cytoplasmic inclusions constipated with immunoglobulins have been called Mott cells or morular cells.

Plasmacytosis

Definition. Increase in circulating plasma cells.

ICD-10 Code D72.8

Pathophysiology. Plasma cells are mature and specialized B lymphocytes. They are not seen in peripheral blood in healthy persons. Increased circulating plasma cells may occur secondary to a reactive process (Moake, 1974; Glassy, 1998) or with malignancy. Conditions and diseases that may be associated with plasmacytosis include chronic infections (viral, bacterial, fungal, and parasitic

infection), inflammatory states, immunization, autoimmune disorders, alcoholic liver disease, cirrhosis, drug reactions, serum sickness, hypersensitivity reactions, sarcoidosis, granulomatous disease, and plasma cell disorders (monoclonal gammopathy of undetermined significance, myeloma, plasma cell leukemia, gamma heavy chain disease, and rarely Waldenstrom's macroglobulinemia) (Bain, 2002).

Clinical Approach. Any increase of plasma cells in a blood smear is abnormal and may be concerning for neoplasia, particularly advanced stages of myeloma. Circulating abnormal plasma cells can be a seen with multiple myeloma, monoclonal gammopathy of undetermined significance, and plasma cell leukemia. Large numbers of immature circulating plasma cells (20% of plasma cells in the differential) are present in plasma cell leukemia. Potential look-alikes include reactive plasmacytoid lymphocytes and lymphoma cells. Morphological features of malignant plasma cells include frequent binucleated and multinucleated forms, large nucleoli, and atypical mitotic figures. Rouleaux formation may be seen on a peripheral blood smear with increased quantities of an M protein. The blood smear may also show a faint purple background when the level of the M protein is very elevated. This background can be demonstrated using the "scratch test," by making a scratch on the slide and comparing the abnormally stained proteinaceous material to the clean colorless glass slide (Pantanowitz, 2004) Circulating nucleated RBCs or a leukoerthrobastic pattern may be seen in some cases with myeloma. Correlation with clinical history, imaging (e.g., bone lesions, underlying chronic inflammatory disease or infection like syphilis, tuberculosis, HIV, or malaria), and where indicated, additional laboratory evaluation (serum protein electrophoresis, immunofixation, Bence–Jones proteins in urine, renal insufficiency, hypercalcemia, flow cytometry, bone marrow assessment, etc.) may be needed to exclude a neoplastic proliferation of plasma cells.

Disorders of Monocytes

Normal Monocyte Physiology

Monocytes originate from the same myeloid stem cell as neutrophils, basophils, and eosinophils. Promonocytes mature under of the influence of granulocyte–macrophage-colony stimulating factor (GM-CSF) or macrophage-colony stimulating factor (M-CSF). Approximately half of all monocytes are stored in the red pulp of the spleen. The bone marrow and the spleen respond to inflammatory signals by releasing monocytes into the peripheral blood. Monocytes differentiate into macrophages and histiocytes as they migrate into the tissue. Monocytes have an important role in the inflammatory response, including phagocytosis with direct pathogen clearance and antibody-mediated cellular cytotoxicity (Silva, 2010). They also contribute to tissue repair and homeostasis.

Normal Monocyte Morphology

On a Wright–Giemsa stained blood film, the monocyte has a diameter of 12 to 15 μm. This is the largest normal cell seen in the peripheral blood smear. The nucleus is eccentrically placed, is reniform to round or irregular in shape, occupies approximately half the area of the cell (Figure 1.14), and has fine reticulated chromatin. Monocytes have a moderate to abundant cytoplasm that is often vacuolated, stains grayish-blue, and contains a variable number of fine, pink-purple granules (so-called ground-glass appearance). Occasionally these cells may contain phagocytosed material (Figure 1.15).

Normal Monocyte Cytochemistry

Nonspecific esterase (NSE) is frequently used as a marker for monocytes. The most useful cytochemical reaction to detect the esterase activity of monocytes is α-naphthyl acetate esterase (ANAE) activity at acid pH. Monocyte esterases are inhibited by sodium fluoride, whereas the esterases of the granulocytic series are not. Monocytes also give a weak but positive periodic acid–Schiff reaction (for polysaccharides) and variable Sudan black B reaction (for lipids) (Hayhoe 1980).

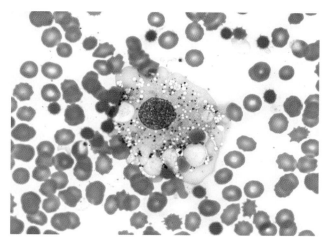

FIGURE 1.15 **Monocyte showing marked erythrophagocytosis**.

Normal Monocyte Immunophenotype

CD11b, an adhesion surface glycoprotein, and CD14, a receptor for endotoxin (LPS), are the most characteristic surface antigens of the monocyte lineage. The CD68 antigen is a specific marker for monocytes/macrophages that is routinely used in paraffin-embedded tissue. A variable percentage of blood monocytes express the CD4 receptor seen in T helper lymphocytes. HIV-1 utilizes CD4 receptors as an entry pathway for infection of monocyte/macrophages.

Monocytosis

Definition. Absolute monocytosis is defined as monocytes in excess of $1.0 \times 10^3/\mathrm{mm}^3$ in adults and $1.2 \times 10^3/\mathrm{mm}^3$ in neonates.

ICD-10 Code D72.8

Pathophysiology. Absolute monocytosis can be secondary to either neoplastic disorders or reactive immune responses (Table 1.8) (Maldonado, 1965). A mild monocytosis commonly accompanies reactive neutrophilia. In neutropenic patients, monocytosis represents a compensatory mechanism (Nguyen, 2000).

Clinical Approach. Reactive monocytes tend to have folded nuclei and vacuolated cytoplasm. Potential look-alikes include monoblasts, atypical lymphocytes, myelocytes, metamyelocytes, and even band neutrophils. In adults, if reactive causes are excluded, absolute monocytosis that is persistent for greater than three months should be considered as a marker of a myelodysplastic/myeloproliferative neoplasm (e.g., chronic myelomonocytic leukemia). The

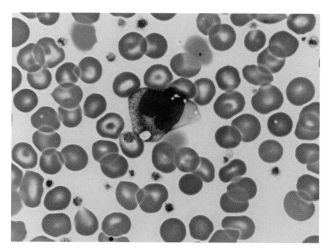

FIGURE 1.14 **Mature monocyte characterized by an indented nucleus and abundant blue-gray cytoplasm containing vacuoles and sparse lilac granules.**

TABLE 1.8 Causes of Monocytosis

Reactive Causes of Monocytosis	
Indolent infection	Bacterial: subacute bacterial endocarditis, tuberculosis, brucellosis, syphilis
	Rickettsial: Rocky Mountain spotted fever, typhus
	Protozoan: malaria, kala azar, trypanosomiasis
Chronic inflammation	Celiac sprue, inflammatory bowel disease, sarcoidosis, rheumatoid arthritis, SLE
Neoplasms	Hodgkin and non-Hodgkin lymphoma, multiple myeloma, cytokine producing carcinoma
Miscellaneous	Recovery from agranulocytosis, tetrachloroethane poisoning, post splenectomy, G-CSF and cytokine therapy, long-term hemodialysis
Neoplastic causes of monocytosis	
Chronic	Chronic myelogenous Leukemia
	Chronic myelomonocytic Leukemia
	Myelodysplastic syndrome
Acute	Acute monoblastic/monocytic leukemia[a]
	Acute myelomonocytic leukemia[a]
	Acute myeloid leukemia with inversion 16[a]

[a]In these disorders the monocytes tend to be immature.

threshold of monocytes greater than $1.0 \times 10^3/\text{mm}^3$ is low and does not help distinguish between reactive and neoplastic causes. A mild monocytosis usually accompanies neutrophilia in reactive conditions, and this may be useful in distinguishing reactive from a neoplastic process. Monocytosis accompanied by cytopenias and other features of myelodysplasia (e.g., hypolobate and hypogranular neutrophils, hypogranular platelets, and dimorphic red blood cells) suggests CMML.

Monocytopenia
Definition. Monocytopenia is a form of leukopenia associated with a deficiency of monocytes.

ICD-10 Code D72.9

Pathophysiology. The causes of monocytopenia include acute infections, stress, treatment with glucocorticoids, aplastic anemia, hairy cell leukemia, acute myeloid leukemia, and treatment with myelotoxic drugs.

Clinical Approach
In the setting of monocytopenia an underlying cause should be sought, particularly hairy cell leukemia.

Disorders of Eosinophils

Normal Eosinophil Physiology
Eosinophils are granulocytes that originate from the same myeloid stem cell precursor that can develop into neutrophils, basophils, or monocytes. Eosinophils are released from the bone marrow into the peripheral blood and tissues in response to interleukins: IL-1, IL-3, and especially IL-5. Degranulation of eosinophils releases major basic protein, histamine, peroxidase, and eosinophil-derived neurotoxin. They have two key roles in the immune system: destroying foreign substances and promoting an inflammatory response. Eosinopenia (reduction in eosinophil count) is usually a nonspecific finding, or it may be attributed to a physiological fall during pregnancy, acute stress, Cushing's syndrome, or drugs.

Normal Eosinophil Morphology
Eosinophils have a diameter of 12 to 17 μm and have a characteristic bilobed nucleus. A small number of normal eosinophils may be trilobed. Their cytoplasm contains a plethora of almost spherical granules that stain reddish orange (Figure 1.16). Immature eosinophils may have fewer granules.

Normal Eosinophil Cytochemistry
Normal eosinophils show positivity for myeloperoxidase and Sudan black and moderate reactivity with naphthol-AS or α-naphthyl esterase. They do not show toluidine blue metachromasia or positivity for alkaline phosphatase, chloroacetate esterase, or periodic acid–Schiff (Hayhoe, 1980).

Eosinophilia
Definition. Absolute eosinophilia is the presence of more than $0.6 \times 10^3/\text{mm}^3$ eosinophils in the circulating blood (Figure 1.17).

ICD-10 Code D72.1

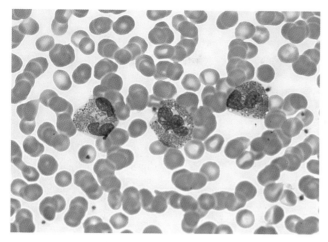

FIGURE 1.16 **Mature eosinophils containing segmented nuclei and cytoplasm filled with coarse orange-red granules**. Note that the central eosinophil has a trilobed nucleus.

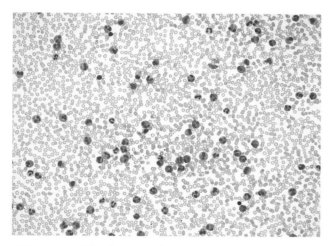

FIGURE 1.17 **Blood smear showing eosinophilia**.

Pathophysiology. Eosinophilia can be divided into mild ($<1.5 \times 10^3/mm^3$), moderate ($1.5–5.0 \times 10^3/mm^3$), or severe ($>5.0 \times 10^3/mm^3$). Absolute blood eosinophilia may be a primary or secondary phenomenon (Lombardi, 2003; Tefferi, 2006; Pardanani, 2008). Refer to Table 1.9 for a list of common causes of eosinophilia. Of note, tumors with tumor-associated tissue eosinophilia appear to have a better prognosis that those without such a response (Lowe, 1981).

- **Primary eosinophilia:** Primary eosinophilia is classified into two categories, clonal and idiopathic. Clonal eosinophilia requires the presence of either cytogenetic evidence or bone marrow histological evidence of an otherwise classified myeloid neoplasm such as acute leukemia or a myeloproliferative neoplasm. Genetic mutations

involving the platelet-derived growth factor receptor genes (PDGFRA, PDGFR-B, and FGFR1) have been pathogenetically linked to clonal eosinophilia, and their presence predicts treatment response to imatinib. Clonal eosinophilia is also associated with chronic myeloid leukemia, chronic eosinophilic leukemia, mastocytosis, and AML with inv (16). Accordingly, cytogenetic and/or molecular investigations for the presence of a molecular/genetic abnormality should accompany the evaluation for primary eosinophilia. Idiopathic eosinophilia (hypereosinophilic syndrome or HES) is a diagnosis of exclusion (i.e., not secondary or clonal). HES refers to a heterogeneous group of disorders (Roufosse, 2003). The diagnosis of HES requires documentation of (1) sustained eosinophilia (i.e., absolute eosinophil count$\geq$1500 cells/μL for at least 6 months), (2) no other etiology for eosinophilia, and (3) target organ damage from eosinophilic infiltration with mediator release (e.g., involvement of the heart, lung, skin, or nerve tissue). There are several variants of HES including myeloproliferative variants, T-lymphocytic variants, familial HES, idiopathic (unclassified) HES, overlap HES, and associated HES (Sheikh, 2007).

- **Secondary eosinophilia:** Causes of secondary (i.e., reactive) eosinophilia include tissue-invasive parasitosis, allergic or inflammatory conditions, drug reactions, and malignancies in which eosinophils are not part of the neoplastic process (Kano, 2009). The level of eosinophilia usually parallels the extent of tissue invasion by parasitic worms. Fungal infections usually associated with eosinophilia include aspergillosis (e.g., allergic bronchopulmonary aspergillosis) and coccidioidomycosis.

Clinical Approach. In a patient with blood eosinophilia, the possibility of secondary eosinophilia must be excluded first. For example, a detailed allergy, drug, and travel history along with stool for ova and parasites are a useful starting point (Checkley, 2010). HIV infection may also be associated with eosinophilia (Skiest, 1997). Once this is accomplished, blood and bone marrow studies should be obtained. The finding of many abnormal eosinophils (e.g., monolobated, hypersegmented, ring forms, hypogranulation, cytoplasmic vacuoles) is non-specific, but often associated with idiopathic HES. An increase in eosinophils with granules that have basophilic staining characteristics (so-called pre-eosinophilic granules or a hybrid

TABLE 1.9 **Reactive Cause of Eosinophilia**

Acquired eosinophilia	
Atopic/allergic diseases	Asthma, urticaria, eczema, rhinitis
Parasitic infestation (with tissue invasion)	Tricninosis, hookworms, Ascaris lumbricoides, schistosomiasis, filariasis, fascioliasis
Drug reaction	Dapsone, allopurinol, sulfa, recombinant human interleukins
Hematopoietic neoplasms	Hodgkin and non-Hodgkin lymphoma
Infectious diseases	Scarlet fever, cat scratch disease, chlamydia, fungi
Inflammatory disease	Colitis, celiac disease, vasculitis, sarcoidosis
Skin diseases	Dermatitis herpetiformis, bullous pemphigus, pemphigoid
Carcinoma	Squamous cell carcinoma, large cell lung carcinoma, adenocarcinoma, bladder transitional cell carcinoma
Miscellaneous	Adrenal insufficiency, atheroembolic disease, hyper-IgE syndrome (Job syndrome), Omenn syndrome
Primary eosinophilia	
Idiopathic	Hypereosinophilic syndrome (HES)
Clonal eosinophilia	Myeloid and lymphoid neoplasms with eosinophilia and abnormalities of PDGFRA, PDGFRB OR FGFR1
	Chronic eosinophilic leukemia, NOS
	Chronic myelogenous leukemia
	Mastocytosis

eosinophilic-basophilic granulocyte) favors leukemia (Weil, 1987; Bain, 2002). Blood studies should include serum tryptase (an increased level suggests systemic mastocytosis), T-cell receptor gene rearrangement analysis (positive test results suggest an underlying clonal T-cell disorder), and serum IL-5 (an elevated level requires careful evaluation of bone marrow studies and T-cell gene rearrangement studies for the presence of a clonal T-cell disease) (Ogbogu, 2009). Bone marrow examination should include cytogenetic studies, tryptase immunostains, and FISH or reverse transcriptase polymerase chain reaction (R-PCR) to screen for FIP1L1-PDGFRA. The last mentioned test can also be performed on peripheral blood. Positive genetic studies suggest a clonal/primary eosinophilic disorder. Persistent eosinophilia with target organ damage can be interpreted as a neoplastic process (chronic eosinophilic leukemia/hypereosinophilic syndrome) even in the absence of genetic abnormalities.

Inherited Abnormalities

Inherited abnormalities of eosinophils are rare. They include the following disorders:

- Absence of peroxidase and phospholipids in eosinophils: An autosomal recessive defect that produces no signs of disease.
- Chédiak–Higashi syndrome (described later): Almost all granulated cells, including eosinophils, contain large abnormal granules

- Neutrophil-specific granule deficiency (described later): This inherited abnormality also involves eosinophils.

Disorders of Basophils

Normal Basophil Physiology

Basophils are granulocytes that originate from the same myeloid stem cell precursor that can develop into neutrophils, eosinophils, or monocytes. Basophils are released from the bone marrow into the peripheral blood and tissues in response to interleukins: GM-CSF, IL-3, and IL-5. Reactive processes lead to degranulation, which releases heparin, histamine, aryl-sulfatase A, and eosinophil chemotactic factor. They have one main role in the immune system: degranulating and promoting an inflammatory response. Some causes of basopenia include acute stress, Cushing's syndrome, ACTH therapy, acute allergic reaction, hyperthyroidism, and progesterone therapy.

Normal Basophil Morphology

Basophils have diameters of 10 to 14 μm and have a characteristic lobated nucleus (Figure 1.18) that is usually obscured by the cytoplasmic granules, which are large and deeply basophilic (dark purple). Hypogranulation of basophils can be seen during an acute allergic attack, in myeloproliferative disorders, and may be an artifact due to the water solubility of these granules (Nguyen, 2000). Eosinophils and neutrophils with marked toxic granulation may mimic

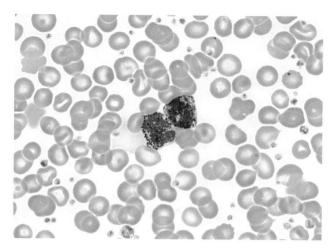

FIGURE 1.18 **Blood smear showing two basophils from a patient with basophilia.** Note that the basophilic granules in these cells overlay and therefore partially obscure the nuclei.

basophils. Mast cells with basophilic granules can also look like basophils. Mast cells are extremely rare in the peripheral blood of healthy individuals (Bain, 2002). Mast cells are larger than basophils, have a small round nucleus and more abundant cytoplasm, and harbor more tightly packed small dark granules.

Basophilia

Definition. Basophilia is the presence of more than $0.2 \times 10^3/\text{mm}^3$ basophils in the circulating blood.

ICD-10 Code D75.8

Pathophysiology. Basophilia can be divided into primary causes, which are associated with chronic myeloid leukemia and basophilic leukemia, and secondary causes, which are reactive. Common causes of basophilia are listed in Table 1.10.

Clinical Approach. Basophil morphology is unremarkable in reactive basophilia. However, basophils in some inherited conditions can have abnormal granules. Abnormal basophils (e.g., hypogranulation) may also indicate MDS or a myeloproliferative disorder. However, degranulation can also occur in acute allergic conditions and during postprandial hyperlipidemia. In patients with suspected primary basophilia, molecular genetic studies for BCR-ABL and JAK2V617F, among others, should be considered to exclude a myeloproliferative neoplasm.

QUALITATIVE DISORDERS OF WBCS

Congenital Disorders of Leukocytes

In addition to the aforementioned quantitative WBC disorders, leukocytes can also have qualitative disorders. There are many constitutional/congenital conditions that may result in dysfunction of neutrophils (Table 1.11). Genetic dysfunctions are rare, but can be severe. Acquired defects are more common, but much less severe. Most of the disorders that will be discussed are associated with neutrophil defects or dysfunction; however, there is a congenital disorder of NK cells that leads to hereditary lymphohistiocytosis (HLH). Familial HLH is an autosomal recessive disease and has a possible gene etiology on chromosomes 9 and 10 (Ohadi, 1999). Secondary HLH occurs in the setting of a strong immunologic response associated with viral (particularly EBV), bacterial, fungal, or parasitic infections and collagen-vascular diseases, as well as T-cell lymphomas. This disease has characteristic findings of fever, splenomegaly, and jaundice. The patient presents with pancytopenia, which is secondary to profound hemophagocytosis within the bone marrow, spleen, and liver (Henter,

TABLE 1.10 **Causes of Basophilia**

Reactive causes of basophilia	
Allergic disease	Chronic sinusitis, hypersensitivity reactions
Infectious disease	Chickenpox, smallpox, tuberculosis
Hematopoietic Neoplasms	Chronic myeloid leukemia, Waldenström's macroglobulinemia, basophilic leukemia, Hodgkin lymphoma, polycythemia vera
Miscellaneous	Radiation, myxedema, chronic hemolytic anemia, post splenectomy, diabetes, increased at onset of menses
Neoplastic causes of basophilia	
Chronic	Chronic myeloid leukemia
Acute	Acute basophilic leukemia

TABLE 1.11 **Congenital Disorders of Leukocytes**

Adhesion defects	Leukocyte adhesion deficiency (types 1, 2, 3)
Granule defects	Neutrophil-specific granule deficiency
	Chediak–Higashi syndrome
	Myeloperoxidase deficiency
Chemotaxis defects	Chediak–Higashi syndrome
	Hyper-IgE (Job) syndrome
	Neutrophil-specific granule deficiency
	Down syndrome
	Neutrophil actin deficiency
	A–mannosidase deficiency
	Severe combined immunodeficiency disease (SCID)
	Wiskott–Aldrich syndrome
	Complement disorders
	Lazy leukocyte syndrome
Phagocytic defects	Chediak–Higashi syndrome
	Neutrophil-specific granule deficiency
	Myeloperoxidase deficiency
	Chronic granulomatous disease
	Immunodeficiency disorders with decreased immunoglobins
	Complement disorders

1991). Hemophagocytosis is observed by the presence of NK cells with perforin release and activated histiocytes that have engulfed erythrocytes, leukocytes, platelets, their precursors, and cellular fragments (Favara, 1992).

The major categories of these neutrophil dysfunctions are adhesion defects, defects in granule structure/function, mobility and chemotaxis defects, and phagocytic or microbicidal defects. Neutrophils have three techniques for combating microorganisms, including phagocytosis, degranulation, and setting neutrophil extracellular traps. The process of phagocytosis consists of the neutrophil internalizing a microbe and killing the microorganism by producing reactive oxygen species (Segal, 2005). As mentioned earlier, neutrophils contain three types of granules. When neutrophils degranulate, the proteins from the three types of granules are able to kill neighboring microbes (Hickey, 2009). Neutrophil extracellular traps are a combination of granule proteins and a chromatin that forms extracellular fibers (Haslett, 1992). The traps bind up microbes and degrade virulence factors. The neutrophils can then phagocytize the microbes or kill them with high concentration degranulation. A breakdown of any of these functions can lead to an increased risk of infection.

There are several laboratory tests that may be used to evaluate neutrophil function (Bogomolski-Yahalom, 1995; Elloumi, 2007). However, most of these are not routinely available in clinical labs. They include the bactericidal killing assay, chemiluminescence assay, superoxide assay, nitroblue tetrazolium (NBT) slide test, and neutrophil chemotaxis assays. Most of these tests rely on the respiratory burst in neutrophils.

Chédiak–Higashi Syndrome

ICD-10 Code E70.3

Chédiak–Higashi is an autosomal recessive disease that is caused by a gene mutation of the CHS1 or LYST protein (part of the BEACH family of vesicle trafficking regulatory proteins), that results in cellular dysfunction and fusion of cytoplasmic granules. Afflicted patients have characteristic giant cytoplasmic granules (Figure 1.19) that result in large secondary lysosomes, which functionally contain less proteinases, elastase, and cathepsin G and, as a result, have slower bactericidal function (Kaplan, 2008; Rezaei, 2009). The giant lysosomal granules are more evident in bone marrow cells than the blood smear. These patients have moderate neutropenia, due to myeloid precursor death while in the marrow and splenic sequestration. They also have thrombocytopenia and perforin-deficient natural killer cells. So these individuals have an increased risk of bacterial and fungal infections due to defects in neutrophil chemotaxis, degranulation, and bactericidal activity. Moreover they are at an increased risk of viral infections due to dysfunctional NK cells. EBV is a classic infection that can lead to EBV-associated lymphoproliferative disorders in this setting (Nargund, 2010).

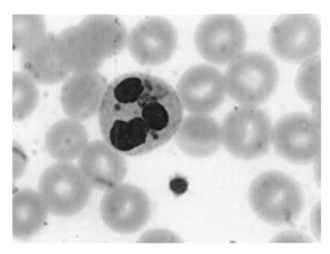

FIGURE 1.19 **Segmented neutrophil from a patient with Chédiak-Higashi syndrome**. Note the large cytoplasmic granules of varying size. (Image courtesy of Dr. Ronald Jaffe, Pittsburgh Children's Hospital.)

Patients with Chédiak–Higashi syndrome also have giant melanosomes that prevent an even distribution of their melanin. Phenotypically they have light silvery hair as well as pale skin and minimal pigment in their iris and optic fundus. They suffer from photophobia and can have horizontal nystagmus. These patients have variable peripheral and cranial neuropathy, ataxia, autonomic dysfunction, muscle weakness, and sensory deficits. They can have prolonged bleeding times with normal platelet counts secondary to impaired platelet aggregation function. Chédiak–Higashi syndrome has an accelerated phase that is characterized by lymphocytic proliferation in the liver, spleen, and bone marrow, and this can result in hepatosplenomegaly, worsening pancytopenia, and an increased susceptibility to infection (Dinauer, 2007). EBV infection in the accelerated phase can display viral-mediated hemophagocytic syndrome, tissue necrosis, and organ failure.

Neutrophil-Specific Granule Deficiency

ICD-10 Code D72.0

Neutrophil-specific granule deficiency (SGD) is an autosomal recessive disorder that is caused by a loss-of-function mutation of CCAAT/enhancer-binding protein ε (Gombart, 2001). The disorder leads to a lack of gelatinolytic activity in the tertiary granules, vitamin B_{12}-binding protein, lactoferrin, as well as a lack of collagenase in specific granules and defensins in primary granules. These neutrophils have a characteristic appearance of absent granules with a bilobed, hyposegmented nucleus (pseudo–Pelger–Huet anomaly). Eosinophils can also be affected and may lack major basic protein, eosinophilic cationic protein, and eosinophil-derived neurotoxin proteins (Rosenberg, 1993). These patients have recurrent pulmonary and cutaneous infections. *Staphylococcus aureus* and *Pseudomonas aeruginosa* are the most commonly involved pathogens.

Chronic Granulomatous Disease

ICD-10 Code D72.0

Chronic granulomatous disease (CGD) is an X-linked (2/3 patients) and autosomal recessive (1/3 patients) disease with defects in expression of glycoproteins (gp91) in the phagocyte membrane. CGD is a primary immunodeficiency disorder of phagocytic cells (neutrophils, monocytes, and macrophages). It comprises five genetic defects impairing one of the five subunits of phagocyte NADPH oxidase (Phox).

Phox normally generates reactive oxygen species (ROS) engaged in intracellular and extracellular microbial killing and resolving accompanying inflammatory processes. The defect can be associated will multiple membrane proteins including p22, p47, and p67. Affected leukocytes are also deficient in C3b receptors. Red blood cells (often acantholytic) bear the McLeod phenotype with absence of Kell antigens Kx and Km. Functionally, the neutrophils cannot activate the respiratory burst process and are not able to kill catalase positive organisms once phagocytosed (Holland, 2010). Consequently these patients have recurrent catalase positive infections with granuloma formation that keep the organisms localized (Heyworth, 2003). The diagnosis is made by neutrophil function testing and mutation analysis. The X-linked recessive inheritance may be confirmed by studying the family history.

Complement Disorders

ICD-10 Code D84.1

Abnormalities in antibodies and complement can result in neutrophil signaling dysfunction (Tedesco, 2008). Affected neutrophils have a break down in their ability to normally apply opsonins and bind chemotatic factors, which results in decreased microbicidal function. C3 deficiency is an autosomal recessive disorder that results in decreased opsonins and consequently can display motility/chemotaxis defects and phagocytic and microbicidal dysfunctions. The severe form of the disease is characterized by recurrent pyogenic infections, and it appears in homozygotes that have undetectable levels of serum C3. Heterozygotes have some functional C3 and can be asymptomatic.

Leukocyte Adhesion Deficiency

ICD-10 Code D72.0

There are two types of genetic leukocyte adhesion deficiency (LAD): type 1 (LAD-1) and II (LAD-II) (Etzioni, 2007). These are autosomal recessive disorders that have adhesion defects that impair cell migration, phagocytosis, and complement- or antibody-dependent cytotoxicity (Arnaout, 1990).

Leukocyte Adhesion Deficiency Type 1. LAD-1 results from an inability of neutrophils to leave the circulation during an infection due to abnormal leukocyte integrins. In LAD-1 there is dysfunction of the CD11/CD18 protein. Patients can have decreased levels of CD11/CD18 cell surface molecules and moderate disease. Patients with complete absence of surface expression of CD11/CD18 proteins have more severe impairment of neutrophil and monocyte adhesion-dependent functions (Foucar, 2006). Although these patients display neutrophilia during infection, due to the decrease in adhesion function they suffer from recurrent sino-pulmonary, skin, and soft-tissue infections, delayed separation of the umbilical cord, poor wound healing, and severely impaired pus formation.

Leukocyte Adhesion Deficiency Type II. LAD-2 results from an inability to appropriately glycosylate another leukocyte adhesion molecule. These individuals have severe cognitive impairment, small stature, and abnormal facies. They have similar but less severe infections than those seen with LAD-1.

Pelger–Huet Anomaly

ICD-10 Code D72.0

Pelger–Huet anomaly (PHA) is an autosomal dominant disorder with mutations in the lamin β-receptor and results in neutrophils that fail to have normal segmentation (Speeckaert, 2009). It was described by Pelger in 1928. Huet recognized the familial nature of this condition in 1931. True PHA is seen in 1 out of 6000 individuals. The characteristic morphology of the neutrophils is of a nonsegmented or a bilobed nucleus, forming a characteristic spectacle or "pince-nez" (dumbbell) shape (Figure 1.20A

and 1.20B). Pince-nez refers to a style of spectacles that are supported without earpieces, by pinching the bridge of the nose. The two lobes are connected by a thin bridge of chromatin. In rare homozygotes with this anomaly, all the neutrophils have round-oval nuclei. The cytoplasm is usually unremarkable in these neutrophils, but it may be accompanied by hypogranulation. Patients with this anomaly tend to be asymptomatic, with no functional deficits of granulocytes (Johnson, 1980) and no other lineage abnormalities. Individuals may show some reduced lobulation of eosinophils and basophils. Pelger–Huet cells can develop multiple lobes with folate or vitamin B_{12} deficiency. The acquired Pelger–Huet anomaly (pseudo–Pelger–Huet) may be induced by drugs (colchicine, sulfonamides), or represent a dysplastic feature seen in myelodysplastic syndrome or other hematologic neoplasms (e.g., AML). The finding of the same anomaly in family members can help confirm the diagnosis. Pelger–Huet cells need to also be distinguished from immature cells observed with a left shift, which have less dense chromatin.

May–Hegglin Anomaly

ICD-10 Code D72.0

May–Hegglin anomaly is a rare autosomal dominant disorder that is associated with a mutation of the MYH9 gene that encodes for nonmuscle myosin heavy chain IIA (Saito, 2008). This mutation results in large, basophilic cytoplasmic inclusions that are

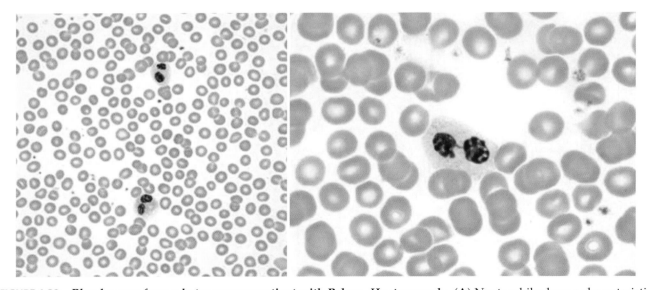

FIGURE 1.20 **Blood smear from a heterozygous patient with Pelger–Huet anomaly.** (A) Neutrophils show a characteristic bilobed appearance. (B) Neutrophil showing a classic bilobed Pelger–Huet nucleus with a "pince-nez" conformation.

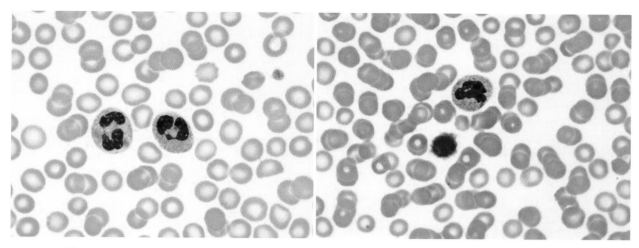

FIGURE 1.21 **Blood smear from a patient with May-Hegglin anomaly.** (**A**) Neutrophils are shown containing light blue Döhle bodies distributed both peripherally and between the nuclear lobes. (**B**) The finding of large cytoplasmic inclusions within a nontoxic neutrophil in association with a giant platelet is pathognomonic.

Döhle-body like (Figure 1.21*A*) (Cawley, 1971; Jenis, 1971). The inclusions are classically identified within neutrophils, but can also be seen in eosinophils, basophils, monocytes, and lymphocytes. The Döhle-like bodies can be abolished by addition of ribonuclease (Mais, 2005). The cytoplasm of neutrophils in this condition do not show other changes (e.g., granules, vacuoles) encountered with toxic or activated neutrophils. They may display other lineage abnormalities, including thrombocytopenia, giant poorly granulated platelets (Figure 1.21*B*), and neutropenia. Thrombocytopenia may be associated with bleeding and purpura (Norris, 1998). Platelet aggregation studies are usually normal.

Alder-Reilly Anomaly

ICD-10 Code D72.0

Alder–Reilly anomaly is an autosomal recessive disorder associated with several genetic mucopolysaccharidoses (i.e., Hurler and Hunter syndromes) (Presentey, 1986). These patients lack the lysozymal enzymes necessary to break down mucopolysaccharides, and they display deeply azurophilic granules in the cytoplasm of all leukocytes (Figure 1.22). The cytoplasmic inclusions are composed of precipitated mucopolysaccharide. Compared to toxic granulation, these bodies are larger and stain positive with metachromatic stains. The abnormality is easier to identify in the bone marrow. Patients often have no functional deficits of their leukocytes or other lineages.

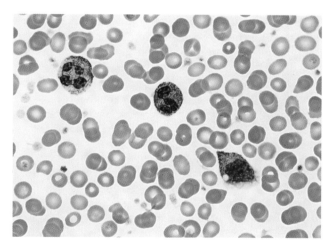

FIGURE 1.22 **Blood smear from an individual with Alder–Reilly anomaly.** Note the segmented neutrophils and a monocyte having many large granules (Alder–Reilly bodies).

Hereditary Hypersegmentation and Giant Neutrophils

ICD-10 Code D72.0

Hereditary hypersegmentation of neutrophils and hereditary giant neutrophils are autosomal dominant inherited disorders of neutrophils. As the name implies, in hereditary hypersegmentation neutrophil nuclei have more than five lobes, but these nuclei display no other abnormalities. Hereditary giant neutrophils have enlarged and hypersegmented nuclei, but not all neutrophils are affected. These patients are asymptomatic and have no abnormalities of other lineages.

Acquired Disorders of Leukocytes

Acquired disorders of leukocytes are more common than congenital disorders. The major categories of neutrophil disorders are the same as the congenital disorders and include adhesion defects, defects in granule structure/function, mobility and chemotaxis defects, and phagocytic and microbicidal defects (Table 1.12). The symptomatology is variable and is dependent on the severity of each patient's defect. Megaloblastic myelopoiesis is a reversible change that can be observed in granulocyte morphology. It arises when DNA synthesis is reduced but RNA synthesis, and hence protein synthesis, remains unaltered. This is seen mainly with vitamin B_{12} and folic acid deficiency, or secondary to alcoholism or a drug-induced effect (e.g., anti-metabolite therapy). The dyssynchrony between nuclear and cytoplasmic development creates large precursors (i.e., giant metamyelocytes and giant bands) and occasionally large neutrophils (macropolyctes). Moreover there is hypersegmentation of neutrophils (Edwin, 1967). Hypersegmentation is defined as exceeding 5% of peripheral blood neutrophils with 5 nuclear lobes, or any neutrophils with 6 or more lobes (Nguyen, 2000). Hypersegmented neutrophils (so-called right shift) can also be seen with infection, uremia, and iron deficiency (Westerman, 1999; Düzgün, 2005), and may resemble dysplastic neutrophils. In the inherited condition known as myelokathexis, neutrophils are also hypersegmented with long chromatin filaments separating the lobes.

TABLE 1.12 Acquired Disorders of Leukocytes

Adhesion defects	Medications (epinephrine, corticosteroids)
	Diabetes
	Renal disorders
	Paraproteinemias
	Sickle cell anemia
Granule defects	Thermal injury
	Trauma/surgery
	Hematologic neoplasms (CML, AML, myelodysplasia)
Chemotaxis defects	Thermal injury
	Medications (colchicine, anti-inflammatory drugs)
	Periodontal disease
	Autoimmune disease (SLE, RA)
	Diabetes
	Malnutrition
	Cirrhosis
	Sepsis
	Viral infections (influenza, HSV, HIV)
	Hematologic/myeloid malignancies
Phagocytic defects	Thermal injury
	Autoimmune disease (SLE, RA)
	Diabetes
	Malnutrition
	Cirrhosis
	Sepsis
	Viral infections-(HIV)
	Sickle cell anemia
	Hematologic neoplasms

REFERENCES

Adams BD, Baker R, Lopez A, Spencer S. 2009. Myeloproliferative disorders and the hyperviscosity syndrome. Emerg Med Clin North Am 27:459–76.

Andrews RG, Briddell RA, Appelbaum FR, McNiece IK. 1994. Stimulation of hematopoiesis in vivo by stem cell factor. Curr Opin Hematol 1:187–96.

Arnaout MA. 1990. Leukocyte adhesion molecules deficiency: its structural basis, pathophysiology and implications for modulating the inflammatory response. Immunol Rev 114:145–80.

Bain BJ. 2002 Blood Cells: A Practical Guide. 3rd ed. Blackwell Science, Oxford.

Bogomolski-Yahalom V, Matzner Y. 1995. Disorders of neutrophil function. Blood Rev 9:183–90.

Brodeur GM, Dahl GV, Williams DL, Tipton RE, Kalwinsky DK. 1980. Transient leukemoid reaction and trisomy 21 mosaicism in a phenotypically normal newborn. Blood 55:691–3.

Buckley RH. 2000 Primary immunodeficiency diseases due to defects in lymphocytes. N Engl J Med 343:1313–24.

Cawley JC, Hayhoe FG. 1972. The inclusions of the May–Hegglin anomaly and Döhle bodies of infection: an ultrastructural comparison. Br J Haematol 22:491–6.

Checkley AM, Chiodini PL, Dockrell DH, Bates I, Thwaites GE, Booth HL, Brown M, Wright SG, Grant AD, Mabey DC, Whitty CJ, Sanderson F. 2010. Eosinophilia in returning travellers and migrants from the tropics: UK recommendations for investigation and initial management. J Infect 60:1–20.

Christensen RD, Rothstein G. 1979. Pitfalls in the interpretation of leukocyte counts of newborn infants. Am J Clin Pathol 72:608–11.

Cianci R, Pagliari D, Pietroni V, Landofi R, Pandolfi F. 2010. Tissue infiltrating lymphocytes: the role of cytokines in their growth and differentiation. J Biol Regul Hemeost Agents 24:239–49.

Datta S, Sarvetnick N. 2009. Lymphocyte proliferation in immune-mediated diseases. Trends Immunol 30:430–8.

Davidson WM, Smith DR. 1954. A morphological sex difference in the polymorphonuclear neutrophil leucocytes. BMJ 2:6–7.

DeSantis DE, Strauss RG. Cell biology and disorders of neutrophils. 1997 In: Clinical Hematology and Fundamentals of Hemostatsis, 3rd ed. FA Davis, Philadelphia,. 16: 265–81.

Dinauer MC. 2007. Disorders of neutrophil function: an overview. Meth Mol Biol 412:489–504.

Düzgün S, Yildirmak Y, Cetinkaya F. 2005. Neutrophil hypersegmentation and thrombocytosis in children with iron deficiency anemia. Turk J Pediatr 47:251–4.

Edwin E. 1967. The segmentation of polymorphonuclear neutrophils. The conditions in hypovitaminosis B$_{12}$ and hypersegmentation. Acta Med Scand 182: 401–10.

Efrati P, Rozenszajn L. 1960. The morphology of buffy coat in normal human adults. Blood 16:1012–9.

Elloumi HZ, Holland SM. 2007. Diagnostic assays for chronic granulomatous disease and other neutrophil disorders. Meth Mol Biol 412:505–23.

Etzioni A. 2007. Leukocyte adhesion deficiencies: molecular basis, clinical findings, and therapeutic options. Adv Exp Med Biol 601:51–60.

Favara B. 1992. Hemophagocytic lymphohistiocytosis: a hemophagocytic syndrome. Semin Diagn Pathol 9:63–74.

Foucar K. 2006. Functional defects of granulocytes. In: Kjeldsberg CR, ed., Practical Diagnosis of Hematologic Disorders. 1. Benign Disorders, 4th ed. ASCP Press, Chicago, 21:239–46.

Gaspar HB, Gilmour KC, Jones AM. 2001. Severe combined immunodeficiency—molecular pathogenesis and diagnosis. Arch Dis Child 84:169–73.

Glassy EF. 1998. Color Atlas of Hematology. CAP, Northfield, IL.

Gombart AF, Shiohara M, Kwok SH, Agematsu K, Komiyama A, Koeffler HP. 2001. Neutrophil-specific granule deficiency: homozygous recessive inheritance of a frameshift mutation in the gene encoding transcription factor CCAAT/enhancer binding protein-epsilon. Blood 97:2561–7.

Gombos MM, Bienkowski RS, Gochman RF, Billett HH. 1998. The absolute neutrophil count: is it the best indicator for occult bacteremia in infants? Am J Clin Pathol 109:221–5.

Groom DA, Kunkel LA, Brynes RK, Parker JW, Johnson CS, Endres D. 1990. Transient stress lymphocytosis during crisis of sickle cell anemia and emergency trauma and medical conditions. An immunophenotyping study. Arch Pathol Lab Med 114:570–6.

Hay BN. 2007. Deletion 22q11: spectrum of associated disorders. Semin Pediatr Neurol 14:136–9.

Hayhoe FGJ, Quaglino D. 1980. Haematological cytochemistry. Churchill Livingstone, London.

Haslett C. 1992. Resolution of acute inflammation and the role of apoptosis in the tissue fate of granulocytes. Clin Sci 83:639–48.

Henter JI, Elinder G, Ost A. 1991. Diagnostic guidelines for hemophagocytic lymphohistiocytosis. Semin Oncol 18:29–33.

Hernandez JA, Aldred SW, Bruce JR, Vanatta PR, Mattingly TL, Sheehan WW. 1980. "Botryoid" nuclei in neutrophils of patients with heatstroke. Lancet 2:642–3.

Heyworth P, Cross A, Curnutte J. 2003. Chronic granulomatous disease. Curr Opin Immunol 15:578–84.

Hickey MJ, Kubes P. 2009. Intravascular immunity: the host–pathogen encounter in blood vessels. Nature Rev Immunol 9: 364–75.

Holland SM. 2010. Chronic granulomatous disease. Clin Rev Allergy Immunol 38:3–10.

Jenis EH, Takeuchi A, Dillon DE, Ruymann FB, Rivkin S. 1971. The May–Hegglin anomaly: ultrastructure of the granulocytic inclusion. Am J Clin Pathol 55:187–96.

Johnson CA, Bass DA, Trillo AA, Snyder MS, DeChatelet LR. 1980. Functional and metabolic studies of polymorphonuclear leukocytes in the congenital Pelger–Huet anomaly. Blood 55:466–9.

Juneja S, Januszewicz E, Wolf M, Cooper I. 1995. Post-splenectomy lymphocytosis. Clin Lab Haematol 17:335–7.

Kano Y, Shiohara T. 2009. The variable clinical picture of drug-induced hypersensitivity syndrome/drug rash with eosinophilia and systemic symptoms in relation to the eliciting drug. Immunol Allergy Clin North Am 29:481–501.

Kaplan J, De Domenico I, Ward DM. 2008. Chediak–Higashi syndrome. Curr Opin Hematol 15:22–9.

Karandikar NJ, Hotchkiss EC, Mckenna RW, Kroft SH. 2002. Transient stress lymphocytosis: an immunophenotypic characterization of the most common cause of newly identified adult lymphocytosis in a tertiary hospital. Am J Clin Pathol 117:819–25.

Klein C. 2009. Congenital neutropenia. Hematology 1:344–50.

Kobrynski LJ, Sullivan KE. 2007. Velocardiofacial syndrome, DiGeorge syndrome: the chromosome 22q11.2 deletion syndromes. Lancet 370(9596):1443–52.

Kubic VL, Kubic PT, Brunning RD. 1991. The morphologic and immunophenotypic assessment of the lymphocytosis accompanying *Bordetella pertussis* infection. Am J Clin Pathol 95:809–15.

Laurence J. 1993. T-cell subsets in health, infectious disease, and idiopathic CD4+ T lymphocytopenia. Ann Intern Med 119:55–62.

Lawrence LW. 1998. The phagocytic leukocytes—morphology, kinetics, and function. In: Stiene-Martin EA, Lotspeich-Steininger CA, Koepke JA, ed. Clinical Hematology: Principles, Procedures, Correlations, 2nd ed., Lippincott, Philadelphia, 22:303–16.

Lombardi C, Passalacqua G. 2003. Eosinophilia and diseases: clinical revision of 1862 cases. Arch Intern Med 163:1371–3.

Lowe D, Jorizzo J, Hutt MS. 1981. Tumour-associated eosinophilia: a review. J Clin Pathol 34:1343–8.

Mais DD. 2005. Quick Compendium of Clinical Pathology. ASCP Press, Chicago, 3.13–3.14.

Malaspina A, Moir S, Chaitt DG, et al. 2007. Idiopathic CD4+ T lymphocytopenia is associated with increases in immature/transitional B cells and serum levels of IL-7. Blood 109:2086–8.

MALDONDAO JE, HANLON DG. 1965. Monocytosis: a current appraisal. Mayo Clin Proc 40:248–59.

MANROE BL, WEINBERG AG, ROSENFELD CR, BROWNE R. 1979. The neonatal blood count in health and disease. I. Reference values for neutrophilic cells. J Pediatr 95(1):89–98.

MARTY J. 1997. Reactive lymphocytosis and infectious mononucleosis. In: Harmening DM, ed., Clinical Hematology and Fundamentals of Hemostatsis, 3rd ed. FA Davis Philadelphia, 17: 283–293.

MITRE E, NUTMAN TB. 2006. Basophils, basophilia and helminth infections. Chem Immunol Allergy 90:141–56.

MOAKE JL, LANDRY PR, OREN ME, SAYER BL, HEFFNER LT. 1974. Transient peripheral plasmacytosis. Am J Clin Pathol 62:8–15.

MORICE, WG. 2007. The immunophenotypic attributes of NK cells and NK-cell lineage lymphoproliferative disorders. AJCP 127:881–6.

NARGUND AR, MADHUMATHI DS, PREMALATHA CS, RAO CR, APPAJI L, LAKSHMIDEVI V. 2010. Accelerated phase of chediak higashi syndrome mimicking lymphoma-a case report. J Pediatr Hematol Oncol 32:e223–6.

NATHAN C. 2006. Neutrophils and immunity: challenges and opportunities. Nature Reviews Immunology. 6:173–82.

NGUYEN DT, DIAMOND LW. 2000. Diagnostic Hematology: A Pattern Approach. Butterworth Heinemann, Oxford.

NKRUMAH FK, ADDY PA. 1973. Acute infectious lymphocytosis. Lancet 1(7814):1257–8.

NORIS P, SPEDINI P, BELLETTI S, MAGRINI U, BALDUINI CL. 1998. Thrombocytopenia, giant platelets, and leukocyte inclusion bodies (May–Hegglin anomaly): clinical and laboratory findings. Am J Med 104:355–60.

OCHS HD, THRASHER AJ. 2006. The Wiskott-Aldrich syndrome. J Allergy Clin Immunol 117:725–38.

OERTEL J, OERTEL B, SCHLEICHER J, HUHN D. 1998. Detection of small numbers of immature cells in the blood of healthy subjects. J Clin Pathol 51:886–90.

OGBOGU PU, BOCHNER BS, BUTTERFIELD JH, GLEICH GJ, HUSS-MARP J, KAHN JE, LEIFERMAN KM, NUTMAN TB, PFAB F, RING J, ROTHENBERG ME, ROUFOSSE F, SAJOUS MH, SHEIKH J, SIMON S, SIMON HU, STEIN ML, WARDLAW A, WELLER PF, KLION AD. 2009. Hypereosinophilic syndrome: a multicenter, retrospective analysis of clinical characteristics and response to therapy. J Allergy Clin Immunol 124:1319–25.

OHADI M, LALLOZ MR, SHAM P, ZHAO J, DEARLOVE AM, SHIACH C, et al. 1999. Localization of a gene for familial hemophagocytic lymphohistiocytosis at chromosome 9q21.3–22 by homozygosity mapping. Am J Hum Genet 64:165–71.

PANTANOWITZ L, MILLER KB, FORD JC, BECKWITH BA. 2004. The scratch test. Arch Path Lab Med 128:598.

PARDANANI A, TEFFERI A. 2008. Primary eosinophilic disorders: a concise review. Curr Hematol Malig Rep 3:37–43.

PATEL KJ, HUGHES CG, PARAPIA LA. 1987. Pseudoleucocytosis and pseudothrombocytosis due to cryoglobulinaemia. J Clin Pathol 40:120–1.

PETERSON L, HRISINKO MA. 1993. Benign lymphocytosis and reactive neutrophilia. Laboratory features provide diagnostic clues. Clin Lab Med 13:863–77.

PETERSON L. Infectious mononucleosis and other reactive disorders of lymphocytes. 2006. In: Kjeldsberg CR, ed. Practical Diagnosis of Hematologic Disorders. 1. Benign Disorders, 4th ed. ASCP Press, Chicago, 23:259–70.

PRESENTEY B. 1986. Alder anomaly accompanied by a mutation of the myeloperoxidase structural gene. Acta Haematol 75:157–9.

RAMPLING, MW. 2003. Hyperviscosity as a complication in a variety of disorders. Semin Thromb Hemost 29(5):459–466.

REZAEI N, MOAZZAMI K, AGHAMOHAMMADI A, KLEIN C. 2009. Neutropenia and primary immunodeficiency diseases. Int Rev Immuno 28:335–66.

ROSENBERG HF, GALLIN JI. 1993. Neutrophil-specific granule deficiency includes eosinophils. Blood. 82:268–73.

ROUFOSSE F, COGAN E, GOLDMAN M. 2003. The hypereosinophilic syndrome revisited. Annu Rev Med 54:169–84.

SAITO H, KUNISHIMA S. 2008. Historical hematology: May–Hegglin anomaly. Am J Hematol 83:304–6.

SAVAGE RA. 1984. Pseudoleukocytosis due to EDTA-induced platelet clumping. Am J Clin Pathol 81:317–22.

SCHMITZ LL, MCCLURE JS, LITZ CE, DAYTON V, WEISDORF DJ, PARKIN JL, BRUNNING RD. 1994. Morphologic and quantitative changes in blood and marrow cells following growth factor therapy. Am J Clin Pathol 101:67–75.

SCHOENTAG RA, CANGIARELLA J. 1993. The nuances of lymphocytopenia. Clin Lab Med 13:923–36.

SCHOFIELD KP, STONE PC, BEDDALL AC, STUART J. 1983. Quantitative cytochemistry of the toxic granulation blood neutrophil. Br J Haematol 53:15–22.

SEEBACH JD, MORANT R, RÜEGG R, SEIFERT B, FEHR J. 1997. The diagnostic value of the neutrophil left shift in predicting inflammatory and infectious disease. Am J Clin Pathol 107:582–91.

SEGAL AW. 2005. How neutrophils kill microbes. Annu Rev Immunol 9:197–223.

SHEIKH J, WELLER PF. 2007. Clinical overview of hypereosinophilic syndromes. Immunol Allergy Clin North Am 27:333–55.

SHIDHAM VB, SWAMI VK. 2000. Evaluation of apoptotic leukocytes in peripheral blood smears. Arch Pathol Lab Med. 124:1291–4.

SILVA MT. 2010. Neutrophils and macrophages work in concert as inducers and effectors of adaptive immunity against extracellular and intracellular microbial pathogens. J Leukoc Biol 87:805–13.

SIMON AK, DESROIS M, SCHMITT-VERHULST AM. 1997. Interferon-regulatory factors during development of CD4 and CD8 thymocytes. Immunology 91:340–5.

SKIEST DJ, KEISER P. 1997. Clinical significance of eosinophilia in HIV-infected individuals. Am J Med 102:449–53.

Speeckaert MM, Verhelst C, Koch A, Speeckaert R, Lacquet F. 2009. Pelger-Huët anomaly: a critical review of the literature. Acta Haematol 121:202–6.

Stiene-Martin EA, Haight V. 1998. Leukocyte abnormalities (nonmalignant). In: Stiene-Martin EA, Lotspeich-Steininger CA, Koepke JA, ed., Clinical Hematology: Principles, Procedures, Correlations, 2nd ed. Lippincott, Philadelphia, 25: 347–63.

Sudo C, Ogawara H, Saleh AW, Nishimoto N, Utsugi T, Ooyama Y, Fukumura Y, Murakami M, Handa H, Tomono S, Murakami H. 2007. Clinical significance of neutrophil apoptosis in peripheral blood of patients with type 2 diabetes mellitus. Lab Hematol 13:108–12.

Tedesco F. 2008. Inherited complement deficiencies and bacterial infections. Vaccine, 26 (suppl 8): I3–8.

Tefferi A, Hanson CA, Inwards DJ. 2005. How to interpret and pursue an abnormal complete blood cell count in adults. Mayo Clin Proc 80:923–36.

Tefferi A, Patnaik MM, Pardanani A. 2006. Eosinophilia: secondary, clonal and idiopathic. Br J Haematol 133: 468–92.

Thomas R, Turner M, Cope AP. 2008. High avidity autoreactive T cells with a low signaling capacity through the T-cell receptor: central to rheumatoid arthritis pathogenesis ? Arthritis Res Ther 10:210–18.

Troussard X, Mossafa H, Valensi F, Maynadie M, Schillinger F, Bulliard G, Malaure H, Flandrin G. 1997. Polyclonal lymphocytosis with binucleated lymphocytes. Morphological, immunological, cytogenetic and molecular analysis in 15 cases (article in French). Presse Med 26:895–9.

Weil SC, Hrisinko MA. 1987. A hybrid eosinophilic-basophilic granulocyte in chronic granulocytic leukemia. Am J Clin Pathol 87:66–70.

Westerman DA, Evans D, Metz J. 1999. Neutrophil hypersegmentation in iron deficiency anaemia: a case-control study. Br J Haematol. 107:512–5.

Witko-Sarsat V, Rieu P, Descamps-Latscha B, Lesavre P, Halbwachs-Mecarelli L. 2000. Neutrophils: molecules, functions and pathophysiological aspects. Lab Invest 80:617–53.

CHAPTER TWO

NON-NEOPLASTIC DISORDERS OF PLATELETS

Lija Joseph

PLATELET PRODUCTION STRUCTURE AND FUNCTION

Production

Pluripotent hematopoietic stem cells, maturing through bipotential erythroid/megakaryocytic precursors, and eventually megakaryoblasts are the precursors of the megakaryocyte, from which the platelets develop. As the name implies, megakaryocytes are the largest hematopoietic cells in the normal bone marrow (100–150 microns in size) (Figures 2.1 and 2.2). Once this cell is committed toward megakaryocytic lineage, it undergoes multiple cycles of endoreduplication of their DNA without cell cytoplasmic division. This leads to the formation of the large cell size often with a DNA ploidy ranging from 4N to 32N. Unlike other elements of the bone marrow, the megakaryocyte remains the earliest identifiable precursor of the platelet under physiologic conditions and routine Hematoxylin and Eosin (H&E) stain. Utilizing special immunohistochemical techniques, one may be able to identify earlier forms of megakaryocytes. Megakaryoblasts express CD34, CD41, c-MPL, and CXCR-4. Once they assume the megakaryocytic form, these cells express CD61 and platelet glycoprotein IIb/IIIa.

In the normal bone marrow the megakaryocytes reside near marrow sinusoids. They develop in the marrow responding to various biochemical and molecular signals to mature into cells that form platelets. Portions of the megakaryocyte cytoplasm project into the sinusoids and bud off into peripheral circulation as platelets. In circulation, platelets survive for about 5 to 9 days. About two-thirds of the platelets remain in circulation and a third remains pooled in the spleen.

Megakaryopoieisis is in primary response to a hormone thrombopoietin. In addition other cytokines, including interleukins, are also involved in thrombopoiesis.

Structure and Function

Platelets are round to oval biconvex anucleate discs about 1.5 to 3.5 microns in size. In routine Romanowsky stained smears they are light purple with a granular cytoplasm (Figure 2.3: normal platelet). The cytoplasm contains mitochondria, Golgi apparatus, microtubules, glycogen granules, as well as enzymes necessary for aerobic and anaerobic respiration.

When evaluated by the electron microscope, there are four types of granules present in the cytoplasm of platelets. The granules contain structures preformed in the megakaryocyte as well as those that are endocytosed from the plasma (Young and Wheater, 2006). They are alpha granules, dense granules, lysosomes,

Non-Neoplastic Hematopathology and Infections, First Edition. Edited by Hernani D. Cualing, Parul Bhargava, and Ramon L. Sandin.
© 2012 Wiley-Blackwell. Published 2012 by John Wiley & Sons, Inc.

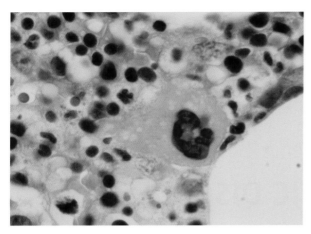

FIGURE 2.1   Normal megakaryocyte biopsy.

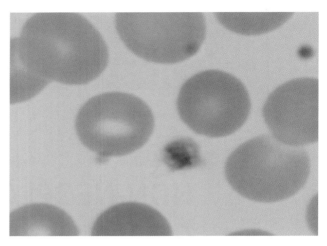

FIGURE 2.3   Normal platelet.

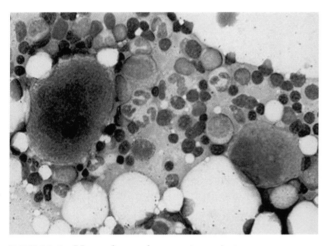

FIGURE 2.2   Normal megakaryocyte aspirate.

TABLE 2.1 **Contents of Platelet Granules**

Alpha granules	Proteoglycans, glycoproteins, coagulation factors, platelet integrin, platelet factor-4, Platelet-derived growth factor, beta thromboglobulin
Dense granules	ATP, ADP, serotonin, histamine, ions (Ca, Mg)

and peroxisomes. Contents of alpha and dense granules are included in Table 2.1.

The primary function of the platelet is in hemostasis. The granules, cytoskeleton of the platelets, and its membrane adhesion molecules participate in normal platelet function. A quiescent platelet is activated by many signals, most importantly thrombin. The platelet primarily achieves its functional role by changes in its structure, adhesion to subendothelial collagen, and secretion of its contents. The platelet secondarily achieves its

effects on hemostasis by activation of endothelial cells and coagulation pathways. Interactions with the endothelial cells help in the process of platelet adhesion even under high shear stress conditions. This step is vWF (von Willebrand factor) dependent, utilizing the platelet receptor GPIb/IX/V. There are other vWF independent mechanisms that aid platelet adhesion under low shear stress conditions, such as the collagen receptor GPIa/IIa. Calcium ions and glycoprotein IIB/IIIA complexes contribute to the platelet aggregation (i.e., platelet-to-platelet interactions forming a platelet plug) processes. A detailed description of the structure and function of platelets can be found in McPherson and Pincus (2006).

The various substances released by the platelets during the process of activation, aggregation, and secretion assist the vasculature to achieve a stable blood clot and control of bleeding. The interaction of platelets with the endothelium is depicted in Figure 2.4. As depicted the interaction with endothelium, circulating coagulation factors, subendothelium, and shear stress factors in vivo are quite complex.

Defects of numbers, structure, or function of platelets leads to various disorders. These disorders will be fully discussed in the next sections.

The reference range of the platelet count is $150-440 \times 10^9/L$. Mild variations in reference ranges do exist among age, gender, racial, and ethnic subgroups, altitudes, and even specific instrument technologies used in the laboratory (Kjeldsberg and Perkins, 2010). For example, the upper limits of normal platelet counts in African American, Latina, and Asian men and women are higher than in Caucasians (Kjeldsberg and Perkins, 2010). In a given clinical context, one may also differentiate degrees of thrombocytopenia into mild

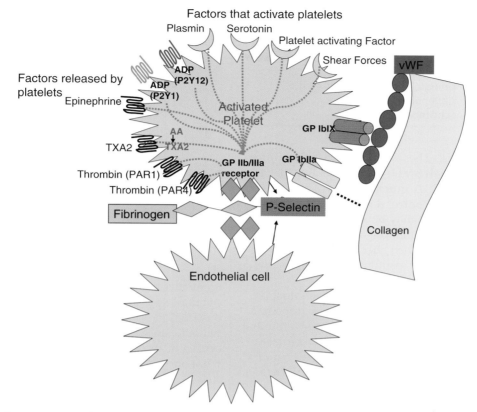

FIGURE 2.4 Platelet receptors & their physiologic interactions. A platelet is activated by thrombin, collagen, plasmin, platelet activating factor, shear stress forces as well as by endothelial cell activation. This leads to morphologic changes as well as activation of several signaling mechanisms, with release of platelet granule contents, as well as expression of various receptors on the platelet membrane. Depicted are simplified schematic representations of GP 1b/IX-vWF interactions in platelet adhesion to subendothelial collagen, non vWF-mediated Gp IbIIa interactions of platelets with collagen, GP IIb/IIIa and fibrinogen mediated platelet-platelet interactions (platelet aggregation) and interactions of platelets with activated endothelial cells. (courtesy Dr. P. Bhargava)

$(100-150 \times 10^9/L)$, moderate $(50-100 \times 10^9/L)$, and severe $(<50 \times 10^9/L)$.

QUANTITATIVE DISORDERS OF PLATELETS

Thrombocytopenia

Definition. Thrombocytopenia refers to a reduction in the platelet count below $150 \times 10^9/L$.

ICD-10 Code D69.6

Clinical Features. Depending on the degree of thrombocytopenia, the patient may manifest with no signs or symptoms, with petechiae, purpura, or hematomas. Bleeding from gums or other mucus membranes may also be seen in severe thrombocytopenia. A complete history (preceding symptoms, family history, dietary history, pharmacologic history, etc.) and a complete physical exam (to evaluate splenomegaly, lymphadenopathy, tumors, infections) are usually helpful in narrowing the diagnostic algorithm.

Lab Diagnosis. A complete blood count (CBC) is the first indication of thrombocytopenia. Evaluation of the peripheral blood smear will often offer additional information that will aid in deciding if a bone marrow examination or additional investigative workup is necessary.

Approach to Evaluation of Thrombobocytopenia
Pseudothrombobocytopenia. Before concluding that a patient has true thrombocytopenia, one needs to make sure that this is not a "spurious" thrombocytopenia due to ex vivo or in vivo factors:

TABLE 2.2 **Ex vivo Conditions Leading to Pseudothrombocytopenia**

Preanalytical	Analytical	Postanalytical
Clotted samples	Instrument derived	Clerical errors
Anticoagulant	Cryoglobulin	LIS errors
Line draw	Clumped platelets	
Clerical errors	Schistocytes	

- Ex vivo Factors: These can be classified into preanaytical, analytical, or postanalytical, as listed in Table 2.2. A quick review of the daily instrument quality control data and evaluation of the peripheral smear may be all that is necessary to make this determination. In routine clinical hematology practice such checks occur regularly before a low platelet count is released in the patient's medical record.

  Platelet clumping is an ex vivo phenomenon that can lead to pseudothrombocytopenia, (Figure 2.5). Platelet satellitism is a unique phenomenon observed in EDTA anticoagulated blood samples at room temperature. In this condition, platelets aggregate around white blood cells [Shahab and Evans, 1998] forming rosette like patterns. Although exact mechanisms have not been elucidated, there appear to be autoantibodies to glycoprotein IIB/IIIA complex which are reactive ex vivo in calcium chelated samples, especially EDTA. In patients demonstrating this phenomenon, platelet counts may require alternative anticoagulants (e.g. heparin), or direct collection of blood into unopettes for phase counts, or bedside fingerstick smears for a smear estimate.

- In vivo factors: In vivo conditions like hemodilution would also lead to thrombocytopenia. Another infrequent, but well-documented phenomenon that can cause pseudothromobocytopenia is plateletphagocytosis or "thrombophagocytosis" (Figure 2.6). In this phenomenon, platelets are ingested by macrophages or neutrophils, probably in response to an immune phenomenon. One case report suggested defects in platelet structure as well as defective platelet function assays in a subject who demonstrated platelet phagocytosis. This phenomenon may occur in vivo or in vitro and is unrelated to hemophagocytic syndrome (Criswell et al., 2001).

True Thrombocytopenia

Although there are many ways of classifying true thrombocytopenia, a practical approach would be to

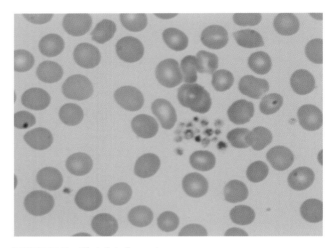

FIGURE 2.5 Platelet clumping.

identify if the cause is due to a defect in platelet production, splenic sequestration, or increased platelet destruction. One must also consider the age of the patient, since many of the congenital or inherited causes of thrombocytopenia are very different from what one would encounter in an adult.

Thrombocytopenia in Children

We list below some of the pediatric syndromes associated with thrombocytopenia. We classified these syndromes into those with large platelet size, those with normal platelet size, and those with small platelets.

Thrombocytopenia with Large Platelets

Large platelet disorders can be identified by evaluating the mean platelet volume on a CBC analyzer or by evaluating a peripheral smear. These disorders include those that have associated neutophilic inclusions as seen in **May–Hegglin anomaly** (ICD-10 Code D72.0), **Epstein syndrome, Sebastian syndrome, and Fechtner syndrome**. Molecular studies have shown that these disorders have a mutation in chromosome 22q12-13 called the MYH 9 gene (myosin heavy chain). Patients with these disorders have mild bleeding tendency and may have associated ocular, auditory, and renal manifestations.

Bernard–Soulier Syndrome

Definition. This syndrome is due to a congenital defect in the platelet glycoprotein 1B-IX complex. It is inherited in an autosomal recessive manner.

ICD-10 Code D69.1

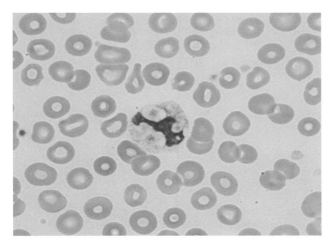

FIGURE 2.6   Platelet phagocytosis.

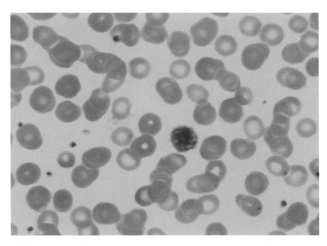

FIGURE 2.7   Giant platelet.

Pathophysiology. The GP 1B-IX complex is necessary for the normal adhesion of platelets to von Willebrand factor (vWF). A defect in this complex thus leads to defects in primary hemostasis.

Clinical Features. This disease manifests as excessive bleeding tendency during surgery.

Lab Diagnosis. Review of peripheral blood smear shows thromobocytopenia and giant platelets (Figure 2.7). Platelet aggregation studies show characteristic lack of aggregation with the agonist ristocetin, with normal response to other agonists such as epinephrine, ADP, collagen, and arachadonic acid. There are newer flow cytometry based assays that evaluate presence of surface glycoprotein GP Ib/IX, as well as genetic assays to evaluate this disorder.

Gray Platelet Syndrome
Definition. Patients with this congenital syndrome have defective alpha granules.

ICD-10 Code D69.1

Pathophysiology. The exact mechanism of this syndrome is not fully described.

Clinical Features. Patients with this type of defective alpha granule contents may manifest with mild symptoms of lifelong bleeding tendency.

Lab Diagnosis. Abnormal responses to thrombin and collagen agonists in a platelet aggregation

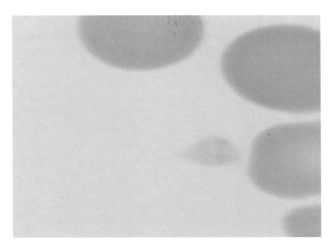

FIGURE 2.8   Gray platelet.

study maybe helpful in identifying this disorder. On a peripheral smear exam one may see large platelets (about 13 microns) with gray or pale appearance without the usual cytoplasmic granularity (Figure 2.8). The bone marrow may show reticulin fibrosis. Electron microscopic studies may show selective lack of alpha granules.

Thrombocytopenia with Decreased Platelet Size
Wiskott–Aldrich Syndrome and X-Linked Thrombocytopenia
Definition. These are congenital disorders related to the Wiskott–Aldrich syndrome gene protein (WASp) gene located on the X chromosome.

ICD-10 Code Wiskott–Aldrich syndrome D82.0 and X-Linked thrombocytopenia D69.1

Pathophysiology. A defective WASp gene leads to a defective hematopoietic stem cell development and function.

Clinical Features. Patients often have the more severe symptoms of thrombocytopenia. They may also have a tendency for frequent infections and other immune dysfunctions.

Lab Diagnosis. The platelets in these syndromes are small, and the platelet function tests show markedly abnormal responses to ADP, epinephrine, and collagen.

Thrombocytopenia with Normal Platelet Size

Both **congenital and acquired thrombocytopenias** can lead to platelet production disorders. The acquired processes include immune thrombocytopenic purpura (ITP), thrombotic thrombocytopenic purpura (TTP), disseminated intravascular coagulation (DIC), HIT hepatin-induced thrombocytopenia (HIT), hemolysis, elevated liver enzymes, and low platelet syndrome (HELLP), neonatal alloimmune thrombocytopenia, congenital rubella syndrome, and drug-induced thrombocytopenia (DIT), among many others. Congenital causes include c-MPL mutations, thrombocytopenia with absent radii (TAR syndrome, ICD-10 Q87.2), Tel-AML-1. One may need to evaluate bone marrow for adequate megakaryocytes in this group of disorders in order to determine if the defect is due to increased destruction or defective production of platelets.

For the rest of this discussion we will focus on adult thrombocytopenia.

Thrombocytopenia in Adults

These can be broadly categorized as due to disorders of platelet production, or increased platelet destruction.

Disorders of Platelet Production

As described earlier, bone marrow megakaryocytes are the primary site of platelet production. A pathogenic process that inhibits or affects megakaryocyte formation or maturation will result in this type of thrombocytopenia. Usually such processes also involve other cell lines especially in cases of chemotherapy, radiation therapy, or other neoplastic or marrow infiltrative disorders. Bone marrow failure, as may be seen in aplastic anemia and other related disorders such as paroxysmal

TABLE 2.3 Common Medications That Cause Thrombocytopenia

Sulfonamides
Phenytoins
Valproic acid
Quinidine
Heparin
Thiazides

nocturnal hemoglobinuria, and myelodysplasia can also cause thromobocytopenia. However, certain drugs or immune responses can be specifically megakaryotoxic. A partial list of drugs that cause isolated thrombocytopenia are included in Table 2.3

Infectious organisms may also be involved in thrombocytopenia. They include human immunodeficiency virus, hepatitis B and C, ehrlichia, leptospirosis, malaria, measles, mumps, Q fever, rubella, syphilis, Ebstein–Barr virus, and cytomegalovirus. The pathogenic mechanisms can be complex and may involve cytokines including interleukin-10.

Other rare immune or idiopathic conditions selectively affecting platelet production include acquired amegakaryocytic thrombocytopenic purpura, which may be due to T-cell aberrancies, MYH-9 related thrombocytopenia syndrome, Mediterranean macrothrombocytopenia and cyclic thrombocytopenia.

Drug-Induced Thrombocytopenia

Definition. This disorder is diagnosed when a definitive association between the thrombocytopenia and the medication can be established

ICD-10 Code D69.5

Pathophysiology The pathogenic mechanisms involved in the thrombocytopenia, may be elusive. However, some well know mechanisms have been identified. They can be broadly categorized as due to (1) increased destruction of the platelets or (2) decreased production in the bone marrow.

The majority of drugs cause thrombocytopenia by an immune-mediated mechanism, leading to increased platelet destruction, and such drugs have recently been reviewed by Kenney and Stack (2009) and Aster and Bougie (2007). Drugs may act as haptens, induce conformational change in platelet receptors, create a neoepitope, or induce alloantibodies. Although heparin is the most often cited (this is discussed under the heparin-induced thrombocytopenia section), many medications have been identified to cause thrombocytopenia.

Specific marrow ablative medications used as part of chemotherapeutic regimens are the primary category of drugs causing thrombocytopenia due to decreased production of platelets. However, certain other drugs, and environmental toxins including alcohol can be directly megakaryoctotoxic.

Clinical Features. Since thrombocytopenia is usually severe (typically <20–30,000/μL), most of the patients have hemorrhagic manifestations, unlike heparin, which causes thrombosis (see discussion in a separate section below). It is important to recognize this etiology, since drug-induced thrombocytopenia may be the one of the most frequent causes of thrombocytopenia in a clinical setting where patients are on multiple medications that may not be usually considered as a cause of thrombocytopenia. One has to have a high index of suspicion in a patient with rapid onset of severe thrombocytopenia usually occurring within a few days (3–10 days) of starting the drug. In patients on multiple medications, one may have to stop one drug at a time to see if the platelet count recovers. If the onset of thrombocytopenia is within 24 hours after administering the new drug, one must consider preexisting antibodies. If it occurs after 2 weeks, most likely the etiology is marrow suppression.

Lab Diagnosis. The diagnosis is generally made on clinical grounds. Some laboratories offer limited testing of drug-dependant antibodies (e.g., flow cytometry based) to evaluate the mechanisms and appropriate therapies can be instituted once identified (Kenney and Stack, 2009).

Heparin-Induced Thrombocytopenia
Definition. Heparin-induced thrombocytopenia is seen in patients who develop thrombocytopenia following heparin therapy.

ICD-10 Code D75.82

Heparin therapy is discussed specifically to highlight the many unique characteristics, as well as its potential life-threatening nature. Thrombocytopena affects about 5 to 8% of patients who are initiated on unfractionated or low-molecular-weight heparin therapy.

Pathophysiology. In patients who are prone to this complication, platelet factor-4 (PF-4) released from platelets form complexes with heparin, and antibodies are developed against this macromolecular complex. The antibody can bind to platelets and activate them as well as activate endothelial cells into a procoagulant surface. These mechanisms thus cascade to cause thrombocytopenia and thrombosis (Arepally and Ortel, 2010).

Clinical Features. Patients usually develop thrombocytopenia at about 5 to 14 days after initiation of therapy; however, since the nadir is generally at about 50–60,000/μL, patients do not bleed spontaneously. They are, however, at significant risk for thrombotic complications. An early onset form (<24 hours) as well as a late onset form (several weeks) has also been described. There are clinical scoring criteria developed (4 T score) to assess probability of HIT. This involves assigning scores of 0, 1, and 2 for degree of thrombocytopenia, the time of onset of thrombocytopenia, thrombotic, or other sequelae, and other factors that may contribute to the thrombocytopenia. Scores of 6 to 8 suggest a high probability of HIT.

Lab Diagnosis. It is critical to be vigilant of decreased platelet production or platelet destruction in patients exposed to heparin, and recently developed laboratory tests that detect the PF-4/heparin antibody can be used along with clinical scoring criteria. Serotonin release assays (considered the gold standard), heparin-induced platelet activation assays, and solid-phase immunoassays are used. A presumptive diagnosis of HIT may initially be made on clinical grounds as laboratory testing might take more time than what a clinically emergent situation would warrant; in such cases heparin must be discontinued and alternative anticoagulant therapy initiated. Specific guidelines for the diagnosis and management of this entity are discussed in a recent review by Arepally and Ortel (2010).

Disorders of Platelet Destruction
Thrombotic Thrombocytopenic Purpura (TTP)
Definition. This is one of a spectrum of thrombotic microangiopathies and is included in this section because of its distinct manifestation of thrombocytopenia.

ICD-10 Code M31.1

Pathophysiology. Recent reviews of the pathogenesis of this entity has specifically identified (often acquired, but rarely congenital) deficiency of, or inhibitor to ADAMTS 13, a protease that cleaves von Willebrand factor (George, 2006).

Clinical Features. The syndrome of TTP is characterized by a classic pentad of fever, microangiopathic hemolytic anemia, thrombocytopenia, and neurologic and renal manifestations. If often affects females between the ages of 10 and 39 years.

Lab Diagnosis. ADAMTS13 protease (activity and inhibitor) can be assayed in the clinical laboratory in patients suspected of having TTP. A peripheral smear examination is useful in identifying and quantifying schistocytes and is often performed on patients suspected of TTP as a quick evaluation and screening. The critical point to remember in this scenario is that such patients should not be transfused with platelets and plasma exchange remains the primary therapy of choice. Moreover one needs to have a high index of clinical suspicion, and in the appropriate clinical context, therapy needs to be initiated without awaiting results of tests such as ADAMTS13 that may not be available on site.

A comprehensive review of thrombotic microangiopathies is reported by Zheng and Sadler (2008).

Immune Thrombocytopenic Purpura (ITP)
Definition. ITP is an immune-mediated acquired thrombocytopenia and currently is a clinical diagnosis of exclusion.

ICD-10 Code D69.3

Although previously termed idiopathic thrombocytopenic purpura, strong evidence of immunologic mechanisms involved in the pathogenesis of this disease has now allowed wide acceptance of this current terminology for patients with acquired thrombocytopenia without other underlying diseases.

Pathophysiology. This disease is considered to develop from immune destruction of platelets due to autosensitization. The etiologic factor that leads to the autosensitization remains controversial; many of the immune responses seem to be directed toward platelet surface glycoprotein. In addition to this there appears to be a role for altered or abnormal immune regulatory pathways that contribute to the destruction of platelets (Cines and Blanchette, 2002; Cines and Bussel, 2005; Provan et al., 2010).

Clinical Features. Commonly seen among 18- to 40-year-old patients with a distinct predilection for women, the disease presents with purpuric lesions. In its classic adult form it presents insidiously in women between the ages of 15 and 40 and presents as a chronic disease. However, older adults or children may also be affected. When it affects children, there is no sex predilection, it is generally acute in onset

and although thrombocytopenia is severe, it resolves spontaneously in over 80% of children.

Lab Diagnosis. Peripheral smear shows normal to larger platelets and a bone marrow study, if performed, will show adequate to increased megakaryocytes.

Consensus guidelines in diagnosis and management of patients with ITP have been recently published (Provan et al., 2010).

Thrombocytosis
Definition. An increase in platelet count (>450,000/μL) is considered thrombocytosis.

Etiology. Increased platelet counts may result from a variety of reactive or neoplastic processes. Differentiating the two processes can be challenging. Careful clinical history and physical examination can give some clues as to the nature of the thrombocytosis. A detailed evaluation of the peripheral smear will often provide additional discriminating details. Table 2.4 lists reactive conditions that lead to elevated platelet counts.

Pseudothrombocytosis
Circulating cryoglobulins, red blood cell fragments, hemoglobin H inclusions, and chronic lymphocytic leukemia fragmentation can lead to pseudothrombocytosis. This is often easily identified by careful clinical history, automated instrument quality control checks, and peripheral blood smear review.

Reactive Thrombocytosis
As shown in Table 2.4, although transient reactive thrombobocytosis can occur after acute blood loss or recovery after chemotherapy, it is the sustained reactive thrombobocytosis that can be difficult to differentiate from neoplastic thrombocytosis. Some

TABLE 2.4 Causes of Reactive Thrombocytosis

Acute stress response
Infection
Hemorrhage
Exercise
Postsurgical
Chronic diseases
Anemia, especially iron deficiency
Neoplasia
Immunological disorders

morphologic clues that may point to the latter include presence of large and giant platelets, basophilia, left-shifted WBCs, and nucleated RBCs with or without dyspoiesis. In equivocal cases, ancillary testing, including marrow examination and molecular testing (e.g. JAK2 mutational analysis), may be needed.

Essential thromobocythemia is a primary neoplastic disorder. It is beyond the scope of this chapter and will not be discussed further in this review.

Clinical Features. Patients with reactive thrombocytosis may have no symptoms, may have a bleeding tendency, or may present with thrombotic episodes, depending on the etiology and additional risk factors (Schafer, 2004).

Lab Diagnosis. Some studies suggest measuring thrombopoietin in differentiating reactive from primary thrombocytosis (Kaushansky, 2008). Additional molecular studies (e.g., BCR-ABL and JAK2) may be warranted in some cases to exclude underlying myeloproliferative disorders.

QUALITATIVE DISORDERS OF PLATELETS

ICD-10 Code D69.1

Although rare, these platelet disorders can cause significant morbidity and diagnostic challenges to the clinical team.

Congenital Causes of Defects in Platelet Function

This category of platelet disorders can be categorized based on the pathophysiologic mechanisms. These mechanisms are discussed in the sequence below.

Defects in Platelet Adhesion

Bernard–Soulier Syndrome This is due to a congenital defect in the Gp Ib/IX receptor on platelets leading to defective adhesion, and is discussed above (see thrombocytopenia in children).

von Willebrand Disease

Definition. This is a group of disorders with either a qualitative of quantitative defect in von Willebrand factor (vWF). Although the defect is not in the platelets per se, it is discussed briefly here as it is a common disorder with an effect on platelet function.

ICD-10 Code D68.0

Pathophysiology. von Willebrand factor (vWF) is a protein that stabilizes factor VIII in circulation. If not adherent to vWF, factor VIII will be rapidly removed from circulation. vWF also allows platelets to adhere to subendothelial collagen. It is present in endothelial cells (in Weibel–Palade bodies), platelets (alpha granules), and megakaryocytes. Defects in quality or quantity of VWF can lead to a group of diseases termed von Willebrand disease and its various subtypes (as listed in Table 2.5). Type 1 vWD, the most common form, is inherited as an autosomal dominant disease.

Clinical Features. Clinical presentation of vWD is often in the form of episodic mucocutaneous bleeding, such as easy bruising, nose bleeds, and menometrorrhagia in a premenopausal woman. Careful family history is important in evaluating patients with vWD.

One must also consider an acquired form of VWD in older patients who have an underlying hematopoietic neoplasia, cardiovascular disease, drug exposures, or autoimmune disorder. Patients with acquired vWD develop autoantibodies to vWF or may have a deficiency of vWF because of adsorption to tumor cells or increased destruction of the factor. Although laboratory testing maybe

TABLE 2.5 Subtypes of von Willebrand Disease (vWD)

Type 1		Quantitatively low amounts of qualitatively normal VWF
Type 2		Qualitatively abnormal VWF
	Type 2A	Selectively low amounts of high-molecular-weight multimers of VWF
	Type 2B	Increased affinity of vWF to platelets leads to thrombocytopenia
	Type 2M	Similar to type 2A, but all multimers are present
	Type 2N	Defective binding to factor VIII
Type 3		Absent vWF
Platelet type		Gain of function mutation on platelet receptor for vWF

helpful in identifying this disorder, one has to have a high index of suspicion because a screening study may not identify this possibility.

Lab Diagnosis. This generally involved measurements of vWF activity (ristocetin based, or collagen based), vWF antigen, and factor VIII levels. Specific laboratory tests incorporating platelet aggregation studies (e.g., ristocetin-induced platelet aggregation assays) as well as vWF multimer analysis may additionally be performed to evaluate a patient with vWD. Mutations responsible for this disease have been documented, and family studies are indicated in patients suspected of this condition.

Defects in Platelet Aggregation

Defective platelet aggregation can lead to abnormal platelet function. Abnormal surface glycoproteins on the platelets are usually involved in the pathogenesis of this group of diseases.

Glanzmann's Thrombasthenia

Definition. This is an autosomal recessive disease that is caused by a defect in the glycoprotein IIb/and/or IIIa complex of the platelet membrane.

ICD-10 Code D69.1

Clinical Features. The patients with this disease may have excessive bleeding usually manifesting in infancy or childhood. Although the platelet count is normal, they are functionally defective.

Lab Diagnosis. This can be identified by specific aggregation pattern in a platelet aggregation study (as shown in Table 2.6) or by more recent flow cytometry based assays (Sebastiano et al., 2010).

Defects in Platelet Granule Secretion

The various granules present in the platelet are secreted when it is activated. Defects in the content of the various platelets granules, their secretion when activated, or its function after activation can lead to this group of disorders. Again specific patterns in platelet aggregation studies can be helpful in identifying this group of disorders.

Storage Pool/Release Defects

This term is used to encompass patient with defects in the various granules in the platelets, or defects in the ability of the platelets to traffic them to

TABLE 2.6 **Comparison of Some Platelet Function Tests**

Method	Principle	Advantages	Limitations
PFA 100	Adhesion and aggregation test using occlusion time of a defined aperture coated with various agonists	Whole blood, not affected by heparin	May be affected by platelet counts, sample volume
Platelet works	Percent aggregation in agonist coated tubes	Whole blood, measures platelet count and aggregation	Testing should be done within 10 minutes, limited clinical application mostly in antiplatelet therapy monitoring
VerifyNow	Fibrinogen-coated beads that respond to proportion of GPIIb/IIIa receptors on platelet surface	Whole blood	Low hematocrit may affect results, does not detect functional disorders or vWD
Thromboelastograph	Measure of mechanical stability and strength of clot as induative of platelet function	Whole blood, graph predicts other coagulation defects including deficient clotting factors, heparin effect, hypercoagulable states	Does not detect vWD or non–thrombin-dependent disorders of platelets
Light transmission aggregometry	Aggregation response to various agonists	Considered gold standard with specific guidelines recently published by CLSI for use and interpretation	Platelet-rich plasma, takes about 4 hours; requires normal blood as quality control

the surface to release contents. Defects of alpha granules, delta granules, as well as other granules have been described. These patients may be asymptomatic or may have mild to moderate bleeding tendencies. Gray platelet syndrome, Chédiak–Higashi syndrome, Hermansky–Pudlasky syndrome and Quebec platelet disorder are some examples of diseases where specific storage pool defects have been identified.

A comprehensive discussion of congenital platelet disorders can be found in Henry's textbook as well as a recent review by Hayward et al. (McPherson and Pincus, 2006; Hayward et al., 2006).

Acquired Defects in Platelet Function

Aspirin is a widely know medication used to inhibit platelet function in patients with cardiovascular diseases. Newer antiplatelet agents like dipyridamole, clopidogrel, and Gp IIB/IIIA inhibitors are also available on the market that specifically inhibits platelet function. Several point-of-care platform tests are now available to test a patient's response to these newer medications.

Dysfunctional platelets maybe present in many chronic diseases like myeloproliferative disorders, diabetes mellitus, hypertension, liver disease, uremia, renal failure, scurvy, and other hematologic and nonhematologic neoplasia. Exact pathophysiologic mechanisms are not fully understood in all of these diseases. However, it is important to recognize that in additional to various coagulation defects, platelet dysfunction contributes to the hematologic manifestations in chronically ill patients. In such patients, a normal platelet count may not be enough to achieve hemostasis, and additional functional studies may be needed.

Laboratory Tests used to Assess Platelet Function

Besides routine CBC studies and bone marrow studies, several new tests that can be used in physician offices as stand-alone testing platforms are now available. We will briefly discuss these tests. Table 2.6 shows a comparison of tests now available to assess platelet function. Detailed discussion of platelet aggregometry is included at the end of this discussion.

Platelet Function Analyzer-100 (PFA-100, Siemens Healthcare, Tarrytown, New York)

This instrument is used to evaluate platelet aggregation and adhesion. Briefly, the instrument utilizes a device that has various agonists coated onto an aperture of defined size. When platelets pass rapidly through this region, they adhere to these agonists, causing closure of the aperture and time to closure can be measured. The test can be performed on whole blood samples. It can be used to evaluate aspirin effect, as well as screen for von Willebrand disease and other intrinsic platelet defects where aggregation responses to various agonists are altered.

Plateletworks (Helena Laboratories, Beaumont, Texas)

This instrument utilizes a method of comparing baseline and residual platelet count after the whole blood is collected in various tubes coated with specific agonists that initiate aggregation. Thus a percentage of platelets that have aggregated is calculated to evaluate the platelet function. This instrument is being marketed as a rapid point-of-care test available to evaluate patient response to platelet Glycoprotein IIb/IIIa (Gp IIb/IIIa) inhibitor therapy.

Verify Now (Accumetrics, San Diego, California)

This point-of-care test is specifically aimed to evaluate platelet function in patients on various antiplatelet medications especially in high risk cardiovascular diseases. Some patients receiving standard doses of antiplatelet medication may not have therapeutic effects or are considered "low reponders" In such patients, monitoring and optimizing platelet function is necessary. This test utilizes fibrinogen-coated beads that are mixed with whole blood samples. The coated beads will aggregate the platelets in direct proportion to available Gp IIb/IIIa on the platelet surface. So, if there is adequate suppression/inhibition of the receptors, the aggregation response will be less.

Thromboelastograph (Haemonetics, Braintree, Massachusetts)

Instead of aggregation assay using light transmittance, this method uses the surrogate of clot formation and its strength as a measure of platelet function. Various instruments are available. This test is mostly being used in patients undergoing cardiothoracic surgery specifically in the immediate postoperative period to determine specific causes of postoperative hematological recovery. Various response patterns can indicate heparin effect, platelet dysfunction, coagulation factor depletion, or hypercoagulability in a given sample. Test can be done on whole blood and after activation of the coagulation system.

Flow Cytometry

This test utilizes the basic principles of flow cytometry and is used to evaluate the specific receptor

TABLE 2.7 Qualitative Abnormalities of Platelet Function as Evaluated by Platelet Aggregation Tests

Syndromes	Aggregation Response to				Special Features
	ADP	Epinephrine	Collagen	Ristocetin—High Dose (1.2 ug/ml)	
Bernard–Soulier disease	Normal	Normal	Normal	• Decreased • Addition of normal plasma (without platelets) fails to correct aggregation • Correction will occur in vWD	• Platelet defect • Large platelets seen on smear • Clinically severe, rare • Deficiency of membrane glycoprotein GP1b • Mild to moderate platelet decrease
Von Willebrand's disease	Normal	Normal	Normal	• Decreased • Type IIB—increased response to low-dose Ristocetin 0.6 ug/ml	• Deficiency or defect in vWF • this is not a platelet defect • Type I, II and III • Normal platelet count (except in IIB)
Glanzmann's thrombasthenia	Absent	Absent	Absent	Normal	• Rare, clinically severe • Deficiency of membrane glycoprotein GPIIb/IIIa • Normal platelet count
Storage pool disease	Normal to decreased primary wave Decreased or absent secondary wave	Normal to decreased primary wave Decreased or absent secondary wave	Decreased	Normal	• Deficiency in dense or alpha Granules • Seen in Chédiak–Higashi, Hermanski–Pudlak, Wiscott–Aldrich, TAR, gray platelet syndrome • Normal platelet count
Aspirin defect	Decreased	Decreased	Normal	Normal	• Aggregation response to arachidonic acid decreased
Myeloproliferative disorders • Polycythemia vera (PV) • Chronic Myelogenous Leukemia (CML) • Myelofibrosis • Essential thrombocythemia (ET)	Normal	Decreased	Normal	Normal	• Aggregation response to arachidonic acid will be normal

Source: Data kindly provided by Kathy White MT (ASCP) Boston Medical Center, Boston, MA 02118.

on the platelet surface. Once the fluorescent labeled markers are bound to the platelet surface, one can gate the platelets and measure the expression of these markers. Thus this test can be used in various scenarios, depending on which surface markers are tested.

For example, if Gp IIb/IIIa markers are being evaluated and there appears to be deficiency of these, one maybe able to diagnose Glanzmann's thrombasthenia in the appropriate clinical setting. Response to specific antiplatelet medication can also be monitored using this methodology. One of the advantages of this test is that it can be done even if the platelet count is low, since many of the other tests described above require a minimum number of platelets.

Platelet Reticulocyte Assay

Flow cytometry principles are also used to evaluate "young platelets" or reticulated platelets. This evaluates the RNA or DNA content of platelets. Some of the newer hematology analyzers have this capability to measure "immature platelet fraction." This maybe used in determining a production versus destruction etiology of thrombocytopenia.

Electron Microscopy

Evaluation of platelet structure, specific granule content, and absence of organelles maybe evaluated using electron microscopy.

Platelet Release Assays

Specific disorders of platelets that are related to alpha or dense granules, can be evaluated either by directly measuring the contents of these granules (see Table 2.1) or by direct evaluation of the specific granules that are released by these granules in an aggregation test platform. Certain secondary waves of the platelet aggregation response curve are directly related to the release of granule content. One may also use flow cytometry or test secondary markers using enzyme-linked immunoassays to evaluate the release of granule content.

Light Transmission Platelet Aggregometry

Platelet aggregation tests performed in a platelet aggregometer utilizes the principle of light transmittance as platelets clump in response to various agonists. The percent light transmittance recorded during a defined timeframe will provide an estimate of platelet function. A primary wave occurs from the initial response to the agonist. A secondary wave in response to the release of platelet granules is recorded for certain agonists. The pattern of aggregation in response to various agonists can be interpreted to identify specific defects of platelet function. The yield as well as sensitivity and specificity of diseases identified by this method will depend on the number of agonists used in a given test as well as predicted reference intervals (CLSI guidelines, 2008; Pai and Hayward, 2009; Kottke-Marchant and Corcoran, 2002). The CLSI standards published in 2008 summarize platelet function testing guidelines, including guidelines of specimen requirements and quality control (CLSI guidelines, 2008). Ideally, if medically possible, the patient should avoid any medication

that affects platelet function for 14 days prior to testing. The platelet collection should be on a fasting sample, and the patient must avoid a fatty meal.

Blood collected with a needle gauge between 19 and 21 and minimal trauma and cuff pressure is suggested. Sodium citrate is the recommended anticoagulant with an anticoagulant to blood ratio of 1:9. It must be transported at room temperature and processed within 4 hours of collection (CLSI guidelines, 2008).

There are various factors that affect platelet function test, including clinical history, pharmacologic history, diet, smoking, fasting status, as well as other systemic diseases. Although not standardized among institutions, aggregometry is currently the most commonly used test used in evaluating platelet function. Table 2.7 summarizes the commonly used agonists and their use in assessing platelet function.

REFERENCES

Arepally GM, Ortel TL. 2010. Heparin-Induced Thrombocytopenia An Rev Med 61:77–90.

Aster RH, Bougie DW 2007. Drug-induced immune thrombocytopenia. N Engl J Med 357:580–7.

Cines DB, Blanchette VS. 2002. Immune thrombocytopenic purpura. N Engl J Med 346:995–1008.

Cines DB, Bussel JB. 2005. How I treat idiopathic thrombocytopenic purpura (ITP). Blood 106:2244–51.

CLSI Document H-58A. Platelet function testing by aggregometry: approved guideline. Vol 28, no.31 Clinical and laboratory Standards Institute, Wayne, PA 2008.

Criswell KA, Breider MA, Bleavins MR. 2001. EDTA-dependent platelet phagocytosis: a cytochemical, ultrastructural, and functional characterization. Am J Clin Pathol 115:376–84.

George JN. 2006. Thrombotic thrombocytopenic purpura. N Engl J Med 354:1927–35.

Hayward CPM, Rao AK, Cattaneo M. 2006, Congenital platelet disorders, overview of their mechanisms, diagnostic evaluation and treatment Hemophilia 12(suppl3):128–36.

Kaushansky K. 2008. Historical review: megakaryopoiesis and thrombopoiesis. Blood 1 (111):981–6.

Kenney B, Stack G. 2009. Drug-induced thrombocytopenia. Arch Pathol Lab Med 133:309–14.

Kjeldsberg CR, Perkins SL. 2010. Practical Diagnosis of Hematologic Disorders, 5th ed. American Society for Clinical Pathology, Chicago, 920–4.

Kottke-Marchant K, Corcoran G. 2002. The laboratory diagnosis of platelet disorders. Arch Pathol Lab Med 126:133–46.

McPherson RA H Pincus MR. 2006, Henry's Clinical Diagnosis and Management by Laboratory Methods. Saunders, philadelphia, 758–60.

McPherson RA H Pincus. 2006. MR Henry's Clinical Diagnosis and Management by Laboratory Methods. Saunders, philadelphia, 747–8.

Pai M, Hayward CPM. 2009. Diagnostic assessment of platelet disorders: what are the challenges to standardization? Semin Thromb Hemost 35:131–8.

Provan D, Stasi R, Newland AC, et al. 2010. International consensus report on the investigation and management of primary immune thrombocytopenia Blood 115:168–86.

Provan D, Stasi R, Newland AC, Blanchette VS, Bolton-Maggs P, Bussel JB, Chong BH, Cines DB, Gernsheimer TB, Godeau B, John Grainger J, Greer I, Hunt BJ, Imbach PA, Lyons G, McMillan R, Rodeghiero F, Sanz MA, Tarantino M, Watson S, Young J, Kuter DS. 2010. International consensus report on the investigation and management of primary immune thrombocytopenia Blood 115:168–86.

Schafer AI. 2004. Thrombocytosis (current concepts). N Engl J Med 350:1211–9.

Sebastiano C, Bromberg M, Breen K, Hurford MT. 2010. Glanzmann's thrombasthenia: report of a case and review of the literature Int J Clin Exp Pathol 3(4): 443–7.

Shahab N, Evans ML. 1998. Platelet satellitism. N Engl J Med 338:591.

Yermiahu T, Shalev H, Hatskelzon L. 1995. Thrombocytosis: misdiagnosis and its prevention. Am J Hematol 48:58–70.

Young B, Wheater PR. 2006. Wheater's Functional Histology: A Text and Colour Atlas. Churchill Livingstone/Elsevier, London, pages 56–57.

Zheng XL, Sadler JE. 2008. Pathogenesis of thrombotic microangiopathies An Rev Pathol 3:249–77.

CHAPTER THREE

APPROACH TO DISORDERS OF RED BLOOD CELLS

Jason C. Ford

INTRODUCTION

Diseases affecting red blood cells (RBCs) are among the most common illnesses worldwide. Red cell disorders are the most common human genetic diseases (Weatherall, 2010a), and acquired anemias affect up to 25% of the world's population (Lewis, 2005). In the United States and Canada the complete blood count (CBC) is the first or second most commonly ordered laboratory test, depending on the patient population (van Walraven, 2003; Tierney, 1988).

Red blood cells are evolved to serve essentially a single function: to carry oxygen from the lungs to the tissues (and on the return journey to carry carbon dioxide from the tissues to the lungs). At the risk of oversimplification, red cells are merely bags of hemoglobin with some supportive enzymes to keep the hemoglobin functional. In disorders of RBCs, oxygen-carrying capacity is usually reduced owing to some combination of reduced red cell numbers and/or dysfunctional hemoglobin. This chapter will focus primarily on the diagnostic approach to these disorders of oxygen carrying capacity, the *anemias*. There are also comparatively rare disorders of increased RBC number, the *polycythemias*: these will be briefly addressed at the end of the chapter.

THE ANEMIAS

Anemia is defined as a low RBC count, low hematocrit, or low hemoglobin concentration. Hematocrit (the proportion of whole blood occupied by RBCs) and hemoglobin concentration (the concentration of hemoglobin in a hemolysate prepared from whole blood) measure essentially the same thing. Given that the volume of a single RBC is occupied almost entirely by hemoglobin, any measurement of a patient's red cell volume (e.g., hematocrit) amounts to a measurement of hemoglobin quantity. In general, the hematocrit (Hct) and the hemoglobin (Hgb) both move up and down together, and in practice, these can be used interchangeably to describe a patient's hematologic status. By contrast, changes in the RBC count do not always parallel changes in Hct or Hgb. It is not uncommon to find a patient with a low Hct or low Hgb and simultaneously a normal or high RBC count (e.g., in thalassemia trait). Such patients are still properly labeled as anemic.

There are two fundamental diagnostic approaches to anemia: the first uses mean cell volume (MCV), and the second is based on pathogenesis. Every clinician and medical student is familiar with the MCV approach, which classifies anemia as microcytic, normocytic, or macrocytic.

Non-Neoplastic Hematopathology and Infections, First Edition. Edited by Hernani D. Cualing, Parul Bhargava, and Ramon L. Sandin.
© 2012 Wiley-Blackwell. Published 2012 by John Wiley & Sons, Inc.

The pathogenetic approach divides anemias into two categories, as being due to either reduced RBC production or increased RBC destruction or loss (or sequestration). Some textbooks combine these two approaches into one elaborate table or chart, but it is much easier and more practical to keep these two approaches separate.

The Complete Blood Count

A typical CBC includes basic assessments of white blood cell and platelet numbers, as well as the following red cell measurements:

- Red blood cell count
- Hemoglobin concentration
- Hematocrit
- Mean cell volume
- Mean cell hemoglobin (MCH)
- Mean cell hemoglobin concentration (MCHC)
- Red cell distribution width (RDW)

(Note that depending on the type of blood analyzer, some of these are direct measurements of RBC properties, while some are calculations. For simplicity's sake, these will all be referred to here as "measurements.")

The MCV is the average RBC size (i.e., volume). In most cases the MCV reflects the size of the majority of the RBCs: the mean cell volume is usually also the mode cell volume (and the median cell volume). However, the MCV may conceal a dual population of RBCs: if a microcytic patient is transfused normocytic blood, for example, the MCV will rise.

MCH and MCHC represent the amount and concentration, respectively, of hemoglobin within the average RBC. Most microcytic anemias are hypochromic (i.e., low MCH), and macrocytic anemias are commonly hyperchromic (i.e., high MCH). MCH is often used simultaneously with MCV to describe an anemia, for example, as being microcytic and hypochromic. Some thalassemia screening programs use MCH either together with or instead of MCV (Vallance, 2003). In contrast, MCHC is only rarely important: the one common condition in which it may be helpful is hereditary spherocytosis (see below), which may demonstrate a high MCHC. Given its limited utility (Mahu, 1990; Ryan, 2006), some laboratories do not report the MCHC.

RDW is the coefficient of variation of red cell volume. It is expressed without units, as either a percentage or a fraction. A high RDW correlates with a wide variation in RBC size, namely anisocytosis. A low RDW would mean *less* variation than normal in RBC size: this is not a diagnostically useful concept, and in practice a "low" RDW is invariably considered to be normal. Some authors cite the RDW as being useful in differentiating iron deficiency from thalassemia trait; this is discussed in more detail in the section on microcytic anemias, below.

The MCV Approach to Anemia: Three Lists of Causes

Every patient with anemia can be classified as microcytic, normocytic, or macrocytic. There are well-known lists of common causes for each type of anemia: one such set of lists is shown in Table 3.1.

These simple lists represent a good starting point for medical students dealing with uncomplicated anemias. Pathologists and hematologists will naturally need to be familiar with the exceptions to these "rules." Some of these special cases include:

- Reticulocytosis (or erythroblastosis, as is commonly seen in neonates) can increase the MCV from low to normal, or from normal to high. For example, hemolytic anemias are usually normocytic, but a brisk reticulocytosis may lead to a macrocytic presentation.
- Many of the microcytic and macrocytic anemias may begin as normocytic anemias, before ultimately developing the classic abnormal MCV. Early iron deficiency, for example, is typically normocytic.
- Patients may have more than one cause for anemia concomitantly. For example, a patient with iron deficiency and folate deficiency may be normocytic (albeit with a very wide RDW).
- Spurious macrocytosis is common enough (e.g., due to rouleaux or RBC agglutination, not to mention reticulocytosis) that it deserves inclusion on the standard list of macrocytic anemias. Spurious microcytosis is very rare, but worth mentioning for subspecialty practitioners. It may be seen in two specific disorders:
  1. Giant platelet syndromes, if the platelets are erroneously classified as RBCs by the automated counter.
  2. Overwhelming extravascular hemolysis, for example, hereditary pyropoikilocytosis in neonates, in which very numerous RBC microfragments lead to a lowered MCV.

Once the MCV is measured and the appropriate anemia differential diagnosis is generated, the next step is often a consideration of the mechanism of the anemia.

TABLE 3.1 MCV Classification of Anemia

Microcytic	Normocytic	Macrocytic
Iron deficiency Thalassemia Anemia of chronic disease Lead poisoning[a] Congenital sideroblastic anemia	Hemorrhage (subacute) Hemolysis: • Immune mediated, e.g., auto- or allo-immune • Extra-erythrocytic causes, e.g., microangiopathic hemolysis, abnormal cardiac valves, malaria, etc. • Membranopathies, e.g., hereditary spherocytosis, hereditary elliptocytosis • Hemoglobinopathies, e.g., sickle cell anemia • Enzymopathies, e.g., G6PD deficiency, PK deficiency Anemia of chronic disease Aplastic anemia and other bone marrow failure syndromes	Megaloblastic: • B_{12} deficiency • Folate deficiency • Intrinsic disorder of erythropoiesis, e.g., MDS Nonmegaloblastic: • Liver disease • Hypothyroidism • Alcohol • Down syndrome • Medication, e.g., AZT • Aplastic anemia and other bone marrow failure syndromes • Spurious macrocytosis

[a]Lead poisoning alone causes normocytic anemia, but in practice it is commonly simultaneous with iron deficiency and therefore presents with microcytosis.

The Pathogenetic Approach to Anemia: Two Possible Mechanisms

Every patient with anemia must have either reduced red cell production or increased red cell destruction or loss (sequestration in the spleen can be considered a special type of RBC loss). Rarely, both mechanisms may be present simultaneously, for example, a patient with acute on chronic GI hemorrhage who has reduced production due to iron deficiency and also simultaneous blood loss.

This same approach to mechanism (production vs. destruction/loss) is equally useful in diagnosing other cytopenias: thrombocytopenia and neutropenia, for example, have the same two possible mechanisms.

The best test for evaluating the mechanism of a patient's anemia is the reticulocyte count. Reticulocytes are slightly immature red cells with remnant RNA and ribosomes. They represent the penultimate stage in red cell maturation from erythroblasts into mature RBCs. The developing erythroid precursor in the bone marrow can be labeled a reticulocyte as soon as it has lost its nucleus. It takes approximately three days for the reticulocyte to lose its RNA and ribosomes, and thereby reach full maturity: typically it lives in the bone marrow for two days, and then circulates in the peripheral blood for one day before it becomes simply a mature erythrocyte.

In anemias due to reduced RBC production (e.g., aplastic anemia or iron deficiency), the number of reticulocytes released into the peripheral blood every day will be lower than normal. In anemia due to increased RBC destruction or loss (e.g., hemolysis or hemorrhage), the kidney identifies the reduced oxygen carriage in the blood, and releases more erythropoietin. The bone marrow responds to this by increasing the amount of erythropoiesis (Hillman, 1971). The increased erythropoietin level also stimulates the marrow to release each reticulocyte earlier than normal: these "early release" reticulocytes will still need three days to mature fully, but may spend (for example) only one day of that time in the marrow, and two days in the blood. Both of these factors—increased erythropoiesis and earlier reticulocyte release—lead to an increased reticulocyte count.

Reticulocytes can be counted by manual or automated methods (Bain, 2001): automated methods are generally preferred because of their greater speed, accuracy, and precision (Zandecki, 2007). The reticulocyte count is reported as either a percentage of circulating RBCs or as an absolute count.

Given that the normal RBC circulates for approximately 120 days, and that it (normally) spends only the first of those days as a reticulocyte, the normal reticulocyte proportion will be approximately 1/120, or roughly 1%. Bain and Bates (Bain, 2001) quote manual ranges of 0.5% to 2.5% for adults and children, and 2% to 5% for infants; automated ranges are often slightly narrower, such as 0.2% to 1.6% for adults. Absolute reticulocyte counts vary by lab and by method, but published ranges (Bain, 2001) include 10–90 or 20–70 ($\times 10^3/mm^3$, or $\times 10^9/L$).

There are several published methods for "correcting" the reticulocyte count for the degree of a patient's anemia. Two of the more commonly used corrections are the Corrected Reticulocyte Count (CRC) and the Reticulocyte Production Index (RPI) (Perkins, 2006). The CRC is used to correct reticulocyte percentages for the degree of a patient's anemia: a reticulocyte count of 1% in a patient with a hematocrit of 0.20 obviously represents half as much absolute reticulocyte production as a count of 1% in a patient with a hematocrit of 0.40.

$$CRC = \text{Reticulocyte } \% \times (\text{patient's Hct} \div 0.45)$$

Children typically have lower hematocrits than adults, so if the CRC is used in pediatrics the "0.45" hematocrit correction should be replaced with a fraction representing the midpoint of the age-specific Hct reference range. Note that the CRC is used only with reticulocyte percentages, and is not required for absolute counts.

The RPI corrects not only for the patient's Hct but also for the presence of "early release" reticulocytes. If a reticulocyte lasts for only one day in the blood, then the reticulocyte count represents the number of reticulocytes released by the bone marrow over the preceding 24 hours. But if (owing to early release) the reticulocyte lasts for two days in the blood, then a reticulocyte count will include 48 hours' worth of reticulocyte release. The RPI corrects for early release by using a correction factor (Table 3.2), as described by Perkins (2006). The correction factor approximates the number of days the reticulocyte persists in the circulation:

$$RPI = (CRC \text{ } or \text{ absolute reticulocyte count})$$
$$\div \text{ Correction factor}$$

Like the CRC, determining the RPI in a pediatric patient requires using slightly lower hematocrit ranges than in adults.

The clinical utility of reticulocyte correction is a subject of debate. Some hematologists and pathologists rely heavily on the CRC or the RPI to improve the specificity of their reticulocyte measurements. Others use an uncorrected reticulocyte count in a more subjective or "big picture" sense: if a patient is severely anemic, for example, one would expect the reticulocyte count to be severely elevated if the anemia were due to hemolysis or hemorrhage.

The reticulocyte count is used in clinical practice to differentiate between the two mechanisms of anemia. Anemia with a low reticulocyte count most likely reflects a reduced production mechanism, while anemia with a high reticulocyte count is consistent with increased RBC destruction or loss. The timing of the reticulocyte count is clinically important: it can take one to two days, or more, for a patient to mount a good reticulocyte response to an acute episode of hemolysis or hemorrhage. It may therefore be necessary to wait one or more days following an acute presentation before a reliable reticulocyte count can be determined.

Medical students occasionally struggle with the fact that the language used to describe reticulocyte counts assumes that a patient's anemia should be due to increased destruction or loss. Reticulocyte counts in anemic patients are often described as "appropriate," meaning raised, or "inappropriate," meaning not raised enough. In a patient with anemia, a "normal" reticulocyte count (i.e., within the reference range) would be considered "inappropriately low": a patient with normal kidneys and a normal bone marrow is expected to develop a high reticulocyte count if he or she becomes anemic owing to blood loss or hemolysis. A failure to raise the reticulocyte count in anemia means the bone marrow is failing to keep up with the increased demands for erythropoiesis. It may help students to remember that the reference ranges for reticulocyte counts are normal only for non-anemic patients. If a patient is anemic, and if the anemia is due to hemorrhage or hemolysis, the appropriate response of the normal bone marrow is an elevated reticulocyte count.

For medical students learning hematology, the pathogenesis should be considered in every case of anemia they encounter. For most practitioners, however, the pathogenesis is only diagnostically relevant in certain cases of anemia.

In a microcytic anemia workup (as in Figure 3.1), pathogenesis is usually not diagnostically important. Although there are five causes of microcytic anemia listed in Table 3.1, only three are common: iron deficiency, thalassemia, and anemia of chronic disease. Theoretically the reticulocyte count could be

TABLE 3.2 Correction Factor for Reticulocyte Production Index

Hematocrit	Correction Factor
0.40–0.45	1.0
0.35–0.39	1.5
0.25–0.34	2.0
0.15–0.24	2.5
< 0.15	3.0

Source: Perkins (2006).

used to help differentiate among these causes: it would be low in iron deficiency and chronic disease, and would often be high in thalassemia. However, in practice, the reticulocyte count is almost never used by experienced specialists in the scenario of microcytic anemia, simply because diagnostic testing for iron deficiency and thalassemia is so straightforward (see Approach to Microcytic Anemia, below).

Reticulocyte counting is most relevant in cases of normocytic or macrocytic anemia, where the differential diagnosis includes hemorrhage or hemolysis, on the one hand, and a variety of marrow failure syndromes, on the other. When the MCV suggests a differential diagnosis in which it is helpful to know the degree of marrow response, the reticulocyte count serves a very practical function.

Peripheral Smear Morphology: The Most Important Test

Review of the peripheral blood smear is the most important single test in diagnosing the cause of a patient's anemia. Peripheral smear review has three components:

1. Confirmation of the CBC findings. Although laboratory error in the CBC is rare, the first step in reviewing the peripheral smear is always to confirm the numbers generated by the automated counter. In the era of direct links between automated counters and laboratory information systems, post-analytical errors are almost impossible—except perhaps for the technologist attaching the wrong blood smear to a CBC printout for pathologist review. Both pre-analytical errors (chiefly specimen mixup) and analytical errors remain possible. The latter include (Cornbleet, 1983; Zandecki, 2007):

- Faulty aspiration of whole blood by the automated counter (e.g., due to a bubble in the specimen or the aspiration tube), leading to spuriously low counts
- Red blood cell agglutination (e.g., due to cold agglutinins) or rouleaux (e.g., due to hypergammaglobulinemia), leading to spurious macrocytosis and a spuriously low RBC count
- Hyperleukocytosis (which may be benign or malignant), leading to spurious macrocytosis and a spuriously elevated RBC count
- Giant platelets (e.g., due to a congenital macrothrombocytopenia such as May–Hegglin syndrome), leading to spurious microcytosis
- Severe hyperglycemia, leading to spurious macrocytosis

2. Overview of white blood cell (WBC) and platelet findings. Any abnormality in these other cell lines should influence the differential diagnosis of anemia. For example:

- Thrombocytosis is common in iron deficiency, and may also be seen in anemia of chronic disease (as an acute phase reaction). It is less likely in the other common microcytic anemia, thalassemia.
- Pancytopenia suggests primary or secondary marrow failure syndromes, including both benign and malignant causes. It would tend to rule out iron deficiency or hemolysis due to an intrinsic RBC defect, although of course more than one diagnosis may coexist.
- Anemia with thrombocytopenia raises the possibility of microangiopathic hemolysis (see below).

3. Identification of poikilocytosis and other relevant RBC findings. The key peripheral smear findings in anemia are usually morphologic abnormalities of the red cells. Red cell morphology has five important aspects:

- **Size**: The automated counter provides the MCV and RDW, but the peripheral smear provides additional information about any variation in RBC size. For example, is there a dual population of microcytic and macrocytic RBCs?
- **Shape**: Poikilocytosis may be the most important RBC finding in anemia. This is discussed further below.
- **Color**: The CBC obviously includes a measurement of the amount of hemoglobin in the average red cell (MCH). The peripheral smear is necessary to reveal any variation in RBC chromicity (anisochromia), an expected finding in iron deficiency that would classically be absent in thalassemia trait and anemia of chronic disease. Polychromasia will also be evident from the smear, which correlates reasonably well with an elevated reticulocyte count.
- **Inclusions**: These include malarial or other parasites, evidence of hyposplenism (e.g., Howell Jolly bodies), and the presence of nucleated RBCs.
- **Arrangement**: RBC agglutination and rouleaux were mentioned above in the context of analytical errors in the CBC. They both also raise specific items in the differential diagnosis (i.e., cold agglutinins and hypergammaglobinemia, respectively).

TABLE 3.3 Common Poikilocytes and Other RBC Findings, and Their Clinical Associations

Peripheral Smear Findings	Clinical Association
Acanthocyte (spur cell)	Advanced liver disease, hyposplenism, some dyslipidemias, pyruvate kinase deficiency
Anisochromia	Iron deficiency, myelodysplasia, hypochromic anemia post transfusion
Anisocytosis	Common nonspecific finding, also seen in iron deficiency, moderate or severe thalassemia, megaloblastic anemia, partially treated anemia of several causes, post-transfusion
Basophilic stippling: coarse	Thalassemia, lead poisoning, myelodysplasia, pyrimidine 5' nucleotidase deficiency, post chemotherapy
Basophilic stippling: fine	Reticulocytosis, normal finding
Bite cell/blister cell	Oxidative hemolysis
Dimorphism	Myelodysplasia, post transfusion
Echinocyte (burr cell)	Artifact, renal failure, post transfusion, phosphate deficiency, burns, dehydration
Elliptocyte	Iron deficiency, megaloblastic anemia, hereditary elliptocytosis, post chemotherapy
Heinz body	Oxidative hemolysis, hyposplenism
Howell Jolly body	Hyposplenism, erythroblastosis, myelodysplasia, megaloblastic anemia, post chemotherapy
Hypochromia	Iron deficiency, thalassemia, anemia of chronic disease
Irregularly contracted cell	Nonspecific finding seen in a variety of conditions including G6PD deficiency, PK deficiency, hemoglobinopathies, normal neonates, etc.
Pappenheimer body	Iron overload, hyposplenism, myelodysplasia
Polychromasia	Reticulocytosis, normal neonate
RBC agglutination	Cold agglutinin, cold autoimmune hemolytic anemia
Rouleaux	Normal finding in the thick part of the blood smear, hypergammaglobulinemia (monoclonal or polyclonal)
Schistocyte	RBC fragmentation syndromes, e.g., microangiopathic hemolytic anemia, hemolysis secondary to cardiac valve, etc.
Sickle cell	Severe sickling syndrome: SS, SC, SD, etc.
Spherocyte	Autoimmune hemolytic anemia, alloimmune hemolytic anemia (e.g., hemolytic disease of the newborn), hereditary spherocytosis
Stomatocyte	Artifact, liver disease, hereditary stomatocytosis, Southeast Asian ovalocytosis
Target cell	Thalassemia, liver disease, hyposplenism, Hgb C disease or SC disease, hereditary xerocytosis; may be seen in iron deficiency
Teardrop cell	Nonspecific finding seen in several conditions including myelofibrosis

Poikilocytosis and Its Clinical Associations

Each patient's MCV (with or without the benefit of the reticulocyte count) suggests a particular list of causes for his or her anemia. The shape of the patient's red cells can often narrow that differential diagnosis considerably. Table 3.3 lists some of the most important RBC findings, and their common clinical associations.

In most cases the MCV and the patient's poikilocytosis will suggest a relatively small number of diagnostic options. Confirmatory testing can follow.

It is worth noting that poikilocytes can be found in very small numbers even in normal patients, and may not be diagnostic by themselves: a single schistocyte in a non-anemic patient is unlikely to be due to microangiopathic hemolysis, for example. This is particularly evident in normal neonates (especially premature infants): newborns very often have a wide variety of poikilocytes even if they are otherwise hematologically normal. It is not unusual for a neonate—particularly a premature baby or an infant in a neonatal ICU—to demonstrate schistocytes, spherocytes, teardrops, targets, and so on. Even nucleated RBCs and Howell Jolly bodies are not necessarily abnormal in a neonate. The finding that suggests significant hematologic pathology in an anemic newborn is not the presence of poikilocytes per se but rather the finding of *one dominant poikilocyte*. In other words, a non-anemic neonate with a long list of poikilocytes is most likely hematologically normal—but an anemic infant with moderate spherocytosis on a background of mild nonspecific poikilocytosis is likely to have hemolysis.

THE APPROACH TO ANEMIA

The laboratory approach to anemia starts with the MCV, which will in turn suggest a specific differential diagnosis. In some cases this list of possible causes will be modified by consideration of the mechanism of anemia, using the reticulocyte count. Findings from the peripheral smear will further limit the differential diagnosis to what is usually a small set of options. Focused laboratory investigations will then typically allow a unifying diagnosis to be made.

This section uses such an approach, focusing on the most common or important anemias. Chapter 4 (by Setoodeh and Kang) provides considerably more detail about each individual entity.

The Approach to Microcytic Anemia

The most common anemias in clinical practice are the microcytic anemias. As every medical student knows, a simple acronym summarizes the causes of microcytic anemia: TAILS.

T (thalassemia and the thalassemic hemoglobino-pathies)

A (anemia of chronic disease)

I (iron deficiency)

L (lead poisoning)

S (congenital sideroblastic anemia)

Expressed in order of frequency, iron deficiency is by far the most common microcytic anemia, followed by (depending on one's patient population) either anemia of chronic disease or thalassemia. Lead poisoning alone causes normocytic anemia: however, as it is classically found in association with iron deficiency, it is usually listed with the microcytic anemias. In any event, lead poisoning remains very uncommon in North America. Congenital sideroblastic anemia is vanishingly rare even at large tertiary care pediatric hospitals.

For the hematologist or pathologist faced with a microcytic anemia, the usual differential diagnosis includes only iron deficiency, thalassemia, and anemia of chronic disease. The latter is a diagnosis of exclusion, so the diagnostic focus almost always targets iron deficiency first; testing for thalassemia is generally limited to at risk patients. One approach to microcytic anemia is outlined in Figure 3.1.

The diagnostic distinction between iron deficiency and anemia of chronic disease is usually straightforward, and is outlined below. Differentiating iron deficiency from thalassemia can be more challenging.

In classic cases, the CBC and peripheral smear morphology may be helpful in differentiating between iron deficiency and thalassemia (see Table 3.4 and Figures 3.2 and 3.3). Unfortunately, most cases are not "classic," and there is considerable laboratory overlap between these two anemias. The spectrum of RBC morphologies in thalassemia trait is particularly broad, ranging from almost normal to severe poikilocytosis with targets, elliptocytes, teardrop cells, and even schistocytes. The only finding from Table 3.4 that is reliable is coarse basophilic

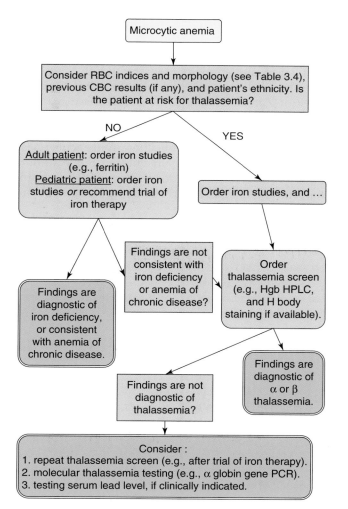

FIGURE 3.1 **Simplified approach to microcytic anemia.**

TABLE 3.4 **Iron Deficiency versus Thalassemia Trait: Typical Laboratory Findings**

Test	Findings in Iron Deficiency	Findings in Thalassemia Trait
RBC count	Decreased[a]	Increased
Hgb or Hct	Decreased[a]	Mildly decreased
MCV	Decreased[a]	Moderately decreased
RDW	Increased	Normal
Morphology	Elliptocytosis, anisocytosis, anisochromia	Target cells, coarse basophilic stippling

[a]These are classically decreased in approximate proportion to one another.

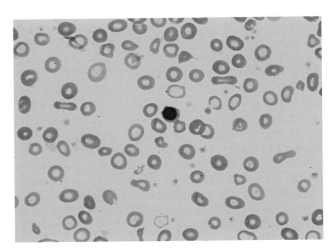

FIGURE 3.2 **Severe iron deficiency shows anisocytosis, anisochromasia, hypochromasia, and elliptocytosis. The poorly hemoglobinized erythroblast in the center of the image reflects the marrow response to elevated erythropoietin.** (Wright–Giemsa, 100×)

There are many published calculations that have been devised to differentiate iron deficiency from the thalassemia trait. Among the simplest and most widely used is the Mentzer index (Mentzer, 1973):

$$\text{Mentzer index} = \text{MCV} \div \text{RBC}$$

If the Mentzer index is less than 13, this is said to indicate thalassemia trait; if the index is greater than 13, this is meant to suggest iron deficiency. Unfortunately, although better than RDW alone (which correctly differentiates iron deficiency from thalassemia in only 59% of cases), the Mentzer index is correct only 76% of the time (Demir, 2002). Recent studies seem to suggest that the RBC count alone is the best predictor of iron deficiency versus thalassemia in both children and adults (Demir, 2002; Beyan, 2007).

Although these various predictors may be of some utility for general practitioners trying to decide which patients to send for diagnostic testing, they remain essentially useless for a hematologist or pathologist charged with providing an actual diagnosis. Differentiating iron deficiency from thalassemia in practice requires some combination of iron studies (Table 3.5) and hemoglobinopathy testing.

The single best outpatient test for adults is serum ferritin (Zanella, 1989): as an acute phase reactant, however, ferritin may be elevated to a falsely normal level in an iron deficient patient with a mild or even clinically silent viral infection. These acute phase changes are more common in children. Some authors have therefore recommended the use of RBC zinc protoporphyrin (Siegel, 1994) or reticulocyte hemoglobin

stippling, which is often present in thalassemia trait (either α or β) and never seen in uncomplicated iron deficiency. However, many thalassemic patients do not demonstrate coarse stippling, and the absence of stippling is not diagnostically useful.

Medical students are often taught that the RDW differentiates between these two conditions: as noted in Table 3.4, it is classically high in iron deficiency and normal in thalassemia. In practice, the RDW is a very weak predictor of diagnosis, and cannot be relied upon (Demir, 2002).

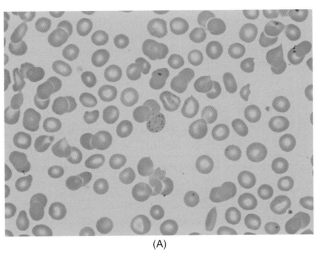

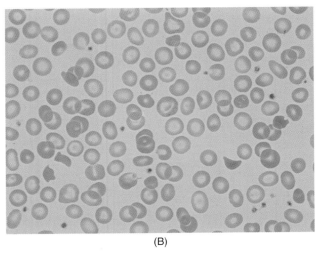

(A)

(B)

FIGURE 3.3 **Coarse basophilic stippling typical of thalassemia.** Image (**A**) shows prominent coarse basophilic stippling with less distinct target cells, and image (**B**) more subtle stippling with distinctive target cell formation. (Wright–Giemsa, 100×)

TABLE 3.5 Laboratory Tests Used in Diagnosing Iron Deficiency

Test	Typical Result
Serum ferritin	Low
RBC zinc protoporphyrin	High
Serum iron	Low
Total iron binding capacity (transferrin)	High
Transferrin saturation	Low
Reticulocyte hemoglobin content	Low

TABLE 3.6 Laboratory tests in Anemia of Chronic Disease

Test	Typical Result
Serum iron	Low
Total iron binding capacity (transferrin)	Low
Iron saturation	Low or normal
Ferritin	Normal or high
RBC zinc protoporphyrin	High

content (Ret-He or CHr) (Brugnara, 1999) in pediatric patients.

Hemoglobinopathy testing is indicated for patients in whom α or β thalassemia is a reasonable likelihood, particularly in patients of reproductive age: some families may wish genetic counseling if both parents carry thalassemia genes. The patient's ethnic group is very important in considering the likelihood of a thalassemia diagnosis. Thalassemia is very uncommon in northern Europeans, American Indians, Canadian First Nations, Inuit, and patients from Japan (Vallance, 2003). Conversely, thalassemia is common in patients from Asia, Africa, the Middle East, and the Mediterranean.

In some patients, thalassemia can be ruled out even without special testing: for example, previously normal CBC results can be used to exclude thalassemia. A patient with α thalassemia should be microcytic from birth, and with β thalassemia the microcytosis should manifest by approximately 6 months of age. New onset microcytosis in an adult cannot be attributed to thalassemia.

A positive diagnosis of thalassemia cannot be made using the CBC and morphology alone, although in some patients the morphologic findings may be highly suggestive. Both coarse basophilic stippling in an ethnically at risk patient and "Fessas bodies" within nucleated RBCs (Fessas, 1963) are consistent with (if not independently diagnostic of) thalassemia.

Hemoglobin electrophoresis is often suggested as an appropriate tool to diagnose thalassemia trait, but in fact this is only rarely helpful. The diagnosis of α thalassemia requires either supravital staining or genetic testing, while the diagnosis of β thalassemia requires a sensitive measurement of the Hgb A_2 fraction, such as by high-pressure liquid chromatography. Densitometric scanning of an electrophoresis gel is not acceptable to diagnose β thalassemia.

The finding of H bodies on supravital staining such as Brilliant Cresyl Blue (Skogerboe, 1992) is highly suggestive of α thalassemia. In an ethnically at risk patient with microcytosis or hypochromia, the presence of H bodies is in practice usually considered diagnostic. Confirmation can be provided using molecular methods such as PCR to interrogate the α globin genome: this approach is usually only required in challenging or complex cases (e.g., compound heterozygosity for α thalassemia and a β chain variant). The sensitivity of H body staining depends on the genotype: with either heterozygous or homozygous single gene deletion (i.e., αα/α- or α-/α-) the sensitivity of H body staining is approximately 40%, while with a double deletion *in cis* (i.e., αα/−) the sensitivity is approximately 90% (Skogerboe, 1992).

A diagnosis of β thalassemia trait is typically suggested by the finding of an elevated Hgb A_2 in an ethnically at risk patient with microcytic anemia. Many β thalassemia patients will also have an elevated Hgb F (i.e., above 1%), but this finding is not diagnostically reliable. As with H bodies, an elevated A_2 is not pathognomonic of thalassemia: the presence of sickle hemoglobin, megaloblastosis, and hyperthyroidism may also elevate the A_2 (Bunn, 1986).

Anemia of chronic disease can be suggested by the results of the iron study investigations (Table 3.6).

The Approach to Normocytic Anemia

Most normocytic anemias occur by one of three main mechanisms:

1. Subacute blood loss
2. Hemolysis
3. Marrow failure or suppression of erythropoiesis

For normocytic anemias, unlike microcytic anemias, the pathogenesis is clinically very important. A normocytic anemia with a high reticulocyte count is almost certainly a case of hemorrhage or hemolysis; with a low reticulocyte count, one would consider marrow failure. The importance of the reticulocyte count is highlighted in Figure 3.4, showing a simplified approach to normocytic anemia.

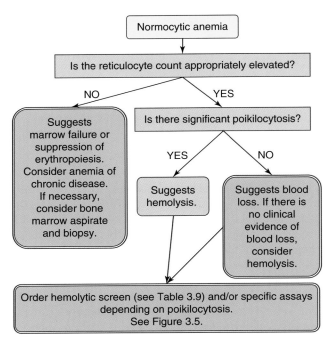

FIGURE 3.4 **Simplified approach to normocytic anemia.**

Even apart from the reticulocyte count, the laboratory presentations of these three mechanisms are usually quite different. Subacute blood loss will typically show a low RBC count, low Hgb (and Hct), and a normal MCV. If there is a very brisk reticulocytosis, the MCV may be mildly elevated. WBC and platelet counts are typically normal. The peripheral smear will show anemia and often polychromasia. There will be no significant poikilocytosis. In practice, the clinicians are usually well aware of a patient's subacute blood loss, and the hematologist or pathologist typically does not play a significant diagnostic role.

(It is worth pointing out that the findings above apply only to *subacute* blood loss, i.e., hemorrhage that is at least several hours old. Blood loss that is *acute* would typically show a totally normal CBC: as a rule it should take several hours for extravascular and intravascular fluid compartments to re-balance following a hemorrhage, and dilute the remaining RBCs to show anemia on the CBC. Blood loss that is *chronic*, however, only leads to anemia via iron deficiency and would therefore be microcytic.)

A patient with hemolysis usually has a similar CBC to a patient with subacute blood loss (i.e., anemia with normal WBCs and platelets; there may be mild macrocytosis if there is brisk reticulocytosis), but would typically show significant poikilocytosis on the peripheral blood smear.

Marrow failure can lead to isolated anemia, or bi- or pancytopenia depending on the specific cause. Marrow failure should be considered in any case of anemia when the reticulocyte count is inappropriately low. If the patient is bi- or pancytopenic, marrow failure should also come to the top of the differential diagnosis because most other causes of anemia do not affect the other cell lines. The MCV can be normal or elevated. The morphology of the red cells is often unremarkable. Making a diagnosis of marrow failure requires a bone marrow aspirate and biopsy.

The Approach to Hemolysis

Hemolysis means red cell death prior to an average of 120 days. One reliable approach to hemolysis is to consider the pathogenesis (see Table 3.7): this approach subdivides hemolysis on the basis of its red blood cell pathology, namely intraerythrocytic, membranous, or extraerythrocytic. Some clinicians prefer

TABLE 3.7 **Pathogenetic Classification of Hemolysis**

Intraerythrocytic	Membranous	Extraerythrocytic
Enzyme • G6PD deficiency • PK deficiency • Other enzyme (rare)	• Hereditary spherocytosis • Hereditary elliptocytosis • Other (rare)	Immune • Warm and cold autoimmune hemolysis • Paroxysmal cold hemoglobinuria • Paroxysmal nocturnal hemoglobinuria • Alloimmune hemolysis
Hemoglobin • α and β Thalassemia • Sickle cell anemia and Sickle—thalassemia compound heterozygosity • Other hemoglobinopathies • Unstable hemoglobin (rare)		Non-immune • Microangiopathic (HUS, TTP, DIC) • RBC trauma • Severe burns • Freshwater drowning • Malaria • Sepsis, e.g., *Clostridium welchii*

TABLE 3.8 Intravascular versus Extravascular Hemolysis: Common Causes

Intravascular	Extravascular
Microangiopathic hemolysis	Hereditary spherocytosis
G6PD deficiency[a]	G6PD deficiency[a]
Warm autoimmune hemolysis[a]	Warm[a] and cold autoimmune hemolysis
PCH	PK deficiency
PNH	Hemoglobinopathies

Source: Tefferi (2003).
[a]Some hemolytic anemias may have both an intravascular and extravascular component.

TABLE 3.9 Intravascular versus Extravascular Hemolysis: Typical Laboratory Findings

Findings	Intravascular	Extravascular
Schistocytes	May be present	Generally absent
Unconjugated bilirubin	Increased	Increased or normal
Lactate dehydrogenase	Increased	Increased
Haptoglobin	Decreased	Decreased
Urine hemosiderin	May be present	Absent

Source: Tefferi (2003).

to subclassify hemolysis on the basis of its vascular location, namely intravascular (within the blood vessels) or extravascular (primarily splenic). Common causes of intravascular and extravascular hemolysis are noted in Table 3.8 (Tefferi, 2003). Laboratory testing may help to differentiate intravascular from extravascular hemolysis (Tefferi, 2003) (Table 3.9).

Most hemolytic patients have significant poikilocytosis, and usually the type of poikilocyte will suggest a specific hemolytic mechanism (see Table 3.3): for example, schistocytes suggest intravascular hemolysis, spherocytes suggest autoimmune hemolysis or hereditary spherocytosis, bite and blister cells suggest oxidative hemolysis, and so on. Where the poikilocytosis suggests specific possible causes for hemolysis, it is appropriate to focus laboratory investigation on those entities. In some cases, particularly in infants, the RBC morphology may not be specific. Here a broader screening approach may be required: one version of a hemolytic screening panel is listed in Table 3.10. A simplified approach to hemolysis that is driven by RBC morphology is shown in Figure 3.5.

Specific approaches to some of the more common hemolytic anemias are outlined below.

RBC Enzyme Defects

The two most common RBC enzyme defects are deficiencies of Glucose-6-phosphate-dehydrogenase (G6PD) and Pyruvate Kinase (PK). G6PD deficiency shows irregularly contracted erythrocytes, bite cells, and blister cells (Figure 3.6) (Bain, 2005). The peripheral smear in PK deficiency often shows only

TABLE 3.10 Tests from a Hemolytic Screening Panel

Test	Purpose
Serum bilirubins (conjugated and unconjugated)	Confirm hemolysis
Serum lactate dehydrogenase	Confirm hemolysis
Serum haptoglobin	Confirm hemolysis
Direct antiglobulin test (DAT)	Detect immune-mediated hemolysis
Eosin-5-maleimide flow cytometry assay or osmotic fragility assay	Detect hereditary spherocytosis
G6PD and pyruvate kinase activity screens	Detect RBC enzyme deficiency
Hgb HPLC or capillary zone electrophoresis	Detect hemoglobinopathy
Isopropanol stability assay or other unstable hemoglobin screen	Detect unstable hemoglobin

nonspecific changes such as irregularly contracted erythrocytes and polychromasia. The classic finding, acanthocytosis (Figure 3.7), is neither sensitive nor specific for PK deficiency.

Clinical features may be helpful in working up a potential RBC enzymopathy: G6PD deficiency classically presents in males as episodic acute hemolysis, while PK deficiency is typically seen in both males and females with continuous hemolysis.

Both of these conditions are usually diagnosed by fluorescent or spectrophotometric demonstration of reduced enzyme activity (Roper, 2001). One proviso is that both enzymes show increased activity in reticulocytes: this increase can push deficient enzyme

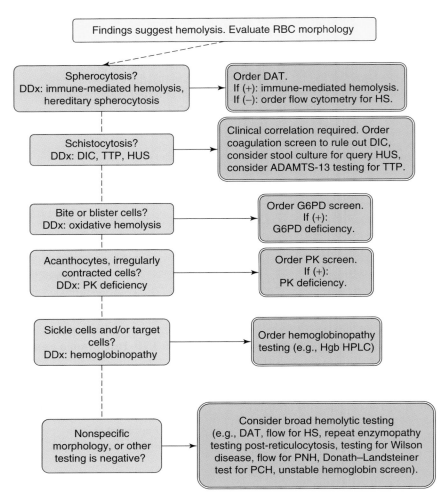

FIGURE 3.5 **Simplified approach to hemolysis**. "DDx" indicates a likely item on the differential diagnosis.

activity up into the normal range. During episodes of very brisk reticulocytosis—namely at the peak of the hemolytic episode—enzyme activity may therefore be falsely normal. Given the episodic nature of hemolysis in G6PD deficiency, in this condition the enzyme activity can be re-tested after the reticulocytosis has normalized. However, in PK deficiency the hemolysis is usually continuous, so it may not be possible to wait until the patient has a normal reticulocyte count before measuring enzyme activity. One helpful feature is that reticulocytosis in a normal patient should lead to a high PK activity: "normal" enzyme levels in the presence of severe reticulocytosis may suggest PK deficiency.

Hemoglobinopathies

Structural abnormalities of the α or β globin chains are properly labeled as *hemoglobinopathies*. These are distinct from the (usually) qualitatively normal but quantitatively reduced chains in the thalassemias. There are a great many

hemoglobinopathies, of varying clinical severity: the most common is sickle cell anemia (also called SS to reflect the homozygous sickle cell mutation) (Weatherall, 2010b). Hemoglobinopathy is too broad a topic to be discussed in detail here (see Chapter 5 by Bhargava for a more detailed description of hemoglobinopathies); this section focuses exclusively on the approach to sickle cell anemia.

The peripheral smear in sickle cell anemia usually shows sickled RBCs in all their morphologic varieties: "sickles," "boats" or "bananas," "holly leaf" cells, and so on. (This is quite unlike the findings in sickle cell trait, which should be completely unremarkable in the vast majority of patients.) By the age of 1 or 2, SS patients should also show morphologic evidence of hyposplenism on the peripheral smear (see Figure 3.8 and Table 3.3). Patients with one of the compound heterozygote sickling syndromes may show somewhat different peripheral smear morphologies: SC disease, for example, shows fewer sickles, more targets, and

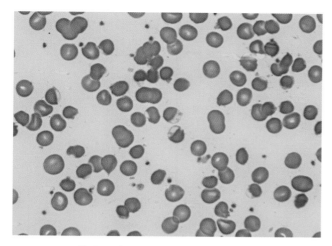

FIGURE 3.6 **G6PD deficiency**. Note the many irregularly contracted cells and blister cells. Three blister cells are in the center of the image. (Wright–Giemsa, 100×)

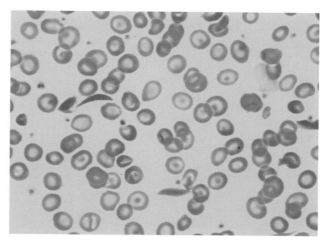

FIGURE 3.8 **Sickle cell anemia and coexisting α thalassemia**. There are prominent sickle cells, as well as a Howell Jolly body owing to splenic infarction. Most patients with sickle cell anemia will have target cells because of hyposplenism; in this patient, targeting is exacerbated because of the concomitant α thalassemia. (Wright–Giemsa, 100×)

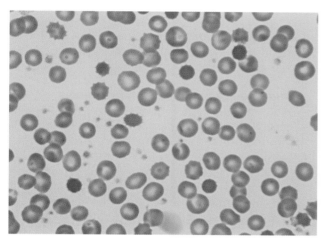

FIGURE 3.7 **Pyruvate kinase deficiency**. The several small acanthocytes in the field are sometimes referred to as "Sputnik cells" after the small spiky Soviet satellite. (Wright–Giemsa, 100×)

less evidence of hyposplenism than sickle cell anemia (Bain, 2002).

Abnormal findings on the peripheral smear, or clinical suspicion, should lead to specific hemoglobinopathy assays: these include hemoglobin high-pressure liquid chromatography (Hgb HPLC) and capillary zone electrophoresis. While alkaline and acid gel electrophoresis can together diagnose S trait or sickle cell anemia, newer methods such as HPLC have many advantages over gel electrophoresis, including ease of quantitation and speed.

RBC Membranopathies

Inherited disorders of RBC structural membrane proteins are important causes of hemolysis. The most common is hereditary spherocytosis (HS), a disorder of so-called vertical RBC membrane elements. Hereditary elliptocytosis (HE), an inherited condition of so-called horizontal RBC membrane proteins, is associated with a much milder clinical phenotype. Other RBC membrane abnormalities such as hereditary xerocytosis and hereditary stomatocytosis are much rarer.

In both HS and HE it is the poikilocytosis that suggests these diagnoses. HS classically presents morphologically with spherocytosis, which can range from mild to severe, as well as polychromasia. HE usually demonstrates severe elliptocytosis (Figure 3.9). Most patients with HE are not anemic, although hemolysis can be particularly severe in neonates who may present with either HE with infantile poikilocytosis (HEIP) or the more severe hereditary pyropoikilocytosis (HPP) (Gallagher, 2004).

Spherocytosis (Figure 3.10) has only two common causes: HS and autoimmune hemolysis (see below). Laboratory testing for autoimmune hemolysis is easier and faster than testing for HS, so a patient with spherocytosis should first have a direct antiglobulin test (DAT). If this is positive, the diagnosis of autoimmunity is essentially established. If the DAT is negative, testing for HS can follow. HS testing traditionally involved the osmotic fragility assay, a time-consuming test of limited value, and one that is difficult to perform in small children given the relatively large volume of blood required. A much

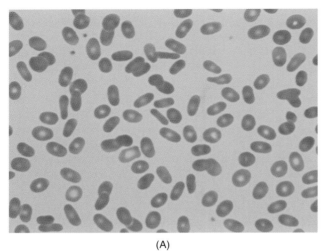

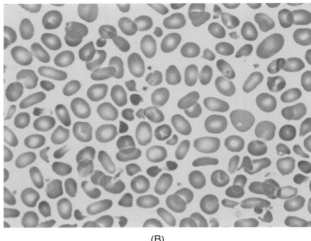

(A)   (B)

FIGURE 3.9   **Hereditary elliptocytosis**. Image (**A**) shows HE in an adult patient, and image (**B**) a newborn with hereditary elliptocytosis with infantile poikilocytosis. Note the presence of schistocytes, pyknocytes, and polychromasia in addition to the elliptocytes in image (**B**). (Wright–Giemsa, 100×)

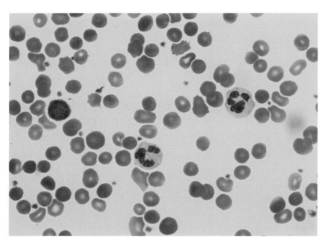

FIGURE 3.10   **Hereditary spherocytosis**. The morphology of warm autoimmune hemolytic anemia is essentially identical. (Wright-Giemsa, 100×)

better assay for HS (King, 2000) uses flow cytometry to measure the amount of band 3 on the surface of the RBCs: this test is positive in HS and negative in AIHA, unlike osmotic fragility which is positive in both conditions.

Elliptocytosis has a much longer differential diagnosis than spherocytosis: in addition to HE, severe elliptocytosis can be caused by iron deficiency, megaloblastic anemia, and a variety of other clinical states, including chemotherapy. In practice, however, the usual approach is to first exclude iron deficiency. If this is ruled out, then the most likely cause of elliptocytosis in an otherwise healthy non-anemic patient with normocytic RBCs is HE. In some patients family

studies can be confirmatory. Specialized diagnostic testing may be available at reference laboratories but is rarely necessary.

Immune-Mediated Hemolytic Anemia

Autoimmune hemolytic anemia (AIHA) involves the targeting of the patient's RBCs by his or her own antibodies and/or complement proteins, leading to the premature clearance of those cells. AIHA is typically divided into warm (WAIHA) and cold (CAIHA) types, which describe the thermal amplitude of the implicated antibodies: the antibodies are either most active at body temperature (warm) or at 4°C (cold). As a rule, WAIHA is IgG mediated, while CAIHA is due to IgM antibodies and complement. Other types of autoimmune hemolysis include drug-induced AIHA, paroxysmal cold hemoglobinuria (PCH) and paroxysmal nocturnal hemoglobinuria (PNH). Immune-mediated hemolysis can also be alloimmune: either the patient's antibodies target nonself RBCs (i.e., acute or delayed hemolytic transfusion reactions) or foreign antibodies target the patient's RBCs (e.g., hemolytic disease of the newborn or immune hemolysis post-IVIG).

Except for PNH, most cases of immune-mediated hemolysis demonstrate spherocytosis and polychromasia. MCV is usually normal.

In PNH, unique among these immune-mediated hemolytic anemias, there is macrocytosis and often pancytopenia; in some cases there is also reticulocytopenia. These findings arise out of the clonal nature of this condition, in which increased sensitivity to complement mediated hemolysis leads to cytopenias. RBCs do not show spherocytosis in PNH.

The direct antiglobulin test (DAT) is the key laboratory tool in diagnosing most cases of immune-mediated hemolysis. In WAIHA the DAT is usually positive for IgG, while in CAIHA there will instead be complement found on the surface of the cells, reflecting the complement-fixing properties of the IgM antibodies. In PCH the DAT may be negative or may identify complement: in this condition a Donath–Landsteiner assay (Regan, 2001) will demonstrate the classic biphasic antibody/complement mediated hemolysis. The DAT in drug-induced immune-mediated hemolysis will usually be negative, unless the test can be performed in the presence of the implicated drug (in which case it may show IgG or complement on the RBCs). The DAT in HDN and in transfusion-associated hemolysis will be positive for IgG, except for cases of ABO mismatch in which cells will carry complement instead.

In most cases of *autoimmune* hemolysis, searching for the specific antigen targeted by the antibody is not helpful. This is not the case in *alloimmune* hemolysis, in which identifying the antigen (e.g., by eluting the antibodies from the affected RBCs and demonstrating their specificity via panel testing) can be a critical part of diagnosis and management.

Testing for PNH is unique: flow cytometry will often show a deficiency of surface RBC complement regulatory proteins (CD55 and CD59), which would normally protect the cell from complement mediated hemolysis (Parker, 2005). Molecular testing may identify mutations in the PIGA (phosphatidylinositolglycan A) gene (Parker, 2005). Bone marrow aspirate and biopsy in PNH may show aplastic changes. Labs without access to flow cytometry may elect to perform the Ham's acidified serum test to demonstrate the RBCs' exaggerated susceptibility to complement-mediated hemolysis (Regan, 2001).

Non-Immune Extraerythrocytic Hemolytic Anemia

There are a wide variety of non-immune causes of extracorpuscular hemolytic anemia, including freshwater drowning, severe burns (Figure 3.11), mechanical membrane damage such as due to a cardiac valvular defect or march hemoglobinuria, and infections such as malaria and Clostridium. Most of these are extremely rare (e.g., hemolysis from freshwater drowning) or are obvious from history (e.g., severe burns). In North America the most important of these extraerythrocytic conditions are the microangiopathic hemolytic anemias (MAHAs).

There are three cardinal microangiopathic hemolytic anemias: thrombotic thrombocytopenic purpura (TTP), hemolytic uremic syndrome (HUS),

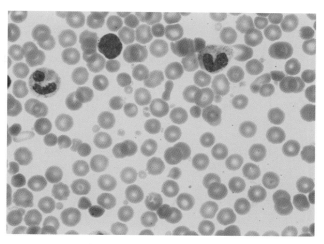

FIGURE 3.11 **Microspherocytosis from a severe thermal burn**. (Wright–Giemsa, 100×)

and disseminated intravascular coagulopathy (DIC). DIC is seen in association with many different clinical syndromes, including sepsis, severe trauma, malignancies (including acute promyelocytic leukemia), obstetrical accidents, and severe hypothermia. Both HUS and TTP may be diagnosed at any age, although HUS is more common in children and TTP is more common in adults. HUS classically presents after exposure to undercooked beef that is contaminated with enterohemorrhagic *Esherichia coli*, serotype O157:H7. In two recent outbreaks in the United States, organic spinach (CDC, 2006) and packaged cookie dough (CDC, 2009) were implicated as *E. coli* sources. TTP has three main subtypes, including an acquired form which is more common in adults, a congenital form that may be diagnosed in childhood, and a drug-induced type linked to certain immunosuppressants (e.g., tacrolimus, cyclosporine).

The three MAHAs are morphologically identical (Figure 3.12): there is schistocytic anemia and thrombocytopenia, often with large platelets (reflecting the generation of new larger platelets to replace the ones consumed). Polychromasia may also be present. The WBC count may be high, normal, or low. Note that the clinical severity of the disease does not correlate well with the degree of morphological abnormality: patients with milder schistocytosis are not necessarily clinically better off than patients with more severe schistocytosis, for example. Clinicians may ask for the schistocytosis to be quantified (e.g., as a percentage of RBCs) over the course of treatment, as a means of tracking their patients' progress: this can be difficult to do with any precision, and is of unclear clinical value.

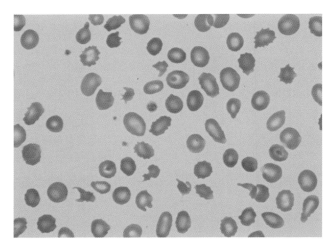

FIGURE 3.12 **Severe hemolytic uremic syndrome.** This example of HUS shows severe schistocytosis as well as thrombocytopenia with large platelets—the latter reflecting the marrow's generation of new (larger) platelets to replace the platelets consumed in the microangiopathy. Moderate echinocytosis is also present, likely due to renal failure. (Wright–Giemsa, 100×)

In DIC there is a consumptive coagulopathy, manifesting in the laboratory as prolongation of the prothrombin time (PT) or international normalized ratio (INR), activated partial thromboplastin time (aPTT), and thrombin time (TT). Fibrinogen activity is reduced, and D-dimer is positive. HUS and TTP lack the coagulation abnormalities of DIC.

In HUS most patients will have enterohemorrhagic *E. coli* demonstrable on a stool culture. Patients will also have biochemical evidence of acute renal failure, such as elevations in blood urea nitrogen (BUN) and creatinine. These renal changes are also often present in TTP.

TTP is often associated with deficiency of or autoantibodies against the ADAMTS-13 enzyme. These can be assayed in specialized reference laboratories (Sadler, 2008), although there remains some controversy whether such testing is clinically helpful.

It should be noted that there are other causes of schistocytosis besides MAHA, including vasculitis, mechanical hemolysis owing to abnormal cardiac valves, and severe thermal burns. Many intravascular hemolytic anemias can also produce schistocytes (e.g., G6PD deficiency), but usually in those conditions the schistocytes are not the most numerous poikilocyte.

Summary

The approach outlined above, and summarized in Figure 3.5, uses poikilocytosis as the starting point for selecting diagnostic laboratory tests. There are other

TABLE 3.11 **Common Megaloblastic and Nonmegaloblastic Causes of Macrocytic Anemia**

Megaloblastic	Nonmegaloblastic
B_{12} deficiency • Dietary limitation • Malabsorption, e.g., intrinsic factor deficiency, celiac sprue • Transport defect, e.g., transcobalamin II deficiency Folate deficiency • Dietary limitation • Malabsorption, e.g., celiac sprue • Increased needs, e.g., hemolytic anemia Folate inhibitors and antimetabolites, e.g., methotrexate, some anticonvulsants Inborn errors of metabolism, e.g., MTHFR deficiency Intrinsic abnormalities of erythropoiesis, either congenital (e.g., congenital dyserythropoietic anemia) or acquired (MDS, HIV, etc.)	Liver disease Hypothyroidism Alcohol Down syndrome Medication, e.g., AZT Aplastic anemia and other bone marrow failure syndromes Reticulocytosis Spurious macrocytosis

approaches to hemolysis that do not rely as heavily on poikilocytosis, such as an intravascular versus extravascular approach (Tefferi, 2003). What these approaches have in common is an initial focus on the more common diagnoses (e.g., DIC), followed only later by testing for rarer entities (e.g., Wilson disease).

The Approach to Macrocytic Anemia

Macrocytic anemias can be divided into *megaloblastic* and *nonmegaloblastic* types. Specific causes of each are shown in Table 3.11. The peripheral smear in megaloblastic anemia classically shows, in the words of Osler (1903), "giant [red cell] forms, megalocytes, which are often ovoid …. Nucleated red blood-corpuscles are almost always present [including] normoblasts and megaloblasts…. Red corpuscles with fragmenting nuclei are common…. The leucocytes are generally normal or diminished in number … [and the] blood-plates are either absent or very scanty."

The typical CBC and peripheral smear findings that suggest a megaloblastic process include:

- Severe macrocytosis (e.g., MCV > 115 fL)
- Oval macrocytes
- Hypersegmented neutrophils

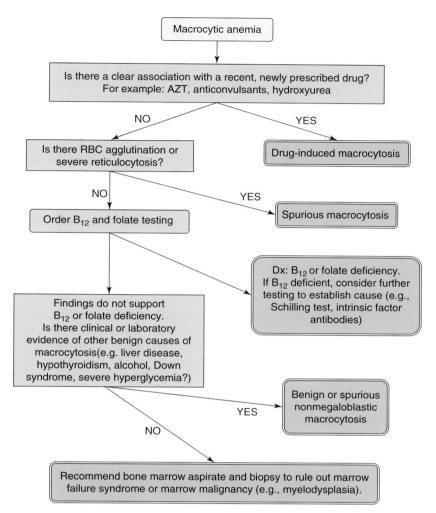

FIGURE 3.13 Simplified approach to macrocytic anemia.

There are several definitions for neutrophilic hyper-segmentation, including > 50% of neutrophils having 4 or more lobes, or > 5% with 5 or more lobes. In practice the term "hypersegmentation" typically refers to the presence of even a single neutrophil with 6 or more nuclear lobes. These must be distinct, separate lobes, joined only by a thin strand of chromatin. Neutrophil hypersegmentation is not pathognomonic of megaloblastic anemia: it may also be seen in myeloproliferative neoplasia or myelodysplastic syndromes.

Nonmegaloblastic macrocytic anemia classically presents with milder macrocytosis (e.g., MCV 100–115 fL), round macrocytes, and normally segmented neutrophils.

In practice, the findings from the CBC and the peripheral smear may be suggestive of either a megaloblastic or nonmegaloblastic process but are often not truly convincing. There can be a great deal of overlap between these two types of macrocytic anemias, and many patients cannot easily be classified as one or the other. Furthermore, although megaloblastic and nonmegaloblastic features should be noted by the pathologist or hematologist, the diagnostic approach to macrocytic anemia is often the same either way. One approach to macrocytic anemia is summarized in Figure 3.13.

The first step in resolving a macrocytic anemia requires attention to the patient's history. Several drugs are well known causes of macrocytosis (Aslinia, 2006), including AZT and many anticonvulsants. If a previously normocytic patient begins a prescription for one of these drugs, and subsequently develops macrocytosis, it may not be necessary to test for other causes.

Review of the peripheral smear should rule out spurious macrocytosis owing to rouleaux or

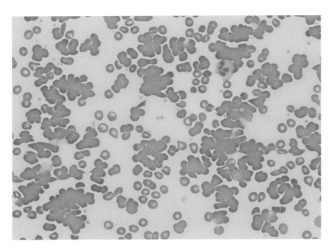

FIGURE 3.14 **RBC agglutination due to a cold agglutinin**. This can cause spurious macrocytosis. (Wright–Giemsa, 50×).

agglutination (Figure 3.14), and reticulocytosis can be excluded by a reticulocyte count.

If neither an obvious pharmaceutical cause nor a spurious cause of macrocytosis is evident, then further testing will usually be required. Deficiencies of folate or B_{12} are the most common causes of megaloblastosis (Babior, 2006). In most macrocytic patients, whether their findings are overtly megaloblastic or not, the best approach is to rule out these easily correctable deficiencies by testing blood levels. Considering folate deficiency is particularly important in woman of childbearing age: inadequate folate stores at the time of conception and pregnancy is strongly associated with severe neural tube defects in the fetus (Blencowe, 2010).

Serum B_{12} is usually low in B_{12} deficiency, and serum and/or RBC folate is low in folate deficiency (Green, 2008). Red blood cell folate (Hoffbrand, 1966) is generally described as a more reliable measurement of body stores than serum folate, which fluctuates more rapidly with diet (Green, 2008). Serum homocysteine will be elevated in both B_{12} and folate deficiency, and serum methylmalonate will be elevated in B_{12} deficiency, but testing these metabolites is not usually necessary (Elghetany, 2006). If a patient is found to be B_{12} deficient, further testing is available to explore the specific cause, including the Schilling test and testing for autoantibodies against intrinsic factor (Ward, 2002).

A bone marrow aspirate is not usually required to diagnose B_{12} or folate deficiency, although it may certainly be part of the investigation of unexplained macrocytic anemia (see below). If the bone marrow is examined, the classic megaloblastic changes will be found in erythroid precursors: namely nuclear-cytoplasmic dyssynchrony, with mature cytoplasm and immature nuclei (Figure 3.15). Abnormal early erythroid precursors—the so-called megaloblasts—are considerably larger than normal proerythroblasts, and contain large, pale nuclei. Other dysplastic nuclear changes are common, including asymmetric nuclear budding and karyorrhexis. Granulocytic morphology is also characteristically abnormal, featuring the so-called giant metamyelocyte: a larger than normal metamyelocyte with an immature and overly large nucleus that wraps

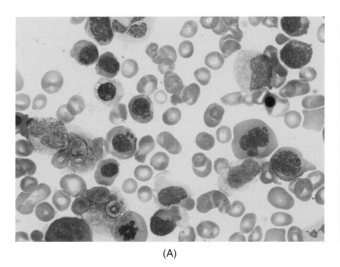

(A)

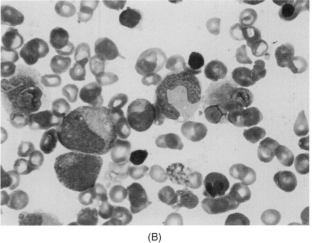

(B)

FIGURE 3.15 **A bone marrow aspirate from a patient with severe megaloblastic anemia**. Image (**A**) shows severely megaloblastic erythropoiesis, with nuclear-cytoplasmic dyssynchrony, nuclear fragmentation, and nuclear multilobation. Image (**B**) shows a giant metamyelocyte with a horseshoe-shaped nucleus. (May Gruenwald Giemsa, 100×)

around the inside of the cell. These megaloblastic changes may be subtle in mild cases, or severe with chronic deficiencies.

B_{12} and folate deficiencies are the most common causes of megaloblastic anemia, but macrocytic anemia overall is more commonly due to nonmegaloblastic causes such as drug therapy, alcohol, and liver disease (Savage, 2000; Snower, 1993). Despite their relative infrequency, initial testing for B_{12} and folate deficiency remains a useful approach if only because those lesions are easily curable.

Myelodysplastic syndrome is another relatively frequent cause of macrocytosis. Other marrow failure syndromes including idiopathic aplastic anemia and Diamond–Blackfan anemia often also present with macrocytic anemia. In patients with macrocytic anemia in whom B_{12} and folate levels are normal, and in whom other convincing causes for macrocytosis are not present, a bone marrow aspirate is required.

THE POLYCYTHEMIAS

Compared to anemia, polycythemia is very rare. Elevations in Hgb or Hct are usually divided into relative and absolute categories.

Relative Polycythemia

In relative polycythemia, the amount of RBCs is normal but the plasma volume is reduced. The two most common examples of relative polycythemia are dehydration and Gaisbock's syndrome (the latter a rare presentation linked to obesity, smoking, and hypertension). Relative polycythemia is usually ruled out clinically.

Absolute Polycythemia

The laboratory approach to polycythemia is focused on absolute polycythemia. An elevation in red cell mass will either be a primary marrow phenomenon or a secondary response. Typical secondary causes of polycythemia include chronic hypoxia (e.g., living at high altitude, chronic cigarette smoking, cyanotic cardiopulmonary disease) and pathologically elevated erythropoietin levels (from renal or other malignancies, renal artery stenosis, blood doping in athletes, etc.). Rarely the lesion will be at the level of the hemoglobin molecule, such as with a high affinity variant.

Primary polycythemia can be a benign familial condition, but more often it is due to a myeloproliferative neoplasm. Primary and secondary polycythemia can be differentiated by testing oxygen saturation and serum erythropoietin level. If O_2 saturation is normal and erythropoietin is low, secondary causes are unlikely. A bone marrow aspirate will then be necessary to diagnose a primary cause. Cytogenetic and/or molecular genetic testing of bone marrow must be a part of this assessment, to rule out chronic myeloid leukemia and polycythemia vera.

REFERENCES

ASLINIA F, MAZZA JJ, YALE SH. 2006. Megaloblastic anemia and other causes of macrocytosis. Clin Med Res 4:236–41.

BABIOR BM. 2006. Folate, cobalamin, and megaloblastic anemias. In: Lichtman MA, Kipps TJ, Kaushansky K, Beutler E, Seligsohn U, Prchal JT, eds., Williams Hematology 7th ed. McGraw-Hill, New York, 477–510.

BAIN BJ, BATES I. 2001. Basic haematological techniques. In: Lewis SM, Bain BJ, Bates I, eds. Dacie and Lewis Practical Hematology, 9th ed. Churchill Livingstone, London, 19–46.

BAIN BJ. 2002. Blood Cells: A Practical Guide, 3rd ed. Blackwell Science, Oxford.

BAIN BJ. 2005. Morphology in the diagnosis of red cell disorders. Hematology 10(suppl 1):178–81.

BEYAN C, KAPTAN K, IFRAN A. 2007. Predictive value of discrimination indices in differential diagnosis of iron deficiency anemia and beta-thalassemia trait. Eur J Haematol 78:524–6.

BLENCOWE H, COUSENS S, MODELL B, LAWN J. 2010. Folic acid to reduce neonatal mortality from neural tube disorders. Int J Epidemiol 39(suppl 1):i110–21.

BRUGNARA C, ZURAKOWSKI D, DICANZIO J, BOYD T, PLATT O. 1999. Reticulocyte hemoglobin content to diagnose iron deficiency in children. JAMA 281:2225–30.

BUNN HF, FORGET BG. 1986. Hemoglobin: Molecular, Genetic and Clinical Aspects. Saunders, Philadelphia.

Centers for Disease Control and Prevention. 2006. Update on multi-state outbreak of *E. coli* O157:H7 infections from fresh spinach. http://www.cdc.gov/foodborne/ecolispinach/100606.htm. Accessed on Nov. 2, 2010.

Centers for Disease Control and Prevention. 2009. Multi-state outbreak of *E. coli* O157:H7 infections linked to eating raw refrigerated, prepackaged cookie dough. http://www.cdc.gov/ecoli/2009/0630.html. Accessed on Nov. 2, 2010.

CORNBLEET J. 1983. Spurious results from automated hematology cell analyzers. Lab Med 14:509–14.

DEMIR A, YARALI N, FISGIN T, DURU F, KARA A. 2002. Most reliable infices in differentiation between thalassemia trait and iron deficiency anemia. Pediatr Int 44:612–6.

ELGHETANY MT, BANKI K. 2006. Erythrocytic disorders. In: McPherson RA, Pincus MR, eds., Henry's Clinical Diagnosis and Management by Laboratory Methods, 21st ed. Saunders, Philadelphia, 1971–2011.

FESSAS P. 1963. Inclusions of hemoglobin in erythroblasts and erythrocytes of thalassemia. Blood 21:21–32.

GALLAGHER PG. 2004. Hereditary elliptocytosis: spectrin and protein 4.1R. Semin Hematol 41:142–64.

GREEN R. 2008. Indicators for assessing folate and vitamin B12 status and for monitoring the efficacy of intervention strategies. Food Nutr Bull 29(suppl 2):S52–63.

HILLMAN RS, FINCH CA. 1971. Erythropoiesis. New Engl J Med 285:99–101.

HOFFBRAND AV, NEWCOMBE FA, MOLLIN DL. 1966. Method of assay of red cell folate activity and the value of the assay as a test for folate deficiency. J Clin Pathol 19:17–28.

KING MJ, BEHRENS J, ROGERS C, FLYNN C, GREENWOOD D, CHAMBERS K. 2000. Rapid flow cytometric test for the diagnosis of membrane cytoskeleton-associated haemolytic anaemia. Br J Haematol 111:924–33.

LEWIS SM. 2005. Introduction—the global problem of nutritional anemias. Hematology 10(suppl 1):224–6.

MAHU JL, LECLERCQ C, SUQUET JP. 1990. Usefulness of red cell distribution width in association with biological parameters in an epidemiological survey of iron deficiency in children. Int J Epidemiol 19:646–54.

MENTZER WC. 1973. Differentiation of iron deficiency from thalassaemia trait. Lancet 1(7808):882.

OSLER W. 1903. The Principles and Practice of Medicine, 5th ed. Appleton, New York.

PARKER C, OMINE M, RICHARDS S, NISHIMURA J, BESSLER M, WARE R, HILLMEN P, LUZZATTO L, YOUNG N, KINOSHITA T, ROSSE W, SOCIÉ G, International PNH Interest Group. 2005. Diagnosis and management of paroxysmal nocturnal hemoglobinuria. Blood 106:3699–709.

PERKINS S. 2006. Diagnosis of anemia. In: Kjeldsberg CR, ed., Practical Diagnosis of Hematologic Disorders, 4th ed., Vol. 1. ASCP Press, Chicago, 3–16.

REGAN F, NEWLANDS M. BAIN BJ. 2001. Acquired hemolytic anemias. In: Lewis SM, Bain BJ, Bates I, eds., Dacie and Lewis Practical Hematology, 9th ed. Churchill Livingstone, London, 199–230.

ROPER D, LAYTON M, LEWIS SM. 2001. Investigation of the hereditary haemolytic anaemias: membrane and enzymatic abnormalities. In: Lewis SM, Bain BJ, Bates I, eds., Dacie and Lewis Practical Hematology, 9th ed. Churchill Livingstone, London, 167–98.

RYAN DH. 2006. Examination of the blood. In: Lichtman MA, Kipps TJ, Kaushansky K, eds., Williams Hematology, 7th ed. McGraw-Hill, New York, 10–9.

SADLER JE. 2008. Von Willebrand factor, ADAMTS13, and thrombotic thrombocytopenic purpura. Blood 112:11–8.

SAVAGE DG, OGUNDIPE A, ALLEN RH, STABLER SP, LINDENBAUM J. 2000. Etiology and diagnostic evaluation of macrocytosis. Am J Med Sci 319:343–52.

SIEGEL RM, LaGRONE DH. 1994. The use of zinc protoporphyrin in screening young children for iron deficiency. Clin Pediatr (Phila) 33:473–9.

SKOGERBOE KJ, WEST SF, SMITH C, TERASHITA ST, LeCRONE CN, DETTER JC, TAIT JF. 1992. Screening for alpha-thalassemia. Correlation of hemoglobin H inclusion bodies with DNA-determined genotype. Arch Pathol Lab Med 116:1012–8.

SNOWER DP, WEIL SC. 1993. Changing etiology of macrocytosis: Zidovudine as a frequent causative factor. Am J Clin Pathol 99:57–60.

TEFFERI A. 2003. Anemia in adults: a contemporary approach to diagnosis. Mayo Clin Proc 78:1274–80.

TIERNEY WM, McDONALD CJ, HUI SL, MARTIN DK. 1988. Computer predictions of abnormal test results. JAMA 259:1194–8.

VALLANCE H, FORD J. 2003. Carrier testing for autosomal-recessive disorders. Crit Rev Clin Lab Sci 40:473–97.

van WALRAVEN C, RAYMOND M. 2003. Population-based study of repeat laboratory testing. Clin Chem 49:1997–2005.

WARD PC. 2002. Modern approaches to the investigation of vitamin B12 deficiency. Clin Lab Med 22:435–45.

WEATHERALL DJ. 2010a. Thalassemia as a global health problem: recent progress toward its control in the developing countries. An NY Acad Sci 1202:17–23.

WEATHERALL DJ. 2010b. The inherited diseases of hemoglobin are an emerging global health burden. Blood 115:4331–6.

ZANDECKI M, GENEVIEVE F, GERARD J, GODON A. 2007. Spurious counts and spurious results on haematology analysers: a review. Part II: White blood cells, red blood cells, haemoglobin, red cell indices and reticulocytes. Int J Lab Hematol 29:21–41.

ZANELLA A, GRIDELLI L, BERZUINI A, COLOTTI MT, MOZZI F, MILANI S, SIRCHIA G. 1989. Sensitivity and predictive value of serum ferritin and free erythrocyte protoporphyrin for iron deficiency. J Lab Clin Med 113:73–8.

CHAPTER FOUR

MICROCYTIC, NORMOCYTIC, AND MACROCYTIC ANEMIAS

Reza Setoodeh and Loveleen C. Kang

MICROCYTIC ANEMIAS

The primary function of the red blood cell is to deliver oxygen to the tissues by reversible binding of hemoglobin in the red cells with oxygen. Anemias are characterized by decrease in red cell mass and are typically associated with a decrease in the oxygen-carrying capacity of the blood. Thus anemia is defined as reduction in the total number of red blood cells, amount of hemoglobin in circulation, or circulating red blood cell mass. Based on red cell mass, anemia can either be relative or absolute. Relative anemia is characterized by a normal red cell mass diluted by an increased plasma volume, brought about by either physiological or pathological plasma volume dysregulation. Relative anemia is seen in pregnancy or excessive hydration. Absolute anemia is characterized as decreased red cell mass. Anemias may be also classified on the basis of morphological criteria (Hussein and Haddad, 2010). Morphological classification subdivides anemia into (1) microcytic anemias, (2) normocytic anemias, and (3) macrocytic anemia. The advantage of morphological classification over other classification is its simplicity and its objective basis derived from red cell indices.

Microcytic anemia is defined by hemoglobin concentration of more than 2 standard deviations below the mean for healthy population adjusted for age and sex (Nathan and Oski, 2003), accompanied by low mean corpuscular volume (i.e., MCV <80 FL) (McPherson, 2007). It is often associated with reduced mean corpuscular hemoglobin (MCH), giving a hypochromic appearance to the red blood cells. In microcytic anemia, cellular proliferation and DNA synthesis is normal, but hemoglobin (Hgb) production is decreased (Kjeldsberg and Perkins, 2010). Given 98% of red blood cell cytoplasmic protein is Hgb, decrease in its synthesis results in production of smaller and paler RBCs (Kjeldsberg and Perkins, 2010). Each Hgb molecule consists of four globin polypeptide chains; one pair of alpha chains and one pair of non-alpha chains. Each globin chain contains a heme group with one attached iron atom (Kumar et al., 2009). Decrease in amount of any of these moieties results in reduced Hgb synthesis. Microcytosis can be visualized in peripheral smear. The diameter of normal RBCs is 6 to 8 microns, close to that of normal lymphocyte nucleus (McPherson, 2007). Pale RBCs with diameter less than that are considered microcytic. Hgb molecules are capable of reversibly binding to oxygen molecules. The main mechanisms leading to microcytic anemia are decreased iron availability as in iron deficiency anemia (IDA), and anemia of chronic disease/inflammation (ACD); defective heme synthesis as in sideroblastic anemia and lead poisoning; and disorders of globin chain production as in thalassemic disorders (Kjeldsberg

Non-Neoplastic Hematopathology and Infections, First Edition. Edited by Hernani D. Cualing, Parul Bhargava, and Ramon L. Sandin.
© 2012 Wiley-Blackwell. Published 2012 by John Wiley & Sons, Inc.

and Perkins, 2010). The three most common causes of microcytic anemia are IDA, ACD, and the alpha or beta thalassemia trait (Benz, 2010). These individual entities and their laboratory diagnosis are covered in detail below. The approach to diagnosis of microcytic anemia is addressed in Chapter 3.

Iron Deficiency Anemia (IDA)

Definition

A very common anemia that occurs due to loss of iron.

ICD-10 Code D50

Epidemiology

IDA is a very common disease worldwide, and the most common treatable anemia. It has the highest prevalence among women and children. Common causes of iron deficiency vary with age (Table 4.1).

Clinical

General clinical manifestations of anemia are a function of hypoxia and include pallor, fatigability, dyspnea on exertion, headache, light headedness, and palpitation. Classic signs specific to iron deficiency are rarely present nowadays and include paresthesia, glossal pain, ulcers at mouth corners (angular stomatitis), chronic gastritis, craving to eat nonfood substances (pica), dysphagia due to esophageal webs, spoon nails, restless legs, and hair loss. Splenomegaly may occur in persistent nontreated patients (Cecil et al., 2007; Fauci et al., 2008; McPherson, 2007; Umbreit, 2005).

Pathobiology

Iron is an essential component of all living cells, playing an important role in electron transfer reactions. In the human body iron is necessary for the production of hemoglobin, myoglobin, and certain enzymes of most body cells. The body conserves iron very efficiently, and there is no specific way for iron excretion. Iron loss is mainly through loss of desquamated cells of the GI tract, GU tract, and the skin. The average amount of daily excreted iron in women (1.5 mg) is more than in men (<1 mg), due to menstrual blood loss (Hoffman, 2008). The balance of iron content in the body is therefore regulated by control of iron absorption. The average dietary iron in the United States is around 15 mg/day, and absorption mostly takes place in the small intestine, especially in the duodenum and proximal jejunum. The rate of iron absorption is usually 5 to 10% of diet iron but varies based on the level of iron demand, and absorption can reach up to 20% in iron deficiency. Minimum daily requirement of iron depends on the sex, age, and stage of growth, the highest in pregnant women (Killip et al., 2007; Adamson, 2008).

Most of the body's total iron is in the erythrocytes; one milliliter of packed red cells contains about one milligram of iron (Fauci et al., 2008). Most of the iron used in the synthesis of hemoglobin is transferred by transferrin to erythrocyte precursor cells from recently degraded hemoglobin in the macrophages. Iron is stored in the form of ferritin or hemosiderin. Ferritin is water soluble and is found in all cells of the body and extra cellular fluids. The serum ferritin concentration is roughly related to the total body iron store, making it important in evaluation of disorders of iron metabolism. Hemosiderin is water insoluble and predominantly found in the macrophages of reticuloendothelial cells. It microscopically appears as golden brown granules (McPherson, 2007).

When demands for iron are not met by iron intake for a long time, deficiency develops through stages. The first stage is iron depletion, characterized by decreased/absent iron storage, decreased ferritin but normal serum iron, transferrin saturation, and blood Hgb. The next step is iron deficiency without anemia, in which serum iron and transferrin saturation are decreased but anemia still not present. In the last stage Hgb is also decreased (iron deficiency anemia) (Fauci et al., 2008).

The development and progression of iron deficiency depends on the individual's initial iron store, which is based on age and gender, being generally lowest in menstruating women. The normal adult male body iron store of 1000 mg will last for three to four years if absorption stops.

TABLE 4.1 Common Causes of Iron Deficiency

Age	Causes of IDA
Children	Inadequate iron intake Rapid growth and increased demand for iron
Women of childbearing age	Menstrual blood loss Pregnancy and increased demand for iron
Men and postmenopausal women	Chronic blood loss Malabsorption

Lab Diagnosis

CBC: In chronic IDA, red blood cell indices show microcytosis (MCV less than lower normal range) and hypochromia (MCH less than lower normal range). Increased platelet count (>450,000/μL) has been attributed to IDA especially in adult patients with active blood loss. Thrombocytopenia has been found and is relatively more common in patients of young age. WBC count is usually within normal ranges or slightly reduced. Granulocytopenia may be seen and presence of hypersegmented neutrophils especially after treatment with iron might be present due to coexistent folate deficiency. Reticulocyte counts are often decreased in number, but become normal after iron therapy (Kjeldsberg and Perkins, 2010; McPherson, 2007; Umbreit, 2005).

Blood smear: In the early stages of iron deficiency anemia erythrocytes are normochromic and normocytic. Anisocytosis is the first recognizable morphologic change of RBCs. As iron becomes more deficient microcytosis, hypochromia, and poikilocytosis develop. RBC membrane is stiff in iron deficient cells, leading to development of cells with abnormal shapes (poikilocytosis), especially elongated hypochromic elliptocytes (pencil cells) (Figure 4.2), and red blood cells with central pallor and sharp-edged, submembranous vacuoles (pre-keratocytes). Anisocytosis may be identified by automated cell counters as increase in red cell distribution width. RBC indices are abnormal when Hgb is at least 2 g/dl below the lower normal limit adjusted for age and sex (Harrington et al., 2008).

Bone marrow: BM aspirate with iron staining is the most direct tool for assessment of iron storage. Absence of stainable iron has been previously considered as the "gold standard" (Phiri et al., 2009), however nowadays not usually required, for the diagnosis of IDA. In early stages of IDA hyperplasia of normoblasts is seen, but as the iron deficiency becomes more severe the erythropoiesis decreases, BM becomes normocellular, and erythroblasts show small size, irregular shape, and decreased hemoglobin in cytoplasm.

Serum iron: Normal range of serum iron is 50 to 160 μg/dl. Iron concentration in serum is usually low in iron deficient patient. All iron in the serum is bound to transferrin, an iron binding protein. Serum iron test measures transferrin bound iron and has a diurnal fluctuation. It increases in the afternoons and decreases in the mornings (Brugnara, 2003). Serum iron concentration decreases in the presence of acute or chronic inflammation, and increases after taking oral iron supplements. These all variables make it less than ideal test for evaluation of iron storage.

Iron binding capacity: Iron binding capacity is an indirect measure of amount of transferrin. Normal range of TIBC is 250 to 400 μg/dl. Since the normal serum iron concentration is about 100 μg/dl, transferrin is only one-third saturated with iron (30%). In IDA, the serum TIBC is increased. However if chronic infection is present, TIBC may not be increased. Transferrin saturation of 16% or less is usually an indicator of IDA.

Serum ferritin: Ferritin is the main intracellular form if iron storage. Serum ferritin, which is in equilibrium with tissue ferritin, correlates with body iron stores, and its measurement is a less invasive test than aspiration of BM for evaluation of total body iron store (Lipschitz et al., 1974). Serum ferritin levels do not show diurnal fluctuations. Normal range for ferritin is 12 to 300 μg/L in adults, and higher in men than in women. Serum ferritin level of less than 12 μg/L is diagnostic of IDA. Ferritin is an acute phase reactant and increased ferritin is seen in diverse variety of inflammatory disorders, independent of body iron stores. In these patients ferritin level cutoff is higher (60 μg/L for rheumatoid arthritis) (Chijiwa et al., 2001).

Erythrocyte zinc protoporphyrin: Protoporphyrin combines with iron and forms the body of heme group of hemoglobin and myoglobin, and so is increased in anemias associated with failure of iron incorporation into heme group. Normal range is 10 to 99 μg/dl. In the absence of iron to bind with protoporphyrin, zinc usually becomes attached and forms zinc protoporphyrin (ZPP). Elevated erythrocyte porphyrin is one of the earliest signs of iron deficiency, present even before changes in RBC indexes.

Transferrin receptor: When iron enters the plasma, transferrin moves it to bone marrow and binds to transferrin receptor (TfR) on the cell surface of erythroblasts. Receptor synthesis is increased in iron deficiency. The levels of soluble form of transferrin receptor (STfR), a truncated receptor produced by shedding from erythrocytes, correlate with amount of membranous receptor (Weiss and Goodnough, 2005; Lee et al., 2002). Normal range for STfR is 4 to 9 μg/L and iron deficiency anemia is associated with increased circulating (soluble) transferrin receptor.

Reticulocyte hemoglobin content: Reticulocyte hemoglobin content (CHr) is a measure of amount of hemoglobin in each reticulocyte which is a 1 to 2-day-old red blood cell. This reflects the amount of iron directly available for hemoglobin synthesis in recent days. CHr is less affected by inflammation and has been shown to be a strong predictor of iron deficiency anemia or functional iron deficiency especially in children and in dialysis patients, for whom the interpretation of transferrin saturation and ferritin level is difficult. In anemic patients with end stage renal disease CHr level is a useful tool for prediction of response to treatment (Singh et al., 2007; Brugnara et al., 1999). The normal range for CHr is 28.9 to 32.9 pg/reticulocyte, and the cutoff point of <26 pg in children and <28 in adults showed optimal sensitivity and specificity for diagnosis of iron deficiency (Mast et al., 2008).

Management

The most important step is finding and correcting the underlying cause of IDA, especially when occult blood loss is suspected. Correction of underlying cause and even surgical intervention for stopping bleeding may then be needed. The goal in treatment of IDA is to supply enough iron to correct the decreased Hgb and replenish the deficit of body iron storage. Severity of anemia is another important issue that determines the approach to treatment of IDA. Oral ferrous sulfate is the therapy of choice for most cases. Intolerance of oral iron is very common and can be solved by taking iron pills with food and modifying amount of iron in each dose. For patients who remain intolerant to oral iron supplement, for IDAs refractory to oral therapy, and patients with gastrointestinal diseases like IBDs, parenteral iron therapy is the treatment of choice. Because of increased risk of adverse reactions (e.g., anaphylactic shock), parenteral iron therapy should be used only after trying oral iron therapy. Response to therapy is seen as increase in reticulocytes which begins within 3 to 5 days and reaches to maximum in 8 to 10 days. Hgb level rises after 5 days and usually becomes normal in 6 weeks if adequate iron replacement is achieved. Iron therapy should be continued for at least 2 months after Hgb has reached to normal value. Complete recovery of MCV value may take about 4 months. Blood transfusion is reserved for critically ill patients with markedly low level of Hgb. Transfused RBCs are sources for iron (200 mg of iron present per unit of packed RBCs).

Anemia of Chronic Disease (ACD)

Definition

ACD is an anemia syndrome typically found in patients with chronic diseases (infectious, inflammatory, or neoplastic) and increased levels of inflammatory cytokines, particularly TNF-alpha, IL-1, IL-6, and INF-gamma (Kjeldsberg and Perkins, 2010).

ICD-10 Code D63

Epidemiology

ACD is a very common cause of anemia, and has been shown to be the most prevalent anemia in hospitalized patients (Kumar et al., 2009). Some studies have shown ACD in patients with severe trauma, diabetes mellitus, and even noninflammatory diseases such as heart failure (McPherson, 2007; Cecil et al., 2007).

Pathobiology

It has been suggested that ACD is a biological response of the human body to inhibit the proliferation of iron-requiring organisms (Weiss and Goodnough, 2005; Zarychanski and Houston, 2008). Affected patients usually develop mild normocytic normochromic anemia, although 20 to 50% of them show microcytosis and hypochromia specially when they are complicated with iron deficiency (Weiss and Goodnough, 2005).

Although the underlying mechanism of anemia of chronic disease/inflammation is not completely understood, some immunity-driven mechanisms are known to be involved in the development of ACD. Abnormal iron retention within macrophages of the reticuloendothelial system leads to reduced serum iron levels and decreased transferrin saturation, resulting in functional iron deficiency (Figure 4.3). Another pathophysiologic mechanism is the inhibition of proliferation and the differentiation of erythroid progenitor cells because of a cytokine-induced decrease in the erythropoietin response and an increased apoptosis of cells. Decreased red cells life span is another underlying cause of ACD (Gardner and Roy, 1961; Fleming and Bacon, 2005).

Hepcidin, an acute phase reactant protein, is the master regulator of iron homeostasis. It controls the expression of a transmembrane iron export protein, ferroportin, on duodenal enterocytes and macrophages (Figure 4.1). Hepcidin by this mean blocks the export of iron from enterocytes and macrophages into the circulation. This pathophysiology is termed "inflammatory block." The synthesis of hepcidin is induced by an iron overload and inflammatory cytokines, and reduced by iron deficiency, most anemias, and hypoxia. An anemic state with many lab features of ACD has been seen after major trauma, myocardial infarction, and surgery that may be secondary to tissue damage and appears to be an acute variant of ACD, and the term "anemia of inflammation" is proposed for both variants (Theurl et al., 2009; Keel and Abkowitz, 2009; Weiss and Goodnough, 2005; Fleming and Bacon, 2005).

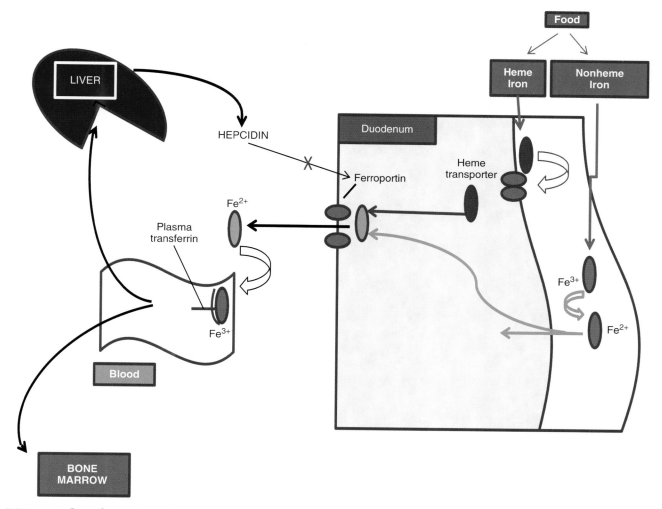

FIGURE 4.1   Iron absorption and transport.

Clinical Features

Anemia of chronic disease is usually mild and develops 1 to 2 months after onset of the underlying disease. In cases of significant anemia, coexistent iron or folate deficiency should be considered. Clinical manifestations of anemia are usually dominated by those of the causative disease. However, anemia negatively affects the quality of life in debilitated patients. (Cecil et al., 2007; Fauci et al., 2008).

Lab Diagnosis

CBC: Leukocytes and platelets are normal. RBCs are usually normochromic and normocytic (Keel and Abkowitz, 2009), but in long-standing cases microcytosis (MCV < 80) and hypochromia (MCHC < 27) is present. RDW is slightly increased (anisocytosis), and slight poikilocytosis is present. Reticulocyte count is inappropriately low, which reflects the decrease

in RBC production. (Kjeldsberg and Perkins, 2010, McPherson, 2007).

Bone marrow: In classic cases of ACD, bone marrow macrophages contain normal or increased iron, reflecting decreased iron export. Marrow is usually normocellular and cell differentiation is not significantly disturbed. Sideroblasts are decreased, reflecting decreased availability of iron for erythropoiesis (Gardner and Roy, 1961).

Iron studies: See Table 4.6. The serum iron concentration and transferrin saturation are decreased resulting from the reduced iron export from macrophages. The transferrin level (TIBC) is decreased or normal. The serum ferritin level and erythrocyte protoporphyrin are elevated. A ferritin level of less than 30 μg/L suggests coexistent iron deficiency. The soluble transferrin receptor (STfR) is normal. The TfR-ferritin index (the ratio of sTfR

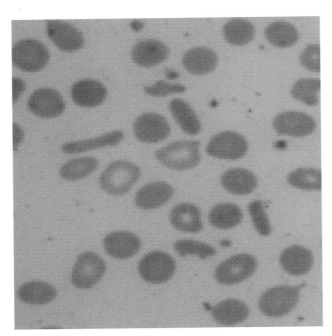

FIGURE 4.2 Red blood cells with anisopoilkilocytosis, including elliptocytes.

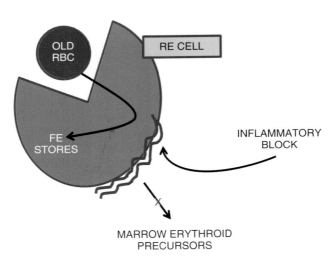

FIGURE 4.3 Functional iron deficiency in anemia of chronic disease.

to the logarithm of the ferritin level) is less than 1 (Punnonen et al., 1997).

Management

Correction of underlying disorder is the treatment of choice. If complete correction is not reachable, the quality of life may improve directly after treatment of anemia. Patients with chronic diseases and EPO levels of less than 500 mU/ml may benefit from EPO administration (Hoffman, 2008; Weiss and Goodnough, 2005).

Thalassemia

Definition

Thalassemia syndromes are inherited autosomal recessive genetic defects that result in absence or underproduction of normal globin chains.

ICD-10 Code D56

Pathobiology

The Hgb molecule consists of four globin polypeptide chains. Two groups of globin polypeptides exist in human hemoglobin: alpha-like globins (alpha and zeta), and beta-like globins (beta, delta, gamma, and epsilon). Combinations of globin chains vary in different Hgbs. Hgb A has one pair of alpha chains and one pair of beta. Hgb A2 consists of two alpha and two delta chains. In Hgb F, the chains are alpha and gamma. For alpha-like globin chains there are two copies of genes on each chromosome 16, and for each type of beta-like globins one encoding gene exists on each chromosome 11.

Thalassemias result from mutations that lead to the absence or reduction of alpha-like or beta-like globin chain synthesis. Alpha thalassemia results from gene deletions and beta thalassemia usually results from point mutations. A reduced amount of one globin chain and relative excess of the other, result in two underlying pathophysiologies of thalassemia syndromes: first, the decrease in Hgb synthesis and its consequent anemia, and second, accumulation and precipitation of unpaired globin chains, which results in the formation of insoluble inclusion bodies and apoptosis of erythroid precursors, and thus ineffective erythropoiesis (Table 4.4).

Epidemiology

Thalassemias are among of the most common genetic disorders worldwide (Rund and Rachmilewitz, 2005). They occur at high frequency throughout the Mediterranean region, the Middle East, and the tropical and subtropical parts of Asia and Africa, regions historically exposed to malaria while the carriers are thus better equipped to survive falciparum malaria (Weatherall and Clegg, 2001).

Clinical Features

Patients who receive transfusions on regular basis develop an iron overload (Table 4.6) that is the cause of most thalassemia-associated mortality and morbidity, with cardiac hemosiderosis as the primary cause of death (Benz, 2010; Hoffman, 2008; Fauci et al., 2008; Cecil et al., 2007).

- **Beta-thalassemia:** Based on clinical severity, beta-thalassemias are classified into three groups: major, intermedia, and minor (Hoffman, 2008). The severity of anemia in these groups is related to the underlying genetic defects. The relationships of clinical phenotypes and genetic defects is summarized in Table 4.2. Clinical findings in β-thalassemia major include jaundice, splenomegaly, bone deformities, and prominent facial bones largely due to expansion of bone marrow, and growth retardation (Rund and Rachmilewitz, 2005).

- **Alpha-thalassemia:** Clinically alpha-thalassemia is classified into four groups: silent carrier, thalassemia trait, Hgb H disease, and Hydrops fetalis. This classification is based on number of deleted alpha globin genes (Table 4.3). Absence of α-chains is incompatible with life, so infants with Bart's Hydops fetalis are stillborn. Hemolysis-induced jaundice and splenomegaly are usually found among less symptomatic patients.

Lab Diagnosis

Serum iron level and transferrin saturation are elevated in major and intermediate forms of thalassemia, however, patients with minor forms or thalassemia trait show decreased or normal levels of serum iron.

- **Beta-thalassemia major:** This disorder produces severe microcytic hypochromic anemia. Without transfusions Hgb levels are typically around 2 to 3 g/dL. Blood smear shows significant

anisopoikilocytosis with bizarrely shaped red blood cells, teardrop red cells, nucleated RBCs, fragmented RBCs, and target cells. After splenectomy, even more deformed microcytes are frequently seen. Precipitates of alpha globins in red blood cells may be apparent as Heinz inclusion bodies. Elevated reticulocytes and basophilic stippling are another finding (see Chapter 3, Figure 3.2A, B). The bone marrow indicates erythroid hyperplasia and aspects of ineffective erythropoiesis. Elevated Hgb F levels are characteristic of this type of thalassemia. Little or no Hgb A is produced. The Hgb A2 level is invariably increased.

- **Beta-thalassemia minor:** These patients have mild to moderate anemia, and the Hgb levels range from 9 to 11 g/dl. The red cells show modest microcytic and hypochromic changes with MCV values of 55 to 70 fL and MCH values of less than 22 pg. Anisopoikilocytosis with target cells, and basophilic stippling may or may not be present. The RBC count is characteristically elevated (5–7 M/μL) and reticulocyte count is twice the normal count. Defected in bone marrow is slight normoblastic erythroid hyperplasia. Hgb A2 is increased to 3.5 to 7%, and Hgb F indicates elevated values (1–3%) in half of the cases (Muncie and Campbell, 2009; Rund and Rachmilewitz, 2005).

- **Alpha-thalassemias:** In Hgb H disease (the absence of three α chains), a chronic hemolytic anemia is present, with Hgb values about 3 g/dL less than normal, MCV values of 60 to 70 fL, and MCH values of 17 to 21 pg. During pregnancy the anemia becomes more severe and more symptomatic. Anisopoikilocytosis with target cells, basophilic stippling, and hypochromia are present in the blood smear. The RBC count is increased (6–6.2 M/μL) and 4 to 5% reticulocytosis is present. Hgb Bart's, which is 2 to 40% at birth, gradually falls to around 4.8%.

TABLE 4.2 **Severity of β-Thalassemia Based on Genotype**

Subtype	Genotype	Severity
Minor	β/β+	Silent
Intermedia	β/β0; β + /β+; β + /β0	Moderate
Major	β0/β0	Severe

Note: β0: No β chain production; β+ : β chain production present but decreased.

TABLE 4.3 **Alpha Thalassemia Types**

Subtype	Genotype	Severity
Carrier	−α/αα	Silent
Trait	−α/ − α; –/αα	Mild hemolytic anemia
HbH dx	–/−α	Mild to moderate
Hydrops	–/–	Incompatible with life

In the α-thalassemia trait (the absence of two α chains) the symptoms of microcytic anemia are mild and can be seen with MCV ranging from 65 to 75 fL. α/β chain ratio is mildly decreased to 0.6 to 0.7, and the Hgb Bart's levels are 5 to 10% in cord blood (normally < 0.5%), show a decrease at birth, and are undetectable in adults. The Hgb electrophoresis is normal, and diagnosis of this subtype in adults is made after excluding other differential diagnoses (Harteveld and Higgs, 2010; McPherson, 2007).

TABLE 4.4 **Hemoglobin Concentration in Thalassemias**

Hgb	β-Major	β-Minor	Hydrops Fetalis	HbH dx	α-Trait	α-Carrier
Hgb A	Absent/reduced	Slightly reduced	Absent	Reduced	Normal	Normal
Hgb A2	May be elevated	Elevated 3.5–7%	Absent	Reduced	Normal/reduced	Normal
Hgb F	Markedly elevated 60–95%	Slightly elevated 1–3%	Absent	Normal	Normal	Normal
Bart's			Main	2–40% at birth	Absent (5–10% in cord blood)	Absent (1–2% in cord blood)
Hgb H			Trace	9% (1–40%)	Inclusions present in –/αα	Absent
Portland			Variable			

The Mentzer index is helpful in differentiating IDA from the thalassemia trait given the presence of microcytosis. The Mentzer index is the quotient of MCV divided by the red blood cell count. If the index is less than 13, thalassemia is likely. If the result is greater than 13, then iron-deficiency anemia is more favored (William, 1973).

Management

Patients with a thalassemia minor or trait do not need any treatment or follow-up. These cases should be diagnosed and documented to prevent treating the patient with iron therapy for possible IDA. Anemia may become severe in pregnancy, so mothers with mild thalassemia need close monitoring during pregnancy.

Supportive therapy is the main treatment in patients with intermediate, major, or HbH forms of the disease. When severe anemia is present, regular blood transfusions along with folate supplementation is the therapy of choice, to maintain Hgb levels. When the need for transfusion becomes markedly apparent due to hypersplenism, splenectomy may be a consideration. Iron-chelating agents like Desferrioxamine are routinely given to patients who are on a regular high transfusion regimen. Serial serum ferritin measuring is the standard route for monitoring the iron overload. Currently the only curative therapy for thalassemia is bone marrow transplantation, and gene therapy, which has shown encouraging results and has opened new horizons in the treatment of thalassemia (Cunningham, 2010; Benz, 2010).

Sideroblastic Anemia

Definition

Sideroblastic anemias include a heterogenous group of disorders characterized by the presence of ring sideroblasts in the bone marrow.

ICD-10 Codes D64.0, D64.1, D64.2, D64.3

Pathobiology

The underlying mechanisms are inherited, or acquired defects disrupting the heme biosynthesis in the mitochondria of the erythroid precursor cells, leading to impaired hemoglobin production and mitochondrial iron accumulation. Sideroblastic anemias are etiologically classified as *acquired* or *congenital* (Table 4.5).

The acquired form is more frequent, and in turn is subclassified into *idiopathic (clonal)* and *secondary (reversible)* sideroblastic anemias. Idiopathic/clonal forms show clonal proliferation of the defective hematopoietic precursor cells, which present as one of the myelodysplastic syndromes (MDS) as refractory anemia with ring sideroblasts (RARS) and RCMD-RS. In the secondary/reversible form, the sideroblastic anemias are associated with removable precipitating factors like drugs, toxins, and nutrient deficiencies that interfere with heme synthesis. Long-term treatment with antituberculosis drugs (e.g., isoniazid), chloramphenicole, penicillamine, lead poisoning, zinc toxicity, copper deficiency, pyridoxine deficiency, and alcohol, as the most common, are potential causes of secondary sideroblastic anemia.

Of the congenital forms, the X-linked sideroblastic anemia is the most common form. Typically the mutations present in the *ALAS2* gene, which encodes delta-aminolevulinate synthase 2, the rate limiting enzyme that catalyzes heme biosynthesis in the presence of pyridoxal phosphate (vitamin B_6).

TABLE 4.5 **Classification of Sideroblastic Anemia**

Congenital	Acquired
X-Linked	MDS
Autosomal recessive	Alcohol
Mitochondrocytic	Drugs
Pearson syndrome	Toxins
	Nutritional deficiency

All the above-mentioned conditions lead to decreased synthesis of heme, which in turn results in accumulation of iron as the mitochondrial ferritin in the erythroblasts and eventually result in ineffective erythropoiesis. Continuous delivery of iron to the erythroid precursor cells and their intramedullary hemolysis, in parallel with the enhanced gastrointestinal iron absorption, results in the systemic iron overload that is a signature feature of sideroblastic anemia, with the hereditary form being more severe than in acquired form.

Clinical Features

Anemia of variable degree is the most common clinical presentation, with Hgb ranging from 4 to 10 g/dl. The age of presentation can vary from early childhood to midlife and even later in life. Other than common symptoms of anemia like pallor, fatigue, and dizziness, specific signs and symptoms of each underlying cause may be present. Mild hepatosplenomegaly is detectable in some cases. The extent of tissue iron deposition increases over time and patients may exhibit manifestations of parenchymal organ damage such as cardiomyopathy, diabetes mellitus, or cirrhosis.

Lab Diagnosis

Blood: The hemoglobin level is low but highly variable. Reticulocytes are not increased and red blood cells are frequently microcytic and hypochromic. The blood smear may show dimorphic red blood cell population, a coexistence of normal and microcytic red blood cells resulting in a bimodal volume distribution curve, a characteristic feature in female carriers of the X-linked disorder (Alcindor and Bridges, 2002). In most cases MCV may be normal but the increased RDW helps differentiate them from normocytic anemia. However, normocytosis and even macrocytosis may present in cases of myelodysplasia. Leukocyte and platelet values are typically normal but may be decreased in the presence of splenomegaly. Occasional red cells with Pappenhaimer bodies and basophilic stippling (siderocytes) are present.

Iron studies: Iron overload results in increased levels of serum iron, serum transferrin saturation, and ferritin and a reduced level of transferrin (TIBC) (Table 4.6). The best way to assess the extent of iron overload is to take a liver biopsy. Ferrokinetic studies have shown serum iron turnover to be rapid. Additional features of ineffective erythropoiesis are mild increase in bilirubin and lactate dehydrogenase, reduced haptoglobin levels, and a relatively normal reticulocyte count. When sideroblastic anemia and

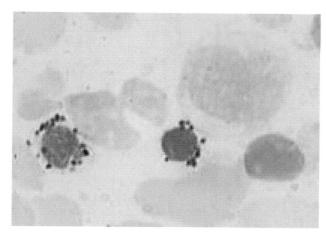

FIGURE 4.4   Ringed sideroblasts.

iron deficiency coexist, the serum iron and ferritin are reduced. This is a condition found in females with excessive menstrual bleeding, or patients with myelodysplastic thrombocytopenia and GI bleeding.

Bone marrow study: The bone marrow should be examined for the presence of ring sideroblasts (Figure 4.4) which is the diagnostic feature. Sideroblasts are erythroblasts with coarse cytoplasmic iron inclusions, and are designated as "ring" when there is a perinuclear localization of inclusions lining around at least one-third of the nucleus circumference. Prussian blue staining is needed to see these changes. Staining also shows a marked increase of iron in marrow macrophages. Coexistent iron deficiency can mask diagnostic bone marrow features of sideroblastic anemia and in this case bone marrow biopsy should be performed after a course of iron therapy. Sideroblastic anemia should also be considered as a possible diagnosis in refractory IDA. Yet another significant indication may be hypochromic erythroid hyperplasia, which along with normal reticulocytes count is a sign of ineffective hematopoiesis.

Molecular studies: Molecular studies are needed to evaluate genetic defects in hereditary sideroblastic anemias. The X-linked form shows mutations in the ALAS2 gene, whereas the autosomal recessive form is identified by mutations in specific mitochondrial transporter genes and other mitochondria proteins. In some cases, defects in the currently implicated genes have not been found.

Management

The first step in the treatment of sideroblastic anemia is identifying and removing the reversible cause if applicable. Supportive therapy is the mainstay of treatment, mainly blood transfusions to relieve the symptomatic anemia. In patients without a history of

TABLE 4.6 Iron Studies in Microcytic Anemias

	Iron Deficiency	Anemia of Chronic Disease	Thalassemia	Sideroblastic Anemia
Serum iron	Decreased	Decreased	Increased/normal	Increased
TIBC	Increased	Decreased	Decreased/normal	Decreased/normal
Serum soluble transferrin receptor	High	Normal	Variable, may be high	Variable, may be high
Bone marrow storage iron	Decreased	Increased	Increased	Increased

transfusion, monitoring of iron values should show progressive iron overload. As well, phlebotomy and iron chelation with Desferrioxamine could be used.

Most patients respond to treatment with pyridoxine, and a complete response has been seen in alcohol-induced cases and anemias resulting from use of pyridoxine antagonists (e.g., anticonvulsants). Administration of folic acid improves the response to pyridoxine therapy and thus compensates for any increase in the erythroid hyperplasia. Among the responsive cases reticulocytosis presents within two weeks, followed by an increase of the Hgb level in the next months and a decrease in transfusion need.

Cytokine therapy combined with erythropoietin and a granulocyte colony stimulating factor (G-CSF) has recently been used to treat acquired sideroblastic anemia, and allogenic bone marrow transplantation has been reported to treat hereditary form of the disease.

Lead Poisoning

Although since 1994 the prevalence of elevated blood lead levels has substantially decreased in the United States, inorganic lead exposure is still an important health problem worldwide. In the United States most elevated blood lead levels observed in adults have been related to occupational exposure. In children lead exposure has to do with ingestion of paint chips in older homes or chewing lead contaminated toys.

ICD-10 Code T56

Pathobiology

Two mechanisms are involved in anemia due to lead poisoning. First, lead interferes with iron absorption and incorporation in the heme production pathway, resulting in a microcytosis that is essentially due to iron deficiency. Second, lead directly inhibits the enzymes of the heme synthesis pathway such as δ-ALA-dehydratase and ferrochelatase. The inhibition of these enzymes leads to an accumulation of protoporphyrin, a precursor of heme, resulting in elevated levels of free and zinc-protoporphyrin in the erythrocytes. Taking a capillary blood sample helps differentiating moderate from severe lead toxicity and distinguishes rebound blood lead levels during therapy from a true acceleration of toxicity.

Lab Diagnosis

A peripheral blood examination should reveal regularly spaced blue dots of RNA in the RBC, basophilic stippling, in the background of a hypochromic micro- or normocytic red blood cells (Bain, 2005). The first step in making a diagnosis is to identify the population at risk and determine the levels of lead in their venous blood (Cecil et al., 2007). The definitive diagnosis is based on finding an elevated blood lead level, with or without clinical signs and symptoms (Woolf et al., 2007). The blood lead level is the best single test for evaluating lead toxicity, and levels at or $>10\ \mu g/dL$ are considered elevated.

Management

The initial treatment for lead poisoning is removal from exposure, which is the only intervention needed for patients with low blood lead levels ($<45\ \mu g/dL$). Increased urinary excretion of lead, or chelation therapy, is the therapy of choice for patients with high blood lead concentrations and symptomatic cases. Chelators include dimercaprol and its water-soluble analogue, Meso-2, 3-dimercaptosuccinic acid (DMSA), calcium disodium ethylenediaminetetraacacetate (CaNa2 EDTA), and D-penicillamine.

NORMOCYTIC ANEMIAS

By definition, anemia is normocytic and normochromic when a patient's Hgb level is low with an MCV and an MCH in the normal range. The classification of normocytic anemia is based on the proliferative status of the erythroid component in the bone marrow and the corresponding number of reticulocytes in peripheral blood. Anemia with decreased red cell production (nonhemolytic normocytic anemia) and anemia with reticulocytosis, due to either increased destruction of red cells or blood loss (hemolytic normocytic anemia), are two subclasses of normocytic normochromic anemia. In the presence of reticulocytosis, blood loss should be first considered due to different approach and treatment compare to other causes of increased reticulocytes.

Hemolytic Anemia

Definition. Anemias with increased red cell destruction are considered hemolytic.

Pathobiology. The main components of red blood cells are the membrane cytoskeleton, Hgb, and metabolic enzymes of the ATP-producing machinery. A defect in any of these intracorpuscular (intrinsic) factors leads to a reduction in the red blood cell's life span and so to hemolysis. Extra corpuscular defects like physical and immune-mediated damage to the red cells result in "extrinsic" hemolysis. Hemolytic anemia disorders are further classified into acquired or hereditary (Table 4.7). Also, based on the location of red cell destruction, the hemolysis could be intravascular or extravascular.

Clinical Findings. The clinical presentation of hemolytic anemia depends largely on the severity and onset of the hemolysis and the compensatory reaction of the bone marrow. When the rate of red cell destruction is low, the bone marrow's response may be enough to keep the hemoglobin level around a normal value. Because other organs may adapt well with slowly progressing anemia, the patient will remain relatively asymptomatic for a long time. However, with rapid onset hemolysis, the bone marrow cannot sufficiently compensate the loss of RBCs, so the patient presents with severe anemia. In addition to general clinical manifestations of anemias (pallor, fatigue, etc.), patients with hemolytic anemia may have specific signs and symptoms related to hemolysis. Jaundice, dark urine, and splenomegaly are among the most common physical findings, but hepatomegaly, pigmented gallstones, and bone deformity may also be seen with severe chronic hemolysis. Rapid onset hemolysis can present with chills, fever, abdominal pain, and low blood pressure.

Lab Diagnosis. The laboratory routine is to study the morphologic features of hemolytic anemia resulting from red cell destruction and the consequent bone marrow response. The different types of hemolytic anemia have specific lab features. Intravascular hemolysis releases RBC components into the serum, causing increased levels of free hemoglobin and its breakdown products, bilirubin, lactate dehydrogenase (LDH), methemalbumin, and methemoglobin in serum and urine. Serum haptoglobin binds to free hemoglobin, and its level shows a reduction in hemolysis. The bone marrow erythropoietic hyperplastic response results in an increased number of reticulocytes in the peripheral blood. This may present as a mild increase in MCV, though the anemia is usually normocytic. Depending on the underlying mechanism of hemolysis, the peripheral blood smear will show the characteristic features. RBC fragments, spherocytes, target cells, and Heinz bodies are frequently encountered morphologic features in the peripheral blood of patients with specific underlying causes of hemolytic anemias. Bone marrow usually shows erythroid hyperplasia.

Intracorpuscular Defects

Among the intracorpuscular defects are hereditary membrane-cytoskeletal defects (e.g., hereditary spherocytosis, hereditary elliptocytosis), enzymopathies (e.g., G-6-PD deficiency, pyruvate kinase deficiency), acquired membrane defects (e.g., paroxysmal nocturanal hemoglobinuria), and certain hemoglobinopathies (discussed in chapter 5 by Bhargava).

Hereditary Membrane–Cytoskeletal Defects

Flexibility is one of the most important features of the red cells and makes them able to pass through the microvasculature without losing their integrity. The deformability and unique biconcave shape of the red cells are largely related to the characteristic structure of their cell membrane, which is composed

TABLE 4.7 **Classification of Hemolytic Anemias**

	Hereditary	Acquired
Intracorpuscular defects	Membranopathies Enzymopathies Hemoglobinopathies	Paroxysmal nocturnal hemoglobinuria (PNH)
Extracorpuscular defects		Environmental: drugs, toxins, infections mechanical Immune mediated: autoimmune, drugs

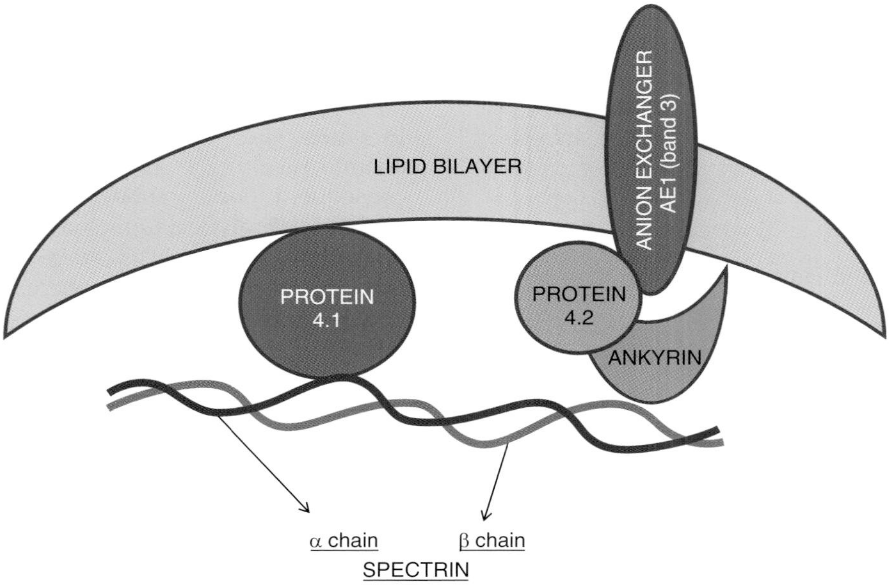

FIGURE 4.5 Erythrocyte Membrane Structure.

of an outer lipid bilayer anchored to the cytoskeleton by transmembrane proteins (Figure 4.5). Loss of any of these components leads to loss of flexibility and discoid shape of the red cells, and eventually early destruction of them in the narrow capillary networks of the splenic microvasculature (hemolysis). Hereditary spherocytosis, hereditary elliptocytosis, and hereditary stomatocytosis are examples of inherited hemolytic anemias with defects in the red cell membrane.

Hereditary Spherocytosis

ICD-10 Code D58.0

Pathobiology. Autosomal and usually dominant mutations affecting different cell membrane proteins like ankyrin, band3, protein 4.2, and most commonly spectrins result in a phenotype known as hereditary spherocytosis (HS) (Agre et al., 1985; Mohandas and Gallagher, 2008). Loss of the connection between the outer lipid layer and the inner cytoskeleton (so-called vertical interactions) leads to a vesiculation of the cell membrane, and the gradual removal of these vesicles in the spleen leads to a reduction of the membrane-to-volume ratio, eventually giving rise to spherocytic RBCs (Stefan and Samuel, 2004; Xiuli and Mohandas, 2008).

Clinical Features . Depending on the severity of the hemolysis, patients present with a variable clinical signs and symptoms, ranging from asymptomatic

hemolysis to severe anemia symptoms. Jaundice and splenomegaly are other common clinical features of HS.

Reactive bone marrow erythroid hyperplasia helps most patients maintain normal hemoglobin levels. However, as in other chronic hemolytic states, exacerbations of anemia may occur from hypersplenism, lack of folate, viral infections (especially parvovirus), or any other stresses to the bone marrow's erythropoiesis.

Cholelithiasis (gallstone) is another complication of HS, and its likelihood increases with age. Rare complications include leg ulcers, gout, priapism, and extramedullary hematopoiesis.

Lab Findings. Anemia, reticulocytosis, and presence of spherocytes in the peripheral blood are common lab features (see Chapter 3, Figure 3.7). Spherocytes are small RBCs that lack central pallor. The number of spherocytes is related to the severity of the defect. The hemolytic nature of anemia causes an elevated serum LDH and unconjugated bilirubin, and decreases the haptoglobin levels. Although spherocytes are smaller than normal red blood cells, their increase in the circulating reticulocytes normalizes the values of MCV. Anisocytosis, presenting as high RDW, is a common finding in peripheral blood smears of these patients. The characteristic red cell index in HS is an elevated MCHC, reflecting the reduced surface-to-volume ratio. The most sensitive test for the detection of spherocytes is the incubated osmotic fragility test, which is based on the increased lysis of fragile spherocytes and the release of hemoglobin in a hypotonic sodium chloride (NaCl) solution (Perrotta et al., 2008; Hassoun and Palek, 1996). However, this finding proves the presence of spherocytes and does not help differentiate HS from other conditions with spherocytosis like AIHA, which can be ruled out by direct coombs test. Flow cytometry has been recently used for diagnosing HS by utilizing florescent dyes that bind to the AE 1 (band 3) cytoskeleton protein (Bolton-Maggs et al., 2004). Decreased florescence indicates low levels of the band 3 protein and so can be used as a screening tool.

Management. Depending on severity of the anemia, the treatment plans can range from supportive care with oral folic acid to blood transfusion and eventually splenectomy in patients with more severe symptoms and complications. Splenectomy allows the red cell life span to increase in HS and other anemias with cytoskeletal defects (Mariani et al., 2008). However, the risks of this procedure and the long-term complications of asplenia should be considered and balanced against its benefits (Bader-Meunier et al., 2001).

Hereditary Elliptocytosis (HE)

Definition HE is a heterogeneous group of genetic disorders with characteristic presence of oval or elliptical red cells (elliptocytes) in the peripheral blood. This characteristic feature was first described by Dresbach in 1904 (Dresbach, 1904).

ICD-10 Code D58.1

Pathobiology. Red blood cells in HE patients lose their capability to keep their biconcave shape when passing through the microvasculature, and this is a membrane-cytoskeletal defect caused by mutations in spectrin α (the most common mutation), spectrin β, glycophorin C, and protein 4.1 genes. Ultimately the defective interactions between the membrane proteins result in the formation of oval shaped red cells (Xiuli and Mohandas, 2008; Gallagher, 2004).

Based on red cell morphology HE is subclassified into three groups: common (mild) HE, spherocytic HE, and Southeast Asian ovalocytosis (McPherson, 2007; Hoffman, 2008).

Clinical Features and Approach to Diagnosis. **Common (mild) HE:** Genetic defects in the α or β spectrin leads to defective horizontal interactions of membrane proteins and thus the most common form of HE. More than 25% of the red cells are elliptocytic (see Chapter 3, Figure 3.6) and the affected persons are mostly asymptomatic and non-anemic; only 10% may show a mild hemolysis that is not related to the extent of blood elliptocytosis. Diagnosis is based on the peripheral blood finding of increased elliptocytic red cells and review of family history; however, specialized testing is also available (Gallagher, 2005).

- **Hereditary pyropoikilocytosis (HPP):** This blood disorder is a subtype of common HE with a homozygous genetic defect and is mostly seen in the African American population. HPP presents with severe congenital transfusion-dependent hemolytic anemia and the peripheral blood smear in these patients shows red cell fragments and poikilocytes. The mutant spectrin is more heat sensitive and denatures in a lower temperature compare to normal forms. Splenectomy can decrease the complications and level of anemia (Medejel et al., 2008); however, for pediatric patients mild HE in neonates can present with moderate to severe hemolysis and peripheral poikilocytosis and splenectomy is better to be postponed.
- **Spherocytic HE:** In this subgroup a molecular defect in the spectrin β chain leads to weakening of both horizontal and vertical interactions between the cell membrane proteins and to the formation of both elliptocytes (due to loss of horizontal interactions) and spherocytes (due to loss of vertical interactions), as revealed using an abnormal osmotic fragility test. Mild hemolytic anemia and splenomegaly are common features of this subtype. As in HS patients, splenectomy could be considered in symptomatic group of patients (Hoffman, 2008).
- **Southeast Asian ovalocytosis:** Aggregation of mutant band 3 proteins along the cell membrane in this group causes rigidity and reduced mobility of the red cell membrane, making them resistant to parasite invasion in malaria. This is found in populations living in malaria endemic areas like Malaysia in Southeast Asia.

Enzymopathies

ICD-10 Code D55

Red blood cells are devoid of nucleus, ribosomes, and mitochondria, and are exclusively dependent on the anaerobic portion of the glycolytic pathway for producing ATP to maintain their functional and structural integrity. Enzyme activity defects in the glycolytic pathway can lead to hemolysis. A hereditary deficiency of enzymes in the glycolytic pathway therefore is the cause of this type of congenital nonspherocytic hemolytic anemia. Pyruvate kinase deficiency and G6PD deficiency are the most common red cell enzyme deficiencies.

Glucose-6-Phosphate Dehydrogenase Deficiency (G6PD)

Definition. G6PD deficiency is an X-linked hereditary caused by mutations that result in highly polymorphic G6PD enzyme variants with variable levels of activity.

ICD-10 Code D55.0

Epidemiology. This disorder affects hundred millions of people around the world. Its distribution is similar to that of malaria in tropical Africa and in tropical and subtropical Asia.

Pathobiology. The G6PD enzyme in the pentose phosphate pathway catalyzes a reduction of the nicotinamide adenine dinucleotide phosphate (NADP) to NADPH, which protects the hemoglobin against oxidative damages. A decrease in G6PD activity is present in all cells of the affected persons, but only RBCs are dependent on pentose phosphate pathway and G6PD as the only source of NADPH (Beutler, 1994; Ronquist and Theodorsson, 2007).

Clinical Features. Based on the extent of enzyme activity, different clinical manifestations may be observed. Most patients are usually found to be asymptomatic with a normal blood smear but develop episodes of acute hemolytic anemia under conditions of oxidative stress triggered by infections, oxidant drugs, and fava beans. The hemolysis is often severe and leads to hemoglobinemia, overt hemoglobinuria, and jaundice. Very rarely when the enzyme activity is less than 10% of the normal level, chronic hemolytic anemia is seen. Neonatal hyperbilirubinemia is more common in G6PD deficient neonates, and neonatal screening test should be performed in male neonates when a positive family history, ethnic origin, or the timing of the jaundice (first 24 hours) is suggestive of the disease (Cappellini and Fiorelli, 2008; Frank, 2005; Beutler, 1994).

Lab Features. The common features of hemolytic anemias, namely reticulocytosis, indirect

bilirubinemia, and decreased serum haptoglobin levels, are present. Heinz bodies, denatured hemoglobin inclusions found in RBCs, are commonly seen and in association with episodic hemolysis support diagnosis of G6PD deficiency. Most of the screening tests for G6PD deficiency work based on a quantitative analysis of NADPH generation. In acute hemolysis the older erythrocytes with lower enzyme activity get hemolyzed, while the quantity of NADPH in most of the remaining younger RBCs and reticulocytes is normal, so false negativity results. G6PD-tetrazolium cytochemical test is the most sensitive test, and only 1 to 5% of the cells with enzyme deficiency are needed to produce an abnormal result, making this test suitable for the diagnosis of enzyme deficiency after hemolytic episodes and even in female heterozygotes. Recently molecular studies have also been applied (Cappellini and Fiorelli, 2008; Ronquist and Theodorsson, 2007).

Management. Identification and avoidance of the precipitating agents is the most effective strategy in management of patients presenting hemolytic anemia. Supportive therapy in episodes of severe hemolytic anemia includes hydration, oxygenation, and transfusions to correct anemia. If the hemoglobinuria induces acute renal failure, hemodialysis might be necessary (Cappellini and Fiorelli, 2008).

Pyruvate Kinase Deficiency

Definition. Deficiency of pyruvate kinase enzyme inherited as an autosomal recessive trait.

ICD-10 Code D55.2

Pathobiology. Pyruvate kinase catalyses the reaction of the second ATP-generating step in the glycolytic pathway. Deficiency of this enzyme gives rise to an imbalance between the erythrocyte energy demand and ATP production, resulting in cell membrane injury and the premature destruction of cells. The anemia ranges from mild or fully compensated to severe life-threatening anemia in icteric neonates, necessitating blood exchange.

Clinical Features and Approach to Diagnosis. Patients with pyruvate kinase deficiency present with usual clinical features of chronic anemia. In contrast to other hemolytic anemias, in patients with PKD, hemolysis and a consequent reticulocytosis may be increased after splenectomy. This is because the spleen sequesters the younger pyruvate kinase deficient erythrocytes and post-splenectomy, although anemia level improves and transfusion requirement is decreased, hemolysis of these normocytic and normochromic red cells continues. The episodes of reticulocytosis increase the MCV. Unlike the "contracted RBCs" and "spiculated" cells described earlier, these cells are nonspecific (see Chapter 3, Figure 3.4). Heinz bodies are absent, and nucleated red cells are rarely seen post splenectomy. Acute infections intensify the degree of hemolysis.

Precise diagnosis is dependent on the quantitative enzyme assays showing decreased activity of the enzyme, or on specific mutations in DNA level being detected.

Management. A safe supportive therapy is folic acid supplementation. A single case of a cure after bone marrow transplantation has been reported in a 5-year-old boy with severe transfusion-dependent hemolytic anemia (Tanphaichitr et al., 2000).

Acquired Membrane Defect

Paroxysmal Nocturnal Hemoglobinuria (PNH)

Definition. PNH is an acquired clonal hematopoietic stem cell disorder resulting from a somatic mutation in the X-linked gene PIG-A.

ICD-10 Code D59.5

Pathobiology. The PIG-A gene mutation gives rise to a deficiency of GPI, a cell surface protein that acts like an anchor and tethers a number of cell surface proteins/antigens to the cell membrane. Among the missing surface proteins in PNH is a group of complement regulators, including a decay accelerating factor (DAF or CD55), a homologous restriction factor (HRF) that acts as a C8 binding protein, and MIRL (CD59), an inhibitor of complement-mediated cell lysis. Lack of these proteins leads to intravascular lysis of RBCs by the complement system proteins.

Three subtypes of defective cells have been described based on the presence of these proteins on the cell surface. PNH type 1 cells have normal amount of proteins, PNH type 2 cells have reduced levels, and PNH type 3 cells are devoid of these proteins (Risitano and Rotoli, 2008; Rotoli et al., 2006).

Clinical Features. PNH is a rare disease with an estimated annual incidence of 4 per million people. The nomenclature for this disease comes from the classical clinical manifestations of intravascular RBC destruction and release of Hgb into the urine, which presents as a dark urine in the morning. Clinical manifestations of PNH are principally due to abnormalities of hematopoietic cells. PNH is classified into three clinical subtypes: classical PNH, PNH with another bone marrow disorder, and subclinical PNH.

The magnitude of hemolysis depends on the number of defective RBCs present in the blood and the subtype of PNH cells (PNH1, 2, or 3). About a third of the cases evolve into aplastic anemia (Cecil et al., 2007); transformation to myelodysplastic syndrome and acute myelogenous leukemia is a rare event (Brodsky et al., 1997).

Lab Features. PNH patients demonstrate common lab features of hemolytic anemias, which include anemia, reticulocytosis, elevated levels of LDH and indirect bilirubin, and decreased haptoglobin levels. The Coombs test is negative. Urine hemosiderin may be demonstrable on Prussian blue staining of urine sediment due to the chronic intravascular hemolysis. The anemia in PNH patients ranges from normal to severe anemia with Hgb <6 g/dl. MCV values can vary from low (due to iron depletion) to high (due to reticulocytosis or folate deficiency). Reticulocytosis, however, is not adequate for determining the severity of anemia in PNH patients due to defective hematopoiesis in the bone marrow (Hoffman, 2008). There is no morphologic finding characteristic for PNH in the peripheral blood. Sucrose promotes the binding and activation of complement on the RBC membrane and hemolysis. This phenomenon is the basis of the sucrose lysis test used for screening of patients suspicious for PNH. The positive acidified serum test (the Ham test) provides a definitive lab diagnosis of PNH; however, the gold standard test is flow cytometry showing the decreased levels of CD55 and/or CD59 on red blood cells and neutrophils (Richards et al., 2000; Madkaikar et al., 2009). A more recently described multiparameter fluorescent aerolysin (FLAER)-based flow assay that identifies PNH monocyte and neutrophil clones has proved to be more sensitive for detecting PNH clones and is the most specific test for diagnosis of PNH (Sutherland et al., 2009; Peghini and Fehr, 2005).

Management. Bone marrow transplant is the ideal and only curative therapy. However, this form of treatment is not realistic for most patients and is reserved for rare cases of malignant transformation or aplastic anemia. Management of PNH has been revolutionized by the anticomplement antibody, eculizumab, which has been shown to markedly reduce intravascular hemolysis and transfusion requirements (Richards et al., 2007; Parker, 2009; Hillmen, 2004). Eculizumab binds to complement C5 and prevents its activation to C5b and MAC formation (Hillmen et al., 2007; Risitano and Rotoli, 2008). Corticosteroids, if administered early in the hemolytic anemias, may improve hemolysis. Continuous lifelong supportive therapy is needed in most of these patients and includes iron and folic acid supply, packed RBCs, anticoagulant agents, and androgenic steroids for stimulation of erythropoiesis.

Extracorpuscula Defects

Nonimmune- and immune-mediated etiologies are responsible for extracorpuscular causes of hemolysis. Nonimmune causes include mechanical (prosthetic valves), infectious (Clostridium sepsis, *E. coli* infection, malaria), microangiopathic hemolytic anemias (disseminated intravascular coagulopathy, thrombotic thrombocytopenia), freshwater drowning, and chemical (disseminated intravascular coagulopathy) etiologies. In immune-mediated hemolytic anemias deposition of antibody or complement on the red cell membrane results in premature destruction of erythrocytes. Classification of immune-mediated hemolytic anemias is based on the presence of autoantibodies, alloantibodies, or drug-related antibodies.

Autoimmune Hemolytic Anemia (AIHA)
Definition. AIHA is a rare immune disorder caused by a defective immune tolerance leading to production of autoantibodies against self RBC antigens resulting in decreased red cell survival.

ICD-10 Code D59.1

Pathobiology. AIHA is subclassified into warm antibody, cold antibody, and mixed type. Warm AIHA is the autoimmune hemolytic anemia associated with IgG, and it has been called warm type because antibodies in this subtype react best with red cells at 37°C. In warm AIHA, which is the most common type, IgG autoantibodies bind to the red cells, and then macrophages in reticuloendothelial system will partially or completely trap these RBCs by recognizing the Fc portion of their coating antibodies (phagocytosis). Most of red cell phagocytoses occur in macrophage-rich organs like spleen and liver, and it is therefore named "extravascular hemolysis." In partial phagocytosis fragments of red cell membrane are taken by macrophages resulting in spherocyte production (McPherson, 2007). Different mechanisms are suggested as the sources of autoantibodies. In

adults sources of warm autoantibodies are autoimmune disorders or malignancies, and pregnancy increases the risk for developing autoantibodies. In pediatric patients AIHA are usually of unknown etiology or antibodies are associated with viral infections (Gehrs and Friedberg, 2002).

AIHA associated with IgM is called cold agglutinin disease because IgM autoantibodies react with red cell antigens at temperatures below 37°C. In this type the antigen–antibody complex activates complement, resulting in the destruction of red cells by the membrane attack complex and thus to "intravascular hemolysis." Cold antibodies are associated with neoplasia (e.g., lymphomas, carcinomas) or infections (e.g., Mycoplasma pneumonia, EBV).

Clinical Features. Signs and symptoms are of the underlying disorders in patients with AIHA. However, clinical manifestations of anemia, jaundice, and sometimes splenomegaly are usually present and associated with hemolysis.

Episodes of hemolysis following cold exposure and Raynaud phenomenon is seen in patients with cold agglutinin disease as the IgM tends to clump together and agglutinate the red cells in small vessels of the extremities where the temperature is low (McPherson, 2007; Kjeldsberg and Perkins, 2010; Lawrence, 2008).

Lab Features. The common lab features of hemolytic anemias are elevated LDH and unconjugated bilirubin, and decreased haptoglobin levels. In patients with warm AIHA, the anemia ranges from moderate to severe and is normocytic and normochromic. Peripheral blood smear shows anisopoikilocytosis including spherocytes, red cell fragments, reticulocytes, and a few nucleated RBCs. Occasionally reticulocytosis leads to an increase in MCV. Cold antibody AIHA demonstrate the same features and an additional finding of red cell clumps (agglutination), which automated machines can falsely show as elevated MCHC. Bone marrow evaluation, if being performed, shows erythroid hyperplasia.

A direct antiglobulin test (DAT), also known as the Coombs test, determines if the red cells are coated by immunoglobulin and/or a complement protein. In this test red cells are incubated with polyclonal antibodies against human immunoglobulins and complement proteins. An agglutination of red cells in this setting leads to positivity of the test. To identify the exact coating protein, a mono-specific antibody can be used. In warm AIHA, the red cells mostly have an IgG with a variable presentation of

C3d. In cold AIHA, C3d is the only coating protein. Special tests are available to detect antibodies when the Coombs is negative in AIHA patients (Hoffman, 2008; Kjeldsberg and Perkins, 2010).

Management. In warm AIHA, mild anemia with compensated hemolysis usually does not require any therapy. When anemia symptoms are severe, red cell transfusion may be considered as a transient supportive therapy. In patients with significant anemia the standard initial treatment is corticosteroid therapy (Hoffman, 2008), which suppresses hemolysis by decreasing autoantibody production and downregulating the Fc receptor expression in macrophages. In cases of refractory hemolysis, IVIg is the next step. Chronic AIHA, refractory to the previously mentioned therapy modalities, may benefit from anti-CD20 agent, Rituximab, which targets immunoglobulin-producing B-cells (Shanafelt et al., 2003; Gupta et al., 2002). Spleen is the major site of red cell destruction so splenectomy may be considered when patient does not respond to conventional treatments (Barros et al., 2010).

Postinfectious cold AIHA is usually self-limited and does not require treatment. In chronic cold AIHA avoidance of cold exposure, treatment of underlying disease, and supportive therapy is usually sufficient.

Drug-Induced Hemolytic Anemia. Hemolytic anemia following drug administration is a rare type of anemia called drug-induced hemolytic anemia (DIHA). The first suspected cases were reported in 1950s and 1960s. Since then the number of hemolysis-inducing drugs have been increased from 15 to more than 125, and the most common causative agents have changed from methyl-dopa and intravenous penicillin to cephalosporins. The antimicrobials, NSAIDs, antineoplastics, and antihypertensive drugs are reported as the most common agents associated with DIHA. Different mechanisms are associated with the disorder. The first mechanism produces antibodies against the drugs (e.g., penicillin) that act as haptens and bind (adsorb) to the RBC membrane, causing the red blood cells to opsonize. Some drugs (e.g., quinidine and NSAIDs) or drug metabolites bind to plasma proteins and form an immunogenic conjugate that can elicit an immune response. The second mechanism of DIHA develops antibodies against the immunogenic conjugate, forming an "immune complex" that adheres to the RBCs and causes hemolysis through the activation of a complement system on the surface of each erythrocyte. The third mechanism induces production of IgG autoantibodies against the

RBCs, and the antibody-coated red blood cells are removed by macrophages in the reticuloendothelial system. Methyldopa is the prototypical drug, and fludarabine is a newer medication that induces this process (Garratty, 2009, 2010; Kjeldsberg and Perkins, 2010).

Patients can present with acute intravascular or a mild extravascular hemolysis with common clinical and lab findings of hemolysis. For suspected cases the result of a direct antiglobulin test (DAT), which is usually positive, is required to diagnose immune hemolytic anemia. The only way to rule out an idiopathic WAIHA is by observing the gradual normalization of hematological findings after the drug's discontinuation (Hoffman, 2008; Garratty, 2010).

Immune hemolysis in DIHA cases is usually mild to moderate. All suspicious drugs should be discontinued immediately, and this is usually enough to stop the hemolysis. However, steroids may be considered in severe or prolonged anemia. Blood transfusion is considered a supportive treatment, and re-exposure to the causative agent should be avoided.

Alloimmune Hemolytic Anemia

Exposure to allogeneic RBCs results in the formation of alloantibodies. These antibodies do not react against a patient's own RBCs. An example is the production of IgG alloantibodies in an Rh(-)ve mother after exposure to Rh(+)ve RBCs of her fetus. These maternal alloantibodies are capable of crossing the placenta, resulting in fetal RBC destruction and hemolytic anemia of the newborn.

Nonhemolytic Normocytic Anemia

This type of anemia is seen in patients with chronic diseases and is referred to as anemia of chronic disease (ACD). In ACD the MCV, MCH, and MCHC may be normal or decreased. So this anemia may present as normocytic normochromic anemia or microcytic hypochromic anemia (as was discussed earlier).

MACROCYTIC ANEMIAS

Macrocytic anemia is defined as anemia with a mean corpuscular volume (MCV) of greater than 100 fl. Some hematologists, however, believe that MCV greater than 96 fl should also be considered as macrocytosis (Rumsey et al., 2007). There are two types of macrocytosis, megaloblastic anemia and macrocytosis with normoblastic marrow (nonmegaloblastic anemia).

Megaloblastic Anemia

Definition. Anemia caused by impaired DNA synthesis.

ICD-10 Codes D51, D52, D53.1

Pathobiology. Megaloblastic anemias are commonly a result of vitamin B_{12} or folate deficiency. A less frequent cause is drugs that interfere with DNA metabolism. Lack of folate and vitamin B_{12} leads to deficiency of a coenzyme essential for DNA synthesis. As a result proliferating cells cannot synthesize enough DNA, which means the cells have prolonged intermitotic resting phase and block in mitosis. Meanwhile RNA and protein synthesis are relatively intact and that leads to nuclear/cytoplasmic maturation asynchrony (Hoffbrand and Provan, 1997). These cells with nuclear/cytoplasmic dissociation are called megaloblasts. In bone marrow the abundance of these gigantic cells with less mature nuclei leads to increased intramedullary cell death, resulting in anemia in the peripheral blood, an early and easily recognizable manifestation of DNA synthesis defect. Since other causes of megaloblastic anemia are extremely rare, we will focus on vitamin B_{12} and folate deficiency anemia.

Vitamin B_{12} (Cobalamin) Deficiency

ICD-10 Code D51

Cobalamin, an essential vitamin for human survival, is exclusively produced by microorganisms. Meats especially from parenchymal organs like liver are the richest sources of cobalamin. It can also be found in dairy products and egg yolk. The adult human body stores 5 mg of cobalamin, of which 2 mg is in the liver. The total body storage of vitamin B_{12} is usually enough for two to five years (Kjeldsberg and Perkins, 2010; McPherson, 2007; Snow, 1999).

Upon ingestion, gastric peptidase releases the cobalamin from food proteins. In the acidic environment of the stomach vitamin B_{12} binds to the R-binders protein secreted in saliva and gastric juice. Gastric parietal cells produce intrinsic factor. In the alkaline environment of second portion of duodenum pancreatic enzymes degrade R-binder-B12 complex, and cobalamin then bind to the intrinsic factor (IF), making a complex very resistant to digestion. There are B12-IF complex receptors on the brush border of the ileum. The complex adheres to the receptor, and within the enterocytes 30% of the released cobalamin binds to transcobalamin II, which has a receptor on the surface of the hepatocytes and the hematopoietic and other dividing cells (Figure 4.6). The remaining 70% binds to transcobalamin I and transcobalamin III and goes to the liver for storage.

Coenzyme B12 (5-deeoxy adenosyl cobalamin) and methylcobalamin are biologically active forms of cobalamin. Adenosylcobalamin mutase is coenzyme for converting methylmalonate to succinate in the mitochondria. Methylcobalamin is a coenzyme for synthesis of methionine from homocystein in the cytoplasm. This pathway is important both in the central nervous system methylation and for the incorporation of the folate into cells. Failure in this pathway is the cause of the neurological deficit in cobalamin deficiency (Reynolds, 2006; Dali-Youcef and Andrès, 2009). Cobalamin excretion occurs through bile and urine.

Cobalamin deficiency is caused either by inadequate intake of cobalamin due to vegetarianism and poverty-induced near-vegetarianism or by an increased need as in pregnancy or a decreased intrinsic factor, seen in pernicious anemia, gastrectomy, total or partial. In pernicious anemia gastric mucosa is unable to secrete the intrinsic factor because in response to the antibodies against the H/K ATPase in their membranes the parietal cells have atrophied. Antiparietal cell antibodies are found in over 90% of patients presenting pernicious anemia (Epstein et al., 1997). Cobalamin deficiency is usually seen in 2 to 10 years after total gastrectomy. Long-term use of H2 blockers or proton pump inhibitors may also cause cobalamin malabsorption. Pancreatic enzymes are essential in breaking down the R-protein cobalamin bound in the small intestine, thereby role of pancreatitis or other causes of pancreatic enzyme insufficiency in vitamin B_{12} is understandable. Other causes of vitamin B_{12} deficiency are bacterial overgrowth in the small intestine and parasites like tapeworms. Since the distalileum has the most important role in vitamin B_{12} absorption, any factor that affects this area, including its removal or a bypass of even 2 feet, can result in cobalamin deficiency. Some drugs like metformin also lower IF (Adams et al., 1983), and others like cholchicine and neomycin can impair the transepithelial transport of cobalamin and lead to vitamin B_{12} deficiency.

Folate Deficiency Anemia

ICD-10 Code D52

Folate is made by both microorganisms and plants. Foods rich in folate include green vegetables,

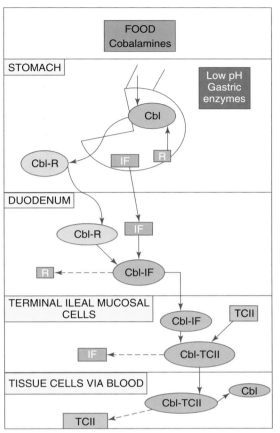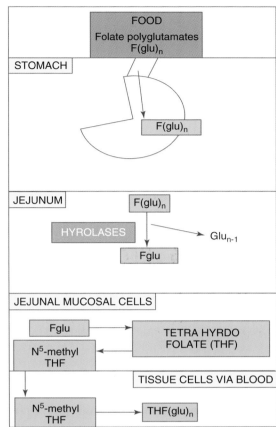

FIGURE 4.6   Cobalamine and folate absorption and transport.

fruits (banana, melon, and lemon), and animal proteins like liver and kidney. In most part of the industrial world, grains are fortified with folate. Adults need approximately 400 µg of folate daily, and the average adult body stores three months' supply of folate (Hoffman, 2008). The folate found in food is mainly in a polyglutamylated form. Conjugase enzymes deconjugate the folate to monoglutamate in the small bowel lumen; it is then absorbed in the duodenum and proximal jejunum. Folate is released into blood plasma in an unbound form as 5-methyl tetrahydro folate (5-methyl THF) which in turn is converted to tetra hydro folate (THF) through methionine synthesis. THF then passes across plasma membrane (Figure 4.6). THF is needed in purine and pyrimidine synthesis (Reynolds, 2006). The excretion of folate is through urine, sweat, saliva, and feces.

The causes of folate deficiency include decreased intake, due to poverty or excessive cooking of vegetables, and alcoholism. In humans with abrupt reduction in folate intake, anemia will appear in three to six months. Alcoholics not only do not take in enough folate-rich food, they cannot absorb folate

because alcohol blocks the enzyme responsible for degranulation of folate. The increased requirement in pregnancy and in infancy can also cause folate deficiency. Pregnancy is a common cause of folate deficiency in developing countries. Providing a folate supplement to pregnant women reduces the risk of a neural tube defect in newborns. In addition any condition associated with rapid cell division like chronic hemolytic anemia, malignancy, sickle cell anemia, and exfoliative skin disease can cause folate deficiency via the increased requirement. Folate deficiency can also occur from impaired absorption, as due to a defect in jejunal mucosa and as in tropical sprue. Celiac disease, regional enteritis, lymphoma, and surgically resected jejunum can also negatively affect folate absorption. Drugs can cause folate deficiency by either reducing absorption (anticonvulsants) or suppressing metabolic enzymes (methotrexate or other antineoplastic and antiretroviral antinucleosides like azidothymidine) (McPherson, 2007).

Clinical Features. The most common presentation of megaloblastic anemia is fatigue and malaise.

The high rate of intramedullary cell death leads to moderate increase in bilirubin and mild jaundice in these patients (Koury et al., 1997). Patients with megaloblastic anemia will experience atrophy of the tongue, GI tract, and vagina as a result of impairment in DNA synthesis. Pancytopenia with megaloblastic marrow is seen in both forms of megaloblastic anemia. Psychiatric problems (depression and flat mood) and infertility are other manifestation of folate deficiency anemia.

Defective methionine synthesis secondary to vitamin B_{12} deficiency results in patchy demyelination, especially in pernicious anemia. The process of demyelinating begins in the dorsal column of the spinal cord and then expands to the corticospinal tract and the spinocerebellar tract. Patients experience gradual numbness and tingling in extremities, decreased vibration and position senses, and ataxia in a later phase. The latest neurologic manifestation is symmetrical paralysis. Other neurologic manifestations include memory impairment and personality change.

Pernicious anemia is one cause of cobalamin deficiency, which is more common in people with northern European ancestry. Among patients 90% are more than 40 years old. When pernicious anemia presents in patients under 30 years old, it is usually associated with other autoimmune diseases like Hashimato thyroiditis and vitiligo (Epstein et al., 1997; Cecil et al., 2007; Reynolds, 2006).

These clinical manifestations never present in a folate deficiency. For a patient with folate deficiency anemia presenting with a neurologic deficit like peripheral neuropathy but without a cobalamin deficiency, para existing conditions such as alcoholism should be considered a cause.

Lab Features. CBC: Macrocytosis is one of the earliest manifestations of megaloblastic anemia. A reticulocyte count can be used to differentiate between megaloblastic and non-megaloblastic macrocytic anemias. The reticulocyte count is low in megaloblastic anemia and high in the case of a hemorrhage or hemolysis. An MCV range of 100 to 150 with normal MCHC is usually seen in megaloblastic patients. An MCV of more than 120 is highly suggestive of megaloblastic anemia, unless the patient is taking a medication that can cause macrocytosis without causing megaloblastic changes. In the presence of coexisting condition like iron deficiency anemia or thalassemia, the MCV can be normal (80–100 FL), or even lower than normal (less than 80 FL). However, in the presence of severe iron deficiency the red cell distribution (RDW) is

markedly elevated (Kjeldsberg and Perkins, 2010; McPherson, 2007; Green et al., 1982).

Blood Smear: When the initial blood cell measurements suggest macrocytic anemia, the next step is to obtain a peripheral blood smear. If there are no megaloblastic features in the peripheral smear, consider another cause of macrocytosis like alcohol, drugs, or thyroid disease. Megaloblastic features in the peripheral smear should include numerous oval macrocytes, spherocytes, and fragmented RBCs. Basophilic stippling and Howell–Jolly bodies may also be seen. Large erythrocytes are more fragile, so they are more prone to damage during their passage through the spleen. This leads to RBC fragmentation. Nucleated RBCs are seen when hematocrit drops below 20%. Hypersegmentation of mature neutrophils is another early manifestation of megaloblastic anemia. This is a result of an abnormal nuclear maturation in the granulocytes. Hypersegmentation is indicated by the presence of 5 lobes in more than 5% of neutrophils or by the presence of cells with 6 or more lobes (McPherson, 2007). Leukopenia and thrombocytopenia may also be indicated. Some patients may even have morphologic changes in blood in the absence of anemia.

The presence of the above mentioned features in the blood smear confirms the diagnosis of megaloblastic anemia, and further tests are required to differentiate folate from vitamin B_{12} deficiency. The next step is to measure the vitamin B_{12} level in serum/plasma (Bain, 2005).

Vitamin B_{12}, homocysteine, methylmalonic acid and folate levels: Because different labs use different methods to measure the cobalamin level (chemiluminescence or radioassay), there are various normal ranges. Cobalamin levels of less than 100 pg/ml are considered diagnostic in vitamin B_{12} deficiency, and no further test is necessary. Cobalamin level more than 300 pg/ml is normal, so vitamin B_{12} deficiency is unlikely. The intermediate or borderline level is between 100 and 300 pg/ml. In the borderline cases the next step is to measure the methylmalanoic acid (MMA) and homocysteine levels. A high level of methylmalonic acid in the serum, plasma, or urine confirms the diagnosis of cobalamin deficiency. The level is normal in the case of folate deficiency. This is a very sensitive and specific test. The total homocysteine level increases in both vitamin B_{12} and folate deficiency anemia. An increased homocysteine level with a normal MMA level suggests folate deficiency anemia. The homocysteine level is helpful in the diagnosis of cobalamin deficiency when the MMA level is borderline. This test is also very sensitive, but in the case of a constitutional enzyme deficiency or transport protein defects, the specificity is low. The MMA and the homocysteine levels rise before the fall in the serum vitamin B_{12} level, so they are the earliest and the most reliable indicator of vitamin B_{12} deficiency in tissue. It is worth noting that testing for the methylmalonic acid level is expensive.

When a borderline vitamin B_{12} level presents with a normal MMA and homocysteine level, consider a bone marrow biopsy evaluation.

In folate deficiency anemia patients with vitamin B_{12} levels at more than 300 pg/ml have a megaloblastic feature in their peripheral smear. In these cases measuring the RBC's folate level is the next step. The serum folate level fluctuates a lot with diet, so this is not reliable to test. It is also falsely negative in severe iron deficiency anemia, and the level is even falsely high in hemolyzed samples. The LDH level is markedly elevated in megaloblastic anemia due to intramedullary cell destruction. Mildly increased indirect bilirubin is also present as a result of both hemolysis of abnormal cells in peripheral blood and high intramedullary cell death. If the folate and vitamin B_{12} levels are both normal and yet blood works and the peripheral blood smear reveal signs of megaloblastic anemia, further evaluation by bone marrow biopsy should be considered for possible diagnosis of myelodysplastic syndrome (McPherson, 2007; Kjeldsberg and Perkins, 2010; Snow, 1999).

Bone marrow exam: A nuclear maturation defect induces intramedullary cell destruction and thus nuclear-cytoplasmic asynchrony with megaloblastic erythropoiesis. The bone marrow examination reveals hypercellularity with trilineage hyperplasia, erythroid predominance, and a reversed myeloid:erythroid ratio. Nuclear hypersegmentation of the mature granulocytes, giant bands/metamyelocytes, and large megakaryocytes are also evident in the bone marrow of patients with megaloblastic anemia (see Chapter 3, Figure 3.11A, 3.11B). Bone marrow biopsy, however, cannot differentiate folate deficiency from vitamin B_{12} deficiency anemia.

Intrinsic factor antibody: For the diagnosis of pernicious anemia, as an etiology of cobalamin deficiency, an intrinsic factor antibody test and a parietal cell antibody test are performed. The intrinsic factor antibody is present in 50 to 70% of patients with pernicious anemia (Carmel, 1992). This test is highly specific. The parietal cell antibody test is a highly sensitive (90%) test with low specificity. It is positive in 5% of the general population. These antibody tests have largely replaced the previously popular Schilling test. For the Schilling test the patient must ingest radio-labeled B_{12}, and the radio-labeled vitamin B_{12} detected in urine confirms the nutritional deficiency. Otherwise, the patient ingests radio-labeled B_{12} bound to the intrinsic factor. If the patient's urine then becomes positive for radio-labeled B_{12}, the diagnosis is an intrinsic factor deficiency or defect; if the urine still remains negative, an abnormal event in small bowl, like bacterial overgrowth or fish tapeworm, may be the cause of the vitamin B_{12} deficiency (Epstein et al., 1997; Kjeldsberg and Perkins, 2010).

Management. When anemia is severe and the etiology is not identified, it may be necessary to treat patients for both cobalamin and folate deficiencies. A therapeutic dose of folate alone should not be started because it might correct the anemia in patients with occult cobalamin deficiency and initiate or exacerbate neurological deficits. Patients should be treated with 1000 µg of parenteral cobalamin for 2 weeks daily, then once a week until the hematocrit value normalizes, and then monthly for life. Within 4 to 6 hours after the initial parenteral treatment, the marrow will show a decrease of the early erythroid precursors and the presence of more mature forms. Hypersegmented neutrophils disappear from the peripheral blood after 12 to 14 days (McPherson, 2007). Oral and parenteral cobalamin therapies have been shown to be similarly as effective (Oh and Brown, 2003; Bolaman et al., 2003). It is reasonable, and more cost-effective, to start with an injection of cobalamin and continue with the oral therapy.

In treating folate deficiency, cobalamin deficiency must be excluded, and corrected if present. Adequate absorption results from treatment with 1 to 5 mg/day oral folic acid. Treatment should be continued until complete hematologic recovery occurs, and the duration of therapy depends on the etiology (Cecil et al., 2007).

Nonmegaloblastic Macrocytic Anemia

This group includes macrocytic anemias with intact DNA synthesis. Alcoholism, hypothyroidism, reticulocytosis, chronic obstructive pulmonary disease (COPD), liver dysfunction, and splenectomy are common causes of nonmegaloblastic macrocytic anemia.

Peripheral blood in these patients shows round macrocytes or macro reticulocytes. Characteristic macro ovalocytes and hypersegmented neutrophils of megaloblastic anemias are absent. The conditions associated with liver and spleen dysfunction produce target cells with an increased red cell membrane surface area. Ethanol and its metabolites directly affect the bone marrow and suppress hematopoiesis. Reticulocytes are immature large erythrocytes and are increased in numbers in blood loss or hemolysis and can be identified in CBC as a high MCV. The macrocytosis of COPD is due to either hypoxemia-induced reticulocytosis or excess cell water. In hypothyroidism the need for oxygen results in a lower hemoglobin regulatory level a concurrent pernicious anemia and erythroid maturational arrest are other underlying mechanisms of anemia in hypothyroid patients. (Cecil et al., 2007; McPherson, 2007; Kaferle and Strzoda, 2009; Aslinia et al., 2006).

REFERENCES

Adams JF, Clark JS, Ireland JT, Kesson CM, Watson WS 1983. Malabsorption of vitamin and intrinsic factor secretion during biguanide therapy. Diabetologia 24:16–18.

Adamson JW. 2008. Iron deficiency and other hypoproliferative anemias. In:Fauci AS, Harrison TR, et al., eds., Harrison's Principles of Internal Medicine, 17th ed. McGraw-Hill, New York, ch. 98.

Agre P, Casella JF, Zinkham WH, McMillan C, Bennett V. 1985. Partial deficiency of erythrocyte spectrin in hereditary spherocytosis. Nature 314:380–3.

Alcindor T, Bridges KR. 2002. Sideroblastic anaemias. Br J Haematol 116:733–43.

Aslinia F, Mazza JJ, Yale SH. 2006. Megaloblastic anemia and other causes of macrocytosis. Clin Med Res 4:236–41.

Bader-Meunier B, Gauthier F, Archambaud F, Cynober T, Mielot F, Dommergues JP, Warszawski J, Mohandas N, Tchernia G. 2001. Long-term evaluation of the beneficial effect of subtotal splenectomy for management of hereditary spherocytosis. Blood 97:399–403.

Bain BJ. 2005. Diagnosis from the blood smear. N Eng J Med 353:498–507.

Barros MMO, Blajchman MA, Bordin JO. 2010. Warm autoimmune hemolytic anemia: recent progress in understanding the immunobiology and the treatment. Transfus Med Rev 24:195–210.

Benz EJ. 2010. Clinical manifestations and diagnosis of the thalassemias. In:Basow DS, ed., UpToDate, Waltham, MA.

Beutler E. 1994. G6PD deficiency. Blood 84:3613–36.

Bolaman Z, Kadikoylu G, Yukselen V, Yavasoglu i, Barutca S, Senturk T. 2003. Oral versus intramuscular cobalamin treatment in megaloblastic anemia: a single-center, prospective, randomized, open-label study. Clin Therapeu 25:3124–34.

Bolton-Maggs PHB, Stevens RF, Dodd NJ, Lamont G, Tittensor P, King MJ. 2004. Guidelines for the diagnosis and management of hereditary spherocytosis. Wiley-Blackwell, Hoboken, NJ.

Brodsky RA, Vala MS, Barber JP, Medof ME, Jones R J. 1997. Resistance to apoptosis caused by PIG-A gene mutations in paroxysmal nocturnal hemoglobinuria. Proc Nat Acad Sci USA 94:8756–60.

Brugnara C. 2003. Iron deficiency and erythropoiesis: new diagnostic approaches. Clin Chem 49:1573–78.

Brugnara C, Zurakowski D, Dicanzio J, Boyd T, Platt O. 1999. Reticulocyte hemoglobin content to diagnose iron deficiency in children. JAMA 281:2225–30.

Cappellini MD, Fiorelli G. 2008. Glucose-6-phosphate dehydrogenase deficiency. Lancet 371:64–74.

Carmel R. 1992. Reassessment of the relative prevalences of antibodies to gastric parietal cell and to intrinsic factor in patients with pernicious anaemia: influence of patient age and race. Clin Exper Immunol 89:74–77.

Cecil RL, Lee G, Ausiello DA. 2007. Cecil Textbook of Medicine, Saunders Elsevier, Philadelphia.

Chijiwa T, Nishiya K, Hashimoto K. 2001. Serum transferrin receptor levels in patients with rheumatoid arthritis are correlated with indicators for anaemia. Clin Rheumatol 20:307–13.

Cunningham MJ. 2010. Update on thalassemia: clinical care and complications. Hematol/Oncol Clin North Am 24:215–27.

Dali-Youcef N, Andrès E. 2009. An update on cobalamin deficiency in adults. QJM 102:17–28.

Dresbach M. 1904. Elliptical human red corpuscles. Science 19:469–70.

Epstein FH, Toh BH, Vandriel IR, Gleeson PA. 1997. Pernicious anemia. N Engl J Med 337:1441–8.

Fauci AS, Harrison TR. 2008. Principles of Internal Medicine, 17th ed. McGraw-Hill, New York.

Fleming RE, Bacon BR. 2005. Orchestration of iron homeostasis. N Engl J Med 352:1741–4.

Frank JE. 2005. Diagnosis and management of G6PD deficiency. Am Fam Physician 72:1277–82.

Gallagher PG. 2004. Hereditary elliptocytosis: spectrin and protein 4.1R. Sem Hematol 41:142–64.

GallagheR PG. 2005. Red cell membrane disorders. Hematology 2005:13–18.

Gardner DL, Roy LMH. 1961. Tissue iron and the reticuloendothelial system in rheumatoid arthritis. An Rheum Dis 20:258–64.

Garratty G. 2009. Drug-induced immune hemolytic anemia. Hematology 2009:73–79.

Garratty G. 2010. Immune hemolytic anemia associated with drug therapy. Blood Rev 24:143–50.

Gehrs BC, Friedberg RC. 2002. Autoimmune hemolytic anemia. Am J Hematol 69:258–71.

Green R, Kuhl W, Jacobson R, Johnson C, Carmel R, Beutler E. 1982. Masking of macrocytosis by α-thalassemia in blacks with pernicious anemia. N Engl J Med 307:1322–5.

Gupta N, Kavuru S, Patel D, Janson D, Driscoll N, Ahmed S, Rai KR. 2002. Rituximab-based chemotherapy for steroid-refractory autoimmune hemolytic anemia of chronic lymphocytic leukemia. Leukemia 16:2092–5.

Harrington AM, Ward PCJ, Kroft SH. 2008. Iron deficiency anemia, β-thalassemia minor, and anemia of chronic disease. Am J Clin Pathol 129:466–71.

Harteveld C, Higgs D. 2010. alpha-thalassaemia. Orphanet Journal of Rare Diseases 5:13.

Hassoun H, Palek J. 1996. Hereditary spherocytosis: a review of the clinical and molecular aspects of the disease. Blood Rev 10:129–47.

Hillmen P, Hall C, Marsh J, Elebute M, Bombara MP, Petro BE, Cullen MJ, Richards SJ, Rollins SA, Mojcik CF, Rother RP. 2004. Effect of Eculizumab on hemolysis and transfusion requirements in patients with paroxysmal nocturnal hemoglobinuria. N Engl J Med 350:552–9.

Hillmen P, Muus P, Duhrsen U, Risitano A M, Schubert J, Luzzatto L, Schrezenmeier H, Szer J, Brodsky RA, Hill A, Socie G, Bessler M, Rollins SA, Bell L, Rother RP, Young NS. 2007. Effect of the complement inhibitor eculizumab on thromboembolism in patients with paroxysmal nocturnal hemoglobinuria. Blood 110:4123–8.

Hoffbrand V, Provan D. 1997. ABC of clinical haematology: macrocytic anaemias. BMJ 314:430.

Hoffman R. 2008. Hematology basic principles and practice [online]. Churchill Livingstone/Elsevier, Philadelphia. https://www.lib.umn.edu/slog.phtml?url=http://www.mdconsult.com/das/book/94258145-2/view/1267.

Hussein M. Haddad RY. 2010. Approach to anemia. Disease-a-Month 56:449–55.

Kaferle J, Strzoda CE. 2009. Evaluation of macrocytosis. Am Fam Physician 79:203–8.

Keel SB, Abkowitz JL. 2009. The Microcytic Red Cell and the Anemia of Inflammation. N Engl J Med 361:1904–6.

Killip S, Bennett JM, Chambers MD. 2007. Iron deficiency anemia. Am Fam Physician 75:671–8.

Kjeldsberg CR, Perkins SL. 2010. Practical diagnosis of hematologic disorders. ASCP Press, Chicago.

Koury MJ, Horne DW, Brown ZA, Pietenpol JA, Blount BC, Ames BN, Hard R, Koury ST. 1997. Apoptosis of late-stage erythroblasts in megaloblastic anemia: association with DNA damage and macrocyte production. Blood 89:4617–23.

Kumar V, Robbins SL. 2009. Robbins and Cotran Pathologic Basis Of Disease. Saunders. Philadelphia.

Lawrence DP. 2008. Cold antibody autoimmune hemolytic anemias. Blood Rev 22:1–15.

Lee EJ, Oh EJ, Park YJ, Lee HK, Kim BK. 2002. Soluble Transferrin Receptor (sTfR), Ferritin, and sTfR/log ferritin index in anemic patients with nonhematologic malignancy and chronic inflammation. Clin Chem 48:1118–21.

Lipschitz DA, Cook JD, Finch CA. 1974. A clinical evaluation of serum ferritin as an index of iron stores. N Engl J Med 290:1213–16.

Madkaikar M, Gupta M, Jijina F, Ghosh K. 2009. Paroxysmal nocturnal haemoglobinuria: diagnostic tests, advantages, and limitations. Eur J Haematol 83:503–11.

Mariani M, Barcellini W, Vercellati C, Marcello AP, Fermo E, Pedotti P, Boschetti C, Zanella A. 2008. Clinical and hematologic features of 300 patients affected by hereditary spherocytosis grouped according to the type of the membrane protein defect. Haematologica 93:1310–7.

Mast AE, Blinder MA, Dietzen DJ. 2008. Reticulocyte hemoglobin content. Am J Hematol 83:307–10.

McPherson RA. 2007. Henry's Clinical Diagnosis and Management by Laboratory Methods. Saunders Elsevier, Philadelphia.

Medejel N Garçon L, Guitton C, Cynober T, Bader-Meunier B. 2008. Effect of subtotal splenectomy for management of hereditary pyropoikilocytosis. Br J Haematol 142:315–7.

Mohandas N, Gallagher PG. 2008. Red cell membrane: past, present, and future. Blood 112:3939–48.

Muncie HL Jr, Campbell J. 2009. Alpha and beta thalassemia. Am Fam Physician 80:339–44.

Nathan DG, Oski FA. 2003. Nathan and Oski's Hematology of Infancy and Childhood. Saunders. Philadelphia.

Oh R, Brown DL. 2003. Vitamin B_{12} deficiency. Am Fam Physician 67:979–86.

Parker CJ. 2009. Bone marrow failure syndromes: paroxysmal nocturnal hemoglobinuria. Hematol/Oncol Clin North Am 23:333–46.

Peghini PE, Fehr J. 2005. Clinical evaluation of an aerolysin-based screening test for paroxysmal nocturnal haemoglobinuria. Clin Cytom 67B:13–18.

Perrotta S, Gallagher PG, Mohandas N. 2008. Hereditary spherocytosis. Lancet 372:1411–26.

Phiri KS, Calis JCJ, Kachala D, Borgstein E, Waluza J, Bates I, Brabin B, Van Hensbroek MB. 2009. Improved method for assessing iron stores in the bone marrow. J Clin Pathol 62:685–9.

Punnonen K, Irjala K, Rajamaki A. 1997. Serum transferrin receptor and its ratio to serum ferritin in the diagnosis of iron deficiency. Blood 89:1052–7.

Reynolds E. 2006. Vitamin B_{12}, folic acid, and the nervous system. Lancet Neurol 5:949–60.

Richards SJ, Hill A, Hillmen P. 2007. Recent advances in the diagnosis, monitoring, and management of patients with paroxysmal nocturnal hemoglobinuria. Clin Cytom 72B:291–8.

Richards SJ, Rawstron AC, Hillmen P. 2000. Application of flow cytometry to the diagnosis of paroxysmal nocturnal hemoglobinuria. Cytometry 42:223–33.

Risitano AM, Rotoli B. 2008. Paroxysmal nocturnal hemoglobinuria: pathophysiology, natural history and treatment options in the era of biological agents. Biologics 2:205–22.

Ronquist G, Theodorsson E. 2007. Inherited, nonspherocytic haemolysis due to deficiency of glucose-6-phosphate dehydrogenase. Scand J Clin Lab Invest 67:105–11.

Rotoli B, Nafa K, Risitano AM. 2006. Paroxysmal nocturnal hemoglobinuria. In:Runge MS, Patterson C, eds., Principles of Molecular Medicine. Humana Press.

Rumsey SE, Hokin B, Magin P J,. & Pond, D. 2007. Macrocytosis—an Australian general practice perspective. Aust Fam Physician 36:571–2.

Rund D, Rachmilewitz E. 2005. β-thalassemia. N Engl J Med 353:1135–46.

Schwartz RS. 2004. Black mornings, yellow sunsets—a day with paroxysmal nocturnal hemoglobinuria. N Engl J Med 350:537–8.

Shanafelt TD, Madueme HL, Wolf RC, Tefferi A. 2003. Rituximab for immune cytopenia in adults: idiopathic thrombocytopenic purpura, autoimmune hemolytic anemia, and Evans syndrome. Mayo Clin Proc 78:1340–6.

Singh AK, Coyne DW, Shapiro W, Rizkala AR. 2007. Predictors of the response to treatment in anemic hemodialysis patients with high serum ferritin and low transferrin saturation. Kidney Int 71:1163–71.

Snow CF. 1999. Laboratory diagnosis of vitamin B_{12} and folate deficiency: a guide for the primary care physician. Arch Intern Med 159:1289–98.

Stefan E, Samuel EL. 2004. Hereditary spherocytosis—defects in proteins that connect the membrane skeleton to the lipid bilayer. Sem Hematol 41:118–41.

Sutherland DR, Kuek N, Azcona-Olivera J, Anderson T, Acton E, Barth D, Keeney M. 2009. Use of a FLAER-based WBC assay in the primary screening of PNH clones. Am J Clin Pathol 132:564–72.

Tanphaichitr VS, Suvatte V, Issaragrisil S, Mahasandana C, Veerakul G, Chongkolwatana V, Waiyawuth W, Ideguchi H. 2000. Successful bone marrow transplantation in a child with red blood cell pyruvate kinase deficiency. Bone Marrow Transpl 26:689–90.

Theurl I, Aigner E, Theurl M, Nairz M, Seifert M, Schroll A, Sonnweber T, Eberwein L, Witcher DR, Murphy AT, Wroblewski VJ, Wurz E, Datz C, Weiss G. 2009. Regulation of iron homeostasis in anemia of chronic disease and iron deficiency anemia: diagnostic and therapeutic implications. Blood 113:5277–86.

Umbreit J. 2005. Iron deficiency: a concise review. Am J Hematol 78:225–231.

Weatherall DJ, Clegg JB. 2001. Inherited haemoglobin disorders: an increasing global health problem. Bull WHO 79:704–12.

Weiss G, Goodnough LT. 2005. Anemia of chronic disease. N Engl J Med 352:1011–23.

William CM. 1973. Differentiation of iron deficiency from thalassæmia trait. Lancet 301:882.

Woolf A, Goldman R, Bellinger D. 2007. Update on the clinical management of childhood lead poisoning. Ped Clin North Am 54:271–94.

Xiuli A, Mohandas N. 2008. Disorders of red cell membrane. Br J Haematol 141:367–75.

Zanella A, Bianchi P, Fermo E. 2007. Pyruvate kinase deficiency. Haematologica 92:721–23.

Zanella A, Fermo E, Bianchi P, Valentini G. 2005. Red cell pyruvate kinase deficiency: molecular and clinical aspects. Br J Haematol 130:11–25.

Zarychanski R, Houston DS. 2008. Anemia of chronic disease: a harmful disorder or an adaptive, beneficial response? CMAJ 179:333–7.

CHAPTER FIVE

DISORDERS OF HEMOGLOBIN

Parul Bhargava

OVERVIEW

Historical Background

Hemeproteins are present in a vast array of species from plants to vertebrates. They have evolved structurally and functionally and are responsible for a wide array of functions (Hardison, 1998). The most abundant form seen in vertebrates is intra-erythrocytic hemoglobin (Hb), a metalloprotein responsible for transport of gases.

Structure

Hemoglobin is a heteroteramer, comprised of a single "heme" moiety attached to four globin chains, typically two alpha and two non–alpha (beta, delta or gamma) subunits. Neonates have a predominance of Hemoglobin F ($\alpha_2\gamma_2$) (70–90%) (Weatherall and Clegg, 1981), with the profile changing to an adult type, typically by 1 year of age. In adults, approximately 97 to 98% is HgA ($\alpha_2\beta_2$), 2 to 3% is HbA2 ($\alpha_2\delta_2$), with trace amounts of HbF.

Synthesis

Hemoglobin production in fetal, neonatal, and adult life are depicted in Figure 5.1 (Hoffbrand and Pettit, 2000).

Genetics

Genetic defects on chromosome 16 (alpha locus) or chromosome 11 (beta, delta, or gamma) may lead to either quantitative defects, namely reduced production of structurally normal hemoglobin, or qualitative defects, namely structurally abnormal hemoglobins. Some structurally abnormal hemoglobins may be synthesized at markedly reduced rates, exhibiting a combined quantitative and qualitative defect. This chapter will review abnormalities of globin structure and synthesis, their clinical manifestations and laboratory diagnosis.

QUANTITATIVE DISORDERS OF HEMOGLOBIN

Disorders of hemoglobin where one of more globin subunits are synthesized at a markedly reduced rate are broadly called thalassemias. Depending on the globin subunit affected, they may be alpha thalassemias, beta thalassemias, gamma thalassemias, delta thalassemias, or larger deletions affecting more than 1 subunits such as delta–beta, delta–beta–gamma delta–beta–gamma–epsilon thalassemias.

Alpha Thalassemia

Definition
A group of disorders resulting from defective production of alpha globin chain.

ICD-10 Code D56.0

Non-Neoplastic Hematopathology and Infections, First Edition. Edited by Hernani D. Cualing, Parul Bhargava, and Ramon L. Sandin.
© 2012 Wiley-Blackwell. Published 2012 by John Wiley & Sons, Inc.

Epidemiology

Thalassemias (Gr. "of the seas") are common in people of Africa, South Asia, the Middle East, and the Mediterranean region.

Etiology

The alpha globin cluster on chromosome 16 (Figure 5.1) consists of two functioning alpha genes, four pseudo-genes, and the embryonic ζ gene. The two functioning α genes are designated $\alpha1$ and $\alpha2$; $\alpha2$ is expressed $1.5\times$ to $3\times$ more than $\alpha1$.

Defects in alpha globin gene production arise most commonly from deletions of variable sizes on chromosome 16, or less commonly from point mutations that inactivate one or more genes. There are two general α-thalassemia haplotypes:

1. α^0, **Complete loss of α-globin production**. This is generally due to deletions of variable sizes.
   a. Deletional, involving both $\alpha1$ and $\alpha2$ genes of a cluster that are deleted in "cis"($-$), (previously called α-thalassemia 1). Examples include THAI, FIL, MED, SEA, $-(\alpha)20.5$; seen in South Asian, Middle Eastern and Mediterranean populations, but uncommon in blacks.
   b. Deletional, 40 to 33 KB upstream of $\alpha1$ and $\alpha2$, with deletion of ζ and minimal consequence sequences (MCS) and sparing of $\alpha1$ and $\alpha2$. MCS contain regulatory elements with transcription factor binding sites critical for α-globin expression.
2. α^+ **Reduced, but not eliminated α-globin production**
   a. Deletional also called α-thalassemia 2, with a $(-\alpha)$ genotype, that is, one of the 2 genes deleted in one cluster. Common deletions involved include (i) $-(\alpha)3.5$ deletion (a 3.7 kB "rightward" deletion spanning $5'$ end of $\alpha1$ and $3'$ end of $\alpha2$ resulting in a fused gene; seen worldwide) or (ii) $(-\alpha)4.2$ (a 4.2 kB "leftward" deletion with loss of $\alpha2$; seen in South Asians and Middle Eastern populations; uncommon in Mediterranean and black populations).
   b. Nondeletional ($\alpha^T\alpha$), generally sporadic with nearly 70 types reported. One of the most frequent is a point mutation in the stop codon of the $\alpha2$ gene resulting in an unusually long α-chain (by 31 amino acids) that is transcribed at a much slower rate than normal, that is, Hb Constant Spring (Hb CS).

Alpha-thalassemia retardation-16 (ATR-16) is a rare syndrome arising from a large deletion from 16p13.3 to the terminus (or subterminus) resulting in deletion of $\alpha1$, $\alpha2$, and contiguous genes. Patients have distinctive facies with variable microcephaly, short stature, low IQ, club foot deformity, and alpha thalassemia (Lindor et al., 1997).

Rarely mutations in Xq13.3 region, through effects on transcriptional regulation, can lead to a syndromic X-linked α-thalassemia and mental retardation syndrome (ATR-X) (Gibbons et al., 1995). Additionally rare cases of acquired α-thalassemia, without mental retardation, have been described associated with myelodysplastic syndromes that are mostly due to acquired somatic mutations in Xp13 region, and occasionally deletions in chromosome 16p.

Pathophysiology

Defects in α-globin production result in an unbalanced excess of β-globin chains. Excess β-chains polymerize to form unstable HbH ($\beta4$ tetramers), which precipitate in aging RBCs. These RBCs, being poorly deformable, are trapped and destroyed in the spleen resulting in a shortened RBC lifespan. Varying degrees of anemia, compensatory erythroid hyperplasia, and increased RBC counts ensue.

Clinical Features

These are dependent on the number of genes deleted.

1. **1-gene deleted** (heterozygous α-thal 2 $\alpha\alpha/-\alpha$): clinically and hematologically silent.
2. **2-genes deleted** (heterozygous α-thal 1 $-/\alpha\alpha$, or homozygous α-thal 2 $-\alpha/-\alpha$) mild asymptomatic microcytic anemia.
3. **3-genes deleted** (compound heterozygosity for α-thal 1 with either α-thal-2, i.e., $-/-\alpha$, or with nondeletional/abnormal α-thal mutations, i.e., $-/\alpha^T\alpha$ or $-/\alpha^{CS}\alpha$): the clinical picture is variable.

   A majority, especially the deletional types, have a mild course with compensated chronic hemolytic anemia, with Hb levels around 9 mg/dL. However, they may develop hemolytic crises during infections or febrile states leading to renal failure and even shock. The nondeletional subtypes tend to have a more severe presentation, with higher rates of growth retardation, need for transfusions, organomegaly, and gallstones.
4. **4-genes deleted** (homozygosity for α-thal 1 or $-/-$): incompatible with life due to requirement of α-globins to make HbF, that is, $\alpha_2\gamma_2$, which constitutes a majority of neonatal Hb. Leads to still birth with marked hypochromic anemia, anasarca, circulating erythroblasts, and Hb Bart's

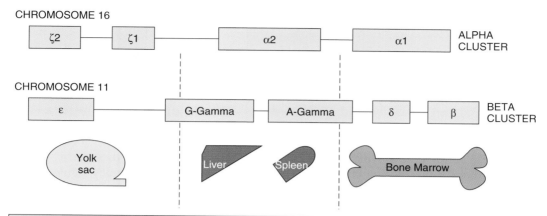

First trimester			2ⁿᵈ, 3ʳᵈ trimester and infancy	Adult	
ζ2ε2	ζ2γ2	α2ε2	α2γ2	α2δ2	α2β2
Gower 1	Portland	Gower 2	Hb F	Hb A2	Hb A
			Predominant type at birth, declines rapidly	2–3%	96–97%

FIGURE 5.1 **Hemoglobin synthesis**. Shown is a simplified version of the alpha globin cluster on chromosome 16, and the beta globin cluster on chromosome 11. The predominant site of hemoglobin synthesis is also depicted. Hb is synthesized largely in the yolk sac up to about 10 weeks of intrauterine life, liver and spleen through the rest of intrauterine life, followed by bone marrow. The table below depicts the major hemoglobin moieties at various stages of development and their relative proportions.

(γ_4), that is, Bart's hydrops fetalis or erythroblastosis fetalis.

Lab Diagnosis

CBC: The RBC indices are normal in single gene deletions. A chronic mild microcytic anemia is seen in patients with the α-thalassemia trait (2-gene deletion), with preserved-to-elevated RBC counts. The average Hb is 13.9 +/− 1.7 g/dl (in males), and 12.0 +/− 1.0 g/dl (females) with a MCV of 72 +/− 4 fl (Galanello and Cao, 2008). RDW is not elevated. Patients with 3-gene deletions have a microcytic anemia with an average Hb of 9 to 10 g/dl and MCV of 61 fl, while those with 4-gene deletions have severe anemia (Hb 3–8 g/dL) with marked reticulocytosis (may be > 60%) and circulating erythroblasts.

Peripheral smear review: A peripheral blood smear is normal in single gene deletion. The α-thalassemia trait (2-gene deletion) shows mild anemia, with a microcytic hypochromic picture. Few targets and teardrop cells are often noted (Figure 5.2). HbH disease shows a moderate anemia, with microcytosis, hypochromasia, and targets. Bart's hydrops fetalis shows marked anemia, with large hypochromic cells, severe anisopoikilocytosis, polychromasia, and nucleated RBCs.

Hb Electrophoresis: No abnormality is seen in single gene deletion. In the deletional α-thalassemia trait, no abnormal band is noted on electrophoresis. The relative proportions of the various Hb moieties (A, A2, F) are also unaltered, since α-chains are

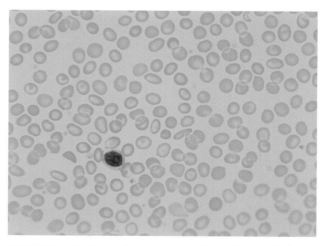

FIGURE 5.2 **Peripheral smear findings in alpha thalassemia (Wright–Giemsa stain, 60×)**. The photomicrograph shows microcytic hypochromic RBCs with targets and rare teardrops.

a component of all these moieties (i.e., HbA $\alpha_2\beta_2$, HbA$_2$ $\alpha_2\delta_2$, HbF $\alpha_2\gamma_2$). However, if the testing is performed at birth, a small proportion of Hb Bart (γ_4) may be detected. In the case of HbCS, a slow moving band (relative proportion 2–3%) is seen cathodal to HbA$_2$ (Figure 5.3A). Three gene deletion, that is, HbH disease (−/-α), can generally be diagnosed through the detection of a fast-moving HbH band (5–40%). Since the clinical presentation may be mild, and H is unstable, careful assessment of alkaline gel for a minor fast band, and/or manual review of HPLC fractions may be needed. Hb Bart's, that is, γ_4 tetramers (20–40%), can be seen at birth. In double heterozygosity for α-thalassemia with Constant

Spring (Hb H Constant Spring, i.e., −/$\alpha^{CS}\alpha$), Hb Bart's (γ_4), Hb H (β_4), and Constant Spring are noted as depicted in Figure 5.3B. In 4-gene deletion, a majority (85–90%) of hemoglobin noted is the fast-moving Hb Bart's (γ_4), with a minor proportion of HbH (β_4) and Hb Portland ($\zeta_2\gamma_2$).

H-body preparation: This is a supravital stain using brilliant cresyl blue. H-inclusions are multiple, fine intra-erythrocytic inclusions in a "golf-ball" like distribution. Rare H-bodies can be seen in 1- or 2-gene deletion alpha thalassemias, while several, involving 5 to 80% of RBCs are noted in HbH disease (Galanello and Cao, 2008; Pan et al., 2005; Skogerboe et al., 1992).

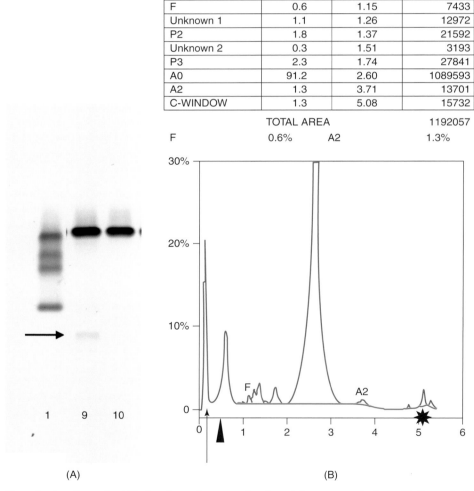

F	0.6	1.15	7433
Unknown 1	1.1	1.26	12972
P2	1.8	1.37	21592
Unknown 2	0.3	1.51	3193
P3	2.3	1.74	27841
A0	91.2	2.60	1089593
A2	1.3	3.71	13701
C-WINDOW	1.3	5.08	15732

TOTAL AREA 1192057

F 0.6% A2 1.3%

(A)   (B)

FIGURE 5.3 **Alkaline electrophoresis.** (A) A minor slow moving band (see arrow in lane 9). Lane 1 shows the standard (from top to bottom: A, F, S, C), and lane 10 is of a normal patient with a dominant band in A position. This adult patient had thalassemic indices and was of Southeast Asian descent; a presumptive diagnosis of Hb Constant Spring was made. (B) HPLC results in a 10-year-old patient with Hb H Constant Spring (i.e., −/$\alpha^{CS}\alpha$). The long arrow marks Hb Bart's (γ_4), the arrow head marks the Hb H (β_4) peak, and the star marks Hb Constant Spring elution peaks. (HPLC image courtesy Dr. J. Ford, Children's Hospital, Vancouver)

Molecular studies: See the section below.

Approach to Diagnosis

Single-gene deletion is silent, both clinically and in laboratory findings. It is generally suspected based on family history, and in the context of antenatal diagnosis/genetic counseling, molecular techniques are necessary for diagnosis. Two gene deletions, namely the α-thalassemia trait, is generally suspected on the basis of unexplained, longstanding microcytic anemia. Being electrophoretically silent, a presumptive diagnosis is typically made in patients with microcytic anemia, without iron deficiency or elevated A2 (see beta thalassemia lab diagnosis) (see Figure 5.4). The presence of Hb Bart at birth, or rare H-bodies, is helpful in making a diagnosis. A molecular diagnosis is employed in situations requiring a more definitive assessment, (e.g., in antenatal workups). HbH disease is diagnosed on the basis of HbH on electrophoresis/HPLC or H-bodies on supravital staining. Decreased HbA_2 levels and elevated ferritin levels support the diagnosis. Hb Bart's hydrops fetalis has characteristic smear findings (see above) and Hb Bart's on electrophoresis.

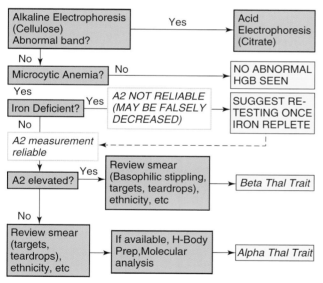

FIGURE 5.4 **Approach to diagnosis of the α-thalassemia trait.** Diagnosis of α-thalassemia is by exclusion as it is electrophoretically silent (i.e., no abnormal bands) and with unaltered relative proportions of adult hemoglobin moieties (i.e., relative proportions of A, A2 and F are generally normal). A patient with thalassemic indices, without an alternative explanation (i.e., iron studies, and/or elevation in A2 indicative of β-thalassemia trait), is presumed to have the α-thalassemia trait. Definitive diagnosis, if necessary, requires molecular testing.

Beta Thalassemia

Definition

A group of disorders results from the defective production of the beta globin chain.

ICD-10 Code D56.1

Epidemiology

Thalassemias (Gr. "of the seas") are common in the Mediterranean region, as well as in Southeast Asia, the Indian subcontinent, and the Middle East.

Etiology

Unlike α-thalassemias that are predominantly due to deletions, β-thalassemias result from point mutations in or near the β-gene cluster on chromosome 11. The β-gene cluster consists of the β gene, δ-gene, γ-gene, a pseudo β-gene, and the fetal ε-gene (Figure 5.1). Nearly 200 mutations have been characterized that may lead to nonsense codons, frameshifts, defective splicing, and so on. Mutations that lead to a complete absence of (beta) globin production are designated β^0, while those that lead to decreased, but not absent β-globin production, are designated β^+. A majority are inherited in an autosomal recessive fashion. A rare autosomal dominant form (with mutations in the third exon) is described that leads to thalassemia intermedia with moderately severe anemia, even in the heterozygous state.

Pathogenesis

Defects in β-globin production lead to a relative excess of α-chains. Alpha chain tetramers (called Fessas bodies) (Fessas, 1963) are insoluble and precipitate early in erythropoiesis, leading to intramedullary destruction. In contrast to α-thalassemia, ineffective erythropoiesis, in addition to the shortened RBC life span due to hemolysis, is a major cause of anemia.

Clinical Features

β-thalassemia minor or trait (β^0/β or β^+/β): Usually the anemia is clinically asymptomatic.

β-thalassemia intermedia (β^+/β^+ or rarely dominant β^+ or β^+/β with ααα/αα): This is an anemia of intermediate severity. Although compatible with normal growth and development, patients develop erythroid hyperplasia with bony deformities, extramedullary hematopoiesis with hepatosplenomegaly, ineffective hematopoiesis with iron overload, and ankle ulcers as a result of anemia.

β-thalassemia major or "Cooley's" anemia (β^0/β^0): Ineffective erythropoiesis causes severe anemia that is transfusion dependent, and fatal if untreated. In patients not adequately supported by transfusions, the marked erythroid hyperplasia leads to bony deformities including an expansion of the flat bones of the skull with the characteristic "hair-on-end" appearance on skull radiographs, frontal bossing, maxillary prominence, and widening of the nasal bridge. Extramedullary hematopoeisis leads to organomegaly. Premature epiphyseal closure, osteoporosis, and fractures may ensue. Despite transfusions and chelation therapy, features of iron toxicity such as diabetes mellitus and hypopituitarism may occur.

Lab Diagnosis

CBC: The β-thalassemia trait is characterized by a mild microcytic anemia, with a low MCV (<79 fl) and preserved-to-elevated RBC counts. RDW is generally not elevated. β-thalassemia major has marked anemia (Hb < 7 g/dL), with low MCV (50–70 fl) and MCH (12–20 pg) (Cao and Galanello, 2010).

Peripheral smear review: The β-thalassemia trait shows a mild anemia, with a microcytic hypochromic picture. Few targets, teardrop cells, and coarse basophilic stippling are often noted (Figure 5.5). Beta-thalassemia major or intermedia shows marked anemia, hypocromasia, polychromasia, and nucleated RBCs. Anisopoikilocytosis, with targets, elliptocytes, fragments, Howell–Jolly bodies, and coarse basophilic stippling are noted.

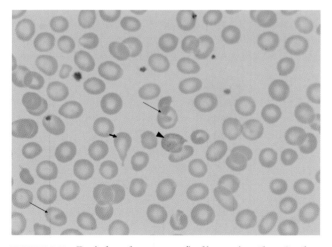

FIGURE 5.5 **Peripheral smear findings in the β thalassemia trait (Wright–Giemsa, 100×).** RBCs are microcytic hypochromic, with targets (long arrows), teardrops (short arrows), and coarse basophilic stippling (arrow head).

Hb Electrophoresis: In the β-thalassemia trait, the relative excess of α-chains combine with δ-chains, leading to an elevation in HbA_2 (typically twice normal; relative proportion 4–6%). In the β-thalassemia major, given the marked deficiency of β-chains, and inherent low transcription rate of δ-chains, the excess α-chains combine with γ leading to markedly increased HbF levels (20–40% in intermedia, 60–98% in major). HbA_2 may or may not be elevated.

Molecular diagnosis (see the section below).

Delta Thalassemia

Definition

The disorder results from defective production of the delta globin chain.

ICD-10 Code D56.8 (other thalassemia)

Epidemiology

Defective δ-globin production is described primarily in Mediterranean (Italian, Greek, Egyptian, Belgian, Sardinian) as well as in Black and Japanese patients.

Etiology

Several mutations have been described that lead to a complete absence (δ^0) or marked reduction (δ^+) in the production of δ chains.

Clinical Features

Since HbA_2 only constitutes approximately 2 to 3% of hemoglobin, defects in δ-globin production have no clinical consequences. The clinical significance of the delta globin defects lies in cases with associated β-thalassemia; in such cases the characteristic elevation of HbA_2 that is used to diagnose the β-thalassemia trait is not seen, and thus a β-thalassemia with associated delta variants may be misdiagnosed as an α-thalassemia trait.

Lab Diagnosis

The CBC parameters and peripheral smear will be normal. It may be incidentally seen on Hb electrophoresis or HPLC as decreased or absent HbA_2. Acquired deficiencies in HbA_2 may also be seen in iron deficiency anemia. A relatively frequent mutation involving δ-globin is HbA', which is seen in 1 to 2% of the black population. It is due to a mutation in the δ-gene leading to a glycine to arginine substitution in the 16th position of the δ-chain. A slow moving faint band is seen on Hb electrophoresis.

Gamma Thalassemia

Definition

The disorder results from defective production of the gamma globin chain.

ICD-10 Code D56.8

Epidemiology

The defective γ-globin production is seen in a minor proportion of infants from Japan, China, India, Europe, and Africa.

Etiology

There are 2 γ-genes on chromosome 11, γG and γA. Unequal crossover, with deletion of the 3′ end of γG and the 5′ end of γA, and a hybrid γGγA-gene formation have been described.

Clinical Features and Lab Diagnosis

Anemia is usually harmless and difficult to detect in adults. It can be detected in newborns due to skewed ratios of γG and γA. Normally this ratio is 7:3 in newborns, changing to 4:6 by three to four months of age. In infants carrying this mutation, a 4:6 ratio was noted at birth (Sukumaran et al., 1983).

Delta-Beta Thalassemias

Definition

The group of disorders results from the defective production of both delta and beta globin chains.

ICD-10 Code D56.2

Epidemiology

The δ-β-thalassemias are common in the Mediterranean region (Sicilian type); other types have been described worldwide. Hb Lepore is most often seen in the Mediterranean region (Spain, Italy, Balkan Peninsula) but is also seen worldwide. Delta-beta-gamma, and delta-beta-gamma-epsilon types are rare, with only a few families described.

Etiology

The deletion of varying sizes involves both delta and beta genes, and less frequently delta-beta-gamma, and delta-beta-gamma-epsilon regions. Delta-beta thalassemias can be divided into four subgroups.

1. Delta-beta thalassemia with deletion spanning delta and beta locus, and sparing of gamma loci [^{G}gamma^{A}gamma(deltabeta)$^\circ$]: The commonest type (Sicilian type) is a −13.4 kB deletion.

2. Hb Lepore: Unequal crossover between delta and beta genes leads to a fusion of delta-beta genes.

3. Delta-beta-gamma thalassemia with a large deletion spanning delta-beta and gamma regions [^{G}gamma(^{A}gammadeltabeta)$^\circ$].

4. Epsilon-gamma-delta-beta thalassemia [(epsilon-gammadeltabeta)$^\circ$].

Pathogenesis

The net effect of all the deletions is a marked underproduction of the beta chains. While A2 production is hampered (due to the involved delta gene), HbF is generally high. Nonetheless, HbF cannot compensate for the loss of the beta allele, leading to an excess of alpha chains, and thus features of beta thalassemia ensue.

Clinical Features and Lab Diagnosis

1. Delta-beta thalassemia [^{G}gamma^{A}gamma(deltabeta)$^\circ$]: Anemia is mild, with a Hb of 10 to 12 g/dl. RBCs are microcytic (MCV 60–65 fl) and hypochromic (MCH 18–24 pg) (Huisman et al., 1996). HbA$_2$ is low, or normal due to the up-regulation of the remaining intact *trans* delta allele. HbF is elevated (5–15%). Homozygous patients have features of thalassemia intermedia with Hb of 8 to 10 g/dL, and 10% HbF. The double heterozygosity for β-thalassemia with δ-β-thalassemia leads to thalassemia major.

2. Hb Lepore: The heterozygotes are mildly anemic (Hb 11–13 g/dl) with thalassemic indices, hypochromasia, and microcytosis (MCV 70–75 fl). An abnormal delta-beta fusion protein band (10–15% of total) is detected on alkaline electrophoresis at position S (Figure 5.6); this co-migrates with A on acid electrophoresis. HbA$_2$ (from the remaining intact delta locus) is generally low normal (2–2.5%). Homozygotes have features of thalassemia major with 80% HbF, 10 to 20% Hb Lepore, and absent HbA and A$_2$. The compound heterozygosity for Lepore with E also leads to a severe transfusion-dependent anemia.

3. Delta-beta-gamma thalassemia [^{G}gamma (^{A}gammadeltabeta)$^\circ$]: The presentation is similar to delta-beta thalassemia, with a mild microcytic hypochromoic anemia in heterozygotes and thalassemia intermedia in homozygotes.

4. Epsilon-gamma-delta-beta thalassemia [(epsilon-gammadeltabeta)$^\circ$]: Heterozygous infants are severely affected, with anemia requiring transfusions. They gradually improve with age, and by 3 to 6 months have mild microcytic hypochromic anemia with low HbF (1–3%) and low normal A2.

Peak Name	Calibrated Area %	Area %	Retention Time (min)	Peak Area
P1	− − −	0.1	0.71	1149
F	15.5*	− − −	1.09	301657
P2	− − −	4.3	1.31	89276
P3	− − −	3.6	1.69	73604
Unknown	− − −	0.2	2.08	3256
A0	− − −	67.5	2.40	1393803
A2	9.5*	− − −	2.43	203345

Total Area: 2,066,090

F Concentration = 15.5* %

A2 Concentration = 9.5* %

*Values outside of expected ranges

Analysis comments:

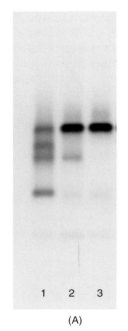

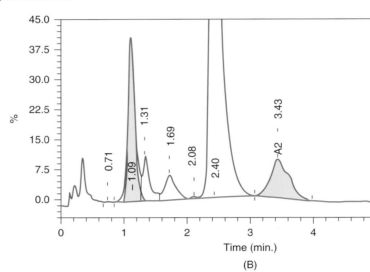

(A)　　　　　　　　　　　　　　(B)

FIGURE 5.6 **Alkaline electrophoresis gel**. (**A**) Lane 1 shows the standard with bands (from top to bottom) A, F, S, C. Lane 2 shows a dominant band in the A-position (83%), and a minor band in the S-position (15%) with 2% Hb A2 (measured separately). The sickledex was negative, and the abnormal Hb migrated to the A-position on the acid (citrate) gel (not shown). The patient had thalassemic indices, which together with the migration pattern and relative proportion of Hb variant is in keeping with a diagnosis of Hb Lepore trait. Lane 3 shows a normal patient with a dominant A band. (**B**) HPLC tracing from a 9-month-old child with Hb Lepore (courtesy Dr. J. Ford, Children's Hospital, Vancouver); Hb Lepore co-elutes with HbA2 on HPLC. HbF level (15.5%) appears mildly higher than expected for a 9-month-old; however, F levels vary widely in first few months of life.

Hereditary Persistence of Fetal Hemoglobin

Definition

A group of disorders leads to persistently elevated levels of HbF in adults.

ICD-10 Code D56.4

Epidemiology

Common deletional types have been described in blacks, Indians, and Southeast Asian families. Others have been described worldwide, with the Swiss-type more prevalent in people of Swiss decent.

Etiology

These can be due to large (∼105–106 kB) deletions spanning β and δ loci (deletional type) or alternatively due to a variety of mutations in the promoter region of one of the gamma loci (nondeletional type). A third type, the so-called Swiss-type, does not involve mutations in the promoter region but may be due to a variety of causes including mutations in trans acting genes (e.g., chromosome 6q, Xp22.2), gene duplications/rearrangements, and mutations that may affect the binding of transcription factors.

Clinical Features
Most cases are asymptomatic.

Lab Diagnosis
CBC and peripheral smear: These are generally unremarkable.

Hb electrophoresis and HPLC: An increased percentage of HbF is demonstrated in adults. The exact quantity varies, depending on the mutation, being the lowest in Swiss (1–5%) and other nondeletional types (1–20%), and highest in deletional types (15–30%). The homozygotes for the deletional types generally have 100% HbF.

Kleihauer–Betke acid elution test: This test was traditionally used to determine the pattern of distribution of HbF, whether pancellular (all RBCs have a similarly increased HbF) or heterocellular (some RBCs have very high HbF, others do not). While deletional forms generally have a pancellular distribution, nondeletional forms may have a pan or a heterocellular distribution (Figure 5.7). Flow cytometric assessment of F-cells is increasingly being used to assess this; while pancellular types will demonstrate a single peak with a fluorescent intensity intermediate to that of A and of F, heterocellular conditions demonstrate two peaks corresponding to A and F, respectively.

Figure 5.7 Kleihauer-Betke acid elution test. A heterocellular distribution is depicted; F-containing RBCs stain pink, while others are unstained 'ghost' cells.

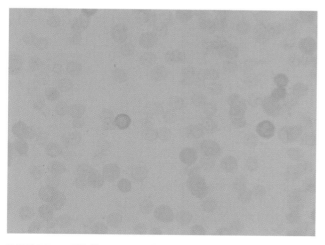

FIGURE 5.7 **Kleihauer–Betke acid elution test**. A heterocellular distribution is depicted; F-containing RBCs stain pink, and others are unstained "ghost" cells.

QUALITATIVE DISORDERS OF HEMOGLOBIN

Mutations in the globin chains that lead to an amino acid substitution and thus to structurally defective hemoglobin are broadly classified under hemoglobinopathies. These structural abnormalities lead may lead to defects in hemoglobin solubility, oxygen binding, stability, and so on (see Table 5.1). These mutants are generally named as uppercase alphabets, or after cities/regions. Although more than 800 variants of alpha and beta globins have been described, some of the clinically significant commonly encountered variants i.e. S, C, E, D and are described below.

Hemoglobin S

Definition
Hemoglobin S is a beta globin chain mutant (Glu → Val at the 6th position of the β-chain) that is insoluble and prone to crystallizing at low oxygen tension.

ICD-10 Codes Sickle cell anemia (HbSS) with crisis D57.0; Sickle cell anemia without crises D57.1; Double heterozygosity of sickle with other disorders D57.2; Sickle cell trait D57.3.

Epidemiology
The highest frequency of S mutation is seen in sub-Saharan Africa, particularly in the central (Gabon, Zaire) and western (Ghana, Nigeria) regions where the gene frequency is reportedly 0.16% (Hoyer and Kroft, 2003). Other high-frequency regions include east central India and northeastern regions of Saudi Arabia and Kuwait, with a gene frequency of 0.1%. Overall, the distribution of this mutation is said to be linked to the distribution of malaria (Piel et al., 2010) because of the protective effect of S mutation on malaria infection.

Etiology
A point mutation in the 17th nucleotide in the beta globin gene leads to a single base pair substitution (GAG → GTG) in the 6th codon, with a resultant substitution of glutamic acid to valine. This substitution creates a hydrophobic tetramer that is prone to polymerization in patients who are homozygous for $β^S$ (i.e., sickle cell anemia) or double heterozygous for $β^S$ with other sickling variants (i.e., sickle cell disease) (Rees et al., 2010). With repeated cycles of deoxygenation, these polymers grow to form elongated crystals. Sickling increases membrane permeability

TABLE 5.1 Examples of Functional Abnormalities and Clinical Effects Seen with Some Hemoglobinopathies

Hemoglobinopathy	Functional Defect	Effect	Clinical Effect
S or C	Low solubility	Hb aggregation	Hemolytic anemia
Unstable hemoglobins	Oxidative susceptibility	Oxidative denaturation	Heinz body hemolytic anemia
High-affinity Hbs (Hb Rahere, Ty Gard, Ypsilante, etc.)	↑ O_2 affinity	↓ O_2 release	Erythrocytosis. +/− cyanosis
Hb Denver	↓ O_2 affinity	Premature O_2 release	Cyanosis/anemia
Hg M (methHg)	Abnormal heme reduction	Inability to carry O_2	Cyanosis
Hb Lepore, Hb Quong-Sze	Variable	↓ Production	Thalassemia

with a loss of intracellular potassium, cellular dehydration, and formation of dense cells. With repeated cycles of sickling, irreversibly sickled cells (ISC) are formed (Brugnara, 2003). Dense cells and ISC occlude small vasculature. Patients have resultant vasocclusive damage, as well as ischemia-reperfusion injuries to several organs and chronic hemolytic anemia.

Clinical Features

Patients heterozygous for β^S (i.e., those with sickle cell trait) are clinically asymptomatic. Patients with sickle cell anemia have features of multi-organ damage, including brain (cognitive impairment in children, infarcts), kidney (papillary necrosis), lung (chest syndrome), bones (dactylitis, pain crisis, deformities including "hand–foot" syndrome), cardiovascular system, and spleen (hyposplenism) (Hoffbrand and Pettit, 2000). They present a chronic hemolytic anemia with associated complications (gall stones, leg ulcers, priapism, etc.) including vasculopathy (pulmonary hypertension) (Rees et al., 2010). Patients have an increased susceptibility to infections, which in children, is the most common cause of death (Platt, 2003). Infection with the Parvovirus can lead to aplastic crises due to poor marrow reserve. SD (predominant in North India) is clinically similar to SS. SO_{ARAB} (rare; reported in North Africa, the Middle East, and the Balkans) have a relatively severe disorder with vasocclusion and chronic hemolysis. SC disease patients typically have mild chronic hemolytic anemia (Hb 10–13 g/dl) but with variable severity of the vasocclusive disease. $S\beta^0$ is comparable to SS (with splenomegaly and low MCV), whereas $S\beta^+$ is milder. Thus sickling disorders in order of severity are SS, $S\beta^0$, SD, $SO_{ARAB} > SC$, $S\beta^0 > SE$.

Lab Diagnosis

Sickle cell trait: the CBC and peripheral blood smear are normal. Hb electrophoresis and HPLC in adults show one A band ($\sim$60%) and one S band ($\sim$40%) (Figure 5.8A). Sickle solubility assay is generally positive in adults but may be negative in newborns, due to predominance of HbF. However, newborn screening by HPLC will demonstrate a "FAS" pattern in babies with S-trait (Figure 5.8B).

Sickle cell anemia: CBC: Anemia develops after the first few months of life (once HbF declines). The typical findings are Hb 7 to 11 g/dL (Platt, 2003), with a normal MCV but a wide RDW. Reticulocytes are generally increased. Peripheral smear shows presence of sickle cells, targets, fragments, spherocytes, hypochromasia and features of hyposplenism (Howell-Jolly-bodies, nucleated RBCs etc) (Figure 5.9A). HPLC or Hb electrophoresis shows a major S-band ($\sim$80–99%), with a variably elevated HbF (2-20%), normal HbA_2 and absent HbA (Figure 5.9B).

Sickle cell disease with compound heterozygosity for S with other hemoglobinopathies: $S\beta$-thal shows a decreased MCV. On HPLC/Hb electrophoresis, $S\beta^0$ have a pattern similar to SS with mostly S, variable HbF and no HbA. $S\beta^+$ has a low proportion of HbA ($\sim$10%), with a predominance of HbS. SC disease has milder anemia (Hb 10–13 g/dL), with increased targets, and irregularly shaped cells (SC poikilocytes, "envelop" or "boat" cells); fewer sickle cells may be noted (Figure 5.10A). HPLC/Hb electrophoresis shows an equal proportion of S and C bands (50% each) (Figure 5.10B, C). SO_{ARAB} or SD-Punjab migrate with the C band on alkaline electrophoresis but can be distinguished on acid electrophoresis. SE demonstrates a mild microcytic anemia with a 65:35 ratio of HbS:HbE on Hb electrophoresis.

Hemoglobin C

Definition

Hemoglobin C is a beta globin mutant caused by a Glu $\rightarrow$ Lys substitution at the 6th position.

ICD-10 Code D58.2

Epidemiology

C mutation is found mostly in people of Western African descent. The HbC trait is found in 25%

people from Ghana, and about 2 to 3% of African Americans (Hoyer and Kroft, 2003). HbC is the 2nd most frequent variant seen in the United States and the 3rd most common worldwide (Bunn and Forget, 1986).

Etiopathogenesis

HbC is less soluble than HbA, and in homozygous individuals, intra-erythrocytic CC crystals are formed. More important, through interactions with cell membranes HbC leads to potassium efflux and red cell dehydration. The increased cell density (high MCHC) together with inclusions leads to poor deformability and reduction in the RBC lifespan (Bunn and Forget, 1986).

Clinical Features

The HbC trait is generally clinically asymptomatic, and patients have a normal RBC lifespan. HbC disease is also clinically mild, with symptoms related to mild to moderate chronic hemolytic anemia. There is generally some splenomegaly noted.

Lab Diagnosis

HbC trait: Patients are generally not anemic; however MCV is low normal or low. Review of peripheral smear shows numerous targets, though crystals are not seen. HPLC/Hb electrophoresis shows a C band (35–40%), along with A band (Figure 5.11A, B, C), both on alkaline and acid agar.

HbC disease: CBC shows a mild to moderate anemia (Hb ~12 g/dL) with a low MCV (~72 fl) (Bunn and Forget, 1986). Peripheral smear review (Figure 5.12) shows numerous targets, microspherocytes and occasional crystals. The latter are rod-like, or polyhedral (sometimes referred to as "Washington monument" shaped) dense eosinophilic bodies present intracellularly in RBCs as well as extracellularly. HPLC/Hb electrophoresis show a dominant C band with absent A band. HbF is generally 0 to 3%, while HbA_2 is difficult to assess on electrophoresis due to co-migration with C. In double heterozygosity

Fractions	%	Ref. %
Hb A	57.7	
HB S	39.1	
Hb A2	3.2	

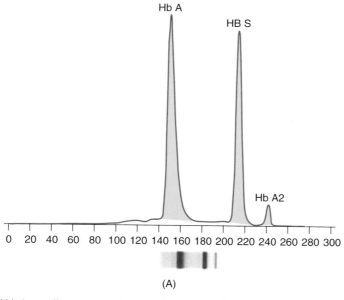

(A)

FIGURE 5.8   **Sickle cell trait**. (**A**) A capillary electrophoresis histogram depicting 57.7% HbA, 39.1% Hb S, and 3.2% HbA2 in an adult patient with the S-trait. (**B**) A neonatal screen performed by HPLC depicted an "FAS" pattern with a dominant F peak and smaller amounts of the A and S diagnostic of the S-trait. (HPLC image courtesy Dr. J. Ford, Children's Hospital, Vancouver)

Peak	Peak Name	Retention Time (min)	Height	Area	Area %
1	FAST	0.118	58034	170125	10.3
2	Unknown	0.306	1626	15346	0.9
3	F1	0.389	3931	20836	1.3
4	F	0.602	499138	1217655	74.0
5	OTHER (1)	0.730	6964	10739	0.7
6	A	0.811	47434	114480	7.0
7	S	1.155	26290	97117	5.9

Pattern: FAS
Total Area: 1646298

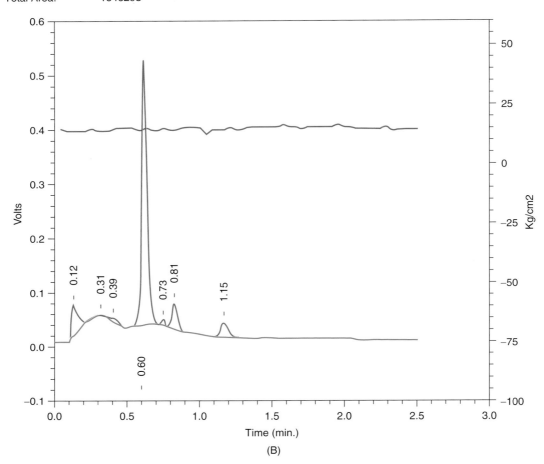

(B)

FIGURE 5.8 *(Continued)*

for $C\beta^0$ thalassemia, the MCV is lower (55–70 fl), with higher F levels (> 5%) (Hoyer and Kroft, 2003).

Hemoglobin E

Definition

Hemoglobin E is a beta globin mutant resulting from the substitution of Glu → Lys at the 26th codon (Hunt and Ingram, 1961).

ICD-10 Code D58.2

Epidemiology

Seen in the Far East and Southeast Asia, the prevalence of Hemoglobin E is estimated to be 13% in Thailand (50% in northeast Thailand) (Sanchaisuriya et al., 2003), 25% in certain tribes of northeast India (Hoyer and Kroft, 2003), and 4% in Cambodia. This is the second most prevalent hemoglobinopathy worldwide (Bunn and Forget, 1996).

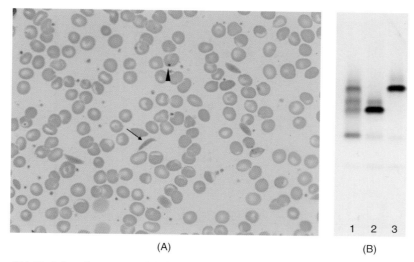

(A) (B)

FIGURE 5.9 **SS-disease.** (A) Peripheral smear in SS disease (Wright-Giemsa stain, 100×) showing targets and sickle cells (arrows). Howell–Jolly bodies (arrow head) suggestive of hyposplenism are also noted. (B) Alkaline electrophoresis gel showing AFSC standard (lane 1), patient with S-disease with a dominant band in the S region (lane 2) and a minor band in the F-position; the absence of HbA is in keeping with SS disease (confirmed by acid electrophoresis). Lane 3 depicts a normal patient with a dominant band in A position.

Etiopathogenesis

The amino acid substitution of lysine for glutamic acid at codon 26 creates a "cryptic" splicing site on exon 1 (Traeger et al., 1980). Alternative splicing at this position leads to nonfunctional mRNA, and thus reduced β-globin production. In addition the HbE that is formed is mildly unstable (Frischer and Bowman, 1975; Macdonald and Charache, 1983). This leads to a β-thalassemia-like phenotype.

Clinical Features

Both the trait and homozygous forms are clinically asymptomatic. Features of hemolysis like icterus or organomegaly are generally not seen. If present, one should consider a diagnosis of Eβ⁰ thalassemia (Fucharoen et al., 2000).

Lab Diagnosis

HbE trait: Hb electrophoresis shows an E band (30–35%) with the remaining Hb being mostly A.

HbE disease: CBC shows no anemia however significant microcytosis. Review of the peripheral smear shows abundant targets (Figure 5.13). HPLC/Hb electrophoresis shows a dominant E band (95–97%) with less than 5% HbF (Tyagi et al., 2004) and absent A.

Eβ⁰ thalassemia generally has a greater proportion of HbF (30–60%) with lesser HbE (40–70%). The peripheral smear may show anisopoikilocytosis with dacryocytes, coarse basophilic stippling, fragments, and nucleated RBCs in addition to targets (Hoyer and Kroft, 2003).

Differential Diagnosis

HbC, C-Harlem, O$_{ARAB}$ comigrate with E on alkaline electrophoresis. However, while E migrates with A on acid electrophoresis, C migrates in the C-position, C-Harlem in the S-position, and O$_{ARAB}$ in between A and S bands. C-Harlem would additionally have a positive sickle solubility test. While HbC is mostly in people of West African descent, C-Harlem is seen in the black population, O$_{ARAB}$ in African Americans and in Bulgaria, and E in Asians.

Hemoglobin D

Definition

Hemoglobin D is a beta globin mutant resulting most commonly from a Glu → Gln substitution at codon 121 (D-Los Angeles, D-Punjab, D-North Carolina, D-Chicago, D-Portugal). Other rarer forms involve different substitutions at codon 121, or substitutions in different codons.

ICD-10 Code D58.2

Epidemiology

This is the fourth most commonly occurring Hb variant. Although primarily found in the Punjab regions of India and Pakistan, it has been reported in several ethnic groups worldwide.

Etiology

This substitution demonstrates no functional abnormalities.

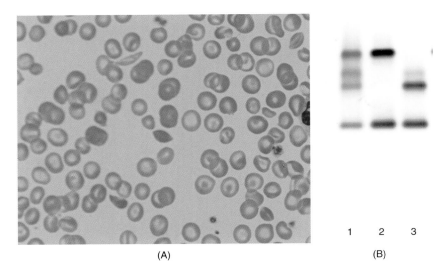

(A)   (B)

Peak Name	Calibrated Area %	Area %	Retention Time (min)	Peak Area
F	1.9*	- - -	1.05	47834
P2	- - -	0.2	1.27	4503
Unknown	- - -	0.0	1.60	1023
P3	- - -	0.1	1.78	1461
Unknown	- - -	0.6	2.17	15491
A0	- - -	1.0	2.34	26418
A2	4.1*	- - -	3.63	112259
S-window	- - -	46.5	4.44	1244478
Unknown	- - -	0.7	4.91	17458
C-window	- - -	45.0	5.15	1203893

Total Area: 2,674,818

F Concentration = 1.9* %

A2 Concentration = 4.1* %

*Values outside of expected ranges

Analysis comments:

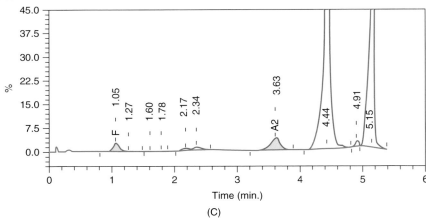

(C)

FIGURE 5.10 **Peripheral smear in SC disease (Wright–Giemsa stain, 100×).** (**A**) Numerous target cells, some hyperchromatic dense irregularly shaped cells, and folded "navicular" cells. (**B**) Alkaline electrophoresis with the standard (A, F, S, C) in lane 1, a patient with C-trait in lane 2, and SC double heterozygosity in lane 3. In lane 3, two dominant bands are noted in the S-position and C-position, respectively (confirmed by acid electrophoresis, not shown). F is mildly increased, and no A band is seen. (**C**) HPLC results in an adult patient with SC disease. (HPLC image courtesy Dr. J. Ford, Children's Hospital, Vancouver)

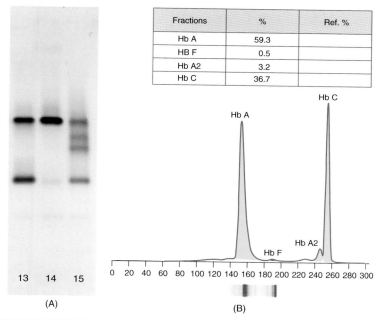

Fractions	%	Ref. %
Hb A	59.3	
HB F	0.5	
Hb A2	3.2	
Hb C	36.7	

(A)

(B)

Peak Name	Calibrated Area %	Area %	Retention Time (min)	Peak Area
F	6.3*	– – –	1.08	143487
P2	– – –	2.9	1.33	70084
P3	– – –	2.6	1.70	62087
Unknown	– – –	0.2	2.11	4654
A0	– – –	50.7	2.45	1215411
A2	3.0	– – –	3.63	81044
S-window	– – –	1.4	4.53	34611
Unknown	– – –	0.5	4.92	11216
C-window	– – –	32.3	5.15	775548

Total Area: 2,398,142

F Concentration = 6.3* %
A2 Concentration = 3.0 %
*Values outside of expected ranges

Analysis comments:

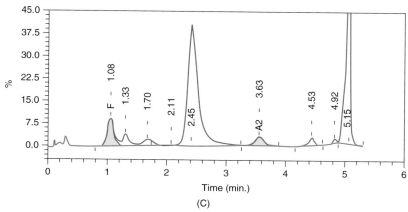

(C)

FIGURE 5.11 **Hemoglobin C-trait**. (**A**) Alkaline electrophoresis gel showing a C-trait in lane 13 with a dominant band in position A and another band in position C (40% by densitometry, confirmed by acid electrophoresis; not shown). (**B**) Capillary electrophoresis histogram from a patient with the C-trait, 59.3% HbA, and 36.7% HbC. Separate small F (0.5%) and A2 (3.5%) peaks are also noted. (**C**) HPLC results in a 10-month old child with the C-trait. The mildly elevated F (6.3%) is within the normal limits for the patient's age. Two dominant peaks (A and C) are depicted. (HPLC image courtesy Dr. J. Ford, Children's Hospital, Vancouver)

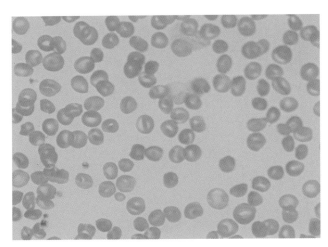

FIGURE 5.12 Peripheral smear in Hb C disease (Wright–Giemsa stain, 100×). The numerous targets and microspherocytes are noted.

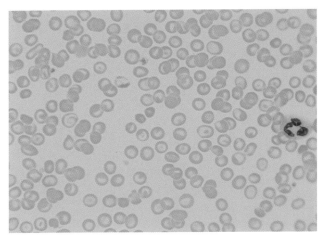

FIGURE 5.13 Peripheral smear in Hb E disease (Wright–Giemsa stain, 100×). The RBCs are hypochromic with numerous targets noted.

Clinical Features and Lab Diagnosis

Patients heterozygous or homozygous for this condition are asymptomatic. They are not anemic, with no evidence of hemolysis, and with normal RBC indices. The peripheral smear review is unremarkable. On electrophoresis/HPLC, the HbD trait shows A (60%), and D (40%) (Figure 5.14). HbD homozygous patients have predominance of D, with absent A. The D band migrates in the S-position on alkaline electrophoresis, and A-position of acid electrophoresis; a sickle solubility test is negative. Double heterozygosity for D with S leads to a severe sickling syndrome.

ANALYTE ID	%	TIME	AREA
F	1.2	1.04	29334
P2	3.4	1.30	88550
Unknown 1	0.4	1.47	11053
P3	2.8	1.68	73612
Unknown 2	2.3	2.07	61090
A0	54.5	2.38	1416555
A2	2.4	3.60	67676
D-WINDOW	33.0	4.08	859107

TOTAL AREA   2606977

F   1.2%   A2   2.4%

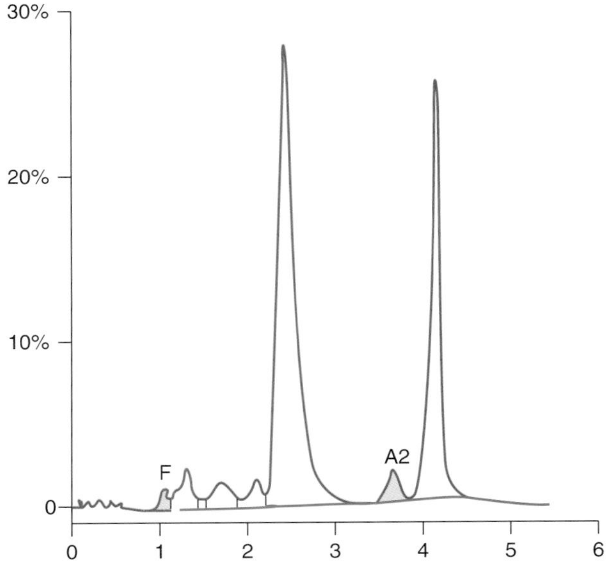

FIGURE 5.14 HPLC results in a patient with the D-trait. (Image courtesy Dr. Jason Ford, Children's Hospital, Vancouver)

Differential Diagnosis

Dβ⁰ thalassemia can resemble D homozygous states; however the former have a mild microcytic anemia, with mild hemolysis. Hb Korle-Bu (Asp → Asn substitution at postion 73) has a similar electrophoretic mobility to D-Los Angeles but can be separated on HPLC. Double heterozygous states for S with Korle-Bu, however, can be distinguished clinically (S–Korle-Bu is aymptomatic), as well as by electrophoresis.

MIXED–QUANTITATIVE QUALITATIVE DISORDERS OF HEMOGLOBIN

These are a heterogeneous group of disorders where the genetic defect leads to structurally defective globin chains that are synthesized at a markedly reduced rate. Examples include Hb Lepore and Hb Quong-Sze. Hb Lepore (see the description above) is a structurally defective hemoglobin due to an unequal crossover of the delta and beta locus, resulting in an abnormally fused delta-beta gene. The beta globin gene thus comes under the influence of the delta promoter and is transcribed at a remarkably low rate (10–15%), with a β-thalassemic outcome. In Hb Quong-Sze a mutated stop codon in the α-globin locus leads to both a qualitative (structurally abnormal α-globin chain that is longer than normal alpha chains by 31 amino acids) and quantitative (transcribed at a much slower rate) defect with an α-thalassemic outcome.

DOUBLE HETEROZYGOUS STATES

Patients may occasionally present with compound heterozygous states for thalassemia and hemoglobinopathy, or alternatively for two hemoglobinopathies or two thalassemias.

Thalassemia-Hemoglobinopathy

In general, co-inheritance of a beta thalassemia with a beta globin hemoglobinopathy trait leads to clinical and lab features resembling the disease state of the hemoglobinopathy. For example, beta thalassemia with sickle trait (a beta mutant), leads to a disease resembling sickle disease, as, of the two beta genes, one is mutated (β^S) while the other is markedly underproducing, with a 90 to 100% production of the mutant beta such as S (see Table 5.2). Similarly co-inheritance of alpha thalassemia with an α-mutant genotype will lead to increased production of the α-mutant (see Table 5.3). Yet inheritance of α-thalassemia with a β-mutant leads to a lower β-mutant proportion than normally observed in the trait (due to decreased availability of alpha chains to combine with the mutant beta chains).

Hemoglobinopathy—Hemoglobinopathy Double Heterozygosity

Double heterozygosity for two beta mutants will lead to the production of two variant hemoglobins in roughly equal proportions with no HbA (since both beta globin genes are mutated). Examples include SC disease (see the preceding section).

Double heterozygosity for an alpha and a beta mutant generally demonstrates multiple (~4) bands on hemoglobin electrophoresis. This is because an $\alpha\alpha^M\alpha\alpha\beta\beta^M$ genotype leads to the following possible combinations: $\alpha\beta, \alpha\beta^M, \alpha^M\beta$, or $\alpha^M\beta^M$. An example of double heterozygosity for C (a β-mutant) with G (an α-mutant) is shown in Figure 5.15.

Thalassemia—Thalassemia Double Heterozygosity

Co-inheritance of two different thalassemia traits leads to the development of thalassemia intermedia or major. Examples include co-inheritance of beta thalassemia with delta-beta thalassemia, Hb Lepore with beta thalassemia, delta-beta thalassemia with HPFH, combinations of beta and alpha thalassemia, or beta thalassemia with alpha triplication.

TABLE 5.2 **Predicted Relative Proportions of Hemoglobin Variants in Double Heterozygosity Involving Beta-Globin Mutants**

	Genotype	Hb A Proportion	Hb Beta-Mutant (β^M) Proportion
Beta mutant trait	$\alpha\alpha\alpha\alpha\beta\beta^M$	60%	40%
Beta mutant with beta-thalassemia	$\alpha\alpha\alpha\alpha\beta^0\beta^M$	0%	100%
	$\alpha\alpha\alpha\alpha\beta^+\beta^M$	10%	90%
Beta mutant with alpha-thalassemia	$\alpha\alpha-\beta\beta^M$	70%	30%

TABLE 5.3 **Predicted Relative Proportions of Hemoglobin Variants in Double Heterozygosity Involving Alpha-Globin Mutants**

	Genotype	Hb A Proportion	Hb Alpha-Mutant (α^M) Proportion
Alpha mutant trait	$\alpha\alpha^M\alpha\alpha\ \beta\beta$	~ 80%	~ 20%
Alpha mutant with alpha-thalassemia	$\alpha\alpha^M-\beta\beta$	~ 50%	~ 50%
Alpha mutant with beta-thalassemia	$\alpha\alpha^M\alpha\alpha\ \beta\beta^0$	~ 90%	~ 10%

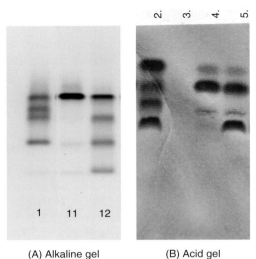

(A) Alkaline gel   (B) Acid gel

FIGURE 5.15 (**A**) Alkaline electrophoresis showing the standard in lane 1 (A, F, S, C bands from top to bottom), a normal patient with dominant A band in lane 11, and a patient with CG disease in lane 12. Four bands are seen, which from top to bottom, are A band ($\alpha\alpha\beta\beta$), G band ($\alpha\alpha$G$\beta\beta$), C band($\alpha\alpha\beta\beta$C), and C-G hybrid band ($\alpha\alpha$G$\beta\beta$C). (**B**) Acid (citrate) electrophoresis shows (patient in lane 5) two bands. A and G migrate to the A-position, while C migrates to the C-position.

APPROACH TO DIAGNOSIS OF HEMOGLOBIN DISORDERS

Generally, the laboratory workup to look for the presence of hemoglobin disorders is initiated based on family history, ethnic background, or otherwise unexplained clinical signs and symptoms such as anemia, cyanosis, or polycythemia. Otherwise asymptomatic individuals may be assessed in the context of antenatal screening, to assess the risk of inherited disorders to the fetus. According to the ACOG practice bulletin (2007), it is reasonable to offer testing for carrier screening to patients from a high-risk ethnic groups, such as of Mediterranean, Southeast Asian, and African descent.

Lab Diagnosis of Thalassemias

With the exception of a notable few (e.g., Hb Lepore), most thalassemias do not have any structurally abnormal hemoglobin moieties and are thus electrophoretically silent. The diagnosis as such is based on a combination of clinical findings, peripheral smear findings, and CBC findings of microcytosis, in the absence of iron deficiency. A diagnosis of the beta thalassemia trait is typically supported by a demonstration of an elevated HbA$_2$ level (>3.5%), which is a very helpful

diagnostic tool in the appropriate clinical/laboratory context. As such, densitometric assessment of such low quantities of Hb variants is inaccurate, and precise quantification by approved methodologies (columns, capillary electrophoresis, etc.) needs to be carried out. The alpha thalassemia trait tends to be a diagnosis of exclusion, in a patient with thalassemic indices, unexplained long-standing microcytosis, in the absence of an abnormal band, elevated A2 or low iron studies (see Figure 5.4). The presence of H-bodies, if demonstrable, is a highly suggestive though definitive, diagnosis that if indicated, requires molecular analysis.

Assays for Quantification of HbA$_2$

Some primary methodologies such as capillary electrophoresis (Figure 5.8A, 5.11B) and HPLC (Figure 5.11C) are approved for quantifying minor bands such as HbA$_2$. However, with other technologies (e.g., alkaline electrophoresis), an accurate quantification of the small Hb bands by densitometry cannot be done, so, where indicated (e.g., for a thalassemia assessment), alternative methods such as microchromatographic columns are often employed for HbA2 quantification. The latter are commercially available columns with an anion exchange resin. The resin has covalently bonded the small positively charged molecules, which then attract the negatively charged Hb. Different Hb fractions are eluted by altering the pH or ionic strength of the buffer. The fraction of the eluted Hb moiety is calculated relative to the total Hb spectrophotometrically.

Assays for Quantification of HbF

HbF quantities may be determined by methods such as capillary electrophoresis and HPLC. While major bands (>10–15%) may be assessed by densitometry measurements of alkaline electrophoresis gels, this is imprecise in the case of minor HbF bands. In such cases, where indicated (e.g., visible band in F region, or thalassemia assessment), alternative methods must be employed. One technique is a radial immunodiffusion assay. In this method, known standards, control samples, and patient samples are inoculated into wells in an agar plate impregnated with anti-F antibodies. After a 24-hour incubation a precipitation ring forms around the wells at the point of equivalence. The square of the diameter of this ring is directly proportional to the amount of HbF in the inoculums. While this quantification method is generally accurate for low quantities of HbF, it may not be accurate once HbF exceeds 10–15%.

Assays to Assess Distribution of HbF

Further assessment of HPFH, if needed, may be done by the following methodologies.

Kleihauer–Betke Test. **Principle** HbF is resistant to acid elution. The patient's peripheral blood film is treated with acid and then stained with acid hematoxylin and eosin B. The cells containing the HbF will stain pink, while those with HbA will remain unstained "ghost" cells (Figure 5.7).

Advantages/usage: This technique is helpful in distinguishing heterocellular versus pancellular distribution of F. In heterocellular distribution of F, some cells will be bright pink, while others will be ghost cells (i.e., with a heterogeneous distribution of F); all RBCs will appear a pale pink in the pancellular distribution.

Flow Cytometry for F-Cells. **Principle**: The RBCs are permeabilized and incubated with fluorescent tagged anti-F antibodies. The cells are analyzed flow cytometrically to determine number and intensity of F-containing RBCs.

Advantages/usage: The presence of two distinct peaks—one with low fluorescent intensity (indicative of non–F cells) and one with bright intensity (F-containing cells)—is indicative of a heterocellular distribution, and a single population of intermediate intensity is indicative of a pancellular distribution.

H-Body Preparation. **Principle**: Hemoglobin H and some unstable hemoglobins precipitate as intraerythrocytic inclusions and can be stained with a supravital stain (brilliant cresyl blue).

Advantages/usage: In a patient with a presumptive diagnosis of an α-thalassemia trait, the detection of H-bodies is highly suggestive of a diagnosis.

Limitations: Sample aging can lead to false positivity. Other unstable hemoglobins may also give a positive H-body test. A negative H-body does not exclude the diagnosis of an α-thalassemia trait.

Molecular Diagnosis of Alpha Thalassemia

As a first screen a targeted mutational analysis via polymerase chain reaction (PCR) studies may be used to detect common alpha-globin deletions (e.g–SEA,–FIL and—THAI,–MED, -alpha20.5, -alpha3.7, and -alpha4.2). In cases where this targeted analysis is negative, a complete sequencing of the alpha globin cluster is used (notably the latter will not detect mutations upstream of the alpha globin

cluster, as those in the HS40 regulatory region). Considered last may be a deletion/duplication analysis using a variety of techniques, such as quantitative PCR, long-range PCR, multiplex ligation-dependent probe amplification (MLPA), or targeted array GH (Galanello and Cao, 2008).

Molecular Diagnosis of Beta Thalassemia

Targeted mutational analysis can be performed based on the known prevalence of beta mutations in the ethnic group that the patient belongs to (Cao and Galanello, 2010). There are more than 200 known beta globin mutations; however, primers/probes targeting commonly occurring mutations can be used. Methods may be based on reverse dot-blot analysis, primer specific amplification, real-time PCR or microarray technology. As well, complete beta globin gene sequencing, and/or deletion/duplication analysis (particularly in suspected δβ-thalassemia or γδβ-thalassemia) may be used. Since alpha globin triplications in association with heterozygosity for beta thalassemia lead to a thalassemia intermedia phenotype, in some patients with this presentation, a separate analysis of the alpha globin cluster may additionally be warranted (Harteveld et al., 2008; Sollaino et al., 2009).

Lab Diagnosis of Hemoglobinopathies

Structurally defective hemoglobins may be distinguishable from normal globin subunits because of differences in their physical characteristics (charge, size, etc.). These differences are utilized in detecting abnormal hemoglobin moieties because of their differential migration on electrophoresis (e.g., alkaline gel electrophoresis, acid gel electrophoresis, capillary electrophoresis), differences in elution times using high performance liquid chromatography (HPLC), differences in isoelectric point using isoelectric focusing, and so on. Commonly used screening methods (per CAP surveys) include cellulose/alkaline gel electrophoresis (with or without citrate/acid gels), and HPLC. The migration patterns of common hemoglobin variants are listed in Figure 5.16. The elution times of abnormal hemoglobins on HPLC are shown in Table 5.4. In rare cases additional testing, such as globin chain electrophoresis, or even molecular sequencing, may be utilized. It is important that to aid the diagnosis of hemoglobin disorders a correlation be made with the clinical findings to ethnic background and family history as well as to other laboratory findings, including CBC, peripheral smear morphology, and where needed ancillary testing (solubility assays, unstable hemoglobin screens, etc.).

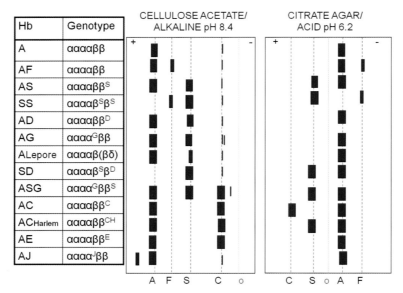

FIGURE 5.16 **Diagrammatic representation of migration patterns of common hemoglobin variants in alkaline (cellulose) and acid (citrate) gel electrophoresis.** The table on the left lists the Hb types and their associated genotypes.

TABLE 5.4 **HPLC: A Representation of Elution Times and Hb Variants**

Retention Time (min)	Manufacturer[a] Assigned Peak Name	Normal Hb Moieties	Hemoglobin Variants[b]
0.63–0.85	P1 window		Hb Barts (γ4), Hb H (β4), HbF1
0.98–1.20	F window	Hb F	
1.24–1.40	P2 window		Hb A1C, Hb Hope
1.40–1.90	P3 window		Hb-Austin, Hb-Camden, Hb Fannin-Lubbock, Hb-Fukuyama, Hb J-Oxford, Hb J-Anatolia, Hb J-Mexico, Hb J-Meerut, Hb N-Baltimore
1.90–3.10	A_0 window	Hb A	Hb J-Toronto, Hb J-Bangkok, Hb Ty Gard, Hb-Koln, Hb-New York, Hb-Twin Peaks
3.30–3.90	A2 window	Hb A2	Hb Lepore, Hb D-Iran, Hb E, Hb Osu-Christiansborg, Hb G-Honolulu
3.90–4.30	D window		Hb Korle-Bu, Hb D-Punjab, Hb G-Philadelphia
4.30–4.70	S window		Hb E-Saskatoon, Hb S, Hb-Manitoba, Hb-Montgomery, Hb Q-thailand, Hb A_2'
(4.70–4.90)			Hb-Hasharon
4.90–5.30	C window		Hb O-Arab, Hb G-Siriraj, Hb C

[a] Bio-Rad Variant II HPLC.
[b] Based on published data by Joutovsky et al. (2004).

Alkaline and Acid Electrophoresis

Alkaline Electrophoresis. In the United States this is one of the most commonly used initial screening method to detect abnormal hemoglobins.

Principle: In this assay, hemolysate from the patient sample is applied to a cellulose acetate or agar gel, and electrophoresed at an alkaline pH of 8.6. At this pH, hemoglobin in being negatively charged moves anodally. Abnormal hemoglobins, with amino acid substitutions, have differences in overall charge and thus migrate differentially. During electrophoretic migration the hemoglobin tetramer dissociates into dimers (i.e., one alpha and one non-alpha chain), which later recombine into tetramers at the site of the band. For example, in a patient with a sickle trait, the possible heteroteramers ($\alpha_2\beta_2, \alpha_2\beta\beta^S, \alpha_2\beta^S_2$), dissociate into dimers $\alpha\beta$ or $\alpha\beta^S$ that migrate differentially, eventually recombining to give two bands, in the A-position ($\alpha_2\beta_2$) and in S-position ($\alpha_2\beta^S_2$). Thus normal samples will results in one major band at position A (97–98%), with a minor band at position C (i.e., HbA_2 at 2–3%). Heterozygous mutations in alpha or beta globin genes generally lead to the formation of two major bands (as in the S example), while homozygous mutations lead to a single abnormal band, without HbA. Given the presence of two beta genes, and the preferential binding of alpha to the non-mutant beta globin, heterozygous beta globin mutations lead to the formation of 40% variant hemoglobin (i.e., slightly less than 50%). However, mutations in one of the normal four alpha genes results in 20% or less of the variant hemoglobin. Additionally a split A2 peak may be discernable in alpha globin mutations, due to the combination of mutant and normal alpha globins with delta subunits.

Advantages: This technique separates most of the common clinically significant mutant hemoglobins from the normal hemoglobin A, and it is therefore a useful initial screen for hemoglobinopathies.

Limitations: Several abnormal hemoglobins have similar migration patterns, generally necessitating a second step to confirm the identity of the abnormal band. Once a major abnormal band is detected on alkaline electrophoresis, its relative proportion can be assessed using densitometry scanning of the gel and calculating the area under the curve for the variant hemoglobin as a proportion of the total area under the curve. While densitometry scanning can be used to obtain an estimate of a major variant band, it is not an accurate assessment of minor bands such as HbA_2 or HbF.

Acid Electrophoresis. A commonly used adjunct to alkaline electrophoresis is acid electrophoresis.

Principle: In this assay, electrophoresis is carried out under altered conditions, namely at an acidic pH of 6.2 using citrate buffer. Under these conditions there is a bidirectional flow of hemoglobin moieties from the point of application on the agar gel. The agar support medium has two components: an immobile matrix made of polymerized agarose and a mobile sulfate polysaccharide agaropectin. Agaropectin, which is negatively charged, complexes with certain hemoglobin moieties and migrates anodally, while uncomplexed hemoglobins migrate cathodally.

Advantages: Some hemoglobins that migrate to the same position on alkaline electrophoresis (e.g., S and D, or C and E) migrate differentially on acid electrophoresis, making acid electrophoresis a useful second step following detection of abnormal bands on alkaline electrophoresis.

Limitations: Since several variant hemoglobins migrate with A in this gel, acid electrophoresis is unsuitable as a primary screen for hemoglobinopathies.

High-Performance Liquid Chromatography (HPLC)

This is an increasingly popular technique used in clinical laboratories as a primary method for detection of hemoglobinopathies and thalassemias.

Principle: Hemolysate from the patient sample is passed through a cartridge containing a weak cation exchange column. As buffers of increasing ionic strength are pumped through the column, hemoglobin variants will elute out at varying retention times, based on their relative polarity. The differentially separated hemoglobin fractions are then detected using techniques such as absorbance at 415 nm. The identity of the various fractions is determined based on retention time (using manufacturer-defined windows), and their relative proportion calculated based on area under the peak as a fraction of total area of all peaks on the chromatogram (Huisman et al., 1975; Ou et al., 1983).

Advantages: The newer generations of analyzers are compact, user-friendly and have a relatively rapid run time (6–7 minutes). They allow precise quantification of hemoglobin moieties, including of minor bands such as A' and are FDA approved for quantification of HbA_2 and F. Unlike in alkaline electrophoresis, HbA_2 can be measured even in the presence of HbC (Figure 5.11C).

Limitations: As with Hb electrophoretic techniques, A2 cannot be measured in the presence of HbE because they co-elute. Occasional hemoglobin variants discernable by electrophoresis may not be detected. For example, Hb-New York is a common β-chain variant seen in the Chinese population, which migrates anodal to A on electrophoresis, but has a retention time similar to A on HPLC. Certain other fast hemoglobins may require electrophoresis in order to be differentiated (Joutovsky et al., 2004). In some systems hemoglobins with a short elution time may not be evaluated, requiring visual evaluation to exclude the presence of Hb Barts or HbH.

Capillary Electrophoresis

Principle: This is a newer FDA-cleared methodology for separating Hb variants. A liquid buffer at an alkaline pH (9.4) is used as a medium along with a negatively charged silica support. High voltage is applied, and the Hb variants migrate differentially based on electroosmotic flow. The separated Hb fractions are detected using absorbance at 415 nm (Louahabi et al., 2006).

Advantages: Capillary electrophoresis offers a high-resolution separation of variants, and allows quantification of A2 and F, even in presence of certain variants like HbS, C etc (Figure 5.8A, 5.11B). It has a relatively short run time, allows automated processing, and has a library of defined zones to allow identification of variant Hb.

Limitations: Abnormal bands need to be confirmed by an alternative method, per CAP guidelines.

Additional Laboratory Testing Methods in the Evaluation of Hemoglobinopathies

Described below are some testing methodologies typically employed additionally as second-line testing. These methods enable further characterization of any variant hemoglobins detected by primary techniques such as electrophoresis or HPLC.

Solubility Test for Sickling Hemoglobins

A simple test based on a principle described in 1953 (Itano, 1953) is still used to determine the presence of sickling hemoglobins.

Principle: Hemoglobin S in a phosphate buffer becomes insoluble and precipitates out of solution when oxygen tension is lowered by the addition of a reducing substance (sodium hydrosulfite). Thus, while test tubes with non–sickling hemoglobins stay transparent, those with sickle hemoglobins turn turbid or opaque.

Advantages/usage: This test is a simple way to screen for sickling hemoglobins.

Limitations: The test is positive when sickle hemoglobin is approximately 10 to 20%. It cannot differentiate the sickle trait from the sickle disease or double heterozygous states of HbS with other hemoglobins. It may be false negative when the proportion of hemoglobin S is lower than 10 to 20% (neonates, hypertransfused patients) or when inadequate quantities of blood are taken from anemic patients. High HbF, or phenothiazines, may also inhibit the reaction. The false-positive test may result from increased nucleated RBCs, Heinz bodies, hypergammaglobulinemia, polycythemia, and some non–S hemoglobins, including Bart's, C-Georgetown, C-Harlem, C-Ziguinchor, Alexandra, Porto Alegre, Memphis/S, and S-Travis. CAP guidelines recommend that all positive sickle solubility assays be confirmed by a second method, so this test should not be used in isolation to diagnose the presence of HbS.

Isoelectric Focusing

Principle: This is an electrophoresis based method in which a pH gradient (pH range 6–8) is established throughout the gel, through the use of small proteins that can carry charge and pH. Hemoglobin moieties from patient samples then travel to their isoelectric point.

Advantages/usage: Hb variants with similar mobility on alkaline electrophoresis (e.g., S, D, G) are all separated on IEF. Minor abnormal variants are also easily identified.

Limitations: Clinically insignificant minor bands, such as due to glycosylation or to sample aging, are seen on IEP, and these may make interpretation difficult.

Globin Chain Electrophoresis

Principle: A hemolysate sample from the patient is treated with hydrochloric acid and acetone. Acetone removes the heme, and the globin precipitates out. The globin is broken into momomers by urea, and the added mercaptoethanol protects chains from denaturation. The momomeric α and β chains are separated using electrophoresis at alkaline (8.9) and acid (6.2) pH using urea-buffered cellulose acetate membranes.

Advantages/usage: This method may be employed as a second line test for variants with a confusing migration pattern in screening methods. It is useful in evaluating compound heterozygosity for α and β mutations. Also has been utilized in analysis of Gγ and Aγ analysis in newborns (Alter et al., 1980).

Unstable Hemoglobinopathy Screen

Principle: Unstable hemoglobins precipitate when exposed to heat (heat denaturation test), or exposed to certain chemicals (isopropanol at 37°C for 20 min) imparting a cloudy appearance, while stable hemoglobins remain clear.

Advantages/usage: This method helps in the evaluation of hemolytic anemia thought to be due to a hemoglobinopathy.

Limitations: Hyper-unstable variants may not be detected. Testing must be performed on fresh samples (ideally within 48 hours of drawing). Other variants, such as sickle, fetal, methhemoglobins, may also precipitate and thus need to be excluded.

Oxygen Dissociation Curve

Principle: This is a curve depicting the relationship between partial pressure of oxygen (x-axis) versus the percent oxygen saturation of hemoglobin (y-axis). There are several methods employed that are beyond the scope of this book. The gold standard method against which most are compared is the gasometric method described by Van Sylke and Neill (1924).

Advantages/usage: This method is helpful in evaluating patients with unexplained polycythemia or cyanosis with a suspected hemoglobinopathy with altered oxygen binding (Imai et al., 2001).

Limitations: Oxygen dissociation is not available in most clinical laboratories.

Mass Spectrometry

Principle: The hemolysate is diluted with a buffer and analyzed by mass spectrometry using a quadrupole-time-of-flight MS and the mass of each variant determined (Zanella-Cleon et al., 2009).

REFERENCES

ACOG Practice Bulletin 78 2007. hemoglobinopathies in pregnancy. Obstet Gynecol 109(1):229–37.

ALTER BP, GOFF SC, EFREMOV GD, GRAVELY ME, HUISMAN TH. 1980. Globin chain electrophoresis: a new approach to the determination of the G gamma/A gamma ratio in fetal haemoglobin and to studies of globin synthesis. Br J Haematol 44(4):527–34.

BRUGNARA C. 2003. Sickle cell disease: from membrane pathophysiology to novel therapies for prevention of erythrocyte dehydration. J Pediatr Hematol Oncol 25(12):927–33.

BUNN HF, FORGET BG. 1986. Human Hemoglobin Variants. Hemoglobin: Molecular, Genetic and Clinical Aspects. Saunders, Philadelphia, 381–450.

CAO A, GALANELLO R. 2010. Beta-thalassemia. In: Pagon RA, Bird TC, Dolan CR, Stephens K, eds. GeneReviews [Internet] http://www.ncbi.nlm.nih.gov/books/NBK1426/. University of Washington, Seattle.

FESSAS P. 1963. Inclusions of hemoglobin erythroblasts and erythrocytes of thalassemia. Blood 21:21–32.

FRISCHER H, BOWMAN J. 1975. Hemoglobin E, an oxidatively unstable mutation. J Lab Clin Med 85(4):531–9.

FUCHAROEN S, KETVICHIT P, POOTRAKUL P, SIRITANARATKUL N, PIANKIJAGUM A, WASI P. 2000. Clinical manifestation of beta-thalassemia/hemoglobin E disease. J Pediatr Hematol Oncol 22(6):552–7.

GALANELLO R, CAO A. 2008. Alpha-thalassemia. In: Pagon RA, Bird TC, Dolan CR, Stephens K, editors. GeneReviews [Internet]. See http://www.ncbi.nlm.nih.gov/books/NBK1435/. University of Washington, Seattle.

GIBBONS RJ, PICKETTS DJ, VILLARD L, HIGGS DR. 1995. Mutations in a putative global transcriptional regulator cause X-linked mental retardation with alpha-thalassemia (ATR-X syndrome). Cell 80(6):837–45.

HARDISON R. 1998. Hemoglobins from bacteria to man: evolution of different patterns of gene expression. J Exp Biol 201(Pt 8):1099–1117.

HARTEVELD CL, REFALDI C, CASSINERIO E, CAPPELLINI MD, GIORDANO PC. 2008. Segmental duplications involving the alpha-globin gene cluster are causing beta-thalassemia intermedia phenotypes in beta-thalassemia heterozygous patients. Blood Cells Mol Dis 40(3):312–6.

HOFFBRAND AV, PETTIT. 2000. Generic disorders of haemoglobin. In: Color Atlas of Clinical Hematology, 3rd ed. Color Atlas of Clinical Hematology. Harcourt, New York, 85–106.

HOYER JD, KROFT SH. 2003. Color Atlas of Hemoglobin Disorders. A Compendium Based oN Proficiency Testing. College of American Pathologists, Northfield, IL.

HUISMAN TH, SCHROEDER WA, BRODIE AN, MAYSON SM, JAKWAY J. 1975. Microchromatography of hemoglobins. II. A simplified procedure for the determination of hemoglobin A2. J Lab Clin Med 86(4):700–2.

HUISMAN THJ, CARVER MFH, EFREMOV GD. 1996. A Syllabus of Human Hemoglobin Variants. Sickle Cell Anemia Foundation, Augusta.

HUNT JA, INGRAM VM. 1961. Abnormal human haemoglobins. VI. The chemical difference between haemoglobins A and E. Biochim Biophys Acta 49:520–36.

IMAI K, TIENTADAKUL P, OPARTKIATTIKUL N, LUENEE P, WINICHAGOON P, SVASTI J, FUCHAROEN S. 2001. Detection of haemoglobin variants and inference of their functional properties using complete oxygen dissociation curve measurements. Br J Haematol 112(2):483–7.

ITANO HA. 1953. Solubilities of naturally occurring mixtures of human hemoglobin. Arch Biochem Biophys 47(1):148–59.

JOUTOVSKY A, HADZI-NESIC J, NARDI MA. 2004. HPLC retention time as a diagnostic tool for hemoglobin variants and hemoglobinopathies: a study of 60000 samples in a clinical diagnostic laboratory. Clin Chem 50(10):1736–47.

LINDOR NM, VALDES MG, WICK M, THIBODEAU SN, JALAL S. 1997. De novo 16p deletion: ATR-16 syndrome. Am J Med Genet 72(4):451–4.

LOUAHABI A, PHILIPPE M, LALI S, WALLEMACQ P, MAISIN D. 2006. Evaluation of a new Sebia kit for analysis of hemoglobin fractions and variants on the capillary system. Clin Chem Lab Med 44(3):340–5.

MACDONALD VW, CHARACHE S. 1983. Differences in the reaction sequences associated with drug-induced oxidation of hemoglobins E, S, A, and F. J Lab Clin Med 102(5):762–72.

OU CN, BUFFONE GJ, REIMER GL, ALPERT AJ. 1983. High-performance liquid chromatography of human hemoglobins on a new cation exchanger. J Chromatogr 266:197–205.

PAN LL, ENG HL, KUO CY, CHEN WJ, HUANG HY. 2005. Usefulness of brilliant cresyl blue staining as an auxiliary method of screening for alpha-thalassemia. J Lab Clin Med 145(2):94–97.

PIEL FB, PATIL AP, HOWES RE, NYANGIRI OA, GETHING PW, WILLIAMS TN, WEATHERALL DJ, HAY SI. 2010. Global distribution of the sickle cell gene and geographical confirmation of the malaria hypothesis. Nat Commun 1(8):104.

PLATT OS. 2003. Sickle syndromes. In: Handin RI, Lux SE, Stossel TP, eds., Blood Principles and Practice of Hematology. Lippincott Williams and Wilkins, Philadelphia, 1655–1708.

REES DC, WILLIAMS TN, GLADWIN MT. 2010. Sickle-cell disease. Lancet 376(9757):2018–31.

SANCHAISURIYA K, FUCHAROEN G, SAE-UNG N, JETSRISUPARB A, FUCHAROEN S. 2003. Molecular and hematologic features of hemoglobin E heterozygotes with different forms of alpha-thalassemia in Thailand. Ann Hematol 82(10):612–6.

SKOGERBOE KJ, WEST SF, SMITH C, TERASHITA ST, LECRONE CN, DETTER JC, TAIT JF. 1992. Screening for alpha-thalassemia: correlation of hemoglobin H inclusion bodies with DNA-determined genotype. Arch Pathol Lab Med 116(10):1012–8.

SOLLAINO MC, PAGLIETTI ME, PERSEU L, GIAGU N, LOI D, GALANELLO R. 2009. Association of alpha globin gene quadruplication and heterozygous beta thalassemia in patients with thalassemia intermedia. Haematologica 94(10):1445–8.

SUKUMARAN PK, NAKATSUJI T, GARDINER MB, REESE AL, GILMAN JG, HUISMAN TH. 1983. Gamma thalassemia resulting from the deletion of a gamma-globin gene. Nucleic Acids Res 11(13):4635–43.

TRAEGER J, WOOD WG, CLEGG JB, WEATHERALL DJ. 1980. Defective synthesis of HbE is due to reduced levels of beta E mRNA. Nature 288(5790):497–9.

TYAGI S, PATI HP, CHOUDHRY VP, SAXENA R. 2004. Clinico-haematological profile of HbE syndrome in adults and children. Hematology 9(1):57–60.

VAN SLYKE DD, NEILL JM. 1924. The determination of gases in blood and other solutions by vacuum extraction and manometric measurement. J Biol Chem 61:523–43.

WEATHERALL DJ, CLEGG JB. 1981. The Thalassemia Syndromes. Blackwell Scientific, Oxford.

ZANELLA-CLEON I, JOLY P, BECCHI M, FRANCINA A. 2009. Phenotype determination of hemoglobinopathies by mass spectrometry. Clin Biochem 42(18):1807–17.

PART II

INFECTIOUS ASPECTS OF HEMATOLOGY

APICOMPLEXAL PARASITES OF PERIPHERAL BLOOD, BONE MARROW, AND SPLEEN: THE GENERA *PLASMODIUM, BABESIA,* AND *TOXOPLASMA*

Lynne S. Garcia

PLASMODIUM

Four species—*P. falciparum, P. vivax, P. ovale,* and *P. malariae*—are well known to infect humans. The fifth species, *P. knowlesi,* which normally infects macaques, is a significant cause of human malaria in Southeast Asia and accounts for more than a quarter of malaria cases in hospitals in Malaysian Borneo (Cox-Singh et al., 2008). Human cases have also been reported from Thailand (Putaporntip et al., 2009), Singapore (Ng et al., 2008), and the Philippines (Luchavez et al., 2008), and in Western travelers returning from Southeast Asia (Bronner et al., 2009; MMWR, 2009c).

Life Cycle

The *Plasmodium* life cycle (Figure 6.1) begins with the injection of sporozoites by the bite of an infected mosquito. These sporozoites almost immediately invade the hepatocytes and undergo the preerythrocytic cycle for 7 to 10 days, producing liver schizonts.

Rupture of each liver schizont releases thousands of free merozoites into the peripheral blood where they invade erythrocytes (RBCs), thus beginning the erythrocytic cycle. In the RBC the early trophozoites (rings) develop into mature trophozoites with an enlarged cytoplasm and an accumulation of malarial pigment. Nuclear and cytoplasmic divisions produce the mature schizont, which ruptures, releasing merozoites and completing the erythrocytic cycle. A few merozoites undergo sexual differentiation into gametocytes, which undergo fertilization and zygote formation following ingestion with a mosquito blood meal. Fertilized gametes develop into ookinetes, which penetrate the intestinal lining and develop into oocysts on the extraluminal wall of the mosquito intestine. Oocysts rupture, releasing sporozoites, which migrate to the salivary glands to complete the life cycle in the female anopheline mosquito.

The time required to complete a single erythrocytic stage cycle is 72 hours in *P. malariae*, 36 to 48 hours in *P. falciparum*, 48 hours in *P. vivax* and

Non-Neoplastic Hematopathology and Infections, First Edition. Edited by Hernani D. Cualing, Parul Bhargava, and Ramon L. Sandin.
© 2012 Wiley-Blackwell. Published 2012 by John Wiley & Sons, Inc.

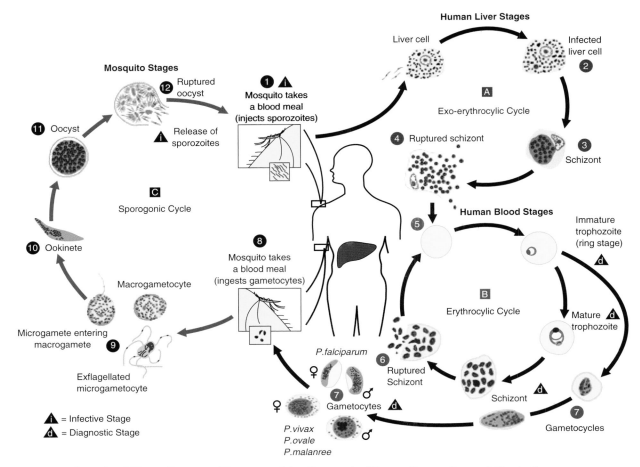

FIGURE 6.1 Life cycle of *Plasmodium* spp. (Courtesy of the Centers for Disease Prevention and Control)

P. ovale, and 24 hours in *P. knowlesi*. In the late trophozoites and schizonts of *P. falciparum*, the RBC membrane is modified, which causes the infected RBCs to adhere to vascular endothelium (Garcia, 2007). Thus these stages of the life cycle do not circulate in the peripheral blood. Some of the *P. vivax* and *P. ovale* original sporozoites may remain dormant in the liver as hypnozoites, which subsequently develop into mature liver schizonts leading to relapse of parasitemia months to a few years later.

ICD-10 Codes

Depending on the species and/or complications, there are a number of relevant ICD-10 Codes that are available. These can be seen in Table 6.1.

Epidemiology

Malaria is endemic in 100 countries with a population of 2.4 billion people, approximately half of whom are located in Africa south of the Sahara. Over 90%

of malaria deaths occur in Africa, primarily among young children. The number of cases outside tropical Africa may reach 20 million, with about 80% being found in Asia. Although the risk of malaria is relatively low in Asia and the Americas, certain areas remain highly endemic. Approximately two-thirds of malaria infections in the Americas occur in the Amazon basin. Also malaria has re-emerged in areas where control had previously been successful; examples include Azerbaijan, Tajikistan, Iraq, and Turkey.

Disease prevention is quite complicated, and no drugs are universally effective. An average number of mosquito bites per person per day must be sustained or the infection gradually dies out. This requirement for sustained infection can be influenced by the vector preference for human blood and habitation and the duration of infection in a specific area in the anopheline mosquito vector and the reservoir of infected humans. Once an area is clear of the infection, the overall population immunity may decline, a situation

TABLE 6.1 ICD-10 Codes for the Genera *Plasmodium, Babesia,* and *Toxoplasma*

Number	Description
B50	**Plasmodium falciparum malaria**; includes mixed infections of Plasmodium falciparum with any other Plasmodium species
B50.0	Plasmodium falciparum malaria with cerebral complications; cerebral malaria NOS
B50.8	Other severe and complicated Plasmodium falciparum malaria; severe or complicated Plasmodium falciparum malaria NOS
B50.9	Plasmodium falciparum malaria, unspecified
B51	**Plasmodium vivax malaria**; includes mixed infections of Plasmodium vivax with other Plasmodium species, except Plasmodium falciparum; excludes 1 when mixed with Plasmodium falciparum (B50.-)
B51.0	Plasmodium vivax malaria with rupture of spleen
B51.8	Plasmodium vivax malaria with other complications
B51.9	Plasmodium vivax malaria without complication; Plasmodium vivax malaria NOS
B52	**Plasmodium malariae malaria**; includes mixed infections of Plasmodium malariae with other Plasmodium species, except Plasmodium falciparum and Plasmodium vivax; excludes 1 when mixed with Plasmodium falciparum (B50.-) or Plasmodium vivax (B51.-)
B52.0	Plasmodium malariae malaria with nephropathy
B52.8	Plasmodium malariae malaria with other complications
B52.9	Plasmodium malariae malaria without complication; Plasmodium malariae malaria NOS
B53	**Other specified malaria**
B53.0	Plasmodium ovale malaria; excludes 1 when mixed with Plasmodium falciparum (B50.-), Plasmodium malariae (B52.-), Plasmodium vivax (B51.-)
B53.1	Malaria due to simian plasmodia (Plasmodium knowlesi); excludes 1 when mixed with Plasmodium falciparum (B50.-), Plasmodium malariae (B52.-), Plasmodium ovale (B53.-), Plasmodium vivax (B51.-)
B53.8	Other parasitologically confirmed malaria, not elsewhere classified; Parasitologically confirmed malaria NOS
B54	**Unspecified malaria**; clinically diagnosed malaria without parasitological confirmation
B58	**Toxoplasmosis**; includes infection due to *Toxoplasma gondii*; excludes 1 congenital toxoplasmosis (P37.1)
B58.00	Toxoplasma oculopathy, unspecified
B58.01	Toxoplasma chorioretinitis
B58.09	Other toxoplasma oculopathy; toxoplasma uveitis
B58.1	Toxoplasma hepatitis
B58.2	Toxoplasma meningoencephalitis
B58.3	Pulmonary toxoplasmosis
B58.8	Toxoplasmosis with other organ involvement
B58.81	Toxoplasma myocarditis
B58.82	Toxoplasma myositis
B58.83	Toxoplasma tubulo-interstitial nephropathy; Toxoplasma pyelonephritis
B58.89	Toxoplasmosis with other organ involvement
B58.9	Toxoplasmosis, unspecified
B60	**Other protozoal diseases, not elsewhere classified**; excludes 1 cryptosporidiosis (A07.2), intestinal microsporidiosis (A07.8), isosporiasis (A07.3)
B60.0	Babesiosis; Piroplasmosis

Source: Site: http://www.cms.gov/ICD10/Downloads/6_I10tab2010.pdf (accessed 6.3.10).

that may lead to a severe epidemic if the infection is reintroduced into the population. Transmission is limited to temperatures within 16 to 33°C or 2000 meters or less in altitude, parameters within which parasite development in the mosquito vector occurs.

In much of sub-Saharan Africa the most severe morbidity and mortality occur in early childhood and the majority of deaths are due to severe anemia. Individuals surviving through early childhood develop partial clinical immunity and are less likely to die from malaria. In areas where transmission is seasonal or unstable, development of clinical immunity is less effective, symptomatic and severe malaria occur at all ages, and cerebral malaria is a common manifestation of severe infection.

Although malaria was eradicated from North America by the midtwentieth century, competent vector species of anopheline mosquitoes are widely present, and small, focal outbreaks of malaria can occur when an immigrant or traveler serves as a reservoir of infection with gametocytes in the blood (MMWR, 2003; Sunstrum et al., 2001).

Clinical Disease

During the first week after infection, the patient remains asymptomatic while the parasites are undergoing multiplication in the preerythrocytic cycle in the liver. Although several broods will begin to develop when the liver merozoites invade the RBCs, one will eventually dominate and suppress the others, thus beginning the process of periodicity. Once the erythrocytic cycle is synchronized, the simultaneous rupture of a large number of RBCs and liberation of metabolic waste by-products into the bloodstream precipitate the typical malaria paroxysms. Before the onset of synchrony, the patient's symptoms may be mild, somewhat vague, and may include a low fever that exhibits no periodicity. This is particularly important for immunologically naïve patients such as travelers who have had no prior exposure to the parasite; in these cases the parasitemia may be extremely low and difficult to detect. Without a typical fever pattern, the disease presentation may mimic many other conditions.

Symptoms include anemia, splenomegaly, and the classic paroxysm, with its cold stage, fever, and sweats. The typical paroxysm begins with the cold stage and rigors lasting 1 to 2 hours. During the next few hours, the patient spikes a high fever and feels very hot, and the skin is warm and dry. The last several hours are characterized by marked sweating and a subsequent drop in body temperature to normal or subnormal. Although the febrile paroxysms strongly suggest a malaria infection, many patients who are seen in medical facilities in the early stages of the infection do not exhibit a typical fever pattern. Patients may have a steady low-grade fever or several small, random peaks each day. Because the symptoms associated with malaria in the early stages are so nonspecific, the diagnosis should be considered in any symptomatic patient with a history of travel to an endemic area.

Anemia can be caused by several mechanisms, such as (1) direct RBC lysis as a function of the parasite life cycle, (2) splenic removal of both infected and uninfected RBCs (coated with immune complexes), (3) autoimmune lysis of coated infected and uninfected RBCs, (4) decreased incorporation of iron into heme, (5) increased fragility of RBCs, and (6) decreased RBC production from bone marrow suppression.

Malaria can mimic many other diseases, such as gastroenteritis, pneumonia, meningitis, encephalitis, or hepatitis. Other possible symptoms include lethargy, anorexia, nausea, vomiting, diarrhea, and headache. Leukopenia can also be seen in malaria, as can an occasional elevated white blood cell count with a left shift. Eosinophilia and thrombocytopenia may be seen but are much less frequent. A comparison of some of the features of the five different malarias is presented in Table 6.2.

Infection with *P. falciparum* may be complicated by various forms of severe malaria. Table 6.3 shows the World Health Organization criteria for severe malaria (WHO, 1990). Severe malaria due to *P. falciparum* may develop rapidly in a patient who initially presents with mild symptoms and a low parasitemia. It is critical to make the diagnosis of *P. falciparum* quickly. *P. knowlesi* has a short erythrocytic cycle time, 24 hours, may therefore reach high parasite densities rapidly, and may also cause severe malaria (Cox-Singh et al., 2008).

P. vivax and *P. ovale* preferentially invade reticulocytes and rarely cause parasitemias greater than 2%. They may relapse from the liver following successful therapy of the blood stage infection and must therefore be treated with primaquine to eradicate hypnozoites in the liver. *P. malariae* preferentially infects older erythrocytes and may cause chronic, asymptomatic parasitemia lasting for many years. Proteinuria is a common finding in *P. malariae* infection and may progress to the nephrotic syndrome in children.

Pathophysiology

Plasmodium falciparum

P. falciparum infects all ages of RBCs, and the percentage of infected cells may exceed 50%. Schizogony occurs in the internal organs (spleen, liver, bone marrow, etc.) rather than in the circulating blood. A decrease in the ability of the RBCs to change shape when passing through capillaries may lead to plugging of the vessels, thus leading to ischemia. Onset of a *P. falciparum* malaria attack occurs 8 to 12 days after infection and is preceded by 3 to 4 days of aches, pains, headache, fatigue, anorexia, or nausea. The onset is characterized by fever, a more severe headache, and nausea and vomiting, with occasional severe epigastric pain. There may be only a feeling of chilliness at the onset of fever. Periodicity of the cycle will not be established during the early stages, and the presumptive diagnosis may be totally unrelated to a possible malaria infection. If the fever does develop a synchronous cycle, it is usually a cycle of somewhat less than 48 hours.

Severe or fatal complications of *P. falciparum* malaria can occur at any time during the infection and are related to the plugging of vessels in the internal

TABLE 6.2 Comparative Information on the Five Species of Human *Plasmodium*

Characteristic	P. falciparum	P. vivax	P. ovale	P. malariae	P. knowlesi
Periodicity (not seen in early infection)	36–48 h	44–48 h	48 h	72 h; more regular in the beginning	24 h
Persistence of extra-erythrocytic cycle	No	Yes	Yes	No	No
True relapses	No	Yes	Yes	No (recrudescence)	No
Size and shape of infected erythrocytes	Normal size and shape; no limit on number of infected RBCs	Enlarged up to 2-fold; may be oval; limited to young RBCs (2–5%)	Normal to enlarged, frequently oval, may be fimbriated; limited to young RBCs (2–5%)	Small to normal size, normal shape; limited to old RBCs (2–5%)	Normal size and shape; no limit on number of infected RBCs
Stippling (best seen with Giemsa stain pH 7.0–7.2)	Occasional Maurer's dots, less numerous than Schüffner's	Schüffner's dots usually present, except in rings	James's stippling, darker than Schüffner's present in all stages, including rings	Ziemann's dots, rarely seen; requires deliberate overstaining	Irregular stippling in late trophozoites and schizonts
Stages seen in peripheral blood	Rings and gametocytes	All	All	All	All
Multiply infected erythrocytes	Common	Occasional	Occasional	Rare	Common
Early trophozoites	Delicate ring, frequently with two small chromatin dots, often at edge of erythrocyte (appliqué form)	Ring up to 1/3 diameter of erythrocyte; larger chromatin dot than P. falciparum	Similar to P. vivax	Smaller than P. vivax; otherwise similar	Double chromatin dots common; infrequent appliqué forms
Mature trophozoites	Not seen in peripheral blood	Ameboid shape, fine golden-brown pigment	Similar to P. vivax except less ameboid, pigment darker brown	Compact cytoplasm, oval, round, or band-shaped, dark brown pigment	Slightly ameboid cytoplasm; band forms common; scattered grains or clumps of golden to brown pigment

(continued)

119

TABLE 6.2 (Continued)

Characteristic	P. falciparum	P. vivax	P. ovale	P. malariae	P. knowlesi
Schizonts	Rarely seen in peripheral blood	12–24 merozoites	8–12 merozoites	6–12 merozoites often radially arranged around central pigment ("daisy-head" schizont)	10–16 merozoites
Gametocytes	Crescent or "banana"-shaped	Round to slightly oval	Round to slightly oval	Round to slightly oval	Round to slightly oval
Most characteristic findings (morphology)	Absence of mature trophozoites and schizonts; normal size of infected erythrocytes; multiple infections; appliqué forms; "banana"-shaped gametocytes	Enlarged infected erythrocytes; Schüffner's dots frequently present; ameboid trophozoite; 12–24 merozoites in each schizont	Normal to enlarged, oval or fimbriated infected erythrocytes; James' stippling may be seen in rings; schizonts with 8–12 merozoites	Normal size of infected erythrocytes; no stippling; "band" trophozoite; "daisy head" schizont with 6–12 merozoites	Rings resemble P. falciparum; trophozoites, schizonts, and gametocytes resemble P. malariae, except that schizonts may contain up to 16 merozoites
Clinical findings	Severe and fatal complications; CNS often involved; plugging of vessels; extreme fevers; cerebral malaria often fatal; all body systems may be involved; drug resistance increasing	Primary attack 3 wks to 2 mo; relapse wks, mo, or years (5) later; severe complications rare; drug resistance documented	Similar to P. vivax; severity of symptoms less; lack of typical rigors	Longer incubation time; more severe paroxysms; linked to kidney problems (nephrotic syndrome); may last 30+ years	Symptoms as severe as those with P. falciparum; no limit on number of infected RBCs and rapid life cycle

TABLE 6.3 World Health Organization Criteria for Severe Malaria

Parasitemia (%)	Number of Parasites/µl	Clinical Correlation[a]
0.0001–0.0004	5–20	Number of organisms required for positive thick film (sensitivity)
		Examination of 100 thick-blood-film (TBF) fields (0.25 µl) may miss up to 20% of infections (sensitivity 80–90%); at least 300 fields should be examined before reporting a negative result
		Examination of 100 thin-blood-film fields (THBF) (0.005 µl); at least 300 fields should be examined before reporting a negative result; **both** thick- and thin-blood films should be examined for every specimen submitted for a suspect malaria case (report final results using 100× oil immersion objective)
		BinaxNOW® rapid lateral flow method (dipstick) (0–100 = 53.9% sensitivity for *P. falciparum*)
		BinaxNOW® rapid lateral flow method (dipstick) (0–100 = 6.2% sensitivity for *P. vivax*))
		One set (TBF + THBF) of negative blood films does not rule out a malaria infection
0.002	100	**Patients may be symptomatic below this level, particularly if they are immunologically naïve** (no prior exposure to malaria; e.g., travelers)
		BinaxNOW® rapid lateral flow method (dipstick) (100–500 = 89.2% sensitivity for *P. falciparum*)
		BinaxNOW® rapid lateral flow method (dipstick) (100–500 = 23.6% sensitivity for *P. vivax*)
0.02	1000	**Level often seen in travelers (immunologically naïve)—results may also be lower than this**
		BinaxNOW® rapid lateral flow method (dipstick) (1000–5000 = 99.2% sensitivity for *P. falciparum*)
		BinaxNOW® rapid lateral flow method (dipstick) (500–1000 = 92.6% sensitivity for *P. falciparum*)
		BinaxNOW® rapid lateral flow method (dipstick) (1000–5000 = 81.0% sensitivity for *P. vivax*) (500–1000 = 47.4% sensitivity for *P. vivax*)
0.1	5000	BinaxNOW® rapid lateral flow method (dipstick) (>5000 = 99.7% sensitivity for *P. falciparum*)
		BinaxNOW® rapid lateral flow method (dipstick) (5000 = 93.5% sensitivity for *P. vivax*)
0.2	10,000	Level above which immune patients will exhibit symptoms
2	100,000	Maximum parasitemia of *P. vivax* and *P. ovale* (which infect young RBCs only)
2–5	100,000–250,000	Hyperparasitemia, severe malaria;[b] increased mortality
10	500,000	Exchange transfusion may be considered; high mortality

Note: Parasitemia determined from conventional light microscopy (clinical correlation).

[a]The BinaxNOW® malaria test (Inverness Medical, Scarborough, ME) is FDA approved. The BinaxNOW® malaria test detects antigen from both viable and nonviable malaria organisms, including gametocytes and sequestered *P. falciparum* parasites. Test performance depends on antigen load in the specimen and may not directly correlate with microscopy performed on the same specimen. Samples with positive rheumatoid factor titers may produce false-positive results. Analytical reactivity testing demonstrates that the pan malarial test line on the BinaxNOW® test is capable of detecting all four malaria species. However, during clinical trials insufficient data were generated to support clinical performance claims for the detection of *P. malariae* or *P. ovale*. Clinical performance claims for this test are made for *P. falciparum* and *P. vivax* detection only. The test is not intended for use in screening asymptomatic populations. (BinaxNOW® malaria test package insert (Inverness Medical, Scarborough, ME). The BinaxNOW Positive Malaria Control, as well as the BinaxNOW® Malaria test, is available commercially (Inverness Medical, Scarborough, ME).

[b]World Health Organization criteria for severe malaria are parasitemia of >10,000/µl and severe anemia (hemoglobin, <5 g/L). Prognosis is poor if >20% of parasites are pigment-containing trophozoites and schizonts and/or if >5% of neutrophils contains visible pigment.

organs. The severity of the complications in a malaria infection may not correlate with the parasitemia seen in the peripheral blood, particularly in *P. falciparum* infections. Acute lung injury is more likely to occur in patients with very severe, multisystemic *P. falciparum* malaria; in these patients with acute lung injury and septic shock, bacterial sepsis should be suspected and treated empirically.

Disseminated intravascular coagulation is rare and is linked to a high parasitemia, pulmonary edema, rapidly developing anemia, and cerebral and renal complications. Small vessel vascular endothelial damage from endotoxins and bound parasitized blood cells may result in clot formation.

Plasmodium vivax

Severe complications are rare, although CNS involvement, coma, and sudden death have been reported. These patients can exhibit cerebral malaria, renal failure, circulatory collapse, severe anemia, hemoglobinuria, abnormal bleeding, acute respiratory distress syndrome, and jaundice. Some cases have been linked to various degrees of primaquine resistance (Spudick, 2005). PCR has confirmed that these were single species infections with *P. vivax*.

Plasmodium ovale

Although *P. ovale* and *P. vivax* infections are clinically similar, *P. ovale* malaria is less severe, tends to relapse less frequently, and usually ends with spontaneous recovery. Although the incubation period is comparable to *P. vivax*, the symptom frequency and severity are much less. *P. ovale* infects only the reticulocytes (as does *P. vivax*), so the parasitemia is generally limited to 2 to 5% of the RBCs.

Plasmodium malariae

P. malariae tends to invade the older RBCs, so the number of infected cells is also limited. The incubation period may range from about 27 to 40 days. A regular periodicity is seen from the beginning, with a more severe paroxysm. Proteinuria is common in *P. malariae* infections and in children may be associated with clinical signs of the nephrotic syndrome, which is unaffected by the administration of steroids. In a chronic infection, kidney problems may result from deposition within the glomeruli of antigen-antibody complexes. A membranoproliferative type of glomerulonephritis with relatively sparse proliferation of endothelial and mesangial cells is the most common lesion seen. Chronic glomerular disease associated with *P. malariae* infections is usually not reversible with therapy. The infection may end with spontaneous recovery, or there may be a recrudescence or series of recrudescences over 30 to 40 or more years.

Plasmodium knowlesi

Patients may be relatively asymptomatic, or may exhibit chills, minor headaches and a daily low-grade fever, while other patients may present with high fevers, mild abdominal problems, leukopenia, and thrombocytopenia (Cox-Singh, 2008; Garcia, 2010). In some cases the microscopy findings initially suggest an infection with *P. falciparum*, while subsequent blood films may suggest a dual infection with *P. falciparum* and *P. malariae*.

A previously healthy 40-year-old male became symptomatic 10 days after spending time in the North Borneo jungle (MMWR, 2009c). Four days later he presented to the hospital, collapsed, and died two hours later. He was hyponatremic and had elevated blood urea, potassium, lactate dehydrogenase, and amino transferase values. He was also thrombocytopenic and eosinophilic. Blood for malaria parasites indicated a high parasitemia, and a *P. knowlesi* infection was confirmed using nested-PCR. Macroscopic examination of the brain and heart revealed multiple petechial hemorrhages, hepato- and splenomegaly, and lungs consistent with acute respiratory distress syndrome. Microscopic pathology demonstrated sequestration of pigmented parasitized red blood cells in the vessels of the cerebrum, cerebellum, heart, and kidney without evidence of chronic inflammatory reaction in the brain or any other organ examined. Spleen and liver histology revealed abundant pigment containing macrophages and parasitized red blood cells, while the kidney showed acute tubular necrosis, and endothelial cells were prominent in cardiac sections.

Diagnosis

Specimen Collection and Patient History

Because *P. falciparum* and *P. knowlesi* can progress rapidly to severe malaria, all requests for malaria diagnosis should be handled on a STAT basis. Using finger-stick blood films or those prepared from EDTA anticoagulant, blood films should be prepared and stained within an hour of drawing the specimen.

Requests for malaria smears should include additional information. If this information is not submitted with the original request, the laboratory must be proactive in obtaining the history. (1) The patient's travel history and date of return or arrival in the United States can suggest infection possibilities and the possible species involved. (2) A history of prophylaxis or treatment for malaria may result in low parasitemia on the blood films. (3) A history of transfusions or shared needles may suggest direct person-to-person transmission, although cases of transfusion related malaria are extremely rare in the United States. (4) A prior history of malaria in the patient suggests the possibility of relapse or recrudescence. (5) Knowledge of the periodicity of the fever pattern and the time in relation to a paroxysm when the specimen was obtained is helpful because in a regularly periodic *P. falciparum* infection the circulating parasitemia can be very low and difficult to detect between paroxysms. Regardless of the presence or absence of a fever pattern, blood should be taken immediately for examination when the patient presents.

Blood Film Examination

Detection and identification of the organisms are performed by examination of thick and thin blood films stained with any of the traditional or rapid blood stains (Figure 6.2). Examination of thick films is the gold standard for detection of organisms, because of the relatively large volume of blood that can be examined directly. Approximately 20 times more blood is examined in each high-power (1000×) field than in a thin film. Early in infection, or following relapse or partial treatment, patients may be symptomatic with low parasitemias so that thick smears are required for parasite detection, while thin films are the gold standard for species identification. Although fewer parasites are present in thin films, fixation preserves erythrocyte morphology, allowing evaluation of infected erythrocyte size and the position of organisms within the erythrocytes. Examination of both thick and thin films is mandatory for a complete blood film examination. Smears should be examined at length using the 100× oil immersion objective; a negative report should not be submitted until 300 oil immersion fields of both thick and thin films have been examined. A single set of negative smears does not exclude malaria. Additional specimens should be examined at 12-hour intervals for the subsequent 36 hours.

The morphology of the five species of *Plasmodium* that infect humans in blood films is reviewed (Garcia, 2007, 2010) and is summarized in Table 6.2 and Figure 6.2. A high parasitemia consisting only of ring forms suggests *P. falciparum*, even if, in early infections, no gametocytes are found. The possibility of mixed infections should be considered, since they are more common than reported. *P. knowlesi* infections in humans have frequently been misdiagnosed as *P. malariae* (Table 6.2), which can be dangerous, as *P. knowlesi*, unlike *P. malariae*, can progress to severe malaria. Therefore patients with a microscopic

diagnosis of *P. malariae* and a recent travel history to Southeast Asia should be considered to have *P. knowlesi* infection.

Although many North American clinicians treat all malaria patients with regimens designed to cover drug-resistant *P. falciparum*, species-specific identification of *Plasmodium* sp. is clinically important for several reasons. *P. falciparum* should be identified because it is both more clinically aggressive and more likely to be multiply drug resistant than the other species. *P. vivax*, and *P. ovale* should be identified because radical cure of these infections requires supplemental treatment with primaquine to eliminate dormant hypnozoites in the liver. Primaquine may cause hemolytic anemia in some patients with G6PD deficiency; correct species identification prevents its unnecessary use in *P. falciparum* or *P. malariae* infection.

Alternative Diagnostic Methods

A number of new approaches to detection of malaria parasites have been described, including staining with acridine orange (Rickman, et al., 1989), PCR (often used for species confirmation) (Barker et al., 1992), loop-mediated isothermal amplification (LAMP) (Han et al., 2007), and antigen detection (Craig and Sharp, 1997). These and other alternative approaches have been recently reviewed (Erdman and Kain, 2008). An immunochromatographic test based on HRP-2 and aldolase, the BinaxNOW Malaria (Binax, Inc., Inverness Medical Professional Diagnostics, Scarborough, ME) has been approved by the FDA for use in the evaluation of symptomatic patients in laboratories that can both (1) acquire a positive external control for *P. falciparum* and (2) perform thick and thin film examination to confirm negative results in the immunochromatographic test.

It is important to remember that automated hematology instrumentation will not reliably detect malaria parasites, particularly in cases of early infection with a low parasitemia. It is mandatory that negative results using alternative diagnostics methods be confirmed by repeated thick film examination. As of 2010, thick film examination remains the gold standard for malaria diagnosis.

Serology

Serologic testing is not a reliable method for species identification, because of cross reactions among the five species. Also it is not recommended for clinical diagnosis because antibodies may be absent in an acute attack and, if present, antibodies may reflect past rather than current infection. Serologies are relevant in the investigation of transfusion

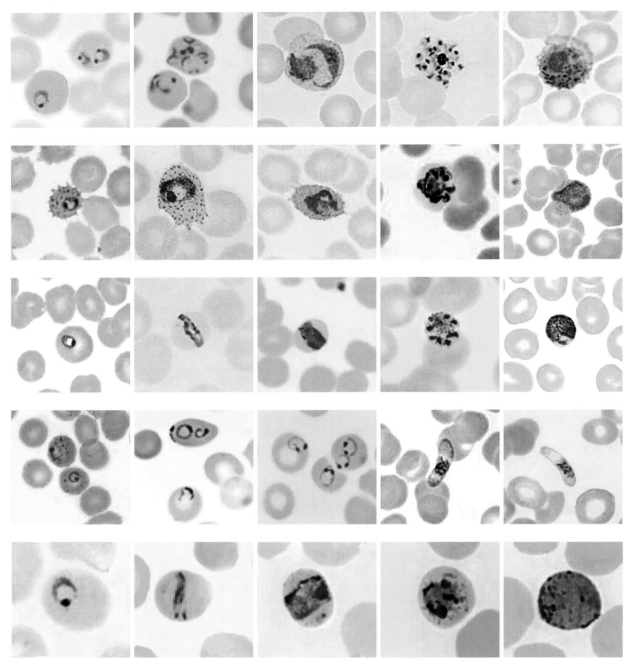

FIGURE 6.2 Examples of the five species of *Plasmodium*. Row 1: *Plasmodium vivax* (top). Left, ring forms (note double rings/RBC—not limited to *P. falciparum*); image 2, early rings (notice the ameboid shape and lack of stippling/from EDTA blood); image 3, developing troph (note the enlarged RBC and ameboid shape); image 4, mature schizont (~12–24 merozoites), last image, mature gametocyte (probably macrogametocyte). Row 2: *Plasmodium ovale*. Left, early ring (note stippling, fimbriated RBC edges and non-ameboid trophozoite); image 2, developing ring (note stippling and fimbriated RBC edges; image 3, older developing troph; image 4, mature schizont (~8–12 merozoites); last image, mature gametocyte (probably macrogametocyte). Row 3: *Plasmodium malariae*. Left, ring form; images 2 and 3, band forms; image 4, mature schizont (~6–12 merozoites); last image, mature gametocyte (probably macrogametocyte). Row 4: *Plasmodium falciparum*. Left, ring forms (note Maurer's clefts/dots); images 2 and 3, multiple rings/RBC (note accolé forms in image 2 and "headphone" rings in image 3); images 4 and 5, mature crescent-shaped gametocytes. Row 5: *Plasmodium knowlesi*. Left, ring form; images 2 and 3, band forms (resemble those seen in *P. malariae*); image 4, developing schizont; last image, mature gametocyte (probably macrogametocyte).

malaria, where results may determine which potential donor was the source of a transfusion-associated case of malaria, and in epidemiological studies, to determine the prevalence of malaria exposure in a population.

Interpretation and Reporting of Results

A positive finding of malaria parasites is a critical result, which must be reported immediately to the clinician. If possible, the report should include the species identification; if not possible, a report comment that *P. falciparum* cannot be excluded is highly recommended. If the microscopic diagnosis is *P. malariae*, but the patient has traveled to Southeast Asia, the clinician should be informed that *P. knowlesi* cannot be excluded. Because patients with high parasitemias (>3–5%) require intensive therapy, quantification of parasitemia is required. Parasitemia may be variously expressed as percent parasitemia (parasites/100 erythrocytes), number of parasites per 200 leukocytes, or parasites/mm3. With high parasitemias, the direct counting of parasites and erythrocytes in a thin film will provide an accurate determination. A negative report should be accompanied by a report comment that a single negative set of smears does not exclude the diagnosis of malaria. Serial malaria smears may be performed to monitor therapy. Parasitemia normally resolves within 2 to 3 days following therapy with an appropriate drug. Continued parasitemia at day 3 or failure of the parasitemia to decrease by 75% within the first 48 hours following treatment is an indication of drug resistance. However, gametocytes may continue to circulate for up to two weeks after successful cure, and their presence is not an indication that treatment has failed.

Treatment and Drug Resistance

Prophylaxis and therapy of malaria have been recently reviewed (Deen, 2008; Freedman, 2008; Griffith et al., 2007). *P. falciparum* resistant to chloroquine is present in all endemic areas with the exception of Central America and the Caribbean. In addition resistance to other drugs, including sulfadoxine/pyrimethamine (Fansidar) and mefloquine, is present in many areas and is expanding rapidly. With expanding drug resistance, many countries in endemic areas have instituted first-line treatment of *P. falciparum* with artemisinin combination therapies (ACT), including artesunate-mefloquine, artemether-lumefantrine, and artesunate-amodiaquine. Unfortunately, resistance to artesunate-mefloquine has already appeared in Southeast Asia (Rogers et al, 2006); widespread

resistance to ACT would pose a serious problem to malaria control. Current information on the distribution of drug resistant *P. falciparum* may be obtained from the Centers for Disease Control and Prevention, Malaria Hotline, in Atlanta (Phone: 770-488-7788). The combinations of quinine or quinidine and doxycycline, or of atovaquone and proguanil remain effective against most strains of *P. falciparum*. Therapy of chloroquine resistant *P. falciparum* is a complex and rapidly evolving field, and consultation with an infectious diseases specialist is essential. Current treatment guidelines from the US CDC are available at www.cdc.gov/malaria/pdf/clinicalguidance.pdf. Chloroquine resistant *P. vivax* emerged in a few areas in the 1990s and has continued to spread (Baird et al., 1991); primaquine tolerance has also been reported (Spudick et al., 2005).

Drug and Vaccine Development

Evidence suggests that a malaria vaccine may be attainable. First, residents of malaria endemic areas who do not succumb to malaria in early childhood develop a limited clinical immunity that greatly reduces their risk of severe disease and death when they become infected. Second, human volunteers immunized with radiation-attenuated sporozoites develop solid sterile immunity to sporozoite challenge. A wide variety of approaches have been used to develop vaccines targeting the pre-erythrocytic or erythrocytic stage of the parasite, including synthetic peptides, recombinant viral particles, DNA vaccines, heterologous prime-boost combinations of DNA and recombinant viral vaccines, and attenuated whole-organism vaccines. The current state of clinical testing of malaria vaccines has been recently reviewed (Takala and Plowe, 2009; Vekemans and Ballou, 2008). No vaccine is yet available for clinical use.

BABESIA

The genus *Babesia* includes approximately 100 species that are transmitted by ticks of the genus *Ixodes* and infect a variety of wild and domestic animals (Vannier and Krause, 2009; Vannier et al., 2008). The taxonomy and phylogeny of *Babesia* has been recently reviewed (Hunfeld et al., 2008). In the United States, *B. microti*, the recently described species *B. duncani*, and MO1 (Herwaldt et al., 1996), a strain closely related to *B. divergens* (Gray, 2006), infect humans. In Europe, the bovine parasites, *B. bovis* and *B. divergens*, have been isolated from human patients. These geographic ranges are not strict; recently infection by *B. microti* has been reported from both Europe and Japan, and infection with a *B. divergens*-like organism was reported in the northwest United States (Herwaldt, 2004).

Life Cycle

While the life cycle of *Babesia* is roughly similar to that of *Plasmodium*, there are a number of important differences (Figure 6.3). No exoerythrocytic stage occurs in *Babesia*; sporozoites injected by the bite of an infected tick invade erythrocytes directly, and the trophozoites reproduce by binary fission rather than schizogony. Also gametocytes have not been morphologically distinguished from trophozoites. As in *Plasmodium*, fertilization of gametes occurs in the insect intestine within the blood meal, and the zygotes pass through the intestinal epithelium to the hemolymph. In *Plasmodium*, sporogony occurs in oocysts attached to the trans-luminal aspect of the mosquito intestine, and sporozoites released from oocysts migrate to the salivary glands; in *Babesia*, fertilized gametes migrate through the tick intestinal wall, through the

hemolymph and on to the salivary glands where they develop into sporoblasts. The production of sporozoites from sporoblasts occurs when the tick begins to take a blood meal; the resulting sporozoites are injected into the host during the final hours of attachment and feeding.

ICD-10 Codes

Depending on the species and/or complications, there are a number of relevant ICD-10 Codes that are available. These can be seen in Table 6.1.

Epidemiology

Babesiosis is transmitted by the bite of infected *Ixodes scapularis* ticks, and outbreaks of human infection have been described in the northeast, midwest, and west coast of the United States, in Europe, and in Japan. Relatively few cases of babesiosis have been reported in the United States, 10 to 12 cases per year in New York and Nantucket over the past 30 years (Homer et al., 1997). However, because babesiosis is

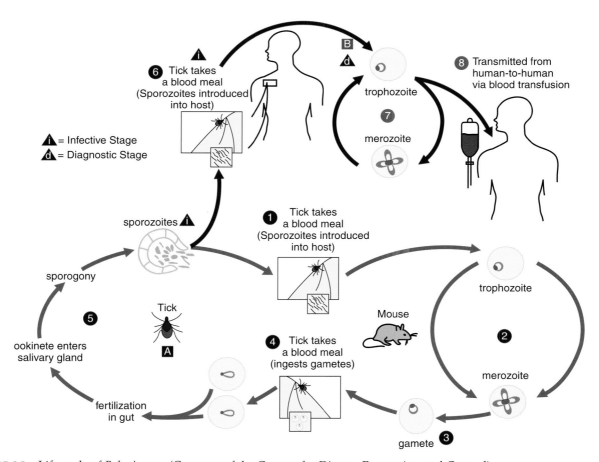

FIGURE 6.3 Life cycle of *Babesia* spp. (Courtesy of the Centers for Disease Prevention and Control)

a mild and self-limiting infection in most persons, the number of unreported infections may be much higher. Serological surveys of blood donors have shown a seroprevalence of 3 to 8% for antibodies to *B. microti* (Homer et al., 1997). With the exception of a few cases attributed to newly described *Babesia* spp. (Herwaldt et al., 1996, 2004; Persing et al., 1995; Quick et al., 1993), babesiosis in the United States is caused by *B. microti*. In Europe, a growing number cases of babesiosis have been reported (Hunfeld et al., 2008), principally infections of splenectomized individuals with *B. divergens*; these infections are clinically serious, with a mortality rate of 42% (Hayman, et al., 2010; Semel et al., 2009). A few cases of transfusion-associated babesiosis, usually involving transmission of *B. microti* from an asymptomatic donor, have been reported from the United States.

The host ranges of *B. microti* and *B. divergens* are wide, and any mammal that is a host for *I. scapularis* ticks can be a reservoir of infection. *Babesia* spp. share both vectors and animal reservoirs, namely *Ixodes* ticks and white-footed mice, with several other tick-borne pathogens, including the agents of Lyme disease and human granulocytic ehrlichiosis. Coinfection with *B. microti* and *Borrelia burgdorferi* occur, and approximately 10% of Lyme disease patients in Babesia-endemic areas may be infected with *B. microti*. Lyme disease patients coinfected with *B. microti* report more severe symptoms than those infected with either agent alone (Krause et al., 1996). *B. venatorum* (formerly EU1) in Europe, together with *B. odocoilei* that infects white-tail deer in the United States, form a sister group to that of *B. divergens*. Three cases with *B. venatorum* have been documented in men beyond 50 years of age who had been splenectomized (Herwaldt et al., 2003; Haselbarth et al., 2007).

Clinical Disease

Clinical presentations range from mild or asymptomatic infection through a fulminant illness clinically similar to malaria and characterized by high fever, myalgias, malaise, fatigue, hepatosplenomegaly, and anemia. Infection with *B. microti* in the United States usually occurs in nonsplenectomized individuals and is relatively mild. However, infections with the more recently described babesias from the United States and with *B. divergens* in Europe occur in splenectomized or immunocompromised individuals and are clinically more severe. Overall, mortality among clinically apparent cases of *B. microti* infection in the United States is 5%, while that in *B. divergens* infection in Europe is 40%. In both the United

States and Europe, risk factors for severe disease include increasing age, splenectomy, and immune compromise.

Pathophysiology

These patients may exhibit fever, pallor, mild splenomegaly or hepatomegaly, and recovery can last over a year. The most common complications of severe babesiosis include jaundice, retinal infarcts, ecchymoses and petechiae, respiratory failure, congestive heart failure, DIC, liver and renal failure, and splenic rupture. In splenectomized patients with *B. divergens* infections in Europe, high fever with severe intravascular hemolysis results in hemoglobinemia, hemoglobinuria, and jaundice. More than half the cases report a rapid onset of renal failure and pulmonary edema; coma has also been reported.

Diagnosis

The diagnosis of babesiosis should be considered based on appropriate clinical symptoms and a travel history to endemic areas, exposure to ticks, or recent blood transfusion. Examination of stained thin blood smears is the most direct approach to diagnosis. The appearance of *Babesia* in thin films is shown in Figure 6.4. Although the trophozoites of *Babesia* can be confused with *Plasmodium* rings, particularly the small-ring trophozoites of *P. falciparum*, *Babesia* can be distinguished from *P. falciparum* by several criteria. *Babesia* trophozoites are quite variable in size and the smallest are smaller than *P. falciparum* rings. Extracellular trophozoites and multiply infected erythrocytes are more common in *Babesia*. Finally, diagnostic tetrads, the Maltese cross, may be present in some cases with *Babesia*. Low parasitemias may occur, particularly in chronic infections in nonsplenectomized patients; in such cases diagnosis may require serologic testing, hamster inoculation, or PCR amplification (Vannier and Krause, 2009).

Treatment

Mild cases with *B. microti* usually resolve spontaneously. In more serious cases treatment with clindamycin and quinine, or atovaquone and azithromycin, is standard. In very severe cases of *B. microti* infection and in *B. divergens* infection in splenectomized or immunosuppressed patients, therapy may be supplemented with exchange transfusion. Appropriate personal protective measures including use of long pants, long sleeved shirts, and insect repellant may reduce the risk of infection when outdoors in endemic areas (Vannier and Krause, 2009).

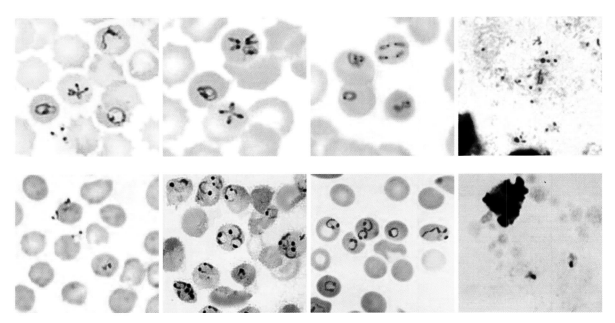

FIGURE 6.4 Thin blood films containing *Babesia* spp. Top row, left, images 1, 2, and 3, trophs/rings of *Babesia* spp. (note the multiple rings/RBC, very pleomorphic organisms); image 4, thick film showing small trophs (often higher parasitemia than seen with *P. falciparum*). Bottom row, Left, images 1, 2, and 3, early rings of *Plasmodium falciparum* (note the similarities, image 2 probably autopsy blood/very heavy infection); image 4, thick film showing two ring forms.

TOXOPLASMA

Toxoplasma gondii is a protozoan parasite that infects humans and most other species of warm blooded animals. Members of the cat family Felidae are the only known definitive hosts for the sexual stages of *T. gondii* and are the main reservoirs of infection. The three stages of this obligate intracellular parasite are (1) tachyzoites (trophozoites), which rapidly proliferate and destroy infected cells during acute infection, (2) bradyzoites, which slowly multiply in tissue cysts, and (3) sporozoites in oocysts. Tachyzoites and bradyzoites occur in body tissues; oocysts are excreted in cat feces.

Life Cycle

Cats become infected with *T. gondii* by the ingestion of infected animals or by ingestion of oocysts (Figure 6.5). Outdoor cats are much more likely to become infected than domestic indoor cats. After tissue cysts or oocysts are ingested by the cat, organisms are released and invade epithelial cells of the small intestine where there is an asexual cycle followed by a sexual cycle with the formation of unsporulated oocysts that are excreted. The oocyst takes 1 to 5 days after excretion to become sporulated (infective). Although cats shed oocysts for 1 to 2 weeks, numbers often exceed 100,000 per g of feces. Oocysts

survive in the environment for several months to more than a year and are very resistant to disinfectants, freezing, and drying; however, they are killed by heating to 70°C for 10 minutes (Remington et al., 2006). Human infection may be acquired by (1) ingestion of undercooked contaminated meat containing *T. gondii* cysts, particularly pork, lamb, and venison; (2) ingestion of oocysts from food, soil, or water contaminated with cat feces; (3) organ transplantation or blood transfusion; (4) transplacental transmission; and (5) accidental inoculation of tachyzoites. The two major routes of infection for humans are oral and congenital. In humans, ingesting either the tissue cyst or the oocyst results in the rupture of the cyst wall, which releases organisms that invade the intestinal epithelium, disseminate throughout the body, and multiply within the cells. The host cell dies and releases tachyzoites that invade adjacent cells, and the process continues. The immune system stimulates the tachyzoites to transform into bradyzoites and form tissue cysts, most commonly in skeletal muscle, myocardium, and brain; these cysts remain throughout the life of the host. The actively proliferating tachyzoites are seen in the early, more acute phases of the infection. The cysts contain the more slowly growing trophozoites or bradyzoites. Bradyzoites encyst approximately 8 to 10 days after entry into the host and differ from tachyzoites in being the only stage to initiate the enteroepithelial cycle

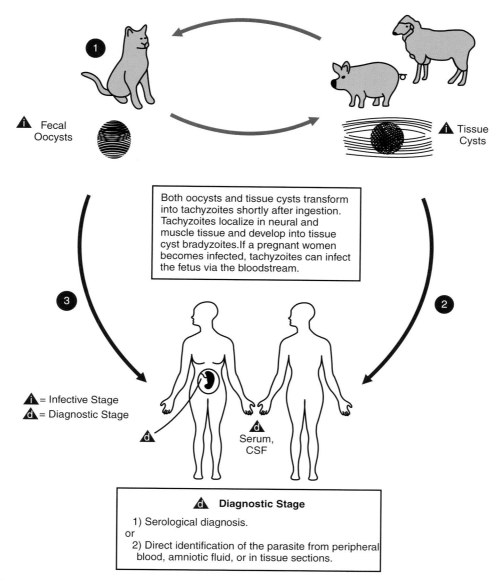

FIGURE 6.5   Life cycle of *Toxoplasma gondii*. (Courtesy of the Centers for Disease Prevention and Control)

and transform into oocysts in the feline intestine. Recrudescence of clinical disease may occur if the host becomes immunosuppressed and the cysts rupture, releasing the parasites.

ICD-10 Codes

Depending on the species and/or complications, there are a number of relevant ICD-10 Codes that are available. These can be seen in Table 6.1.

Epidemiology

Serologic prevalence data indicate that toxoplasmosis is one of the most common infections of humans throughout the world. Since *T. gondii* organisms are rarely detected in humans with infection, serologic examination is used to confirm infection by detecting *Toxoplasma*-specific antibodies. The prevalence of positive serologic titers increases with age. Infection tends to be more common in warm climates and at lower altitudes than in cold climates and mountainous regions. Distribution is probably related to conditions favoring the sporulation and survival of oocysts. Differences in the infection prevalence within the same locale are also probably due to differences in exposure. A high prevalence of infection in France (50–85%) is related to a preference for eating raw or undercooked meat. However, a high prevalence in

Central America is related to the number of stray cats in a climate favoring oocyst survival. Data comparing antibody prevalence in US military recruits in 1962 and 1989 indicated a one-third decrease in seropositivity (Smith et al., 1996). The overall seroprevalence in the United States as determined with specimens collected by the Third National Health and Nutritional Assessment Survey (NHANES III) between 1988 and 1994 among persons 12 or more years of age was found to be 22.5%, with seroprevalence among women of childbearing age (15–44 years) of 15% (Jones et al., 2001). More recently NHANES data showed that *T. gondii* seroprevalence declined in US-born persons 12 to 49 years old from 14.1% in 1988 to 1994 to 9.0% in 1999 to 2004 (Jones et al., 2007).

Risk factors for *T. gondii* infection identified include eating raw or undercooked pork, mutton, lamb, beef, mince meat products, oysters, clams, or mussels, and wild game meat, kitten ownership, cleaning the cat litter box, contact with soil (gardening and yard work), and eating raw or unwashed vegetables or fruits (Elmore et al., 2010; Jones et al., 2009). Recommendations for prevention of toxoplasmosis in pregnant women include (1) food should be cooked to safe temperatures (beef, lamb, and veal roasts and steaks to at least 145°F; pork, ground meat, and wild game to 160°F; poultry to 180°F); (2) fruits and vegetables should be peeled or washed thoroughly before eating; (3) cutting boards, dishes, counters, utensils, and hands should always be washed with hot soapy water after they have contacted raw meat, poultry, seafood, or unwashed fruits or vegetables; (4) pregnant women should wear gloves when gardening and during any contact with soil or sand because cat waste might be in soil or sand, and wash hands afterward; and (5) pregnant women should avoid changing cat litter if possible. If no one else is available to change the cat litter, pregnant women should use gloves, then wash their hands thoroughly. The litter box should be changed daily because *T. gondii* oocysts require more than one day to become infectious. Pregnant women should keep their cats inside and not adopt or handle stray cats. Cats should be fed only canned or dried commercial food or well-cooked table food, not raw or undercooked meats.

Clinical Disease

Toxoplasmosis can be categorized into four groups: (1) acquired in the immunocompetent patient, (2) acquired or reactivated in the immunodeficient patient, (3) congenital, and (4) ocular.

Acquired infection with *Toxoplasma* in immunocompetent individuals is generally an asymptomatic infection. However, 10 to 20% of patients with acute infection may develop cervical lymphadenopathy and/or a flu-like illness. The clinical course is benign and self-limited with symptoms resolving within weeks to months.

Immunodeficient patients often have central nervous system (CNS) disease but may have myocarditis or pneumonitis. In patients with AIDS, toxoplasmic encephalitis is the most common cause of intracerebral mass lesions and is probably due to reactivation of chronic infection (Pereira-Chioccola et al., 2009). Toxoplasmosis in patients being treated with immunosuppressive drugs may be due to either newly acquired or reactivated latent infection (Schmidt-Hieber at al., 2009).

Congenital toxoplasmosis results from an acute primary infection acquired by the mother during pregnancy. The incidence and severity of congenital toxoplasmosis vary with the trimester during which infection was acquired. Because treatment of the mother may reduce the severity of symptoms in the infant due to congenital infection, prompt and accurate diagnosis is extremely important. Many infants with subclinical infection at birth will subsequently develop signs or symptoms of congenital toxoplasmosis; however, treatment may help prevent subsequent symptoms.

Ocular toxoplasmosis, an important cause of chorioretinitis in the United States, may result from congenital or acquired infection, which is more common than congenital infection. Congenitally infected patients are often asymptomatic until the second or third decade of life, when lesions develop in the eye presumably due to cyst rupture and subsequent release of tachyzoites and bradyzoites. Chorioretinitis is characteristically bilateral with congenital infection but is often unilateral in individuals with acute acquired *T. gondii* infection.

Pathophysiology

Acquired Infections in Immunocompetent Individuals

In approximately 90% of cases, no clinical symptoms are seen during the acute infection. However, 10 to 20% of patients with acute infection may develop painless cervical lymphadenopathy. This presentation is benign and self-limited, with symptoms resolving within weeks to months. In some rare cases acute visceral manifestations are seen. In reviewing the possible link between *T. gondii* and schizophrenia, some cases of acute toxoplasmosis in adults are associated with psychiatric symptoms such as delusions and hallucinations (Torrey and Yolken, 2003).

Infections in the Immunocompromised Patient

Infections in the compromised patient can result in severe complications. Conditions that may influence the course of the disease include various malignancies (e.g., Hodgkin's disease, non-Hodgkin's lymphomas, leukemias, and solid tumors), collagen vascular disease, organ transplantation, and AIDS. In the immunocompromised patient, the CNS is primarily involved, with diffuse encephalopathy, meningoencephalitis, or cerebral mass lesions. More than half of these patients will show altered mental state, motor impairment, seizures, abnormal reflexes, and other neurologic sequelae. In these groups, studies indicate that most patients receiving chemotherapy for toxoplasmosis will improve significantly or have complete remission. However, in those with AIDS, therapy must be continued for long periods to maintain a clinical response (Pereira-Chioccola et al., 2009).

Transplant Recipients. Disease severity depends on prior exposure to *T. gondii* by the donor and recipient, the type of organ transplanted, and the level of immunosuppression of the patient. Reactivation of a latent infection or an acute primary infection acquired directly from the transplanted organ are primary causes of disease. Stem cell transplant (SCT) recipients are particularly susceptible to severe toxoplasmosis, primarily due to reactivation of a previously acquired latent infection. If SCT patients have a positive serology prior to transplantation, they are at risk for severe disseminated toxoplasmosis (Menotti, 2003). All potential transplant recipients should be tested for *Toxoplasma*-specific IgG antibodies to determine their antibody status. Individuals with acute acquired infection often produce detectable IgG and IgM antibodies, while those with reactivation may or may not have an increase in IgG antibodies and normally will not demonstrate an IgM response. Seronegative cardiac transplant recipients who receive an organ from a seropositive donor may develop toxoplasmic myocarditis; this disease presentation may also mimic organ rejection.

AIDS Patients. Patients who are infected with *T. gondii* risk developing disease when their CD4$^+$ T-lymphocyte count falls below 100,000/ ml. Fever and malaise usually precede the first neurologic symptoms; headache, confusion, seizures, or other focal signs strongly suggest the diagnosis of toxoplasmosis. *Toxoplasma* encephalitis (TE) has been reported as a life-threatening opportunistic infection among patients with AIDS prior to the use of highly active antiretroviral therapies (HAART). This condition is fatal if untreated.

Congenital Infections

Congenital infections may be severe if the mother acquires the infection during the first or second trimester of pregnancy. At birth or soon thereafter, symptoms in these infants may include retinochoroiditis, cerebral calcification, and occasionally hydrocephalus or microcephaly. Symptoms of congenital central nervous system (CNS) involvement may not appear until several years later. The characteristic symptoms of hydrocephalus, cerebral calcifications, and chorioretinitis resulting in mental retardation, epilepsy, and impaired vision represent the most severe form of the disease. Cerebral lesions may calcify, providing retrospective signs of congenital infection.

Ocular Infections

Chorioretinitis in immunocompetent patients is generally due to an earlier congenital infection. Patients may be asymptomatic until the second or third decade when cysts may rupture with lesions then developing in the eye. The number of people who develop chorioretinitis later in life is unknown but may represent over two-thirds. Chorioretinitis is usually bilateral in patients with congenitally acquired infection, and is generally unilateral in patients with recently acquired infection.

Diagnosis

The diagnosis of toxoplasmosis is critical in these four groups: pregnant women with infection during gestation, congenitally infected newborns, patients with chorioretinitis, and immunosuppressed individuals. Diagnosis is usually made using serologic procedures. A guideline for the clinical use and interpretation of serologic tests for *Toxoplasma gondii* was published (Wilson and McAuley, 2003) by the Clinical and Laboratory Standards Institute (formerly called the National Committee for Clinical Laboratory Standards or NCCLS) and is available for purchase on their website at www.clsi.org. Other diagnostic procedures include PCR, examining biopsy specimens, buffy coat cells, or cerebrospinal fluid or isolating the organism in tissue culture or in laboratory animals. Because many individuals have been exposed to *T. gondii* and might have cysts within the tissues, recovery of organisms from tissue culture or animal inoculation may be misleading, since the organisms may be isolated but may not be the etiologic agent of disease (Figure 6.6). For this reason serologic tests are often recommended as the diagnostic approach

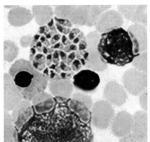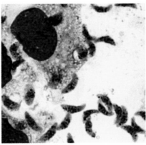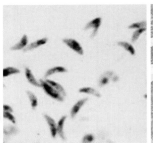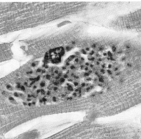

FIGURE 6.6 *Toxoplasma gondii*. Left, tachyzoites in bone marrow; image 2, tachyzoites in bone marrow; image 3, tachyzoites isolated from body fluid; image 4, bradyzoites in tissue (resting cyst forms) (image 4, Courtesy of the Centers for Disease Prevention and Control).

of choice. However, two representative situations in which the detection of organisms may be very significant are (1) tachyzoite-positive smears and/or tissue cultures inoculated from cerebrospinal fluid and (2) in patients with acute pulmonary disease, the demonstration of tachyzoites in smears of bronchoalveolar lavage (BAL) fluid stained with any of the blood stains, some tachyzoites being extracellular and some intracellular.

Determination of Immune Status

Baseline information about an individual's immune status is useful in the following situations: (1) before conception, (2) before receiving immunosuppressive therapy, and (3) after the initial determination of positive HIV-1 status. Screening one serum specimen with a sensitive test for IgG antibodies, such as DT, IFA, or EIA, is sufficient. A negative test result indicates that the patient has not been infected. A positive result of any degree indicates infection with *T. gondii* at some undetermined time.

Acute Acquired Infections

If an acute acquired infection is suspected, the patient's serum should be tested for *Toxoplasma*-specific antibodies. In an immunocompetent individual a negative result in the Sabin–Feldman dye test (DT), IgG IFA test, or IgG EIA essentially excludes the diagnosis of acute *Toxoplasma* infection. Seroconversion from a negative titer to a positive titer or of more than a fourfold increase in titer confirms the diagnosis of recent infection when specimens drawn several weeks apart are tested in parallel using the same test. However, often specimens are drawn after titers have peaked; thus it is too late to observe titer changes after initial infection. The presence of typical lymphadenopathy, the presence of a high DT or IgG IFA titer ($\geq$300 IU/ml or $\geq$1:1000) and the presence of specific IgM is indicative of acute infection. If the

patient has symptoms compatible with toxoplasmosis but the IgG titer is low, a follow-up test 3 weeks later should show an increase in the antibody titer if the illness is due to acute toxoplasmosis and the host is not severely immunosuppressed.

Results of an EIA for IgM and an IgG avidity assay can provide additional evidence for or against acute infection when IgG antibodies are present (Montoya and Remington, 1995; Roberts et al., 2001). A negative IgM test essentially rules out infection in the previous 6 months. A positive IgM titer combined with a positive IgG titer may be suggestive of acute infection, due to persistent IgM antibodies, or may be a false-positive reaction.

Pregnancy

Congenital toxoplasmosis occurs when a woman passes the infection to her fetus after acquiring a primary infection during pregnancy or, more rarely, when a pregnant woman is immunocompromised and a previously acquired infection is reactivated. The rate of transmission of infection to the fetus ranges from 11% in the first trimester to 90% in the late third trimester, with an overall transmission rate of approximately 40 to 50%.

Immunocompetent women who have the IgG antibody before conception are considered immune and have very little risk for transmission of infection to the fetus, while women who are seronegative are considered at risk for infection. If a woman is first tested after conception and has *Toxoplasma*-specific IgG antibodies, IgM and IgG avidity testing should be done to determine if acute infection has occurred during pregnancy (Roberts et al., 2001). A high avidity result in the first 12 weeks of pregnancy essentially rules out an infection acquired during gestation. A low IgG avidity result cannot be used as an indicator of recent infection because some individuals have persistent low IgG avidity for many months after infection. Immunodiagnosis of acute infection in a pregnant woman should be confirmed by a toxoplasmosis reference laboratory prior to intervention (Montoya and Remington, 2008).

Newborn

Diagnosis of *Toxoplasma* infection in the newborn often requires a combination of serologic testing, parasite isolation, and nonspecific findings (McLeod et al., 2009). A child suspected of having congenital toxoplasmosis should have a thorough general, neurologic, and ophthalmologic examination and a computed tomographic scan of the head (magnetic resonance imaging does not demonstrate calcifications). Because the diagnosis can take several months to confirm, clinicians may have to treat patients based on early signs, symptoms, and serology while awaiting definitive confirmation.

Persistent or increasing IgG antibody levels in the infant compared with the mother as measured by the DT or IFA test, and/or positive result for *Toxoplasma*-specific IgM or IgA are diagnostic of congenital infection. Demonstration by IgG and IgM Western blots in the newborn of serum antibodies that are directed against unique *Toxoplasma* epitopes not found in the mother's serum is also evidence of congenital infection (Montoya and Remington, 2009).

Placental leak can lead to false-positive IgM or IgA measurements in the newborn. Positive tests usually must be confirmed by repeat testing of IgM at 2 to 4 days of life and repeat testing for IgA at 10 days of life. Passively transferred maternal IgG has a half life of approximately 1 month. Maternal antibodies can be detected for several months and have been reported up to 1 year of age. The untreated congenitally infected newborn will begin to produce *Toxoplasma*-specific IgG antibody within approximately 3 months. Treatment of the infected child may delay antibody production until 9 months of age and on rare occasion may prevent production altogether. Persistence of a positive IgG result at 12 months of life in the child confirms infection. Demonstration of a decrease in antibody load (*Toxoplasma*-specific IgG antibody divided by total IgG) can be helpful in differentiating maternal antibody from fetal antibody.

Although rarely performed, demonstration of IgM antibody or local *Toxoplasma*-specific IgG antibody production in CSF not contaminated with peripheral blood can help confirm the diagnosis of congenital toxoplasmosis.

A long-term prospective study is currently under way in the United States to define optimal therapeutic regimens for the treatment of congenital toxoplasmosis (Boyer et al., 2005; McAuley et al., 1994).

Ocular Infection

Toxoplasma chorioretinitis results from both acute infection and congenital infection (Holland, 2003, 2004). In addition to demonstrating IgG antibody to *Toxoplasma* in the serum of a person with compatible eye lesions, demonstration of the local production of antibody and detection of parasite DNA in aqueous humor have been used to document active ocular toxoplasmosis (Fekkar et al.; Garweg, 2005; Talabani et al., 2009).

Immunocompromised Host

Immunosuppressed hosts with lymphoma, leukemia, multiple myeloma, carcinoma, neuroblastoma, thymoma, systemic lupus erythematosus, scleroderma, autoimmune hemolytic anemia, and kidney, liver, and heart transplants can have severe, often fatal, toxoplasmosis. The disease is usually associated with reactivation of a latent infection and commonly involves the CNS. Diagnosis can be difficult, since IgM antibody is usually not detectable and the presence of IgG antibody only confirms chronic infection. However, diagnosis can be confirmed by demonstration of the organism histologically or cytologically as replicating within tissue or by isolation or identification of its nucleic acids in a site such as amniotic fluid, CSF, bronchoalveolar fluid, or placenta, in which the encysted organism would not be present as part of a latent infection.

Prior to organ or bone marrow transplantation, patients should be tested for *Toxoplasma*-specific IgG antibodies to determine immune status; they are at risk for either acute acquired infection if they are seronegative before transplantation or at risk for reactivation if they are seropositive before transplantation (Schaffner, 2001). Serial measurement of *Toxoplasma* DNA in peripheral blood by PCR has been advocated by some as a means of monitoring for development of toxoplasmosis in bone marrow transplant patients (Derouin et al., 2008; Edvinsson et al., 2008). Those with acute acquired infection will usually develop detectable *Toxoplasma*-specific IgG and IgM antibodies, while those with reactivation will not have a detectable *Toxoplasma*-specific IgM response. Seronegative transplant recipients of hearts from seropositive donors can develop toxoplasmic myocarditis that mimics organ rejection.

Toxoplasmic encephalitis is the most frequent CNS opportunistic infection of AIDS patients and is fatal if untreated. All HIV-infected persons should be tested for *Toxoplasma*-specific IgG antibodies soon after the diagnosis of HIV infection to detect latent infection (Calderaro et al., 2009). If *Toxoplasma*-seropositive, adult/adolescent patients who have a

CD4+ T-lymphocyte count of under 100/μl should be administered prophylaxis against toxoplasmic encephalitis with trimethoprim-sulfamethoxazole (TMP-SMZ). Most AIDS patients with toxoplasmic encephalitis have demonstrable IgG antibodies to *T. gondii*. However, approximately 3% of AIDS patients with toxoplasmic encephalitis do not have *Toxoplasma*-specific antibody in their serum. Disseminated toxoplasmosis should be considered in the differential diagnosis of immunocompromised patients with culture-negative sepsis, particularly if combined with neurologic, respiratory, or unexplained skin lesions.

Evaluation, Interpretation, and Result Reporting

Situations in which the laboratory will need to provide interpretation of results include acute primary infection in pregnant women and active disease in hosts who are unable to mount the typical immune response, such as fetuses, neonates, or immunosuppressed individuals. Rarely is the mere presence or absence of *Toxoplasma* IgG sufficient to guide the clinician. The laboratory will need to use additional testing (avidity, IgM, IgA, etc.) in an attempt to define the timing of infection in the case of pregnant women, or the presence of actively replicating parasites (PCR, tachyzoites, etc.) in the case of the fetus/neonate or immunosuppressed host.

Treatment

In general, physicians treat *T. gondii* infection in four circumstances: (1) pregnant women with acute infection to prevent fetal infection, (2) congenitally infected infants, (3) immune-suppressed persons, usually with reactivated disease, and (4) acute and recurrent ocular disease (Holland, 2003, 2004). Drugs are also prescribed for preventive or suppressive treatment in HIV-infected persons (MMWR, 2009a, b). The currently recommended drugs work primarily against the actively dividing tachyzoite form of *T. gondii* and do not eradicate encysted organisms (bradyzoites).

The most common drug combination for congenital toxoplasmosis consists of pyrimethamine and a sulfonamide (sulfadiazine is recommended in the United States), plus folinic acid in the form of leucovorin calcium to protect the bone marrow from the toxic effects of pyrimethamine. Spiramycin (available through the FDA, phone 301-796-1600) is recommended for pregnant women with acute toxoplasmosis when fetal infection has not been confirmed in an attempt to prevent transmission of *T. gondii*

from the mother to the fetus (Montoya and Liesenfeld, 2004). Pyrimethamine and sulfadiazine (plus leucovorin) are used to treat infants with congenital toxoplasmosis with improved outcomes compared with historic controls (Remington et al., 2006).

In immunosuppressed persons with toxoplasmosis, pyrimethamine and sulfadiazine plus leucovorin is the preferred treatment (MMWR, 2009a, b). Clindamycin is a second alternative for use in combination with pyrimethamine and leucovorin in those who cannot tolerate sulfonamides. Atovaquone in combination with either pyrimethamine or sulfadiazine can be considered for treatment in some less severely affected adult patients (Montoya and Leisenfeld, 2004). In general, alternative drugs such as azithromycin, clarithromycin, and dapsone should be used in combination with another drug, preferably pyrimethamine for patients intolerant to first-line therapy (Montoya and Remington, 2008).

Because relapse often occurs in HIV-infected patients, maintenance therapy with pyrimethamine plus sulfadiazine (first choice) or pyrimethamine plus clindamycin (alternative) is recommended (MMWR, 2009a, b). For prophylaxis to prevent an initial episode of *T. gondii* in *Toxoplasma*-seropositive persons with a CD4+ T-lymphocyte counts less than 100 cells/μl, trimethoprim-sulfamethoxazole is recommended as the first choice with alternatives of dapsone plus pyrimethamine, or atovaquone with or without pyrimethamine. Leucovorin is given with all regimens including pyrimethamine (MMWR, 2009a, b).

Pyrimethamine and sulfadiazine are often used for ocular disease (Holland, 2004). Clindamycin, in combination with other antiparasitic medications, is also prescribed for ocular disease. In addition to antiparasitic drugs, physicians may add corticosteroids to reduce ocular inflammation.

REFERENCES

BAIRD JK. 2004. Chloroquine resistance in *Plasmodium vivax*. Antimicrob Agents Chemother 48:4075–83.

BOYER KM., HOLFELS E, ROIZEN N, SWISHER C, MACK D, REMINGTON J, WITHERS S, MEIER P, MCLEOD R. 2005. Risk factors for *Toxoplasma gondii* infection in mothers of infants with congenital toxoplasmosis: Implications for prenatal management and screening. Am J Obstet Gynecol 192:564–71.

BARKER RH, BANCHONGAKSORN T, COURVAL JM, SUWONKERD W, RIMWUNGTRAGOON K, WIRTH DF. 1992. A simple method to detect *Plasmodium falciparum* directly from blood using the polymerase chain reaction. Am J Trop Med Hyg 46:416–26.

BRONNER U, DIVIS PC, FARNERT A, SINGH B. 2009. Swedish traveler with *Plasmodium knowlesi* malaria after visiting Malaysian Borneo. Malar J 8:15.

CALDERARO A, PERUZZI S, PICCOLO G, GORRINI C, MONTECCHINI S, ROSSI S, CHEZZI C, DETTORI G. 2009. Laboratory diagnosis of *Toxoplasma gondii* infection. Int J Med Sci 6:135–6.

Centers for Disease Control and Prevention. 2003. Local transmission of *Plasmodium vivax* malaria—Palm Beach County, Florida. MMWR 52:908–11.

Centers for Disease Control and Prevention. 2009a. Guidelines for prevention and treatment of opportunistic infections among HIV-infected adults and adolescents. MMWR 58(RR-04):1–216.

Centers for Disease Control and Prevention. 2009b. Guidelines for prevention and treatment of opportunistic infections among HIV-exposed and infected children. MMWR 58(RR-11):1–166.

Centers for Disease Control and Prevention. 2009c. Simian malaria in a U.S. traveler—New York, 2008. MMWR 58:229–32.

COX-SINGH J., DAVIS TM, LEE KS, SHAMSUL SS, MATUSOP A, RATNAM S, RAHMAN HA, CONWAY DJ, SINGH B. 2008. *Plasmodium knowlesi* malaria in humans is widely distributed and potentially life threatening. Clin Infect Dis 46:165–71.

CRAIG MH, SHARP BL. 1997. Comparative evaluation of four techniques for the diagnosis of *Plasmodium falciparum* infections. Trans R Soc Trop Med Hyg 91:279–82.

DEEN JL, VON SEIDLEIN L, DONDORP A. 2008. Therapy of uncomplicated malaria in children: a review of treatment principles, essential drugs and current recommendations. Trop Med Int Health 13:1111–30.

DEROUIN F, PELLOUX H, on behalf of the ESCMID Study Group on Clinical Parasitology. 2008. Prevention of toxoplasmosis in transplant patients. Clin Microbiol Infect 14:1089–1101.

EDVINSSON B, LUNDQUIST J, LJUNGMAN P, RINGDEN O, EVENGARD B. 2008. Prevention of toxoplasmosis in transplant patients. APMIS. 116:1965–67.

ELMORE SA, JONES JL, CONRAD PA, PATTON S, LINDSAY DS, DUBEY JP. 2010. *Toxoplasma gondii*: epidemiology, feline clinical aspects, and prevention. Trends Parasitol 26:190–6.

ERDMAN L K, KAIN KC. 2008. Molecular diagnostic and surveillance tools for global malaria control. Travel Med Infect Dis 6:82–99.

FEKKAR A, BODAGHI B, TOUAFEK F, LE HOANG P, MAZIER D, PARIS L. 2008. Comparison of immunoblotting, calculation of the Goldmann–Witmer coefficient, and real-time PCR using aqueous humor samples for diagnosis of ocular toxoplasmosis. J Clin Microbiol 46:1965–7.

FREEDMAN D O. 2008. Clinical practice. Malaria prevention in short-term travelers. N Engl J Med 359:603–12.

GARCIA LS. 2010 Malaria. Clin Lab Med 30:93–129.

GARCIA LS. 2007. Diagnostic Medical Parasitology, 5th ed. ASM Press, Washington, DC.

GARWEG J G. 2005. Determinants of immunodiagnostic success in human ocular toxoplasmosis. Parasite Immunol 27:61–8.

GRAY J S. 2006. Identity of the causal agents of human babesiosis in Europe. Int J Med Microbiol 296(suppl 40):131–6.

GRIFFITH K S., LEWIS LS, MALI S, PARISE ME. 2007. Treatment of malaria in the United States: a systematic review. JAMA 297:2264–77.

HAN ET, WATANABE R, SATTABONGKOT J, KHUNTIRAT B, SIRICHAISINTHOP J, IRIKO H, JIN L, TAKEO S, TSUBOI T. 2007. Detection of four *Plasmodium* species by genus- and species-specific loop-mediated isothermal amplification for clinical diagnosis. J Clin Microbiol 45:2521–8.

HASELBARTH A, TENTER M, BRADE V, KRIEGER G, HUNFELD KP. 2007. First case of human babesiosis in Germany—clinical presentation and molecular characterization of the pathogen. Inter J Med Microbiol 297:197–204.

HAYMAN P, COCHEZ, C, HOFHUIS A, VANDER GLESSEN J, SPRONG H, PORTER SR, LOSSON B, SAEGERMAN, C, DONOSO-MANTKE O, NIEDRIG M, PAPA A. 2010. A clear and present danger: tick-borne diseases in Europe. Expert Rev Anti Infect Ther 8:33–50

HERWALDT BL, CACCIÒ S, GHERLINZONI F, ASPOCK H, SLEMENDA SB, PICCALUGA P, MARTINELLI G, EDELHOFER R, HOLLENSTEIN U, POLETTI G, PAMPIGLIONE S, LOSCHENBERGER K, TURA S, PIENIAZEK NJ. 2003. Molecular characterization of a non-*Babesia divergens* organism causing zoonotic babesiosis in Europe. Emerg Infect Dis 9(8):942–8.

HERWALDT BL, DE BRUYN G, PIENIAZEK NJ, HOMER M, LOFY KH, SLEMENDA SB, FRITSCHE TR, PERSING DH, LIMAYE AP. 2004. *Babesia divergens*-like infection, Washington State. Emerg Infect Dis 10:622–9.

HERWALDT BL, PERSING DH, PRECIGOUT EA, GOFF WL, MATHIESEN DA, TAYLOR PW, EBERHARD ML, GORENFLOT AF. 1996. A fatal case of babesiosis in Missouri: identification of another piroplasm that infects humans. Ann Intern Med 124:643–50.

HOLLAND GN. 2003. Ocular toxoplasmosis: a global reassessment. Part I: Epidemiology and course of disease. Am J Ophthalmol 136:973–88.

HOLLAND GN. 2004. Ocular toxoplasmosis: a global reassessment. Part II: Disease manifestations and management. Am J Ophthalmol 137:1–17.

HOMER M J, AGUILAR-DELFIN I, TELFORD SR III KRAUS PJ, PERSING DH. 2000. Babesiosis. Clin Microbiol Rev 13:451–69.

HUNFELD K P, HILDEBRANDT A, GRAY JS. 2008. Babesiosis: recent insights into an ancient disease. Int J Parasitol 38:1219–37.

JONES JL, DARGELAS V, ROBERTS J, PRESS C, REMINGTON JS, MONTOYA JG. 2009. Risk factors for *Toxoplasma gondii* infection in the United States. Clin Infect Dis 49:878–84.

JONES JL, KRUSZON-MORAN D, SANDERS-LEWIS K, WILSON M. 2007. *Toxoplasma gondii* infection in the United States, 1999–2004, decline from the prior decade. Am J Trop Med Hyg 77:405–10.

JONES JL, KRUSZON-MORAN D, WILSON M, MCQUILLAN G, NAVIN T, MCAULEY JB. 2001. *Toxoplasma gondii* infection in the United States: seroprevalence and risk factors. Am J Epidemiol 154:357–65.

KRAUSE PJ, TELFORD, III SR, SPIELMAN A, SIKAND V, CHRISTIANSON D, BURKE G, BRASSARD P, POLLACK R, PECK J, PERSING DH. 1996. Concurrent Lyme disease and babesiosis. Evidence for increased severity and duration of illness. JAMA 275:1657–60.

KYRONSEPPA H, TIULA E, REPO H, LAHDEVIRTA J. 1989. Diagnosis of *falciparum* malaria delayed by long incubation period and misleading presenting systems: life-saving role of manual leucocyte differential count. Scand J Infect Dis 21:117–8.

LUCHAVEZ J, ESPINO F, CURAMENG P, ESPINA R, BELL D, CHIODINI P, NOLDER D, SUTHERLAND C, LEE KS, SINGH B. 2008. Human Infections with *Plasmodium knowlesi*, the Philippines. Emerg Infect Dis 14:811–3.

MCAULEY J, BOYER KM, PATEL D, METS M, SWISHER C, ROIZEN N, WOLTERS C, STEIN L, STEIN M, SCHEY W, et al. 1994. Early and longitudinal evaluations of treated infants and children and untreated historical patients with congenital toxoplasmosis: the Chicago Collaborative Treatment Trial. Clin Infect Dis 18:38–72.

MCLEOD R, KIEFFER F, SAUTTER M, HOSTEN T, PELLOUX H. 2009. Why prevent, diagnose, and treat congenital toxoplasmosis? Mem Inst Oswaldo Cruz 104:320–44.

MENOTTI J, VILELA G, ROMAND S, GARIN YJ, ADES L, GLUCKMAN E, DEROUIN F, RIBAUD P. 2003. Comparison of PCR-enzyme-linked immunosorbent assay and real-time PCR assay for diagnosis of an unusual case of cerebral toxoplasmosis in a stem cell transplant recipient. J Clin Microbiol 41:5313–6.

MONTOYA JF, REMINGTON JS. 2008. Management of *Toxoplasma gondii* infection during pregnancy. Clin Infect Dis 47:554–66.

MONTOYA JF, REMINGTON JS. 2009. *Toxoplasma gondii*, chapter 279. In: Mandell GL, Bennett JE, Dolin R, (eds., Principles and Practice of Infectious Diseases, 7th ed. Churchill Livingstone, New York.

MONTOYA JG, LIESENFELD O. 2004. Toxoplasmosis. Lancet 363:1965–76.

NG OT, OOI EE, LEE CC, LEE PJ, NG LC, PEI SW, TU TM, LOH JP, LEO YS. 2008. Naturally acquired human *Plasmodium knowlesi* infection, Singapore. Emerg Infect Dis 14:814–6.

PEREIRA-CHIOCCOLA VL, VIDAL JE, SU C. 2009. *Toxoplasma gondii* infection and cerebral toxoplasmosis in HIV-infected patients. Future Microbiol 4:1363–79.

PERSING DH, HERWALDT BL, GLASER C, LANE RS, THOMFORD JW, MATHIESEN D, KRAUSE PJ, PHILLIP DF, CONRAD PA. 1995. Infection with a *Babesia*-like organism in northern California. N Engl J Med 332:298–303.

PUTAPORNTI, C, HONGSRIMUANG T, SEETHAMCHAI S, KOBASA T, LIMKITTIKUL K, CUI L, JONGWUTIWES S. 2009. Differential prevalence of *Plasmodium* infections and cryptic *Plasmodium knowlesi* malaria in humans in Thailand. J Infect Dis 199:1143–50.

QUICK RE, HERWALDT BL, THOMFORD JW, GARNETT ME, EBERHARD ML, WILSON M, SPACH DH, DICKERSON JW, TELFORD, III SR, STEINGART KR, POLLOCK R, PERSING DH, KOBAYASHI JM, JURANEK DD, CONRAD PA. 1993.

Babesiosis in Washington State: a new species of *Babesia*? An Intern Med 119:284–90.

REMINGTON JS, MCLEOD R, THULLIEZ P, DESMONTS G. 2006. Toxoplasmosis, p. 947–1092. In: Remington JS, Klein, JO, eds., Infectious Diseases of the Fetus and Newborn Infant, 6th ed. Saunders, Philadelphia.

RICKMAN LS, LONG GW, OBERST R, CABANBAN A, SANGALANG R, SMITH JI, CHULAY JD,. HOFFMAN SL. 1989. Rapid diagnosis of malaria by acridine orange staining of centrifuged parasites. Lancet 1:68–71.

ROBERTS A, HEDMAN K, LUYASU V, ZUFFEREY J, BESSIERES MH, BLATZ RM, CANDOLFI E, DECOSTER A, ENDERS G, GROSS U, GUY E, HAYDE M, HO-YEN D, JOHNSON J, LECOLIER B, NAESSENS A, PELLOUX H, THULLIEZ P, PETERSEN E. 2001. Multicenter evaluation of strategies for serodiagnosis of primary infection with *Toxoplasma gondii*. Eur J Clin Microbiol Infect Dis 20:467–74.

ROGERS WO, ATUGUBA F, ODURO AR, HODGSON A, KORAM KA. 2006. Clinical case definitions and malaria vaccine efficacy. J Infect Dis 193:467–73.

SCHAFFNER A. 2001. Pretransplant evaluation for infections in donors and recipients of solid organs. Clin Infect Dis 33 (Suppl 1):S9–14.

SCHMIDT-HIEBER M, ZWEIGNER J, UHAREK L, BLAU IW, THIEL E. 2009. Central nervous system infections in immunocompromised patients—update on diagnosis and therapy. Leuk Lymph 50:24–36.

SEMEL ME, TAVAKKOLIZADEH A, GATES JD. 2009. Babesiosis in the immediate postoperative period after splenectomy for trauma. Surg Infect 10:553–6

SMITH KL, WILSON M, HIGHTOWER AW, KELLEY PW, STRUEWING JP, JURANEK DD, MCAULEY JB. 1996. Prevalence of *Toxoplasma gondii* antibodies in US military recruits in 1989: comparison with data published in 1965. Clin Infect Dis 23:1182–3.

SPUDICK JM, GARCIA LS, GRAHAM DM, HAAKE DA. 2005. Diagnostic and therapeutic pitfalls associated with primaquine-tolerant *Plasmodium vivax*. J Clin Microbiol 43:978–81.

SUNSTRUM J, ELLIOTT LJ, BARAT LM, WALKER ED, ZUCKER JR. 2001. Probable autochthonous *Plasmodium vivax* malaria transmission in Michigan: case report and epidemiological investigation. Am J Trop Med Hyg 65:949–53.

TAKALA SL, PLOWE CV. 2009. Genetic diversity and malaria vaccine design, testing, and efficacy: preventing and overcoming "vaccine resistant malaria." Parasite Immunol 31:560–73.

TALABANI H, ASSERAF M, YER H, DELAIR E, ANCELLE T, THULLIEZ P, BREZIN AP, DUPOUY-CAMET J. 2009. Contributions of immunoblotting, real-time PCR, and the Goldmann–Witmer coefficient to diagnosis of atypical toxoplasmic retinochoroiditis. J Clin Microbiol 47:2131–5.

TORREY EF, YOLKEN RH. 2003. *Toxoplasma gondii* and schizophrenia. Emerg Inf Dis 9:1375–80.

VANNIER E, GEWURZ BE, KRAUSE PT. 2008. Human babesiosis. Infect Dis Clin North Am 22:469–88.

Vannier E, Krause PT. 2009. Update on babesiosis. Interdiscip Perspect Infect Dis 2009:984568.

Vekemans J, Ballou WR. 2008. *Plasmodium falciparum* malaria vaccines in development. Expert Rev Vaccines 7:223–40.

Wilson M, McAuley JB. 2003. Clinical use and interpretation of serologic tests for *Toxoplasma gondii*. M36-A, NCCLS, Wayne, PA.

World Health Organization. 1990. Severe and complicated malaria. Trans R Soc Trop Med Hyg 84(suppl 2):1–65.

CHAPTER SEVEN

BLOOD AND TISSUE FLAGELLATES OF THE CLASS KINETOPLASTIDEA: THE GENERA *LEISHMANIA* AND *TRYPANOSOMA*

Raul E. Villanueva and Stephen D. Allen

LEISHMANIASIS

The genus *Leishmania* contains more than 20 different species that are known to be associated with disease in humans and animals and can cause different patterns of disease based on species and mode of infection. Lesions of the skin, mucous membranes, mouth, and internal organs may all be seen in Leishmania infections (Banuls, Hide et al. 2007; Lukes, Mauricio, et al. 2007; Rougeron, De Meeus, et al. 2009).

Life Cycle

The life cycle of the *Leishmania* species involves two stages (Figures 7.1 and 7.2). The first occurs within sandfly vectors and the other in the affected mammals. In the first stage, the organisms are located in the digestive tracts of the sandfly vectors (Genus *Phlebotomus* in the old world and *Lutzomyia* in the new world). In this stage of development the organisms exist in a flagellated form known as a promastigote. When the sandfly takes a blood meal from the mammalian host, the organisms are injected through the proboscis into the human or other host (Murray, Berman, et al.

2005). Once inside the mammalian host the *Leishmania* promastigotes find and infect cells from the reticuloendothelial system (e.g., monocytes/macrophages, tissue histiocytes). They then lose their flagella and are referred to as amastigotes, also sometimes called ''leishmanial forms.'' The amastigotes are intracellular pathogens that replicate within the cells and can reach several hundred organisms per cell. The infected cells eventually burst, releasing the organisms to infect the surrounding cells as well as the blood stream (Alexander, Satoskar, et al. 1999). If the infected host is then bitten by a sandfly, the ingested amastigote will become the flagellated promastigote in the insect's gut. They reproduce by binary fission before migrating to the pharynx and mouth and starting the cycle over again.

Epidemiology

Leishmaniasis is endemic in every continent except Australia and Antarctica, and infections can be found in more than 88 countries worldwide. It is estimated there are about 2 million new cases each year with a prevalence of about 12 million (Choi and Lerner,

Non-Neoplastic Hematopathology and Infections, First Edition. Edited by Hernani D. Cualing, Parul Bhargava, and Ramon L. Sandin.
© 2012 Wiley-Blackwell. Published 2012 by John Wiley & Sons, Inc.

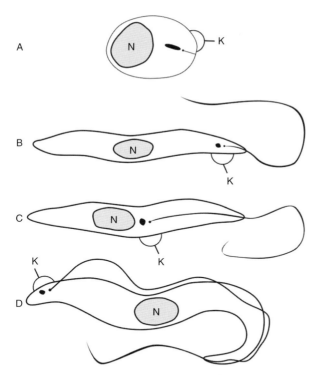

FIGURE 7.1 **Life cycle stages of blood and tissue flagellates**. (**A**) amastigote stage (leishmanial form), (**B**) promastigote, (**C**) epimastigote, (**D**) trypomastigote (trypanosomal form), (N) nucleus, (K) kinetoplast. (Illustration by Fredrik Hans Skarstedt)

2001). Most cases of leishmaniasis are due to infections affecting people living in the endemic areas; however, an increasing number of cases are due to infections of travelers to these areas. Traditionally, leishmaniasis has been divided into cutaneous leishmaniasis and visceral leishmaniasis. Cutaneous leishmaniasis is further subdivided into "old world" leishmaniasis associated with the species *L. tropica, L. major,* and *L. aethiopica* and "new world" leishmaniasis, which is caused by the *L. braziliensis* complex and the *L. mexicana* complex. Visceral leishmaniasis is caused by *L. donovani* and *L. infantum* (Desjeux, 2001). Epidemics tend to occur when susceptible individuals move into endemic areas or when sandfly habitats are disturbed. In recent years there has been a significant increase in leishmania infections in US military personnel stationed in Iraq and Afghanistan. In all of the cases where an organism was successfully isolated, the involved species was identified as *L. major* (CDC, 2004).

Clinical Syndromes

Leishmaniasis can range from asymptomatic infections to disseminated infections involving the skin or visceral organs. The majority of patients infected with *Leishmania sp.* are asymptomatic. Symptoms usually occur around a week after infection, but development of symptoms can occur years after the original infection. There are between 1 million and 1.5 million new cases of cutaneous leishmaniasis each year, and upward of 90% are limited to the countries of Brazil, Peru, Saudi Arabia, Iran, and Afghanistan. There are four main cutaneous syndromes: localized cutaneous leishmaniasis (LCL), diffuse cutaneous leishmaniasis (DCL), mucosal leishmaniasis (ML), and leishmania recidivans (LR).

Usually occurring on exposed skin, LCL starts off as a pink or red papule which then grows into an ulcer (Figure 7.3). The ulcer itself is painless and shows raised margins with granulomatous tissue at the base. There can be localized lymphadenopathy and rarely multiple ulcers arise along the area of lymphatic drainage. These ulcers usually resolve spontaneously with only a hypopigmented depressed scar at the ulcer site. The speed at which the ulcers heal depends both on the species causing the infection and the host's immune response (Markle and Makhoul, 2004).

DCL is uncommon and is usually associated with the species *L. aethiopica, L. mexicana, and L. amazonensis.* In this condition, when the organism first enters the host, it does not cause an ulcer. The organisms spread and invade macrophages in the skin throughout the body and cause the formation of plaques and nodules in the affected areas. The lesions are most common on the face and extensor surfaces of the arms and legs. Patients with DCL usually show a remitting-relapsing or a chronically progressive disease. These nodules can continue to grow for years and, due both to the appearance and distribution on the cooler areas of the body, can be mistaken for lepromatous leprosy. Most patients presenting with DCL have a defect in cell-mediated immunity and are thus unable to mount an effective immune response against the *Leishmania* parasites, allowing for unrestrained infection and spread (Convit, Ulrich, et al. 1993).

ML is found exclusively in the new world, and the vast majority of cases are due to infection with *L. braziliensis.* After formation of a primary ulcer at the site of infection, *L. braziliensis* can spread to the host's mucosal surfaces. This disease is commonly known as "espundia" in the endemic regions found mainly in Brazil and Bolivia. About 50% of ML cases occur in the first 2 to 3 years following primary infection; however, clinical manifestations can recur at mucosal sites months or even years after the primary ulcers heals. The route of spread is not direct contact but rather by dissemination through the blood or lymphatics. It is estimated that patients contracting infection by

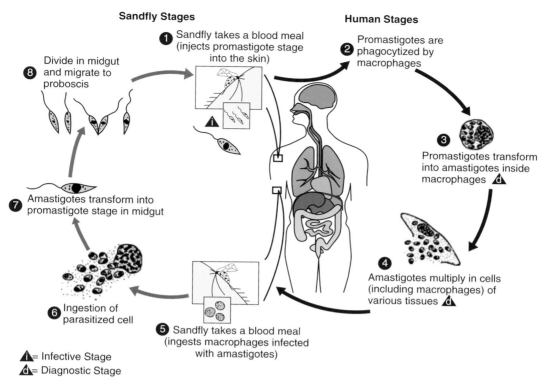

Sandfly Stages

Human Stages

❶ Sandfly takes a blood meal (injects promastigote stage into the skin)

❷ Promastigotes are phagocytized by macrophages

❽ Divide in midgut and migrate to proboscis

❸ Promastigotes transform into amastigotes inside macrophages

❼ Amastigotes transform into promastigote stage in midgut

❹ Amastigotes multiply in cells (including macrophages) of various tissues

❻ Ingestion of parasitized cell

❺ Sandfly takes a blood meal (ingests macrophages infected with amastigotes)

▲ = Infective Stage
▲ᵈ = Diagnostic Stage

FIGURE 7.2 *Leishmania* **species life cycle**. (Courtesy of the Centers for Disease Control and Prevention)

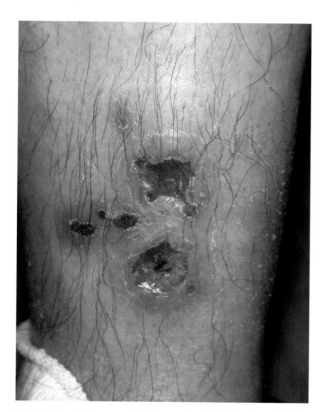

FIGURE 7.3 **Cutaneous leishmaniasis (skin ulcer).** (Photo courtesy of Diane Janovics, MD)

L. braziliensis have a 1 to 5% lifetime risk of developing mucosal disease.

ML usually involves the nose, nasal septum, or mouth, but other areas such as the palate, pharynx, larynx, trachea, and even the genitals can become involved. The infection is destructive and often leads to destruction of the nasal septum, with perforation or loss of the palate with the associated consequences. Unlike the skin ulcers of leishmaniasis, which are usually painless and asymptomatic, mucosal lesions often present with bleeding. The condition can range from mild, with only nasal congestion, to severe, with associated dysphonia, odynophagia, respiratory distress, and—in extreme cases—even death (Lessa, Lessa, et al. 2007).

The final cutaneous manifestation of leishmaniasis, LR, is found mainly in the Middle East and is caused by *L. tropica*. When the original ulcer heals, new lesions can appear in the skin surrounding the scar, which will then in turn ulcerate and heal; the same thing will happen again in the tissue surrounding the new scars. This cycle can continue for decades with new lesions appearing and disappearing or with a single slowly enlarging lesion that heals at the center while continuing to expand along the periphery. Unlike DCL, in LR the hosts usually have normal cellular immunity, and not many organisms are present in the lesions (Marovich, Lira, et al. 2001).

Visceral leishmaniasis (VL) is a more serious condition caused by *Leishmania* species and is most often associated with infection with *L. donovani* or *L. infantum/L. chagasi*. There have been rare cases of VL associated with *L. mexicana* and *L. tropica*, two species that are usually encountered only in cutaneous disease. The two commonly seen species cause a nearly identical clinical syndrome and cannot be differentiated simply on clinical grounds. Treatment is not dependent on the actual species but is based on the area of infection, severity of disease, and presence of any other conditions (Guerin, Olliaro, et al. 2002).

In VL the organisms bypass the cellular and humoral immune systems and replicate inside host macrophages. Mechanisms used include suppression of CD4+ T cells, interference with complement activity, and prevention of release from the affected macrophages of reactive oxygen or nitrogen intermediates (Bogdan and Rollinghoff, 1998). The condition remains even after the primary infection has apparently been cured; recovery is rare without medical intervention. The most serious form of VL is known as kala-azar syndrome in which patients have abdominal discomfort and fullness. Hepatosplenomegaly is commonly observed but the splenomegaly is usually more prominent than the hepatic enlargement. The spleen is usually enlarged, firm, and can range from somewhat tender to exquisitely painful due to rapid enlargement with distention of the capsule. Lymphadenopathy is another manifestation observed in East African cases but uncommon in cases seen elsewhere.

Development of kala-azar syndrome can range from 2 weeks to a few years after primary infection; however, most cases develop within 2 to 6 months from exposure. Symptoms are subacute and develop over time. They include feelings of malaise, fever, weight loss, and splenomegaly/hepatosplenomegaly. This syndrome is associated with high levels of parasites that accumulate in the cells of the reticuloendothelial system (e.g., spleen, liver, bone marrow). Involvement of the bone marrow can cause suppression of normal hematopoiesis and lead to severe anemia and thrombocytopenia. Intravascular hemolysis and splenic sequestration can further exacerbate the anemia, and spontaneous mucosal bleeding is a common finding. Damage to the liver leads to development of cachexia, edema, and hypoalbuminemia, which can later progress to development of jaundice and ascites. On rare occasions infection of the GI tract can occur and lead to malabsorption and chronic diarrhea (Baba, Makharia, et al. 2006).

Kala-azar literally means "black fever" due to darkening of the skin of infected individuals, which is common in cases seen is South Asia but uncommon in cases seen in other parts of the world (Joshi, Bajracharya, et al. 2006). The immunosuppression caused by bone marrow involvement can lead to development of secondary bacterial infections. Infection during pregnancy can lead to spontaneous abortions. Without treatment, most patients suffering from Kala-azar will die. Treatment is still associated with a 10% mortality, which is worse in patients showing wasting, severe anemia, jaundice, or additional immunosuppression (HIV) (Peters, Fish, et al. 1990).

Viscerotropic disease is a form of systemic leishmaniasis that shares several characteristics with kala-azar but is significantly milder. It is associated with fever, malaise, cough, diarrhea, abdominal pain, and adenopathy, as well as mild hepatosplenomegaly. First seen in veterans of the 1991 Gulf War, it was linked with *L. tropica* infections and responded well to therapy (Magill, Grogl, et al. 1993).

Differential Diagnosis

The ulcers encountered in leishmaniasis must be differentiated from other ulcers caused by infectious and noninfectious etiologies. However, leishmanial ulcers are not painful or pruritic, which is helpful in excluding most other etiologies. The differential diagnosis of visceral leishmaniasis includes Chagas disease, malaria, tuberculosis, typhoid fever, histoplasmosis, brucellosis, amoebic liver abscess, and lymphoma. Wasting, fever, and splenomegaly can be associated with schistosomiasis, chronic malaria, or a myeloproliferative disease.

Diagnosis

For the diagnosis of cutaneous leishmaniasis, the preferred specimen is a skin scraping or aspirate. A relatively simple skin scraping consists of using a sterile blade or scalpel and scraping the surface of an open lesion suspected of being caused by leishmaniasis. A skin aspirate is obtained by injecting sterile saline into the wound followed by aspirating the fluid. Ideally three to five aspirates should be obtained per lesion to maximize chances of detection. The gold standard specimen for diagnosis is a skin biopsy. The punch should be taken from the raised border at the edge of the lesion and not the ulcer base that would yield only necrotic tissue. The punch biopsy should be divided into three parts and used for microbiologic culture, touch preparations, and histology (Markle and Makhoul, 2004).

In most cases leishmaniae are relatively easily identified in the skin biopsy specimens. Difficulty in identification of any organisms can be encountered in cases of LR or in infections by *L. braziliensis*. Findings in skin biopsies range from aggregates of macrophages filled with leishmanial parasites to granulomas with many lymphocytes but few organisms (Figure 7.4). The organisms are visible on H&E, Giemsa, or Wright stains; they appear as small amastigotes that average 1 to 2 μm in diameter in tissue sections and are located within macrophages or extracellularly. *Leishmania sp.* have a prominent nucleus and a smaller rod- or dot-shaped kinetoplast that consists of abundant mitochondrial DNA. The nucleus is usually black to dark blue or purple, large, and eccentric in location; the kinetoplast is smaller and usually stains red to black (Figure 7.5). The kinetoplast is usually harder to find in tissue sections than in stained touch preparations or aspirates where cells tend to flatten out and the amastigotes appear larger. Morphologically, *Leishmania sp.* have a very similar appearance to *Histoplasma capsulatum*, and differentiation relies on identification of the kinetoplast as well as the staining pattern on GMS and other fungal stains. In contrast, *H. capsulatum*, which forms narrow-necked buds, is usually 2 to 4 μm in

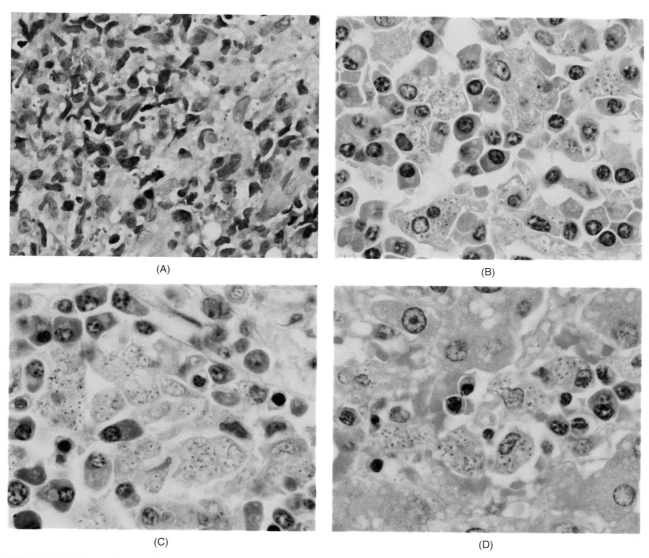

(A)

(B)

(C)

(D)

FIGURE 7.4 *Leishmania* **species in histologic sections.** (A) cutaneous leishmaniasis; biopsy taken from cutaneous ulcer shown grossly in Figure 7.3 (H&E, 100× objective), (**B**) visceral leishmaniasis (VL) in spleen (H&E, 100× objective), (**C**) VL in spleen (Giemsa stain, 100× objective), (**D**) VL in Kuppfer cells of liver (H&E, 100× objective).

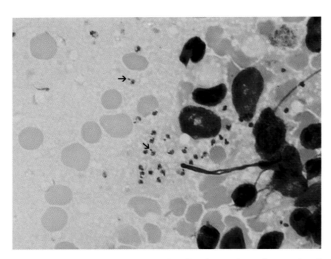

FIGURE 7.5 *Leishmania* **species in tissue imprint stained with Giemsa**. Arrows point to kinetoplasts of amastigotes (100× objective).

diameter; in our experience it is slightly larger than the amastigote forms of *Leishmania* in histologic sections.

Attempts to culture *Leishmania sp.* usually use Novy, MacNeal, Nicolle (NNN), or another medium containing calf serum (e.g., Schnider's medium). The ideal temperature for growth is 26 to 28°C. Cultures should be kept for at least four weeks because the appearance of growth will be delayed if the inoculum contains limited numbers of organisms; however, growth may be apparent in a few days if the inoculum contains many organisms (Dedet, Pratlong, et al. 1999).

Ideally, *Leishmania* should be identified to the species level as different species are associated with different patterns of disease and prognostic implications. However, in most cases the organism is only identified to genus, and the species name is assumed based on epidemiological grounds. Specific identification can be accomplished via PCR testing, DNA hybridization, DNA probes for the kinetoplast, species-specific monoclonal antibodies, and isoenzyme pattern analysis. However, most of these techniques remain limited to research use. Only PCR is widely used as a diagnostic tool; PCR allows for both detection as well as identification to the species level of the *Leishmania* causing the infection (Schonian, Nasereddin, et al. 2003). Although some studies suggested that PCR did not have high enough sensitivity to be used in cases of suspected cutaneous infections, later studies showed that PCR sensitivity was actually superior to all other diagnostic modalities utilized. However, studies of the specificity of PCR diagnosis of leishmaniasis have been lacking. (de Oliveira, Bafica, et al. 2003)

Serology has marginal diagnostic utility as only about 50% of patients with cutaneous leishmaniasis manifest an antibody response against the parasite. However, the Montenegro skin test (Leishmanin skin test) is useful. In it, killed promastigotes are injected into the skin in an attempt to induce a cutaneous delayed-type hypersensitivity reaction similar to a tuberculin skin test. After 48 hours the injection site is examined; an area of induration greater than 5 mm is considered a positive reaction. This technique is not approved for use in the United States (Manzur and Bari, 2006).

Numerous nonspecific findings can be seen in VL such as anemia, thrombocytopenia, and neutropenia as well as elevated bilirubin and elevated liver enzymes. Isolation of the organism from a tissue biopsy or smear is necessary for definitive diagnosis. The specimen is usually collected from the spleen or bone marrow (Sundar and Rai, 2002). Bone marrow aspiration or biopsy is preferred to splenic sampling due to the risk of splenic laceration and bleeding or accidental bowel perforation associated with the later. After the specimen is obtained, both touch preparations and histologic sections should be prepared and, ideally, an appropriate culture should be set up (e.g., using NNN medium). Culture, however, is not practical for hospital laboratories that rarely receive specimens from patients suspected of having leishmaniasis; if clinically warranted, such specimens could be sent to an outside referral laboratory. Touch preparations, in addition to tissue sections, should be made and stained with Giemsa stain because intracellular Leishmaniae and their kinetoplasts might be easier to see in touch preps having a single cell layer (Figure 7.5).

Unlike cases of cutaneous leishmaniasis in which antibodies are seen in only about half of all cases, in VL there is a marked stimulation of the humoral immune system with polyclonal B-cell stimulation and antibody production. This allows the use of enzyme-linked immunosorbent assays (ELISAs), indirect fluorescent antibody tests (IFA), or direct agglutination test (DAT) procedures to test for the presence of anti-leishmanial antibodies (el Harith, Kolk, et al. 1988). In endemic areas for VL people can have positive serologic test results but remain asymptomatic. Additionally serologic assays remain positive for several months after successful therapy and thus are not useful for rapid assessment of cure. Thus a positive serologic test cannot be used as definitive evidence of active VL.

A relatively newer ELISA test uses rK39, a recombinant kinesin antigen that is the cloned antigen of 39 amino acid repeats of a kinesin-like gene found in *L. chagasi*. Antibodies to rK39 could be detected in nearly 98% of sera from patients with visceral leishmaniasis in Brazil, Sudan, China, and Pakistan but were virtually absent in South American patients with mucocutaneous leishmaniasis and cutaneous leishmaniasis. This antigen can also be used in an immunochromatographic procedure for rapid testing in developing countries where access to advanced equipment is limited (Zijlstra, Daifalla, et al. 1998).

An additional method of identification is the leishmania urine antigen test. One of the most widely used in endemic regions, and not commercially available in the United States, is the kala-azar latex agglutination test (KATEX, Kalon Biological Ltd-UK), which detects leishmanial antigens in voided urine. The test is limited by low sensitivity (<70%) but has a relatively high specificity. Additionally it becomes negative after treatment, making it a viable alternative for evaluation of efficacy of treatment (Sundar, Agrawal, et al. 2005; Diro, Techane, et al. 2007).

Therapy

Cutaneous leishmaniasis can be treated with a variety of drugs. In cases of mild disease where there is little chance of spread to the mucosal surfaces, topical paromomycin is used. Alternative drugs include topical imiquimod cream, ketoconazole, itraconazole, allopurinol, or miltefosine. Other options include cryotherapy or heat therapy (radiofrequency). For more invasive lesions and those involving lymph nodes, joints, or mucosal surfaces, sodium stibogluconate or pentamidine can be used.

Treatment of VL is limited by the small number of available drugs. The most commonly used therapeutic agents are the pentavalent antimonials (Sbs), amphotericin B deoxycholate, amphotericin B in lipid formulations, miltefosine, and paromomycin. All of these drugs are relatively toxic, and costly, and with the exception of miltefosine are parenteral. The most commonly used drugs are the Sbs; however, resistance has developed to these drugs, and they now are mostly ineffective in northern India. India accounts for about 50% of the cases of kala-azar disease in the world. Even in areas of susceptible populations, the required IM injections of the Sb compounds are quite painful and the regimen requires 30 days of administration. Amphotericin B is an option in areas where Sb resistance is high; however, amphotericin B also needs a 30-day treatment schedule and has serious side effects necessitating hospitalization for administration and monitoring. The use of amphotericin B in lipid formulations allows for highly effective short-course treatments; unfortunately, the cost is prohibitively high in most endemic areas (Sundar, 2001).

Of the final two options for treating leishmaniasis, miltefosine has the advantage of being the only drug that can be administered orally, although it also has a long treatment course (28 days) and close observation is necessary to check for compliance and ensure that no resistance develops (Sundar, Jha, et al. 2002). Paromomycin is affordable and very effective, but the treatment course consists of 21 days of IM injections (Sundar, Jha, et al. 2007).

CHAGAS' DISEASE

Trypanosoma cruzi is the causative agent of Chagas' disease (or American trypanosomiasis), a condition affecting millions of people in Central and South America. In addition an ever-increasing number of people in the United States, immigrants from Latin America and people dwelling along the border with Mexico where the organism and the vector are endemic, are at risk for the disease (Barrett, Burchmore, et al. 2003).

Life Cycle

T. cruzi has three stages in its life cycle (Figure 7.6). The organism is spread by infected bugs called triatomines, also known as triatomid, reduviid, conenose, or kissing bugs (Figure 7.7). Infection of the bug occurs when it takes a blood meal from a human host who has organisms circulating in the blood. In the infected insect *T. cruzi* exists in the epimastigote form (previously known as crithidial form) in the midgut. In the midgut the organism goes through various cycles of replication, increasing in number before migrating to the insect's hindgut. Once there, it changes into a metacyclic trypomastigote that is the infectious stage. *T. cruzi* transmission is initiated when the triatomine bug takes a blood meal and defecates on the skin, usually while the victim is sleeping. The bite site itches and bug feces are introduced into the wound when the host rubs or scratches the area. After the trypomastigotes are introduced through a bite site, wound, or abrasion of the skin, mucous membranes of the nose or mouth, or into conjunctivae, the trypomastigotes enter into a variety of cell types in different organ systems, including muscle (especially cardiac), neurons, and glia. Once inside cells the organisms become amastigotes, which are oval shaped, averaging

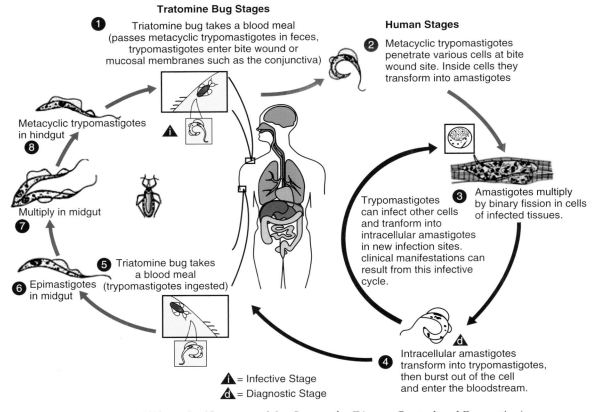

Tratomine Bug Stages

1 Triatomine bug takes a blood meal (passes metacyclic trypomastigotes in feces, trypomastigotes enter bite wound or mucosal membranes such as the conjunctiva)

Human Stages

2 Metacyclic trypomastigotes penetrate various cells at bite wound site. Inside cells they transform into amastigotes

Metacyclic trypomastigotes in hindgut **8**

Multiply in midgut **7**

5 Triatomine bug takes a blood meal (trypomastigotes ingested)

6 Epimastigotes in midgut

3 Amastigotes multiply by binary fission in cells of infected tissues.

Trypomastigotes can infect other cells and tranform into intracellular amastigotes in new infection sites. clinical manifestations can result from this infective cycle.

4 Intracellular amastigotes transform into trypomastigotes, then burst out of the cell and enter the bloodstream.

▲**i** = Infective Stage
▲**d** = Diagnostic Stage

FIGURE 7.6 *Trypanosoma cruzi* **life cycle.** (Courtesy of the Centers for Disease Control and Prevention)

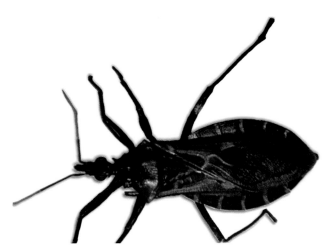

FIGURE 7.7 **Triatomine bug vector for *Trypanosoma cruzi*.** Modified image is from the collection of Herman Zaiman, "A Pictorial Presentation of Parasites."

about 2 to 4 μm with a nucleus and kinetoplast but no flagellum or undulating membrane. These amastigotes are morphologically indistinguishable from the amastigotes of Leishmaniae. As the amastigotes multiply and fill the cells, they transform

into trypomastigotes and the cells lyse, releasing the trypomastigotes into the blood stream where they circulate to distant sites and infect new cells. If the host is bitten by a reduviid bug while the trypomastigotes are present in the blood, the bug will become infected and start the cycle over again (Lack and Filie, 1997).

Epidemiology

Chagas' disease is most commonly acquired through contact with the feces of an infected triatomine bug. Infection can also be acquired through receipt of contaminated blood products (transfusions), organ transplantation from an infected donor, congenital transmission (mother to baby), a laboratory accident, or contaminated food or drink (rare).

Chagas' disease is endemic throughout Mexico and Central and South America. A recent report estimates 8 to 10 million people in Latin America are infected with *T. cruzi* (Stimpert and Montgomery, 2010); in addition approximately 300,000 infected persons live in the United States (Bern and Montgomery, 2009). Infection can occur at any age; however, the mean age of infection is believed to be around 4 years old. The vast majority of those infected (70–90%) become asymptomatic carriers with no clinical manifestations.

Clinical Syndromes

Chagas' disease has an acute and a chronic stage of disease. The acute phase usually lasts between 4 to 8 weeks, and most patients are asymptomatic for the duration. In those who do show clinical manifestations, the most commonly observed signs are the chagomas, which are areas of inflammatory swelling that are associated with regional lymphadenopathy if the site of inoculation is on the skin, or Romaña's sign, which involves periorbital swelling as well as conjunctivitis when the organisms penetrate the conjunctiva (often in conjunction with rubbing the eye; Figure 7.8). More systemic manifestations include splenomegaly, hepatomegaly, and cardiomegaly. In patients with cardiomegaly there can be dilation of all chambers with marked myocarditis with extensive myocyte necrosis and acute and chronic inflammatory cell infiltration. Additionally there is extensive interstitial edema and vascular dilation as well as involvement of the cardiac conduction system (Koberle, 1968).

Besides involvement of the heart, spleen, and liver, *T. cruzi* may infect the esophagus and colon; the organism can also invade the central nervous sytem. In the heart, amastigote forms of the parasite are usually seen in infected myofibers in association with prominent inflammatory cell infiltrates and varying amounts of edema and fibrosis. Clusters of *T. cruzi* amastigotes within myofibers have been referred to as "pseudocysts." In contrast to amastigotes of *Leishmania* species, amastigotes of *T. cruzi* have no special predisposition to phagocytosis by macrophages (or histiocytes) (Lack and Filie, 1997).

Manifestations of chronic Chagas' disease usually do not present until 5 to 15 years or longer after infection. The most common complication of chronic Chagas' disease is cardiac, with cardiomegaly (up to 800 g) and chamber dilation, which is usually more prominent on the right side leading to signs of systemic congestion rather than pulmonary congestion. Relatively often dilation leads to formation of an apical ventricular aneurysm or apical ventricular malformation that has been identified in just over half of patients at autopsy. Morphologically the lesions are thin, with myocardial atrophy and fibrosis, and they seldom rupture. Additionally in approximately one-third of the cases of Chagas' disease, mural thrombi are present, with an equal distribution between the right and left heart. Approximately half of all patients also have thrombi in both the pulmonary and systemic circulations (Samuel, Oliveira, et al. 1983).

Mechanisms that have been suggested to explain the cardiac manifestations of chronic Chagas' disease include direct inflammation, neuronal damage, damage to the cardiac microvasculature, and immune-mediated cardiac damage. Although chronic Chagas' disease is not associated with the high parasitemia and significant inflammation that is seen in the acute form, inflammatory foci can be present in specimens obtained from these patients. The inflammatory foci contain *T. cruzi* antigenic material, suggesting a continued role of the parasite in the persistent inflammatory response. Therapy aimed at reducing the parasite load resulted in less severe cardiomyopathy; patients with Chagas' disease who died from cardiomyopathy consistently showed the presence of *T. cruzi* DNA, while those who were seropositive but showed no sign of cardiac disease did not show *T. cruzi* DNA (Jones, Colley, et al. 1992). In addition evidence from experimental models has shown that the intensity of cardiac inflammation is directly correlated with the parasite burden (Zhang and Tarleton, 1999).

Trypanosomal infection results in extensive involvement of the cardiac conduction system leading to cell death and reactive fibrosis, particularly involving the right bundle branch and the left anterior fascicle of the left bundle branch where right bundle branch block and left anterior fascicular block occur (Rossi, 1991). Studies have shown significant loss of autonomic control over the heart with both sympathetic and parasympathetic functions being affected; however, it is not clear whether this is a cause or an effect of the cardiac dysfunction (Marin-Neto, Bromberg-Marin, et al. 1998).

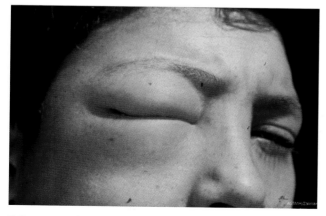

FIGURE 7.8 **Romaña's sign**. (Image is from the collection of Herman Zaiman, "A Pictorial Presentation of Parasites.")

Some studies have shown Chagas' disease to be associated with a dysfunction in the coronary microvasculature that may act in conjunction with the inflammation to damage the myocardial tissue. These findings have been correlated with limited studies in animal models that have shown similar findings. Abnormal responses to both vasodilatory and vasoconstrictive impulses may explain the EKG changes, ischemic-like symptoms, and perfusion defects often associated with Chagas' cardiomyopathy (Rossi, 1990).

An additional mechanism of myocardial damage associated with Chagas' disease is immune-mediated injury. Reports have indicated that infected cardiac cells secrete cytokines and chemokines, resulting in leukocyte aggregation and subsequent localized inflammation. In addition to their effect on parasite replication in infected cells, cytokines and chemokines appear to cause lysis of cells that are not infected by the parasites, leading to cardiac injury and cell loss (Andrade, Andrade, et al. 1994). More specifically, other findings have aided in the identification of Cha, a dominant autoantigen present in myocardiocytes. The Cha antigen contains epitopes that can crossreact, with both T cells and B cells stimulating the production of anti-Cha antibodies that attack and damage the myocardiocytes. If T cells from infected animals are given to animals not infected with *T. cruzi*, the activated T cells will lead to production of the anti-Cha antibodies and development of cardiac pathology identical to that seen in animals with Chagas' disease. Additionally there is significant crossreactivity between the myosin heavy chain of heart muscle and several *T. cruzi* antigens (Girones, Rodriguez, et al. 2001). In patients suffering from Chagasic cardiomyopathy there was crossreactivity between the cardiac myosin heavy chain and the B13 protein of *T. cruzi* in 100% of the cases. However, in patients positive for Chagas' disease but not suffering from any cardiac issues, the crossreactivity was only 14%.

The other major complications of chronic Chagas' disease are megaesophagus and megacolon. Although there might be some direct damage to the smooth muscle of these organs, the main cause is the destruction of the neurons forming the submucosal plexus that regulate relaxation. The destruction of these neurons leads to constriction and dilation of the organ in the segments preceding the affected section. (Meneghelli, 1985) While the manifestations are characteristic of the chronic form of the disease, the actual damage to the neurons happens in the acute stages of infection.

Differential Diagnosis

Acute Chagas' disease is usually asymptomatic. In cases of chronic Chagas' disease the Chagasic cardiomyopathy is often difficult to differentiate from ischemic, hypertensive, or idiopathic causes. In addition the differential diagnosis includes conditions that cause high-output heart failure (e.g., anemia, hyperthyroidism, beriberi, acute rheumatic fever, valvular disease, congenital abnormalities, pericardial disorders, and sequelae of acute myocarditis). Megaesophagus due to Chagas' disease is easily confused with achalasia; blockage due to tumors or strictures should also be taken into consideration. Finally, megacolon in Chagas' disease may need to be differentiated from a number of other conditions including Hirschsprung's disease, diabetic neuropathy, strictures, neurological diseases (Parkinson's disease, myotonic dystrophy), scleroderma, amyloidosis, and even psychogenic causes (schizophrenia).

Diagnosis

It is important for blood-borne pathogens that biosafety precautions be followed by health care personnel working with blood samples drawn from patients suspected of having Chagas' disease as trypomastigotes are highly infectious. The method of diagnosis depends on the stage of the disease. In the acute phase (i.e., during the first 90 days of infection) the parasites are present in high numbers and microscopic identification of motile trypomastigotes in anticoagulated blood or buffy coat samples can be of diagnostic utility (Strout, 1962; Bern, Montgomery, et al. 2007). In addition Giemsa-stained thick and thin smears should be prepared and examined. Thick smears concentrate the blood and aid in confirmation of the diagnosis, particularly in cases of low-level parasitemia. Thin smears allow for clear visualization of the parasite and are especially useful for purposes of identification (Figure 7.9). (Winn, Allen et al. 2006) For even higher yields, the microhematocrit concentration method (MH) is useful. It involves centrifugation of the patient's blood in six 50 μl tubes followed by examination of the buffy coat. This concentrates the parasites in a small area and increases sensitivity over simple microscopic examination (Feilij, Muller, et al. 1983). Although PCR methods are available for the diagnosis of the acute phase of Chagas' disease and have high specificity and sensitivity when used during this stage, these methods are not FDA cleared and access to PCR remains limited to research and highly specialized referral laboratories. (Kirchhoff, Votava, et al. 1996; Castro,

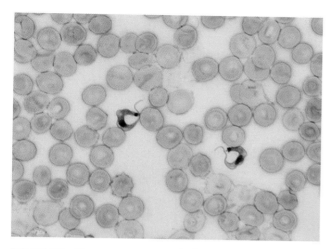

FIGURE 7.9 *Trypanosoma cruzi* **C- or U- shaped typo-mastigotes in peripheral blood thin smear (Giemsa stain, 100× objective).** (Photo courtesy of Linda M. Marler and Jean A. Siders)

Luquetti, et al. 2002) In the acute phase serology is of limited usefulness due to the low levels of antibodies present.

Other methods for diagnosis are used both in the early stages of the disease as well as during the more chronic stages. These include hemoculture and xenodiagnosis. In hemoculture, packed red blood cells prepared from the patient suspected of having the infection are placed into LIT medium and incubated at 28°C, and they are observed for the growth of any organisms (Chiari, Días, et al. 1989). Xenodiagnosis is a unique method for the detection of *Trypanosoma cruzi*; in this procedure uninfected reduviid bugs are placed in a jar that is then placed on the skin of the patient being tested. The insects are allowed to feed, and after 25 to 30 days of incubation the animal's feces are examined microscopically for the presence of the parasite. Since the insects were known to be uninfected prior to contact with the patient's skin, its presence in the insect indicates the parasite must have come from the patient (Días, 1940).

In chronic Chagas' disease, serology plays a much more prominent role in diagnosis than it does in acute Chagas' disease. Although not FDA cleared, a variety of serological tests are available for identification of antibodies against *T. cruzi*, and it is recommended that two different modalities be used as these methods lack sensitivity and specificity. Over 30 different serologic assays have been used for identification over the years; currently the most widely utilized methods are IFA, ELISA, and indirect hemaglutination. Most of the tests use epimastigote antigens;

however, some of the newer tests utilize recombinant proteins. PCR techniques are also available for use in suspected chronic cases; however, they have shown variable sensitivity and specificity and are not commercially available (Brasil, De Castro, et al. 2010).

In tissue or aspirated samples, the amastigote forms of *T. cruzi* and *L. donovani* share a similar morphologic appearance, and it may be necessary to differentiate between them. The finding of amastigotes in striated muscle (but not in macrophages) in a cardiac biopsy from a patient with consistent travel or geographic history would be considered diagnostic for *T. cruzi* and would exclude *L. donovani* (Figure 7.10). Other means of differentiating between Chagas' disease and VL include PCR, serology, culture using NNN agar (for epimastigotes of *T. cruzi* or promastigotes of *Leishmania* spp.), and xenodiagnosis (Chiaramonte, Frank, et al. 1999; Chiari, 1999; Castro, Luquetti, et al. 2002; Maldonado, Albano, et al. 2004).

Therapy

Pharmacologic drug therapy of Chagas' disease varies with the phase of the disease and age of the patient. As reviewed by Bern and colleagues, antitrypanosomal treatment is currently indicated for patients with acute infection, congenital infection, reactivated infection in patients with AIDS or other immunosuppression (e.g., organ transplantation), and in children younger than 18 years old with chronic Chagas' disease (Bern, Montgomery, et al. 2007). Only two drugs are known to be effective against *T. cruzi*: benznidazole and nifurtimox. Both are active against trypomastigotes and amastigotes. Benznidazole is generally better tolerated and is thus viewed as the drug of choice (Rodriques Coura and de Castro, 2002). For individuals who are 19 to 50 years of age with Chagas' disease and do not have advanced cardiac involvement, Bern and colleagues recommend that treatment be offered, but for individuals older than 50 years, the risk of drug toxicity is substantial and treatment is considered optional. For patients with chronic Chagas' disease, antitrypanosomal drug treatment is generally ineffective in curing the infection and thus any treatment is mostly supportive and geared toward dealing with secondary complications that develop, such as cardiac failure or arrhythmias in patients with cardiomyopathy or the development of megacolon or megaesophagus (Pinto Dias, 2006; Bern, Montgomery, et al. 2007; Viotti, Vigliano, et al. 2009).

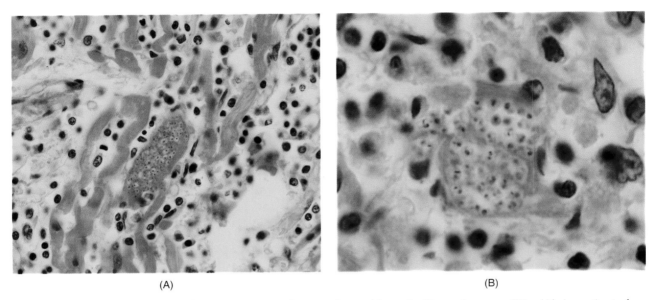

(A)   (B)

FIGURE 7.10   **Histologic section of heart at necropsy from patient with acute Chagas' myocarditis**. (**A**) Amastigote forms of *Trypanosoma cruzi* in cardiac myofiber (but not in macrophages or histiocytes; H&E section, 50× objective) (**B**) Same case as (**A**) showing a large cluster of *T. cruzi* amastigotes in a cardiac myofiber that appears lysed (H&E, 100× objective).

AFRICAN TRYPANOSOMIASIS

African trypanosomiasis, also known as human African trypanosomiasis (HAT) or African sleeping sickness, is caused by the hemoflagellate protozoan *Trypanosoma brucei*. Spread by the tsetse fly, the disease occurs in two forms, the more severe form largely confined to east and southern Africa caused by *Trypanosoma brucei* subspecies *rhodesiense* and the less severe form seen in west and central Africa that is associated with *Trypanosoma brucei* subspecies *gambiense*. An additional subspecies, *Trypanosoma brucei brucei*, does not cause disease in humans (Barrett, Burchmore, et al. 2003).

Life Cycle

Both subspecies of *T. brucei* pathogenic to humans are morphologically indistinguishable, and both are transmitted by tsetse flies of more than 30 species and subspecies of the genus *Glossina*, blood-sucking insects found only in Africa. In the fly's salivary glands, epimastigotes transform into the nondividing metacyclic trypomastigote form. When an infected male or female fly bites the host and takes a blood meal, it injects metacyclic trypomastigotes into the bite site. The first sign of infection can be the development of a chancre where the bite occurred and the parasites multiply. After a few days to a few weeks, the parasites enter the lymphatics and disseminate in the bloodstream. They differentiate into trypomastigotes that are longer and more slender than the metacyclic trypomastigotes injected in the bite of the tsetse fly (Figure 7.11). These motile parasites are able to divide in the blood stream. They disseminate to lymph nodes and have the ability to cross the blood–brain barrier, enter the cerebrospinal fluid (CSF), and invade the brain itself. If an uninfected tsetse fly takes a blood meal from a host suffering from African trypanosomiasis, it will ingest the active trypomastigotes, which then migrate toward the midgut of the fly where they differentiate into procyclic trypomastigotes and undergo replication. Three weeks after ingestion, they migrate to the salivary glands where they progress through the epimastigote stage before finally progressing once more to the infective metacyclic trypomastigote (Smith, Pepin, et al. 1998; Brun, Blum, et al. 2010).

Epidemiology

HAT is largely restricted geographically to sub-Saharan Africa; it is acquired mostly in rural areas in relation to the habitats for tsetse flies. Tsetse flies tend to prefer shady warm areas and appear to be attracted to moving objects as well as the color blue. Once they pick up the parasite, tsetse flies can pass on the infection for the rest of their lives, which average 1 to 6 months in duration. Although both subspecies have a tsetse fly vector, *T. b. gambiense* is transmitted by the *Glossina palpalis* fly while *T. b. rhodesiense*

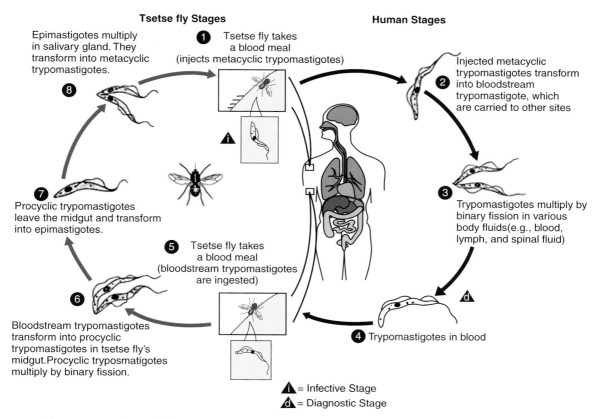

Tsetse fly Stages

Human Stages

Epimastigotes multiply in salivary gland. They transform into metacyclic trypomastigotes.

8

1 Tsetse fly takes a blood meal (injects metacyclic trypomastigotes)

2 Injected metacyclic trypomastigotes transform into bloodstream trypomastigote, which are carried to other sites

7 Procyclic trypomastigotes leave the midgut and transform into epimastigotes.

3 Trypomastigotes multiply by binary fission in various body fluids(e.g., blood, lymph, and spinal fluid)

5 Tsetse fly takes a blood meal (bloodstream trypomastigotes are ingested)

6 Bloodstream trypomastigotes transform into procyclic trypomastigotes in tsetse fly's midgut.Procyclic tryposmatigotes multiply by binary fission.

4 Trypomastigotes in blood

i = Infective Stage
d = Diagnostic Stage

FIGURE 7.11   *Trypanosoma brucei* **life cycle**. (Courtesy of the Centers for Disease Control and Prevention)

is transmitted by the *Glossina morsitans* fly. These two species vary slightly in their preferred habitats and biting patterns leading to a slight difference in epidemiology between the two trypanosomal subspecies (Fevre, Picozzi, et al. 2006).

Tsetse flies of the *Glossina palpalis* group (i.e., *G. palpalis, G. fuscipes,* and *G. tachinoides*), the vectors for *T. b. gambiense*, are responsible for transmitting most trypanosomal infections acquired in western and central Africa. These flies prefer more humid climates and are often found in forested areas surrounding rivers. Although the flies bite both animals and humans who live in the area, they preferentially affect humans, and thus humans are the primary reservoir of these parasites. Mainly *T. b. gambiense* infections affect people living in rural areas that frequent the water sources where the flies live and are bitten as they bathe or wash their clothes (Brun, Blum, et al. 2010).

Tsetse flies of the *Glossina morsitans* group (*G. morsitans, G. pallidipes,* etc.), which transmit *T. b. rhodesiense* and African trypanosomiasis in eastern and southern Africa, tend to favor a drier climate of the savannahs and woodlands not associated with water. These flies are mainly zoophilic and most of their meals come from wild or domestic animals, including warthogs, bushpigs, buffalo, kudu, and cattle. Thus, in contrast to *T. b. gambiense*, which relies on a human reservoir, the main reservoir for *T. b. rhodesiense* is the wild animal population. Human infection is usually due to accidental bites and is usually limited to hunters or farmers who wander into the affected areas (Smith, Pepin, et al. 1998; Brun, Blum, et al. 2010).

While most cases of African trypanosomiasis occur among locals in the areas of endemic tsetse fly habitation, trypanosomiasis involving visitors and tourists in Africa as well as those returning to the United States or Europe have been reported (Spencer, Gibson, et al. 1975; Hanly, 1997; Jelinek, Bisoffi, et al. 2002; Moore, Edwards, et al. 2002; Gautret, Clerinx, et al. 2009). *T. brucei* has also been acquired rarely by transplacental transmission, from blood transfusion, or from other biting insects (Hanly, 1997).

Clinical Syndromes

Trypanosoma brucei has a unique method for evading the host's immune system known as antigenic variation. The extracellular trypomastigotes found in the bloodstream are covered with a very dense coat of glycoproteins, known as variant surface glycoproteins (VSG), that are constantly being altered and prevent the immune system from mounting an adequate immunologic response. Approximately 1000 genes have been reported to code for the VSGs; these genes are spread throughout the parasite's genome. Only a single VSG gene is expressed at a time so only one VSG protein is present on the trypomastigote cell surface. By sequentially expressing these genes, the parasites are able to elude the immune system and cause a persistent infection. As many as 100 different serotypes have been identified in a single infection, and it is thought that the switch occurs every 5 to 7 days, thus accounting for waves of parasitemia that are seen every 7 to 14 days. The VSG is also found inside the trypomastigote itself as well as released into the blood; this is thought to explain the findings of immune dysfunction that is often seen in those infected with *T. brucei*. The circulating VSGs lead to release of γ-interferon, suppression of interleukin-2, and hypergammaglobulinemia, which affect the hosts ability to mount an effective immune response (Pays, 2005; Garcia, 2007; Navarro, Penate, et al. 2007).

HAT occurs in three stages: (1) the chancre, (2) the hemolymphatic stage, and (3) the meningoencephalitic stage. The stages are more clearly defined in infections by *T. b. gambiense* than they are in the more rapidly progressive disease due to *T. b. rhodesiense*. Within a few days to 2 weeks after the tsetse fly bite, about 20% of patients infected by *T. b. rhodesiense* develop a trypanosomal chancre. This is a well-circumscribed, rubbery, inflammatory lesion. It is usually quite painful and measures anywhere from 2 to 5 cm across. The chancre can ulcerate but usually will resolve on its own after a few weeks. The development of a trypanosomal chancre is rare in patients infected with *T. b. gambiense*. In addition rashes develop after infection that can be urticarial, macular, or even erythematous (Uslan, Jacobson, et al. 2006).

Relatively early in the infection, the trypanosomes can be found in large numbers in blood and in lymph nodes where they proliferate. Lymph node involvement leads to lymphadenitis. This phenomenon is evident in infections by *T. b. gambiense* in which the parasites tend to preferentially involve posterior cervical lymph nodes. When present, the enlarged lymph nodes are referred to as "Winterbottom's sign" and are usually soft and painless. When lymph node involvement occurs in infections by *T. b. rhodesiense*, the cervical lymph nodes are usually spared; instead, axillary, or inguinal nodes may be involved (Kirchhoff, 2010).

Infections by the two different subspecies vary in other ways. *T. b. gambiense* has a long progressive course with worsening of the symptoms over months to years. It tends to present with fevers, malaise, headache, and arthralgias intermittently in its early stages. The intermittent nature of the symptoms is thought to be due to waves of parasites being released into the circulation. Organomegaly, and especially splenomegaly, is common as is the previously mentioned lymphadenopathy. On occasion, the parasites can infiltrate the vasculature of the heart, leading to pancarditis with associated arrhythmias and even cardiac failure (Hanly, 1997; Brun, Blum, et al. 2010; Kirchhoff, 2010).

As the disease progresses there is diffuse meningoencephalitis as well as edema of the brain parenchyma. The damage leads to multifocal demyelination of the white matter as well as diffuse cerebral hemorrhages. The patient at first complains of severe headaches and difficulty in concentrating. As the symptoms progress caretakers will note changes in personality, which progress to frank psychosis. There are also sensory and motor symptoms with loss of sensation as well as ataxia and tremor. The reason for the commonly used name of "sleeping sickness" is the fact that the parasites cause an alteration in the circadian cycles of the affected individuals leading to excessive somnolence, particularly in the daytime. The somnolence gets more pronounced as the disease progresses, and the patient will become stuporous and unable to perform activities of daily living. As they are unable to eat, they develop malnutrition and wasting, and they are also at increased risk of aspiration pneumonia due to the neurologic dysfunction. In the final stages, patients may suffer convulsions, especially if they are infants or children (Wery, Mulumba, et al. 1982).

In infections with *T. b. rhodesiense*, the signs and symptoms share similarity to those of patients infected with *T. b. gambiense*. However, in contrast to the longer timeline for disease due to *T. b. gambiense*, the course is much more accelerated, and the condition progresses more rapidly when due to *T. b. rhodesiense*. Without treatment, trypanosomiasis due to *T. b. rhodesiense* is lethal within weeks or months, although both conditions eventually lead to development of coma and death in untreated individuals. Infection with *T. b. gambiense* can lie dormant and appear years after the original exposure; therefore testing should be done on patients with a travel history to endemic areas who are having any sort of neurological symptoms (Fevre, Picozzi, et al. 2006).

Differential Diagnosis

In the early stages of the disease, the differential includes common causes of fevers of unknown origin (e.g., typhoid fever, early HIV infection, malaria, and Epstein–Barr virus). The lymphadenopathy should raise suspicion for TB, HIV infection, or malignancy (lymphoma, metastatic cancer). Differential diagnoses of mental status changes include, again TB and HIV-related symptoms, and meningitis as well as multiple other infections and inflammatory CNS diseases. The differential in late stage HAT includes meningoencephalitis due to other infectious agents or psychiatric illnesses (Maguire, 2004).

Diagnosis

Due to the limited geographic area of HAT, a combination of epidemiologic information (e.g., history of travel to an endemic region) coupled with clinical findings should suggest the possibility of African trypanosomiasis and the need for further workup. Unfortunately, most cases of HAT occur in regions with limited resources, and most of those afflicted with the disease die before an accurate diagnosis is made. Some nonspecific laboratory findings include hypoalbuminemia, hypocomplementemia, and hypergammaglobulinemia along with a high erythrocyte sedimentation rate (ESR). Leukocytosis is common, and both anemia and thrombocytopenia are frequently encountered. The anemia is believed to be due to immune-mediated hemolysis while the thrombocytopenia is probably attributable to splenic sequestration. In the late stage after neurological symptoms have begun, an electroencephalogram can aid in detecting decreased brain activity as well as slow wave oscillations (Chimelli and Scaravilli, 1997; Chappuis, Loutan, et al. 2005).

Definitive diagnosis can be established by direct demonstration of the parasite in fluid expressed from chancres (early stage), blood (Figure 7.12), lymph node aspirates, bone marrow aspirates, biopsy material (hemolymphatic stage), and CSF (late stages). As is true for Chagas' disease, it is important that blood-borne pathogen biosafety precautions be followed by health care personnel working with specimens collected from patients suspected of having HAT; the trypomastigotes are highly infectious. Wet mounts (for motile trypomastigotes) and Giemsa-stained thick and thin smears (i.e., of blood, CSF, lymph node aspirates, and bone marrow aspirates) should be prepared for microscopic examination. Thin smears of peripheral blood are relatively easy to read and interpret (Figure 7.12), but the thick smears concentrate the organisms and increase the sensitivity

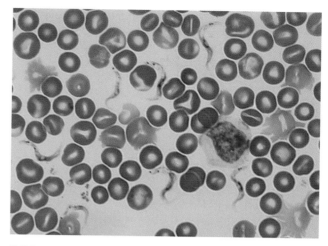

FIGURE 7.12 *Trypanosoma brucei* **trypomastigotes in peripheral blood thin smear (Giemsa stain, 100× objective)**. (Photo courtesy of Linda M. Marler and Jean A. Siders)

of the test. Thick smears can detect trypomastigotes at concentrations above 2000/ml. In addition to an increased likelihood of finding trypomastigotes in the hemolympatic stage, the sensitivity of direct microscopic examination depends on which of the two species is causing the disease. In the hemolymphatic stage of HAT due to *T. b. rhodesiense*, the concentration of blood stream trypomastigotes is greater than in infections by *T. b. gambiense*, thus making it more likely that the parasites will be seen in peripheral blood smears from patients infected by *T. b. rhodesiense*. However, the levels of parasitemia fluctuate, and as in cases of malaria, a single negative result is not sufficient to completely rule out infection if the index of suspicion is sufficiently high. Thus repeated blood smears should be examined (Chappuis, Loutan, et al. 2005).

Concentration methods are used to increase the yield of blood specimen examinations and may facilitate the diagnosis. Techniques include the micro-hematocrit centrifugation technique (also called the capillary tube centrifugation technique or the "Woo test") in which motile trypomastigotes are concentrated among the white cells between the erythrocytes and plasma and can be seen directly under the microscope. Also there is a very sensitive quantitative buffy coat (QBC) procedure involving centrifugation and use of a fluorescent stain to identify trypomastigotes in the concentrated sample (Bailey and Smith 1992). Another method uses a mini-anion exchange column (mAECT) in which the blood is passed through a column containing a resin that tends to bind the blood but does not have significant affinity for the trypanosomes. The resulting parasite-rich eluate can then be centrifuged and microscopically examined for the presence of trypanosomes and can detect levels as low as 5/ ml (Lumsden, Kimber, et al. 1979). While resulting in higher positive results, these concentration techniques are not widely available in the endemic areas where they would be of greatest utility (Chappuis, Loutan, et al. 2005).

In all cases of HAT or suspected HAT, it is imperative that the CSF be screened for the presence of parasites, even if positive identification is made from blood samples (Kennedy, 2008). The CSF examination is necessary not just for diagnosis of trypanosomal infection but also is used in the staging of the disease to determine whether the illness has entered the late or meningoencepalitic stage of HAT. According to the World Health Organization, the main diagnostic criteria are a WBC count higher than 5 cells per μl, increased levels of protein, over 370 mg/L, or the identification of trypanosomes in the CSF (WHO 1998). Additional uncommon diagnostic criteria include the presence of large eosinophilic plasma cells which contain antiparasitic IgM that has not been secreted. These characteristic cells are known as "Mott cells," and their presence is highly characteristic of CNS involvement (Greenwood and Whittle, 1973). It should be noted that trypomastigotes do not have to be identified in the CSF in order for a diagnosis of CNS disease to be made. Although it may be helpful if they are seen, the absence of trypomastigotes in a sample of CSF in the presence of other diagnostic criteria is not sufficient to rule out CNS involvement (Chappuis, Loutan, et al. 2005).

Aspiration or biopsy of enlarged lymph nodes can yield motile trypomastigotes on direct examination or can reveal trypomastigotes after fixation and staining with Giemsa or Wright stains. Aspiration can also be useful at the site of the chancre formation as well as in cases of suspected bone marrow involvement. *T. b. gambiense* infections tend to have lymphadenopathy relatively frequently, and the examination of lymph node aspirates has traditionally been useful for screening and diagnosis of West African trypanosomiasis (Simarro, Louis, et al. 2003).

Specimens of blood, CSF, bone marrow, or lymph node aspirates can be inoculated into liquid culture media; trypanosomes have grown in some cases where no parasites were identified in the original sample. A kit for in vitro isolation of trypanosomes in the field has been described. PCR testing is possible in research settings and referral laboratories but not widely available, particularly in endemic countries (Chappuis, Loutan, et al. 2005).

Serology is of limited use in the diagnosis of sleeping sickness as there is no commercially available test for *T.b.rhodesiense* antibodies. In cases of *T. b. gambiense*, several antibody tests are available, but they are not definitive for diagnosis as they have variable sensitivities and specificities. The most common test used is the so-called card agglutination test for trypanosomes (CATT; available in kit form for field use from the Institute of Tropical Medicine in Antwerp, Belgium). The CATT/*T. b. gambiense* was introduced for population screening but is now considered a rapid and simple means of diagnosing *T. b. gambiense* HAT. The CATT method uses freeze-dried trypanosomes that agglutinate in the presence of variant-specific antibodies. Sensitivity is generally good in the 94 to 98% range, but it can vary depending on the geographical area in which the testing is being performed. The specificity of the test depends on whether the patient's whole blood is being used or whether a plasma dilution is being used. False-positive reactions with malaria and with past exposure to zoonotic trypanosomes that are nonpathogenic for humans are among the specificity issues (Simarro, Ruiz, et al. 1999; Garcia, Jamonneau, et al. 2000; Truc, Lejon, et al. 2002). An alternative test is the detection of trypanosomal antigens via an ELISA test; however, the studies have shown variable results and these tests are not readily available (Lejon, Buscher, et al. 1998). Tests have been developed to measure antitrypanosomal antibodies in the CSF to test for neurological involvement; however, these do not have the sensitivity required to be useful. Increased intrathecal synthesis of antitrypanosomal IgM is believed to be the most sensitive measure of CNS involvement (Lejon, Reiber, et al. 2003).

Although *T. brucei* infection is most commonly diagnosed by examination of the blood and CSF, it can affect many different organs; there are few pathognomonic findings associated with it. When biopsied, the chancre can rarely show trypomastigotes, but usually it only shows a perivascular lymphocytic vasculitis that is generally limited to the dermal blood vessels. The affected lymph nodes are usually large and rubbery and show follicular hyperplasia, plasmacytosis, and sinus histiocytosis. Parasites are only occasionally seen in the biopsied nodes; however, touch imprints of the nodes often show numerous organisms, a finding that can greatly aid in diagnosis. The other organ commonly showing significant findings is the brain, which can appear hyperemic and edematous grossly, and which is often covered with thickened, opaque meninges. When examined microscopically, small ring hemorrhages, similar in appearance to the Durk granulomas in cerebral malaria and multiple small infarcts, may be seen. Another characteristic finding is a mononuclear cell infiltrate involving Virchow–Robins spaces that is composed mainly of plasma cells, including the IgM filled Mott cells. Also the heart can show evidence of pancarditis with mild cardiac enlargement, pericardial effusions, endocardial fibrosis, and myocardial infiltration with lymphocytes, histiocytes, and plasma cells, plus associated areas of myocyte death. In addition the spleen may be enlarged with congested red pulp, localized areas of necrosis with giant cells sometimes present, or irregular areas of fibrosis may be seen (Hanly 1997).

Therapy

Treatment recommendations for HAT vary depending on whether the infection is caused by *T. b. gambiense* or *T. b. rhodesiense*. Additionally the treatment is determined by the stage of the disease. Treatment for early disease in the presence of undiagnosed neurological involvement can lead to treatment failure. For treatment of early *T. b. gambiense* infection, it is recommended that the clinician use pentamidine with suramin reserved as an alternative agent. In cases of CNS disease, melarsoprol is recommended; however, its significant toxicity limits its effective use. In cases of late disease, it is recommended that eflornithine be utilized due to its less toxic effects although it is significantly more costly. After treatment, patients should receive close follow-up and monitoring for 2 years, and receive lumbar punctures and CSF analysis every 6 months. Any rise in CSF WBC count or identification of trypanosomes in any of the patient's samples is proof of relapse, and treatment should be reinitialized.

For patients with *T. b. rhodesiense* infection, suramin should be used in the early stage of disease. For later stages, the only drug to show any effect is melarsoprol. If there is a successful recovery, follow-up with observation for a year is recommended and screening lumbar puncture should be performed every 3 months (Pepin and Milord, 1994; Denise and Barrett, 2001; Kennedy, 2008).

REFERENCES

ALEXANDER J, SATOSKAR AR, et al. 1999. Leishmania species: models of intracellular parasitism. J Cell Sci 112(18):2993–3002.

ANDRADE ZA, ANDRADE SG, et al. 1994. Myocardial changes in acute *Trypanosoma cruzi* infection. Ultrastructural evidence of immune damage and the role of microangiopathy. Am J Pathol 144(6):1403–11.

BABA CS, MAKHARIA GK, et al. 2006. Chronic diarrhea and malabsorption caused by *Leishmania donovani*. Ind J Gastroenterol 25(6):309–10.

BAILEY JW, SMITH DH 1992. The use of the acridine orange QBC technique in the diagnosis of African trypanosomiasis. Trans R Soc Trop Med Hyg 86(6):630.

BANULS AL, HIDE M, et al. 2007. Leishmania and the leishmaniases: a parasite genetic update and advances in taxonomy, epidemiology and pathogenicity in humans. Adv Parasitol 64:1–109.

BARRETT MP, BURCHMORE RJ, et al. 2003. The trypanosomiases. Lancet 362(9394):1469–80.

BERN C, MONTGOMERY SP. 2009. An estimate of the burden of Chagas disease in the United States. Clin Infect Dis 49(5):e52–4.

BERN C, MONTGOMERY SP, et al. 2007. Evaluation and treatment of chagas disease in the United States: a systematic review. JAMA 298(18):2171–81.

BOGDAN C, ROLLINGHOFF M. 1998. The immune response to Leishmania: mechanisms of parasite control and evasion. Int J Parasitol 28(1):121–34.

BRASIL P, DE CASTRO L, et al. 2010. ELISA versus PCR for diagnosis of chronic Chagas' disease: systematic review and meta-analysis. BMC Infect Dis 10: 337–354.

BRUN R, BLUM J, et al. 2010. Human African trypanosomiasis. Lancet 375(9709):148–59.

CASTRO AM, LUQUETTI AO, et al. 2002. Blood culture and polymerase chain reaction for the diagnosis of the chronic phase of human infection with *Trypanosoma cruzi*. Parasitol Res 88(10):894–900.

CDC 2004. Update: cutaneous leishmaniasis in U.S. military personnel—Southwest/Central Asia, 2002–2004. MMWR Morb Mortal Wkly Rep 53(12):264–5.

CHAPPUIS F, LOUTAN L, et al. 2005. Options for field diagnosis of human african trypanosomiasis. Clin Microbiol Rev 18(1):133–46.

CHIARAMONTE MG, FRANK FM, et al. 1999. Polymerase chain reaction reveals *Trypanosoma cruzi* infection suspected by serology in cutaneous and mucocutaneous leishmaniasis patients. Acta Trop 72(3):295–308.

CHIARI E. 1999. Chagas disease diagnosis using polymerase chain reaction, hemoculture and serologic methods. Mem Inst Oswaldo Cruz 94 (suppl 1): 299–300.

CHIARI E, DIAS JC, et al. 1989. Hemocultures for the parasitological diagnosis of human chronic Chagas' disease. Rev Soc Bras Med Trop 22(1):19–23.

CHIMELLI L, SCARAVILLI F. 1997. Trypanosomiasis. Brain Pathol 7(1):599–611.

CHOI CM, LERNER EA. 2001. Leishmaniasis as an emerging infection. J Investig Dermatol Symp Proc 6(3):175–82.

CONVIT J, ULRICH M, et al. 1993. The clinical and immunological spectrum of American cutaneous leishmaniasis. Trans R Soc Trop Med Hyg 87(4):444–8.

DE OLIVEIRA CI, BAFICA A, et al. 2003. Clinical utility of polymerase chain reaction-based detection of Leishmania in the diagnosis of American cutaneous leishmaniasis. Clin Infect Dis 37(11):e149–53.

DEDET JP, F PRATLONG, et al. 1999. Delayed culture of Leishmania in skin biopsies. Trans R Soc Trop Med Hyg 93(6):673–4.

DENISE H, BARRETT MP. 2001. Uptake and mode of action of drugs used against sleeping sickness. Biochem Pharmacol 61(1):1–5.

DESJEUX P. 2001. The increase in risk factors for leishmaniasis worldwide. Trans R Soc Trop Med Hyg 95(3):239–43.

DIAS, E. 1940. The technique of xenodiagnosis of Chagas' disease. Memorias do Instituto Oswaldo Cruz 35: 335–342.

DIRO E, TECHANE Y, et al. 2007. Field evaluation of FD-DAT, rK39 dipstick and KATEX (urine latex agglutination) for diagnosis of visceral leishmaniasis in northwest Ethiopia. Trans R Soc Trop Med Hyg 101(9):908–14.

EL HARITH, A, KOLK AH, et al. 1988. Improvement of a direct agglutination test for field studies of visceral leishmaniasis. J Clin Microbiol 26(7):1321–5.

FEILIJ H, MULLER L, et al. 1983. Direct micromethod for diagnosis of acute and congenital Chagas' disease. J Clin Microbiol 18(2):327–30.

FEVRE EM, PICOZZI K, et al. 2006. Human African trypanosomiasis: epidemiology and control. Adv Parasitol 61:167–221.

GARCIA A, JAMONNEAU V, et al. 2000. Follow-up of card agglutination trypanosomiasis test (CATT) positive but apparently aparasitaemic individuals in Cote d'Ivoire: evidence for a complex and heterogeneous population. Trop Med Int Health 5(11):786–93.

GARCIA, L. (2007). Diagnostic Medical Parasitology. ASM Press, Washington, DC.

GAUTRET P, CLERINX J, et al. 2009. Imported human African trypanosomiasis in Europe, 2005–2009. Euro Surveill 14(36):1–3.

GIRONES N, RODRIGUEZ CI, et al. 2001. Dominant T- and B-cell epitopes in an autoantigen linked to Chagas' disease. J Clin Invest 107(8):985–93.

GREENWOOD BM, WHITTLE HC. 1973. Cerebrospinal-fluid IgM in patients with sleeping-sickness. Lancet 2(7828):525–7.

GUERIN PJ, OLLIARO P, et al. 2002. Visceral leishmaniasis: current status of control, diagnosis, and treatment, and a proposed research and development agenda. Lancet Infect Dis 2(8):494–501.

HANLY MG. 1997. African trypanosomiasis. Vol 2. In: CONNOR DH, F. W. CHANDLER FW, D. A. SCHWARTZET DA, et al., eds., Pathology of Infectious Diseases, Appleton and Lange, Stamford, CT, 1285–95

JELINEK T, BISOFFI Z, et al. 2002. Cluster of African trypanosomiasis in travelers to Tanzanian national parks. Emerg Infect Dis 8(6):634–5.

JONES EM, COLLEY DG, et al. 1992. A *Trypanosoma cruzi* DNA sequence amplified from inflammatory lesions in human chagasic cardiomyopathy. Trans Assoc Am Physicians 105:182–9.

JOSHI S, BAJRACHARYA BL, et al. 2006. Kala-azar (visceral Leishmaniasis) from Khotang. Kathmandu Univ Med J (KUMJ) 4(2):232–4.

KENNEDY PG. 2008. The continuing problem of human African trypanosomiasis (sleeping sickness). Ann Neurol 64(2):116–26.

KIRCHHOFF LV. 2010. Agents of African trypanosomiasis. In: Mandell, Douglas, and Bennett's Principles and Practice of Infectious Diseases Vol 2. Mandell GL, Bennett JE, Dolin R, eds., Churchill-Livingstone-Elsevier, Philadelphia, 3489–94.

KIRCHHOFF LV, VOTAVA JR, et al. 1996. Comparison of PCR and microscopic methods for detecting *Trypanosoma cruzi*. J Clin Microbiol 34(5):1171–5.

KOBERLE F. 1968. Chagas' disease and Chagas' syndromes: the pathology of American trypanosomiasis. Adv Parasitol 6:63–116.

LACK E, FILIE A. 1997. American trypanosomiasis. Pathol Infect Dis 2:1297–1304.

LEJON V, BUSCHER P, et al. 1998. A semi-quantitative ELISA for detection of Trypanosoma brucei gambiense specific antibodies in serum and cerebrospinal fluid of sleeping sickness patients. Acta Trop 69(2):151–64.

LEJON V, REIBER H, et al. 2003. Intrathecal immune response pattern for improved diagnosis of central nervous system involvement in trypanosomiasis. J Infect Dis 187(9):1475–83.

LESSA MM, LESSA HA, et al. 2007. Mucosal leishmaniasis: epidemiological and clinical aspects. Braz J Otorhinolaryngol 73(6):843–7.

LUKES J, MAURICIO IL, et al. 2007. Evolutionary and geographical history of the Leishmania donovani complex with a revision of current taxonomy. Proc Natl Acad Sci USA 104(22):9375–80.

LUMSDEN WH, KIMBER CD, et al. 1979. Trypanosoma brucei: miniature anion-exchange centrifugation technique for detection of low parasitaemias: Adaptation for field use. Trans R Soc Trop Med Hyg 73(3):312–7.

MAGILL AJ, GROGL M, et al. 1993. Visceral infection caused by *Leishmania tropica* in veterans of Operation Desert Storm. N Engl J Med 328(19):1383–7.

MAGUIRE JH. 2004. Trypanosoma. In: Infectious Diseases. Lippincott Williams and Wilkins, Philadelphia, 2327–2334.

MALDONADO C, ALBANO S, et al. 2004. Using polymerase chain reaction in early diagnosis of re-activated *Trypanosoma cruzi* infection after heart transplantation. J Heart Lung Transplant 23(12):1345–8.

MANZUR A, BARI A. 2006. Sensitivity of leishmanin skin test in patients of acute cutaneous leishmaniasis. Dermatol Online J 12(4):2.

MARIN-NETO JA, BROMBERG-MARIN G, et al. 1998. Cardiac autonomic impairment and early myocardial damage involving the right ventricle are independent phenomena in Chagas' disease. Int J Cardiol 65(3):261–9.

MARKLE WH, MAKHOUL K. 2004. Cutaneous leishmaniasis: recognition and treatment. Am Fam Physician 69(6):1455–60.

MAROVICH MA, LIRA R, et al. 2001. *Leishmaniasis recidivans* recurrence after 43 years: a clinical and immunologic report after successful treatment. Clin Infect Dis 33(7):1076–9.

MENEGHELLI UG. 1985. Chagas' disease: a model of denervation in the study of digestive tract motility. Braz J Med Biol Res 18(3):255–64.

MOORE DA, EDWARDS M, et al. 2002. African trypanosomiasis in travelers returning to the United Kingdom. Emerg Infect Dis 8(1):74–6.

MURRAY HW, BERMAN JD, et al. 2005. Advances in leishmaniasis. Lancet 366(9496):1561–77.

NAVARRO M, PENATE X, et al. 2007. Nuclear architecture underlying gene expression in Trypanosoma brucei. Trends Microbiol 15(6):263–70.

PAYS E. 2005. Regulation of antigen gene expression in *Trypanosoma brucei*. Trends Parasitol 21(11):517–20.

PEPIN J, MILORD F. 1994. The treatment of human African trypanosomiasis. Adv Parasitol 33:1–47.

PETERS BS, FISH D, et al. 1990. Visceral leishmaniasis in HIV infection and AIDS: clinical features and response to therapy. Q J Med 77(283):1101–11.

PINTO DIAS JC. 2006. The treatment of Chagas disease (South American trypanosomiasis). An Intern Med 144(10):772–4.

RODRIQUES COURA J, DE CASTRO S. 2002. A critical review on Chagas' disease chemotherapy. Mem Inst Oswaldo Cruz 97: 3–24.

ROSSI MA. 1990. Microvascular changes as a cause of chronic cardiomyopathy in Chagas' disease. Am Heart J 120(1):233–6.

ROSSI MA. 1991. Patterns of myocardial fibrosis in idiopathic cardiomyopathies and chronic Chagasic cardiopathy. Can J Cardiol 7(7):287–94.

ROUGERON V, DE MEEUS T, et al. 2009. Extreme inbreeding in *Leishmania braziliensis*. Proc Natl Acad Sci USA 106(25):10224–9.

SAMUEL J, OLIVEIRA M, et al. 1983. Cardiac thrombosis and thromboembolism in chronic Chagas' heart disease. Am J Cardiol 52(1):147–51.

SCHONIAN G, NASEREDDIN A, et al. 2003. PCR diagnosis and characterization of Leishmania in local and imported clinical samples. Diagn Microbiol Infect Dis 47(1):349–58.

SIMARRO PP, LOUIS FJ, et al. 2003. Sleeping sickness, forgotten illness: what are the consequences in the field ? Med Trop (Mars) 63(3):231–5.

SIMARRO PP, RUIZ JA, et al. 1999. Attitude towards CATT-positive individuals without parasitological confirmation in the African Trypanosomiasis (*T.b. gambiense*) focus of Quicama (Angola). Trop Med Int Health 4(12):858–61.

SMITH DH, PEPIN J, et al. 1998. Human African trypanosomiasis: an emerging public health crisis. Br Med Bull 54(2):341–55.

SPENCER HC Jr, GIBSON JJ Jr, et al. 1975. Imported African trypanosomiasis in the United States. Ann Intern Med 82(5):633–8.

STIMPERT KK, MONTGOMERY SP 2010. Physician awareness of Chagas disease, USA. Emerg Infect Dis 16(5): 871–2.

STROUT RG. 1962. A method for concentrating hemoflagellates. J Parasitol 48:100.

SUNDAR S. 2001. Drug resistance in Indian visceral leishmaniasis. Trop Med Int Health 6(11):849–54.

SUNDAR S, AGRAWAL S, et al. 2005. Detection of leishmanial antigen in the urine of patients with visceral leishmaniasis by a latex agglutination test. Am J Trop Med Hyg 73(2):269–71.

SUNDAR S, JHA TK, et al. 2002. Oral miltefosine for Indian visceral leishmaniasis. N Engl J Med 347(22): 1739–46.

SUNDAR S, JHA TK, et al. 2007. Injectable paromomycin for *Visceral leishmaniasis* in India. N Engl J Med 356(25): 2571–81.

SUNDAR S, RAI M. 2002. Laboratory diagnosis of visceral leishmaniasis. Clin Diagn Lab Immunol 9(5):951–8.

TRUC P, LEJON V, et al. (2002). Evaluation of the micro-CATT, CATT/*Trypanosoma brucei gambiense*, and LATEX/*T. b. gambiense* methods for serodiagnosis and surveillance of human African trypanosomiasis in West and Central Africa. *Bull WHO* 80(11):882–6.

USLAN DZ, JACOBSON KM, et al. 2006. A woman with fever and rash after African safari. Clin Infect Dis 43(5):609, 661–2.

VIOTTI R, VIGLIANO C, et al. 2009. Side effects of benznidazole as treatment in chronic Chagas disease: fears and realities. Expert Rev Anti Infect Ther 7(2):157–63.

WERY M, MULUMBA PM, et al. 1982. Hematologic manifestations, diagnosis, and immunopathology of African trypanosomiasis. Semin Hematol 19(2):83–92.

WHO. 1998. Control and surveillance of African trypanosomiasis: report of a WHO expert committee. WHO, Geneva.

WINN WC Jr, ALLEN SD, et al. 2006. Koneman's Color Atlas and Textbook of Diagnostic Microbiology, 6th ed. Lippincott Williams and Wilkins, Philadelphia.

ZHANG L, TARLETON RL. 1999. Parasite persistence correlates with disease severity and localization in chronic Chagas' disease. J Infect Dis 180(2):480–6.

ZIJLSTRA EE, DAIFALLA NS, et al. 1998. rK39 enzyme-linked immunosorbent assay for diagnosis of *Leishmania donovani* infection. Clin Diagn Lab Immunol 5(5): 717–20.

CHAPTER EIGHT

PROTEOBACTERIA AND RICKETTSIAL AGENTS: HUMAN GRANULOCYTIC ANAPLASMOSIS AND HUMAN MONOCYTIC EHRLICHIOSIS

Sheldon Campbell and Tal Oren

MICROBIOLOGY AND EPIDEMIOLOGY OF HGA AND HME

Human granulocytic anaplasmosis (HGA) is caused by *Anaplasma phagocytophilum* (formerly *Ehrlichia phagocytophilum*). Human Monocytic Ehrlichiosis (HME) is caused by Ehrlichia *chaffeensis*. Both are tick-borne bacterial pathogens that, as their names imply, infect human leukocytes. They cause similar, but not identical, acute infectious syndromes.

ICD-10 Codes

A79.9 Rickettsiosis, unspecified: Rickettsial infection NOS

Both organisms are bacterial pathogens in the family Rickettsiaceae in the α-proteobacteria group. Both are obligate intracellular pathogens that are phagocytosed, then proliferate within a phagocytic vacuole in the infected cells; the infected vacuoles are referred to as "morulae." Both have minimal cell walls and, while taxonomically related to other Gram-negative organisms in phylum Proteobacteria, are not typically visualized by Gram stain.

Anaplasma phagocytophilum combines the species formerly known as *Ehrlichia phagocytophilum* and *Ehrlichia equi*. Transmitted by the *Ixodes* ticks that also transmit Lyme disease and *Babesia microti*, HGA is endemic in the northeastern and north-central United States, and has also been described in parts of Europe. *Anaplasma* primarily infects neutrophils; monocytes appear to be relatively nonpermissive for both invasion and intracellular survival. Infected neutrophils have reduced adhesion, migration, and phagocytic capabilities. The cytopenias produced in *A. phagocytophilum* infection appear to be related to increased peripheral destruction, but not to direct cytolysis by *Anaplasma*.

Ehrlichia chaffeensis is primarily transmitted by *Amblyomma americanum*, the Lone Star tick, and is prevalent in the United States in the southeast, south-central, and mid-Atlantic states. Seroprevalence studies suggest that it is also transmitted in Mexico, Central, and South America. *E. chaffeensis*

Non-Neoplastic Hematopathology and Infections, First Edition. Edited by Hernani D. Cualing, Parul Bhargava, and Ramon L. Sandin.
© 2012 Wiley-Blackwell. Published 2012 by John Wiley & Sons, Inc.

preferentially infect monocytes and macrophages. Both species are exquisitely adapted pathogens; both possess genetic mechanisms for expression of variant surface antigens, allowing for potential persistent and repeat infections (Ohashi et al 1998; Yu et al 2000; Asanovich et al 1997; Ijdo et al 2002).

CLINICAL SYNDROMES

Both HGA and HME present as acute, febrile illnesses, usually with relatively nonspecific presentations. Signs, symptoms, and laboratory findings are shown in Table 8.1. The combination of fever, leukopenia or thrombocytopenia, and elevated transaminases, while not unique to HME/HGA, is typical and fairly unusual, and should prompt the clinician to think of these illnesses in persons with tick exposure in an endemic area. Note that discrimination of HGA and HME on clinical grounds is difficult, although the presence of rash in suspected HGA should prompt investigation of other etiologies.

Disease can vary from mild to critical; immuno-compromised patients are particularly at risk for severe, life-threatening HME infection. Severe complications may include adult respiratory distress syndrome, acute renal insufficiency, central nervous system (CNS) complications, including menin-goencephalitis, coagulopathy, and gastrointestinal hemorrhage (Walker and Dumler 1997). Failure to recognize pulmonary and cerebral involvement is associated with poor outcomes (Hamburg et al. 2008).

CNS involvement has rarely been observed in HGA, with significant sequelae. In addition opportunistic bacterial and viral infections may occur, associated with the profound neutropenia seen in some patients.

Seroprevalence surveys in endemic regions suggest that many *Ehrlichia* and *Anaplasma* infections are mild or asymptomatic; seropositivity rates of up to 39% have been observed in endemic areas (Aguero-Rosenfeld et al. 2002).

DIFFERENTIAL DIAGNOSIS

Because of the typically nonspecific presentation of HME/HGA, the initial differential diagnosis is broad and includes a variety of febrile infectious, rheumatological, and neoplastic syndromes. Viral syndromes, sepsis of any etiology, pneumonia, or gastroenteritis may be considered, depending on the clinical presentation. A history of outdoor activity or tick exposure will cause Rocky Mountain Spotted fever, Lyme disease, babesiosis, or rarer diseases to be added to the list; altered mental status or other CNS findings, or CSF pleocytosis, will raise concern for bacterial or viral meningitis or meningoencephalitis. A variety of other infectious etiologies may be considered, depending on exposure and risk histories. Collagen-vascular disease and hematologic malignancies, particularly in the presence of cytopenias, may be investigated.

TABLE 8.1 Signs, Symptoms, and Laboratory Findings in HGA and HME

Clinical Finding	Prevalence in HGA (%)	Prevalence in HME (%)
Signs and symptoms		
Fever	94–100	97
Headache	61–85	81
Myalgias	68	78–98
Malaise	98	84
Chills/rigors	39–98	67
Anorexia	37	66
Nausea	39	48
Cough	29	26
Abdominal pain	20	22
Confusion	17	20
Rash	2–11	36
Laboratory findings		
Leukopenia	50–59	60
Thrombocytopenia	59–92	68
Elevated AST	69–91	86
Elevated creatinine	70	29

Source: Adapted from Dumler and Walker (2009) and from Baken and Dumler (2008).

DIAGNOSTIC APPROACH

The laboratory workup of a patient in whom a diagnosis of HGA or HME is clinically suspected begins with a routine laboratory evaluation, including a complete blood count (Figures 8.1 and 8.2). The most common and reproducible CBC abnormalities seen in patients with HGA include variable degrees of leukopenia and thrombocytopenia. In a large study of 144 patients with HGA (Bakken et al., 2001), the mean WBC concentration was 5.0×10^9 cells/L (control patients 7.2×10^9 cells/L) and the mean platelet count was 124×10^9 cells/L (control patients 213×10^9 cells/L). Patients infected with HGA also harbored a significantly increased number of band neutrophils (0.83×10^9 cells/L for infected patients compared to 0.42×10^9 cells/L for control patients).

Absolute and relative monocyte counts were not significantly different between infected and control patients. A large meta analysis of multiple studies of patients with HGA demonstrated that 49% and 71% of infected patients demonstrated leukopenia and thrombocytopenia, respectively, at some point in their clinical course (Dumler et al 2005, 2007).

Leukopenia and thrombocytopenia are also seen in patients infected with HME, with a mean WBC concentration of 4.5×10^9 cells/L (reference $4-10 \times 10^9$ cells/L) and a mean platelet count of 98.5×10^9 cells/L (reference $150-340 \times 10^9$ cells/L) in one recent retrospective study (Olano et al., 2003). A small percentage of these cases had an appreciable monocytosis (8%), a finding that may serve as a small distinguishing point between patients infected with HME versus those infected with HGA. The same

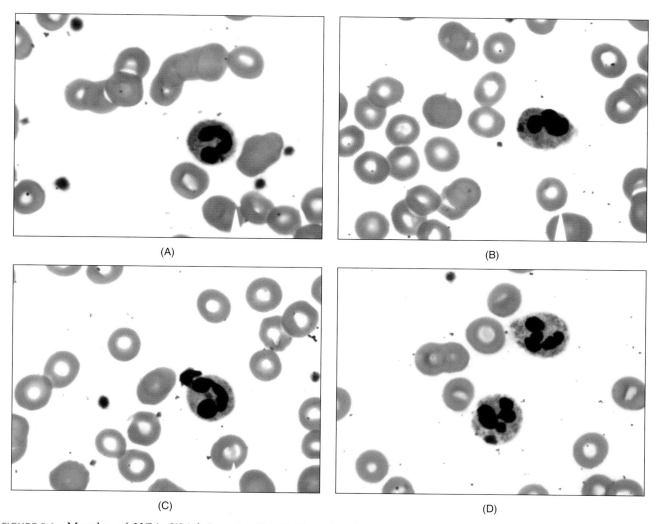

(A)

(B)

(C)

(D)

FIGURE 8.1 Morulae of HGA, Wright's stain. (**A–D**) Cytoplasmic inclusions. These are discrete, pale-blue, and either blob-like or grouped in clusters ("morulae" comes from the Greek word for grapes).

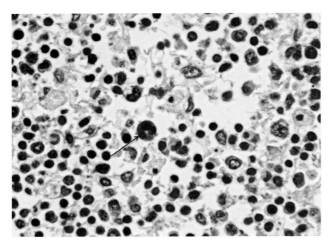

FIGURE 8.2   HME morula in bone marrow, H&E. (Courtesy of Drs. Sherif R. Zaki and Wun-Ju Shieh, Infectious Diseases Pathology Branch, Centers for Disease Control and Prevention)

meta analysis referenced above demonstrated that 62% and 71% of patients infected with HME demonstrated leukopenia and thrombocytopenia (Dumler 2005; Dumler et al., 2007). Another helpful, albeit not entirely specific, laboratory finding in patients with HME or HGA is an elevated serum AST or ALT, having been reported in 83% of patients with HME and 71% of patients with HGA (Dumler et al., 2007).

Although these laboratory findings are clearly not specific for infection by HGA or HME, they are seen with enough frequency to provide justification to proceed with more specific testing in patients with a compatible clinical presentation (fever, headache, myalgias, rigors, etc.). The easiest logical next step in the laboratory workup is examination of a Wright- or Giemsa-stained peripheral blood smear for the characteristic findings of HGA or HME. Identification of stippled blue morulae within granulocytes (HGA) or monocytes (HME) is the most rapid means by which to make a presumptive diagnosis of infection. False positives would be unusual and relatively rare in the hands of experienced hematologists and hematopathologists. However, false negatives are common, and a peripheral smear examination is not a very sensitive diagnostic modality, particularly for HME, for fewer than half of patients will demonstrate diagnostic findings on peripheral smear examination (Standaert et al 2000; Hamilton et al., 2004). Although a reactive monocytosis is often seen in the patients suffering from HME, this finding is nonspecific. The sensitivity of blood smear examination for identifying HGA infection is better (approximately 60% in one study from Bakken et al., 2001), but this approach will

still miss a significant number of clinical infections. It is important to recognize that the sensitivity of peripheral blood examination is influenced by both the administration of doxycycline for therapy and the duration from the time of onset of clinical symptoms (Dumler et al., 2007). Accordingly, although peripheral smear examination has the potential to represent a rapid and cost effective means by which to make a diagnosis of HGA or HME, the number of false negatives requires other diagnostic modalities in smear negative cases.

Serologic testing can be helpful in the setting of a false-negative peripheral smear result and can also serve as confirmation of a positive peripheral smear result. It is the most sensitive method by which to detect infection by either organism. Testing serum for either seroconversion or a fourfold increase in antibody levels in convalescence would represent serologic confirmation of infection (Bakken et al, 2000, 2002; Olano et al., 2003; Bakken et al., 1996). However, a number of caveats need to be kept in mind when interpreting serologic evidence of infection. First, seroprevalence rates are high in certain parts of the country, even in the absence of clinical signs of infection, emphasizing the importance of a *change* in titer levels rather than an absolute level. Second, IgG antibodies can persist for months to years in the absence of any clinical evidence of persistent infection. Despite these limitations, prudent use of serologic testing in a patient with a high clinical probability of harboring HGA or HME results in positive and negative predictive values in excess of 90% (Dumler et al., 2007). However, false positive serologic tests do occur in a variety of clinical settings, including bacterial infections, certain viral infections (particularly Epstein–Barr virus), and a variety of autoimmune disorders.

Although identification of the offending organisms by culture is the most specific methodology available, its clinical utility is limited by both the small number of laboratories capable of providing this service and the long delay before a result is obtained (in vitro assays can take up to 6 weeks before infected cells can be detected). Accordingly, this approach has not reached widespread clinical acceptance and is rarely used in the routine workup of patients. Nevertheless, culture isolation of *E. chaffeensis* (grown in DH82 canine histiocytic cells) and *A. phagocytophilum* (grown in human promyelocytic HL-60 cells) can be performed in those rare situations where culture is deemed clinically useful.

Molecular diagnostics is a relatively recent addition to the diagnostic armamentarium and has the potential to be both rapid and relatively specific.

As such, it has quickly attained widespread acceptance and is now an important diagnostic tool for the diagnosis of both HGA and HME. A positive result with primers specific for a particular organism should be considered to be diagnostic of infection in a patient with the appropriate clinical presentation. Unfortunately, although these assays are relatively sensitive, false negatives with PCR-based assays are not unusual; sensitivity for HME has been reported to range between 60% and 85% (Standaert et al., 2000; Olana et al., 2003), while sensitivity for HGA has been reported to range between 67% and 90% (Bakken et al., 2000; Horowitz et al., 1998). As with other diagnostic modalities, PCR-based assays are prone to false-negative results with antecedent doxycycline treatment, likely serving as a plausible explanation for at least some of the false-negative results seen with this approach. Accordingly, a negative PCR study does not exclude a diagnosis of either HGA or HME, and alternative methodologies, such as serology, should be employed in a patient with a significant likelihood of infection.

PREVENTION AND TREATMENT

The main means of prevention of HME and HGA is tick avoidance, using protective clothing, DEET-based repellants, and inspecting for and removing ticks. The drug of choice for both infections is doxycycline or tetracycline, based on in vitro studies. Chloramphenicol, effective against other rickettsiae, is likely to be ineffective; rifampin has been used effectively during pregnancy and in young children, but experience with this drug is limited (Wormser et al., 2006).

REFERENCES

Aguero-Rosenfeld ME, Donnarumma L, Zentmaier L, Jacob J, Frey M, Noto R, Carbonaro CA, Wormser GP. 2002. Seroprevalence of antibodies that react with Anaplasma phagocytophila, the agent of human granulocytic ehrlichiosis, in different populations in Westchester County, New York. J Clin Microbiol 40:2612–5.

Asanovich KM, Bakken JS, Madigan JE, Aguero-Rosenfeld M, Wormser GP, Dumler JS. 1997. Antigenic diversity of granulocytic Ehrlichia isolates from humans in Wisconsin and New York and a horse in California. J Infect Dis 176:1029–34.

Bakken JS, Dumler S. 2008. Human granulocytic anaplasmosis. Infect Dis Clin N Am 22:433–48.

Bakken JS, Aguero-Rosenfeld ME, Tilden RL, Wormser GP, Horowitz HW, Raffalli JT, Baluch M, Riddell D, Walls JJ, Dumler JS. 2001. Serial measurements of hematologic counts during the active phase of human granulocytic ehrlichiosis. Clin Infect Dis 2:862–70.

Bakken JS, Krueth J, Wilson-Nordskog C, Tilden RL, Asanovich K, Dumler JS. 1996. Clinical and laboratory characteristics of human granulocytic ehrlichiosis. JAMA 275:199–205.

Dumler JS, Choi KS, Garcia-Garcia JC, Barat NS, Scorpio DG, Garyu JW, Grab DJ, Bakken JS. 2005. Human granulocytic anaplasmosis and Anaplasma phagocytophilum. Emerg Infect Dis 11(12):1828–34.

Dumler JS, Madigan JE, Pusterla N, Bakken JS. 2007. Ehrlichioses in humans: epidemiology, clinical presentation, diagnosis, and treatment. Clin Infect Dis 45 (suppl 1): S45–51.

Dumler S, Walker JH. 2009. Ehrlichia chaffeensis (human monocytotropic ehrlichiosis), Anaplasma phagocytophilum (human granulocytotropic anaplasmosis), and other anaplasmataceae. In Mandell, Douglas, and Bennett's Principles and Practice of Infectious Diseases, 7th ed. Churchill-Livingstone, Philadelphia, ch. 193.

Hamburg BJ, Storch GA, Micek ST, Kollef MH. 2008. The importance of early treatment with doxycycline in human ehrlichiosis. Medicine (Baltimore) 87:53–60.

Hamilton KS, Standaert SM, Kinney MC. 2004. Characteristic peripheral blood findings in human ehrlichiosis. Mod Pathol 17:512–7.

Horowitz HW, Aguero-Rosenfeld ME, McKenna DF, Holmgren D, Hsieh TC, Varde SA, Dumler SJ, Wu JM, Schwartz I, Rikihisa Y, Wormser GP. 1998. Clinical and laboratory spectrum of culture-proven human granulocytic ehrlichiosis: comparison with culture-negative cases. Clin Infect Dis. 27:1314–7.

Ijdo JW, Wu C, Telford SR III, Fikrig E. 2002. Differential expression of the p44 gene family in the agent of human granulocytic ehrlichiosis. Infect Immun 70:5295–8.

Ohashi N, Zhi N, Zhang Y, Rikihisa Y. 1998. Immunodominant major outer membrane proteins of Ehrlichia chaffeensis are encoded by a polymorphic multigene family. Infect Immun 66:132–9.

Olano JP, Hogrefe W, Seaton B, Walker DH. 2003. Clinical manifestations, epidemiology, and laboratory diagnosis of human monocytotropic ehrlichiosis in a commercial laboratory setting. Clin Diag Lab Immunol 10:891–6.

Standaert SM, Yu T. Scott MA, Childs JE, Paddock CD, Nicholson WL, Singleton J Jr, Blaser MJ. 2000. Primary isolation of Ehrlichia chaffeensis from patients with febrile illnesses: clinical and molecular characteristics. J Infect Dis 181:1082–8.

Walker DH, Dumler JS. 1997. Human monocytic and granulocytic ehrlichioses: discovery and diagnosis of emerging tick-borne infections and the critical role of the pathologist. Arch Pathol Lab Med 121:785–91.

Wormser GP, Dattwyler RJ, Shapiro ED, Halperin JJ, Steere AC, Klempner MS, Krause PJ, Bakken JS, Strle F, Stanek G, Bockenstedt L, Fish D, Dumler JS,

NADELMAN RB. 2006. The clinical assessment, treatment, and prevention of Lyme disease, human granulocytic anaplasmosis, and babesiosis: clinical practice guidelines by the Infectious Diseases Society of America. Clin Infect Dis43:1089.

YU X, MCBRIDE JW, ZHANG X, WALKER DH. 2000. Characterization of the complete transcriptionally active *Ehrlichia chaffeensis* 28-kDa outer membrane protein multigene family. Gene 248:59–68.

CHAPTER NINE

CLINICALLY SIGNIFICANT FUNGAL YEASTS

Ramon L. Sandin

INTRODUCTION

Fungi are eukaryotes that can be divided morphologically into two basic groups: yeasts and molds (Beneke and Rogers, 1980). Yeasts are unicellular budding fungi that can reproduce sexually and/or asexually. On the culture plate in the microbiology laboratory, yeast colonies are often described as slimy, mucoid, or less commonly as dry. Molds are filamentous fungi that grow by forming long chains of cells called "hyphae" (Kern, 1985). A mass of hyphae is called a "mycelium." On the culture plate, mold colonies are often described using terms such as downy, fluffy, granular, cottony, or wooly. Table 9.1 lists the most clinically relevant mycoses and the corresponding fungal agents, arranged according to the extent of fungal involvement and body site affected.

Some fungi are "dimorphic" or "diphasic," which means that they exhibit two forms or phases when they grow in different environments (Beneke et al., 1984). One phase is the mycelial or filamentous form that is found as the free-living or "saprophytic" form in nature, as well as when the agent is growing at 30°C (equivalent to room temperature) on the culture plate. The other phase is the yeast or yeast-like "parasitic" phase that the agent assumes when growing at 37°C on a culture plate, or at body temperature and as seen in histopathological slides prepared from patient tissue or body fluid samples (Bulmer, 1978). Since the form switch in most (albeit not all) of these agents occurs in response to changes in temperature, it is customary to refer to them as "thermodimorphic" agents. Seven clinically relevant thermodimorphic agents are *Histoplasma capsulatum*, *Blastomyces dermatitidis*, *Coccidioides immitis*, *Paracoccidioides brasiliensis*, *Sporothrix schenckii*, *Penicillium marneffei*, and the dematiaceous molds that are causative agents of Chromoblastomycosis (Larone, 2002; Rippon, 1982).

Several of these dimorphic agents may be encountered by hematopathologists during the examination of peripheral blood or bone marrow specimens as part of differential diagnostic considerations. Other nondimorphic agents also are on that list. Table 9.2 lists the six genera of yeast or yeast-like clinical agents most frequently encountered by hematopathologists in peripheral blood or bone marrow samples. The remainder of this chapter will emphasize only the six agents listed on Table 9.2.

Non-Neoplastic Hematopathology and Infections, First Edition. Edited by Hernani D. Cualing, Parul Bhargava, and Ramon L. Sandin.
© 2012 Wiley-Blackwell. Published 2012 by John Wiley & Sons, Inc.

TABLE 9.1 Clinically Most Relevant Human Mycoses and Their Fungal Agents, Arranged by Extent of Body Involvement

Type	Disease	Agent(s)
Deep or systemic	Histoplasmosis	*Histoplasma capsulatum*
	Blastomycosis	*Blastomyces dermatitidis*
	Coccidioidomycosis	*Coccidioides immitis*
	Paracoccidioidomycosis	*Paracoccidioides brasiliensis*
Subcutaneous	Eumycotic mycetoma	*Pseudallescheria boydii* and other dematiaceous or hyaline molds
	Chromoblastomycosis	*Fonsecaea pedrosoi* and other dematiaceous molds
	Sporothrichosis	*Sporothrix schenckii*
	Rhinosporidiosis (disease now considered among the parasitoses)	*Rhinosporidium seeberi* (agent now reclassified as aquatic protistan parasite)
	Lobomycosis	*Lacazia* (Loboa) *loboi*
Cutaneous/superficial	Candidiasis	*Candida albicans* and other species
	Tinea versicolor	*Malassezia furfur*
	Tineas ("ringworms")	Species of *Microsporum, Epidermophyton, Trichophyton*
Opportunistic	Cryptococcosis	*Cryptococcus neoformans, C. gattii*
	Hyalohyphomycosis	*Aspergillus spp. Fusarium,* and many other hyaline genera of molds
	Phaeohyphomycosis	*Scedosporium, Curvularia,* and many other dematiaceous genera of molds
	Zygomycosis	*Rhizopus, Mucor, Absidia,* and other genera of zygomycetous fungi

TABLE 9.2 Yeast or Yeast-like Clinical Agents Frequently Encountered in Smears from Peripheral Blood or Bone Marrow Specimens

Histoplasma capsulatum var. capsulatum
Blastomyces dermatitidis
Coccidioides immitis
Cryptococcus neoformans
Candida albicans and other *Candida* species
Malassezia furfur

HISTOPLASMA CAPSULATUM VAR. CAPSULATUM (H. CAPSULATUM)

Histoplasmosis capsulati (histoplasmosis) is a very common granulomatous disease of worldwide distribution caused by the dimorphic fungus *H. capsulatum*. Approximately 95% of cases are inapparent, subclinical, or completely benign. The remaining patients have a chronic progressive lung disease, a chronic systemic or cutaneous disease, or an acute fulminating, rapidly fatal, systemic infection (Amstrong and Cohen, 1999; Rippon, 1982). It is

this acute systemic infection—which may affect any severely immunocompromised patient—that is of particular importance to the hematopathologist (Kang and Sandin, 2004; Sandin, 1996). In such scenarios, the agent resides inside various cell types of the reticuloendothelial system in clinical samples that a hematopathologist may be asked to review. The yeast forms of *H. capsulatum* may be present in various types of peripheral blood leucocytes, in macrophages or lymphocytes of the spleen or liver, within lymph nodes (see Chapter 20) as well as clumped together in groups on bone marrow aspirates, touch preps, or fixed bone marrow biopsy tissue.

While there is also a clinically distinct form of disease, histoplasmosis duboisii, common in Africa, caused by *H. capsulatum var. duboisii* (Rippon,1982), this chapter will not expand on that form of the disease. See Chapter 20 for *H. capsulatum var. duboisii*. All material covered in this chapter will refer to histoplasmosis caused by *H. capsulatum var. capsulatum*.

Definition

Histoplasmosis is a self-limited or progressive pulmonary mycosis with a marked proclivity to disseminate via the mononuclear phagocyte system. The natural habitat of the fungus is fecal-enriched soil found in avian and chiropteran habitats such as roosting shelters, chicken coops, caves, and attics. There is no evidence that this disease is contagious from person to person and about half of all patients have no apparent immunologic defects (Chandler and Watts, 1987; Connor and Chandler, 1997).

ICD-10 Codes B39.0-B39.9

B39   **Histoplasmosis**
B39.0 Acute pulmonary histoplasmosis capsulati
B39.1 Chronic pulmonary histoplasmosis capsulati
B39.2 Pulmonary histoplasmosis capsulati, unspecified
B39.3 Disseminated histoplasmosis capsulati
    Generalized histoplasmosis capsulati
B39.4 Histoplasmosis capsulati, unspecified
    American histoplasmosis
B39.5 Histoplasmosis duboisii
    African histoplasmosis
B39.9 Histoplasmosis, unspecified

Synonyms

Darling's disease, reticuloendotheliosis, reticuloendothelial cytomycosis, cave disease, Ohio River Valley disease, Tingo Maria fever (Rippon, 1982).

Epidemiology

The etiologic agent has been found in practically all habitable areas of the earth in which it has been sought. Its growth is particularly associated with the presence of guano and debris of birds and bats. The fungus can survive and be transmitted from one location to another in the dermal appendages of both and also in the intestinal contents of bats, but wind is probably the most important agent of dissemination. The infection is also very common in wild and domestic animals in endemic areas. In the Western Hemisphere, hyperendemic areas include Guatemala, Mexico, Peru, Venezuela, and the broad region of the Ohio and Mississippi River valleys in the United States (Chandler and Watts, 1987; DiSalvo, 1983; Rippon, 1982).

Clinical Aspects and Pathophysiology

About a half million new cases of histoplasmosis occur each year in the United States. However, 90 to 95% of these cases are asymptomatic, self-limited infections, but such patients would have positive reactions to the histoplasmin skin test. In time, many of these individuals develop residual pulmonary lesions that may calcify and be discovered inadvertently on chest radiological tests or at autopsy. Symptomatic infection in the remaining 5 to 10% of patients can be divided into three major clinical forms: acute pulmonary, disseminated, and chronic pulmonary (Chandler and Watts, 1987; Mujeeb et al., 2002).

In acute pulmonary disease, patients develop a mild flu-like respiratory syndrome 3 to 14 days after exposure to aerosolized conidia of the fungus. However, in rapidly progressive manifestations of this acute pulmonary form of infection, bilateral and often miliary reticulo-nodular infiltrates evolve. The severity and duration of disease depend on host resistance and the number of fungal conidia inhaled. Most infections resolve within 1 to 4 weeks with supportive therapy, though at times antifungal administration may be required (Chandler and Watts, 1987).

In a minority of patients with the acute pulmonary form, infection is progressive and disseminates via the mononuclear phagocyte system. This is the stage that is of particular relevance to the hematopathologist. Cell-mediated immunity is thought to play a major role in preventing replication of the agent in tissue. The sites most commonly involved in the course of disseminated disease are lymph nodes, spleen, liver, bone marrow, lungs, gastrointestinal tract, adrenals, and mucous membranes of the oral cavity. Due to hematogenous dissemination, the agent may be found in smears from peripheral blood during this stage. In addition to flu-like and several other generalized symptoms, the patient may have weight loss, leucopenia, anemia, purpura, generalized lymphadenopathy, hepatosplenomegaly, and other symptoms that resemble those of a rapidly progressive lymphoproliferative disease. The fatality rate of this form of histoplasmosis is potentially great and prompt treatment with antifungals is imperative (Chandler and Watts, 1987).

Chronic pulmonary histoplasmosis is primarily a disease of adults that may follow the acute form of the disease or become clinically apparent after a long period of dormancy. Symptoms include productive cough, weight loss, dyspnea, fever, chest pain, and hemoptysis. Two roentgenographic patterns predominate among several others: cavitary lesions that result from endogenous reinfection and are most often seen in the upper lung lobes, and the residual solitary nodule or histoplasmoma that present as a "coin lesion." These are single or solitary, discrete, subpleural nodules that are frequently calcified and may be accompanied by enlarged, caseated and calcified hilar lymph nodes. Fibrosing mediastinitis may complicate chronic infection of hilar and mediastinal lymph nodes (Chandler and Watts, 1987).

Differential Diagnosis

At all stages of its pathogenesis, histoplasmosis mimics tuberculosis. Only culture and adequate serologic evidence provide the correct diagnosis. Histoplasmosis may coexist with any number of granulomatous diseases of the lung, including TB, sarcoidosis, actinomycosis, and other mycotic infections (Rippon, 1982).

Primary histoplasmosis in its acute stage closely resembles the acute infection produced by other mycoses, viral and bacterial pneumonias, lipoid pneumonia, and Hamman-rich syndrome (diffuse interstitial pulmonary fibrosis) (Rippon, 1982).

Acute disseminated histoplasmosis with its accompanying hepatosplenomegaly, lymphadenopathy, anemia, and leucopenia resembles the acute stage of visceral leishmaniasis as well as many of the lymphoproliferative diseases. In most forms of histoplasmosis, thick blood smears or material from sternal punctures often reveal the organism more readily than culture or direct sputum examination. The blood smears can be prepared from the buffy coat of centrifuged citrated blood or from the bottom of the tube where sedimented, heavily infested cells are found. Other diseases to be considered in the differential diagnosis of histoplasmosis are infectious mononucleosis, brucellosis, malaria, and Gaucher's disease. When cutaneous or mucocutaneous lesions are present, they may suggest neoplasias, sporotrichosis, syphilis, toxoplasmosis, bacterial cellulitis, tuberculosis cutis, or other systemic mycotic infection (Rippon, 1982).

Treatment of Choice and Prognosis

Amphotericin B and its lipid formulations have considerable activity against most endemic fungal pathogens in vitro. Amphotericin B deoxycholate (AmBd) is recommended as initial therapy in the management of severe forms of histoplasmosis, including acute and chronic pulmonary disease, disseminated disease, CNS disease, and granulomatous mediastinitis. If high dosages of AmBd are not tolerated, substitution with a lipid formulation can be considered. After the initial induction period, usually 2 weeks, treatment for most patients can be changed to an azole or an extended-interval dose of a polyene for the maintenance phase of therapy (Mohr et al., 2008).

Approach to Diagnosis

Clinical Workup

A thorough history and physical examination is key to developing an early suspicion for histoplasmosis. X-ray or CT scan evaluation for pulmonary lesions is routinely ordered. This would be accompanied by routine blood testing for hematological and chemical markers. If acute disseminated disease is suspected, evaluation of peripheral blood smears or formalin-fixed and stained sections from bone marrow or biopsy tissues should be performed and may be accompanied by serological evaluation for markers of seroconversion.

Morphologic Aspects

Histoplasma capsulatum is a thermo-dimorphic fungus that exhibits quite different morphologies when found at 30°C and 37°C. From any type of infected fluid or tissue sample derived from a patient for hematologic, cytologic, or histopathologic evaluation, the agent will be found in its 37°C "parasitic" form, which is a yeast form, just as it would appear on a smear from a culture plate incubated at 37°C (Figure 9.1).

The yeast-like cells of this fungus are spherical to oval, 2 to 4 μm in diameter, uninucleate, have single buds, and are often clustered within large mononuclear phagocytes, which accounts for the term used at times of "histiocytomycotic" or "reticuloendothelial cytomycotic" disease (Figures 9.2 and 9.3). When stained with H&E, the basophilic cytoplasm of the fungal cell is retracted from the thin, poorly stained cell wall, which creates a clear space that gives the false impression of an unstained capsule or halo (pseudocapsule). With the special stains for fungi, however, the cell walls are intensely colored and the halo effect is abolished. In addition to typical organisms, hyphae and huge, bizarre yeast forms are occasionally found on or near the surface of valvular vegetations in endocarditis by *Histoplasma* (Chandler and Watts, 1987; Salfelder, 1980; Salfelder, 1990). Table 9.3 summarizes the morphologic findings of *H. capsulatum* when it is found as yeasts in tissues and body fluids.

TABLE 9.3 Morphologic Diagnostic Features of *Histoplasma capsulatum var. capsulatum* in Blood, Bone Marrow, Body Fluids, or Histopathological Slides, or in Synthetic Culture Media at 37°C

Single or budding yeast cells; if budding, with one daughter yeast attached

Small yeast size, 2–5 μm per cell, and round to oval shape

Thin-neck between mother and daughter yeast cell

In acute disease, located inside cells of the RES (reticuloendothelial system)

In chronic pulmonary disease, located inside fibrocaseous or fibrocalcific lesions

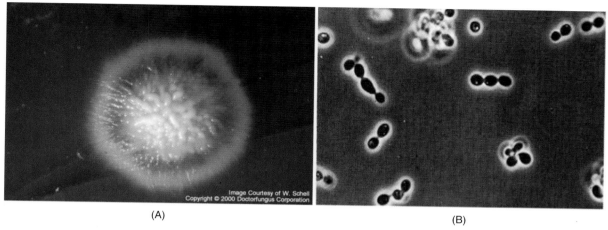

(A)   (B)

FIGURE 9.1   *Histoplasma capsulatum* **on the culture plate at 37°C, gross and microscopic morphology.** (A) Colonies are dry, coral-like, and cerebriform. (B) A smear reveals small budding yeasts, 2 to 5 μm in size, with a narrow neck between mother and daughter yeasts and usually a single bud per adult cell. (http://botit.botany.wisc.edu/toms_fungi/images/hcapyeast.jpg)

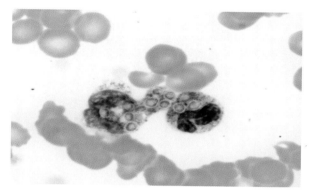

FIGURE 9.2   *Histoplasma capsulatum* **yeast phase.** Several intracellular fungi, including budding yeasts, are evident within polymorphonucleate neutrophils on a peripheral blood smear. Wright stain, oil immersion 1000×. (ASCP Hematology Check Sample H 2005-3 (H-294))

Several microbial agents may resemble *H. capsulatum* in smears and sections from clinical samples. Intracellular microforms of *Blastomyces dermatitidis* are rare but could be confused with *Histoplasma* organisms. However, they would be multinucleate, with broad-based budding and thick walls. The yeast-like cells of *Candida* (*Torulopsis*) *glabrata* are comparable in size to *Histoplasma* and are often sequestered within phagocytes, but there is no halo or pseudocapsular effect. Amastigotes of *Leishmania* spp. and *Trypanosoma cruzi*, when located within mononuclear phagocytes, appear similar to *Histoplasma* yeast cells. However, these parasites have bar-shaped kinetoplasts next to their nuclei. Calcific bodies, which are often found in the caseated centers of granulomas of diverse etiology, are readily stained with H&E and the PAS stain and may resemble yeast-like cells.

However, they do not stain with GMS or Gridley stains (Chandler and Watts, 1987).

"Wet" Diagnosis in the Clinical Microbiology Laboratory

Histoplasma capsulatum is a thermodimorphic fungus that exhibits different morphologies when cultured at 30°C and 37°C. When growing at 30°C on fungal media such as blood-brain heart infusion agar (BBHI) or Sabouraud's fungal media (Sab), the organism is a slow-grower and manifests itself as a cottony, white to brown mycelium that is not fully pathognomonic. A microscopic examination of a smear in lactophenol cotton blue reveals the presence of large, tuberculated (echinulate or spiny) macroconidia as well as microconidia. The macroconidia are large and round, 8 to 16 μm and are the diagnostic feature. The saprophytic fungus *Sepedonium* produces tuberculated macroconidia like *Histoplasma* at 30°C but has no microconidia. It is also not a dimorphic organism (Beneke and Rogers, 1980; Koneman and Roberts, 1985; Koneman et al., 1997; Sutton et al., 1998).

When it grows at 37°C on artificial media, the colony switches its appearance from that of mold-like to moist and pasty, at times dry, coral-like or "cerebriform." A lactophenol cotton blue smear would show small budding yeasts identical to those described already as seen at 37°C in tissues or body fluids. Conversion to the yeast phase in synthetic media is slow, and sometimes may fail to occur and require several trials (Beneke and Rogers, 1980).

Newer Diagnostic Modalities

There are commercially available kits for extracting, concentrating, and testing exoantigens derived from

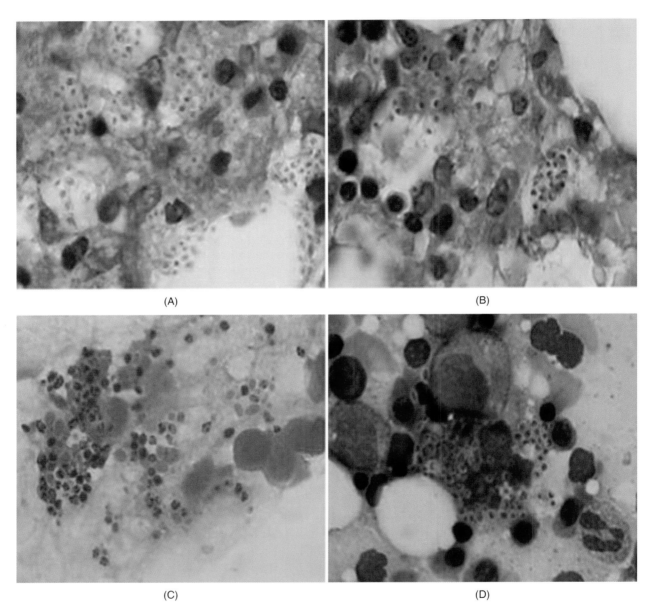

(A)

(B)

(C)

(D)

FIGURE 9.3 *Histoplasma capsulatum* **yeast phase**. The bone marrow biopsy specimen shows numerous oval-shaped intracellular and extracellular microorganisms (A, B). The bone marrow aspiration smear shows numerous yeast-like organisms (C, D). (A) Hematoxylin and eosin stain, 1000×; (B) periodic acid-Schiff stain, 1000×; (C) Gram's stain, 1000×; (D) Wright stain, 1000×. (http://www.cdc.gov/ncidod/EID/13/1/127-G1.htm Lai et al., *Emerging Infect Dis*, 13(1), 2007)

cultural isolates for confirmation of suspected fungal morphologic identity. However, it is toward the new frontier of nucleic acid probes and molecular amplification techniques that the field is moving rapidly in the quest to provide sensitive and specific confirmatory tools for fungal diagnosis, and *Histoplasma* is no exception (Alkan et al., 1995; Mitchell et al., 1994; Sandin, 2002). There are commercially available DNA probes for culture confirmation of *Histoplasma* (Sandin et al., 1993a) and reports of in-house or home-brew

reagent combinations for PCR detection of gene targets by conventional or real-time approaches, and this can be done directly from clinical samples (Sandin, 2002).

BLASTOMYCES DERMATITIDIS

North American blastomycosis is a chronic granulomatous and suppurative disease having a primary pulmonary stage that is frequently followed by dissemination to other body sites, chiefly the skin and bone. The primary infection in the lung is often inapparent. The causative agent is the dimorphic fungus *Blastomyces dermatitidis*, formerly thought to be restricted to the North American continent, but subsequently described from divergent parts of Africa, Asia, and Europe. Unlike the other common systemic mycoses, it does not appear to have a common mild subclinical form, and the frequency of the self-limited, spontaneously resolving infection is as yet unknown (Rippon, 1982).

Definition

North American Blastomycosis is a chronic granulomatous and suppurative infection caused by the dimorphic fungus *Blastomyces dermatitidis*, which occurs in the central and southeastern areas of the United States as a sporadic disease, with rare episodes of epidemics, and in the Middle East and several African countries. Most infections result from inhalation of airborne conidia of the mycelial form of the fungus growing as a saprophyte in soil. In rare instances, however, a primary cutaneous infection results from the accidental direct inoculation of the fungus; thus inoculation blastomycosis could be considered an occupational hazard for pathologists (Chandler and Watts, 1987; Connor and Chandler, 1997).

ICD-10 Codes B40.0-B40.9

B40	**Blastomycosis**
	Excludes: Brazilian blastomycosis (B41.-)
	keloidal blastomycosis (B48.0)
B40.0	**Acute pulmonary blastomycosis**
B40.1	**Chronic pulmonary blastomycosis**
B40.2	**Pulmonary blastomycosis, unspecified**
B40.3	**Cutaneous blastomycosis**
B40.7	**Disseminated blastomycosis**
	Generalized blastomycosis
B40.8	**Other forms of blastomycosis**
B40.9	**Blastomycosis, unspecified**

Synonyms

North American Blastomycosis, Gilchrist's disease, Chicago disease (Rippon, 1982).

Epidemiology

The natural habitat of *B. dermatitidis* remains an enigma. Since essentially all infections are acquired by inhalation of conidia into the lungs, the organism should be a saprophyte in soil, producing mycelium and airborne conidia. Most attempts to isolate the organism from soil in endemic areas have failed, with only a few exceptions. It appears that conidia from this organism that are placed in the soil, survive for a few weeks only. These may be unable to compete with the normal flora of soil and perhaps survive only in a very restricted ecologic environment. It does grow on decaying organic material. The overall range of autochthonous cases in the American continent includes the middle western states, the southeastern states, and the Appalachian states, which is the general drainage pattern for the Mississippi and Ohio River basins (Chandler and Watts, 1987; DiSalvo, 1983; Rippon, 1982).

Infections in dogs often serve as a harbinger of the outbreak of human case clusters. As has been established by analysis of numerous case reports and autopsies, blastomycosis is acquired by the inhalation of fungal conidia and is not considered contagious from human to human. However, very rarely and under extraordinary circumstances, such transmission has apparently occurred, such as during some cases of conjugal transmission of yeast cells in semen (Rippon, 1982).

Clinical Aspects and Pathophysiology

Sporadic blastomycosis occurs most often in persons 30 to 50 years old who spend much of their time outdoors. However, epidemic blastomycosis is usually a disease of young persons of either sex. Clinically apparent blastomycosis can be either systemic or cutaneous. Both clinical forms have a pulmonary inception, but their presentation, clinical course, and prognosis differ. The systemic form is primarily a pulmonary disease that either remains confined to the lungs or disseminates hematogenously to other organs, specially the skin, bones, lymph nodes, mucosal surfaces, adrenal glands, and central nervous system. When the fungus disseminates to the skin only, it produces ulcerative and verrucous lesions in a chronic pattern marked by remissions and exacerbations with gradually enlarging lesions. While untreated systemic blastomycosis is a serious, progressive, and often fatal disease, the general health of the patient with lesions confined to the skin and without apparent visceral involvement is not impaired. In addition to these two manifestations, and just as it may occur with any of the deep or systemic fungal pathogens, there are the rare reports of primary cutaneous blastomycosis that appear to occur solely as inoculation into the skin of fungal conidia from the environment (Chandler and Watts, 1987; Mujeeb et al., 2002).

Differential Diagnosis

Blastomycosis must be differentiated from any chronic granulomatous or suppurative pulmonary disease. The list includes histoplasmosis, because of the overlap of endemic areas, tuberculosis, silicosis, sarcoidosis, and to a lesser extent actinomycosis, nocardiosis, and other bacterial diseases. High on the list of differentials are pulmonary neoplasms. Cutaneous lesions resemble scrofuloderma, lupus vulgaris, epitheliomas, bromoderma, iododerma, nodular syphilids, granuloma inguinale, fishtank granuloma, and similar diseases (Rippon, 1982).

There does not seem to be an association of blastomycosis with underlying or debilitating disease. In the many reviews of complications that occur in patients with neoplasias and leukemias, and of those receiving steroids, no increase in incidence of blastomycosis was found. It is possible that subtle immunologic differences are present in the patient who develops the disease. This is particularly true in patients with the systemic form rather than the chronic cutaneous form of the disease. Blastomycosis may coexist with tuberculosis, histoplasmosis, and bronchogenic carcinoma, as well as other diseases with severe pulmonary involvement (Rippon, 1982).

Treatment of Choice and Prognosis

Amphotericin B and its lipid formulations have considerable activity against most endemic fungal pathogens in vitro. Amphotericin B deoxycholate (AmBd) is the preferred treatment for pulmonary disease, life-threatening disseminated non-CNS disease, and any disseminated CNS blastomycosis. As an alternative to AmBd, lipid formulations of amphotericin B can be prescribed, but no comparative trials have evaluated them in patiens with blastomycosis. Alternative therapies in use by selected medical groups include several of the azole group of drugs, including itraconazole (Mohr et al., 2008).

Approach to Diagnosis

Clinical Workup

A thorough history and physical examination is key to developing an early suspicion for blastomycosis. X-ray or CT scan evaluation for determination of any systemic extent of the lesions may be ordered. This would be accompanied by routine blood testing for hematological and chemical markers. Biopsy and culture evaluation of any accessible skin lesion would be diagnostic. If there are pulmonary symptoms including a productive cough, then a sputum sample should be submitted to microbiology for smear and culture, as could a bronchoalveolar lavage sample that is collected during a bronchoscopic examination. Peripheral blood may be inoculated into blood culture bottles if the systemic stage of the disease is suspected.

Morphologic Aspects

B. dermatitidis is found in both suppurative and granulomatous lesions as intra- and extracellular, spherical to oval, large, multinucleate yeast-like cells, 8 to 15 µm in diameter (Figure 9.4). Some organisms may be as large as 20 to 30 µm in diameter. The cells have thick, doubly contoured refractile walls (best demonstrated with H&E) and single, broad-based buds. The persistent broad-based budding of *B. dermatitidis* is diagnostic. It helps to differentiate this fungus from yeast forms of similar size, especially the African variety of histoplasmosis termed *Histoplasma capsulatum var duboisii*. The presence of multiple nuclei within the centrally retracted cytoplasm is also helpful (Chandler and Watts, 1987; Rippon, 1982). Table 9.4 summarizes the morphologic findings of *B. dermatitidis* as it is found in tissues and body fluids. A hematopathologist who is asked to review a peripheral blood smear or bone marrow biopsy during the dissemination phase of a systemic infection, would use these features for diagnosis.

Occasionally very small (2–4 µm) but morphologically typical forms of *B. dermatitidis* are found in the lesions of blastomycosis. These are called "microforms" and are almost always found as part of a continuous series of sizes and in the presence of the larger more pathognomonic yeast forms. Germ tubes, pseudohyphae, and hyphae are formed rarely in tissues (Chandler and Watts, 1987).

In both localized and systemic infections, the fungus characteristically incites a mixed suppurative and granulomatous inflammatory reaction. In early lesions, neutrophils predominate, but eosinophils

TABLE 9.4 Morphologic Diagnostic Features of *Blastomyces dermatitidis* in Blood, Bone Marrow, Body Fluids, or Histopathological Slides, or in Synthetic Culture Media at 37°C

Single or budding yeasts, 8–15 µm in diameter per cell
Some larger rare yeasts (20–30 µm)
Thick and rigid, "doubly-contoured" (or doubly refractile) cell wall
Multinucleate cytoplasm
Broad-based budding between mother and daughter yeast cells
Rare microforms have been described (2–5 µm), the size of *Histoplasma*

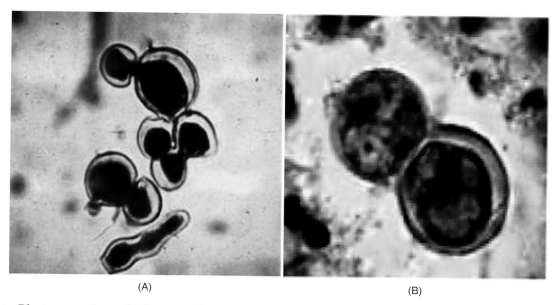

(A)   (B)

FIGURE 9.4 *Blastomyces dermatitidis*, **yeast phase, as found in infected cells and tissues or in culture at 37°C.** (A) Large mother yeasts, 7 to 15 μm, with thick double-contoured walls, as appreciated by phase-microscopy at 400×. (B) A single bud can be appreciated, with a broad base between mother and daughter yeast. H&E 1000×. (Courtesy of the teaching collections of E.S. Beneke and A.L. Rogers; Beneke ES, Rogers AL. 1980. *Medical Mycology Manual.* 4th ed. Minneapolis: Burgess Publishing Company)

may also be present. Older lesions appear as focal and confluent epithelioid and giant cell granulomas, some of which have central abscesses or caseation or both. Unless the yeast-like cells of *B. dermatitidis* are identified, it is often difficult to distinguish these lesions from those of chronic active tuberculosis or, at times, from those of histoplasmosis. Acute, rapidly expanding lesions sometimes contain enormous numbers of proliferating intra-alveolar yeast forms, whereas fungal cells are usually sparse in the chronic lesions. Fibrosis is common and may be accompanied by cavitation. However, solitary residual fibrocaseous nodules, commonly seen in histoplasmosis, are rare, and calcification of such lesions is even rarer. Florid pseudoepitheliomatous hyperplasia characterizes cutaneous blastomycosis, which can mimic squamous cell carcinoma (Chandler and Watts, 1987; Salfelder, 1980; Salfelder, 1990).

The differential diagnosis of this agent in histopathologic sections or smears from body fluids will now be described. When typical budding forms with the diagnostic broad base are found, this agent can be identified with confidence, but otherwise, the agent may be confused with others, especially nonbudding, hypocapsular ("capsule deficient") cells of *Cryptococcus neoformans*. In such cases mucin stains should be used to demonstrate an attenuated mucopolysaccharide capsule in *C. neoformans*. However, the cell walls of *B. dermatitidis* may also

react positively with mucin stains, but it is the wall that stains in such cases, not any capsular material, and the intensity of staining is never as great as that of typical capsular staining in *Cryptococcus* cells. Also *C. neoformans* daughter cells are attached by narrow necks, not by broad bases as is *B. dermatitidis* (Chandler and Watts, 1987; Salfelder, 1980; Salfelder, 1990).

Last, large, nonbudding cells of *B. dermatitidis* that are empty-looking may be mistaken for immature spherules of *Coccidioides immitis*. Tissue-form cells of *H. capsulatum var duboisii* are comparable in size to *B. dermatitidis*, but the former contain a single nucleus and undergo narrow-base budding like *H. capsulatum var capsulatum*, as described in the earlier section of this chapter. Intracellular microforms of *B. dermatitidis*, 2 to 4 μm in diameter, may also be confused with *H. capsulatum var. capsulatum* as far as size. A mixture of microforms and the large, typical forms of *B. dermatitidis* could potentially be mistaken for coexisting mycoses (Chandler and Watts, 1987; Rippon, 1982).

"Wet" Diagnosis in the Clinical Microbiology Laboratory

B. dermatitidis is a thermodimorphic fungus that exhibits quite different morphologies when cultured at 30°C and 37°C. When growing at 30°C on fungal media such as BBHI or Sab, the organism may first manifest itself as a yeast-like growth, then develops the "prickly stage" with surface hyphal projections termed coremia, and finally the entire surface becomes downy or fluffy white. Older cultures become tan to brown. A microscopic examination of a smear in lactophenol cotton blue reveals the presence of numerous round to pyriform (pear-shaped), one-celled conidia, 2 to 10 μm in diameter, attached directly to the hyphae or on short conidiophores. These structures are not wholly pathognomonic for *B. dermatitidis* since agents such as *Pseudallescheria boydii* or *Chrysosporium* spp., among others, may produce similar "lollipop" or pyriform conidia. Older cultures may have chlamydospores with thickened walls (Beneke and Rogers, 1980; Koneman and Roberts, 1985; Koneman et al., 1997; Sutton et al., 1998).

When it grows at 37°C on artificial media, the colony switches its appearance from that of mold-like to moist and pasty, at times dry, coral-like or "cerebriform." A lactophenol cotton blue smear would show large, thick-walled, single and budding yeast cells with broad-based budding identical to those described already as seen at 37°C in tissues or body fluids. Short mycelial fragments will also be present (Beneke and Rogers, 1980).

Newer Diagnostic Modalities

There are commercially available kits for extracting, concentrating, and testing exoantigens derived from cultural isolates for confirmation of suspected fungal morphologic identity. However, it is toward the new frontier of nucleic acid probes and molecular amplification techniques that the field is moving rapidly, in the quest to provide sensitive and specific confirmatory tools for fungal diagnosis, and *Blastomyces* is no exception (Alkan et al., 1995; Mitchell et al., 1994; Sandin, 2002). There are commercially available DNA probes for culture confirmation of *Blastomyces* (Sandin, 1991; Sandin et al., 1993b) and reports of in-house or home-brew reagent combinations for PCR detection of gene targets by conventional or real-time approaches, and this can be done directly from clinical samples (Sandin, 2002).

COCCIDIOIDES IMMITIS

Coccidioidomycosis is an acute self-limited or progressive pulmonary mycosis caused by the dimorphic pathogen *Coccidioides immitis*. The mycelial form of this fungus inhabits desert soil throughout the Lower Sonoran Life Zone, a semi-arid climatic zone with a brief, intense rainy season. The disease is hyperendemic in the southwestern United States (southern California, Arizona, New Mexico, western Texas, Nevada, and Utah), northern and central Mexico, and parts of Central America and South America, where these climatic conditions prevail (Chandler and Watts, 1987; Connor and Chandler, 1997).

Definition

Coccidioidomycosis is a benign, inapparent, or mildly severe upper respiratory infection that usually resolves quickly. It was the first of the severe fatal mycoses in which an inapparent or mild form of disease was found to occur commonly in inhabitants of its endemic region. Rarely the disease is an acute or chronic, severe disseminating, fatal mycosis. If infection is established, the disease may progress as a chronic pulmonary condition or as a systemic disease involving the meninges, bones, joints, and subcutaneous and cutaneous tissues. During dissemination to any of these sites, the agent gains importance to the hematopathologist since it may be encountered during review of peripheral blood smears, bone marrow aspirates or biopsies, or fixed sections of tissue from lymph nodes, spleen, or liver (Rippon, 1982).

ICD-10 Codes B38.0-B38.9

B38	**Coccidioidomycosis**
B38.0	**Acute pulmonary coccidioidomycosis**
B38.1	**Chronic pulmonary coccidioidomycosis**
B38.2	**Pulmonary coccidioidomycosis, unspecified**
B38.3	**Cutaneous coccidioidomycosis**
B38.4+	**Coccidioidomycosis meningitis** (G02.1*)
B38.7	**Disseminated coccidioidomycosis**
	Generalized coccidioidomycosis
B38.8	**Other forms of coccidioidomycosis**
B38.9	**Coccidioidomycosis, unspecified**

Synonyms

Posadas's disease, coccidioidal granuloma, Valley Fever, desert rheumatism, Valley bumps, California disease (Rippon, 1982).

Epidemiology

An essentially unique feature of coccidioidomycosis is the purported increased susceptibility of persons with pigmented skin. Most of all cases of the disseminated disease in the early literature were among Portuguese and Filipino farm laborers. Equalizing as much as possible for occupational exposure and socioeconomic conditions, Filipinos and Negroes run the highest risk of dissemination, with the rate considerably less for

Native Americans and Mexican-Indians. Caucasians have the lowest incidence of dissemination. Some studies indicate an association of severe disease with group B blood type and HLA-A9; both parameters are more common in persons of black and Filipino origin than in those of Caucasian background (Rippon, 1982; DiSalvo, 1983).

Clinical Aspects and Pathophysiology

Primary pulmonary coccidioidomycosis is initiated by inhalation of highly infectious, aerosolized arthroconidia produced by the mycelial form of the fungus in soil. About 40% of patients develop a mild, flu-like respiratory syndrome or frank pneumonia following a 1 to 4 weeks incubation period; the remaining 60% have an asymptomatic infection that resolves spontaneously. The mildly symptomatic form is referred to as the San Joaquin Valley Fever. Allergic manifestations such as cutaneous erythemas occur in about 10% of patients with symptomatic primary pulmonary disease. Most cases of primary pulmonary infection resolve spontaneously. About 1% of patients with symptomatic primary pulmonary infection develop chronic progressive coccidioidal pneumonia, a chronic fibrocavitary infection that resembles chronic tuberculosis. Miliary pulmonary and extrapulmonary hematogenous dissemination of infection are serious sequelae of coccidioidomycosis that occur in <1% of patients. Disseminated infection is virtually restricted to members of certain high-risk groups such as the ethnic groups mentioned earlier, as well as pregnant females, infants, the elderly, and patients immunocompromised by chemotherapy, or by solid organ or bone marrow transplantation. Organs frequently involved include the skin, meninges, bones and joints, liver, spleen, lymph nodes, genitourinary tract, and adrenal glands. Mortality in such cases, even with treatment, is high (Chandler and Watts, 1987; Mujeeb et al., 2002).

Differential Diagnosis

In the endemic areas, coccidioidomycosis should be considered in the differential diagnosis of any nonspecific illness. This is also true with persons who have visited these areas at any time prior to onset of symptoms, particularly when the signs and symptoms are vague and nonspecific.

Primary disease is often confused with other acute pulmonary infections, such as influenza, primary atypical pneumonia, bronchitis, bronchopneumonia, or simply a "cold." Since this form of disease most often resolves uneventfully and without treatment,

the patient is none the worse. Secondary coccidioidomycosis, however, requires therapy so that it is imperative to make a specific diagnosis. The disease must be differentiated from tuberculosis, neoplasias, other mycotic infections, syphilis, tularemia, melioidosis, and bacterial osteomyelitis (Rippon, 1982).

Treatment of Choice and Prognosis

Use of polyenes for management of chronic pulmonary or disseminated coccidioidomycosis has been supplanted mainly by azoles such as fluconazole and itraconazole. Amphotericin B is now typically reserved for patients with hypoxia and/or respiratory failure, those with rapidly progressing coccidioidal infections, or women during pregnancy because azoles are teratogenic. Lipid formulations of amphotericin B are alternatives to amphotericin B, but data supporting administration of lipid formulations are limited to open-label experience (Mohr et al., 2008).

Approach to Diagnosis

Clinical Workup

A thorough history and physical examination is key to developing an early suspicion for coccidioidomycosis. X-ray or CT scan evaluation for determination of any systemic extent of the lesions may be ordered. This would be accompanied by routine blood testing for hematological and chemical markers. Biopsy and culture evaluation of any accessible skin lesion would be diagnostic. If there are pulmonary symptoms including a productive cough, then a sputum sample should be submitted to microbiology for smear and culture, as could a bronchoalveolar lavage sample that is collected during a bronchoscopic examination. Peripheral blood may be inoculated into blood culture bottles if the systemic stage of the disease is suspected.

Morphologic Aspects

The asexual developmental forms produced by *C. immitis* in host tissues consist of immature spherules, mature spherules, and endospores (Figure 9.5). Only the endosporulating spherules are diagnostic. Immature, nonendosporulating, spherules, 5 to 30 μm in diameter, develop directly in the lungs from exogenous, inhaled arthroconidia. Once the infection is established, however, immature spherules develop mainly from endogenously released endospores. The walls and granular internal contents of the immature spherules are PAS positive. Mature, endosporulating, spherules range in diameter from 30 to 100 μm or more, with occasional ones reaching a diameter

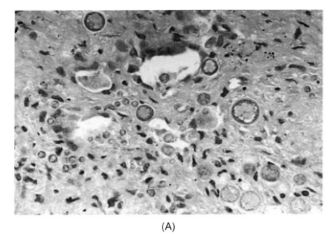

(A)

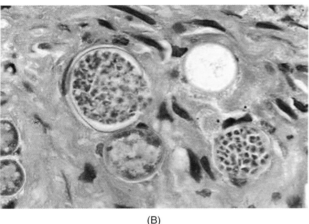

(B)

FIGURE 9.5 *Coccidioides immitis,* **yeast phase, as found in infected cells and tissues or in specialized broth conversion media at 40°C.** (A) This case of acute pneumonitis reveals the presence in tissue of multiple spherules of various sizes and at various stages of development. H&E stain, 400×. (B) Several mature spherules (approximately 50 μm) with endospores are present. Intraspherular cytoplasm compartmentalizes into individual endospores that, once mature, are released into the surrounding parenchyma. The wall of one spherule can be seen breaking down as it begins to release its content. H&E 1000×. (Courtesy of Ramon L. Sandin, MD, MS)

of 200 μm. Their thin, refractile walls are GMS variable but PAS negative. Uninucleate endospores, 2 to 5 μm in diameter, have walls and punctate cytoplasmic inclusions that are GMS and PAS positive. A hematopathologist reviewing a clinical sample during the dissemination stage of the disease may encounter all of the aforementioned structures during the evaluation. Spherules and clusters of endospores may be surrounded by a radiating, eosinophililc corona of Splendore–Hoeppli material in tissue sections, which indicates an immunologic host reaction to fungal

TABLE 9.5 Morphologic Diagnostic Features of *Coccidioides immitis* **in Blood, Bone Marrow, Body fluids or histopathological slides, or in specialized broth conversion media at 40°C**

Mature (endosporulating) spherules in multiple stages of development are diagnostic
These Spherules measure 30–100 μm in diameter, with an average of 50 μm
Their thin refractile walls may stain with GMS but are PAS negative
Mature spherules contain multiple uninucleate endospores
Endospores measure 2–5 μm in diameter
Their walls and internal contents are PAS positive
Immature spherules are usually present and measure 5–30 μm
Their walls and internal contents are also PAS positive

antigens (Chandler and Watts, 1987; Salfelder, 1980; Salfelder, 1990). Table 9.5 summarizes the diagnostic morphologic features of *Coccidioides immitis* in blood, bone marrow, body fluids, or histopathological slides.

Pulmonary nodules consist of either active granulomas or residual fibrocaseous nodules (Figure 9.6). The latter are discrete, subpleural nodules detected radiographically as "coin lesions" in asymptomatic individuals. They are sharply demarcated peripherally by a fibrous capsule, and their centers consist of caseous, necrotic tissue that is amorphous. Typical endosporulating spherules are found in only about half of these nodules; the rest are either devoid of fungal elements entirely or contain scattered immature spherules and distorted fragments of spherule walls. These atypical fungal elements are sufficient to establish a histopathologic diagnosis in the appropriate clinical and geographic setting, but the diagnosis should be confirmed, if possible, by culture, serology, or immunofluorescence staining (Chandler and Watts, 1987).

Differential diagnosis of the 37°C tissue phase of *C. immitis* includes the sporangia of *Rhinosporidium seeberi*. This is an aquatic protistan parasite with spherule-like structures containing endospores. However, the spherules, on the average, measure 200 μm in diameter and vary from 50 to 300 μm, which makes them much larger than the average 50-μm coccidioidal spherules. The endospores and the internal aspect of the sporangial wall of *R. seeberi* would stain positive with the mucicarmine stain, while those structures are negative in *C. immitis.* Myospherulosis is a pseudomycosis, but it is also in the differential diagnostic list of *C. immitis.* This condition follows local trauma or a previous surgical procedure of the soft tissues, upper respiratory

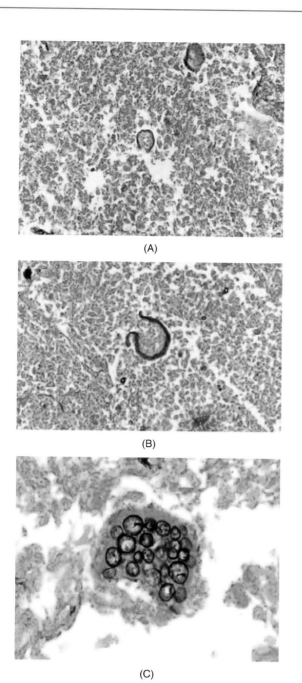

(A)

(B)

(C)

FIGURE 9.6 *Coccidioides immitis*, **old coccidioidoma (fibrocaseous or fibrocalcific lesion) in pulmonary parenchyma**. (A) Shown are typically old lesions where the agent has been walled off and what remains are broken down remnants from the agent (100×). (B) GMS fungal stained sections show empty and broken down remnants of spherule walls (400×). (C) GMS fungal stained section reveals remnants from an old mature spherule with complete absence of the spherule wall and presence of a clustered group of endospores (1000×). (Courtesy of Ramon L. Sandin, MD; http://img.medscape.com/fullsize/migrated/474/677/iim474677.fig3b.jpg)

tract, or middle ear. The lesion consists of altered erythrocytes forming a micelle within a fatty covering which could be supplied by the ointment vehicle of an applied antibiotic or other medication (Chandler and Watts, 1987).

"Wet" Diagnosis in the Clinical Microbiology Laboratory

Coccidioides immitis is a thermodimorphic fungus that exhibits quite different morphologies when growing at 30°C and 37°C. When growing at 30°C on fungal media such as blood-brain heart infusion agar (BBHI) or Sabouraud's fungal media (Sab), the mycelial form of the fungus is manifest. The colony develops moderately fast in 3 to 5 days with abundant aerial mycelia that turns white and is easily airborne. This entity is extremely infectious when large amounts of conidia are breathed in, so all cultural manipulations must be carried out under a laboratory safety hood. A lactophenol cotton blue prep from the colony would show septate hyphae, 2 to 4 μm in width, that produce alternating thick-walled, barrel-shaped arthroconidia up to 10 μm in diameter. As the colony matures, dead cells form in between those arthroconidia. At that point, the conidia separate from each other and are free to be released, thus making them very infectious (Beneke and Rogers, 1980; Koneman and Roberts, 1985; Koneman et al., 1997; Sutton et al., 1998).

The 37°C stage of this organism requires special liquid conversion media and culture at 40°C, but several other culture methods, including tissue culture, have been developed to produce spherules from the mycelial phase. The microscopic evaluation of smears from such cultures would show the same morphology as has already been described for the tissue phase of this organism (Beneke and Rogers, 1980).

Newer Diagnostic Modalities

There are commercially available kits for extracting, concentrating, and testing exoantigens derived from cultural isolates for confirmation of suspected fungal morphologic identity. However, it is toward the new frontier of nucleic acid probes and molecular amplification techniques that the field is moving rapidly in the quest to provide sensitive and specific confirmatory tools for fungal diagnosis, and *Coccidioides* is no exception (Alkan et al., 1995; Mitchell et al., 1994; Sandin, 2002). There are commercially available DNA probes for culture confirmation of *Coccidioides* and reports of in-house or home-brew reagent combinations for PCR detection of gene targets by conventional or real-time approaches, and this can be done directly from clinical samples (Sandin, 2002).

CRYPTOCOCCUS NEOFORMANS

Cryptococcosis is a self-limited or progressive pulmonary mycosis with a marked propensity for cerebromeningeal dissemination caused by the yeast-like fungus, *Cryptococcus neoformans* (Chandler and Watts, 1987). Dermatotropicity is manifested by this agent also, which can be considered a true opportunistic mycosis affecting the immunocompromised patient. A related species has received much attention of recent, namely *Cryptococcus gattii*, an agent that has the capacity to affect nonimmunocompromised individuals and has reportedly been cultured from geographic sites far away from its originally described habitat of Asia and Australia. However, as the great majority of infections requiring diagnosis by a hematopathologist would still be expected to be caused by *C. neoformans*, only the latter species of this genus will be emphasized in the remainder of this chapter.

Definition

Cryptococcosis is a chronic, subacute or rarely acute pulmonary, systemic, or meningitic infection caused by the yeast *Cryptococcus neoformans*. The primary infection in human is almost always pulmonary following inhalation of the yeast; in animal it may follow implantation or ingestion. Pulmonary infection in human is usually subclinical and transitory; however, it may arise as a complication of other diseases in debilitated patients and become rapidly systemic or even fulminant. In Europe it has been known for a long time as the signal disease (malade signal), as it signals an underlying debilitating disease. It has a predilection for the central nervous system. The tissue reaction is sparse, with few macrophages appearing in active infection, but the focus of infection may evolve into tuberculoid granulomas in chronic and healing disease. Suppuration and caseation necrosis are infrequent. The etiologic agent is unique among pathogenic fungi because of its production of a mucinous capsule in tissue and culture (Rippon, 1982; Amstrong and Cohen, 1999).

ICD-10 Codes B45.0-B45.9

B45   **Cryptococcosis**
B45.0 **Pulmonary cryptococcosis**
B45.1 **Cerebral cryptococcosis**
          Cryptococcal meningitis+ (G02.1*)
          Cryptococcosis meningocerebralis
B45.2 **Cutaneous cryptococcosis**
B45.3 **Osseous cryptococcosis**

B45.7 **Disseminated cryptococcosis**
          Generalized cryptococcosis
B45.8 **Other forms of cryptococcosis**
B45.9 **Cryptococcosis, unspecified**

Synonyms

Torulosis, Busse-Buschke's disease, European blastomycosis, malade signal (Rippon, 1982).

Epidemiology

C. neoformans is a soil-inhabiting yeast that is abundant in avian habitats, particularly those heavily contaminated with pigeon excreta. The fungus has a global distribution and has been shown by surveys of pigeon nests to be present in both urban and rural settings. Almost all human infections have a pulmonary inception after inhalation of aerosolized cells of *C. neoformans* that grow as saprophytes in nature. Primary skin infections, which result from accidental percutaneous inoculation, are rare. The disease is not contagious (Rippon, 1982; DiSalvo, 1983).

Cryptococcosis occurs worldwide in temperate as well as tropical climates, but the prevalence of clinically apparent disease is highest in the United States and Australia. Although it may occur in healthy, immunocompetent subjects, it is encountered much more frequently and with greater severity as an opportunistic infection. Up to 85% of patients with this mycosis have severe underlying diseases or immunodeficiencies including hematologic malignancies, long-term corticosteroid therapy, diabetes mellitus, and sarcoidosis. Disseminated cryptococcosis may also be a complicating infection in patients with AIDS (Chandler and Watts, 1987; DiSalvo, 1983; Rippon, 1982).

Clinical Aspects and Pathophysiology

There are two major clinical forms of cryptococcosis: pulmonary and, by hematogenous dissemination from a primary pulmonary focus, cerebromeningeal. Sites less often involved in disseminated infection include the skin, bones and joints, lymph nodes, kidneys, spleen, liver, prostate, and other internal organs. Cutaneous lesions, encountered in 10 to 20% of cases, usually consist of papules and pustules (Chandler and Watts, 1987; Haight et al., 1994; Mujeeb et al., 2002).

Most pulmonary infections in apparently healthy subjects are asymptomatic or mildly symptomatic but self-limited. Infections usually remain localized and either resolve spontaneously or encapsulate. When encapsulation occurs, residual lesions may be detected months to years later by radiologic chest studies or incidentally at autopsy as fibrocaseous nodules known as cryptococcomas. These nodules are similar to those that develop in residual pulmonary histoplasmosis and coccidioidomycosis, but unlike those, they rarely calcify (Chandler and Watts, 1987).

Patients with progressive pulmonary cryptococcosis usually present with chronic cough, low-grade fever, chest pain, malaise, and weight loss. The clinical course is sub-acute or chronic and frequently complicated by concomitant extrapulmonary infection (Hamilton et al., 1998). The predominant clinical form of cryptococcosis, however, is cerebromeningeal. This agent is extremely neurotropic and frequently disseminates to the central nervous system from a primary pulmonary focus of infection that may not be clinically apparent. Some patients undergo exploratory craniotomy because they have symptoms of an expanding intracranial lesion that mimic those of a neoplasm. The duration of the disease varies from a few days to 20 years or more, although the clinical course is usually fulminant and, if untreated, is almost invariably fatal (Chandler and Watts, 1987).

Differential Diagnosis

Several points are considered important in differentiating cryptococcal disease from other mycotic and bacterial infections. In cryptococcosis there is marked predilection for disease to become established in the lower lung fields. Cavitation, fibrosis or calcification, hilar lymphadenopathy, and pulmonary collapse are rare occurrences. Coin lesions, which are so common in old histoplasmosis or coccidioidomycosis, are uncommon in cryptococcosis. Thin-walled cavities usually do not develop. "Crab-claw" shadows, so called because they extend from a focal lesion and emulate carcinoma, are found in blastomycosis but not in cryptococcosis. Definitive diagnosis of the disease depends on the isolation of the organism. Although *C. neoformans* is not part of the regular resident human flora, it may be a transient colonizer. It is necessary to identify specifically any encapsulated yeast isolated from sputum to establish the diagnosis of cryptococcosis. In some infections, particularly low-grade infections, however, the capsule may be absent or very small (Rippon, 1982).

Treatment of Choice and Prognosis

Amphotericin B (AmB) plus flucytosine is the gold standard of induction therapy for cryptococcal meningitis in patients with and without HIV infection. A combination of AmB plus flucytosine for 6 weeks is more efficacious than AmB alone for 10 weeks. Alternatively, when AmB cannot be tolerated, lipid formulations of AmB may be substituted, although the clinical response is similar with either treatment. Among the azoles, fluconazole has been found to be efficacious as continuation therapy following induction therapy with a formulation of AmB plus flucytosine (Mohr et al., 2008).

Approach to Diagnosis

Clinical Workup

A thorough history and physical examination are important in developing an early suspicion for cryptococcal meningitis and cryptococcosis. As already mentioned in the section on differential diagnosis, this disease does not produce some of the typical findings of several of the other mycoses. X-ray or CT scan evaluation for determination of any systemic extent of the lesions may be ordered; however, cavitation, fibrosis, calcification, hylar lymphadenopathy, or coin lesions are rare findings with pulmonary cryptococcosis. Routine blood testing for hematological and chemical markers is important, but definitive diagnosis depends on isolation of the organism in culture. Accessible skin lesions may be biopsed for culture and histopathology. If there are pulmonary symptoms including a productive cough, then a sputum sample should be submitted to microbiology for smear and culture, as could a bronchoalveolar lavage sample that is collected during a bronchoscopic examination. Peripheral blood may be inoculated into blood culture bottles if the systemic stage of the disease is suspected. CSF should be evaluated by the cryptococcal antigen latex agglutination test, which is more sensitive than the time-honored India Ink test (Koneman and Roberts, 1985; Koneman et al., 1997; Larone, 2002; Mujeeb et al., 2002).

Morphologic Aspects

In H&E-stained tissue sections, as well as in smears from peripheral blood or bone marrow aspirates, *C. neoformans* appears as eosinophilic or lightly basophilic, uninucleate, thin-walled, spherical, oval or elliptical yeast-like cells that vary in size from 2 to 20 μm but commonly measure 4 to 10 μm in diameter (Figures 9.7 and 9.8). Typically the yeasts are surrounded by wide, clear to faintly stained spherical zones, or halos, that represent mucopolysaccharide capsular material which is readily demonstrated with mucin stains such as Alcian blue, colloidal iron, and Mayer's mucicarmine and often has a spinous or crenated appearance because of irregular shrinkage

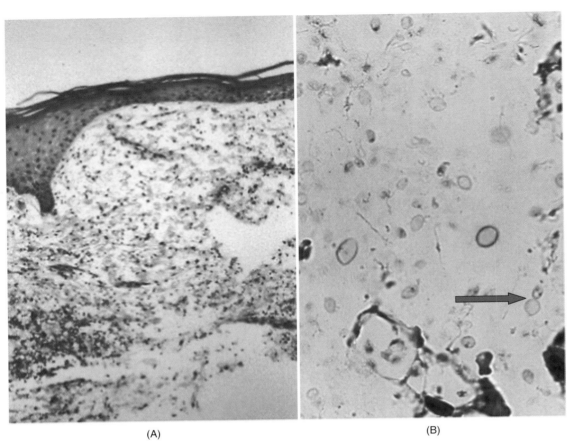

(A)   (B)

FIGURE 9.7 *Cryptococcus neoformans*, a monomorphic yeast, in sections of a skin nodule from an HIV positive patient with disseminated cryptococcosis. (A) Low-power view reveals the rarefied appearance of the dermis with abundant intervening empty-looking spaces. H&E stain, 100×. (B) Yeasts with variability in size and shape are present in the midst of empty-looking spaces. An arrow points to the thin neck that unites a mother and daughter yeast pair. H&E stain, oil immersion, 1000×. (Courtesy of Ramon L. Sandin, MD, MS)

TABLE 9.6 **Morphologic Diagnostic Features of *Cryptococcus neoformans* in Blood, Bone Marrow, Body Fluids, or Histopathological Slides, or in Synthetic Culture Media**

Thin-walled, uninucleate, monomorphic, single or budding yeast cells
Usually one, maybe two, daughter yeasts are attached
Daughter yeasts attached by a narrow neck
Large variability in yeast size and shape
Yeast size varying from 2–20 μm, with averages of 4–10 μm
Shapes varying from round to oval to elliptical
Yeast cell bodies usually staining well with H&E stain
Yeasts surrounded by mucopolysaccharide capsules of various sizes
Infrequently capsules appearing as "halos" but staining avidly with mucin stains such as mucicarmine
Infrequently capsules deficient or absent and staining weakly or not at all[a]

[a] A modified Fontana–Masson stain may be used to identify such capsule-deficient strains.

during processing of the tissue for histopathological examination (Figures 9.9 and 9.10). The staining reaction may be absent or equivocal if the capsules are attenuated or have been digested by phagocytes. *C. neoformans* is the only pathogenic fungus that has a mucinous capsule. In lesions containing abundant, proliferating cryptococci, budding is frequent. Single budding by a narrow neck is common, and chains of budding cells may also be observed. Germ tubes, pseudohyphae, and branched septate hyphae are

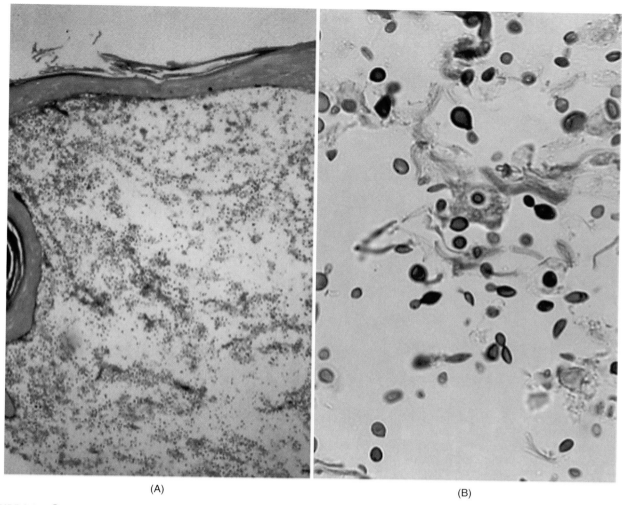

(A)   (B)

FIGURE 9.8 *Cryptococcus neoformans* **patient from Figure 9.7.** (A) Low-power view reveals an abundance of black dots in the dermis that represent individual yeast forms of *Cryptococcus neoformans*. GMS (Grocott–Gomori methenamine silver) stain, 100×. (B) Yeasts with variability in size (2–20 μm) and shape (round to crescentic) are present in the midst of empty-looking spaces. Buds occur at an average of one or two per mother yeast and are attached by thin necks. GMS stain, oil immersion, 1000×. (Courtesy of Ramon L. Sandin, MD, MS)

occasionally produced in tissues. The cell walls of *C. neoformans* are colored intensely with any of the special stains for fungi, such as GMS and PAS (Chandler and Watts, 1987; Salfelder, 1980; Salfelder, 1990). The morphologic pearls for diagnosis of cryptococcosis are summarized in Table 9.6.

Differential diagnostic histologic features of importance to cryptococcosis will now be mentioned. Because *C. neoformans* varies greatly in size and shape, and its encapsulated forms are not always evident, cryptococcosis should be considered in the histologic differential diagnosis of virtually any yeast-form mycosis. Occasionally the cell walls of *B. dermatitidis* and *Rhinosporidium seeberi* also react positively with mucin stains. However, both agents

are nonencapsulated and morphologically distinct from *C. neoformans*. A modified Fontana–Masson stain can be used to identify capsule-deficient cryptococci in tissue sections because a positive reaction does not depend on the presence of a capsular polysaccharide. Corpora amylacea in the aged brain and spinal cord may be mistaken for cryptococci, especially when present in perivascular or subpial locations. These amorphous, lightly basophilic structures are spherical, well-demarcated, 15 μm or more in diameter, PAS and GMS positive, and frequently have a more deeply stained spherical core that gives the false appearance of a dense cell body surrounded by a lightly stained capsule. When apposed, corpora amylacea may look like

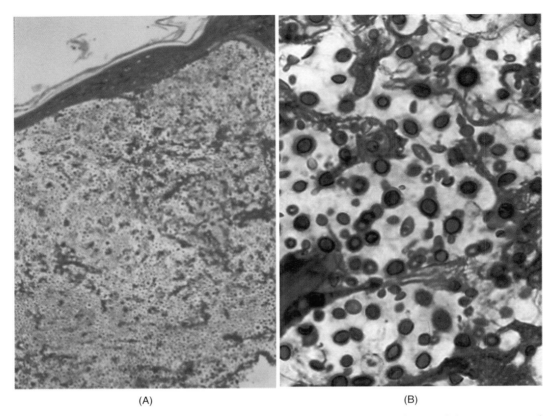

(A)   (B)

FIGURE 9.9 *Cryptococcus neoformans* **patient from Figure 9.7.** (A) Individual yeast forms of *Cryptococcus neoformans* stain pink to red. PAS (Periodic acid-Schiff) stain, 100×. (B) Just like with GMS, PAS stains the "body" of the organism and not its capsule. Yeasts with variability in size (2–20 μm) and shape (round to crescentic) are present. PAS stain, oil immersion, 1000×. (Courtesy of Ramon L. Sandin, MD, MS)

budding yeast forms. In malakoplakia, the spherical, laminated, PAS-positive and sometimes mineralized concretions known as Michaelis–Gutmann bodies may also mimic cryptococci, especially the small, poorly encapsulated forms. These entities correspond to giant phagosomes that contain particulate and membranous profiles, usually of bacterial origin (Chandler and Watts, 1987).

"Wet" Diagnosis in the Clinical Microbiology Laboratory

Isolation of *C. neoformans* from clinical specimens generally is not difficult. On standard synthetic fungal media that does not contain cycloheximide (it inhibits growth of *C. neoformans*), the fungus grows rapidly at either 30°C or 37°C and develops a moist, convex, white to pale yellow colony. The colony is composed entirely of pleomorphic yeast-like cells, as described in Table 9.6. A smear prepared with a drop of India Ink will highlight the capsule of the yeasts against a dark background. Unlike most yeast-form pathogens, *C. neoformans* is not dimorphic.

Two ordinarily nonpathogenic *Cryptococcus* species, *C. albidus* and *C. laurentii*, have rarely been reported to cause invasive infection, and they look just like *C. neoformans* in histopathologic sections. Cultural isolation followed by biochemical identification will confirm their identity (Beneke and Rogers, 1980; Koneman and Roberts, 1985; Koneman et al., 1997; Sutton et al., 1998).

The new emerging pathogen, *Cryptococcus gattii*, resembles *C. neoformans* morphologically and biochemically and will also react positively in the cryptococcal antigen latex agglutination test. It is also urea positive and fails to grow on cycloheximide-containing media. To tell them apart, two selective and differential agar media are used: Niger seed agar and the CGB (canavanine-glycine-bromothymol blue) agar (Klein et al., 2009). On Niger seed agar (also known as caffeic acid agar or Staib agar), dark brown colonies will form from growth of either *C. neoformans* or *C. gattii*, but not from any of the other species of *Cryptococcus* or any other noncryptococcal yeast-like fungus, most of which do not even grow

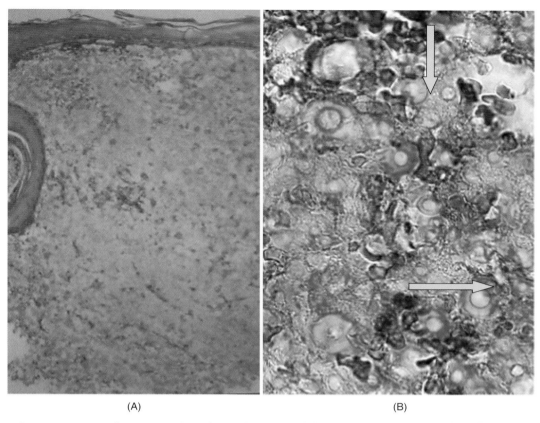

(A)   (B)

FIGURE 9.10   *Cryptococcus neoformans,* **patient from Figure 9.7.** (A) Low-power view reveals diffuse and intense pink staining of *Cryptococcus* capsular material in the dermis. No individual yeast forms of *Cryptococcus neoformans* can be discerned at the present magnification. Meyer's mucicarmine capsular stain, 100X. (B) Capsules of individual yeasts stain strongly pink and surround the unstained central "body" of the organism. Arrows point at capsular material. Meyer's mucicarmine capsular stain, oil immersion, 1000X. (Courtesy of Ramon L. Sandin, MD, MS)

on the media. The color is due to the production of melanin by way of a phenol oxidase enzyme. Inoculation of *C. gattii* on CGB media will show growth and a deep cobalt blue discoloration of the media (which is originally yellow) within 2 to 5 days at room temperature; *C. neoformans* on CGB media shows either poor or no growth, and the medium remains yellow. Other *Cryptococcus* species that may produce false positives on CGB would all fail to grow on Niger seed agar, and thus they should not be misidentified as either *C. gattii* or *C. neoformans* (Klein et al., 2009).

Newer Diagnostic Modalities

There are commercially available kits for extracting, concentrating, and testing exoantigens derived from cultural isolates for confirmation of suspected fungal morphologic identity. The cryptococcal antigen latex agglutination test is also very sensitive as a diagnostic tool and can be used in plasma, CSF, and urine (Koneman et al., 1997; Mujeeb et al., 2002; Sutton et al., 1998). However, it is toward

the new frontier of nucleic acid probes, molecular amplification techniques, and sequencing that the field is moving rapidly in the quest to provide sensitive and specific confirmatory tools for fungal diagnosis, and *Cryptococcus* is no exception (Klein et al., 2009). There are reports of in-house or homebrew reagent combinations for PCR detection of gene targets by conventional or real-time approaches, and even more recently, of the use of DNA sequencing for identification of *C. neoformans* and *C. gattii* (Klein et al., 2009).

CANDIDA ALBICANS AND OTHER *CANDIDA* SPECIES

The *Candida* spp. are responsible for a diverse assortment of infectious diseases, which range from chronic superficial infections of the skin and mucosal surfaces to invasive and disseminated infections of severely compromised hosts. *Candida albicans*, the leading agent of candidiasis, is an endogenous commensal that constitutes part of the normal flora of the oral cavity, upper respiratory tract, gastrointestinal tract, and vagina but is seldom isolated from normal skin or from the environment (Chandler and Watts, 1987; Connor and Chandler, 1997). Other species of the genus *Candida* have gained prominence in recent years as causes of fungemia due to their innate or acquired resistance to various antifungals. Included in that list are *C. krusei*, *C. tropicalis*, and *C. glabrata* (Figure 9.11).

Definition

Candidiasis is a primary or secondary infection involving a member of the genus *Candida*. The clinical manifestations of the disease are extremely varied, ranging from acute, subacute, and chronic to episodic. Involvement may be localized to the mouth, throat, skin, scalp, vagina, fingers, nails, bronchi, lungs, or the gastrointestinal tract, or become systemic as in septicemia, endocarditis, and meningitis. The pathologic processes evoked are also diverse and vary from irritation and inflammation to chronic and acute suppuration or granulomatous

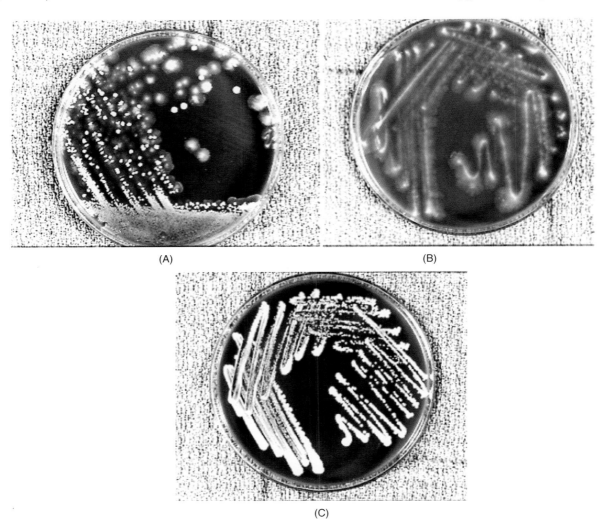

(A)

(B)

(C)

FIGURE 9.11 *Candida spp.* **in culture**. An elderly neutropenic cancer patient status postchemotherapy develops fever and hypotension. From multiple blood cultures during the patient's hospital stay, there is growth of the same two species of *Candida*. (A) Sabouraud's (Sab) agar plate shows growth of colonies following a subculture from a positive blood culture bottle. Two different colonial morphologies are observed on the agar. (B) One colony type is streaked onto a separate plate and reveals the mold-like growth of colonies with feet-like extensions. The agent was identified biochemically as *Candida krusei*. (C) The second colony type in pure culture was yeast-like: moist, pasty, and cream colored and typed biochemically as *Candida tropicalis*. Both agents were found to be resistant to fluconazole in vitro. (Courtesy of Ramon L. Sandin, MD, MS)

response. Since *C. albicans* is an endogenous species, the disease represents an opportunistic infection (Rippon, 1982).

ICD-10 Codes B37.0-B37.9

B37   **Candidiasis**
Includes: candidosis
           moniliasis
Excludes: neonatal candidiasis (P37.5)
B37.0   **Candidal stomatitis**
Oral thrush
B37.1   **Pulmonary candidiasis**
B37.2   **Candidiasis of skin and nail**
Candidal:
· onychia
· paronychia
Excludes: diaper [napkin] dermatitis (L22)
B37.3+**Candidiasis of vulva and vagina** (N77.1*)
Candidal vulvovaginitis
Monilial vulvovaginitis
Vaginal thrush
B37.4   **Candidiasis of other urogenital sites**
Candidal:
· balanitis+ (N51.2*)
· urethritis+ (N37.0*)
B37.5+**Candidal meningitis** (G02.1*)
B37.6+**Candidal endocarditis** (I39.8*)
B37.7   **Candidal septicaemia**
B37.8   **Candidiasis of other sites**
Candidal:
· cheilitis
· enteritis
B37.9   **Candidiasis, unspecified**
Thrush NOS

Synonyms

Candidosis, thrush, dermatocandidiasis, bronchomycosis, mycotic vulvovaginitis, muguet, moniliasis (Rippon, 1982).

Epidemiology

Although the etiologic agent *Candida albicans* is usually encountered in most of the clinical forms of candidiasis, in some of the less common clinical conditions, such as endocarditis, other species are more frequently isolated. These other species represent normal flora of the cutaneous and mucocutaneous areas and are of very limited pathogenicity. All species may be involved in any form of candidiasis, but some are regularly encountered in one particular type. These include *C. parapsilosis* from paronychias, endocarditis, and otitis externa; *C. tropicalis* from vaginitis, intestinal disease, bronchopulmonary, and systemic infections, and onychomycosis; *C. stellatoidea* from vaginitis; *C. guilliermondii* from endocarditis, cutaneous candidiasis, and onychomycosis; *C. pseudotropicalis* from vaginitis; *C. glabrata* from esophageal and vaginal lesions; *C. krusei* very rarely from endocarditis and vaginitis; and *C. zeylanoides* from onychomycosis (Chandler and Watts, 1987; DiSalvo, 1983; Rippon, 1982).

Clinical Aspects and Pathophysiology

Although under normal circumstances the *Candida spp.* are harmless saprophytes or commensals, they may become superficial or invasive pathogens whenever host defense mechanisms are compromised. Factors or diseases that predispose to candidiasis include disruption of cutaneous or mucosal barriers, alteration of normal endogenous microflora by broad-spectrum antibiotics, metabolic abnormalities such as diabetes mellitus, indwelling vascular catheters, neutropenia or defective leukocyte function caused by neoplasia or its therapy, corticosteroid therapy, and abnormalities of cell-mediated immunity (Bodey, 1993; Chandler and Watts, 1987; Mujeeb et al., 2002; Sanders et al., 1999; Sandin et al., 1993; Strickland-Marmol et al., 2004).

Superficial candidiasis involves the skin and the mucosal surfaces of the oral cavity and vagina. Thrush, or pseudomembranous candidiasis, is the most frequent clinical form of oral and genital infection. Obese patients or those with diabetes may develop intertriginous infections of glabrous skin. Paronychia or onychomycosis complicate prolonged, repeated immersion of the hands or feet in water. In all such scenarios the fungal elements remain largely confined to the epidermis or mucosa, and they do not invade subepithelial tissues (Chandler and Watts, 1987).

Chronic mucocutaneous candidiasis is a special type of superficial candidiasis that affects patients, usually children, whose cell-mediated immunity is defective. Patients develop chronic, persistent Candida infections of the skin, nails, and mucous membranes that are notoriously refractory to treatment. The cutaneous lesions are warty, hyperkeratotic papules and plaques, termed Candida granulomas, that may become quite disfiguring. Microscopically, the epidermis is hyperkeratotic and acanthotic, and the dermis contains a mixed cellular infiltrate with multinucleate giant cells. Despite the severity of these lesions, the fungal elements usually remain confined to the epidermis (Chandler and Watts, 1987).

Systemic candidiasis is the type of Candida infection of importance to the hematopathologist. It may involve a single organ system, such as the gastrointestinal or urinary tract, or in more severely compromised patients, may involve multiple organs by hematogenous dissemination. It is during this dissemination phase that a hematopathologist may encounter the morphologic elements of *Candida spp.* in blood, bone marrow, or other body fluids submitted for hematologic evaluation. One example of the latter is hematogenous renal candidiasis where bilateral miliary nodules are produced that are more numerous in the cortex than in the medulla. Hematogenous pulmonary candidiasis in neutropenic patients produces angiocentric nodular infarcts, similar to those produced in the lungs by *Aspergillus spp.*, and each contain a microcolony of yeast-like cells and mycelial elements growing in a radial pattern from a central nidus (Chandler and Watts, 1987).

Differential Diagnosis

In all cases of suspected candidiasis, complete cultural confirmation is necessary. A negative mycologic examination is significant, but a positive one is not unassailable proof of candidal involvement. Consideration of the numbers and morphology of the organisms present, as well as exclusion of other etiologies, is necessary before Candida is implicated as the sole inciting agent of any pathologic process. Isolation of Candida from the blood is usually significant and warrants attention. Thrush in the newborn is pathognomonic in its appearance and presents little diagnostic problems. In other patients, leukoplakia, lichen planus, tertiary syphilis, and other lesions resemble cutaneous candidiasis. The differential diagnosis of systemic infection must include other mycoses, tuberculosis, neoplasms, or chronic bacterial infections. Since Candida may colonize any preexisting cutaneous, mucocutaneous, or respiratory condition, it is very difficult to assess the contribution, if any, of isolated yeasts to the observed pathology (Rippon, 1982).

Treatment of Choice and Prognosis

Caspofungin and micafungin have been found efficacious in multicenter studies for the treatment of esophageal candidiasis in HIV positive patients, and for treatment of invasive candidiasis and candidemia. Micafungin has been found comparable to fluconazole in another multicenter study of HIV+ patients with esophageal candidiasis. In general, various studies have shown the efficacy of echinocandins, azoles, and amphotericin B in the treatment of various manifestations of systemic Candida infection (Mohr et al., 2008).

Approach to Diagnosis

Clinical Workup

A thorough history and physical examination are important in developing an early suspicion for candidal involvement. As already mentioned in the section on differential diagnosis, this disease does not produce some of the pathognomonic findings of some of the other mycoses. X-ray or CT scan evaluation for determination of systemic candidiasis may be ordered, but the findings may be nonspecific for this particular agent. Routine blood testing for markers in hematology and chemistry is important, but definitive diagnosis depends on isolation of the organism in culture. Accessible skin lesions may be biopsied for culture and histopathology. If there is productive cough, a sputum sample should be submitted to microbiology for smear and culture. Peripheral blood may be inoculated into blood culture bottles, but the percentage of negative blood cultures associated with an eventual biopsy positive result of affected systemic organs is high. "Tissue is the issue" is a phrase that applies quite well to the diagnosis of systemic candidiasis. (Koneman and Roberts, 1985; Koneman et al., 1997; Larone, 2002; Mujeeb et al., 2002; Sandin et al., 1993; Strickland-Marmol et al., 2004).

Morphologic Aspects

The microscopic morphology of the individual *Candida spp.* is so similar that they cannot be reliably differentiated from one another in histopathologic sections. With the exception of *C. glabrata*, *Candida spp.* produce oval yeast-like cells, 3 to 7 μm in diameter, and mycelial elements composed of pseudohyphae and true hyphae. Pseudohyphae are composed of elongated yeast-like cells that remain attached end-to-end in chains. They are distinguished from true hyphae by the presence of prominent constrictions at points of attachment between adjacent cells, whereas true septate hyphae, 3 to 5 μm in width, are tubular and have parallel contours. Pseudohyphae and true hyphae of Candida may be referred to collectively as mycelial elements. When compared to the true hyphae of *Aspergillus spp.*, and of most other members of the hyalo- and phaeohyphomycetes, the true hyphae of *Candida spp.* are thinner in width and do not bifurcate at 45-degree angulations (Chandler and Watts, 1987; Salfelder, 1980, 1990).

The combination of yeast-like cells, pseudohyphae, and true hyphae distinguishes the *Candida spp.*

from most other yeast-like pathogens in histopathologic sections. The *Trichosporon spp.*, which produce both yeast-like and mycelial elements, may provide a vexing problem in differential diagnosis (Figure 9.12). The yeast-like cells of the *Trichosporon spp.* are somewhat larger and more pleomorphic than those of the *Candida spp.*, and their hyphae produce rectangular arthroconidia that in turn may give rise to small oval-shaped buds. Weakly pigmented agents of phaeohyphomycosis can also be mistaken for a *Candida spp.* in histopathologic sections. In difficult cases a provisional diagnosis of candidiasis can be confirmed by culture or direct immunofluorescence (Chandler and Watts, 1987). Diagnostic morphologic features of *Candida spp.* of importance to the hematopathologist

when the agent is found in blood, bone marrow, body fluids, or histopathologic tissue slides, are included in Table 9.7.

"Wet" Diagnosis in the Clinical Microbiology Laboratory

The *Candida spp.* grow rapidly on standard synthetic media at either room temperature or 37°C. *C. krusei*, *C. tropicalis*, and *C. parapsilosis* are inhibited by cycloxehimide. Only *C. albicans* (and more rarely its variant *C. stellatoidea*, as well as *C. tropicalis*) produce germ tubes and terminal chlamydoconidia under special conditions of growth. Cornmeal agar with added Tween 80 is used most commonly for chlamydospore formation, and germ tube formation is detected in human or sheep serum at 37°C. Identification of the

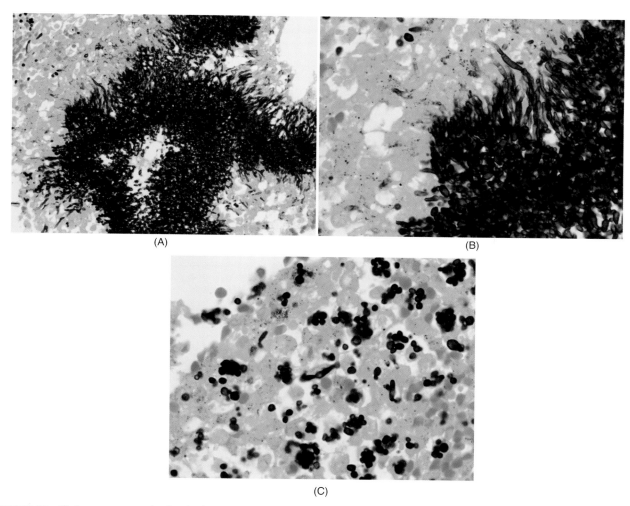

(A)

(B)

(C)

FIGURE 9.12 **Cutaneous pannicular lesions of** *Candida* **present as a manifestation of disseminated disease**. From the patient described in Figure 9.11. Sections from the biopsy are shown at various magnifications. (A) Cluster of filamentous and yeast forms is seen on GMS stain, 100×. (B) Pseudohyphal forms are seen at the edge of the growth with slight "pinching" between attached cells on GMS stain, 400×. (C) Abundant scattered single and budding yeast forms are seen in the midst of a few pseudohyphae on GMS stain, 1000×. (Courtesy of Ramon L. Sandin, MD, MS)

TABLE 9.7 Morphologic Diagnostic Features of *Candida spp.* in Blood, Bone Marrow, Body Fluids, or Histopathological Slides

Combination of yeast-like cells, pseudohyphae, and true hyphae manifest
Oval to round yeast-like cells, 3–7 μm in diameter, single or budding
Pseudohyphae with end-to-end attachment of cells and "pinching" (constrictions) in between them
True hyphae are tubular with parallel contours and measure 3–5 μm in width[a]

[a]Both true hyphae and pseudohyphae are thinner in width than *Aspergillus* hyphae, and do not show the diagnostic bifurcations at 45-degree angulations.

other *Candida spp.* is based predominantly on patterns of carbohydrate fermentation and assimilation (Beneke and Rogers, 1980; Koneman and Roberts, 1985; Koneman et al., 1997; Sutton et al., 1998).

Newer Diagnostic Modalities

It is toward the new frontier of nucleic acid probes, molecular amplification techniques, and sequencing that the field is moving rapidly in the quest to provide sensitive and specific confirmatory tools for fungal diagnosis, and Candida is no exception (Mujeeb et al., 2002). There are now commercially available PNA-FISH probes (Peptide Nucleic Acid–Fluorescence In Situ Hybridization) for detection of various *Candida spp.* in positive blood culture bottles (Reller et al., 2007; Shepard et al., 2008). There are reports of in-house or home-brew reagent combinations for PCR detection of gene targets by conventional or real-time approaches, although to date no FDA-approved kits are available for PCR amplification of *Candida spp.* from normally sterile body fluids.

MALASSEZIA FURFUR

Yeasts of the genus Malassezia are obligatory or nonobligatory lipophilic, normal flora organisms of the skin of warm-blooded hosts. Under appropriate conditions they cause superficial infections of the skin and associated structures. The most commonly described human infection is pityriasis versicolor, a chronic, superficial disease of the stratum corneum layer of the epidermis. Recently data from several institutions have implicated both *M. furfur* and *M. pachydermatis* as causing a number of more invasive human infections, including intravascular catheter-associated sepsis (Larone, 2002; Marcon and Powell, 1992; Sandin et al., 1993). It is during such hematogenous, disseminated episodes that a hematopathologist may encounter yeasts of this agent in the peripheral blood, bone marrow, or in histopathologic review of sections from the spleen. Although rare, such episodes require knowledge of the morphologic

characteristics that distinguish this genus from other more commonly encountered yeasts in the blood.

Definition

Malassezia organisms are globose to ellipsoidal, unipolar budding, lipophilic yeasts that appear to be basidiomycetes. The genus contains at least three species: *M. furfur*, an obligatory lipophilic organism commonly found on human skin; *M. sympodialis*, a second and more rare obligatory lipophilic species; and *M. pachydermatis*, a nonobligatory lipophilic species most often isolated from dogs.

The rest of the discussion on Malassezia in this chapter will be limited to *M. furfur*, the best described species. Likewise we will expound on the particular clinical scenario of *M. furfur*-associated sepsis in patients with intravascular catheters, and folliculitis in cancer patients.

ICD-10 Codes B36

B36   Other superficial mycoses
B36.0 Pityriasis versicolor
        Tinea:
        · flava
        · versicolor

Synonyms

Pityrosporum orbiculare, pityrosporum ovale for the organism; for the condition of tinea versicolor, other synonyms include pityriasis versicolor, dermatomycosis furfuracea, chromophytosis, tinea flava, liver spots (Rippon, 1982).

Epidemiology

The etiologic agent *M. furfur* has been shown to be a common endogenous saprophyte of normal skin. Older and sexually mature children yield more positive cultures of this agent than younger groups. It appears that the organism is universally present as a member of the normal flora of skin, and can elicit disease only under special systemic or local conditions when an overgrowth of the organism occurs (Rippon,

1982). The factors responsible for such overgrowth resulting in tinea versicolor are not yet known but a slowed rate of squamous cell turnover of skin may propitiate the condition. It has been suggested that a genetic predisposition, poor nutritional state, or the accumulation of extracellular glycogen in patients prone to the disease may give rise to the condition. Once *M. furfur* catheter-associated sepsis in newborn infants was described, investigators examined the incidence of *M. furfur* colonization in hospitalized infants. Several studies have reported a colonization rate of 28 to 32% in that population (Marcon and Powell, 1992).

Clinical Aspects and Pathophysiology

The manifestation of disease by *M. furfur* of greatest importance to a hematopathologist is its association with catheter-related sepsis. This is an iatrogenic infection, primarily of low-birth-weight infants, that occurs infrequently as a complication of placement of central venous catheters for long-term venous access coupled with administration of hyperalimentation fluids containing lipid emulsions (Larone, 2002; Marcon and Powell, 1992; Sandin et al., 1993). Exactly how the organism gains access to the catheter is unclear. It is possible that the catheter becomes contaminated with the organism at the time of surgical placement, by administration of a contaminated infusate through the catheter, or by hematogenous seeding of the catheter from a distant point of bloodstream invasion.

Another manifestation of importance to the practicing pathologist is *M. furfur* folliculitis. It was first described around 1970 and is an erythematous papulopustular rash that most often affects adults and may be more common than recognized. Underlying

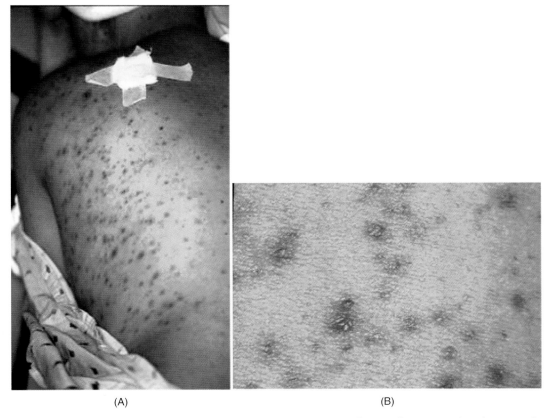

(A)   (B)

FIGURE 9.13   Follicular rash on back and shoulders of a bone marrow transplant patient soon after the transplant. Biopsies of representative lesions are taken and sent to histology for morphologic diagnosis and to microbiology for culture and smear examination. **(A)** Gross picture of multiple follicular lesions on the patient's back. One of the biopsy sites is covered with gauze and tape. **(B)** Close-up of several follicular back lesions. **(C)** Microscopic review of section from skin biopsy at low power shows a disrupted hair follicle containing abundant debris (H&E, 100×). **(D)** Medium-power view reveals an abundance of small, round, single, and budding yeast forms (H&E, 400×). 13E: High-power view from section stained with special fungal stain reveals small (approx. 2–5 μm) single and budding yeast with a broad base between mother and daughter yeasts (PAS stain, 1000×). (Courtesy of Ramon L. Sandin, MD, MS)

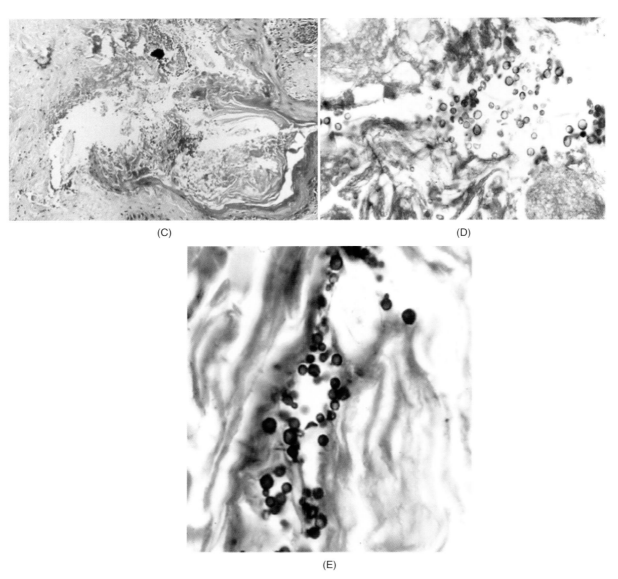

(C)

(D)

(E)

FIGURE 9.13 (*Continued*)

conditions that may predispose to it include diabetes mellitus, Cushing's syndrome, multiple trauma, chronic renal failure, renal transplantation, bone marrow transplantation, malignancy, and the administration of broad-spectrum antibiotics or corticosteroids (Marcon and Powell, 1992). Figures 9.13, 9.14, and 9.15 present the clinical, histopathological, microbiological, and electron microscopic characteristics of a case of *M. furfur* folliculitis in a patient who underwent bone marrow transplantation.

Differential Diagnosis

The diagnosis of catheter-related sepsis by this lipophilic yeast can be suspected in any inmunocompromised patient—especially the premature newborn or transplant patient—from whom yeasts have been detected in blood and who is undergoing hyperalimentation with fluids containing lipid emulsions. The morphology of the yeasts in a peripheral blood smear can provide a preliminary identification but the only definitive way to arrive at final diagnosis is by way of culture and some biochemical testing in the microbiology laboratory (Sandin et al, 1993).

Treatment of Choice and Prognosis

Treatment of *M. furfur* sepsis has varied greatly from center to center (Marcon and Powell, 1992). Therapy has generally involved one of the following four approaches: discontinuation of lipids while the central venous catheter (CVC) is left in place, removal of

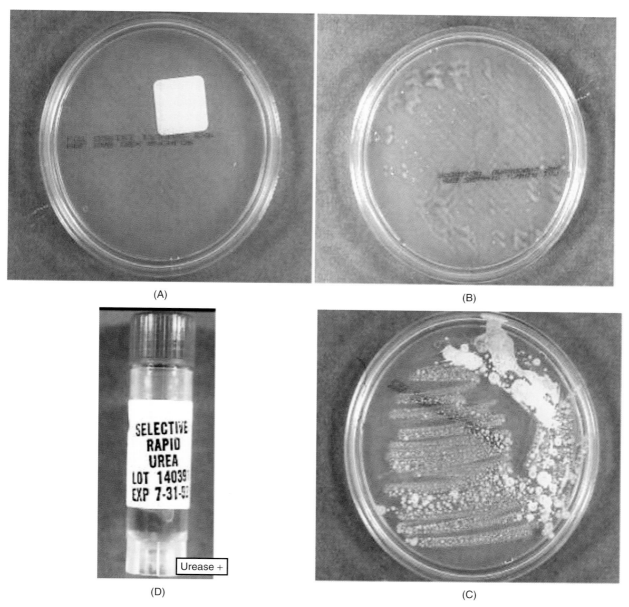

(A)

(B)

(D)

(C)

FIGURE 9.14   **Biopsy results from culture in the previous bone marrow transplant patient**. The agent that grew is *Malassezia furfur*. It is a lipophilic yeast that requires an exogenous source of medium to long-chain fatty acids to able to grow on synthetic media, as well as when causing folliculitis in a patient. It is also a urease producing yeast. **(A)** Sabouraud's fungal agar medium was inoculated with a portion of the homegenized biopsy tissue received in microbiology. Following culture at 30° C in an incubator for 2 days, there is no growth on the plate, as shown. **(B)** An olive oil overlay is added to the plate shown on **(A)**, and it is placed back in the incubator. **(C)** The same plate is now shown 2 days after being overlaid with olive oil and re-incubated. The plate is teeming with yeast colonies. Microscopic examination of smears from the colonies showed yeasts of 2 to 4 μm sizes, with thickened collaretes around the budding sites and broad-based buds between mother and daughter yeasts. **(D)** A selective rapid urea slant is stabbed with colonies from the plate and shows a strong pink color formation after 20-min incubation, denoting a urease-positive organism such as the genus *Malassezia*. (Courtesy of Ramon L. Sandin, MD, MS)

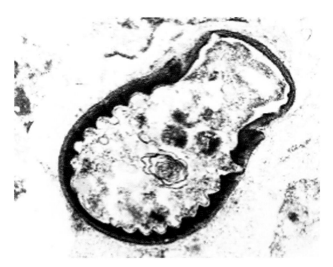

FIGURE 9.15 **Transmission electron micrograph of** *Malassezia furfur.* Shown are five pathognomonic features: thick, multilayered walls; broad-based budding; unipolar budding; "corrugations" of the yeast's cell membrane as it contacts the organism's cell wall; and "collarettes," which are thickenings that form at the budding site on the mother yeast. (Courtesy of the teaching collection of Ramon L. Sandin, MD, MS)

the CVC with or without continuation of lipid emulsions, antifungal therapy without CVC removal, or, antifungal therapy with CVC removal. The most successful mode of treatment seems to be removal of the infected CVC, with or without concomitant administration of antifungal therapy (Marcon and Powell, 1992).

Approach to Diagnosis

Clinical Workup

A thorough history and physical examination are very important in developing a suspicion for *M. furfur* catheter-associated sepsis as it would reveal the most important underlying predisposing conditions: debilitation, presence of a venous access catheter, with infusion of lipid-containing fluids. Review of

a peripheral blood smear flagged by a technologist for the presence of yeasts with the appropriate morphology would lead to a preliminary diagnosis, but definitive identification depends on the isolation and identification of the organism in culture. Peripheral blood may be inoculated into blood culture bottles or lysis-centrifugation tubes for retrieval of the agent (Larone, 2002; Marcon and Powell, 1992; Sandin et al., 1993).

Morphologic Aspects

The morphologic diagnostic features of *Malassezia furfur* in a peripheral blood smear, bone marrow aspirate or biopsy, body fluid smear, or histopathological tissue slide are summarized in Table 9.8.

"Wet" Diagnosis in the Clinical Microbiology Laboratory. *M. furfur* is a lipophilic yeast with a need for external supplementation with medium to long-chain fatty acids, such as can be supplied by the use of olive or other oils. The organism can be recovered best with the use of blood collected through the catheter suspected of being infected and placed in Isolator tubes (Wampole Labs., Cranbury, NJ). The sediment from such tubes can be plated onto fungal media such as Sabouraud's dextrose agar to which an olive oil overlay is added. Most modern automated noninvasive, continuous-monitoring blood culture systems should also support growth of the agent in their blood culture bottle media if such blood is drawn through the infected catheters. The subculture of blood from bottles with a suspicious gram stain that is plated onto fungal media should also be accompanied by an olive oil overlay. Plates are incubated at 35 to 37°C and held for at least 1 week. Most *M. furfur* isolates are detected after 2 to 4 days of incubation. The morphology of the agent growing in culture at that temperature is described in Table 9.8. Evaluation of a smear under oil immersion should reveal the presence of "collarettes." In our laboratory we perform a urease test by stabbing a

TABLE 9.8 **Morphologic Diagnostic Features of** *Malassezia furfur* **in Blood, Bone Marrow, Body Fluids or Histopathological Slides, or in Synthetic Culture Media at 35–37°C**

Small single or budding yeasts, 2–4 μm in diameter

Each single bud attached to the mother yeast by a broad base

Agent of similar in size to *Histoplasma capsulatum*, but with daughter yeasts of this dimorphic agent connected by thin necks

Unipolar budding (all buds are produced from the same site in the mother cell)

A small circumferential thickening formed at the budding site on the mother cell described as a "collarette"

Walls relatively thick and multilayered

In sepsis or folliculitis, only yeasts found

In tinea versicolor, short hyphal fragments and round spores seen, described as "spaguetti and meatballs"

urea-containing medium and evaluating the change in color of the indicator. We provide a preliminary diagnosis based on all of the above. Malassezia does not grow well in the liquid media used in standard assimilation tests or in common commercial yeast identification systems, unless an external source of oil is added, which is not practical for most laboratories (Beneke and Rogers, 1980; Koneman and Roberts, 1985; Koneman et al., 1997; Larone, 2002; Marcon and Powell, 1992; Rippon, 1982; Sandin et al, 1993; Sutton et al., 1998).

REFERENCES

ALKAN S, DIAZ JI, SANDIN RL. 1995. Techniques of diagnostic molecular pathology. Cancer Contr 2(2):149–54.

ARMSTRONG D, COHEN J. 1999. Infectious Diseases: Fungal Infections. Mosby–Wolfe Medical Communications, London.

BENEKE ES, ROGERS AL. 1980. Medical Mycology Manual, 4th ed. Burgess, Minneapolis.

BENEKE ES, RIPPON JW, ROGERS AL. 1984. Human Mycoses, A Scope Publication, 8th ed. Upjohn, Kalamazoo.

BODEY GP. 1993. Candidiasis: Pathogenesis, Diagnosis and Treatment, 2nd ed. Raven Press, New York.

BULMER GS. 1978. Medical Mycology, A Scope Publication. Upjohn, Kalamazoo.

CHANDLER FW, WATTS JC. 1987. Pathologic Diagnosis of Fungal Infections. ASCP Press, Chicago.

Connor DH, Chandler FW, ed. 1997. Part Four: Fungal and algal infections. In: Pathology of Infectious Diseases, Appleton and Lange, Stamford, CT, 927–1113.

DiSalvo AF. 1983. Occupational Mycoses. Lea and Febiger, Philadelphia.

HAIGHT DO, ESPERANZA LE, GREENE JN, SANDIN RL, DeGREGORIO R, SPIERS ASD. 1994. Case report: cutaneous manifestations of cryptococcosis. Am J Med Sci 308(3):192–5.

HAMILTON RA, SANDIN RL, PFALZGRAF R. 1998. Disseminated cryptococcosis as cause of sudden death in a medical examiner case. ASCP Forensic Path Check Sample, FP 98-3(FP-234):33–45.

KANG L, SANDIN RL. 2004. Role of the Microbiology Laboratory. In: Greene JN, ed., Infections in Cancer Patients. Dekker, New York, ch. 39: 509–522.

KERN ME. 1985. Medical Mycology. A Self-instructional Text. Davis, Philadelphia.

KLEIN KR, HALL L, DEML SM, RYSAVY JM, WOHLFIEL SL, WENGENACK NL. 2009. Identification of *Cryptococcus gattii* by use of L-canavanine glycine bromothymol blue medium and DNA sequencing. J Clin Microbiol 47(11):3669–72.

KONEMAN EW, ROBERTS GD. 1985. Practical Laboratory Mycology, 3rd ed. Williams and Wilkins, Baltimore.

KONEMAN EW, ALLEN SD, JANDA WM, SCHRECKENBERGER PC, WINN WC. 1997. Mycology. In: Color Atlas and Textbook of Diagnostic Microbiology, 5th ed. Lippincott–Raven, Philadelphia, 983–1057.

LARONE DH. 2002. Medically Important Fungi, a Guide to Identification. 4th ed. Washington DC: ASM Press.

MARCON MJ, POWELL DA. 1992. Human Infections due to *Malassezia spp*. Clin Microbiol Rev 5(2):101–19.

MITCHELL TG, SANDIN RL, BOWMAN BH, MEYER W, MERZ WG. 1994. Molecular mycology: DNA probes and applications of PCR technology. J Med Vet Mycol 32(suppl 1):351–66.

MOHR J, JOHNSON M, COOPER T, LEWIS JS, OSTROSKY-ZEICHNER L. 2008. Current options in antifungal pharmacotherapy. Pharmacotherapy 28(5):614–45.

MUJEEB IB, SUTTON DA, FOTHERGILL AW, RINALDI MG, PFALLER MA. 2002. Fungi and fungal infections. In: McClatchey KD, ed., Clinical Laboratory Medicine, 2nd ed. Lippincott, Williams and Wilkins, Philadelphia, 1125–56.

RELLER ME, MALLONEE AB, KWIATKOWSKI NP, MERZ WG. 2007. Use of peptide nucleic acid-fluorescence in situ hybridization for definitive, rapid identification of five common Candida species. J Clin Microbiol 45(11):3802–3.

RIPPON JW. 1982. Medical Mycology. The Pathogenic Fungi and the Pathogenic Actinomycetes, 2nd ed. Saunders, Philadelphia.

SALFELDER K. 1980. Atlas of Deep Mycoses. Saunders Philadephia.

SALFELDER K. 1990. Atlas of Fungal Pathology. Kluwer Academic, Lancaster.

SANDERS SL, GREENE JN, SANDIN RL. 1999. Disseminated candidiasis complicating treatment of acute leukemia. Infect Medic 16(6):403–15.

SANDIN RL. 1991. DNA probe for *Blastomyces dermatitidis* is sensitive and specific. Mycol Obs 2(6):8.

SANDIN RL, ISADA CM, HALL GS, RUTHERFORD I, TOMFORD JW, ROGERS AL, WASHINGTON JA. 1993a. Aberrant *Histoplasma capsulatum*: confirmation of identity by a chemiluminescence-labelled DNA probe. Diag Microbiol Infect Dis 17:235–8.

SANDIN RL, HALL GS, LONGWORTH DL, WASHINGTON JA. 1993b. Unpredictability of commercially-available exoantigen culture confirmation tests in confirming the identity of five *Blastomyces dermatitidis* isolates. Am J Clin Pathol, 1993, 99:542–5.

SANDIN RL, FANG T, HIEMENZ JW, GREENE JN, CARD L, KALIK A, SZAKACS JE. 1993c. *Malassezia furfur* folliculitis in cancer patients: the need for interaction of microbiologist, surgical pathologist and clinician in facilitating identification by the clinical microbiology laboratory. An Clin Lab Science 23(5):377–84.

SANDIN RL. 1996. Special considerations for the clinical microbiology laboratory in the diagnosis of infections in the cancer patient. In: Greene JN, Hiemenz JW, eds., Infectious Disease Clinics of North America. Saunders, Philadelphia.

SANDIN RL. 2002. Molecular biology of infectious diseases. In: McClatchey KD, ed., Clinical Laboratory Medicine,

2nd ed. Lippincott, Williams and Wilkins, Philadelphia, 186–210.

SHEPARD JR, ADDISON RM, ALEXANDER BD, DELLA-LATTA P, GHERNA M, HAASE G, HALL G, JOHNSON JK, MERZ WG, PELTROCHE-LIACSAHUANGA H, STENDER H, VENEZIA RA, WILSON D, PROCOP GW, WU F, FIANDACA MJ. 2008. Multicenter evaluation of the *Candida albicans/Candida glabrata* peptide nucleic acid fluorescent in situ hybridization method for simultaneous dual-color identification of *C. albicans* and *C. glabrata* directly from blood culture bottles. J Clin Microbiol 46(1):50–5.

STRICKLAND-MARMOL LB, VINCENT AL, LAARTZ BW, SANDIN RL, GREENE JN. 2004. Candidemia in cancer and bone marrow transplant patients: a 10-year retrospective analysis. Infect Med 21(1):37–42.

SUTTON DA, FOTHERGILL AW, RINALDI MG. 1998. Guide to Clinically-Significant Fungi. Williams and Wilkins, Baltimore.

CHAPTER TEN

HEMATOLOGIC ASPECTS OF TROPICAL INFECTIONS

Deniz Peker

ANEMIA IN TROPICAL INFECTIONS

Malaria

Malaria affects more than 2 billion people, mostly in tropical and subtropical areas where temperature and rainfall are most suitable for the development of the malaria-causing *Plasmodium* parasites within *Anopheles* mosquitoes. The disease has been eradicated in the United States and Western Europe with the use of preventive medicine and vector control.

Epidemiology

Malaria in humans is generally caused by five *Plasmodium* species, *P. malaria, P. ovale, P. vivax, P. knowlesi, and P. falciparum*. See Chapter 6 for more discussion. Infection of the human host with a *Plasmodium* parasite begins with the bite of an infected *Anopheles* mosquito that inoculates the individual with sporozoites. The sporozoites are believed to reach the blood stream from skin and eventually invades hepatocytes to form the exoerythrocytic merozoites (tissue schizogony). For *P. vivax* and *P. ovale*, dormant forms called hypnozoites typically remain latent in the liver. Once merozoites leave the liver, they invade erythrocytes and develop into early ring-shaped trophozoites.

Once the parasite begins to divide, the trophozoites are called schizonts, consisting of many daughter merozoites (blood schizogony). The erythrocytes are lysed by merozoites and then infect other red cells.

Clinical Manifestations

The incubation period ranges from 10 to 15 days depending on the plasmodial species and the host immunity. Clinical signs and symptoms are associated with release of merozoites into the circulation following destruction of infected erythrocytes. Prodromal symptoms include malaise, myalgia, headache, anorexia, and low fever. An acute paroxysm presents with chills followed by high temperatures of 40° to 41°C (104°–106°F) in primary falciparum infections and 39° to 40°C (102–104°F) in other three species. The fever lasts from 2 to 6 hours. The sweating stage, in which the temperature falls rapidly, lasts 2 to 3 hours. In addition to fever and sweats, other constitutional symptoms may be seen including gastrointestinal symptoms (i.e., nausea, vomiting, diarrhea, and abdominal pain). The patients usually have tachycardia, warm and flushed skin. The spleen is often palpable, soft and tender in acute malaria and later attacks. The liver is usually enlarged and tender. The laboratory findings usually consist of anemia, leukopenia, and thrombocytopenia. Impaired liver and renal functions are also seen.

Non-Neoplastic Hematopathology and Infections, First Edition. Edited by Hernani D. Cualing, Parul Bhargava, and Ramon L. Sandin.
© 2012 Wiley-Blackwell. Published 2012 by John Wiley & Sons, Inc.

Anemia in Malaria

The degree of anemia in acute or recurrent phases is related with severity of disease, endemicity, and sometimes treatment. In acute malaria, rapid fall in hemoglobin and hematocrit and decreased red cell mass are the usual findings. Sequestration and destruction of erythrocytes occur in spleen and correlate with spleen size and the intensity of the parasitemia. Hemolysis of the noninfected cells is a result of reticuloendothelial system macrophage activation and Fc-receptor mediated uptake. The anemia is normochromic normocytic. The reticulocyte count is often low despite an erythroid hyperplasia in bone marrow. During the acute phase, iron sequestration, erythrophagocytosis, and dyserythropoiesis may occur. Elevated total and indirect bilirubin levels are common due to hemolysis. The low hemoglobin and hematocrit levels may remain for 7 to 21 days due to continued hemolysis and bone marrow suppression.

Recurrent attacks of malaria are usually seen in chronic re-infection by *P. falciparum* and common in children in the endemic areas and is associated with the tropical splenomegaly syndrome. They have moderate splenomegaly with chronic normochromic normocytic anemia. The anemia is a result of both hypersplenism and impaired bone marrow function. The reticulocyte count is persistantly low.

The chemotherapy may also result in anemia in malaria patients with G-6-PD deficiency. Primaquine may cause intravascular hemolysis due to oxidative destruction of erythrocytes.

In falciparum malaria, a severe hemolytic anemia can occur as a complication, also called "blackwater fever." This is a state of acute intravascular hemolysis accompanied by hemoglobinuria, oliguria, and jaundice. It may also cause impairement of renal function, for example, hemoglobin casts and proteinuria.

Diagnosis

Light microscopy of thick and thin Giemsa-stained blood smears are the gold standard for diagnosing malaria. See Chapter 6 for detailed discussion on blood smear diagnosis. For the diagnosis of the presence of the parasite, a thick blood smear examination is the gold standard. The identification of the species must be confirmed by examination of the thin film. On thin film, *P. falciparum* is often numerous with more than 10% red cells infected. Ring forms are most common with one or two chromatin dots. Infected erythrocytes are not enlarged. *P. vivax* parasites are usually few on thin blood smear infecting not more than 2% of the red cells. Rings are large. There is usually one chromatin

dot. Large pigmented schizonts (containing about 12 merozoites) are common. Infected erythrocytes are usually enlarged. Large irregular trophozoites with finely granular, yellow-brown pigment may be seen. Gametocytes are round and usually fill the cell. *P. malaria* can be seen as ring forms, pigmented trophozoites, schizonts, and gametocytes on thin films. Rings are small with one chromatin dot. Trophozoites are usually in band forms with coarse, dark-brown pigment. In schizonts, the merozoites may be seen forming a rosette around a central pigment. Gametocytes are rounded with pigment granules and central chromatin. The infected red cells are usually normal in size. *P. ovale* resembles *P. vivax* (see Chapter 6 for images).

Advanced diagnostic methods are also available, including fluorescence microscopy of parasite nuclei stained with acridine orange, rapid dipstick immunoassay, and polymerase chain reaction assays (Trampuz et al., 2003).

Treatment

In all forms, particularly falciparum malaria, the therapy must be started as soon as the diagnosis is made. Chloroquine, quinine, proguanil, pyrimethamine, primaquine, mepacrine, sulphonamides, and dapsone are some of the choices of treatment.

Babesiosis

Epidemiology

Human babesiosis is a tick-borne infectious disease caused by Babesia, an intraerythrocytic protozoan. *Ixodes dammini* has been identified as the tick vector. The disease has many similar features to those of malaria. Elderly individuals, immunocompromised, and splenectomized patients are particularly at the highest risk for severe disease. *B. microti, B. duncani, B. divergens*, and *B. venatorum* are the species that most commonly infect people.

The organism multiplies in the erythrocytes asexually by budding, usually forming 2 or 4 daughter parasites. Following the rupture of the infected cells, other red cells are invaded and the cycle is repeated. The major clinicopathologic features of babesiosis including hemoglobinemia, hemoglobinuria, jaundice, and renal dysfunction are the result of destruction of the red cells by the organism following the multiplication within the cells. The incubation period varies from 1 to 4 weeks.

Clinical Manifestations

The clinical presentation ranges from asymptomatic infection to fulminant disease resulting in death, although the majority of healthy adults experience a mild-to-moderate illness. Most asymptomatic patients are presented with chills, fever, nausea, vomiting, and hemolytic anemia, which may progress to hemoglobinemia, hemoglobinuria, jaundice, and renal dysfunction. The anemia is mild to moderate in *B. microti* infections but severe in *B. divergens* infections. The reticulocyte count is often high. Nucleated red blood cells may be seen on peripheral blood smears depending on the degree of the anemia. The leukocyte count may be normal to slightly decreased as well as thrombocytopenia. In severe hemolytic anemia, markedly elevated bilirubin, liver enzymes, blood urea nitrogen, and creatinine levels are common.

Diagnosis

Microscopic identification of the organism is made by Giemsa-stained thin blood smears. *B. microti* and other *Babesia spp.* are round, oval, or pear-shaped and have a blue cytoplasm with a red chromatin. The ring form is most common and can be mistaken for early stage ring forms of *Plasmodium falciparum*. See Chapter 6 for images. PCR and serology may be performed if the ring-like structures are observed.

Treatment

The standard treatment is clindamycin and quinine. Atovaquone and azithromycin are also used as alternative chemotherapy.

Visceral Leishmaniasis (Kala-Azar)

Kala-azar, or VL, is also known as tropical splenomegaly, black sickness, or burdwan fever, and is mainly caused by *Leishmania donovani* (Reithinger R et al. 2007). It is found in North, East, West, and Central Africa; the Middle East; India; China; and Central and South America.

The transmission is from a reservoir animal (e.g., dogs, foxes, rodents) to human or human to human by the bites of *Phlebotomus* (sandfly). The incubation period between the sandfly bite and clinical symptoms lies between 2 weeks and 18 months.

The onset may be gradual or abrupt as in falciparum malaria. There may be irregular fever, a low blood pressure, and a high pulse rate. The disease is due to infection of reticuloendothelial cells diffusely in the body with *L. donovoni*, which leads to reticuloendothelial hyperplasia. As a result the liver and especially the spleen enlarge, and there is bone marrow hyperplasia as well. The enlarged spleen and liver are not painful or tender. The lab findings include leukopenia (2000–4000 per mm^3), thrombocytopenia and a slowly progressing anemia as a result

of hemolysis and sequestration in the enlarged spleen. The red cell count falls between 2 and 3 million per mm^3. The red cells may be hyperchromic and macrocytic (usually secondary to the high demands of the folic acid) and the fragility is increased. The sedimentation rate is always high. Total albumin is low and the globulin fraction is increased due to the increased IgG levels.

The diagnosis of visceral leishmaniasis is based on the recovery and recognition of the parasite. Direct visualization of amastigotes in the spleen, bone marrow, lymph node aspirate smears, or liver or skin biopsy is the gold standard for diagnosis of VL (Artan et al., (2006); Herwaldt, 1999). Giemsa stain demonstrates intracellular amastigotes better than routine stains. See Chapter 20 for figures. Dursun et al. reported that a Leishmania hemagglutination test could be used, but it proved to have low sensitivity (Dursun, (2009)).

Liposomal amphotericin B recently became the first and only drug approved by the US Food and Drug Administration for the treatment of VL with high effect and significantly less side effects (Pearson et al., 2000). Sodium stibogluconate, meglumine antimoniate, and paromomycin are the therapy choices.

Trypanosomiasis

Trypanosomiasis is an endemic infectious disease in the tropics caused by a protozoan Trypanosoma. *Trypanosoma brucei gambiense* and *rhodesiense* are endemic in sub-Saharan Africa and cause African trypanosomiasis (sleeping sickness), whereas the disease form *T. b. cruzi* causes American trypanosomiasis (Chagas disease) in Central and South America and in the US southeast. Tsetse flies (*Glossina sp.*) and Triatomine bugs (e.g., *Rhodnius sp*) are the vectors of African and American trypanosomiasis, respectively. Transmission via blood transfusion and shared needle is also described.

American trypanosomiasis is characterized with systemic disease including fever, myalgia, skin rash, lymphadenopathy, and edema as well as acute myocarditis and encephalitis.

The diagnostic symptoms of African trypanosomiasis include fever, lymphadenopathy, heatosplenomegaly and delayed sensation. Moderate to severe anemia is also a common lab finding as well as neutropenia, increased sedimentation rate, and increased serum IgM levels. The anemia is normocytic with increased reticulocytes and usually due to hemolysis. The parasite effect and certain immunologic mechanisms are responsible for the destruction of erythrocytes. In addition Maclean et al. showed that IL-10 levels are significantly elevated during the disease (Maclean et al., 2001). IL-10 inhibits the hematopoietic growth factors GM-CSF and G-CSF (de Waal Malefyt, (1991)). Bone marrow failure is a feature in severe disease.

The diagnosis is based on detection of parasite in the thick blood smears stained by Giemsa. Pentamidine, suramin, melarsoprol, and eflornithine are the treatment choices.

Amoebiasis

Ameobiasis is an infection caused by *Entamoeba histolytica*, the most important intestinal amoeba for humans. *E. histolytica* has worldwide distribution but is more common in tropical and subtropical regions. The three life-cycle stages of the organism are the trophozoite, precyst, and cyst. The cyst is the infective form, and it is transmitted by ingestion of contaminated food or water. It causes amoebic dysentery, which is characterized by dysenteric stools with or without blood appearing within a few days to 2 weeks. Usually amoebic ulcers are seen in the rectal mucosa. Pain and tenderness may depend on the severity of the disease. Severe amoebic dysentery is a fatal disease that most often afflicts African children. Onset is sudden, presenting as severe, diffuse, necrotizing colitis. The stool usually contains dark blood with mucus. The patients often have normocytic anemia due to blood loss and neutrophilia in addition to poor general nutrition. Hemorrhage from a destructed blood vessel in the intestinal ulcer area is a complication of the dysentery and, when massive, may require immediate blood transfusion.

Another manifestation of *E. histolytica* is liver abscess, which may be associated with the intestinal disease. The usual symptoms are fever and right upper quadrant pain. A majority of these patients have leukocytosis and normochromic normocytic anemia. Iron-deficiency anemia has also been described in patients with amoebic liver abscess (Mayett and Powell, 1964). It has also been shown that hemolytic uremic syndrome may be associated with *E. histolytica* (Cavagnaro et al., 2006).

Diagnosis is often made by an examination of the patient's stool for trophozoites and cysts. Serologic tests, an indirect hemagglutination test, immunofluorescence testing (IFA), and ELISA are also used as diagnostic tools. Radiologic studies and, if necessary, the examination of the aspiration material for trophozoites and cysts can be used for diagnosis of amoebic liver abscess.

Chloroquine phosphate, emetine hydrochloride, iodoquinol, metronidazol, and paramomycin are the classic therapy agents. Dehydroemetine and diloxanide furoate are also in use for treatment.

Giardiasis

Giardiasis is a small intestinal infection caused by a flagellate protozoan, *Giardia intestinalis*. It has a worldwide distribution, with higher endemicity in areas with poor sanitation. Colorado is the most endemic area in the United States due to the waterborne transmission of the organism. In the tropics, children are especially prone to infection where nutrition and sanitation conditions are poor. Person to person transmission is a frequent occurrence among children at day care and among homosexual individuals. The infection usually presents following ingestion of cyst forms in contaminated food or water. The excysted trophozoites in the alkaline duodenal contents locate in the duodenal and proximal jejunal mucosal surface without invading the epithelium.

The infection is usually self-limiting. About 20% the infected individuals are symptomatic with acute diarrheal disease. A minority of the patients may develop chronic disease causing malabsorbtion, weight loss, and anemia. Iron deficiency is the major cause of anemia in both children and adults infected by Giardia (De Vizia et al., (1986); Gonen et al., (2007)). Vitamin B_{12} deficiency, and consequent anemia, may also be a manifestation in Giardiasis due to its malabsorbtion (Cowen and Campbell, 1973; Cordingley and Crawford, 1986).

The diagnosis is usually made by the identifying cysts in stool samples. Histopathologic examination of a mucosal biopsy or a string test is indicated if the stool test is negative. Serologic tests, including IFA and ELISA, are also among other diagnostic tools for Giardiasis. The choice of treatment is antibiotic therapy most of with metronidazol.

Tuberculosis

Tuberculosis is still a major public health problem and one of the leading causes of death from infectious diseases worldwide. The most common agent is *Mycobacterium tuberculosis*, an acid-fast bacteria that is a member of mycobacterium tuberculosis complex. Other mycobacterium species (e.g., *M. bovis*) can also cause clinical tuberculosis in humans.

Primary tuberculosis is usually seen in young adults and children. The clinical presentation is frequently with pulmonary symptoms. Secondary tuberculosis is a late generalized infection usually seen in older patients with pulmonary symptoms and also as an occasionally disseminated disease. After the introduction of the antituberculosis therapy, the clinical presentation of late infection dramatically changed. It often is a disseminated infection but less often with the pulmonary symptoms that afflict immuno-supressed individuals (Madkour, 2004). Tuberculosis is the cause of 11% of adult deaths in the HIV positive population (Corbett et al., (2003)).

Culture from sputum or tissue is the gold standard method for detection of mycobacteria. Histopathologic examination of tissue-supported stains including acid fast bacilli stain (Ziehl–Nielsen or Kinyoun's method) and Fite stain is also helpful for diagnosis. In addition nucleic acid amplification assays can be used for direct detection of the organism. Lymphadenopathy and lymph node histopathology, along with tissue stains, is the common specimen seen in surgical pathology (see the discussion of lymph node pathology in Chapter 20).

Anemia in Tuberculosis

Although hematologic manifestations are not common in a pulmonary tuberculosis infection, some patients may present with anemia, leukocytosis, thrombocytopenia, and myelofibrosis in addition to other lab findings including an increased erythrocyte sedimentation rate, a low serum albumin level, and an abnormal liver function (Cameron, 1974). The anemia is usually associated with nutritional deficiency, malabsorbtion, iron deficiency, and bone marrow failure or hemolysis.

Severe anemia is seen in majority of the patients with the disseminated disease (Mandell et al., 2004). The anemia is normocytic and normochromic in most patients with hemoglobin level of less than 10 mg/dL. Several reported cases showed that tuberculosis may also cause immune hemolytic anemia in adults and children (Kuo et al., 2001; Bakhshi et al., 2004). It has been shown that the severity of the hematologic symptoms, including hemoglobin level, white cell count, and erythrocyte sedimentation rate, correlates with the prognosis of the disease (Bozoky et al., 1997).

Anemia in tuberculosis responds well to antituberculosis therapy. The therapy commonly used is a combination of rifampicin, isoniazid, pyrazinamid, and ethambutol.

Human Immune Deficiency Virus

The human immunodeficiency virus (HIV) is an RNA virus within the retrovirus family that causes the acquired immunodeficiency syndrome (AIDS). Two major types are important for infections in humans, HIV-1 and HIV-2. The distribution of HIV-1 is worldwide. HIV-2 related infections are predominantly reported in West Africa. At the end of 2007, 40 million persons worldwide were living with HIV or AIDS (UNAIDS, 2006).

The virus contains a reverse transcriptase enzyme, also known as RNA-dependent DNA polymerase, that allows the transcription of single-stranded RNA into double-stranded DNA and integration into the host cell. T-helper lymphocytes (CD4 + T cells) are the usual host cells infected by the virus, as are additionally the macrophages (Volberding, Baker, and Levine, 2003).

The transmission of the virus is usually by sexual contact, by transfusion of blood products, or by transplacental or contaminated needles. The virus compromises the immune system in humans and thus makes the afflicted individuals prone to opportunistic infections.

The spectrum of clinical disease associated with HIV ranges from asymptomatic carrier state to full disease, AIDS, with opportunistic infections, malignancies and neurodegenerative disorders.

Anemia in HIV Infection

Hematological complications are a common manifestation of HIV infection. The hematopoietic abnormalities are due to the impaired generation and function of blood cells of all lineages, and these present as various degrees of cytopenia in infected individuals (Kirchoff and Silvestri, (2008)). Cytopenia frequently is a result of ineffective hematopoiesis, which is most probably due to released cytokines such as interleukin-1, a tumor necrosis factor-alpha and transforming growth factor. Infections, malignancies involving the bone marrow, and chemotherapy agents may cause cytopenias in HIV-infected patients. The viral load appears to be related to the severity of the hematologic abnormalities.

Anemia is a common hematologic manifestation in 63 to 95% of HIV-infected individuals with increased incidence in the advanced stages (Sullivan, Hanson, Chu, et al., 1998). It may accompanied by granulocytopenia and/or thrombocytopenia. The etiology of anemia remains unclear, however, so different etiologic factors are considered to be cause of anemia (Table 10.1). The most common form of HIV-related anemia is the anemia of chronic disease (Volberding, Baker, and Levine, 2003).

Treatment of Choice

The degree of anemia in HIV-infected patients is strongly associated with prognosis independent of the CD4 levels. Furthermore the recovery from anemia is associated with good response to therapy and decreased mortality. Mocroft et al. showed that the hemoglobin level in HIV-infected patients is correlated with disease progression and is an independent prognostic factor for death after adjustment

TABLE 10.1 **Causes of Anemia**

Decreased production
- Drugs
  - Zidovudine
  - Trimethoprim-sulfamethoxazole
  - Amphotericin B
  - Ganciclovir
  - Dapsone
  - Delavirdine
- Deficiencies
  - Erythropoietin
  - Iron
  - Folate
  - Vitamin B12
- Infection
  - HIV
  - Parvovirus B19
  - Mycobacterium avium complex (MAC)
  - Mycobacterium tuberculosis
  - Histoplasma capsulatum
- Neoplasia
  - Non-Hodgkin's lymphoma
  - Multiple myeloma
  - Castleman's disease
  - Hodgkin's disease
- Miscellaneous
  - Anemia of chronic disease
  - Preexisting condition (sickle cell disease, thalassemia,etc.)

Increased loss
- Hemolysis
  - Thrombotic thrombocytopenic purpura
  - Glucose-6-phosphate dehydrogenase deficiency (trimethoprim-sulfamethoxazole [TMP-SMX], dapsone,primaquine)
  - Autoimmune hemolytic anemia
- Idiopathic
- Drugs (ceftriaxone, indinavir, "Ecstasy")
- Infection (cytomegalovirus [CMV])
- Gastrointestinal bleeding
  - Kaposi's sarcoma
  - Non-Hodgkin's lymphoma
  - Infection (CMV, Candida)
- Hypersplenism
  - Infection
  - Lymphoma
  - Hemophagocytosis
  - Cirrhosis (hepatitis B virus [HBV], hepatitis C virus

Source: Volberding, Baker, and Levine (2003).

for CD4 count and viral load (Mocroft, Kirk, Barton, et al., 1999). The symptoms of the anemia are also the most common constitutional symptoms of the HIV infection.

Anemia should be investigated if the hemoglobin level is less than 10 g/dl. Blood and bone marrow examination should be performed as well as blood cultures. Iron, folate, and vitamin B_{12} studies should be done if clinically suspected. Anisocytosis with fragments and macrocytosis are common findings in the blood films of patients on antiviral therapy (e.g., Zidovudine and Ganciclovir).

The treatment of the underlying cause of anemia is the treatment of choice. The retroviral therapy is effective in most patients in the treatment of anemia. Interventions to prevent anaemia may lead to improved health and survival potential of HIV-infected individuals (Doukas, 1992).

Hookworms

Hookworm infection is a parasitic infection caused by *Necator americanus* and *Ancylostoma duodenale*. It has a widespread distribution in tropics and subtropics. *N. americanus* is the most prevelant hookworm with high incidence in sub-Saharan Africa, South and Central America, and Southeast Asia while *A. duodenale* is found more often in the Middle East, North Africa, and India.

Hookworms are intestinal nematodes from Ancylostomidae family. Humans are the natural hosts. The eggs are passed in the feces (diagnostic stage) and develop to rhabditiform larva and subsequently filariform larva (infective stage) in the soil. The filariform larvae penetrate through the host skin, and are carried to the lungs via venous circulation. The larvae move to the pharynx through bronchial tree. The larvae are swallowed in pharynx and arrive in small intestine where they complete the life circle and become adults (Strickland, 1991).

The most important clinical manifestation of hookworm infection is anemia due to iron deficiency. The degree of anemia is related to the number of parasites and hemoglobin level of the host (Latham, Stephenson; Hall et al., (1983)). Iron deficiency occurs mainly due to consumption of blood directly by the parasite from intestinal circulation. Bleeding at the site of parasite due to mucosal damage also contributes to anemia (Kalkofen, 1974) as well as nutritional deficiencies (Table 10.2). The hemoglobin level ranges from 4 to 10 mg/dl. The differentiation of hookworm-related anemia and nutritional anemia may be challenging, especially in developing countries. Additional clinical and laboratory findings, including skin pigmentation, zinc, and hypoalbuminemia due to deacreased absorbtion and eosinophilia, may alert the clinician to a hookworm infection (Strickland, 1991).

Additional clinical manifestations include dermatitis at the penetration site, pulmonary symptoms, Loeffler syndrome, and gastrointestinal symptoms, including epigastric pain and abdominal distention.

TABLE 10.2 **Etiology of Anemia**

1. Malaria	Hemolytic, tropical splenomegaly
2. Babesiosis	Hemolytic
3. Visceral leishmaniasis (Kala-Azar)	Hemolysis, blood loss, splenic sequestration
4. Trypanosomiasis	Anemia of chronic disease
5. Amoebiasis	Blood loss
6. Giardiasis	Blood loss
7. Tuberculosis	Anemia of chronic disease
8. HIV	Anemia of chronic disease
9. Hookworms	Blood loss, microcytic,
10. Schistosomiasis	Hypersplenic sequestration syndrome
11. Trichuriasis	Blood loss

Malnutrition associated with protein deficiency is also a frequent manifestation that causes hypoalbuminaemia (Tandon, Saraya, et al., 1969).

The laboratory findings are usually combination of hypochromic and microcytic anemia, decreased iron and ferritin levels, and increased iron-binding capacity. Eosinophilia and decreased albumin levels are also common. The treatment of hookworm infections consist of iron replacement therapy and anti-helmintic medication including mebendazole, alben-dazole, pyrantel pamoate, and levamizole (WHO, 2007).

Blood transfusion is rarely required in patients with severe anemia.

Schistosomiasis

Schistosomiasis (also called bilharziasis) is a parasitic infection caused by *Schistosoma spp.* of the class Trematoda. The disease is endemic in the tropical and subtropical regions. It is estimated that more than 200 million people worldwide are infected (Mahmoud, 2001).

Schistosoma mansoni, Schistosoma japonicum, Schistosoma mekongi, Schistosoma intercalatum, and *Schistosoma haematobium* are the more common medically important infections caused in humans and characterized by a specific geographical distribution. *S. mansoni* is endemic in the Middle East, Africa, South America, and the Caribbean. *S. japonicum* is endemic in Asia, and *S. haematobium* is found in North Africa and Middle East. *S. mekongi* and *S. intercalatum* are endemic in Southeast Asia and Central Africa, respectively.

Pathology

Although the parasites are prevalent in animals, humans are the major hosts for all *schistosoma* species. The adult forms are diecious, living as two separate sexes. The adult foms of all infective species except *haematobium* inhabit the hepatic, portal, and mesenteric vessels while the vesical plexus, the urinary tract, and bladder are the major habitat for *S. haematobium*.

The humans propagate the disease as the eggs of the mature parasites by excretion via feces or urine. If the egss come in contact with fresh water, ciliated motile miracidia are released from the hatched eggs and penetrate the snail, which are the intermediate hosts. The miracidia multiply asexually in the body of the snail and motile cercariae are released from the snail. The infective cercariae can penetrate the human host skin and develop schistosomulae. These migrate to lungs and liver, where they develop into mature worms and further relocate to their final anatomical habitats.

The clinical manifestations could be characterized as acute and chronic disease. Acute disease manifests as dermatitis at the site of penetration, as allergic pneumonitis and as Katayama fever. The latter form of disease occurs more often with the *S. japonicum* infection. Katayama fever occurs at the time of maturing of adult forms and onset of egg release and is akin to serum sickness in symptoms. It has an acute onset of fever accompanied by chills, sweating, headache, and cough. Generalized lymphadenopathy and hepatosplenomegaly occur in majority of patients. There may be hypersplenism with splenic sequestration of blood leading to extravascular hemolysis. The exact etiology of anemia is not entirely clear, although the disease's pathology could lead to blood loss from extra-corporeal iron loss, splenomegaly leading to red blood cell sequestration, autoimmune hemolysis, and anemia of inflammation (Farid, Patwardhan, and Darby, 1969).

The chronic disease is a result of constant release of the eggs by the parasite. It causes a strong antigen-specific cell-mediated granulomatous response to the antigens. Abdominal pain and bloody diarrhea due to release of the eggs and focal inflammation of the intestines are common symptoms of infection especially with *S. mansoni* and *S.japonicum*. Release of *S. haematobium* eggs results in the inflammation and thickening of the bladder wall. Patients usually present with hematuria and dysuria. The diagnosis requires detailed clinical history including traveling history and examination of feces and urine for parasitic eggs.

Hematologic Manifestations

The patients infected by *Schistosoma sp.* may develop iron deficiency anemia due to blood loss from intestinal and urinary tracts. Hypersplenism also causes mild anemia due to the red cell pooling in the spleen as well as red cell destruction in infected individuals with an enlarged spleen (Farid, Patwardhan, and Darby, 1969).

The anemia in Schistosomiasis is usually morphologically hypochromic and slightly macrocytic. An elevated white blood cell count and eosinophilia are common hematologic findings. Anemia usually responds to iron replacement treatment and also, if necessary, splenectomy.

Praziquantel, broad spectrum antihelmintic agent, is the primary choice of therapy. Metrifonate against *S. haematobium* and Oxaminiquine against *S. mansoni* are alternative agent-specific drugs.

Trichuriasis

Trichuriasis is one of the most common intestinal helmintic infection caused by *Trichuris trichura* (whipworm).

T. trichura is a nematode that infects humans as the primary hosts. It is distributed worldwide, but the worm prefers warm and moist soil prevalent in the tropics. It is transmitted by ingestion of eggs from the infective soil. The ingested embryonated eggs are infective and release the larvae in the bowel. The young worms penetrate the intestinal mucosa through their whip-like anterior end and eventually mature. The adults could measure from 30 to 50 mm in length and prefer the cecal mucosa. A female adult may produce 2000 to 6000 eggs per day. The eggs are passed in feces to soil where they mature in 10 to 14 days (Strickland, 1991).

Most infected individuals are asymptomatic. In symptomatic patients, abdominal pain with nausea and vomiting are frequent symptoms. The worms may incite local inflammation, characterized as mucositis with eosinophils. The disrupted mucosa may lead to blood loss resulting in iron deficiency anemia, which are especially noted in young children in endemic areas. The infection is also associated with malnutrition and diarrhea as well as iron deficiency (Stephenson, 1987). Rectal prolapse is a rare complication. A rare condition of trichuriasis associated Coomb's negative anemia has also been reported (Huicho, 1995). The diagnosis is made by demonstrating eggs in the stool. Mebendazole and albendazole are the treatment of choice.

VASCULAR PURPURAS

Viral Hemorrhagic Fever—Yellow Fever

Yellow fever is an acute viral hemorrhagic disease usually transmitted by *Aedes aegypti* mosquito. The virus is a 20 μm, spherical, enveloped RNA virus from Flaviviridae family. The disease is endemic in subSaharan Africa and South America and spreads rapidly. The dissemination is attributed to the increasingly accessible endemic areas because of population demographics, widening urbanization, and global travel. Transmission can be vector-borne (via the bite of an infected mosquito) or anthroponotic (human-to-vector-to-human).

Two epidemic forms of yellow fever can be distinguished on the basis of different mosquito vectors and vertebrate hosts involved in the cycle of virus transmission: urban and jungle. In the urban form, the virus is passed by *Aedes aegypti* mosquito directly to humans. In the jungle yellow fever, the bite of forest mosquito is a zoonotic infection acquired and maintained via the monkey–mosquito–monkey cycle. These forms are clinically and pathologically identical (Strickland, 1991). The incubation period is usually 3 to 8 days.

Clinical manifestations vary from mild disease to fatal disease. Mild disease is characterized by indolent mild fever. Severe disease initially presents with fever, headache, back pain, fatigue, and generalized myalgia. During this phase the patients experience congested conjunctivae, reddened tongue, and flushed face. The virus can be detected in the blood during this period. A short symptomatic remission may be seen following the initial disease. When the toxic phase develops, fever and symptoms reoccur with vomiting, abdominal pain, and jaundice. Hematemesis, epistaxis, gum bleeding, melena, metrrhoragia, petechiaa, ecchymosis, and easy bruising may occur due to hepatic coagulopathy. Dehydration and renal insufficiency with proteinuria are common complications. The pulse is usually low despite high fever. The recovery follows the toxic phase in 3 days up to 2 weeks. Some patients may develop hypotension, shock, acute tubular necrosis, and heart failure. When an epidemic occurs in unvaccinated populations, fatality rates range from 15% to more than 50% (CDC, 2007).

Diagnosis is often based on clinical findings and travel history. Laboratory findings include coagulopathy with low platelets, increase in bleeding time (prothrombin and partial thromboplastin times), in fibrin split products, and in serum bilirubin levels, as well as elevated serum alanine and aspartate aminotransferases. Normocytic normochromic anemia from blood loss due to bleeding may occur in patients with hepatic injury. Definitive diagnosis includes complement fixation and IgM enzyme-linked immunosorbent assay (ELISA) performed in serum or cerebrospinal fluid. Nucleic acid amplification testing and immunofluorescence assay (IFA) for IgM and IgG antibodies are also used (Koraka, (2002)). Histopathological diagnosis with immunocytochemical techniques may also be a method used in liver tissue biopsy.

There is no specific treatment for yellow fever. Supportive care to treat dehydration and other complications is required. Prevention is key in control of disease. Vaccination with live-attenuated yellow fever 17D vaccine is available for individuals living in the endemic areas or travelers.

Defective Platelet Function—Lassa Fever

Lassa fever is caused by the Lassa virus, an arenavirus. The Lassa virus is a single-stranded enveloped RNA virus with a mean diameter of 50 to 300 nm. The virus is a natural parasite of *Mastomys* rodents and can be excreted in the urine of the rodent; humans can be infected as accidental hosts. Human-to-human transmission is also possible, although the risk is lower.

Lassa fever is an acute viral disease that is endemic throughout West Africa. The infection affects 100,000 to 300,000 people every year with approximately 5000 deaths (CDC, 2004).

Following an incubation period of 1 to 3 weeks after contact with the virus, patients develop fever, weakness, malaise, sore throat, back and chest pain, cough, and abdominal pain. Most patients also have vomiting, diarrhea, proteinuria, conjunctivitis, and coagulopathy due to hepatic injury. Some patients may experience severe pulmonary and cardiac symptoms, including pneumonitis and cardiac failure and neurologic signs varying from tremor to severe encephalitis.

Hematologic manifestations are often due to platelet dysfunction and possibly endothelial cell dysfunction. See Chapter 22 on Lassa virus lymphadenopathy. The platelet defect appears to be mediated by an inhibitory factor in blood plasma that specifically inhibits platelet dense granules and adenosine triphosphate release (Strickland, 1991; Chen, (2007)).

The diagnosis is most often made by using ELISA, which detects IgM and IgG antibodies as well as Lassa virus antigen or virus isolation in cell culture. IFA and real-time polymerase chain reaction (RT-PCR) are sensitive techniques for rapid detection of the virus. A new technique using reverse transcription-loop-mediated isothermal amplification is investigation as an alterate method (Fukuma (2011)).

Ribavirin is the first line treatment of Lassa fever. Vaccines are also available for prevention.

REFERENCES

Artan R, Yilmaz A, Akçam M, et al. 2006. 'Liver biopsy in the diagnosis of visceral leishmaniasis.' J Gastroenterol Hepatol 21:101–4.

Bakhshi S, Rao IS, Jain V, Arya LS. 2007. Autoimmune hemolytic anemia complication disseminated childhood tuberculosis. Ind J Pediatr 71 (6):549–51.

Bozoky G, Ruby E, Goher I, Toth J, Mohos A. 1997. Hematologic abnormalities in pulmonary tuberculosis. Orvil Hetil 138:1053–6.

Cameron SJ. 1974. Tuberculosis and the blood: a special relationship. Tubercle 5:65–72.

Cavagnaro F, Guzman C, Harris P. 2006. Hemolytic uremic syndrome associated with Entamoeba histolytica intestinal infection. Pediatr Nephrol 21(1):126–8.

Centers for Disease Control and Prevention. 2007.

Chen JP, Cosgriff TM. 2001. Hemorrhagic Yellow fever virus-induced changes in hemostasis and vascular biology. Blood Coagul Fibrinolysis 11(5):461–83.

Corbett EL, Watt CJ, Walker N, et al. 2003. The growing burden of tuberculosis: global trends and interactions with the HIV epidemic. Arch Intern Med 163:1009–21.

Cordingley FT, Crawford GP. 1986. Giardia infection causes vitamin B_{12} deficiency. Aust NZ J Med 16(1):78–9.

Cowen AE, Campbell CB. 1973. Giardiasis—a cause of vitamin B_{12} malabsorption. Am J Dig Dis 18(5):384–90.

De Vizia B, Poggi V, Vajro P, Cucchiara S, Acampora A. 1986. Iron malabsorption in giardiasis. J Pediatr 107(1):75–8.

De Waal Malefyt R, Abrams J, Bennett B, Figdor CG, de Vries JE. 1991. Interleukin 10(IL-10) inhibits cytokine synthesis by human monocytes: an autoregulatory role of IL-10 produced by monocytes. J Exp Med 174(5):1209–20.

Doukas M. 1992. Human immunodeficiency virus associated anemia. Med Clin North Am 76:699.

Dursun O, Erisir S, Yesilipek A. 2009. Visceral childhood leishmaniasis in southern Turkey: experience of twenty years. Turk J Pediatr 51(1):1–5.

Farid Z, Patwardhan VN, Darby WJ. 1969. Parasitism and anemia. Am J Clin Nut 22(5):498–503.

Fukuma A, Kurosaki Y, Morikawa Y, Grolla A, Feldmann H, Yasuda J. 2011. Rapid detection of Lassa virus by reverse transcription-loop-mediated isothermal amplification. Microbiol Immunol 55(1):44–50.

Gonen C, Yilmaz N, Yalcin M et al. 2007. Diagnostic yield of routine duodenal biopsies in iron deficiency anaemia: a study from Western Anatolia. Eur J Gastroenterol Hepatol 19(1):37–41.

Herwaldt BL. 1999. Leishmaniasis. Lancet 354:1191–99.

Huicho L. 1995. Trichuriasis associated to severe transient Coomb's-negative hemolytic anemia and macroscopic hematuria. Wilderness Enviro Med 6:247.

Kalkofen UP. 1974. Intestinal trauma resulting from feeding activities of *Ancylostoma caninum*. Am J Trop Med Hyg 23(6):1046–53.

Kirchhoff F, Silvestri G. 2008. Is Nef the elusive cause of HIV-associated hematopoietic dysfunction? J Clin Invest 118:1622–5.

Koraka P, Zeller H, Niedrig M, et al. 2002. Reactivity of serum samples from patients with a flavivirus infection measured by immunofluorescense assay and ELISA. Microbes Infect 4(12):1209–15.

Kuo PH, Yang PC, Kou SS, Luh KT. 2001. Severe immune hemolytic anemia in disseminated tuberculosis with response to antituberculosis therapy. Chest 119:1961–3.

Latham MC, Stephenson LS, Hall A, Wolgemuth JC, Elliot TC, Crompton DW. 1983. Parasitic infections, anaemia and nutritional status: a study of their interrelationships and the effect of prophylaxis and treatment on workers in Kwale District, Kenya. Trans R Soc Trop Med Hyg 77:41–8.

Madkour MM (ed.). 2004. Tuberculosis. Springer, Heidelberg.

Mahmoud AF. 2001. Schistosomiasis. World Scientific, Singapore, 9–13.

Mandell GL, Bennett JE, Dolin R (eds.). 2004. Principals and Practice of Infectious Diseases, 6th ed. Elsevier Churchill Livingstone, Edinburgh.

Mandell GL, Bennett JE, Dolin R. 2000. Mandell, Douglas, and Bennett's Principle and Practice of Infectious Diseases, 5th ed. Churchill Livingstone, Philadelphia, 2950–3.

Mayett FG, Powel SJ. 1964. Anemia, hypochromic; blood chemical analysis; bone marrow examination; hemoglobinometry; iron; liver abscess, amebic. Am J Trop Med Hyg 13(6):790–3.

McLean L, Odiit M, Sternberg JM 2001. Nitric oxide and cytokine synthesis in human African trypanosomiasis. J Infect Dis 184:1086–90.

Mocroft A, Kirk O, Simon B, et al. 1999. Anaemia is an independent predictive marker for clinical prognosis in HIV-infected patients from across Europe. AIDS 13(8):943–50.

Pearson RD, Queiroz SA, Jeronimo SM. 2000. Leishmania species: visceral (kala-azar), cutaneous, and mucosal leishmaniasis. In: Mandell GL, Bennett JE, Dolin R, eds., Mandell: Principles and Practice of Infectious Diseases, 5th ed. Churchill Livingstone, Philadelphia, 2831–41.

Reithinger R, Brooker S, Kolaczinski JH. 2007. Visceral leishmaniasis in eastern Africa—current status. Trans R Soc Trop Med Hyg 101(12):1169–70.

Stephenson LS. 1987. The Impact of Helminth Infections of Human Nutrition. Taylor and Francis, London, 691–4.

Strickland T. 1991. Hunter's Tropical Medicine, 7th ed. W.B. Saunders, Philadelphia, 700–6.

Sullivan PS, Hanson DL, Chu SY, Jones JL, Ward JW, the Adult/Adolescent Spectrum of Disease Group. 1998. Epidemiology of anemia in human immunodeficiency virus (HIV)-infected persons: results from the multistate adult and adolescentspectrum of HIV disease surveillance project. Blood 91:301–8.

Tandon BN, Saraya AK, Ramachandran K, Sama SK. 1969. Relationship of anemia and hypoproteinemia to the functional and structural changes in the small bowel in hookworm disease. Gut 10:360–5.

Trampuz A, Jereb M, Muzlovic I, Prabhu RM. 2003. Clinical review: severe malaria. Crit Care 7:315–23.

UNAIDS. 2006. Report on the Global AIDS Epidemic. Geneva.

Volberding P, Baker K, Levine A. 2003. Human immunodeficiency virus hematology. Am Soc of Hemat 1:294–313.

WHO. 2009. Essential Medicines: WHO Model List. Geneva.

PART III

NON-NEOPLASTIC LYMPH NODE PATHOLOGY AND INFECTIONS

CHAPTER ELEVEN

CLASSIFICATION OF REACTIVE LYMPHADENOPATHY

Hernani D. Cualing

INTRODUCTION

The difficulty in diagnosis of reactive lymphadenopathy rivals, if not exceeds, that of lymphomas. The ease of recognizing a reactive lymph node belies its complexity, and contributes to the generally nonchalant attention it receives compared to its malignant cousin. Just like the lymphomas, there is an approach that makes sense of the numerous entities under its roof (see Table 11.1) as well as a framework to formulate diagnosis. There have been many ways to classify its entities, and like the lymphomas, historical artifice hinders easy understanding and simple diagnosis. Partly to blame is the aspect that "it is just benign, who cares what kind" until the lymphoma is mistaken for a benign diagnosis, or a treatable infection, or one that is highly contagious is missed. Often the lack of clinical history compounds the limited microscopic window that a pathologist initially sees. Hence we use an approach used by many hematopathologists, in their approach to diagnose lymphomas: widen this microscopic window by knowing what are the pitfalls, the clinical milieu, and the subtle histologic features that differentiate entities.

Non-neoplastic hematopathology is difficult to diagnose not only because of its mimicry of lymphomas, but also because it has received less studious attention than its neoplastic counterpart. Inherently, reactive lymph nodes are also difficult to classify because lymph nodes, upon stimulation, display a dynamic variability that depends on the patient's age, immune status, phase or duration of reaction, and whether the etiology is infectious or noninfectious. About 30 to 40% of reactive lymph nodes have specific histologic features leading to a definite diagnosis: features in histology suggest a pattern that requires ancillary serology, phenotypic or serologic tests that may lead to a specific diagnosis. The rest of lymph nodes seen in pathology practice may show a nonspecific histology, but its pattern needs to be stated to initiate a pattern-based differential diagnosis. Even for a nonspecific reactive hyperplasia, such as a mixed follicular and paracortical reaction, diagnosis is important because of the implicit concern for a lymphoma is considered and not favored. A specific reactive lymphadenopathy diagnosis, when suggested by a constellation of clues, needs to be given so that confirmatory tests can be performed. A diagnosis of infection is furthermore of emergent nature since a therapy could be started, surveillance for endemic and communicable disease performed, and malignancy ruled out.

Since many excellent texts have been written on reactive splenic, skin, bone marrow, and extranodal disorders, we limited the section largely to lymph nodes. We begin with low-power recognition

Non-Neoplastic Hematopathology and Infections, First Edition. Edited by Hernani D. Cualing, Parul Bhargava, and Ramon L. Sandin.
© 2012 Wiley-Blackwell. Published 2012 by John Wiley & Sons, Inc.

TABLE 11.1 Patterns of Reactive Lymphadenopathies

I. Reactive follicular patterns

Follicle (germinal) center hyperplasia
    Florid follicular hyperplasia, nonspecific
    Reactive follicular and paracortical
      hyperplasia
    HIV-related progressive generalized
      lymphadenopathy
Progressive transformation of germinal centers
Marginal zone hyperplasia
Mantle zone hyperplasia
Regressed (atrophic) germinal centers
    Involuted phase of HIV-related lymphadenopathy
    Castleman's disease, hyaline vascular
    Primary immune deficiency lymph nodes
Reactive follicles, mixed with other patterns, specific
  entities
    Kimura's lymphadenopathy
    Allergic lymphadenopathy
    Angio-lymphoid hyperplasia with eosinophila
    Autoimmune lymphadenopathy
      Rheumatoid arthritis lymphadenopathy
      Sjogren's syndrome lymphadenopathy
      Systemic lupus lymphadenopathy,
    Toxoplasmic lymphadenopathy,
    Syphilis lymphadenopathy

II. Reactive interfollicular or paracortical hyperplasia
*   including diffuse immunoblastic reactions*

Paracortical hyperplasia, nonspecific common
Dermatopathic lymphadenopathy
Postimmune (vaccine) reactive paracortical hyperplasia
Drug-induced reactive paracortical hyperplasia
    Methotrexate drug lymphadenopathy
    Anticonvulsant drug
      lymphadenopathy
Reactive immunoblastic proliferations
    Reactive immunoblastic proliferation,
      nonspecific
    Interfollicular Hodgkinoid lymphadenopathy
    Acute infectious mononucleosis
    CMV lymphadenitis
    Herpes simplex lymphadenitis
    Herpes zoster lymphadenitis

III. Sinus hyperplasia patterns

Sinus histiocytosis, nonspecific
Sinus histiocytosis, secondary to adjacent tumor drainage
Signet ring histiocytosis
Sinus histiocytosis with massive lymphadenopathy
Pigmented sinus histiocytic pattern
Histiocytic reactions to foreign materials
    Lymphangiography lymphadenopathy
    Mucicarminophilic histiocytosis (PVP
      lymphadenopathy)
    Histiocytosis postmetallic joint prosthesis
Sinus histiocytosis pattern of extramedullary
  hematopoieisis

Immature "sinus histiocytosis" or monocytoid B-cell
  hyperplasia
Histiocytic hemophagocytic syndromes
Vascular transformation of sinuses
Whipple (*T. whipelli*) lymphadenopathy

IV. Mixed reactive patterns

Necrotizing lymphadenopathies
    Fine needle aspiration lymphadenopathy
    Infarcted lymph node
    Radiation necrosis lymphadenopathy
    Kikuchi necrotizing lymphadenopathy
    Kawasaki's necrotizing lymphadenopathy
    Systemic lupus necrotizing lymphadenopathy
Granulomatous lymphadenopathy,
    noninfectious
    Sarcoidosis
    Berylliosis
    Tumor reactive granulomatous lymphadenopathy
    Granulomas adjacent carcinomas
    Reactive granulomas associated with lymphomas
Deposition lymphadenopathhy
    Proteinaceous lymphadenopathy
    Immunoglobulin deposition lymphadenopathy
Vascular and stromal reactive
    lymphadenopathy
    Inflammatory pseudotumor
    Bacillary angiomatosis
Granulomatous lymphadenopathy,
    infectious
Suppurative granulomas
    Cat-scratch (*Bartonella henselae*)
    Tularemia Francisella tularensis
    Lymphogranuloma venereum (*Chlamydia
      trachomatis*)
    Chancroid (*H. ducrei*)
    Yersiniosis (*Yersinia enterocolitical
      pseudotuberculosis*)
    Brucellosis lymphadenitis
    Melioidosis (*Burkholderia pseudomallei*)
    Typhoid lymphadenitis (*Salmonella typhi*)
Granulomas and diagnostic microorganisms
    Filarial lymphadenopathy

      Dirofilaria lymphadenitis

      Brugia spp. lymphadenitis
      Bancroftian spp. lymphadenitis
      Loa Loa lymphaditis
      Tropical eosinophilic lymphadenopathy
    Schistosomiasis lymphadenitis
    Leismaniasis spp. lymphadenitis
Granulomas with foamy histiocytosis—leprosy
Mixed pattern with deposition of interstitial
  substance—pneumocystiis jiroveci Lymphadenitis
Mixed Pattern with granulomas and caseation necrosis
    Mycobacteria tuberculosis lymphadenopathy

TABLE 11.1 (Continued)

BCG lymphadenitis
Systemic fungal lymphadenitis
Mixed pattern with angiomatoid
pattern
Bartonella bacilliformis and *R. henselae* bacillary
angiomatosis
Lymphadenopathy not otherwise
characterized/provisional patterns
Hemorrhagic lymphadenopathy
Bacillus anthracis (anthrax) lymphadenopathy
Rocky Mountain spotted fever
Sinus pattern
Yersinia pestis (bubonic plaque) lymphadenopathy

Leptospira interogans lymphadenopathy
Scrub typhus lymphadenopathy
Diffuse pattern with depletion and atypical immunoblastic
reaction
Dengue hemorrhagic fever
lymphadenopathy
Ehrlichiosis
lymphadenopathy
Lassa hemorrhagic fever
Nipah virus
Ring granulomas
Q fever

of the histology patterns and proceed from there. We also take lessons from a Family Circus cartoon by Bil Keane: kids overlooking an adult reading a book say "Grown-up books are harder to read … they make you think up your own pictures!!!" We incorporate many color pictures, and in this and subsequent chapters, we try to fill in with more guideposts, the map of non-neoplastic hematopathology, which is already dotted with classic landmarks. We are indebted to hematopathology pioneers who described reactive lymphadenopathy and its classic patterns. (Schnitzer, 1992; Weiss, 2008). We further extend this exploration into the realm of the infectious diseases. We are indeed excited and thrilled navigating unexplored seas and wondrous terra incognita as the fictional sailors of Lewis Carroll and hope the readers will be as excited as well to fill in the blanks:

> He had brought a large map representing the sea,
> Without the least vestige of land:
> And the crew were much pleased when they found it to be
> A map they could all understand.
> … "Other maps are such shapes, with their islands and capes!
> But we've got our brave Captain to thank"
> (So the crew would protest) "that he's brought us the best—
> A perfect and absolute blank!"
>
> Lewis Carroll, *Fit The Second, The Hunting of the Snark*

Definition

Lymphadenopathy is enlargement or swelling of the lymphatic nodes of wide-ranging causes, but can be more broadly defined as an abnormality in character,

TABLE 11.2 Examples of Lymphadenopathy

Infectious
Cat-scratch disease
Toxoplasmosis
Histoplasmosis
Infectious mononucleousis
Tuberculosis
HIV
Leishmaniasis
Ricketssial (TIBOLA)
Tropical Infections
Autoimmune/Allergic
SLE
Rheumatoid arthritis
Allergic granulomatosis
Neoplasms
Lymphoma
Metastasis
Leukemia
Exogenous
Medications
Silicosis
Beryllium
Prosthetic substances
Idiopathic
Sarcoidosis
Kikuchi's disease
Kawasaki's disease
Kimura's disease
Castleman's disease (HV variant)

or size, caused by inflammation, infection, or neoplastic cells (see Table 11.2). Lymphadenitis refers to a swollen, inflamed lymph node, while lymphangitis relates to an inflammation of lymph vessels.

Synonyms

Lymph node hyperplasia, reactive lymph node, or nonspecific reactive hyperplasia, enlarged gland,

---

> **BOX 11.1 To biopsy or Not to Biopsy**
>
> Whether to perform a biopsy or empirically treat, it is the clinician's task to determine the correct diagnosis. Diagnosis is often arrived at by referring the biopsied materials to experts in histopathology or cytopathology of lymphadenopathy.

gland hypertrophy, swollen glands, or hyperplastic glands.

Epidemiology

An enlarged lymph node is a common sign of a variety of infectious and malignant conditions (Figure 11.1). It is a recognized manifestation of many diseases including inflammatory disorders, autoimmune diseases, acute or chronic infection, metastatic disease, or lymphomas. An annual incidence of 0.6 to 0.7% has been estimated for the general population in Western societies (Allhiser, McKnight, and Shank, 1981a,b; Fijten and Blijham, 1988). In tropical and subtropical countries benign causes exceed malignant causes, and of the benign causes, infections account for about one-third of the cases. In a retrospective study of lymphadenopathy in India, non-neoplastic etiology comprise 67.6% and neoplastic lymph nodes comprise 32.4%; of non-neoplastic causes, 25% were due to specific causes: broken down into 65.6% non-infectious and 34% infectious etiology (Chhabra et al., 2006) (see

Table 11.3). Although the prevalence of malignancy in patients presenting to the primary care office with unexplained lymphadenopathy is only 1.1% (Chau, 2003), the incidence of malignant diagnosis in a tertiary center is much higher. In a referral institution study using aspirate of lymph nodes, 75% of the diagnosis was malignant, with the most common diagnosis as carcinoma or lymphoma, with reactive lymph nodes or granulomas accounting for 20% of the diagnosis (Schafernak, 2003). Whatever the etiology, a lymph node biopsy or cytologic aspiration are key procedures to ascertain and confirm a benign or malignant diagnosis (see Box 11.1).

Clinically, several risk factors for malignancy are identified: duration, age, location, immunologic status, and specific immunosuppressive treatments. Patients with lymphadenopathy presenting for more than one month requires a biopsy to rule out malignancy (Bazemore, 2002). Although, lymphadenopathy presents in patients of all ages, the incidence of malignancy differs according to patient age: there is a higher incidence of malignant lymphadenopathy in adults than in children. In adults, generalized lymphadenopathy is a sign of a hematological or systemic disease. In children, the incidence of reactive lymph node was 60% and malignancy only accounted for 18% of the cases. Malignant lymph node is generally diagnosed associated with four conditions: lymph nodes bigger than 3 cm, high lactate dehydrogenase

REACTION PATTERNS

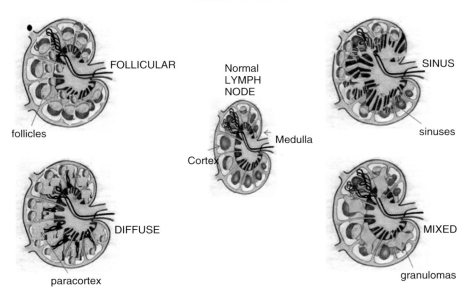

FIGURE 11.1 Patterns of lymph node reactions. Four patterns are seen in reactive lymph nodes. Each pattern has a corresponding nonneoplastic and neoplastic differential diagnoses.

TABLE 11.3 **Causes of Reactive Noninfectious Lymphadenopathy**

Diagnosis: Reactive Noninfectious N = 164		Percent
Reactive follicular hyperplasia-	115	70.0
Sinus histiocytosis	7	4.2
Dermatopathic lymphadenitis	15	9.2
Kikuchi's disease	7	4.2
Sarcoidosis	4	2.5
Granulomas, non-specific	3	1.8
Kimura's disease	3	1.8
Castleman's disease, Hyaline vascular	3	1.8
Histiocytosis, Langerhan's	1	0.6
Necrotic lymph node	1	0.6
Eosinophilic lymphadenitis	1	0.6
Others, descriptive	4	2.5

Source: Adapted from Chhabra et al. (2006) data from Chandigar, India.

levels, the presence of hepatosplenomegaly or generalized lymphadenopathy (Yaris et al., 2006). Caution should be exercised, however, when children present with generalized lymphadenopathy, since viral infections is the most common etiology (Leung and Robson, 2004). In addition the incidence of low-grade lymphoma is rare in persons below 20 years old. In children, supraclavicular fixed lymphadenopathy is most worrisome for malignancy and that of cervical lymph node less likely to be malignant (Soldes, Younger, and Hirschl, 1999). In a study of 1877 cervical lymphadenopathies in children of developing countries, in contrast to children of developed countries, there was a higher incidence of infective cause, chiefly tuberculosis. About 12% showed neoplastic causes; enough to argue for diagnostic surgical biopsy and 48% had nonspecific lymph node hyperplasia, 36% with granulomatous disease, with tuberculosis as the cause in 25%. Other less common findings include pyogenic adenitis, Rosai–Dorfman disease, cat-scratch disease, syphilis, yaws, and toxoplasmosis (Moore, Schneider, and Schaaf, 2003). Immunosuppression or an immunocompromise state from any cause is a risk factor in the development of malignant lymphoma: in HIV, the risk is up to 200 times a normal individual and in post-transplant patients, the incidence is up 26% (Swerdlow et al., 2008).

Processing of a Lymph Node

A well-prepared histological and cytological workup that begins upon receiving a fresh lymph node is essential for an accurate interpretation. A protocol is required to standardize the processing of the specimen. The pathologist usually examines a fresh unfixed lymph node for intraoperative consultation suspected of neoplasm. The physician or surgeon are instructed to send the specimen in a sterile container with steripad. The steripad is moistened with sterile saline solution, especially important in core or biopsy fragments, to prevent the drying artifacts. A careful measurement of the node then should occur and, if intact, oriented, and the hilum identified. The pathologist sections the lymph node along the long sagittal plane, carefully transecting through the hilum, to demonstrate the normal anatomical structures and to carefully examine the node for color and texture. Touch imprints or frozen sections are made on selected sections. Although the prefered technic is cytologic imprints, the pathologist may easily find carcinoma or melanoma, especially if faced with a sclerotic lymph node, by doing an intraoperative frozen section examination.

The pathologist can avoid suboptimally prepared cytologic imprints by paying attention to a few simple and easy to follow rules. Gently press the dry microscopic slides onto cut surfaces of a lymph node; other extranodal tissue such as a bisected skin biopsy should yield good cytologic details and preserve tissue integrity. In small biopsy or thru-cut needle cores, forceps are not optimal because of their tendency to crush fragile cores. An alternate way of lifting the tissue is by using a pointed end of a broken Q-tip wood stick that has been snapped into two pieces. Gently lift the core biopsy fragments with the pointed cut end of the stick, and slide the fragments on the surface of a glass slide to allow for a good cellular imprint. Spleen sections or any tissue with hemorrhagic cut surface requires blotting with absorbent paper to remove blood until the surface becomes reddish matte-dry. After this simple step, the imprint should yield the lymphocyte imprints instead of cells obscured by blood.

Wright–Giemsa or Diff Quick stained slides on air-dried cytologic touch imprints are examined next. This procedure is a standard for intraoperative evaluation of lymph node obtained to determine the cause of lymphadenopathy and to rule out malignant lymphoma. It has advantages over a frozen section histology in that touch imprints help conserve precious tissue later needed for flow cytometry, molecular gene rearrangement, or cytogenetic tests. Cytologic imprints provide higher microscopic resolution compared with a histostained frozen sectioned tissue slide. The imprint findings should provide enough information to determine whether a microbiologic or lymphoma workup is warranted. The imprints will show if there are extensive necrosis, pus, or paucicellularity that may jeopardize the adequacy of the surgical specimen for a complete workup. The surgeon is particularly interested in obtaining an volume of specimen adequate for all the required tests, so the pathologist should communicate the adequacy of a specimen: to prevent unwanted rebiopsy, patient inconvenience, and additional medical expenses.

The pathologist needs to carefully evaluate the cytology on low power for adequacy, staining quality, and field to focus. This evaluation should provide much of the information that would be of use to the surgeon and the pathologist in the intraoperative workup. A lymphoma of Hodgkin type or a large cell or follicular center cell category is more easily recognized using these preparations than a frozen section. A high-power view allows examination of nuclear contours and cytoplasmic details for the presence of inflammatory complements: all of which are features important in determining whether the lymphocytes are neoplastic. The adequacy of the specimen and the presence of granulomas, clusters of histiocytes, or stacks of neutrophils are important clues that would prompt a microbiological or infectious disease workup. Once a microbiological or infectious disease workup is determined based on the clinical history and the intraoperative cytological examination, a sterile kit is essential to obtain the tissue for microbiological analysis. A sterile culture medium such as RPMI is often required for microbiological, cytogenetic, or flow cytometric analysis. A gram stain, fungal, or Wright–Giemsa stain on the touch imprint will show bacteria, hyphae, or protozoal organisms and, in immunocompromized patients, any number of microorganisms. A communication with your microbiologist facilitates diagnosis, especially in a clinical setting of an immunocompromised state and sepsis.

Gross Appearance

Bean-shaped, 2 mm to 2 cm in size, lymph nodes are soft, glistening with pale thin capsule when freshly excised. Surgeons, who examine their specimen in the frozen section room, should be welcome to provide orientation, clinical status, and timely feedback on intraoperative consultation. They are generally satisfied with cytologic imprint evaluation when their concern is lymphoma or leukemia.

The cut section should be oriented along the long or sagittal axis of the node preferably transecting the hilum, which appears often as an indentation in a properly excised node (see Figure 11.2). Section appearance provides clues to pathology. A reactive lymph node looks reddish-tan and uniform in color with a soft fleshy texture (see Figure 11.3). The

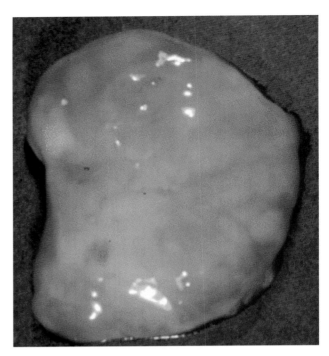

FIGURE 11.2 **Intact capsulated properly excised lymph node with glistening capsule**. The prominent vascularity that points toward the indented hilum. Note the wet saline, which is important in preventing drying artifacts that interfere with optimal histology.

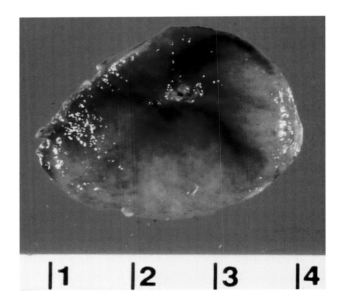

FIGURE 11.3 **Reddish tan cut surface of an enlarged lymph node (3 cm) showing the nonspecific follicular center hyperplasia**. Note the vague nodularities on the glistening cut surface and the vascularity toward the hilar vessels (sectioned sagitally, but the hilum vessels are not transected along the capsule edge).

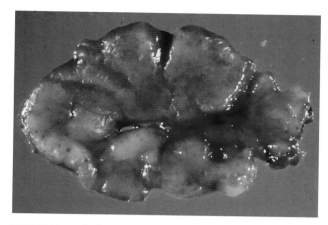

FIGURE 11.4 A 2.5-cm cut section of an infectious lymphadenopathy of "cat-scratch disease." Note the pale whitish patches of suppurative necrotizing granulomas on a background of reddish-tan reactive pulp.

presence of pale white or grayish-yellow pus or exudates should prompt a microbiologic or infectious disease workup and touch imprints and microbiology sample separately submitted in a sterile prep kit (see Figure 11.4).

A pale or fish-flesh cut section indicate an abnormality, often that of a lymphoma. Discrete yellow or red discolorations, nodularities, hemorrhages, or focal firmness or chalky granularities are abnormal and would indicate a pathology (see Figure 11.6). A nodularity seen on cut section could be a gross picture of a florid follicular hyperplasia, Hodgkin lymphoma, or follicular lymphoma—elicited by varying the angle of light (see Figure 11.6). Hemorrhages, yellowish whitish exudate or frank fibrosis could be observed in cases suspected of acute infection.

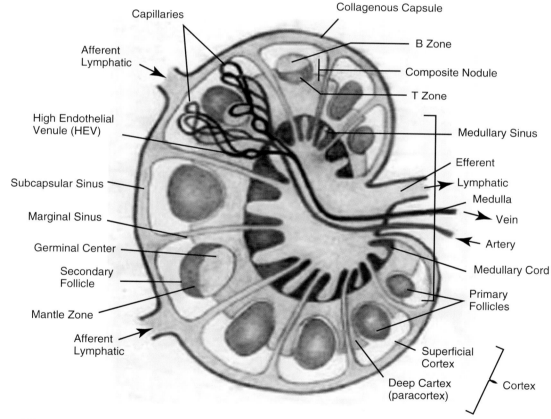

FIGURE 11.5 **Diagram of a lymph node showing normal histological and functional compartments.** The cortex and medulla are the two major areas where functional structures of the follicles, paracortex (deep cortex), sinuses, and medullary components are futher delineated and identified. Also shown is the lymphatic and arteriovenous supply. The superficial cortex is also called the diffuse or interfollicular cortex. The paracortex shows the high endothelial venules, while the capillaries are in the superficial cortex and germinal centers. The collagenous capsule shows the afferent lymphatic inflow to the sinuses and the medulla shows the efferent sinus and lymphatic outflow along with arterial supply and venous drainage. Immunologic reactions elicit the formation of B and T cell zones—also called a composite nodule. Adapted from droid.cuhk.edu.hk.

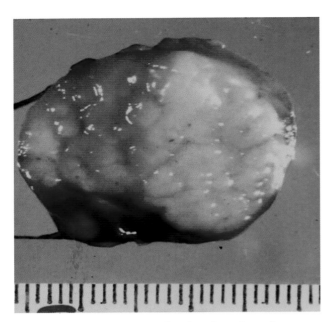

FIGURE 11.6 **In contrast to benign lymph nodes, a cut section of a lymphoma showing a fish-flesh coloration.** In this case a Hodgkin lymphoma was identified on histology. Notice the visible nodularity and thickened capsule that contrast with the reddish-tan cut surface of reactive lymph node cut section in previous figures.

Morphologic Approach

To appreciate the background information presented in the following topics knowledge is necessary of the approach the pathologist routinely uses when presented with lymph node touch imprints or lymph node histopathology for benign or malignant differential diagnosis. This approach applies to both intraoperative consultation and evaluation of touch imprints.

To begin, the tissue that comes to the histopathology lab is usually in response to a patient's concern that has been brought to the attention of the patient's doctor. The primary doctor may initiate treatment empirically based on the clinical symptomatology or the results of a serology and, after finding nondiagnostic information, may order a direct examination of the enlarged lymph node/s. An aspiration or surgical excision of the lymph node then allows for a histologic evaluation. After recording the gross features of a specimen, the pathologist sections the node and performs about five air dried touch imprints. The cut sections are examined for texture and color, selecting lymph node proper from fatty stroma, and abnormalities noted that offer clues to the pathology (see Figure 11.3). Sections are alloted for possible flow cytometry, cytogenetics, microbiology, and other

ancillary tests. One air-dried imprint is stained with Diff-Quick, the other four are saved for microbiology or in situ hybridization studies. It is important to keep the tissue covered under a moist sterile pad while performing these procedures to prevent drying artifacts.

The pathologist sections tissue in the fresh state on the long sagittal plane of an intact lymph node, making the thickness 2 to 3 mm (which is about as thin as a scalpel holder) to ensure adequate fixation using standard formalin-based fixative. A B5-based fixative offers a higher histological definition but is less often used because it contains mercury, which is toxic.

Cytomorphology

This cytologic touch imprints approach can be used for both intraoperative consultation and routine evaluation. The examination of the Diff-Quick stained slide starts at low-power scan. The low-power scan is then used to select areas that are optimal, avoiding dark clumps, smeared edges, or pale suboptimal stained areas. The pathologist uses a medium-power view on a selected area for the presence of large cells, epithelial clusters of histiocytes, or endothelia, as well as for Reed–Sternberg cells if included as a plausible disease for age and location. If there is none of the above, further examination proceeds to the high-power view to identify macrophages with the size of the nuclei as the benchmark for small and large cells. To elaborate, the rule of thumb is "small" means small as small lymphocytes or small as intermediate sized lymphoblasts or small noncleaved centroblasts. For small or intermediate size predominant cell imprints, the pathologist looks at nuclei for contours, clefting, and irregularity. An increased presence of clefted or notched nuclei indicative of follicular lymphoma, especially if large centroblasts or noncleaved cells with marginalized nucleoli are present. Predominant small nuclei with round contours, clumped, or soccer ball chromatin with minimal centroblasts, few mast cells, and few plasma cells would support neoplastic lymphoid imprints, and the pathologist has to consider small lymphocytic lymphoma or mantle cell lymphoma if slightly larger nuclei with peppery nuclear chromatin are evident. Predominance of small centroblast nuclei with moderately dispersed chromatin and marginalized nucleoli and deep blue vacuolated cytoplasm indicates Burkitt lymphoma, especially if a lot of mitosis is identified. Lymphoblasts have small to intermediate size nuclei with dusty and finely dispersed chromatin and small nucleoli (see Chapter 21 cytomorphology of reactive lymph nodes).

The presence of reactive inflammatory cells in the form of clusters of neutrophils and plasma cells, especially on a background of necrotic cytology would require a microbiologic workup, provided that other malignant features such as Hodgkin cells, large cell lymphoma, or atypical lymphocytes are not present. If pus or a necrotic node is present, the pathologist should send several touch imprints for rapid microbiological screening for bacterial or fungal or, in endemic areas, for parasitic or protozoan microorganisms. At this point involvement of microbiology laboratory and personnel is an essential step in the workup, for obtaining culture or early diagnosis based on the direct microscopic identification of the bacteria or fungi, parasites, or other microorganisms. In all instances the pathologist should preserve a piece of tissue in RPMI, if equipped, for potential cytogenetic, flow cytometry, or microbiologic culture.

Histology

After processing, the histology of the lymph node is examined systematically. The goal is to determine if the normal architecture is intact and if ancillary tests will be useful. The ancillary tests are contemplated based on the features present. The architecture is examined at low power and the cells at high power. A normal non-effaced and intact lymph node architecture is recognized if the distinction between the cortex and medulla is present. Although the normal lymph node histology changes dynamically, certain structures are relatively constant: the capsule, hilum, and medullary cords; the sinuses, the cortex, and the paracortex. In a high-power view, cellular heterogeneity, the presence of plasma cells and histiocytes, and the absence of atypical or dysplastic cells support a benign process. Each of the lymph node structures is described below.

The capsule and hilum are identified first. Attention should be paid to its thickness and whether there is fibrosis or capsulitis. While exceptions occur, normal lymph nodes have a thin capsule. A fibrotic or inflamed capsule is abnormal. An indented hilum is normal in benign nodes but may bulge or flattened in florid hyperplasia or malignant lymphoma. If a lymph node is correctly sectioned through the hilum along the longer or sagittal plane, a hilum will be visible on an edge and not in the center of the section (see Figure 11.3 for an incorrectly sectioned hilum).

The pathologist next scans the subcapsular sinuses, then the marginal or intermediate sinuses located along trabeculae all the way to the medullary sinuses, looking for foreign cells or normal occupants, including sinus histiocytes, lymphocytes, or inflammatory cells. Sinuses may be distended and numerous, secondary to an increased number of histiocytes or other cells indicating a sinus pattern. The sinus pattern is seen in a number of nonneoplastic and neoplastic processes (see Chapter 16). Paracortical sinuses are different and should not be confused with lymph node sinuses occupied by histiocytes; paracortical sinuses may be recognized as leaf-shaped lymphocyte-filled structures confined to the paracortex. These are located between superficial and deep cortex just underneath the follicles. These are rarely found except in the lymph node with florid reactive hyperplasia or as a feature associated with low-grade lymphomas. Similarly, in an intense early immune response, expanded medullary cords with nodules of plasma cells or lymphocytes are sometimes seen between medullary sinuses.

On a low-power examination, subtle color hues indicate collections of certain type of cells: dark blue are small cells, pale blue are large cells, pink areas are occupied by cells with much cytoplasm such as histiocytes, purple sheets are plasma cells, orange collections are eosinophils, and violet granulated metachromasia are normal round mast cells and oblong pale blue cytoplasm signify abnormal mast cells. The classic way to see patterns and hues optimally is by using a low-power objective, 4× or below, decreasing the light intensity and shifting the focus back and forth.

The cortex and paracortex are examined as a next step to see if their components have increased in size and number. The cortex is examined for size, shape, and distribution of follicles. Follicles are normally present in the cortex but, when additionally present in the medullary areas, a florid follicle center hyperplasia is indicated. Primary and secondary follicles are identified. The primary follicles are small nodules of small lymphocytes, located in the cortex or medulla, that lack pale germinal centers. Secondary follicles acquire germinal centers and appear to have a central pale area with a mantle of darker small lymphocytes. The secondary follicles are examined for polarity, which should be present in at least a number of the follicles in the reactive lymph node but is largely absent in follicular lymphoma.

The paracortex is normally increased in area more than the cortex, but when the paracortex shows nodules, usually associated with mottled patterns along many high endothelial venules, primary, secondary, or tertiary paracortical hyperplasia is present. Tertiary nodules are obvious as paler dermatopathic interfollicular or paracortical areas. The paracortex lies between adjacent follicles, and in between the follicles and medulla and normally appear diffuse. The paracortex is composed of small cells, several types of dendritic cells, histiocytes, and scattered high endothelial venules. A predominance of T cells is present along with scattered B cells and plasma cells. When the paracortex appears vaguely nodular and mottled at low-power view, along with prominent high endothelial venules (HEVs) and increase number of dendritic cells, paracortical hyperplasia is present. Primary T-zone nodules are mottled but lack HEVs and secondary T-zone nodules additionally show prominent HEVs. Tertiary nodules are synonymous with dermatopathic lymphadenopathy and appear in the interfollicular or paracortical areas as pale structures with increased pigmented histiocytes and sheets of dendritic reticulum cells.

A paracortical hyperplasia with a diffuse pattern may reveal, in addition to the usual cells in the paracortex, increased plasma cells with sheets of immunoblasts. This is also called diffuse polymorphic hyperplasia because of the mixture of lymphocytes, plasma cells, and large transformed cells. Another name is reactive or diffuse immunoblastic proliferation. Because of increase in transformed lymphocytes, along with focal necrosis, this is the most common reactive pattern that is histologically confused with lymphomas. Medullary cords may be prominent with the increase in medullary plasma cells. In between the medullary–cortical junction and the subcapsular compartments, the presence of necrosis, granulomas, plasmacytoid monocytes, monocytoid hyperplasia, vascularity, fibrosis, neutrophils and plasma cells, along with the other previously mentioned patterns, would indicate a mixed pattern.

Normal Lymph Node Histology

Diseases of the lymph nodes show as tenderness or enlargement, pain from expansion of capsule or compression of adjacent organs, and systemic symptoms including fever, night sweats, or weight loss. As principal physical processing units of the immune system, lymph nodes can be the site of infections and immune response to inflammation, injury, and intrinsic or secondary diseases. Reactive lymphadenopathies are generally self-limited, polyclonal proliferation of mature T and B cells, sometimes with mononuclear or polymorphonuclear leucocytes, in response to a variety of antigens or infectious agents.

This proliferation leads to expansion of compartments, where B cells, T cells, macrophages, and vascular elements normally exist. As these cells proliferate, normal histological compartments become defined as the basic patterns that we can recognize. The most common of these patterns is a nonspecific reactive lymph node hyperplasia; comprised of mild or hyperplastic follicular and paracortical reaction (see Figure 11.13). One of these patterns may be predominant and minimize the other compartments. For example, in a predominant pattern of florid follicular hyperplasia, the other compartments such as the sinuses and paracortical venules are compressed and inconspicuous. This low-power pattern is what prompts assignment of entities under one or more of four classic reactive patterns, discussed in more detail below. The classic patterns include follicular, diffuse, sinus, and mixed type. If there are co-dominant patterns, then one may assign a reaction to a mixed pattern category. A histology tour of a lymph node follows.

Let us review the histology of an optimally sectioned lymph node with the capsule and the hilum intact and present. The normal lymph node hilum shows a characteristic central adipose and fibrous tissue with prominent blood and lymphatic vessels usually located at an edge of a section. Single or multiple arteries or veins supply and drain the lymph node, respectively, usually located at the hilum in superficial nodes. In deeply situated nodes like the mesenteric chain, vessels may be found beyond the hilum and penetrate the node in the surrounding capsule (Semeraro and Davies, 1986). Inside the pulp, thick-walled arterioles give way to small arterioles terminating in capillaries at the cortex and inside follicles. The capillaries give way to postcapillary venules or HEVs at the paracortex. The HEVs terminate in thicker walled venules at the hilum. A thin capsule surrounds the lymph node in a normal unstimulated state, but the capsule may be thickened, edematous, inflamed, or fibrosed in highly reactive or neoplastic conditions. The capsule and trabecular branches become prominent in inflammatory fibrous tumor, certain infections, and certain lymphomas.

The fibrous capsule continues into the pulp normally as inconspicuous trabeculae partitioning a lymph node into inverted pyramidal compartments. The base contains a subcapsular sinus that receives many afferent lymphatics, and the apex comprises an efferent lymphatic together with hilar structures. The subcapsular sinus continues into the pulp along trabecula as marginal or intermediate sinus. Between the capsule and hilar vessels, four regions undergo marked changes during an immune response: cortex, paracortex, sinuses, and medulla (see Figure 11.1). Just below the cortex is the paracortex, which is an area underneath and between follicles. The paracortex is also called deep cortex, and the part of the cortex in between the follicles is also called

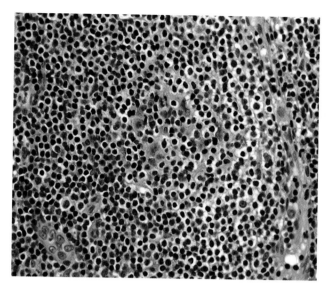

FIGURE 11.7 **Primary follicle with small lymphocytes and with few follicular dendritic cells.** Note the lack of centroblasts.

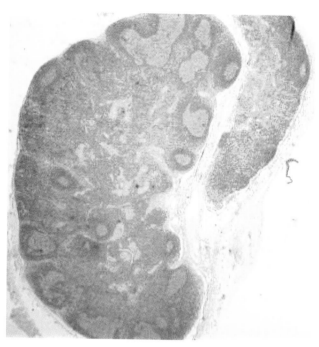

FIGURE 11.8 **Intact normal reactive lymph node histologic architecture with thin capsule.** Note the indented hilum, stimulated cortex, mottled paracortex, and dilated sinuses.

superficial cortex, vestiges of terms dividing the lymph node into two compartments: cortex and medulla (see Figure 11.5).

In normal unstimulated lymph nodes, the architecture of the cortex and medulla is visible with more primary follicles present than that of secondary follicles. Primary follicles appear in low-power view as nondescript darkly colored small nodules located in the cortex or in the medullary cords (see Figure 11.7). B lymphocytes home in to follicles in the superficial cortex and medulla, and T cells home in to the deep cortex or paracortex. The paracortex lies below the follicles and above the medullary cords and sinuses and is identified with their characteristic HEVs structures. Plasma cells are normally present in the medulla in normal lymph nodes while histiocytes normally appear in the sinuses.

An intact lymph node showing all the reactive components in a nonspecific reactive lymphoid hyperplasia is shown in Figure 11.8. In this histology there is no single predominant pattern since the follicles, paracortex, and sinuses are all stimulated. Based on the classic reactive patterns, a cortical reaction can show as a follicular pattern, paracortical as a diffuse or interfollicular pattern, sinus hyperplasia as a sinus pattern, and medullary–cortical reaction admixed with any of the three patterns above, with other features such as necrosis, granulomas, hemorrhages, and vascularity as belonging to the mixed classic pattern (see Figure 11.1). The entities under each pattern is shown in Table 11.1. We discuss details of each compartment in the following text.

Cortex

The cortex is located beneath the capsule and contains primary and secondary follicles. Primary follicles are unstimulated by antigen, while secondary follicles have been stimulated by an antigen. Both structures are rich in follicular dendritic networks and is supplied by capillaries (see Figure 11.9). The secondary follicles push out the small lymphocytes of the primary follicle to form the mantle zone or corona, visible as dark-blue staining small lymphocytes around pale staining germinal centers with larger lymphocytes. The earliest appearnce of secondary follicles could be recognized as a primary follicle with a centrally located cluster of centroblasts and few follicular dendritic cells. The transformation of primary to secondary follicles follows a series of morphologic and phenotypic changes that increase and expand the number and size of secondary follicles.

Polarity of Follicles. In the secondary follicle, as the germinal center area expands in size, the centroblasts migrate to one pole of the follicular dendritic network, generating a polarized secondary follicle. At this stage the germinal centers and mantle zones in reactive lymph nodes usually demonstrate polarity. Hence in normal reactive germinal center, in contrast to follicular lymphoma follicle, there is a definite

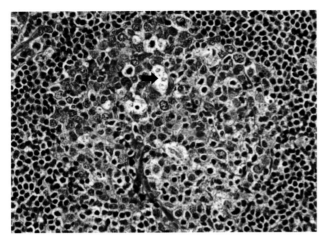

FIGURE 11.9 **Capillaries piercing the basal light zone of germinal center supply needs for proliferative activity.** Arrow indicates presence of tingible body macrophages.

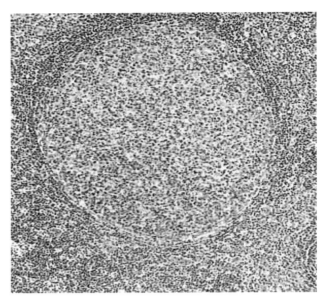

FIGURE 11.10 **Polarized benign reactive follicle with both biphasic germinal center and biphasic mantle zone.**

biphasic appearance known as polarity of the follicle: the germinal center appears biphasic with a dark and a light zone and the mantle zone adjacent to the dark zone and is thin, and the mantle zone abutting the light zone is prominent. The mantle layer on the light zone may be so thick that it resembles a dark crown ("corona"). Hence, in some sections, a four-phase polarity is evident (see Figure 11.10). In high-power view the dark zone contains sheets of centroblasts, with an increase in mitosis and apoptosis (see Figure 11.11). Tingible body macrophages also comprise the dark zone: performing cytophagic action by swallowing up cells that fail selection, lost antibody binding, or have developed autoreactivity. A follicular dendritic reticulum cell network and small centrocytes(cleaved) populate the light zone imparting a pale appearance (see Figure 11.12). The light zone faces the site of antigen source and is usually toward the sinus.

Hence normal reactive germinal centers, in contrast to follicular lymphomas, should show a definite biphasic appearance known as polarity. The polarity of follicle centers appears in the tonsils, spleen, appendix, and the Peyer's patches in the small bowel. In the spleen, the light zone is proximal to the marginal sinus where the blood carries the antigen. In the Peyer's patches, appendix, and tonsils, the light zone is oriented toward the mucosa. Polarity is largely absent in follicular lymphomas. Caution should be exercised in evaluating lymph nodes with florid follicular hyperplasia, like that seen in HIV lymphadenopathy, as the follicles are often composed of germinal centers with a diffuse, inconspicuous pale zone and seemingly all dark zone. Often these follicles

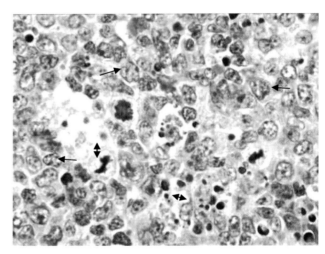

FIGURE 11.11 **Dark zone with numerous tingible body macrophages (double arrow).** Mitotically active small and large centroblasts (arrows) show marginated nucleoli on the vesicular nuclei.

lack mantle zone lymphocytes and appear as large naked germinal centers with a misshapen confluent or dumbbell appearance. Follicular large cell or grade III follicle center cell lymphoma often lacks polarity, shows tingible body macrophages, and therefore may pose a diagnostic challenge that often requires ancillary tests to distinguish from reactive follicles.

Follicle Zones and Their Phenotypes. The microenvironment of the germinal center is well

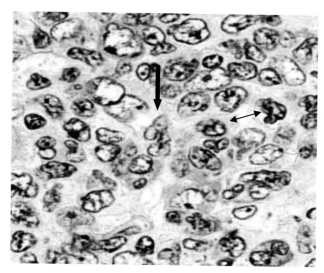

FIGURE 11.12 Light zone with many hyperlobated crinkled dendritic reticulum cells (arrow) and background of small cleaved cells (double-tip arrows).

suited to the task of expanding and selecting memory B cells of high affinity for the inducing antigen and functions as a cell development nursery. Real time imaging with two photon microscopy confirms that centroblast in the dark zone give rise to centrocytes in the light zones. Both cells migrate between the two zone in competition for antigen and T-cell help (Allen, Okada, and Cyster, 2007). The end result is the generation of germinal center-derived long lived plasma cells and memory B cells. Centroblasts give rise to centrocytes, historically so called because of their germinal center origin. Four morphologically distinct cells develop in the germinal center—containing both types of small and large lymphocytes, which have either cleaved (centrocytes) and noncleaved nuclei (centroblasts). There are also the relatively obscure follicular dendritic cells and the more visible tingible body macrophages (named for nuclear detritus in their cytoplasm) (Figure 11.11). There are also few small lymphocytes, which may correspond to the follicular T helper cells, as well as a few plasma cells (see Table 11.4 for the phenotypes of germinal center cells and Table 11.5 for cell type or function and cell markers).

Paracortex

The prominence of the paracortex varies according to the site, with cervical and axillary nodes displaying a prominent paracortex. The paracortex may be the largest area in a normal nonreactive node. Mostly CD4+ T cells populate the paracortex, but that population may be inverted and show more CD8+ T

TABLE 11.4 Phenotype of Cells Comprising Follicles

Germinal centers comprise a mixture of cell types:

- follicle center B cells (CD20+, CD79a+, CD10+, bcl-6+, bcl-2−, IgD−)
- small T-lymphocytes (most with a peculiar CD4+, CD57+, CD279(PD1)+ immunophenotype)
- tingible-body macrophages (CD68+)
- follicular dendritic cells (CD21+, CD35+)
- occasional plasma cells (CD138+, CD20−)

Mantle zone small B lymphocytes (CD20+, CD79a+, CD10−, IgD+, IgM+). They are Bcl-2+, often CD5+.

Marginal zone cells are often absent or inconspicuous, except in intraabdominal lymph nodes: (CD20+, CD5−, CD10−)

TABLE 11.5 Useful Antibodies for Lymph Nodes Fixed in paraffin

B lineage	CD20
T lineage	CD3
NK lineage	CD56
Apoptosis-blocker	Bcl2
Follicle center cell	CD10 (or bcl-6)
Mantle zone cell	IgD
Naïve B	IgM
Plasma cell	CD20−, CD138+
Histiocyte	CD68
Follicle dendritic cell	CD21 + CD35
Langerhans cell	S100, CD1a

cells in lymph nodes affected by primary or secondary immunodeficiency syndromes.

High Endothelial Venules. The most common nonspecific reaction manifests as the prominent paracortex together with variable hyperplasia of germinal centers (Figure 11.13). The paracortical reaction is often a less recognized reaction by pathologists when compared to germinal center reaction, although its features are very distinct and easily seen in low-power view. Once recognized, they are as easy to spot as germinal centers. The high endothelial venules are visible in a normal paracortex. These are noted underneath the cortical follicles and as far down as on the cortical medullary junction. Most of the lining cells of high endothelial venules show a large amount of cytoplasm that is cuboidal, hence the name "high," in contrast to the flattened endothelium of capillaries (Figure 11.15). The histological appearance is secondary to activation by many cytokines and inflammatory mediators. In reactive states, prominent transmigration of small lymphocytes appear in

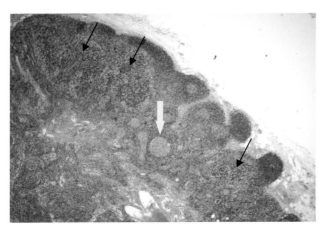

FIGURE 11.13 **Common nonspecific reactive pattern.** Note the pale follicles (open arrow) and mottled nodules of paracortical hyperplasia (arrow).

the surrounding wall and spaces and may obscure and compress the lumen. In the medulla, the arterioles and venules show thickened walls.

Paracortical Hyperplasia. Similar to the cortical follicles, rapid expansion of T lymphocytes generate mottled nodules called T-zone nodules or florid paracortical hyperplasia (Figure 11.14). The mottling results largely from an increase in interdigitating reticulum cells, which are a common antigen-presenting cell in the paracortex. These are S100+ but lack CD1a. Langerhans cells possesing S100 and CD1a are also present. A predominance of small T lymphocytes, sometimes showing atypical

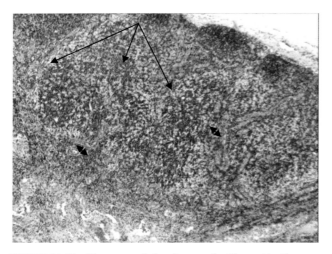

FIGURE 11.14 **T zone nodules (arrows) adjacent to the cortex and capsule with numerous high endothelial venules (double arrows).** Nonspecific paracortical hyperplasia is visible as a mottled nodular subcapsular or subcortical pattern, although sometimes they appear to coalesce.

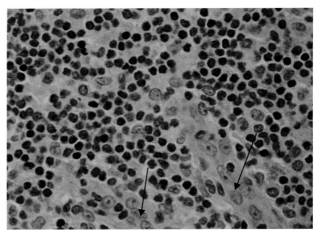

FIGURE 11.15 **Presence of postcapillary or high endothelial venules (HEVs) that identify the paracortex.** The paracortex population consists of small cells, plasma cells, pale dendritic cells and Langherhans cells, and rare immunoblasts. The high endothelia refers to the large oval plump lining cells of the venule and obscuring the lumen (arrows).

clefted or convoluted contours, also appears in reactive lymph nodes. The T zones are vaguely nodular, can coalesce, and can progress to large, pale nodules of dermatopathic lymphadenopathy (Figure 11.16). The presence of dermatopathic lymphadenopathy on a clinical background of dermatitis should prompt an investigation of any underlying Mycosis fungoides if no history is given. Dermatopathic lymphadenopathy, on low and high power, shows as pale structures between and under the follicles (Figure 11.16). Dense interdigitating interfollicular dendritic cells and histiocytes with pigments comprise the population, together with small lymphocytes, scattered plasma cells, eosinophils, and rare immunoblasts. Pigments in the macrophages could be melanin or other exogenous materials like lipofuscin (see Figure 11.17).

In humans, there are two types of dendritic cells, the myeloid dendritic cells (DC) and plasmacytoid dendritic cells. Myeloid DCs give rise to Langerhan's dendritic cells of the skin. These cells are S100B+ but fascin negative. These cells are prominent in skin inflammation and migrate to the lymph node to become transformed S100B+, CD1a+, CD68 weakly positive, and Fascin positive interdigitating reticulum cells (Nishikawa et al., 2009; Facchetti et al., 1988a). In contrast, sinus and pulp histiocytes are CD68+ but lack both S100 and CD1a. Plasmacytoid monocytes are dendritic cells that populate the paracortex in a number of reactive and inflammatory disorders, and

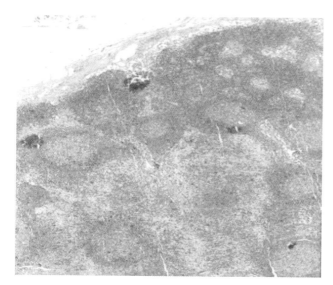

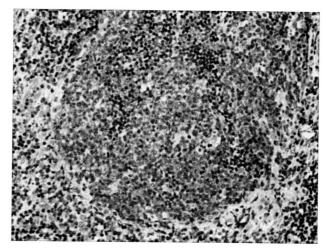

FIGURE 11.16 **Tertiary paracortical T zone hyperplasia or dermatopathic lymphadenopathy from a lymph node draining adjacent skin with excoriating dermatitis.**

FIGURE 11.18 **Plasmacytoid monocyte cluster in low power view showing characteristic violaceous hue and associated tingible body macrophages.** Unlike the germinal centers that it resembles, there is no mantle zone. Often early collections can be seen around the high endothelial venules, as shown.

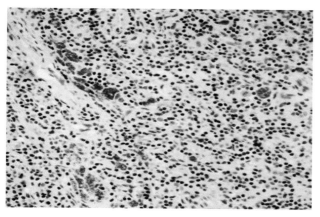

FIGURE 11.17 **Pigmented macrophages in dermatopathic lymphadenopathy.**

they differ from the interdigitating reticulum cells or sinus-derived histiocytes.

Plasmacytoid Dendritic Cells (pDC). Initially thought of as plasmacytoid T cells, plasmacytoid dendritic cells, also known as plasmacytoid monocytes, are associated with epithelioid granulomas, high endothelial venules, and T cells in the paracortex and may represent precursor of epithelioid histiocytes (Facchetti et al., 1989). These cells appear in about one of every six cases of nonspecific lymphadenitis but in the majority of lymph nodes if immunomarkers are used (Facchetti et al., 1988b). In lymph nodes, plasmacytoid dendritic cell clusters appear as

violaceous nodules with tangible body macrophages (Figure 11.18). Plasmacytoid dendritic cell clusters are prominent in many lymphadenopathies including Kikuchi lymphadenitis, hyaline vascular Castleman's disease, autoimmune diseases, and in neoplasms such as carcinomas, classic Hodgkin lymphoma, and blastic plasmacytoid dendritic cell leukemia (Jegalian, Facchetti, and Jaffe, 2009). While Fascin is a marker for mature plasmacytoid dendritic cells, CD123 is a marker of mature and immature pDC, and CD123 appears in blastic plasmacytoid dendritic cell leukemia along with expression of CD56 and CD4. In the lymph nodes, pDC express CD123 (Vermi et al., 2005) (Figure 11.19). In certain reactive conditions like Kikuchi's lymphadenitis, Kimura's, SLE, and other granulomatous lymphadenitis, plasmacytoid dendritic cells are prominent reactive component. In lupus, and viral infection, secretion of interferon alpha by the pDC is implicated in pathogenesis (Colonna, Trinchieri, and Liu, 2004). These are CD123 positive, S100 negative cells.

Diffuse Immunoblastic Reaction. When a diffuse pattern is present in the paracortex or interfollicular areas on low- and high-power examination, with an increase in immunoblasts and plasma cells along with eosinophils as well as increased endothelial vessels and histiocytes, a diffuse reactive immunoblastic hyperplasia may be present (Figure 11.20). The presence of immunoblasts and plasma cells is easily evinced with methyl green

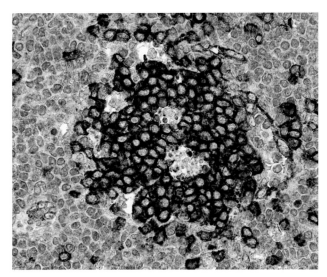

FIGURE 11.19 **CD123 positive cluster of plasmacytoid dendritic cells adjacent HEV**. Courtesy of Dr. Fabio Facchetti, University of Brecia, Italy.

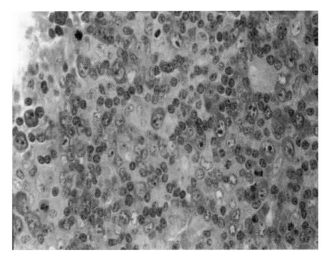

FIGURE 11.21 **MGP stain showing numerous magenta-stained immunoblasts and plasma cells in a florid diffuse immunoblastic reaction**.

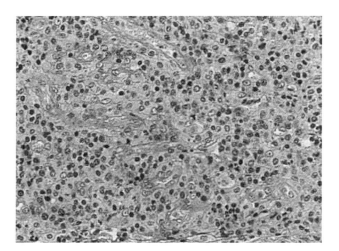

FIGURE 11.20 **PAS stain highlighting venules that are hyperplastic in a florid immunoblastic reaction**.

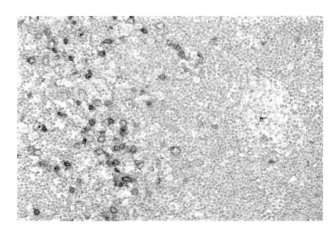

FIGURE 11.22 **CD30 positive cells increased in paracortex in diffuse immunoblastic reaction**.

pyronin stain (Figure 11.21). The immunoblasts can also be highlighted by antiCD30 stain (Figure 11.22). A low pattern view will show an interfollicular pattern that is rather diffuse, somewhat paler than mantle zone in color, owing to the presence of many larger cells such as immunoblasts and histiocytes (Figure 11.23). This pattern may be drug or virally induced and is the pattern most likely to be confused with malignant lymphoma. Mottling is present in both the diffuse and nodular forms of paracortical hyperplasia, and is a feature that suggests a diagnosis of a reactive T-cell response instead of a lymphoma. The presence of Reed–Sternberg-like cells will be

evident along with focal necrosis in the most intense viral- or drug-induced reactions, typically from EBV or diphenylhydantoin, respectively.

Sinus Lining Cells and Reticular Framework

Flattened fibroblastic reticular cells (FRCs) line the sinuses and express fibronectin, at least in lower mammals, have some characteristics of epithelial cell, fibroblasts, and endothelium, and express cytokeratins 8 and 18 and form reticular fibers. Reticular fibers are composed of a core of collagen fibrils enveloped in a basement membrane containing collagens types I, III, and IV, elastin, entactin, fibronectin, laminin-1, tenascin, vitronectin, and heparan sulfate. (Sainte-Marie and Peng, 1986). Macrophages, referred to as sinus histiocytes, reside on the reticular meshwork

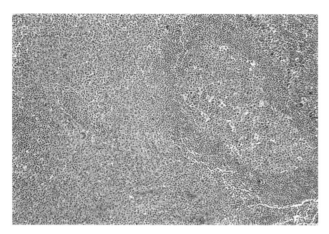

FIGURE 11.23 **Paracortical hyperplasia**. Adjacent to germinal center is the pink area with diffuse large cell immunoblastic proliferation, nonspecific.

like spiders on a web of channels composing the sinuses (Willard-Mack, 2006).

Sinuses and Medulla

Subcapsular sinuses lie immediately below the capsule are continuous with intermediate sinuses which are seen adjacent to trabeculae within the lymph nodes (Figure 11.24). The sinuses appear as pale pink surrounded by a sea of dark blue lymphocytes on low power. When the sinuses are prominent, dilated, and filled with cells, we have a sinus pattern of reaction. Focal sinus histiocytosis is a common reaction identified by presence of reactive histiocytes. The

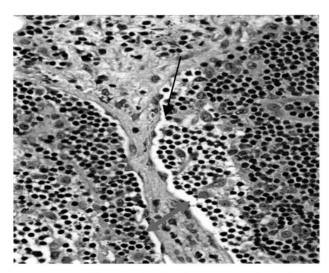

FIGURE 11.24 **Sinuses**. Trabecular sinuses (arrow) and adjacent intermediate sinus space (double arrows) filled with tethered sinus histiocytes and lymphocytes, and lined by fibroblastic reticular sinus lining cells.

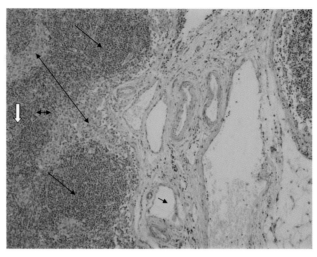

FIGURE 11.25 **Sinuses**. Hilum or medulla identified with associated with thin walled venules and efferent lymphatics. Medullary cords (arrows) in between medullary sinuses (long double arrows). Medullary sinus with sinus histiocytes (left) and corticomedullary junction (small double arrow). Note the high endothelial venules (open arrow) of the deep cortex or paracortex. Lymph fluid and debris empty into efferent lymphatic vessels (small arrow).

lymphs contents in the medulla directly empty into an efferent lymphatic vessel located in medulla. The medulla of lymph node is easily identified by its associated vessels, the thick-walled arterioles, the thin-walled elongated venules, and efferent lymphatic (Figure 11.25). It is often indented in reactive lymph nodes and usually pushed out and inconspicuous in florid lymphadenopathy or lymphomas. The hilum and blood vessels may be conspicuous in congested lymph nodes (Figure 11.26). Trabecular sinuses are continuous with medullary sinuses, and these sinuses show as labyrinthine spaces (Figure 11.27):

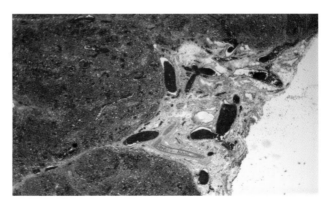

FIGURE 11.26 **Medullary structures with congestion and dilated venules, capillaries filled with RBCs, and empty-looking lumina of the efferent lymphatic vessel.**

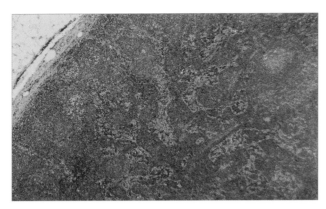

FIGURE 11.27 **Sinus histiocytosis showing labyrinthine subcapsular sinuses coursing toward the medullary sinuses.**

Afferent and Efferent Lymphatics

Afferent lymphatics supply the lymph nodes and enter the capsule from many directions. They show on the cut section as either with a clear lumen or filled with pale amorphous pink fluid. Lymphatic fluid and lymphatic contents enter the lymph node via the afferent lymphatics that pierce the capsule just above the cortex (Figure 11.28). Lymphatics are located above sites of cortical reaction and contribute to the formation of lymphoid reactive lobules, which are composed of cortical follicles made up of B cells and associated paracortex made up of T cells. The sinus fluid carries solutes, antigen-presenting cells, chemokines, and lymphocytes. A single afferent vessel may incite a number of composite lobules. The subcapsular sinus is compartmentalized, bounded by fibrous trabeculae, and its sinus content flows in and around the composite nodule into the medullary sinuses. Sinus spaces could be filled

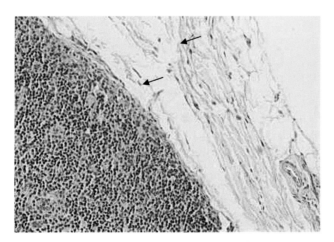

FIGURE 11.28 **Afferent lymphatics (arrows) piercing the capsule and joining the subcapsular sinus.**

by macrophages, antigen-presenting cells, lymphocytes, and sometimes plasma cells. A distinct type of sinus pattern is comprised of monocytoid cells, which are identified in sinusoidal spaces as arc-shaped bands, composed of small to medium size cells with large amount of clear cytoplasm. A single efferent lymphatic drains the node and exits the hilum.

Capillaries

The capillaries are associated with the cortical elements. The subcapsular and interfollicular cortex as well as the follicles are supplied with capillaries. Cortical capillaries are not easily visualized but are evident in congested lymph nodes.

Patterns of Reactions

In this chapter we introduce these patterns of reaction based on the four classic patterns. A discussion of the diseases classified under the different patterns is covered in subsequent chapters. Each pattern suggests a set of diseases in the differential diagnosis and may include other reactive patterns or other neoplasms or lymphomas.

Assigning a Pattern

Interpretation of the pattern type is best done by those familiar with microanatomic areas and the different cell types in a normal lymph node. The diagnosis and differential diagnosis then proceeds from the recognition of compartments or cell types that are atypical, hyperplastic, or abnormal. Using the classic categories as initial point of analysis, we could more or less place each pattern in one or more of four patterns.

The reader is cautioned that these patterns and the entities under them are not written in stone. Some of the diseases under one pattern may be classified in another pattern. The appearance of a reactive lymph node depends on the duration of reaction, immunocompetence status, and presence or absence of specific morphogic features such as necrosis, granulomas, and type of reactive cells. For example, early HIV may show as a florid germinal center hyperplasia but later on show an involuted or regressed germinal center pattern. Similarly early CMV may show follicular hyperplasia but later on show a diffuse immunoblastic reaction. A lymph node adjacent to a primary or secondary syphilis infection in the genital area may show the typical follicular hyperplasia, plasmacytosis, vasculitis, or even granulomatous pattern that easily could be assigned to the mixed pattern but lymph nodes away from infection may show only a follicular pattern under nonspecific germinal center hyperplasia. The key is identifying other features, whether morphological, cytochemical, or immunohistochemical results, and combining them with the salient clinical, epidemiological, as well as serological findings, that allow congruence in a diagnosis of a current presenting histological pattern.

Follicular Pattern

Florid Follicular Hyperplasia, Nonspecific. This is a follicular pattern seen in infections, autoimmune disorders, and nonspecific reactions. The pattern can be generated by any of the normal components of the follicle and leads to hyperplasia of germinal centers, mantle zones, and marginal zones.

Follicular hyperplasia is, in practice, synonymous with follicle center hyperplasia, or more specifically, with germinal center hyperplasia (see Table 11.8). This pattern is the most common and is often admixed with other patterns. Both progressive and regressive transformations of follicles generate a follicular pattern. Some entities that are special forms of follicular pattern admixed with other findings include toxoplasmosis or syphilis (see Chapter 13). These and other examples may be also categorized into a mixed type of pattern depending on the stage of reaction, and the increasing amount of nonfollicular pattern present. These other co-dominant patterns include a paracortical sinus pattern and the presence of a specific pathology such as necrosis, granulomas, monocytoid cells, plasma cells, eosinophils, or any number of neutrophilic components. The differential diagnosis includes follicular lymphoma.

The most common is follicle center hyperplasia, nonspecific, and it comprises 76% of noninfectious reactive lymph nodes (Chhabra et al., 2006). The pattern almost always shows small partial areas with a paracortical or sinus pattern. Reactive follicular and paracortical hyperplasia may belong this group since a follicular hyperplasia has invariably associated with one or more paracortical nodules of the T zones. Florid follicular hyperplasia, nonspecific presents with hyperplastic germinal centers that extend to the paracortical and medullary areas. The nonspecific type is common in young adults and children and typically presents as a solitary nontender mass.

Although more children show this type of pattern than adults, has a more ominous significance in older people above 60 years old. In this age group, 63% show nonspecific etiology and in 37% a diagnosis is present (Kojima et al., 2005). The most common specific diseases include autoimmune, cancer-associated reactions, and lastly EBV induced in 15%. Among the nonspecific causes, the most

TABLE 11.6 Malignant Differential Diagnosis of Follicular Patterns

Benign	Malignant
Follicle center hyperplasia	Follicular large-cell lymphoma
Mantle cell hyperplasia	Mantle cell lymphoma, Lymphocyte rich HL
Involuted germinal center	Angioimmunoblastic T-cell lymphoma
Progressive transformation of GC	Nodular LPHL Follicular lymphoma
Marginal zone hyperplasia	Marginal zone lymphoma Extranodal marginal zone lymphoma

frequent finding is progressive transformation of germinal centers. Malignant lymphoma developed in 2.1%, and this warrants a careful examination of interfollicular areas for atypical cells and atypical patterns (Osborne and Butler, 1991) (see Table 11.6, and Figures 11.29–11.31). An example of a follicular pattern that mimics follicular hyperplasia is follicular large cell lymphoma with inconspicuous mantle zones (Figure 11.29). In high-power view, the neoplastic follicles show numerous large cells as well as scattered tangible body macrophages, features also seen in follicular hyperplasia (Figure 11.30). A low-power view of a bilobed follicles with expanded germinal centers, lacking mantle zone, and with feature of polarity, is shown as dark zone present on both lateral edges and lighter centers of (Figure 11.31).

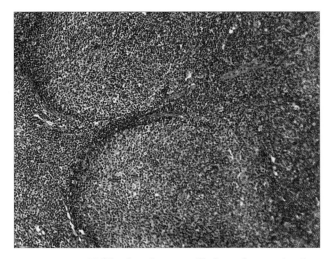

FIGURE 11.29 **Follicular large cell lymphoma in low power with no polarity, wispy mantle zone.**

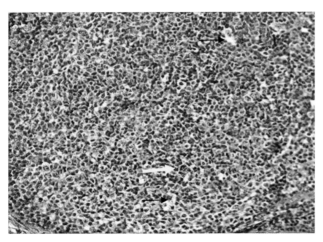

FIGURE 11.30   Follicular large cell lymphoma with monomorphic large cells and tingible bodies (arrows).

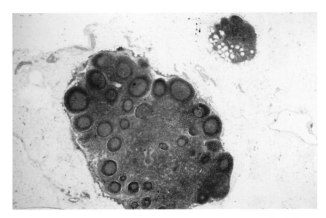

FIGURE 11.33   Follicular hyperplasia mixed with follicular involution. Follicular hyperplasia is seen in patients with a longer standing HIV-related persistent generalized lymph node.

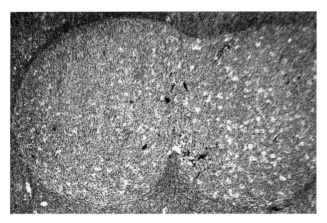

FIGURE 11.31   Follicle center hyperplasia, bilobed with dark zonal polarities at both ends.

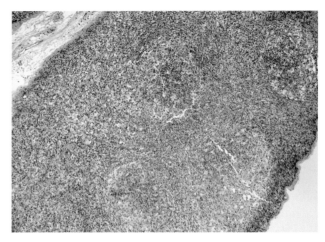

FIGURE 11.34   Follicular hyperplasia with back-to-back misshapen naked follicles. This pattern is seen in patients with longer standing HIV-related persistent generalized lymph node.

Follicular involution is another name for regressed follicles or regressive transformation of germinal centers. These are seen in Castleman's disease (Figure 11.35), an involuted phase of HIV, and congenital immune deficiency; regressed follicle with residual follicle dendritic meshwork (Figure 11.32); follicular hyperplasia and involution in intermediate HIV adenopathy (Figure 11.33); and hyperplastic follicles with inconspicuous mantle zone and follicle lysis (Figure 11.34).

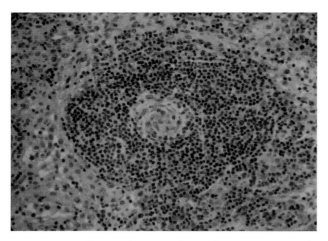

FIGURE 11.32   Regressive transformation pattern seen in long-standing HIV adenopathy. The pattern is also called depleted or burnt out, and sometimes epithelioid follicle center cells because of residual follicle dendritic meshwork.

Progressive Transformation of Germinal Centers. Progressive transformation of germinal centers (PTGC) is a morphologic feature of reactive hyperplasia initially described by Lennert as germinal centers obscured by lymphocytes. PTGC is

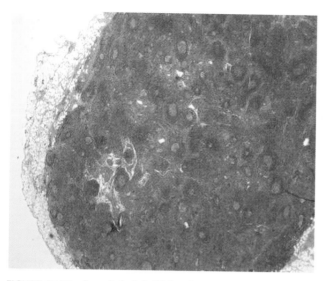

FIGURE 11.35 **Involuted follicles in Castleman's disease,** **Hyaline vascular variant**.

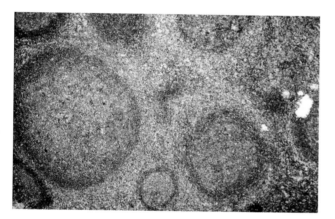

FIGURE 11.36 **Progressive transformation pattern**. The rim of normal tissue above with no definite "mass" effect raises a differential for NLPHL.

seen in 3.5 to 10% of reactive lymph nodes with chronic nonspecific lymphadenitis (Ferry, 1992; Osborne, 1984). The transformed follicles are about three times the size of normal follicles (Figure 11.36). Sometimes a large follicle with a germinal center can be mistaken for PTGC and care must be taken not to confuse the two because of clinical implications. Persistent or recurring PTGC is seen particularly in pediatric cases (Osborne, 1992). PTGC also may occur as a predominant pattern in lymph node hyperplasia, designated as florid PTGC. The risk of developing nodular lymphocyte predominant Hodgkin lymphoma (LPHL) in lymph node with florid PTGC is less than 5% (Ferry, 1992; Osborne, 1992). Nodular LPHL is delineated from florid PTGC

by the lymphoma's formation of coalescent nodules exerting a mass pushing out or distorting the normal lymph node architecture.

Mantle Cell Hyperplasia. Mantle cell hyperplasia may be seen in reactive lymph nodes as a solitary, enlarged lymph node in young patient or an incidental finding with nonspecific etiology. A study of 35 cases with mantle cell/marginal zone hyperplasia pattern showed this as uncommon and identified very rare incidence of non-Hodgkin lymphoma over a long term follow-up (Hunt et al., 2001). Distinction from mantle cell lymphoma is critical, with mantle cell lymphoma morphologically showing in the mantle zone subtype, nodules of mantle zones distributed beyond the cortex, and monotypic light chains with aberrant expression of CD43, CD5, and cyclin D1. (See Chapter 13.)

Monocytoid cell nuclei have twice the diameter of small lymphocytes and show generous cytoplasm. They are almost indistinguishable from marginal

TABLE 11.7 **Malignant Differential Diagnosis** **of Paracortical or Diffuse Pattern**

Benign	Malignant
Dermatopathic change	Mycosis fungoides
Paracortical nodules	T zone lymphoma
Viral lymphadenitis	PTLD
Reactive immunoblastic proliferation	Peripheral T-cell lymphoma, DLBCL
Interfollicular infiltrate, NOS	Metastatic disease, granulocytic sarcoma, mast cell disease, anaplastic large-cell lymphoma, interfollicular Hodgkin lymphoma, Langerhan's cell histiocytosis, Kaposi's sarcoma, monocytoid B cell lymphoma, Immunoblastic diffuse large B-cell lymphoma, plasmacytoma, lymphoplasmacytic lymphoma

TABLE 11.8 **Follicular Patterns**

Follicle Center Hyperplasia
Mantle zone pattern
Marginal zone patttern
Progressive transformation
Regressive transformation

zone B cells but may differ in having more cytoplasm, with less plasmacytic differentiation and presence of neutrophilic clusters. Marginal zone B cells may be different from monocytoid B cells in lineage, origin, and certain immunophenotypic markers (Falini et al., 2003). Monocytoid B cells can be seen in any number of reactive follicular hyperplasia and could be found in about 14% of reactive lymph nodes (Plank, Hansmann, and Fischer, 1993). The reaction however is particularly prominent in a few specific lymphadenopathies, which include cat-scratch disease, toxoplasmic adenitis, HIV lymphadenopathy, CMV, and lymphogranuloma venereum (Sheibani et al. 1990; Sohn et al., 1985). (See Chapter 13 and Chapter 16.)

Paracortical Pattern

A paracortical or diffuse pattern is seen in viral infections, lymph node draining skin pathology, and nonspecific reactions. Nodular paracortical zones often are in degrees from primary to tertiary T zone nodules. Diffuse interfollicular or paracortical reactions often involve the diffuse cortex with plasmacytic and immunoblastic proliferation, such as those seen in vacinnial, drug, or viral reactive immunobllastic proliferation (see Table 11.7) (Figure 11.37). (See Chapter 14 and Chapter 15.)

Sinus Pattern

A sinus pattern is seen in lymph nodes draining limbs, inflammatory lesions, and malignancies. Entrapped marrow cells such as extramedullary hematopoieisis, histiocytosis, vascular proliferation, fibrous proliferation can also generate a sinus pattern. (See Chapter 16.)

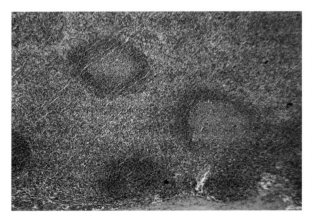

FIGURE 11.37 **Paracortical hyperplasia pattern in patient with mycosis fungoides with lymph node grade LN3 involved by lymphoma**.

Sinus histiocytosis of a nonspecific type is quite common and is often seen in association with other reactive patterns. When florid and prominent, this is typically seen in the reactive lymph node draining an inflamed or infected site, a foreign body reaction to prosthesis, or in lymph nodes adjacent to carcinoma, lymphoma, or other neoplasms. The mesenteric and abdominal lymph node often displays this reaction as it drains the gut. Sinus histiocytosis is typically seen in lymph node dissection of axillary contents in breast carcinoma mastectomy, even without evidence of metastasis (Black, 1958).

Histiocytes are tissue macrophages with delicate nuclear membrane, small nucleoli, fine to cleared chromatin, and abundant cytoplasm. Histiocytes are positive for CD68 and CD163 (Lau, Chu, and Weiss, 2004). The CD163 antibody reacts with interfollicular macrophages and sinus histiocytes. Occasional histiocytes may show cytophagic debris or even mimic a signet ring appearance of metastatic carcinoma or other malignancies (Gould et al., 1989). Recognition of nonspecific sinus histiocytosis is often not a diagnostic problem unless the cells appear atypical and have not the usual polygonal or round appearance. Some histiocytes show signet ring morphology and therefore invoke a differential of carcinoma, melanoma, or lymphoma as discussed in the Chapter 16 on sinus patterns. Several specific findings may be considered as summarized in Tables 11.9 for sinus pattern

TABLE 11.9 Sinus Pattern

Benign	Malignant
Sinus histiocytosis	Metastatic disease, anaplastic large cell lymphoma
	Langerhan cell histiocytosis
Signet ring histiocytosis	Carcinoma, lymphoma, melanoma
Pigmented sinus histiocytosis	Metastatic melanoma
Spindly histiocytosis	Interdigitating reticulum cell tumor
Histiocytic reaction to foreign matter	Metastasis
Extramedullary hematopoieisis	Granulocytic sarcoma
Sinus histiocytosis with massive lymphadenopathy	Malignant lymphoma with hemophagocytosis
Monocytoid hyperplasia	Monocytoid lymphoma
Hemophagocytic histiocytes	Malignant lymphoma with hemophagocytosis
Vascular transformation	Kaposi's sarcoma
	Vascular neoplasm

TABLE 11.10 Mixed Pattern

Benign	Malignant
Kikuchi–Fujimoto	Large-cell lymphoma
SLE	Large-cell lymphoma
Bacterial Lymphadenitis with prominent microgranulomas	Lennert's lymphoma, Hodgkin lymphoma
Epithelioid granulomas	Malignancy, NHL, HL, carcinoma
Prominent necrosis, subtotal or total	NHL with infarction, post-transplant lymphomas
Plasmacytoid monocytic proliferation	Large-cell lymphoma
Monocytoid hyperplasia	Monocytoid B-cell lymphoma, marginal zone lymphoma, MALToma: nodal or splenic
Nodules of suppurative epithelioid granulomas	Nodular sclerosing Hodgkin lymphoma
Depleted pattern	Hodgkin lymphoma, lymphoid depletion type

Abbreviations: NHL (non-Hodgkin lymphoma), HL (Hodgkin lymphoma), MALT (mucosa-associated lymphoid tissue), DLBCL (diffuse large B-cell lymphoma), PTLD (post-transplant lymphoproliferative disorder), LPHL (lymphocyte predominant Hodgkin lymphoma).

and 11.10 for mixed pattern and their malignant differential diagnosis, respectively.

The mixed pattern comprises any combination of the dominant patterns and co-dominant patterns noted above. A mixed pattern may also be associated with specific features of infection or inflammation: necrosis, granulomas, eosinophilia suppuration, hemorrhages, and histiocytosis other than granulomas such as plasmacytoid monocytosis or monocytoid hyperplasia. The mixed pattern with granuloma and necrosis may be seen in infections, autoimmune reactions, and, foreign body rejection as well as in cancer: lymphoma, carcinoma, melanoma, and sarcoma (more on this in Chapters 18 and 19).

REFERENCES

Allen CD, Okada T, Cyster JG. 2007. Germinal-Center Organization and cellular dynamics. Immunity 27:190–202.

Allhiser JN, McKnight TA, Shank JC. 1981. Lymphadenopathy in a family practice. J Fam Pract 12:27–32.

Colonna M, Trinchieri G, Liu YJ. 2004. Plasmacytoid dendritic cells in immunity. Nat Immunol 5: 1219–26.

Facchetti F, de Wolf-Peeters C, De VR, van den Oord JJ, Pulford KA, Desmet VJ. 1989. Plasmacytoid monocytes (so-called plasmacytoid T cells) in granulomatous lymphadenitis. Hum Pathol 20:588–93.

Facchetti F, de Wolf-Peeters C, Mason DY, Pulford K, van den Oord JJ, Desmet VJ. 1988a. Plasmacytoid T cells: immunohistochemical evidence for their monocyte/macrophage origin. Am J Pathol 133:15–21.

Facchetti F, de Wolf-Peeters C, van den Oord JJ, De VR, Desmet VJ. 1988b. Plasmacytoid T cells: a cell population normally present in the reactive lymph node. An immunohistochemical and electronmicroscopic study. Hum Pathol 19:1085–92.

Falini B, Tiacci E, Pucciarini A, Bigerna B, Kurth J, Hatzivassiliou G, Droetto S, Galletti BV, Gambacorta M, Orazi A, Pasqualucci L, Miller I, Kuppers R, la-Favera R, Cattoretti G. 2003. Expression of the IRTA1 receptor identifies intraepithelial and subepithelial marginal zone B cells of the mucosa-associated lymphoid tissue (MALT). Blood 102:3684–92.

Fijten GH, Blijham GH. 1988. Unexplained lymphadenopathy in family practice: an evaluation of the probability of malignant causes and the effectiveness of physicians' workup. J Fam Pract 27:373–6.

Gould E, Perez J, bores-Saavedra J, Legaspi A. 1989; Signet ring cell sinus histiocytosis: a previously unrecognized histologic condition mimicking metastatic adenocarcinoma in lymph nodes. Am J Clin Pathol 92:509–12.

Hunt JP, Chan JA, Samoszuk M, Brynes RK, Hernandez AM, Bass R, Weisenburger DD, Muller-Hermelink K, Nathwani BN. 2001. Hyperplasia of mantle/marginal zone B cells with clear cytoplasm in peripheral lymph nodes. A clinicopathologic study of 35 cases. Am J Clin Pathol 116:550–9.

Jegalian AG, Facchetti F, Jaffe ES. 2009. Plasmacytoid dendritic cells: physiologic roles and pathologic states. Adv Anat Pathol 16:392–404.

Kojima M, Nakamura S, Itoh H, Shimizu K, Murayama K, Iijima M, Hosomura Y, Ohno Y, Yoshida K, Motoori T, Sakata N, Masawa N. 2005. Clinical implication of florid reactive follicular hyperplasia in Japanese patients 60 years or older: A study of 46 cases. Int J Surg Pathol 13:175–80.

Lau SK, Chu PG, Weiss LM. 2004. CD163: a Specific marker of macrophages in paraffin-embedded tissue samples. Am J Clin Pathol 122:794–801.

Leung AK, Robson WL. 2004. Childhood cervical lymphadenopathy. J Pediatr Health Care 18:3–7.

Moore SW, Schneider JW, Schaaf HS. 2003. Diagnostic aspects of cervical lymphadenopathy in children in the developing world: a study of 1,877 surgical specimens. Ped Surg Int 19:240–4.

Nishikawa Y, Sato H, Oka T, Yoshino T, Takahashi K. 2009. Immunohistochemical discrimination of plasmacytoid dendritic cells from myeloid dendritic cells in human pathological tissues. J Clin Exp Hematop 49:23–31.

Osborne BM, Butler JJ. 1991. Clinical implications of nodal reactive follicular hyperplasia in the elderly patient with enlarged lymph nodes. Mod Pathol 4:24–30.

Plank L, Hansmann ML, Fischer R. 1993. The cytological spectrum of the monocytoid B-cell reaction: recognition of its large cell type. Histopathology 23:425–31.

Sainte-Marie G, Peng FS. 1986. Diffusion of a lymph-carried antigen in the fiber network of the lymph node of the rat. Cell Tissue Res 245:481–6.

Schnitzer B. 1992. Reactive lymphadenopathies. In: Knowles DM, ed. Neoplastic Hematopathology. Baltimore, Md: Williams & Wilkins; 435–438.

Semeraro D, Davies JD. 1986. The arterial blood supply of human inguinal and mesenteric lymph nodes. J Anat 144:221–33.

Sheibani K, Ben-Ezra J, Swartz WG, Rossi J, Kezirian J, Koo CH, Winberg CD. 1990. Monocytoid B-cell lymphoma in a patient with human immunodeficiency virus infection: demonstration of human immunodeficiency virus sequences in paraffin-embedded lymph node sections by polymerase chain reaction amplification. Arch Pathol Lab Med 114:1264–7.

Sohn CC, Sheibani K, Winberg CD, Rappaport H. 1985. Monocytoid B lymphocytes: their relation to the patterns of the acquired immunodeficiency syndrome (AIDS) and AIDS-related lymphadenopathy. Hum Pathol 16:979–85.

Soldes OS, Younger JG, Hirschl RB. 1999. Predictors of malignancy in childhood peripheral lymphadenopathy. J Pediatr Surg 34:1447–52.

Vermi W, Riboldi E, Wittamer V, Gentili F, Luini W, Marrelli S, Vecchi A, Franssen JD, Communi D, Massardi L, Sironi M, Mantovani A, Parmentier M, Facchetti F, Sozzani S. 2005. Role of chemR23 in directing the migration of myeloid and plasmacytoid dendritic cells to lymphoid organs and inflamed skin. J Exp Med 201:509–15.

Weiss L. Lymph Nodes. New York: Cambridge Univ Press. 2008.

Yaris N, Cakir M, Sozen E, Cobanoglu U. 2006. Analysis of children with peripheral lymphadenopathy. Clin Pediatr (Phila) 45:544–9.

CHAPTER TWELVE

LYMPH NODE BIOLOGY, MARKERS AND DISEASE

Hernani D. Cualing

PERIPHERAL LYMPHOID TISSUE

Lymph nodes form an integral component of the secondary lymphoreticular system, which includes spleen, mucosa-associated lymphoid tissue (gastrointestinal, bronchopulmonary) and other extranodal sites. The primary lymphoid organs, where initial development of precursor and immature cells take place, are the bone marrow and the thymus.

Lymph nodes (LN) develop into competent organs starting at birth. Embyonal lymph nodes show structures after 20 weeks of gestation, but fetal LNs do not approach the adult pattern until 2 g fetal weight. At this stage, LNs are devoid of plasma cells and show scant reticular framework. At birth, the LNs show a medulla with paracortex but no germinal centers. The histology is similar to LNs in patients with aggammaglobulinemia. The follicles and germinal centers develop only after infection or immunologic challenge. The sinuses and medullary cords are, however, well formed.

In adults, lymph nodes are located in key regions draining specific anatomical areas: the cervical, axillary, mediastinal, abdominal, mesenteric, pelvic, inguinal, with anastomosing lymphatic vasculatures that link drainage of bowels, spleen, lung, and all other extranodal organs. The adult human body is radiographically imaged to contain up to 1200 LNs (Qatarneh et al., 2006) based on the 3D visible human data set, although the often cited nodes number is lower. Thus it is not easy to select which LN to sample. The clinical observation and imaging method may be useful in centrally located nodes. Evaluation of intact LN vessels by endoscopic ultrasound may suggest which node to biopsy, in that decreased intranodal vessels signal metastasis or a tumor infiltrate (Sawhney et al., 2007).

PATHOPHYSIOLOGY

A branching system of lymphatic tubes drains the lymph fluid from tissue to LNs. These vessels terminally converge to LNs, but the cells carried by lymphatic fluids return to systemic circulation. The plasma fluid drains tissue interstitial spaces and transports a host of elements such as biomolecules, infectious agents, and cells. The cells are lymphocytes, monocytes, and dendritic cells, which putatively contain biological information from the tissue milieu. The lymphatic system function carrying the information is thought to be similar to the information superhighway (von Andrian and Mempel, 2003); a counterpart biologic highway brings the immune response information and cellular effectors to the lymph nodes.

The immune response takes one of two forms: immediate or delayed, corresponding to innate and adaptive responses. The innate type of response is the

Non-Neoplastic Hematopathology and Infections, First Edition. Edited by Hernani D. Cualing, Parul Bhargava, and Ramon L. Sandin.
© 2012 Wiley-Blackwell. Published 2012 by John Wiley & Sons, Inc.

first line of defense; akin to a "knee-jerk" response. The adaptive immune response follows the innate defense and suggests "intelligence." While the innate response is often localized on the barrier lining the mucosa or skin, adaptive immunity is centralized. The lymph nodes are the archetype central hub orchestrating, screening, and directing the response. While the innate response is not specific and forgets its antigen, the adaptive response is tailored to a specific antigen and recalls. This response keeps this information stored in memory subsets of mature T and B cells. Dendritic cells are mobile cellular bridges functioning as carriers of information relaying the microbial invasion signal to the lymph nodes. These cells recognize microbial antigens via toll-like surface receptors, which are pattern recognition molecules for specific microbes. These cells leave the blood and mature as well as differentiate as antigen-presenting cells in the lymph nodes.

Antigen-presenting cells, such as dendritic cells and B cells, neutrophils "present" antigen to lymphocytes. On encountering the antigen that specifically fits T- and B-cell surface receptors, these cells undergo a defined series of maturation, transformation, and migration that ultimately carries out each cell's specific immune role. In the process these cells, along with other leucocytes, multiply and in lymph nodes display histological reaction as follicular, paracortical, sinusoidal, or mixed patterns. In addition to these classic patterns, a perspective based on functional anatomy divides lymph nodes into composite nodules and extranodular compartments, to be discussed more below. Classic histology, however, divides the lymph node into a cortex and medulla and their subcompartments.

The cortex contains primary and secondary follicles, interfollicular or diffuse cortex, and deep cortex or paracortex. The primary follicles contain resting B cells which become part of the mantle in secondary follicles. Mantle cells are small lymphocytes with nuclei showing clumped chromatin and scant cytoplasm. In low-power view these cells appear as dark blue dots. High-power view, best appreciated on oil immersion, shows more of the nuclear texture: variously described as "soccer ball," "cracked earth," "fish-scale," and just plain "clumped" or "mature" (see Table 12.1)

During primary immune response to stimuli, the naïve lymphocytes in the interfollicular or diffuse cortex and the activated naïve B cells in primary follicles undergo blastic change, rapid cell division, and differentiation to form germinal centers and generate short-lived IgM secreting plasma cells, respectively. The latter cells migrate to the medulla to form medullary cords and secrete IgM antibodies that circulate as antigen–antibody complexes. These complexes are conveyed to and trapped in the germinal center follicular dendritic cells (FDCs). FDCs possess antibody and complement receptors enabling trapping of immune complex. The antigen presenting FDCs in contact with naïve lymphocytes generate a secondary follicle—a follicle with a germinal center.

CORTEX

Generation of Germinal Centers

B cells home in to primary follicles where they interact with FDCs. Within 24 hours of encountering its antigen attached to the FDC, B lymphocyte clonal expansion and proliferation happen, giving rise to germinal center centroblasts. Germinal center B cells undergo a series of phenotypic, genotypic, and morphologic transformation, generating three progenies: memory B cells, plasma cells, and recycling cells to more centroblasts (Casamayor-Palleja et al., 1996). They lose surface IgD, undergo heavy chain class switching to high-affinity IgG and IgA memory B cells or preplasma cells and exit the germinal centers (MacLennan et al., 2000). Genotypically, the centroblast genetic machinery is shuffled to generate somatic mutation to enhance antigen affinity. Hypervariable gene region mutation can result in production of B cells with high-affinity B cell receptor and corresponding neutralizing antibodies to viruses and other infections.

The germinal center reaction happens 2 to 4 days after antigen exposure, identified as a group of dividing centroblasts. Tingible body macrophages are the phagocytic cells containing lysosomes and cell debris. B cells also die by apoptosis and engulfed by macrophages (Figure 12.1). By day 7, a dense network of follicular dendritic cells are present in the pale or light zone, making them appear less densely packed than the centroblasts populating the dark zone. Between 7 to 10 days, polarity of the germinal center is apparent with migration of cells to opposite poles. Migration of centrocytes and centroblasts forms the light and dark zones. A prominent polarized germinal center reaction persists for 2 to 3 weeks and, without further stimulation, will subside to atrophic germinal centers with small dark zones or residual follicle dendritic cells.

Cytology

Conceptually two types of small and large lymphocytes comprise germinal center cells: morphologically

TABLE 12.1 Cells and Immunophenotypic Markers

Table of Romanowsky and H&E Stained Cells

	Small lymphocyte	Large non-cleaved	Small cleaved	Marginal zone cells	Immunoblast	Plasma cells
Macrophage-Tingible body						
Monocyte-blood Histiocytes-tissue	Naïve B-cell-mantle/prim follicle	Centroblasts-Germinal center-dark zone	Centrocytes-Germinal center-light zone	Memory B cell-perifollicular, sinuses	Transformed large B cell- interfollicular	Medulla, interfollicular, bone marrow
Yardstick nuclear size cutoff for small and large	Small cell, round nucleus, clumped "soccer ball" chromatin	Large cell, round vesicular nucleus, peripheralized nucleoli,pyroninophilic cytoplasm	Small cell, irregularcleaved, dark membrane chromocenters	Small Medium round, cleaved nucleus, copius cytoplasm	Very large, vesicular nucleus, prominent nucleous, pyroninophilic cytoplasm	Small medium, clock face nucleus, pyroninophilic cytoplasm
Phenotype CD68, CD64, CD163	IgM, IgD double+, Bcl2+	CD20+, CD10+, BCL6+, Ki67+	CD20+, CD10+, BCL6+, Ki67-	CD20+, CD5-, CD10-	CD20+, CD5-, CD10-	CD20-, CD38+, CD138+
Genotype-Germline	Unmutated rearranged Ig	Ongoing Mutation with Mutated Ig	Ongoing Mutation with Mutated Ig	Mutated Ig	Mutated Ig	Mutated Ig
Neoplastic couterpart-Histiocytic Neoplasms	MCL, CLL	DLBC, FL, NLPHL	DLBC, FL	Marginal zone lymphoma, CLL	DLBCL	Plasmacytoma, Myeloma

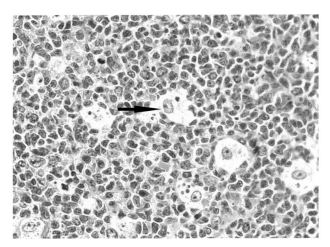

FIGURE 12.1 **Germinal center cells with characteristic tingible body macrophages (arrow).** Tingible bodies within macrophages are cell debris.

appearing cleaved and noncleaved, the former corresponding to centrocytes and the latter to centroblasts. The size of nuclei can be varied by type of fixation, but the size yardstick cutoff for small and large cells is the size of a macrophage or endothelial nucleus. The average macrophage nuclear diameter is the historical and rough microscopic gauge to assign a cutoff size for small and large cells; with intermediate size cells approximating the size of macrophage or endothelial cell nuclei. Other cell size comparators on the small size spectrum are small lymphocyte nucleus or red blood cells. Macrophages show as oval to round nucleis with pale chromatin, small pinkish nucleoli, and a generous rim of cytoplasm. These cells are easily identified as large cells with "tingible bodies" of dead, apoptotic, or pyknotic nuclear debris, often seen inside the germinal centers.

Centrocytes show cleaved or folded nuclear contours with dark chromocenters, absent nucleoli, and scant cytoplasm. Small or large centroblast shows a single central to several peripheralized nucleoli, round to slightly folded membrane, and moderate amount of pale cytoplasm. Centroblasts, in methyl green pyronin stain, show a dull magenta color, bluish in Giemsa, and creamy pink in PAS stain. Intermediate size cells inside germinal centers are often comprised of small noncleaved cells with fewer large noncleaved cells or large centroblasts. The small cleaved cell or centrocyte has a slightly larger nucleus than small lymphocytes, and the former has dark chromocenters instead of the membrane-associated nucleolus. Marginalized nucleoli are characteristic of noncleaved or centroblast cells. In routine stains, the nucleoli appear as round, amphophilic to

pink intranuclear bodies. This contrasts with the intranuclear chromocenters, which are dark blue with irregular chromatin condensation, a characteristic of nuclei of cleaved cells or centrocytes. It has to be pointed out that reactive lymph nodes show as well a few scattered cleaved cells, which are generally associated with germinal centers and tingible body macrophages. If centrocytes are numerous in many fields, examined on cytologic preps for intraoperative cytology, this finding generally suggests a follicular lymphoma. Small lymphocytes are few inside germinal centers and show as lymphocytes with small round nuclei displaying clumped or "soccer ball" chromatin and scant cytoplasm (see Table 12.1).

On touch imprints, small lymphocytes are the most common cell observed in a lymph node outside of germinal centers. The small lymphocyte is also the most nondescript, and its bland appearance hides its phenotypic heterogeneity. Larger cells, when prominent on low-power examination, may signal the presence of Hodgkin cells, especially when seen with prominent nucleolus. Large cells other than Hodgkin cell could be metastatic cells, especially if clustered, but more commonly seen are macrophages, endothelial cells, or transformed lymphocytes such as immunoblasts. Histiocyte clusters suggest granulomas. Endothelial cells show as an elongated array of spindled cells with pale chromatin and oblong nuclei with small nucleoli. Immunoblasts are large cells with eccentric amphophilic or pyroninophilic cytoplasm, vesicular nuclei with single prominent nucleolus. Large centroblasts show nuclei with a few membrane-bound nucleoli and pyroninophilic cytoplasm. Plasma cells are rarely increased, but if found in sheets, or with atypical lymphoplasmacytes and large forms with intranuclear inclusions, may suggest plasma cell tumors. Plasma cells with few pink cytoplasmic globules (Russell bodies) or plasma cells with "bunch-balloons" pink inclusions (Mott plasma cells) favor reactive plasma cells. A marked reactive plasmacytosis may be seen in autoimmune disorders like rheumatoid arthritis or lupus lymphadenopathy or lymphadenopathy secondary to infection, such as syphilis.

Eosinophils are relatively rare in reactive lymph nodes but when present, in a setting of peripheral eosinophilia, should raise concern for allergic lymphadenopathy secondary to drugs, immune reaction, or parasitic infections. Reactive lymph nodes with prominent eosinophils bring up a diagnosis of Kimura's disease, angiolymphoid hyperplasia with eosinophilia or in the proper settings, drug or autoimmune lymphadenopathy. Table 12.1 shows the high-power cytology of Wright–Giemsa and H&E stained cells normally found in lymph nodes.

Immunophenotypic Markers

Primary follicles show small lymphocytes that mark with Bcl-2, CD20, and surface IgM and IgD. They do not express BCL-6 or CD10. These cells comprise the majority of circulating B lymphocytes that has not encountered the antigen. They are also called "virgin" or "naïve" B cells. When they form adjacent nodules that stain with Bcl-2, they may be mistaken for nodular or mantle cell lymphoma. Unlike these lymphomas, primary follicle nodules are CD10, CD43, and cyclin-D1 negative.

Primary follicles can form as nodules in medullary cords in reactive lymph nodes that may sometimes be concerning for nodular lymphoma Figure 12.2. A high-power magnification view readily shows these nodules to be composed of small lymphocytes with round nuclei, instead of small cleaved or irregular cells typical of follicular lymphomas or mantle cell lymphomas.

Germinal center B cells express CD20, co-express bcl-6 and CD10, but lack Bcl-2 and CD5 staining. Unlike follicular lymphoma follicles, reactive germinal centers are Bcl-2 negative Figure 12.3. Care must be taken when interpreting scattered positivity inside benign germinal centers where Bcl-2 positive germinal center T helper cells are present. Sometimes numerous T cells are present inside benign germinal centers forming a ridge of follicular T helper cells at the interface of mantle and germinal center

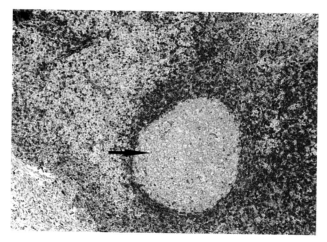

FIGURE 12.3 **Bcl-2 negative benign germinal centers B cells (arrow) contrasts with Bcl-2 positive T cells.** AEC red chromogen.

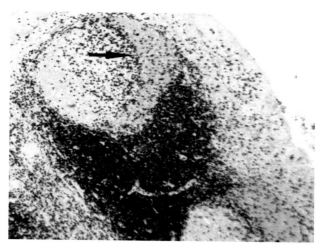

FIGURE 12.4 **T cells in germinal centers.** Follicular helper T cells expressing CD3+ CD57+ CD279+ CD4+ form a ridge visible between light zone and mantle zone (arrows).

Figure 12.4. The majority of the mantle zone corona and germinal center cells express CD20 Figure 12.5.

Germinal center cells are thought to transform from primary follicle B cells upon expression of CD38 surface marker. These cells are thought to be "founder" cells because they still have IgM, IgD, and immunoglobulin variable genes that have yet to carry mutation. In addition these cells soon lose IgD, acquire CD10, CD71, FAS, and Ki67 but lose Bcl-2 (antiapoptosis), indicating a propensity to die by apoptosis unless rescued by an appropriate antigen or CD40 ligand (Lebecque et al., 1997). The centroblasts and centrocytes both show germinal center phenotype, but the centroblasts show higher Ki67 and express CD77 while the centrocytes lack both.

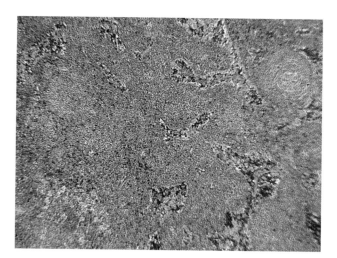

FIGURE 12.2 **Prominent medullary cords and primary follicles and early secondary follicles in a reactive lymph node**.

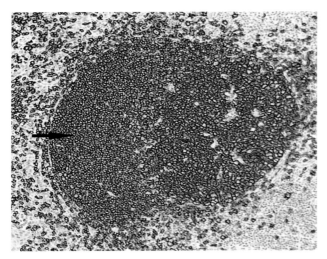

FIGURE 12.5   CD20 in mantle corona (arrow) and germinal center (right).

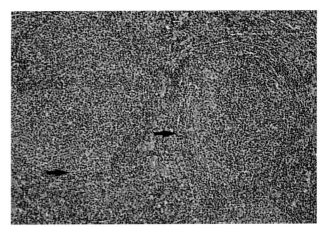

FIGURE 12.6   **Follicular lymphoma with back-to-back follicles, without polarity, and indistinct mantle zones borders (arrows).**

Flow Cytometry

Although there is no distinctive immunophenotypic result that helps in classifying reactive lymphoid hyperplasia, the presence of a light chain restriction or an aberrancy of the antigen expression help exclude any polyclonal hyperplastic reactions. Polyclonal plasmacytosis is, however, an exception and can be seen in association with either a clonal T, B cell lymphoma, or Hodgkin lymphoma. The flow cytometry results of a reactive lymph node typically show that the CD3+ T cells predominate, with a 58 to 73% range, and that the CD19 B cells are a minority, with a 24 to 42% range. The typical CD4/CD8 ratio is 1.4 to 3.9 with a kappa to lambda ratio of 1.5 to 2.0. CD10 range from 2.2 to 12% and CD71 from 3.8 to 20% (Westermann et al., 1990).

Follicular Lymphoma versus Follicular Hyperplasia

The most reliable criterion for diagnosing follicular lymphoma from hyperplasia is the low-power pattern of the follicles. Follicles back to back in a lymph node with insignificant intervening tissue are diagnostic of lymphoma and are rarely seen in follicular hyperplasia (Nathwani et al., 1981) Figures 12.6, 12.7. Moreover lack of polarity and vague demarcation of follicles favor lymphoma. The caveat is florid follicle center hyperplasia in HIV lymphadenopathy, which may lack polarity and show back-to-back germinal centers lacking prominent mantle zones. Immunohistochemistry is standard workup, typically showing reactive germinal centers lacking bcl-2 staining in contrast with bcl-2 positive follicular lymphoma follicles (Utz and Swerdlow, 1993),

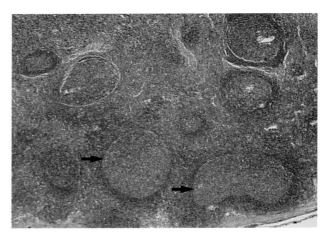

FIGURE 12.7   **Follicular hyperplasia with well separated, varied sized follicles.** Note the four-phase polarity and distinct mantle zone demarcation (arrows).

with the caveat that 10 to 15% of follicular lymphomas lack bcl-2. The utility of flow cytometry in differentiating lymphoma from hyperplasia is also evident when evaluating coexpression of CD10 or bcl-2 in association with CD20 (Cook, Craig, and Swerdlow, 2003). In the bcl-2 negative lymphoma cases, the strong expression of CD19+ CD10+ B cells, along with monotypic light chains, would be diagnostic. See Figure 12.8 and 12.9, which show weak and strong expressions of CD10 in follicular hyperplasia and lymphoma, respectively (Almasri, Iturraspe, and Braylan, 1998). In Figure 12.8 histogram, a large population of CD3 T cells is present in the follicular hyperplasia, virtually displayed as a large cluster of CD19 negative population in quadrant three. It is

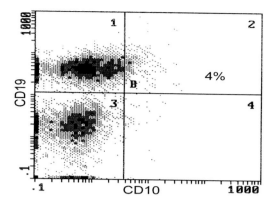

FIGURE 12.8 **Follicular hyperplasia**. Weak intensity CD10+ CD19+ B cells. Note the presence of increased CD19 negative population, in this case these are CD3+ reactive T cells, in contrast to the relatively decreased reactive component in follicular lymphoma.(Interpretation: Quadrant 2 shows CD19 CD10 double positive cells; Quadrant 3 double negative cells; Quadrant 1 CD19 positive CD10 negative; Quadrant 4 CD10 positive CD19 negative cells).

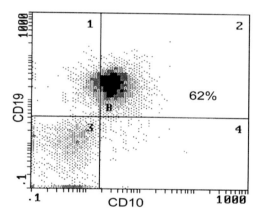

FIGURE 12.9 **Follicular lymphoma flow cytometry dot plot histogram showing increased CD10+ CD19+ B cells**.

to be noted that reactive T cells are present in both the follicular lymphoma and follicular hyperplasia when flow cytometry or immunohistochemistry is performed. Follicular lymphoma T cells may comprise as much as 60% of the node. In flow cytometry, caution is advised when interpreting results from scant tissue or specimen from small biopsy. In those cases a finding suggestive of a light chain excess may either be an oligoclonal artifact or a true clonal population so small that it raises an issue of mono-clonal lymphocytes of unknown significance (MLUS). Similarly the absence of CD10 or light chain restriction in flow cytometry does rule out a follicle center cell lymphoma, since some follicular large cell lymphoma may not express CD10 or some large cell

lymphoma lack surface immunoglobulins (Eshoa et al., 2001). In those cases B-cell clonality by gene rearrangement assay need be performed to confirm monoclonality.

Mantle Zones

The crown or corona of a mantle zone of a follicle is oriented toward the source of antigen, which is the sinus in a lymph node or the epithelial surface in mucosal lymphoid tissue. The typical mantle zone lymphocytes are small lymphocytes and appear homogeneous. However, mantle cells are heterogeneous by immunophenotype. The mantle is composed of at least two types of cells: resting naïve B cells and memory B cells. Whereas resting naïve mantle B-cell follicles express IgD+, IgM+, CD5weak+, Bcl-2+, CD38−, and lack CD23; the B-cell subset with CD23 expression likely reflect's memory B cells post-antigen selection (De Wolf-Peeters, 2001). The naïve B cells present in primary follicles and mantle zones are described often as CD5+ and thought to be the putative origin of mantle cell lymphomas (Hummel et al., 1994; Inghirami et al., 1991; Kips, 1989; De Wolf-Peeters, 2001). These cell generate the short-lived primary IgM immune response. In normal lymph nodes using paraffin immunohistochemistry, mantle zone cells show as weak CD5 positive B-cells compared to distinct darker staining CD3+ T cells (see Figure 12.10).

Monocytoid B Cell and Marginal Zones B Cells

Monocytoid B cells typically form pale crescentic sheets. They are medium sized and have slightly

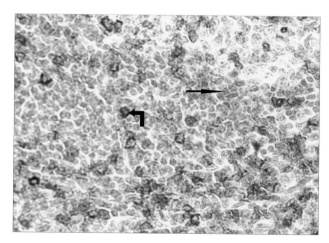

FIGURE 12.10 **CD5 immunostained mantle cells showing the weak staining mantle cells (arrow) and stronger staining T cells (bent arrow)**.

indented notched basophilic nuclei with inconspicuous nucleoli and open chromatin; their abundant pinkish cytoplasm is about 1.5× the size of small lymphocytes. Monocytoid B cells are often inconspicuous in lymph nodes except in certain types of lymphadenopathies such as toxoplasmosis, human immune deficiency virus (HIV), cytomegalovirus (CMV), cat-scratch disease (CSD), and lymphogranuloma venereum (LGV) (Plank, Hansmann, and Fischer, 1993; Hernandez et al. 1995; Sohn et al. 1985). These cells are recognized by their large amount of cytoplasm akin to that of monocytes but are really B cells. Monocytoid B cells express CD19 and CD20, and most express surface IgG, Ki-B3 and are negative for CD5, CD10, CD21, CD23, bcl-2, IgM, and IgD.

Immunoglobulin gene mutation and isotype expression studies have produced incongruous results because approximately 75% of the monocytoid B cells lack point mutations in the immunoglobulin genes, and therefore their molecular genetic structure is that of naïve B cells (Stein et al., 1999, 2000). This finding is in apparent paradox to the uniform expression of IgG by the monocytoid B cells (Cardoso De, Harris, and Bhan, 1984; Stein et al., 1999). IgG is generally expressed by post-follicular B cells. The exact role of monocytoid B cells is not clear, although it is apparent that these cells are induced in many immune stimulations of the lymph node. Phenotypically monocytoid B cells appear to be immunocompetent B cells despite the naïve pattern of their genes and the absence of CD21. Since monocytoid B cells are prominent after antigenic stimulation, a short-lived recirculating B-cell pool from lymph nodes may be postulated. Monocytoid B cells may not be the nodal counterpart of splenic marginal zone B cells. Monocytoid B cells may not be the same as marginal zone B cells in lymph nodes (Johrens et al., 2005).

Marginal zone lymphocytes are often prominent in normal activated splenic follicles (Figure 12.11) as well as in intra-abdominal lymph nodes or underneath the surface of the mucosal membrane of the intestinal tract in Peyer's patches, where antigen stimulation is constant. They are readily identified as small cells with abundant cytoplasm, round or cleaved nuclei, with or without nucleolus and may have associated plasma cells (Figure 12.12). These cells constitute a distinct B-cell subset that show an antigenic profile different from monocytoid B cells. Marginal zone lymphocytes express pan B-cell markers, surface IgM, and CD25 but, unlike germinal center cells or mantle cells, lack CD10, Bcl-6, and CD5, respectively. These cells also normally lack CD23, and express CD43 and Ki67 as an antigen aberrancy only

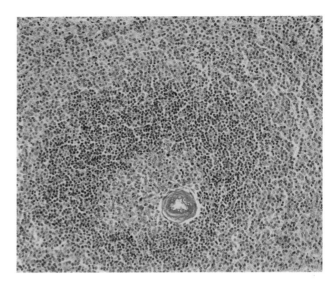

FIGURE 12.11 **Splenic marginal zone as a pale layer surrounding the darker mantle cell lymphocytes and whitish center of a white pulp follicle adjacent to a central arteriole (PAS stain).** Normal white pulp follicle is composed of three layers or a tripartite architecture composed of germinal center, mantle zone and marginal zone.

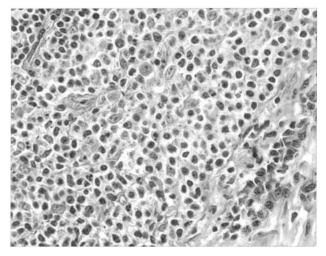

FIGURE 12.12 **Marginal zone B cells adjacent to mantle cells on left and plasma cells on right.**

in marginal zone lymphomas (Weiss, 2008). Marginal zone B cells express CD19 and CD20 as well and have the phenotypic features of memory B cells. They are strongly positive for IgM, IgG, and IgA, and a subpopulation exhibits weak IgD staining. They also express bcl-2, CD21, and CD27, and they are negative for CD5, CD10, CD23, CD43, and Ki-B3 (an antibody that recognizes aglycosylation-independent epitope of CD45RA, expressed by B lymphocytes that are immunocompetent but that have not yet responded to antigen) (Pileri et al., 2004). CD27 is a marker of memory B cells (Klein 1998, 1999; Agematsu 2000).

Conditions where one can recognize an expanded splenic marginal zone population include chronic infections, autoimmune disorders (including autoimmune hemolysis and autoimmune thrombocytopenia), polyclonal B-cell lymphocytosis, and the autoimmune lymphoproliferative syndrome (van Krieken et al., 1989).

The idea that marginal zone cells may contribute to the generation of monocytoid B cells in association with either follicles or sinuses is unresolved (Camacho, 2001; Kojima, 2006). Because of the expression of similar markers in both monocytoid B cells and marginal zone B cells derived from MALT, a view has held these cells to be similar if not identical (Nizze, 1991). When inside the sinus, monocytoid B cells are initially thought as immature sinus histiocytes owing to their appearance in low-power view as band-shaped pale areas composed of cells with clear cytoplasm. Dendritic cells, along with neutrophils, and monocytoid cells are admixed with sinus histiocytes in a reactive monocytoid B-cell reaction. Monocytoid B cells express IgG, T-bet, IRTA1, PCA-1, and KiB3 as well as CD11c, CD22, CD25, CD45RA, and CD75. Most monocytoid B cells do not express IgM and IgD and show absence of CD2, CD5, CD8a, CD9, CD10, CD21, CD24, CD27, CD38, and Bcl2.

Some of these markers may have direct practical utility, but the issue remains complex. Nodal marginal zone B-cell lymphoma is Bcl-2 positive, in contrast to monocytoid B-cell hyperplasia, which are bcl-2 negative. The caveat is that the normal marginal zone B cells are bcl-2 positive, and these cells may be also be present in normal lymph nodes (Jöhrens et al., 2005). There is also a subset of monocytoid B cells that may express the memory B cell marker CD27. Lazzi et al. have reported that IRTA1(+) monocytoid B cells are located predominantly in the subcapsular and intermediary sinuses but are observed also scattered within germinal centres in all lymphadenitis cases examined. IRTA1(+) monocytoid B cells in germinal centers express the memory B-cell marker CD27 (Lassi et al., 2006). IRTA1 is a receptor that is also associated with MALT marginal zone B cells (Jöhrens et al., 2005).

Germinal Center T Cells

T cells comprise 5 to 20% of germinal centers cells, particularly prominent in the apical light zone (see Figure 12.4). The presence of T helper cells in germinal centers are required for the development of memory B cells (Arnold, 2007). CD279 or PD1 is also a recently recognized marker of follicular T helper and is useful in classifying some T-cell lymphomas, like angioimmunoblastic T-cell lymphoma, that originate from follicular T helper cells.

Follicular Dendritic Cells

B cells are nestled in a cellular meshwork composed of follicular dendritic cells, the fixed or stationary antigen-presenting cells found only in follicles. These cells show intricate cytoplasmic processes, retaining and presenting immune complex bodies—called icosomes. The cells may originate from hematopoieitic or mesenchymal progenitors. They are not easily identified but at high-power and electron microscopic view, they have large, irregular or lobated nuclei, open vesicular chromatin that contrast with the closed, darker chromatin of surrounding lymphoid nuclei. They have dendritic cytoplasmic extensions with desmosomes, express monocytic markers CD14, complement receptors CD35 and CD21, along with immunoglobulin Fc receptor CD32, and CD23 IgE receptor, consistent with their immune complex scavenger role. They express adhesion molecules enabling lymphocyte attachment. In tissue stained with CD23, dendritic follicular networks are readily seen. The marker S100 is less strongly expressed when compared with the strong expression in interdigitating reticulum cells. These meshwork mirror the pathology, becoming well formed and hyperplastic in HIV-related follicular hyperplasia but involutes in time. The involuted germinal centers show concentric layers of follicular dendritic cells, rimmed by onion-skinned mantle zone, sometimes with hyalinized blood vessels, imparting a "lollipop" pattern similar to that seen in Castleman's disease (Figure 12.13). Pathology showing involuted follicles with follicular dendritic cells include angioimmunoblastic T-cell lymphoma, atypical lymphoproliferative disorders including Castleman's disease, both nodal and extranodal in skin (Naghashpour et al., 2010) and terminal depleted phase in HIV lymph nodes.

Warthin–Finkeldy giant cells or polykaryotes are identified more easily in HIV-related involution phase than in hyperplastic phase. These cells express follicular dendritic-specific markers CD21, CD23, clusterin, and CD35. The polykaryotes are identified as large multinucleated cells with grapelike clustered nuclei (Figure 12.14). These cells could be seen additionally in measles lymphadenopathy and Kimura's disease. Tumor derived from follicular dendritic cells include follicular dendritic cell sarcoma—a spindle cell neoplasm—with markers identical to its normal counterpart.

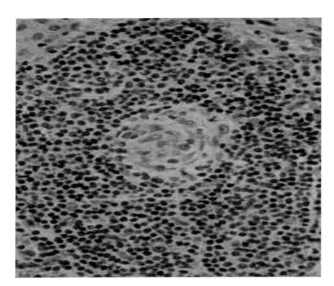

FIGURE 12.13 **Involuted follicle with follicular dendritic cell follicle center remnant rimmed by mantle zone cells.**

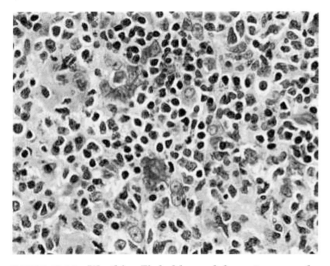

FIGURE 12.14 **Warthin–Finkeldy polykaryotes can be seen in follicle center or interfollicular area.**

PARACORTEX

T-Cell Reaction

T cells are stimulated to proliferate 1 to 2 days after antigen exposure. This reaction is manifest by increased paracortical size characteristically by increased proliferation of T cells into T-cell immunoblasts along with an increase in antigen presenting cells: the interdigitating reticulum cells. These reactions give rise to the characteristic nodule of T zone recognized as paracortex hyperplasia. On high-power view, the cell milieu is heterogeneous and polymorphic with small and large cells admixed with high endothelial venules. This histology and cellular pattern is recapitulated in T-cell neoplasms that originate from this compartment. Plasma cells, eosinophils, immunoblasts, admixed interdigitation reticulum cells, as well as vessels comprise the cellular milieu.

Perivenular Sinus

A perivenular sinus is present alongside paracortical cords surrounding the HEVs (Figure 12.15). This arrangement allows incoming lymphocytes from systemic circulation to be in close contact with the antigen and immune complex, as well as inflammatory mediators that originate from afferent lymphatics by the way of subcapsular sinuses route. The entry of lymphocytes and other cells are facilitated by proteins such as CCR7 recognized by ligand on lymphatic endothelial cells, which carry CXC21. These perivenular sinuses are also called paracortical sinuses, can sometimes be prominent in reactive or neoplastic lymph nodes as dark elliplical lymphocyte-rich structures or empty pinnate-shaped spaces, and are seen on low-power view. Dilated sinus spaces devoid of lymphocytes can sometimes be seen paradoxically in some low-grade B-cell lymphomas.

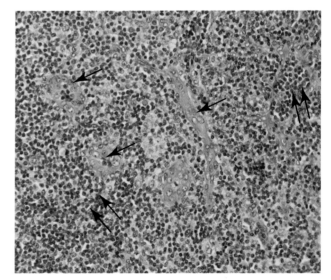

FIGURE 12.15 **Oval structures of high endothelial venules or post capillary venules in cross section and tangential cut.** Identified are high endothelial cells, narrow lumina, and the presence of lymphocytes transmigrating within its walls. Dark layers of paracortical cords (double arrow) surround the HEVs (arrows).

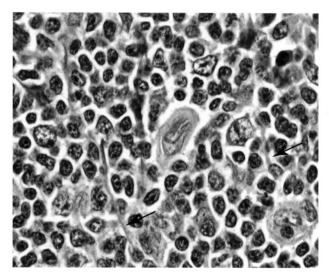

FIGURE 12.16 **Interdigiditating reticulum cells with its highly convoluted nucleus and pink cytoplasm with dendrites.** Fibroblastic reticular network conduits are seen in between cells as hyaline thin anastomosing fibrous network (arrows).

Dendritic Cells

Dendritic cells enter via the subcapsular lymph spaces or HEVs to reside in lymph node pulp specifically in interfollicular and paracortical areas (see Chapter 11 on dendritic cell types). Dendritic cells reside in strategic locations to further intercept microbes, foreign cells, antigens, immune complexes, and solutes. In the lymph node they capture and present these reactants to the surface of "crawling" lymphocytes via their dendritic cell processes. These cells may reside in scattered fashion in the paracortex or interfollicular areas and may form clusters in granulomatous adenopathy. Other types of dendritic cells also enter directly from blood via the portals of the high endothelial venules. They form a network of interdigitating dendritic reticulum cells (IDRCs) with dendrites that interdigitate around lymphocytes (Figure 12.16). An IDRC presents a specific antigen to a T lymphocyte that bear a corresponding specific receptor. Lymphocytes, in their search for unique cognate antigen, crawl and move circumferentially inside the lymph channels after entering the portals of the high endothelial venules (HEV) and, if successfully activated by its antigen, will commence cellular transformation. Otherwise, these cells exit via efferent lymphatic in continued search for its antigen in other lymph nodes. High endothelial venules characterize the paracortex and are the portal for lymphocytes and cells from blood to lymph nodes. Trafficking lymphocytes are easily seen. (More discussion of HEV follows below).

Pathogens and Dendritic Cells

Pathogen-associated molecular patterns are recognized by receptors on dendritic cells. The receptors on these cells, called toll-like receptors (TLRs), recognize molecular patterns unique to microorganisms. The dendritic cell's role of early recognition defines its place in the initial or innate immune system. Ten different TLRs have been identified, and these are receptors to viral RNA, bacterial lipoproteins, yeast cell wall sugars, toxoplasma profilin, bacterial flagellin, and parasites G proteins (Janssens, 2003). Dendritic cells upon activation by TLRs relay this information of microbial presence to lymph nodes, and facilitate the secondary or specific immune response.

However, microbes also cause decrease in dendritic cell functions. Viral targeting of antigen-presenting cells contributes to immunosuppression during chronic infection (Mueller et al., 2007; Sevilla et al., 2003). Viruses known to cause immunosuppression include HIV, measles, Lassa virus, and lymphocytic choriomeningitis virus (see chapter 22 on examples of lymphoid depletion secondary to virus). These viruses interact with alpha-dystroglycan, which is a receptor present in CD11c+ mature interdigitating dendritic reticulum cells.

NK Cells

Natural killer (NK) cells are also mediators of the innate response. NK cells circulate and enter the lymph nodes via HEVs and home into the paracortex and medulla (Bajenoff et al., 2006). CD56 positive NK cells interact with the dendritic cells and produce cytokines. NK cells target microbial and diseased cells directly without the need of major histocompatibility complex recognition. NK cells rapidly recruited from the blood enter via HEVs upon infection, and accumulate under the B-cell follicles, where they produce cytokines such as interferon gamma.

Plasmacytoid Dendritic Cells

As a reaction to infections and in autoimmune diseases, nodules of plasmacytoid dendritic cells, may be seen as well. Plasmacytoid dendritic cells (pDCs), also called plasmacytoid monocytes, have emerged as a principal subset of dendritic cells. They represent 0.2 to 0.8% of peripheral blood mononuclear cells in humans, display eccentric plasmacytoid morphology, express toll-like receptors 7 and 9, and secrete type 1 interferon, following viral contact. In lymph nodes they mature as fixed dendritic cells that directly regulate the function of T cells and thus link innate

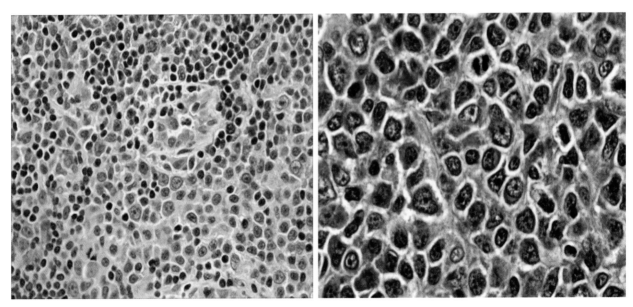

FIGURE 12.17 **HEVs seen in certain reactive lymphadenopathies**. HEVs are seen often in association with plasmacytoid monocytes or plasmacytoid dendritic cells. In high-power view their eccentric purple violet cytoplasm mimic plasma cells.

and adaptive immune responses. In low-power view, plasmacytoid dendritic cluster may be associated with HEVs or isolated as violaceous clusters and, at high power, display eccentric violet cytoplasm mimicking plasma cells (Figure 12.17). These may show tingible bodies simulating a germinal center, but unlike a reactive germinal center, PDCs show no polarity.

SINUS HISTIOCYTES

Foamy Histiocytosis

Dilated sinuses with histiocytes is characteristic of sinus histiocytosis. Normal histiocytes in the sinuses show a large amount of pink cytoplasm. Certain infections induce a foamy histiocyte appearance. These include infection by *T. whippelii, Leismania spp., Leprosy, Legionella*, as well as *Rhodococcus*. Noninfectious etiology include storage disease, hyperlipidemia, cholegranulomas, lymphangiography effect, and histiocytic reaction to foreign materials like hip replacement, metal prosthesis, silicone, polyethyl or polyvinyl materials, gold, cobalt, and chromium. (See Chapter 16 on sinus patterns).

Signet Ring Histiocytosis

Histiocytes rarely assume a signet ring morphology that mimics carcinoma or other cancers (Guerrero-

Medrano et al., 1997). See the sinus patterns in Chapter 16.

Pigmented Histiocytes

The presence of increased melanophages in sinuses are seen in dermatopathic lymphadenopathy (see Chapter 14 on paracortical hyperplasia). When extensive and with increased melanin pigments, the differential diagnosis of metastatic melanoma should be entertained. Hemochromatosis is one of the most common genetic disorders in the United States and can produce iron-pigmented histiocytosis along with some acquired conditions secondary to frequent blood transfusion and blood hemolysis.

Parasitophorous Vacuoles

Most intracellular pathogens avoid lysing their host cells during invasion by wrapping themselves in a vacuolar membrane of macrophages. This is the strategy of parasites that actively penetrate their respective mammalian host. During the process of invasion, they initiate the formation of a membrane, called a parasitophorous vacuole. This membrane, which surrounds the intracellular parasite differs from endosomal membranes or the membrane of phagolysosomes. The parasitophorous vacuole thus serves as a critical transport interface between the parasite and the host cell cytoplasm. Plasmodium and toxoplasma belong to a group of microorganisms wrapped by parasitophorous vacuoles of macrophage.

EPITHELIOID HISTIOCYTES AND GRANULOMAS

Granulomas are compact, organized nodular collections of epithelioid histiocytes, a mature type of macrophage. Epithelioid histiocytes have elongated nuclei, with larger nuclei than ordinary macrophages, and pink cytoplasm; they resemble epithelial cells in appearance. The borders of histiocytes are difficult to delineate. Granulomas are a tight, ball-like clusters and not a loose or dispersed collection of histiocytes. All granulomas may contain cells and a matrix of neutrophils, eosinophils, lymphocytes, and fused histiocytes: multinucleated giant cells. Fibroblasts or a collagen matrix may be seen in long-standing granulomas.

The most common disease associated with epithelioid granulomas is sarcoidosis. The presence of other features like necrosis is important because most infections have associated necrosis. A common type of necrosis associated with *Mycobacteria spp.* is caseation necrosis—a gross feature resembling cheese in color and consistency.

Most infectious granulomas also show a collection of neutrophils or abscess: called suppurative granulomas. Absence of suppuration in the presence of necrosis is an important feature of certain specific granulomatous lymphadenopathy such as Lupus or Kikuchi–Fujimoto disease. In contrast, suppurative necrotizing lymphadenitis is a pattern associated with certain specific diseases such as cat-scratch lymphadenitis, and tularemia (see Chapter 19 on infectious granulomas). Eosinophils, within and outside granulomas, are also features of certain specific entities, namely Kimura's disease and similar entities (see Chapter 18 for noninfectious granulomas).

The localization of granulomas is not well studied but may be associated with both B-cell areas and T-cell areas of the lymph node. A possible origin of granulomas is in the functional area that overlaps with the location of the paracortex and medullary cords, also called the *extranodular compartment*.

NODAL FRAMEWORK

The fibroblastic reticular framework supports the lymph node parenchyma. These are not readily seen on routine stains but may be highlighted by staining with vimentin, smooth muscle actin, desmin, keratin, and factor XIII. Collagen II distribution follows the distribution of this network, which can also be are outlined by silver stain such as Gomori's reticulin.

The Composite Nodule and Extranodular Compartment Concept

In addition to the classic pattern based on histology, there is a lymph node compartmentalization based on functional domains. This conception of a lymph node divides it into a composite nodule compartment and an extranodular compartment (van de Oord, 1996) bordered by the sinusoidal-vascular boundaries. About 50% of reactive lymph nodes show a composite of germinal centers admixed with cortical T zones—comprising the so-called composite nodule. In the remaining 50%, a predominant follicle center or paracortical reaction can be seen.

In the composite nodule compartment are included the germinal center B cells plus the cortical T cells. Hence the classic follicular pattern may be generated by expansion of the B-cell component of the composite nodules. The extranodule comprises everything else that do not belong to the composite nodule and may include the paracortex and medullary cords as well as the histiocytic reactions associated with these reactions. The paracortical and mixed reaction patterns may originate from the extranodular compartment, but this issue remains to be investigated.

The extranodule compartment has sinuses as boundaries. It is limited by subcapsular sinuses at the top, by intermediate or marginal sinuses along the trabeculae, and by the medullary junction sinuses and perhaps paracortical sinuses (Van Den Oord et al., 1986). The composite nodule, in this scheme, would have included nodules bounded by these sinuses and hence both primary follicles and secondary follicles with its germinal centers, its mantle coronas, and its adjacent rim of superficial cortical T cells (cortical ridge) (Figure 12.18, 12.20). This functional rim may be difficult to see in relation to the overlying germinal centers but becomes evident in low power after T-cell staining (Figure 12.21), when it expands to become a primary T-cell nodule. In this scheme, one may interpret the classic follicular patterns as a composite nodule response and the paracortical and medullary pattern as extranodule responses.

Transformation in Extranodule

If an interdigitating dendritic reticulum cell has the cognate antigen and encounters the T cell bearing the receptor, then this cell undergoes a series of transformations from a small lymphocyte to a large T immunoblast. Reactive paracortical hyperplasia or diffuse immunoblastic proliferation may be seen. The mottling pattern is characteristic of an interfollicular or paracortical reaction (Figure 12.19). Histologically

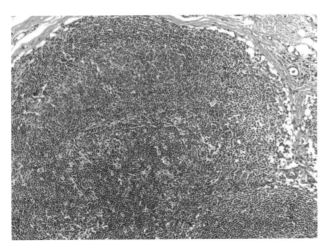

FIGURE 12.18 **Composite nodule.** The germinal center is at top and the mottled paracortical T zone below.

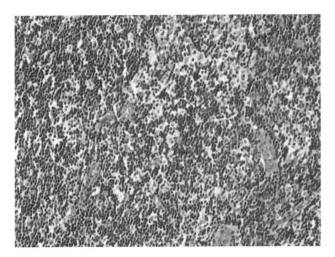

FIGURE 12.19 **Mottling and HEV characteristic of T paracortical reaction.**

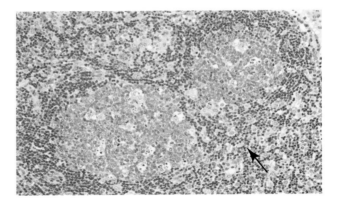

FIGURE 12.20 **Composite nodules with two secondary follicles and cortical T cell ridges (arrow).** Note the absence of high endothelial venules in the early T-cell response.

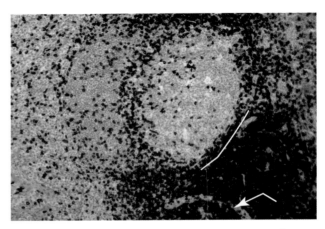

FIGURE 12.21 **Cortical T ridge stained by CD3 with overlying unstained germinal center component (line).** The paracortex begins immediately below identified by HEVs (bent arrow).

the mottled nodular structure is composed of a polymorphic population composed of a collection of reactive T cells with mottling of dendritic cells and histiocytes. Histiocytes could at times be a prominent component.

Granulomas

The extranodule compartment may expand after infections and noninfectious reactions, displaying granulomas, plasmacytoid dendritic cells along with plasma cells, neutrophils, eosinophils, and vessels. Plasmacytoid monocytes may arise in the extranodular compartment of the functional lymph node (personal communication, F. Faccheti). Examples include Kikuchi–Fujimoto, which shows prominent

nodules of plasmacytoid dendritic cells (Fachetti 2003). Lupus lymphadenopathy similarly shows extranodule collections of plasmacytoid dendritic cells, associated with HEVs, and often associated with tingible bodies. Suppurative necrotizing granulomas such as cat-scratch disease show collections of nodules of plasmacytoid dendritic cells as well in the extranodular compartment. The extranodule may correspond to the historical classic term lymph node pulp.

The extranodule also has paracortical cords. The paracortical cords functional structure was previously described (Gretz, Anderson, and Shaw, 1997). The paracortical cords are centered on HEVs, and circumferentially bordered by sinuses and channels (Figure 12.15). The paracortical cord is the tubular repeating unit structure of the paracortical compartment. Stacks of paracortical cords are layered side to side, like tubular arrays oriented end to end from the cortex to the medulla. Histologically, and at low-power view, the paracortical sinuses are normally not obvious but become highly visible as dark pinnate or lobate structures when filled with small lymphocytes in certain reactive and neoplastic lymph nodes. These are supplied by tubular conduits: fibroblastic reticulum channels that convey information-rich fluid from subcapsular sinus into the HEVs of paracortical cords. This way, as antigen rich fluid flows toward the HEVs, the cells that enter the HEVs move into the paracortex against this current. Hence T cells, B cells, and mononuclear dendritic cells from blood get bathed with cytokines and other chemotactic signals, as well as antigen-bearing solutes from tissue drained by lymphatics.

Extranodal or Ectopic Lymphoid Tissue

The bone marrow and thymus are the primary immune organs and the lymph nodes and spleen are secondary immune sites. Tertiary organs like gastrointestinal (GI), salivary glands, thyroid, and skin do not usually carry lymphoid structures but are induced to generate lymphoid follicles by antigen or infection: this is the physiologic basis of mucosa-associated lymphoid tissue (MALT), bronchial-associated lymphoid tissue (BALT), and skin-associated lymphoid tissue (SALT).

Tonsillitis

Bilateral enlargement of tonsils are usually not biopsied unless there is abscess or with marked inflammation that is not responsive to therapy. Most are secondary to viral infections, but about a third are secondary to Staph/Streptococcus infections. When there is unilateral enlargement, a concern for diseases other than infectious, prompts an excision. The histology is often uniformly follicle center hyperplasia with occasional commensal actinomyces in crypts. Interlobular fibrosis is seen in chronic tonsillitis. Involvement by viral infections like CMV and EBV show similar findings as in the lymphadenopathy secondary to those agents.

Lymphoepithelial lesions in Waldeyer's ring and increased B cells in the epithelia are not necessarily a sign of MALTOMA, unlike that seen in gastric or duodenal mucosa (Figure 12.22).

Thymic Hyperplasia

The inflammatory reaction in thymus is called thymic hyperplasia, a pathology found in the majority of patients with myasthenia gravis without

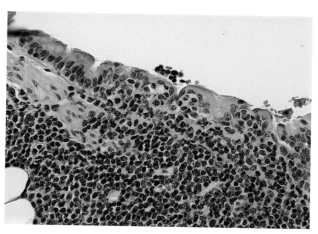

FIGURE 12.22 **Reactive lymphoepithelial lesion.** This is a normal finding in Waldeyer's ring mucosae.

thymoma. The gross appearance of excised thymus is lobated and its shape is generally preserved. Histology shows a characteristic displacement of thymic medulla with reactive germinal centers in close association with thymic remnants. The lobular and medullary thymic epithelial pattern is preserved. Medulla is often expanded with scattered Hassall's corpuscles in between hyperplastic germinal centers with follicular mantles. The epithelium of the reactive thymus can be hyperplastic or involuted. Increased vascularity around the Hassal's corpuscles or germinal centers may be seen. Masts cells may be seen scattered. Plasmacytosis could also be prominent, including presence of Russell's bodies, especially when associated with other symptoms. In the absence of myasthenia, plasmacytosis may associated with systemic lupus erythematosus.

The polarity of germinal centers may be seen, indicating its benign provenance. Other diseases showing less prominent reactive follicles in thymus may be seen in rheumatoid arthritis, Sjögren's, Addison's, Graves diseases, and as mentioned, lupus erythematosus.

Rectal Tonsil or Polypoid Lymphoid Hyperplasia

The presence of a polypoid lymphoid lesion that is reactive with florid follicular hyperplasia may be seen in rectal tonsil (also called polypoid localized lymphoid hyperplasia) as non-specific inflammatory response or putatively associated with specific infection like *Chlamydia sp.* (Cramer et al., 2009) (Figure 12.23). Awareness of this localized polypoid reactive proliferation of lymphoid tissue can prevent a misdiagnosis of lymphoma (Farris et al., 2008). Sometimes polypoid-localized lymphoid hyperplasia

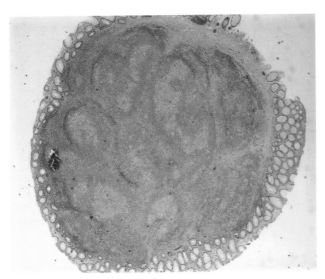

FIGURE 12.23 **Rectal tonsil or polypoid localized lymphoid hyperplasia**. The polyclonal reactive extranodal mass can be mistaken for lymphoma. Note the reactive follicles underneath the benign mucosa. Eosinophils and follicle fragmentation present.

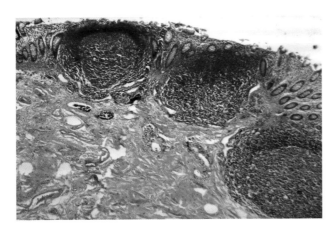

FIGURE 12.24 **Prominent Peyer's patch**. The patch expresses as a nonspecific reactive follicle center hyperplasia in the ileum.

have marginal zone hyperplasia, raising concern for MALTOMA (Kojima et al., 2008).

Peyer's Patch

Polarized follicles are seen in mucosa of the small intestinal ileum segment. These are sites for antigen induction of mucosal secretory IgA antibody responses mediated through the microfold cells or M cells: the antigen presenting cells in this area. These cells transports antigens and even microbes. M cells transport *Salmonella, Yersinia,* and *Escherichia coli*—for

induction of antigen-specific immune responses. The patch usually contain more than 5 prominent germinal centers and the patch number about 30 in humans (Figure 12.24). These are not usually hypertrophic unless there is a structural anomaly like intussusception or infections. Salmonella infection preferentially involve the Peyer's patches, some develop ulceration, and induce adjacent mesenteric lymphadenitis. Prominent hyperplasia of the Peyer's patch is typical of early Salmonella enteritis.

These B-cell sites are also called epithelial-associated B cells. The B cells underneath tonsil epithelia and in the dome epithelium of Peyer's patches have a memory B-cell phenotype with expression of CD27 and BCL-2 antigens (Falini et al., 2003).

REFERENCES

AGEMATSU K. 2000. Memory B cells and CD27. Histol Histopathol 15:573–6.

ALMASRI NM, ITURRASPE JA, BRAYLAN RC. 1998. CD10 expression in follicular lymphoma and large cell lymphoma is different from that of reactive lymph node follicles. Arch Pathol Lab Med 122:539–44.

ARNOLD C, CAMPBELL D, LIPP M, BUTCHER E. The germinal center response is impaired in the absence of T-cell expressed CXCR5. Eur J Immunol 37:100–109.

BAJENOFF M, BREART B, HUANG AY, QI H, CAZARETH J, BRAUD VM, GERMAIN RN, GLAICHENHAUS N. 2006. Natural killer cell behavior in lymph nodes revealed by static and real-time imaging. J Exp Med 203:619–31.

CAMACHO FI, GARCIA, JF, SÁNCHEZ-VERDE L, SÁEZ AI, SÁNCHEZ-BEATO M, MOLLEJO M, PIRIS M A. 2001. Unique phenotypic profile of monocytoid B cells differences in comparison with the phenotypic profile observed in marginal zone B cells and so-called monocytoid B cell lymphoma. Am J Pathol 158:1363–9.

CARDOSO DE AP, HARRIS NL, BHAN AK. 1984. Characterization of immature sinus histiocytes (monocytoid cells) in reactive lymph nodes by use of monoclonal antibodies. Hum Pathol 15:330–5.

CASAMAYOR-PALLEJA M, FEUILLARD J, BALL J, DREW M, MACLENNA ICM. 1996. Cemtrocytes rapidly adopt a memory B cell phenotype on coculture with autologous germinal center T cell enriched preparations. Int Immunol 8:737–44.

COOK JR, CRAIG FE, SWERDLOW SH. 2003. Bcl-2 Expression by multicolor flow cytometric analysis assists in the diagnosis of follicular lymphoma in lymph node and bone marrow. Am J Clin Pathol 119:145–51.

CRAMER SF, ROMANSKY S, HULBERT B, RAUH S, PAPP JR, CASIANO-COLON AE. 2009. The rectal tonsil: a reaction to chlamydial infection ? Am J Surg Pathol 33:483–5.

De Wolf-Peeters C, Tierens A, Achten R. 2001. Normal histology and immunoarchitecture of the lymphohematopoietic system. In: Knowles DM, ed., Neoplastic Hematopathology, 2nd ed. Lippincott William and Wilkins, New York, 271–305.

Eshoa C, Perkins S, Kampalath B, Shidham V, Juckett M, Chang CC. 2001. Decreased CD10 expression in grade III and in interfollicular infiltrates of follicular lymphomas. Am J Clin Pathol 115:862–7.

Fachetti F, Vermi W, Mason D, Colonna M. 2003. The plasmacytoid monocytte/interferon producing cells. Virch Arch 443:703–17.

Falini B, Tiacci E, Pucciarini A, Bigerna B, Kurth J, Hatzivassiliou G, Droetto S, Galletti BV, Gambacorta M, Orazi A, Pasqualucci L, Miller I, Kuppers R, la-Favera R, Cattoretti G. 2003. Expression of the IRTA1 receptor identifies intraepithelial and subepithelial marginal zone B cells of the mucosa-associated lymphoid tissue (MALT). Blood 102:3684–92.

Farris AB, Lauwers GY, Ferry JA, Zukerberg LR. 2008. The rectal tonsil: a reactive lymphoid proliferation that may mimic lymphoma. Am J Surg Pathol 32:1075–9.

Gretz JE, Anderson AO, Shaw S. 1997. Cords, channels, corridors and conduits: critical architectural elements facilitating cell interactions in the lymph node cortex. Immunol Rev 156:11–24.

Guerrero-Medrano J, Delgado R, bores-Saavedra J. 1997. Signet-ring sinus histiocytosis: a reactive disorder that mimics metastatic adenocarcinoma. Cancer 80:277–85.

Hernandez AM, Nathwani BN, Nguyen D, Shibata D, Chuan W, Nichols P, Taylor CR. 1995. Nodal benign and malignant monocytoid B cells with and without follicular lymphomas: a comparative study of follicular colonization, light chain restriction, Bcl-2, and T(14;18) in 39 cases. Hum Pathol 26:625–32.

Hummel M, Tamaru J, Kalvelage B, Stein H. 1994. Mantle cell lymphomas express VH genes with no or very little somatic mutations like the physiologic cells of the follicle mantle. Blood 84:403–7.

Inghirami G, Foitl DR, Sabichi A, Zhu BY, Knowles DM. 1991. Autoantibody-associated cross-reactive idiotype-bearing human B lymphocytes: distribution and characterization, including Ig VH gene and CD5 antigen expression. Blood 78:1503–15.

Janssens S, Beyaert R. 2003. Role of toll-like receptors in pathogen recognition. Clin Microbial Rev. 1:637–46.

Johrens K, Shimizu Y, Anagnostopoulos I, Schiffmann S, Tiacci E, Falini B, Stein H. 2005. T-beta-positive and IRTA1-positive monocytoid B cells differ from marginal zone B cells and epithelial-associated B cells in their antigen profile and topographical distribution. Haematologica 90:1070–7.

Kipps TJ. 1989. The CD5 B cell. Adv Immunol 47:117–85.

Klein U, Goossens T, Fischer M, Kanzler H, Braeuninger A, Rajewsky K, Kuppers R. 1998. Somatic hypermutation in normal and transformed human B cells. Immunol Rev 162:261–80.

Klein U, Rajewsky K, Kuppers R. 1998. Human immunoglobulin (Ig)M+IgD+ peripheral blood B cells expressing the CD27 cell surface antigen carry somatically mutated variable region genes: CD27 as a general marker for somatically mutated (memory) B cells. J Exp Med 188:1679–89.

Kojima M, Motoori T, Iijima M, Ono T, Yoshizumi T, Matsumoto M, Masawa N, Nakamura S. 2006. Florid monocytoid B-cell hyperplasia resembling nodal marginal zone B-cell lymphoma of mucosa associated lymphoid tissue type: a histological and immunohistochemical study of four cases. Pathol Res Pract 202(12): 877–82.

Kojima M, Shimizu K, Sameshima S, Saruki N, Nakamura N. 2008. Focal lymphoid hyperplasia of the terminal ileum presenting mantle zone hyperplasia with clear cytoplasm: a report of three cases. Pathol Oncol Res 14:337–40.

Lazzi S, Bellan C, Tiacci E, Palummo N, Vatti R, Oggioni M, Amato T, Schuerfeld K, Tonini T, Tosi P, Falini B, Leoncini L. 2006. IRTA1+ monocytoid B cells in reactive lymphadenitis show a unique topographic distribution and immunophenotype and a peculiar usage and mutational pattern of IgVH genes. J Pathol 209:56–66.

Lebecque S, de BO, Arpin C, Banchereau J, Liu YJ. 1997. Germinal Center founder cells display propensity for apoptosis before onset of somatic mutation. J Exp Med 185:563–71.

MacLennan IC, de Vinuesa CG, Casamayor-Palleja M. 2000. B cell memory and the persistence of antibody responses. Proc Tans R Soc Lond B 355:345–50.

Mueller SN, Matloubian M, Clemens DM, Sharpe AH, Freeman GJ, Gangappa S, Larsen CP, Ahmed R. 2007. Viral targeting of fibroblastic reticular cells contributes to immunosuppression and persistence during chronic infection. Proc Natl Acad Sci USA 104:15430–35.

Naghashpour M, Cualing H, Szabunio M, Bui M. 2010. Haline-vascular Castleman disease: a rare cause of solitary subcutaneous soft tissue mass. Am J of Dermatopath 32:293–7.

Nathwani BN, Winberg CD, Diamond LW, Bearman RM, Kim H. 1981. Morphologic criteria for the differentiation of follicular lymphoma from florid reactive follicular hyperplasia: a study of 80 cases. Cancer 48:1794–1806.

Nizze H, Cogliatti SB, von SC, Feller AC, Lennert K. 1991. Monocytoid B-cell lymphoma: morphological variants and relationship to low-grade B-cell lymphoma of the mucosa-associated lymphoid tissue. Histopathology 18:403–14.

Pileri S, Kikuchi M, Helbron D, Lennert K. 1982. Histiocytic necrotizing lymphadenitis without granulocytic infiltration. Virchows Arch (A) 395:257–71.

Plank L, Hansmann ML, Fischer R. 1993. The cytological spectrum of the monocytoid B-cell reaction: recognition of its large cell type. Histopathology 23:425–31.

QATARNEH SM, KIRICUTA IC, BRAHME A, TIEDE U, LIND BK. 2006. Three-dimensional atlas of lymph node topography based on the visible human data set. Anat Record (Part B) 289b:98–111,

SAWHNEY MS, DEBOLD SM, KRATZKE RA, LEDERLE FA, NELSON DB, KELLY RF. 2007. Central intranodal blood vessel: a new EUS sign described in mediastinal lymph nodes. Gastrointest Endosc 65:602–8.

SEVILLA N, KUNZ S, McGAVERN D, OLDSTONE MB. 2003. Infection of dendritic cells by lymphocytic choriomeningitis virus. Curr Top Microbiol Immunol 276:125–44.

SOHN CC, SHEIBANI K, WINBERG CD, RAPPAPORT H. 1985. Monocytoid B lymphocytes: their relation to the patterns of the acquired immunodeficiency syndrome (AIDS) and AIDS-related lymphadenopathy. Hum Pathol 16:979–85.

STEIN K, HUMMEL M, KORBJUHN P, FOSS HD, ANAGNOSTOPOULOS I, MARAFIOTI T, STEIN H. 1999. Monocytoid B cells are distinct from splenic marginal zone cells and commonly derive from unmutated naive B cells and less frequently from postgerminal center B cells by polyclonal transformation. Blood 94:2800–8.

STEIN K, HUMMEL M, KORBJUHN P, FOSS HD, ANAGNOSTOPOULOS I, MARAFIOTI T, STEIN H. 2000. [Monocytic B-cells represent a new cell population that is mainly recruited from unmutated polyconal naive B-cells]. Verh Dtsch Ges Pathol 84:151–2.

UTZ GL, SWERDLOW SH. 1993. Distinction of follicular hyperplasia from follicular lymphoma in B5-fixed tissues: comparison of MT2 and Bcl-2 antibodies. Hum Pathol 24:1155–8.

VAN DEN OORD JJ. DE WOLF-PEETERS C, DESMET VJ. 1986. The composite nodule, a structural and functional unit of the reactive human lymph node. Am J Pathol 122:83–91.

VAN KRIEKEN JH, VON SC, KLUIN PM, LENNERT K. 1989. Splenic marginal zone lymphocytes and related cells in the lymph node: a morphologic and immunohistochemical study. Hum Pathol 20:320–5.

VON ANDRIAN UH, MEMPEL TR. 2003. Homing and cellular traffic in lymph nodes. Nat Rev Immunol 3:867–78.

WEISS L. 2008. Lymph Nodes. Cambridge University Press, New York.

WESTERMANN CD, HURTUBISE PE, LINNEMANN CC, SWERDLOW SH. 1990. Comparison of histologic nodal reactive patterns, cell suspension immunophenotypic data, and HIV status. Mod Pathol 3:54–60

WILLARD-MACK C. 2006. Normal structure, function, and histology of lymph nodes. Toxicol Pathol 34:409–24.

VAN KRIEKEN JH, VON SC, KLUIN PM, LENNERT K. 1989. Splenic marginal zone lymphocytes and related cells in the lymph node: a morphologic and immunohistochemical study. Hum Pathol 20:320–5.

VON ANDRIAN UH, MEMPEL TR. 2003. Homing and cellular traffic in lymph nodes. Nat Rev Immunol 3:867–78.

CHAPTER THIRTEEN

LYMPHADENOPATHY WITH PREDOMINANT FOLLICULAR PATTERNS

Shohreh Iravani Dickinson, Jun Mo, and Hernani D. Cualing

GERMINAL CENTER HYPERPLASIA

Florid Follicular Hyperplasia, Nonspecific

Follicular hyperplasia (FH) is a structural and immunological pattern recognized as part of reactive lymphoid hyperplasia. Reactive lymphoid hyperplasia encompasses proliferations occurring in all compartments of the lymph node including the B-cell follicles, T-cell paracortical or interfollicular areas, plasma cell medullary regions, and the monocyte/macrophage containing sinuses. Hyperplasia may involve the lymph node in a diffuse pattern with compression of normal architecture by numerous lymphocytes, immunoblasts, and macrophages. Hyperplasia can also present more commonly in mixed patterns involving in varying degrees the follicles, interfollicular areas, and sinuses. Reactive FH is a benign nonspecific reaction occurring in follicles of primarily enlarged lymph nodes. It is one of the most common causes of lymph node enlargement. Most cases of FH are idiopathic without an identifiable cause. However, FH can be seen consequentially in association with various disorders including viral, bacterial and parasitic infections, autoimmune disorders, inflammatory states, multicentric Castleman's disease, and immune deficiencies such as early stage human immunodeficiency virus infection. Furthermore Hodgkin's lymphoma, early involvement by a variety of B- and T-cell lymphomas, and progressive transformation of germinal centers (PTGC) may show reactive FH within the same lymph node. Benign conditions overall rather than malignancies are nonetheless the most common cause of lymph node enlargement. Certain stimuli may produce characteristic morphologic findings, suggesting a specific diagnosis or differential diagnosis. Recognition of the morphologic patterns of reactive FH can assist in distinguishing it from various lymphomas and perhaps identify in some cases, the etiology for the proliferation (Vakiani et al., 2007; Ioachim et al., 1990; Schnitzer, 2001).

Definition

Reactive FH is a polyclonal B-cell response to antigenic stimuli, resulting in the reversible proliferation of polymorphous activated lymphocytes within lymphoid follicles.

ICD-10 Codes R59.9 Enlarged lymph node, unspecified
R59.1 Lymphadenopathy, NOS

Non-Neoplastic Hematopathology and Infections, First Edition. Edited by Hernani D. Cualing, Parul Bhargava, and Ramon L. Sandin.
© 2012 Wiley-Blackwell. Published 2012 by John Wiley & Sons, Inc.

Synonyms

Benign follicular hyperplasia, benign lymphoid hyperplasia, follicular hyperplasia, lymphadenomegaly, pseudolymphoma, reactive lymphoid follicular hyperplasia, reactive lymphoid hyperplasia, reactive lymph node hyperplasia with giant follicles, lymphadenopathy NOS, enlarged lymph node, unspecified.

Epidemiology

FH is more frequent in children and younger individuals. Florid reactive FH is uncommon in patients over 50 years old, since humoral responses are comparatively suppressed in this age group (Kojima et al., 1998; Osborne et al., 1991).

Clinical Aspects

Reactive FH can occur anywhere lymphoid tissue is present. It may affect all ages but is more common in children and younger individuals. FH can also present in extranodal sites including the gastrointestinal tract, orbit, lung, skin, and rarely in the liver and peripheral nerves. The term pseudolymphoma has been given to lymphoid hyperplasia occurring in visceral organs and extranodal sites. The presence of florid FH in individuals over 50 years of age may indicate the presence of concurrent malignancy. Occasionally FH is seen concomitantly with or subsequent to various B- and T-cell lymphomas as well as Hodgkin lymphoma. Therefore the exclusion of lymphoma is essential in cases of reactive FH, specifically in patients over 50 years of age (Ioachim et al., 1990; Kojima et al., 1998; Osborne et al., 1991; Snover et al., 1981).

Reactive FH can be present, particularly in adults, in association with various disorders including infections, immune deficiencies such as primary immunodeficiency, autoimmune disorders (rheumatoid arthritis, systemic lupus erythematosus, autoimmune thyroiditis, Sjögren's syndrome, and primary biliary cirrhosis), and inflammatory states such as thrombophlebitis. Florid FH is commonly seen in patients with early stage human immunodeficiency virus infection, multicentric Castleman's disease, and progressive transformation of germinal centers. FH may also be evident in lymph nodes draining sites of infection such as in tonsillitis. FH is frequently present in conjunction with various viral infections, including Epstein–Barr virus, infectious mononucleosis, cytomegalovirus, herpes virus, and hepatitis B and hepatitis C virus infections. Florid FH may also occur in association with post-transplant lymphoproliferative disorder. Rare cases of florid reactive FH have been reported as a post-therapy

reaction in patients treated for hematologic malignancies such as acute myeloid leukemia and diffuse large B-cell lymphoma. In these cases it is postulated that the florid FH transpires consequentially as a result of chronic stimulation in an altered immune post-therapy state. Florid FH following subsequent to therapy for carcinoma can also occur but is exceedingly rare (Vakiani et al., 2007; Kojima et al., 1998, 2006).

Pathophysiology

The cause of reactive FH remains largely unknown in the vast majority of cases. Particularly in children and younger individuals, the etiology of reactive FH is often without a known cause. Occasional cases are linked to antigenic activation of the immune system by various stimuli. Inflammatory states and infectious agents as well as their by-products can antigenically stimulate and promote B lymphocyte activation within the lymphoid follicles. Activated lymphoid cells within the follicles then undergo somatic hypermutation and clonal selection, leading to secondary germinal center formation. Ultimately the result is humoral immunity with the production of plasma cells secreting antibody specific to the antigen involved. In adults, reactive FH is additionally linked to systemic or local immune imbalance and dysfunction (Kojima et al., 1998).

Morphologic Aspects

The morphologic features of reactive FH are contingent on the age of the patient, specific causative agent, past exposure to the agent, capacity of the immune system to response, period of time following exposure, and the duration of exposure to the antigenic stimuli. Reactive FH is characterized by the presence of numerous enlarged hyperplastic follicles that vary considerable in size and shape (Figure 13.1). There is both an increase in the number and size of the germinal centers in FH. The hyperplastic follicles may occasionally involve the entire lymph node appearing to distort and compress the paracortical regions, medulla, and/or sinuses. However, there is preservation of lymph node architecture without effacement. In reactive FH there is typically no extracapsular extension of lymphoid cells into the surrounding fat. However, occasional cases may show numerous lymphoid cells within the capsule and surrounding adipose fat, lymphatic channels, and blood vessels, thereby mimicking neoplastic proliferations (Henry, 1992; Dorfman et al., 1974).

Hyperplastic germinal centers generally are well demarcated, circumscribed, and round to oval. Occasionally there is coalescence of germinal centers

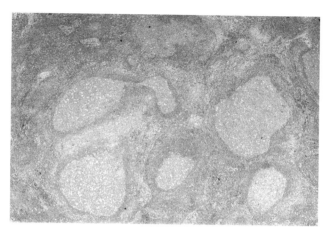

FIGURE 13.1 Nonspecific follicular hyperplasia with sharply demarcated follicles of variable shapes and sizes.

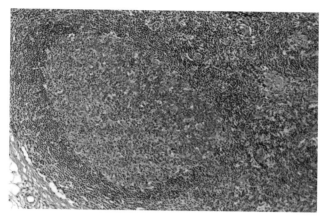

FIGURE 13.2 Nonspecific follicular hyperplasia with polarization of germinal centers and mantle zones. A light zone abuts a thick mantle, while dark zone forms an attenuated mantle zone.

forming hourglass, dumbbell, serpentine or irregular shapes (Figure 13.1). An admixture of polymorphic and polyclonal lymphoid cells including centroblasts, centrocytes, occasional immunoblasts, plasmacytoid lymphocytes, and plasma cells is present in the germinal centers. Plasma cells occasionally may be numerous in the germinal centers. Centroblasts are activated large cells containing scant basophilic cytoplasm and large oval vesicular nuclei with prominent one to multiple nucleoli. Centrocytes are small sized and have scant cytoplasm, cleaved nuclei and inconspicuous nucleoli. See Chapter 12 for figures. Polarity is the hallmark of reactive germinal centers and is not seen in neoplastic follicles. Polarity refers to the unique appearance of isolated dark zones containing centroblasts exhibiting abundant mitosis and apoptosis situated adjacent to light zones composed of centrocytes, T helper cells, and follicular dendritic cells. Numerous tingible body macrophages are present in the dark zones. The light zones face the sinus, where antigens enter into the node, and the dark zones are farthest from the sinus at the opposite end (Figure 13.2). Centroblasts in the dark zones undergo rapid proliferation and mitosis as well as somatic hypermutation and class switching of their immunoglobulin genes. Centroblasts that can no longer divide transform to smaller nondividing centrocytes and migrate into the light zones. In the light zones the centrocytes are selected based on their affinity of their surface antibody for the antigenic stimulus. Helper T cells and a network of follicular dendritic cells in the light zones aid in the sequestration of antigen. Centrocytes that can effectively bind antigen and obtain T-cell assistance survive. The surviving centrocytes subsequently transform to plasma cells or memory B cells and eventually egress

from the germinal centers. Centrocytes that do not survive, due to failure to bind antigen and/or receive T-cell help, undergo apoptosis and are cleared from the germinal centers by macrophages. Consequently numerous tingible body macrophages indicative of a high proliferation rate, and containing apoptotic phagocytized cellular debris, produce a starry-sky pattern characteristic of a reactive follicle. Follicular dendritic cell networks are hyperplastic, may be slightly compressed in the adjacent mantle zones, but do not show prominent disruption (Berek et al., 1991; Katayanagi et al., 1994; Swerdlow, 2004; Schnitzer, 2001).

Mantle zones of hyperplastic follicles have sharp distinct borders and are well delineated from the surrounding germinal centers. Mantle zones are often of normal size or slightly enlarged. Rarely, mantle zones may be hyperplastic, prominent and expanded in reactive FH (Figure 13.3). The differential diagnosis includes mantle cell lymphoma. Larger follicles may be surrounded by an attenuated thin mantle zone. Mantle zone cells are primarily small sized with scant cytoplasm, slightly indented or irregular nuclei and inconspicuous nucleoli. Rarely, mantle zone B cells of both primary and secondary follicles may appear larger and contain moderate amounts of pale clear cytoplasm, thereby mimicking marginal zone cells morphologically.

FH containing foci of marginal zone hyperplasia is exceedingly rare in peripheral lymph nodes but is commonly seen in a reactive spleen (Figure 13.4). Marginal zones are commonly well defined from mantle zones in FH. Marginal zone B cells are small to medium sized with round to oval nuclei and have finely dispersed nuclear chromatin, inconspicuous nucleoli, and moderate amounts of pale clear

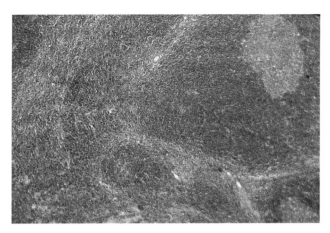

FIGURE 13.3 **Mantle zone hyperplasia (on the top) with normal mantle zones (on the bottom right)**.

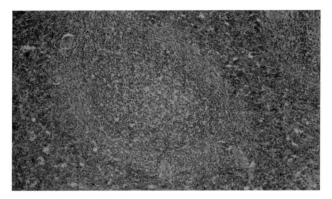

FIGURE 13.4 **Hyperplastic marginal zone in splenic white pulp**. Note the pale zone around the darker mantle zone surrounding this germinal center.

cytoplasm. In general, marginal zone B cells are loosely packed, larger, and have finer chromatin than mantle zone B cells (Katayanagi et al., 1994; Swerdlow, 2004).

Interfollicular areas frequently contain a proliferation of predominantly mature T cells, and occasional scattered immunoblasts, plasmacytoid lymphocytes, plasma cells, and occasional eosinophils among histiocytes, dendritic cells, and other stromal cells. Vascularity may be prominent with hyperplastic endothelial cells. B lymphocytes are exceedingly rare and tend to be scattered in the interfollicular areas. The dendritic cell networks within the interfollicular areas do not show prominent disruption but may be slightly compressed particularly in areas adjacent to the hyperplastic follicles. There may be prominent aggregates of sinus histiocytes. Stromal fibrosis may be evident.

Immunophenotyping

The immunophenotype of reactive FH is distinct. Well-demarcated secondary follicle germinal centers contain predominantly polytypic B lymphocytes that express CD20, CD79a, PAX5, focally express Bcl-6 and CD10, and are classically negative for Bcl-2, IgD and CD43. In FH, reactivity for Bcl-6 and CD10 is mostly restricted to within the secondary follicle germinal centers. The interfollicular regions in FH do not contain broad or expansive areas of Bcl-6, CD10, or CD20 positive cells. Only rare scattered interfollicular cells express Bcl-6, CD10, and CD20 in FH. In contrast, primary follicles contain predominantly mantle zone naïve B cells that express Bcl-2 and lack expression for the germinal center markers Bcl-6 and CD10. Bcl-2 is also characteristically expressed on T cells, hence necessitating the use of T-cell markers when assessing for Bcl-2 expression.

Mantle zone lymphocytes of primary and secondary follicles are predominantly small B cells expressing CD20, CD79a, PAX5, Bcl-2, and surface IgM and IgD heavy chains. Mantle zone B lymphocytes also weakly express CD5 but are negative for CD3 and CD43. Marginal zone B cells, although rare, surrounding the distinct mantle zones, characteristically also express CD20, CD79a, and PAX5. Bcl-2 is usually negative on marginal zone B cells; however, a subpopulation of marginal zone cells can be Bcl-2 positive. Bcl-2 reactivity therefore is not likely to aid in distinguishing reactive marginal zone cells from marginal zone B cell lymphoma since both can express Bcl-2. Marginal zone B cells in FH may express surface IgM and may weakly express surface IgD, but classically lack expression of CD5, CD10, CD21, CD23, CD43, and CD45RO. Cyclin D1 is characteristically negative in both mantle and marginal zone cells in FH (Dogan et al., 2000; Spencer et al., 1998; Van den Ord et al., 1986; Hunt et al., 2001).

Admixed T lymphocytes in germinal centers and interfollicular areas express Bcl-2, PD-1 (CD279, programmed death-1), CD3, CD5, CD43, CD45RO, and CD45. Germinal center and interfollicular T cells are predominantly helper phenotype expressing CD4. Plasma cells can be outlined by Bcl-2, CD43, CD79a, and CD138. Plasma cells and plasmacytoid lymphocytes show a polyclonal kappa and lambda light chain staining pattern. Tingible body macrophages can be outlined by lysozyme, CD43, CD68, and CD163. The hyperplastic follicular dendritic cell networks are outlined by antibodies to CD21, CD23, CD35, EGFR (epidermal growth factor receptor), CAN.42, R4/23 (DRC-1), and LNGFR/p75. The LNGFR/p75 antibody also outlines other stromal cells including fibroblasts and fibroblastic reticular cells.

Occasional immunoblasts within the follicles are predominantly B immunoblasts expressing CD20, CD30, and CD45. Scattered immunoblasts in the interfollicular areas are an admixture of CD20/CD45 positive B immunoblasts and CD3/CD45 positive T immunoblasts, both of which can express CD30 but classically lack expression for CD15. B immunoblasts show polyclonal kappa and lambda light chains. In contrast, interfollicular Hodgkin's cells express CD30 as well as CD15, may co-express CD20 and PAX5, but are characteristically negative for CD45. Hodgkin's lymphoma can also express both kappa and lambda light chains. A potential pitfall is the expression of CD15 by cytomegalovirus infected benign cells, thereby mimicking CD15 positive Hodgkin's cells (Rushin et al., 1990).

Laboratory Diagnosis

Complete history and physical exam, laboratory investigation including microbiology cultures, serology, and molecular studies such as polymerase chain reaction may be helpful in excluding certain infections, inflammatory states, autoimmune disorders, and other disorders related to immune dysfunction. Immunohistochemistry, flow cytometry, and cytogenetic and immunoglobulin gene rearrangement studies may be critical to exclude the possibility of lymphoma. However, exceedingly rare cases of light chain restricted monoclonal lymphoid cells have been reported in reactive germinal centers (Nam-Cha et al., 2008). Therefore the presence of a monoclonal population does not necessarily denote a malignant lymphoma, particularly in cases where the morphologic features are conventional for FH. Clonal T-cell proliferations have also been reported in viral infections associated with FH (Farhi et al., 1993; Yasuda et al., 1996; Mathew et al., 2001).

Differential Diagnosis

The morphologic features of reactive and florid FH are distinctive. However, there is a broad range of disorders that show reactive hyperplastic follicles as a dominant morphologic pattern, thereby mimicking otherwise idiopathic FH. These disorders include autoimmune disorders (rheumatoid arthritis, systemic lupus erythematosus, Sjögren's syndrome), immune deficiencies (primary immunodeficiency [see below] and early stage human immunodeficiency virus infection), multicentric Castleman's disease, infections, interfollicular Hodgkin lymphoma, early involvement by various B- and T-cell lymphomas, as well as progressive transformation of germinal centers (PTGC). Rare cases of florid FH may represent a post-transplant lymphoproliferative disorder. Viral infections mimicking florid FH include Epstein–Barr virus, infectious mononucleosis, cytomegalovirus, herpes virus, and rarely hepatitis B and hepatitis C infections. There is no correlation between Epstein–Barr virus infection and the incidence of florid reactive FH. Syphilis, toxoplasmosis, and numerous bacterial and fungal infections can show florid RH as a prevailing morphologic pattern. In toxoplasmosis, however, there are in addition clusters of epithelioid histiocytes within or surrounding germinal centers as well as monocytoid B lymphocytes distending the sinuses. In children and younger individuals, additional entities included in the differential include autoimmune lymphoproliferative syndrome, Kimura's disease, and necrotizing histiocytic lymphadenitis (Kikuchi–Fujimoto disease) (Dorfman et al., 1973; Dorfman et al., 1975; Symmers, 1978; Henry, 1972; Vakiani et al., 2007; Tanizawa et al., 1996).

Reactive FH can also morphologically mimic lymphoma, especially in cases showing prominent nodular pattern, florid hyperplasia, expanded mantle or marginal zones, follicular lysis, and cells containing pale clear cytoplasm. Although the basic architecture of a reactive lymph node is maintained, there is always a possibility of partial or focal involvement by lymphoma. Preserved follicular architecture is most notably seen in interfollicular Hodgkin lymphoma, follicular lymphoma in situ, and focal involvement of paracortical areas by T cell lymphoma. Interfollicular Hodgkin's lymphoma may be concealed amongst numerous hyperplastic lymphoid follicles (Figure 13.5). Partial involvement by follicular lymphoma and follicular lymphoma in situ are challenging to differentiate from reactive FH and may require the aid of monoclonality, cytogenetic, and/or molecular studies. The nodular variant of lymphocyte predominant Hodgkin's lymphoma may mimic the nodular pattern of FH as well. Various B cell lymphomas, particularly those exhibiting a mantle or marginal pattern can also mimic reactive FH. In patients over the age of 50 years, the presence of reactive FH promptly obligates a search for B-cell lymphoma, T-cell lymphoma, or interfollicular Hodgkin's lymphoma (Campo et al., 1999; Kojima et al., 2002; Spencer et al., 1998; van Krieken et al., 1989; Van Krieken et al., 1990; Schnitzer, 2001).

It is often necessary to differentiate between follicular lymphoma and florid reactive FH. The most reliable feature in distinguishing benign from neoplastic follicles is the density and distribution of the follicles in the lymph node, best seen on low-power

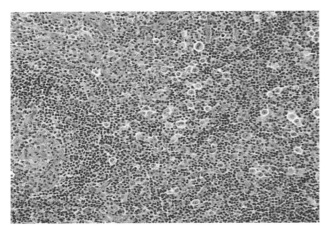

FIGURE 13.5 **Classic Reed–Sternberg cells dotting the interfollicular areas to the right adjacent to residual follicle on the left**.

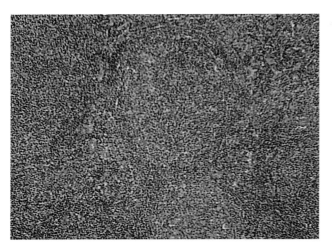

FIGURE 13.6 **Follicular lymphoma showing back-to-back follicles that are similar in size and without polarity**. The neoplastic cells are monomorphous and spill into the interfollicular areas. The mantle zones (bottom) are indistinct, attenuated and broken in areas where lymphoma coalesces beyond the round contours.

magnification. Neoplastic follicles of follicular lymphoma are generally densely packed, back to back and tend to efface lymph node architecture (Figure 13.6). Reactive follicles are not as densely packed and do not obliterate lymph node architecture and show polarization. Commonly in reactive FH the follicles are not as uniform and are more irregular than in follicular lymphoma. Moreover in follicular lymphoma the B cells are not only in the follicles but also in the interfollicular areas. In contrast, in reactive FH, B cells are rare in the interfollicular regions. Reactive germinal centers contain a polymorphic population of variably sized small to large lymphocytes, macrophages,

and dendritic cells. In contrast, neoplastic follicles are primarily monomorphic and may contain vast number of small cleaved cells. The amount of mitotic figures, tingible body macrophages, and apoptotic debris is generally greater in reactive follicles than in neoplastic follicles. However, neoplastic follicles in rare cases may contain prominent tingible body macrophages, numerous T cells, numerous plasma cells, and/or mitotic figures, mimicking reactive FH. Interfollicular plasmacytosis may also rarely involve the interfollicular areas in follicular lymphoma. Thus additional studies such as flow cytometry, cytogenetics, and/or molecular analysis may be warranted in these cases.

In follicular patterns, Bcl-2 is widely utilized to distinguish follicular lymphoma from follicular hyperplasia. The Bcl-2 protein prolongs cell survival by inhibiting apoptosis. It is overexpressed in follicular lymphoma primarily as a result of the t(14;18)(q32;q21) translocation. Bcl-2 can also be overexpressed in most other small B cell non-Hodgkin's lymphomas, and occasionally in diffuse large B-cell and peripheral T-cell lymphomas. The majority of follicular lymphomas contain neoplastic B cells expressing Bcl-2, Bcl-6, CD10, CD20, CD79a, and PAX5. Only approximately 10 to 15% of cases of follicular lymphoma are Bcl-2 negative by immunohistochemistry. In contrast, reactive follicle B cells are characteristically Bcl-2 negative by immunohistochemistry. Similar to follicular lymphoma, reactive follicles also can express Bcl-6 and CD10. Given that T cells in germinal centers are also Bcl-2 positive, it is advisable to perform a T-cell marker such as CD3 in conjunction with Bcl-2. CD10, Bcl-6, PAX5, and specific B cell markers (CD20 and CD79a) can aid in outlining large clusters and sheets of neoplastic cells in the interfollicular and/or extracapsular areas. The presence of monoclonal B-cell population by flow cytometry often showing co-expression of Bcl-2 and strong expression of CD10 is supportive of follicular lymphoma (Lai et al., 1998; Zutter et al., 1991; Dogan et al., 2000).

The lymphocytes of benign primary follicles are uniform and may appear monomorphic, thus deceptively mimicking the monomorphism of neoplastic follicles of low-grade lymphomas with a prominent nodular pattern such as follicular lymphoma, mantle cell lymphoma, marginal zone lymphoma, and small lymphocytic lymphoma. Primary follicles in FH contain predominantly unstimulated naïve small mantle zone B lymphocytes admixed with follicular dendritic cell networks. Primary follicles are not as densely packed as lymphoma and lack centroblasts. Furthermore primary follicles express B-cell markers and are Bcl-2 positive but lack expression of germinal center markers such as Bcl-6 and CD10. Primary follicles can also express CD5, surface IgM, and surface IgD. In contrast, neoplastic follicles may show co-expression of Bcl-2, Bcl-6, and/or CD10.

Reactive FH exhibiting hyperplasia of the marginal and mantle zones is exceedingly rare in peripheral lymph nodes. The spleen and frequently mesenteric lymph nodes normally can contain well-formed marginal zones surrounding the mantle zones. In peripheral lymph nodes, the marginal zones are typically absent, indiscernible and/or admixed with small mantle zone B lymphocytes (Isaacson, 2001; van Krieken et al., 1990; Van den Ord et al., 1986). FH with marginal zone hyperplasia can mimic lymphomas exhibiting a marginal zone distribution pattern. Likewise FH with prominent mantle zone hyperplasia can mimic mantle cell lymphoma. B-cell lymphomas exhibiting a marginal zone distribution pattern include nodal and extranodal marginal zone lymphoma, mantle zone lymphoma with marginal zone differentiation, follicular lymphoma with marginal zone differentiation, floral variant of follicular lymphoma with marginal zone differentiation, and small lymphocytic lymphoma with proliferation centers. The proliferation centers of small lymphocytic lymphoma can infrequently surround mantle zones imitating a marginal zone pattern. Hyperplastic mantle zone cells containing cells with moderate amounts of pale clear cytoplasm can also resemble marginal zone B cells, thus mimicking lymphomas with a marginal zone pattern. Additionally perifollicular lymphocytes with pale clear cytoplasm may signify partial involved by hairy cell leukemia, T-cell lymphoma, and mastocytosis. Therefore nodal cells with clear cytoplasm may represent B cells, T cells, leukemic cells, or mast cells. FH with a prominent marginal zone pattern may also be seen in association with human immunodeficiency virus infection, toxoplasmosis, cat-scratch disease and various viral (Epstein-Barr virus) and bacterial infections. There may be concomitant FH with a prominent mantle zone pattern in lymph nodes of patients with Castleman's disease (Hsu et al., 1983; Hunt et al., 2001; Van Krieken et al., 1990; Kojima et al., 2005).

In follicular lysis, clusters of small lymphocytes dissolve and disaggregate the germinal centers (see Figure 13.7). FH showing follicular lysis can mimic morphologically certain autoimmune disorders such as systemic lupus erythematosus, immunodeficiencies such as human immunodeficiency virus infection, and lymphomas such as the floral variant of follicular lymphoma or the floral variant of marginal zone B-cell

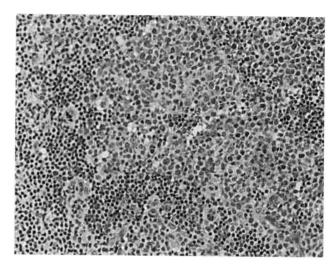

FIGURE 13.7 **Follicle lysis with disaggregated germinal center showing hemorrhage and follicular fragmentation**.

lymphoma. The floral variant of marginal zone lymphoma is exceedingly rare and characterized by the proliferation of neoplastic marginal zone cells surrounding expanded mantle zones and hyperplastic follicles, some of which have undergone follicular lysis. Progressively transformed germinal centers may be evident in the floral variant of marginal zone lymphoma as well (Karube et al., 2005; Kojima et al., 2005; Goates et al., 1994; Osborne et al., 1982).

FH with associated paracortical hyperplasia may inadvertently resemble early involvement by angioimmunoblastic T-cell lymphoma (AITL), especially if there are regressed follicles and increased vascularity. AITL should be suspected in patients with unusual symptoms and signs such as high fever, autoantibodies (rheumatoid factor), polyclonal hypergammaglobulinemia, edema, ascites, pleural effusion, circulating immune complexes, or other immune reactions such as autoimmune hemolytic anemia, immune thrombocytopenic purpura, itchy skin rash, or arthritis. The interfollicular neoplastic T cells of AITL often express CD5, CD10, Bcl-6, and PD-1 (CD279) indicating follicular T helper subset derivation. There is variable expression of CD4, CD8, CD30, and Epstein–Barr virus and lack expression of CD20 and CD15 on the neoplastic T cells. In contrast, in reactive FH there are no large aggregates of CD10 or Bcl-6 positive cells in the interfollicular regions. A characteristic feature of AITL is the expanded and disrupted dendritic cell networks around the neoplastic proliferation (Kojima et al., 2001).

Treatment and Prognosis

Idiopathic reactive FH is a benign and does not require treatment. However, in cases where an underlying disorder (infection, autoimmune, immunodeficiency, malignancy) is evident, treatment of the underlying disorder is warranted. In individuals older than 50 years of age who present with follicular hyperplasia, an increased risk of lymphomas is reported and additional studies may be needed to exclude presence of malignancy.

REGRESSIVE TRANSFORMATION OF GERMINAL CENTER (ATROPHIC) PATTERN

Castleman's Hyaline Vascular Pattern

Castleman's disease (CD) is a rare atypical lymphoproliferative disorder with a diversity of clinical presentations and morphologic variants. CD encompasses mainly three morphologic variants (hyaline vascular, plasma cell, and mixed) and two clinical manifestations (unicentric or multicentric). Unicentric (unifocal) CD is localized and solitary, usually asymptomatic and presents as an isolated mass, regional adenopathy or swelling. Unicentric CD is considered a benign disorder usually with an indolent course and may present with or without systemic symptoms. Complete resection of unicentric CD is considered curative and typically confers resolution of any clinical symptoms. Only rare cases of hyaline vascular CD recur subsequent to complete excision. Multicentric (multifocal) CD is a generalized multiorgan systemic disorder with constitutional symptoms characterized by fever, anemia, cytopenias, fatigue, night sweats, weight loss, anorexia, pain, hypergammaglobulinemia, generalized lymphadenopathy, and hepatosplenomegaly. Multicentric CD often requires more aggressive therapy and signifies a poorer prognosis often with disease recurrences. Multicentric CD also has an increased risk of progression to malignant neoplasms including lymphoma and Kaposi's sarcoma. Mixed type of CD presents with characteristics of both Hyaline Vascular and plasma cell types; although the clinical features are more frequently multicentric resembling PC type (Fazakas et al., 2009; Newlon et al., 2007).

Benjamin Castleman et al. in 1956 first described CD as a new disease entity in patients who presented with asymptomatic localized enlarged mediastinal lymph nodes in which there was involution of germinal centers associated with striking capillary proliferation. (Castleman et al., 1956). In 1969, Flendrig et al. (Flendrig et al., 1969) and in 1972, Keller et al. (Keller et al., 1972) elaborated on the various morphologic

and clinical features to further subclassify CD and introduce the plasma cell type. In the 1980s, Frizzera et al. (Frizzera et al., 1983) subsequently defined the clinical subtypes and morphologic variants of CD into localized HV, localized PC, and multicentric types.

The most common variant is the unicentric (localized) HV type, accounting for 72 to 91% of all cases of CD. Approximately 90% of unicentric (localized) CD is of the HV type. The HV type is further classified into the lymphoid subtype and stroma-rich subtype. Multicentric variant accounts for up to 20% of cases of CD and consists primarily of the PC type and rarely of the plasmablastic (PB) type. Multicentric CD of the HV type is exceedingly rare. The mixed variant comprises 2 to 10% of CD cases and is more commonly multicentric. Unicentric and multicentric CD have similar overlapping morphologic features in common despite their dissimilar clinical presentations. CD is a clinicopathologic diagnosis of exclusion since other diseases can show identical morphologic features (Roca et al., 2009; Martino et al., 2004).

Definition

Castleman disease (CD) is a polyclonal B-cell lymphoproliferative disorder characterized by unique morphology of follicular involution or hyperplasia associated with prominent vascularity, plasmacytosis, and by a variant associated with human herpesvirus type 8(HHV-8) infection. CD may occur in any location in which there is lymphoid tissue.

ICD-10 Codes Hyaline Vascular type   D21.9
            Plasma cell   D47.9

Neoplasm of uncertain or unknown behavior of lymphoid haematoporietic and related tissue, unspecified M8000/1.

Synonyms

Angiofollicular hyperplasia, angiofollicular lymph node hyperplasia, angiofollicular lymphoid hyperplasia, angiomatous lymphoid hamartoma, angiomatous lymphoid hamartoma, angiomatous lymphoid hyperplasia, angiofollicular mediastinal lymph node hyperplasia, angiofollicular and plasmacytic polyadenopathy, benign giant lymphoma, benign giant lymphoma, Castleman's lymphoma, follicular lymphoreticuloma, giant lymph node hyperplasia, idiopathic plasmacytic lymphadenopathy with polyclonal hypergammaglobulinemia, lymphoid hamartoma, lymph node harmatoma, lymph nodal harmartoma, localized hamartoma, multicentric angiofollicular hyperplasia (Ghosh et al., 2010; Newlon, 2007).

Epidemiology

The incidence of CD in the general population is unknown. However, in the United States, the case population prevalence of CD is estimated as ranging from 30,000 to 100,000 cases (Casper, 2005).

Clinical Aspects

CD can be found any body regions where lymphoid tissue is normally present such as in the mediastinum, retroperitoneal, abdomen, mesentery, and inguinal regions. Rarely, CD may affect a number of extranodal sites, including the cranium and brain, classically as a meningeal rooted intracranial lesion, spine, orbit, lung, nasopharynx, adrenal, paraadrenal, pararenal, face, skin, buccal mucosa, parotid gland, submandibular, pericardium, head and neck, chest wall, pelvis, thorax, shoulder, vulva, pancreas, stomach, colorectal, liver, spleen, muscle, broad ligament, and soft tissues of the extremities. The clinical manifestations of CD depend on the morphologic variant (Ghosh et al., 2010; Liang et al., 2009; McCarty et al., 1995).

Unicentric CD of the HV type presents most commonly as a slow-growing mass found as an incidental finding on imaging studies. It is typically benign and self-limiting with a five-year survival reported as nearly 100%. HV occurs predominantly in young adults, mostly between the second and fourth decades, though the age ranges from 2 months to the eight decade of life. There is no gender predominance (Roca, 2009). Most patients are asymptomatic frequently presenting with a mass in the mediastinum, abdomen, pelvis, cervical neck, axilla, or peripheral lymph nodes. Mediastinal presentation is the most common, occurring in up to two-thirds of patients. Node-based disease is significantly more common than disease in extranodal sites. Occasional patients exhibit symptoms related to compression of adjacent organs or mass effect such as postprandial discomfort, vomiting, weight loss, urinary retention, cough, dyspnea, hemoptysis, respiratory infection, gastric or colonic erosions, gastric outlet obstruction, or intestinal obstruction; back and chest pain may exist as well. (Liang et al., 2009). Other systems related to inflammation—B-cell hyperactivity, and immune dysregulation occur but are uncommon. Fever, weight loss, anemia, elevated erythrocyte sedimentation rate, lymphadenopathy, and polyclonal hypergammaglobulinemia—are more common in patients with unicentric CD of the PC type but may be seen in the unicentric HV type. While similar symptoms may be detected in multicentric CD, patients with multicentric CD exhibit a more aggressive, sometimes fatal clinical course (Ghosh et al., 2010; Martino et al., 2004; Newlon et al., 2007).

Multicentric CD develops in an array of clinical settings. Multicentric CD more frequently presents in mesenteric and/or retroperitoneal nodal or extranodal tissues. It is more common in extranodal sites such as the retroperitoneum, mesentery, chest wall, and viscera organs than the unicentric type. Patients with multicentric CD of the PC type are, in general, older than patients with unicentric CD, presenting in the fifth to sixth decades of life. The clinical course is usually unpredictable from indolent cases with flocculating clinical symptoms to more aggressive cases with a fulminant clinical course. Symptoms and signs are related to chronic inflammatory and immunologic stimuli manifesting as fatigue, fever, anemia, elevated erythrocyte sedimentation rate, increased acute phase proteins (C-reactive protein, fibrinogen), and polyclonal hyperglobulinemia. The majority of patients with multicentric CD of the PC type have polyclonal hyperimmunoglobulinemia; however, rare cases of monoclonal immunoglobulins have also been reported. (Fazakas et al., 2009). Rarely, patients may be asymptomatic. Additionally multicentric CD patients exhibit symptoms of renal dysfunction including proteinuria, hematuria, renal insufficiency, and nephrotic syndrome. Secondary systemic amyloidosis, central nervous system involvement with pseudotumor cerebri, peripheral neuropathy, growth retardation, gynecomastia, pure red cell aplasia, skin hyperpigmentation, thrombocytosis, coagulopathy, hypogammaglobulinemia, hypoalbuminemia, and IgA paraproteinemia may be associated findings. Central nervous system involvement in some patients may result in death (Newlon et al., 2007; McCarty et al., 1995 Peterson et al., 1993). Both the PC and HV types may be associated with autoimmune related disorders such as systemic lupus erythematosus (SLE), secondary amyloidosis of AA type, Sjögren's syndrome, myasthenia gravis, autoimmune hemolytic anemia, thrombotic thrombocytopenic purpura, cytopenias, rheumatoid arthritis with Raynaud's phenomenon and joint effusions, Bechet's disease, lymphoid interstitial pneumonitis, bronchiolitis obliterans, and a variety of renal disorders such as membranous nephropathy, temporal arteritis, pemphigus vulgaris, and paraneoplastic pemphigus (PNP). PNP is a rare autoimmune mucocutaneous disorder frequently seen in association with lymphoid neoplasms. (Hung et al., 2006; Menenakos et al., 2007; Hsiao et al., 2001; Martino et al., 2004).

In patients with human immunodeficiency virus (HIV) there is an increased prevalence of CD, usually of the multicentric PC or mixed types. The incidence of CD shows no relation to the CD4 cell count, degree of immunodeficiency or viral load in HIV positive patients. Patients with HIV also often have concomitant Kaposi's sarcoma. The Kaposi sarcoma-associated herpesvirus (KSHV) also known as the human herpesvirus-8 (HHV-8) is associated with almost all of the HIV positive CD and over 50% of HIV negative multicentric CD. Kaposi's sarcoma may also present in a minor population of unicentric cases. Interleukin-6 (IL-6) levels are remarkably elevated in multicentric CD. Since HHV-8 encodes a homologue of IL-6, it is postulated that IL-6 mediates the systemic manifestations of multicentric CD. Clinical symptoms in HIV positive patients with CD have a tendency to be more aggressive with considerable morbidity and mortality (Stebbing, 2008; Mylona, 2008; Barbounis et al., 1996; Waterston et al., 2004).

CD does coexist with and/or progresses to a variety of malignancies. These include Kaposi's sarcoma, other sarcomas such as dendritic cell sarcoma, vascular tumors, non-Hodgkin's lymphoma, Hodgkin's lymphoma, peripheral T-cell lymphoma, Waldenström macroglobulinemia, and other Kaposi's sarcoma associated herpes virus (KSHV)/HHV-8 related neoplasms such as primary effusion lymphoma and multicentric CD-associated plasmablastic lymphoma. In HIV positive patients the progression to lymphoma is significantly higher in those with CD than in HIV patients who do not have CD. Progression to Hodgkin's lymphoma occurs most commonly in CD of the PC type and may involve interfollicular regions. Thymoma has also been reported in patients with CD (Stebbing et al., 2008; Amin et al., 2003; Casper, 2005).

POEMS syndrome is an infrequent paraneoplastic disorder caused by an underlying plasma cell dyscrasia. Even though a variety of plasma cell disorders can occur in patients with POEMS syndrome, the majority of patients have either osteosclerotic myeloma or monoclonal gammopathy of unknown significance. Approximately 11 to 30% of POEMS patients have CD or a CD-like disorder. POEMS was initially recognized by Scheinker in 1938, and the term POEMS was used in 1980 by Bardwick et al. to describe the disease. POEMS is also known as Takatsuki syndrome, or Crow–Fukasa syndrome. It is defined as the presence of (P)polyneuropathy, (O)organomegaly [splenomegaly, hepatomegaly, or lymphadenopathy], (E)endocrinopathy [adrenal, thyroid, pituitary, gonadal, parathyroid, pancreatic], (M) monoclonal protein, and (S) skin changes. The neuropathy is regarded as required to render a diagnosis of POEMS. POEMS syndrome is also associated with other clinical features manifestations including

sclerotic or mixed sclerotic and lytic bone lesions, increased vascular endothelial growth factor (VEGF) levels, fever, anasarca, papilledema, finger clubbing, hyperhidrosis, extravascular volume excess (edema, pleural effusions, ascites), hematologic disorders (thrombocytosis, polycythemia), cardiomyopathy, pulmonary dysfunction, thrombosis, hypercalcemia, renal insufficiency, gynecomastia, diarrhea, arthralgias, low vitamin B_{12} values, and muscular atrophy. Patients may also present with hypothalamic dysfunction. Up to 95% of patients with POEMS will have a monoclonal lambda-restricted plasmacytoma and/or increased bone marrow plasma cells. Typically the bone marrow reveals up to 5% plasma cells. Patients with concomitant multicentric MCD and POEMS are more likely to be infected with HHV-8 (Dispenzieri, 2007; Huang et al., 2007; Dispenzieri et al., 2004; Leiti et al., 2007; Kreft et al., 2007).

In children, CD is primarily unicentric and benign. It is more frequent in the mesentery and less common in the thorax in children than in adults. Anemia, hypergammaglobulinemia, and failure to thrive denote the main clinical presentations of CD in children. Children with CD have better prognosis than adults (Baserga et al., 2005; Buesing et al., 2009).

Pathophysiology

The pathogenesis of CD of PC type remains not entirely elucidated; however, immune dysregulation, chronic inflammatory processes, infection, and immunodeficiency states have been implicated as causative factors. Human herpesvirus-8 (HHV-8) infection plays an important role in the pathogenesis of multicentric CD. HHV-8, particularly in immunocompromised individuals, also is a cause of Kaposi's sarcoma, primary effusion lymphoma, and multicentric CD-associated plasmablastic lymphoma. The genome of HHV-8 encodes an analogue of the interleulin-6 (IL-6) gene, which can induce endogenous human IL-6 secretion. HHV-8 infection can also stimulate B lymphocytes and immunoblasts to produce IL-6 especially in nodal mantle zones (Roca, 2009; Newlon et al., 2007; Good et al., 2009; Martino et al., 2004). Abnormal production of IL-6, either as a result of stimulation by HHV-8 infection or less commonly by other cytokines, seems to mediate the initial phase of induction of multicentric CD. IL-6, either by autocrine or by paracrine stimulation, promotes proliferation of lymphoid cells, resulting in polyclonal hypergammaglobulinemia with plasma cell hyperplasia. Plasma cells consequently produce a vascular endothelial growth factor (VEGF) that in turn promotes angiogenesis, resulting in CD's attributing hypervascularity (Oksenhendler et al., 2002; Choi et al., 2008).

In HHV-8 negative CD, other exogenous or endogenous factors may promote production of IL-6 by B lymphocytes. Circulating IL-6 most likely is responsible for the systemic symptoms of CD (Casper, 2005). IL-6 also plays a role in amyloid precursor serum amyloid A protein production in the liver, which may result in systemic amyloidosis (Androulaki et al., 2007) Other viruses such as Epstein–Barr virus (EBV) are also highly associated with CD of either PC or HV types. EBV within germinal cells and interfollicular areas is reported to stimulate B cells to produce IL-6 and other cytokines, thereby promoting angiogenesis (Casper, 2005; Hung et al., 2006; Chen et al., 2009).

CD of HV type is postulated to be a disorder of aberrant stromal cells and may represent a developmental or hamartomatous disorder. Follicular dendritic cells (FDCs) play a critical role in the pathogenesis of HV. FDC are essential in maintaining and developing normal nodal architecture. FDC have been shown to harbor clonal cytogenetic abnormalities, suggesting that genetic aberrations in stromal cells may be the initial step in HV development. It is unclear whether these clonal aberrations signal a primary or secondary phenomenon in the pathogenesis of HV CD. Abnormalities of FDC are related to poor follicle formation and stromal overgrowth. Neoplastic FDC proliferations, including FDC sarcoma, are also known to coexist with HV CD. HHV-8 and IL-6 are not considered to be significant in the pathogenesis of HV CD (Vasudev Rao et al., 2007; Lee et al., 2008).

Clinical Workup and Approach to Diagnosis

Surgical resection with morphologic evaluation is recommended for a definitive diagnosis of CD. Other causes of lymphadenopathy with similar morphology to CD such as malignancy, rheumatoid arthritis, lupus, Sjögren's and drug sensitivity should be clinically excluded. Disease activity may be followed by assessing for serum IgG, C reactive protein, erythrocyte sedimentation rate, and lactate dehydrogenase. Serum interleukin-6 and HHV-8 levels in patients with systemic symptoms may aid in determining treatment modalities. Close clinical follow-up is recommended for patients with multicentric CD. Follow-up radiological evaluation within 6 to 12 months post therapy may be helpful in assessing for disease cure (Roca, 2009; Casper, 2005).

Although radiologic findings are nonspecific and not pathognomonic for CD, CT scans can aid in differentiating unicentric versus multicentric forms.

The CT scan typically reveals a solid, homogeneous, hypervascular, well-demarcated mass with or without microcalcifications that enhances with intravenous contrast. Typically there is no necrosis or liquefaction. The PC type shows lesser enhancement due to the reduced vascularity. Magnetic resonance imaging of CD reveals an isointense or low intensity on T1-weighted images and higher signal intensity on T2-weighted images. Angiography shows a highly vascular tumor with distinct arterial supply and irregular vascular channels without arteriovenous shunting (Jongsma et al., 2007).

Morphologic Aspects

The gross appearance of CD is characteristically fleshy to granular, tan-yellow to gray-red, firm, partially encapsulated, and well circumscribed. Every compartment of a lymph node is affected in CD. The term hyaline vascular (HV) entails the distinctive morphology of penetrating thickened hyalinized vessels entering the follicles from the mantle zones and interfollicular areas. In HV CD the lymph node architecture is partially effaced and distorted by increased numbers of variably sized, poorly formed follicles with an abnormal morphology exhibiting a lollipop-like and/or targetoid appearance, with or without germinal center formation. Lymph node sinuses are often compressed and rarely discernable (Figure 13.8). The follicles are often hypervascular and involuted (burned-out) or regressively transformed with lymphoid depletion and obliteration by dense hyalinization. A characteristic feature of CD is larger follicles containing double or triple atrophic

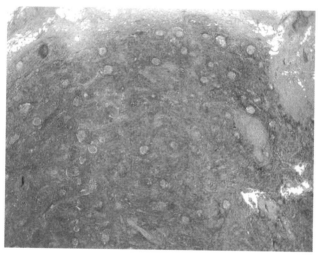

FIGURE 13.8 Enlarged lymph node with numerous small germinal centers with surrounding pink hypervascular interfollicular areas.

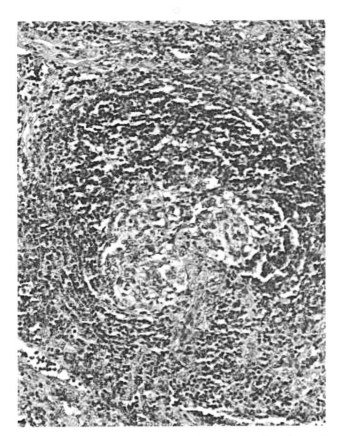

FIGURE 13.9 "Lollipop" germinal center with sclerosed vessel penetrating its center and surrounding rim of small mantle zone lymphocytes vessels.

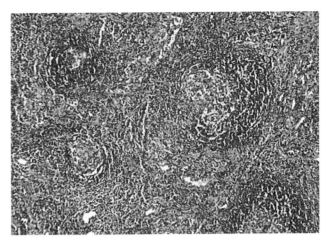

FIGURE 13.10 Slightly thickened mantle zones surrounding atrophic or regressed germinal centers containing sclerosed vessels.

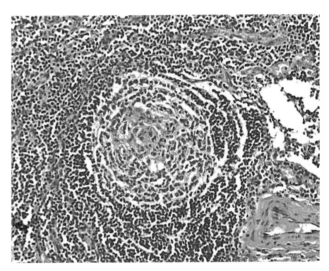

FIGURE 13.11 Targetoid or onion skin tightly packed layer mantle cells surrounding a regressed germinal center.

germinal centers. Occasionally the eosinophilic material within the follicles may denote apoptotic cellular debris of follicle-derived lymphocytes. Thick-walled hyalinized branching vessels, capillaries, and arterioles, with hypertrophic endothelium, perpendicularly penetrate the regressed follicles and mantle zones, imparting a lollipop-like appearance (Figure 13.9). Broadened and expanded, often thickened, mantle zones often rim the follicles. The mantle zones are often arranged in orderly concentric tightly packed layers, composed of small to medium size lymphocytes without significant cytologic atypia (Figure 13.10). This layering of lymphocytes forms a prominent targetoid or onion skin or onion bulb or stadium seating appearance (Figure 13.11). Occasionally B cells with clear cytoplasm are present within the hyperplastic marginal zones and mantle zones (Ghosh et al., 2010; Peh et al., 2003; Stebbing et al., 2008; Chen et al., 2006).

Follicular dendritic cells within the regressively transformed follicles are prominent, showing large vesicular nuclei and a disrupted disorganized pattern. These follicular dendritic cells proliferate to form an extrafollicular expanded meshwork radiating from the follicles into the mantle zones. Interfollicular areas are frequently hypervascular and expanded by a striking proliferation of arborizing vessels including capillaries and high endothelial (postcapillary) venules. These branching vessels display hyalinized walls containing hyperplastic plump endothelial cells. Interfollicular regions are commonly hypocellular and may be stromal rich, containing a proliferation of stromal elements such as plasmacytoid dendritic cells (also known as plasmacytoid monocytes) showing CD68, CD45RA and CD123 expression, follicular dendritic cells, and/or fibroblastic reticulum cells (myofibroblastic cells). Foci of calcification and significant fibrosis or sclerosis may also be present. Other inflammatory cells including small lymphocytes, predominantly T cells, polyclonal plasma cells, eosinophils, immunoblasts, monocytes, and histiocytes are frequently present but are few in numbers. Intervening area of normal lymph node morphology may be present. Adjacent lymph nodes may also demonstrate occasional follicles with hyaline vascular morphology (Ghosh et al., 2010; Lee et al., 2008; Baserga et al., 2005).

The HV type is further subdivided into a lymphoid subtype in which there is marked expansion of the mantle zones and a stroma-rich subtype with a predominance of the vascular and stromal components. The lymphoid variant of HV refers to cases where there is marked expansion of the mantle zones with medium size lymphocytes containing moderate amounts of clear cytoplasm and round or slightly indented nuclei. Germinal centers are small and inconspicuous in the lymphoid subtype of HV (Kojima et al., 2008). Follicular dendritic cell networks are densely packed. Small foci of plasmacytoid monocytes may be present, and there is minimum interfollicular vascularity. The morphologic features of the lymphoid subtype of HV demonstrating mantle zone hyperplasia composed of clear cells is similar to nodal marginal zone B-cell lymphoma, mantle cell lymphoma, and follicular lymphoma. Therefore in this subtype immunophenotypic and genotypic studies may be essential to rule out lymphoma. Reactive lymph nodes only infrequently show mantle cell hyperplasia with clear cytoplasm (Ghosh, 2010; Kojima, 2005; Hunz et al., 2001).

In CD of the PC type there is striking follicular hyperplasia associated with plasmacytosis, expansion of interfollicular and paracortical areas, as well as dilatation of sinuses At varying times there may be either a proliferative period with very florid proliferation of interfollicular plasma cells, immunoblasts and hyalinized high endothelial venules, or an accumulative period with normal amounts of plasma cells and vascularity. There is no associated immunoblastic proliferation in the accumulative stage classically. Rarely, a burned-out period is present with regressively transformed germinal centers, collapsed vessels, and sparse plasmacytosis, mimicking CD of the HV type. There is less prominent vascular proliferation in the PC CD than in the HV type. The follicle dendritic cell networks of the PC CD are reported as analogous to that of normal and/or reactive lymph nodes. The bone marrow of patients with CD of the PC type often shows plasmacytosis. Within the spleen there is reactive follicular hyperplasia associated with white pulp polyclonal plasmacytosis, and frequent focal fibrosis. Plasmacytoid lymphocytes surrounding splenic follicles and subcapsular areas may also appear prominent (Peterson, 1993; Good et al., 2009; McCarty et al., 1995; Roca, 2009; Peh et al., 2003; Lee et al., 2008).

In lymph nodes of CD of the PC type, the germinal centers are often prominent and hyperplastic, with ill-defined borders and expanded vascularity. The majority of follicles appears large but may be of variable size. Regressed hyalinized follicles may also occasionally occur. Amorphous acidophilic deposits most likely consisting of fibrin and immune complexes, numerous mitotic figures, nuclear fragments, and histiocytes can be seen within the follicles. Florid polyclonal plasmacytosis intermittently occurring with an immunoblastic proliferation is a characteristic striking feature in CD of the PC type.

Plasmacytosis occurs in surrounding intact follicles, in interfollicular and perisinusoidal areas, as well as in the medulla of lymph nodes. Occasional histiocytes, lymphocytes, and immunoblasts are mingled with the plasma cells. Numerous Russell bodies may be evident. Mantle zones appear partially dissolved and narrower as well as mostly replaced by plasma cells. Rarely, there is a light chain restricted or a predominant plasma cell population. The monoclonal plasma cells of CD may not necessarily undergo progression to widespread disease and may be confined to the lymph nodes. In rare cases, germinal centers may also contain light chain restriction plasmablasts. Nevertheless, the presence of monoclonality, connotes the necessity to further investigate for transformation to a B-cell lymphoma with plasmacytic differentiation or a plasma cell dyscrasia (Peterson, 1993; Amin et al., 2003; Good et al., 2009).

Multicentric CD of the plasmablastic type is most commonly seen in patients with HIV infection and/or POEMS. It is associated mainly with an aggressive clinical course. It is distinguished by increased numbers of plasmablasts morphologically resembling immunoblasts within expanded mantle zones and in germinal centers. The plasmablasts are medium to large size with moderate amounts of amphophilic cytoplasm, large vesicular nuclei, and single or multiple prominent nucleoli. The plasmablasts are scattered or arranged in small clusters without sheeting out and may comprise up to one-half of mantle zone elements. Sheets of plasmablasts are concerning and raise the possibility of progression to plasmablastic lymphoma. Germinal centers are often regressed or dissolved. Mantle zones typically appear indistinct with blurred borders with the interfollicular regions. Sinuses are commonly dilated. Follicular dendritic cells are frequently prominent.

There is an associated marked vascular proliferation with endothelial hyperplasia in both follicular and interfollicular areas (Dupin et al., 2000; Stebbing et al., 2008). In nearly all patients the plasmablasts are positive for HHV-8 latent nuclear antigen 1 (LANA1) and the IgM heavy chain. A lambda light chain restricted plasmablast population is common; however, the vast majority of cases do not show clonal immunoglobulin gene rearrangements by molecular analysis. This implies that the HHV-8 infection evokes a monoclonal plasmablastic phenotype but is a polyclonal molecular B-cell proliferation. Plasmablasts can also co-express CD20 and are negative for CD138. IgM positive immunoblasts are also present in the interfollicular areas. Mature plasma cells are HHV-8 negative and do not show lambda light chain predominance or restriction. HHV-8 is also positive in the expanded follicular dendritic cells. Co-infection with EBV has also been detected in these cases (El-Daly et al., 2010; Good et al., 2009).

CD of the mixed type shows a hybrid morphology with features of both the HV and PC subtypes. It is characterized by the presence of atrophic regressed germinal centers with the central sclerosis cuffed by an onion skin pattern of lymphocytes. There is expansion and disruption of follicular dendritic cell networks within germinal centers and mantle zones with abnormal clustering. Prominent marked vascularity with occasional vessels radially piercing the germinal centers is a characteristic finding. A predominance of plasma cells rim the vasculature (Waterston et al., 2004).

Immunophenotyping/Cytochemistry

Germinal centers generally contain predominantly CD20 positive, CD10 positive, and Bcl-2 negative B lymphocytes. In atrophic germinal centers and their mantle zones, there is a corresponding discernible decrease of Bcl-6 positive B cells and a concomitant striking increase of CD21 positive follicular dendritic cells (FDC). There is also a paucity of CD57 (Leu-7) positive T cells with only few CD57 positive T cells, both of CD4 and CD8 types in atrophic follicles. In contrast, reactive enlarged follicles show increased numbers of both Bcl-6 positive B cells and CD57 positive T cells (Peterson et al., 1993). Polyclonal small lymphocytes composing the expanded mantle zones of the HV type are predominantly B cells positive for CD20, CD22, CD79a, PAX5, Bcl-2 (an apoptosis inhibiting protein), HLA-DR, and IgM and IgD surface heavy chains. In contrast, the mantle zones of the PC type contain both B cells and T cells, similar to that of reactive lymph nodes. Both variants of CD show lower levels of CD5 and Bcl-2 expression in the

mantle zones than that seen in reactive lymph nodes (McCarty et al., 1995).

Atrophic germinal centers and expanded mantle zones of CD of HV type typically show strong reactivity to a variety of FDC markers such as CD21, CD23, CD35, and EGFR. The epidermal growth factor receptor (EGFR) is a novel marker for follicular dendritic cells (FDCs). EGFR is a receptor tyrosine kinase often amplified in human cancers that is responsible for altering proliferative and/or cellular differentiation. These markers outline the abundance of tight concentric FDC networks in these germinal centers and expanded mantle zones. Other antibodies highlighting FDC that show strong reactivity in the HV type include R4/23 (DRC-1), CNA.42, and LNGFR/p75. The LNGFR/p75 antibody outlines both FDC networks as well as other stromal cells including fibroblasts and fibroblastic reticular cells. In contrast, the expression of FDC markers in the PC type tends to be similar to that of normal and/or reactive lymph nodes (Vasudev Rao et al., 2007; Chen et al., 2006; Kojima et al., 2005).

Anti-interleukin-6 (IL-6) antibody stains detect copious amounts of IL-6 in the germinal centers of CD of the PC type. In contrast, reactive and normal lymph nodes lack this IL-6 staining pattern. The IL-6 gene is expressed in large amounts by follicular dendritic cells (FDCs) in CD of the PC type as well. IL-6 is also expressed in all variants of CD in interfollicular areas by macrophages, interdigitating reticulum cells, lymphocytes, and endothelial cells (Peterson et al., 1993).

A diagnosis of CD also can be supported by positive staining for the HHV-8 antibody. Polyclonal plasma cells can be highlighted by CD138, CD79a, Bcl-2, and CD43 as well as kappa and lambda light chains. Small clusters of plasmacytoid monocytes in the HV type show positive staining for CD4, CD45RA, CD45, and CD68 (PGM-1) and CD123. Hyperplastic endothelial cells can be outlined by factor VIII-related antigen, Ulex europaeus lectin, CD31, CD34 as well as laminin (Pauwels et al., 2000).

Laboratory Diagnosis

A wide variety of laboratory abnormalities can be detected. These include anemia, immune hemolysis, cytopenias (leucopenia and immune thrombocytopenia), thrombocytosis, eosinophilia, lymphocytosis, and plasmacytosis. An elevated erythrocyte sedimentation rate, polyclonal hypergammaglobulins of the IgG, IgM, and IgA types, hypoalbumenia, abnormal liver tests, antinuclear antibodies, the rheumatoid factor, a positive VDRL, cryoglobulins, and inhibitors of factors VII and VIII have been reported. Proteinuria, hematuria, and signs of renal insufficiency and nephrotic syndrome may also be evident (Sato et al., 2009).

Differential Diagnosis

The pathologic features of CD are nonspecific and often overlap with various other benign and malignant disorders. Therefore CD is considered a diagnosis of exclusion. Multicentric CD may morphologically mimic numerous other disorders, including primary immunodeficiencies, autoimmune disorders (systemic lupus erythematosus, Sjogren's and IgG4-related disease), rheumatologic diseases (rheumatoid arthritis), presence of an adjacent neoplasm, idiopathic plasmacytic lymphadenopathy with polyclonal hyperimmunoglobulinemia, POEMS syndrome, drug sensitivity, vaccination site, inflammatory bowel disease, angioimmunoblastic lymphadenopathy, non-Hodgkin's lymphoma, plasma cell dyscrasias, and peripheral T-cell lymphoma. Among these, multicentric CD is comparatively rare. Frequently patients with systemic lupus erythematosus (SLE) show multicentric adenopathy and morphologic features similar to that of either the mixed type or the HV type of CD. Furthermore lymph nodes of patients with SLE also show an altered follicular dendritic cell (FDC) networks. It is imperative to distinguish between SLE and CD clinically due to their therapeutic dissimilarities.

When polyneuropathy is present, distinction between CD and POEMS syndrome can be challenging. Systemic IgG4-related disease and multicentric CD display somewhat similar overlapping pathologic features as well. The systemic IgG4-related disease is a systemic disease, frequently associated with lymphadenopathy, characterized by the diffuse tissue infiltration of various organs by abundant polyclonal IgG4-positive plasma cells and numerous T lymphocytes, in a background of sclerosis and fibrosis. However, serum C-reactive protein and interleukin-6 (IL-6) are generally not elevated in systemic IgG4-related disease. In contrast, serum C-reactive protein and IL-6 are usually increased in multicentric CD (van den Berge et al., 2002; Sato et al., 2009; Barbounis et al., 1996). CD of the PC type frequently coexists in patients with rheumatoid arthritis and angioimmunoblastic lymphadenopathy. Reactive lymphadenopathy due to infectious causes such as human immunodeficiency virus (HIV) infection, syphilis, toxoplasmosis, cytomegalovirus, Epstein–Barr virus infections such as mononucleosis, cat-scratch disease, mycobacterium tuberculosis,

and tularemia are also considered in the differential diagnosis of multicentric CD. However, in cat-scratch disease, tuberculosis, and tularemia, there is also necrotizing granulomatous lymphadenitis (Kojima et al., 2005; Barbounis et al., 1996). Toxic substance ingestion may also be included in the differential diagnosis of CD. Cases of CD like reactions associated with toxic substance ingestion may present with eosinophilia. Rarely, sarcoidosis, thymoma and Kikuchi disease may also enter into the morphologic differential diagnosis of CD (Peterson, 1993; Kojima et al., 2005; van den Berge et al., 2002; Paydas et al., 2009).

The pathologic features of the HV CD can be similar to autoimmune diseases, primary immunodeficiencies, disseminated Kaposi's sarcoma, angioimmunoblastic lymphadenopathy, and the late phase of the HIV infection, since these also can contain regressively transformed germinal centers. Clinical and serologic findings can aid in these distinctions. Likewise several nonspecific reactive lymphadenopathies may show HV like features as well. Calcifying fibrous pseudotumor and inflammatory myofibroblastic tumor may also enter into the morphologic differential diagnosis of the HV type (Peterson, 1993; Azam et al., 2009; Good, et al., 2009).

Both multicentric and unicentric variants of CD are associated with lymphoma. Lymphoma may occur either several years after the onset of CD and/or concurrently with CD (Choi et al., 2008). The most common are low-grade B-cell lymphomas, including extranodal and nodal marginal zone B-cell lymphoma (MALToma), mantle cell lymphoma, follicular lymphoma, and small lymphocytic lymphoma. The lymphoid subtype of HV CD should be morphologically distinguished from lymphomas with a follicular pattern composed of clear cells such as mantle cell lymphoma, marginal zone lymphoma, and follicular lymphoma with marginal zone differentiation. Mantle cell lymphoma is considered in the morphologic differential diagnosis of the lymphoid subtype of the HV CD in view of the expanded mantle zones comprised of clear cells. Furthermore about 5% of cases of mantle cell lymphoma show marginal zone differentiation (Kojima et al., 2008 Kojima et al., 2005). Nodal marginal zone lymphoma may sporadically show a mixed type of CD-like morphology with many regressively transformed germinal centers and interfollicular plasmacytosis mimicking CD.

Moreover classical Hodgkin's disease may have areas showing CD-like germinal centers. Multicentric CD of the PC type may coexist in the same lymph node with interfollicular type of classic Hodgkin's disease. The plasmablastic type of multicentric CD may morphologically mimic HHV-8 positive plasmablastic lymphoma if sheets of monoclonal plasmablasts are present by immunohistochemistry. However, a molecular analysis showing lack of clonal immunoglobulin gene rearrangements can be helpful in the distinction (Dupin et al., 2000; Vasudev Rao et al., 2007). In the skin the differential diagnosis includes various disorders exhibiting increased vascularity including angiolymphoid hyperplasia with eosinophilia, Kimura's disease, sinus histiocytosis, and angioimmunoblastic lymphadenopathy. Low-grade cutaneous B-cell lymphomas such as primary cutaneous marginal zone lymphoma and primary cutaneous follicle center cell lymphoma are also in the differential diagnosis of CD involving the skin (Tomasini et al., 2009).

Treatment of Choice and Prognosis

There is no definite gold standard therapy for CD. Generally, unicentric CD is benign and has excellent prognosis. Complete surgical removal of the lesion is considered nearly always curative for unicentric CD of either the HV and/or PC types. Five-year survival rates of 100% have been reported with only rare recurrences (Martino et al., 2004). Clinical symptoms improve and amyloid deposits partially regress with removal of the mass (Androulaki et al., 2007). There is no consensus on the most effective treatment for incompletely resectable or inoperable cases of unicentric CD. However, prognosis is excellent still for patients with incompletely resectable masses. Radiotherapy has been shown to be efficacious in patients with incomplete excision, unresectable lesions, recurrences, and poor surgical candidates. Chemotherapy is typically not necessary for unicentric CD. However, anti-EGFR agents have been reported as useful adjunctively for patients who can not undergo complete resection. Treatment of CD is imperative due to its progressive course, growing size impinging on adjacent structures, and/or systemic effects. Clinical follow-up monitoring for recurrences should also be considered. Moreover screening for coexisting or subsequent malignancies is prudent due to the increased risk of lymphoma and Kaposi's sarcoma (Disperizieri et al., 2005).

The treatment of multicentric CD is controversial. The clinical course is unpredictable and extremely variable. However, generally, multicentric CD is more aggressive with frequent exacerbations. Some patients quickly progress and may even die within weeks. Prognosis is generally poor with patients frequently showing resistance to therapy (McCarty et al., 1995; Roca, 2009). Nonetheless, the median survival is reported as 2 to 3 years in patients with multicentric CD. Approximately 20 to 30% of patients develop either lymphoma or Kaposi's sarcoma during the course of their disease. The majority of patients with multicentric CD die of sepsis, progression of disease leading to multi-organ system failure, or related malignancies. Children tend to have a more favorable prognosis and clinical outcome with better response to therapy than adults. Recurrences have not been reported in children (Parez et al., 1999; Buesing et al., 2009).

A variety of modalities including chemotherapy, radiation, plasmapheresis, hematopoietic stem cell transplant, immune modulators—corticosteroids, antiviral agents (ganciclovir, foscarnet, cidofovir), interferon-alpha, intravenous immunoglobulin, all-trans retinoic acid, thalidomide—methotrexate, and specific monoclonal anti-IL-6 antibody (tocilizumab, atlizumab) and/or anti-CD20 monoclonal antibody (rituximab) have been utilized in the treatment of multicentric CD. Systemic symptoms variably improve with therapy. Serum IL-6 correlates with disease activity in patients with multicentric CD. Treatment with the humanized anti–IL-6 receptor (tocilizumab, atlizumab) has been shown to resolve and/or improve clinical symptoms and laboratory abnormalities in patients with increased serum IL-6 levels (Choi et al., 2008). Anti-CD 20 monoclonal antibodies (rituximab) may be useful in recurrences (Vasudev Rao et al., 2007). Anti-EGFR therapeutic agents may be adjunctively used in both the HV and PC types of CD (Lee et al., 2008). In patients with systemic manifestations, corticosteroids have been shown to transiently alleviate symptoms. Patients with the multicentric variant of CD are not generally offered surgery; however, some patients may undergo splenectomy.

In patients with POEMS, treatment modalities reported to improve neurologic and clinical symptoms include radiation, surgical removal of solitary lesions, corticosteroids, alkylators, interferon alpha, azathioprine, intravenous immunoglobulin, plasmapheresis, and peripheral blood stem cell transplantation (Leiti et al., 2007). In HIV patients, the prognosis is poor, with an average survival of 8 to 14 months and mortality rates reaching 85%. Most patients die of fulminant infections and/or malignant tumors. Combined chemotherapy, corticosteroid, and radiation therapy may be used as adjuvant therapy along with antiviral drugs in HIV-positive patients (Bowne et al., 1999).

Atrophic Follicular or Germinal Center Pattern in Primary Immunodeficiency Diseases

Depending on the type of primary immunodeficiency diseases (PID), the morphological features of lymph nodes in PID range from lymphoid depletion with poorly formed follicle or germinal centers, to nonspecific lymphoid hyperplasia, to atypical lymphoid hyperplasia (Frizzera et al., 2001). In the major types, the morphology is characterized by atrophic or depleted lymphoid follicles. In some cases, malignant lymphoma is identified in lieu of reactive lymphadenopathy.

ICD-10 Codes

Hyper IgM syndrome D80.5
X-linked agammaglobulinemia D80.0
Severe combined immunodeficiency D81.2
Ataxia-telangiectasia G11.3
Wiskott-Aldrich syndrome D82.0
Autoimmune lymphoprolifertive syndrome D89.82

The atrophic follicular or germinal center pattern is most commonly seen in patients with the hyper IgM syndrome (HIGM) associated with CD40L or CD40 deficiency, X-linked agammaglobulinemia, and severe combined immunodeficiency (SCID), but to a lesser extent also encountered in Ataxia-telangiectasia (A-T), Wiskott–Aldrich syndrome (WAS), and autoimmune lymphoprolifertive syndrome (ALPS).

Morphologically, in the atrophic follicular pattern, the follicles are characterized by hypoplastic, involuted or aplastic (completely absent) germinal centers with prominent lymphocyte depletion. The atrophic germinal centers may show hypervascularity with hyalinization, mimicking hyaline-vascular Castleman's disease.

Hyper IgM (HIGM) Syndrome

Hyper IgM (HIGM) syndrome is a heterogeneous group of PIDs characterized by decreased serum IgG, IgA, and IgE and normal or elevated IgM. The morphological features of the lymphoid tissue in HIGM vary according to the type of defective gene product. The atrophic pattern is usually seen in HIGM associated with either the CD40 ligand (CD40L) or CD40 deficiency (Facchetti et al., 1995). CD40L deficiency is the most common cause of HIGM and accounts for 65 to 70% of the reported cases; it is inherited in an X-linked recessive form. CD40L is primarily expressed on activated T helper cells and binds the CD40 molecule expressed on B cells, dendritic cells,

and macrophages. Defective CD40–CD40L interaction results in severely impaired T-cell-dependent B-cell development, immunoglobulin-class switching, and germinal center formation (Vassilios et al., 2005; Notarangelo et al., 2007). In contrast, in HIGM associated with deficiency of activation-induced cytidine deaminase (AICD) or Uracil-DNA glycosylase (UNG), there is lymphoid hyperplasia with enlarged lymph nodes and hypertrophic tonsils; the lymph nodes and tonsils have with massive germinal center enlargement due to proliferation of B cells that coexpress IgM and IgD (Revy et al., 2000; Kavli et al., 2005).

X-Linked Agammaglobulinemia

X-linked agammaglobulinemia (XLA, also called Bruton's agammaglobulinemia) is the first known PID caused by a defect in early B-cell development. It is characterized by low numbers of B cells, or absent B cells and a severe reduction in all classes of immunoglobulins (C.I. Edvard Smith et al., 1998). In patients with XLA, lymph nodes, tonsils, and adenoids are usually absent or hypoplastic with small and atrophic follicles containing absent or poorly developed germinal centers. There is absence or marked paucity of plasma cells. The paracortical areas are expanded and the T-cell function and cellular immunity are intact.

Severe Combined Immunodeficiency (SCID)

Severe combined immunodeficiency (SCID) is a heterogeneous group of rare inherited disorders characterized by severe combined deficits of cellular and humoral immunity. As many as 15 different genes have been associated with SCID. Molecular defects in those genes block the differentiation and proliferation of T cells, always associated with a direct or indirect impairment of B-cell immunity and, in some types, of NK cells. The resulting combined immunodeficiency is responsible for the clinical severity of SCID.

The morphology of lymphoid tissue in SCID is associated with different genetic and molecular defects. Typically there is a marked depletion of lymphoid cells (Cotter et al., 1991). In the T-B+ SCID group, patients usually have B cells, present either as scattered cells or remnants of follicles without germinal centers (Huber et al., 1992); see Figure 13.12A and 13.12b. However, the presence of follicles with fully developed germinal centers has also been observed in this group (Facchetti et al., 1998). In the T-B− SCID group, one typically sees "stromal" nodes containing fibroblasts, endothelial cells, macrophages, and interdigitating reticulum

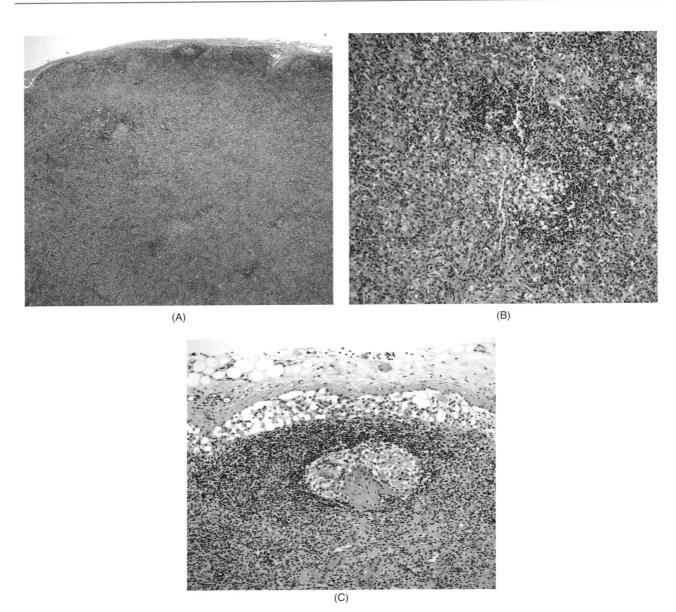

(A)

(B)

(C)

FIGURE 13.12 **Primary immune deficiency, SCID.** (**A**) Rare follicles and expanded paracortex with prominent vascularity and stroma. Two poorly formed follicles are seen and few small lymphoid aggregates in a sea of stroma with prominent framework in lieu of paracortex. (**B**) Dysorganized hypoplastic follicle with poorly formed germinal center and skewed mantle zone. The paracortical region is hypoplastic and replaced by stroma and vessels. (**C**) Poorly formed germinal center with hypoplasia of normal cells and prominent hyaline sclerosis and fibroblastic reticular meshwork. A loose zone resembling mantle zone lymphocytes is noted as well as subcapsular sinus with reticular meshwork. The paracortical area shows hyaline sclerosis and hypocellularity.

cells with severe depletion of T cells and B cells. There is lack of follicles or germinal centers or lymph nodes may contain rare small primary follicles (Facchetti et al., 1998); see Figure 13.12C. It also has been observed that all T-B+ SCID patient's lymph nodes with preserved follicles are from patients with relatively intact immune functions, higher numbers of T cells in the peripheral blood and normal serum immunoglobulin level.

Some variation occurs and Facchetti et al. also reported that in patients of T-B+ SCID due to γ-chain and Jak 3 deficiency, there was complete absence of lymphoid tissue (Heymer et al., 1976). The histological findings in lymphoid tissue may be further complicated by the presence of coexisting opportunistic infections including bacterial, viral, and fungal infections. In some cases the nodal morphology resembles that observed in Omenn's syndrome (OS). OS is a form of SCID characterized by erythroderma, lymphadenopathy, and hypereosinophilia. Lymph nodes of OS reveal total effacement of the architecture, either lacking a distinct cortex or with a severe depletion of B lymphocytes with no follicle formation, and a diffuse proliferation of interdigitating reticulum cells with numerous eosinophils (Martin et al., 1995; Facchetti et al., 1998). Hemophagocytic lymphohistiocytosis has been reported in X-linked SCID and cartilage-hair hypoplasia.

Ataxia-Telangiectasia (A-T)

Ataxia-telangiectasia (A-T) is a recessive genetic disorder with progressive neurodegeneration and immunodeficiency. The disorder is characterized by recurrent infections, telangiectasia, progressive ataxia, and hypersensitivity to ionizing radiation with increased incidence of hematological malignancy. Lymph nodes in A-T tend to be hypoplastic due to depletion of B lymphocytes in follicles (Peterson et al., 1966). There is a progressive decrease in CD4-positive T cells with poorly defined follicles and paracortical regions. The germinal centers may be absent or small and fibrotic, and they may also show reactive enlargement.

Wiskott–Aldrich Syndrome (WAS)

Wiskott–Aldrich syndrome (WAS) is a severe X-linked immunodeficiency disorder characterized by thrombocytopenia, eczema, and immunodeficiency with increased risk of developing autoimmunity and malignancy. It is caused by mutations in WAS gene, located on Xp11.22–23. The immune defect in WAS involves both B and T lymphocytes. The main histopathologic findings are in lymphoid tissue and thymus, which are usually hypoplastic to a variable degree and show a gradual loss of cellular elements. Follicle formation is poor or absent. There is progressive depletion of T cells in the interfollicular areas (Cooper et al., 1968; Wolff, 1967).

Autoimmune Lymphoproliferative Syndrome (ALPS)

The atrophic pattern may also be encountered in the lymphoid tissue of patients with the autoimmune lymphoproliferative syndrome (ALPS). Lymphoid tissue in ALPS typically reveals prominent interfollicular/paracortical expansion, with the follicles showing a spectrum of reactive changes: florid follicular hyperplasia to focal progressive transformation of germinal centers to involuted (atrophic) germinal centers (Lim et al.,1998). ALPS is a disorder associated with defective Fas-mediated lymphocyte apoptosis (Jackson et al., 1999). The impaired apoptosis causes abnormal proliferation of lymphocytes with an increased number of CD4 and CD8 double-negative T cells. Clinical manifestations include lymphadenopathy, enlarged spleen, autoimmunity, and a significantly increased risk of malignant lymphoma (Puck et al., 1997; Straus et al., 2001).

PROGRESSIVE TRANSFORMATION OF GERMINAL CENTER PATTERN

Progressive transformation of the germinal center (PTGC) is a benign reactive pattern often associated with reactive follicular hyperplasia. It is most frequently seen in patients with asymptomatic, persistent or recurrent lymphadenopathy showing nonspecific reactive follicular hyperplasia. The term PTGC was introduced in 1975 by Lennert and Müller-Hermelink as representing "germinal centers that are lost in a mass of lymphocytes" (Müller-Hermelink et al., 1978). In general, 2 to 15% of the lymph nodes with reactive hyperplasia show one or more germinal centers with PTGC (Chang et al., 2003; Verma et al., 2002).

ICD-10 Code R59.9 Enlarged lymph node, unspecified.

Definition

PTGC is a morphologic pattern seen as a consequence of persistent lymph node enlargement. Germinal centers are usually 2 to 5 times the size of reactive follicles and have expanded mantle zones (Hicks et al., 2002).

Epidemiology

Overall, PTGC occurs in up to 15% of enlarged lymph nodes with reactive follicular hyperplasia. Recurrences of PTGC are significantly higher in children, occurring in 50%, than in individuals over the age of 16 years, occurring in 23% of cases (Lennert et al., 1987; Poppema, 1992; Chan, 1999; Segal et al., 1995).

Clinical Aspects

PTGC is localized and without significant clinical consequences in the majority of cases. It may be self-limited or persistent with durations of less than 1 year to over 10 years. It is most frequently encountered in areas involved by reactive follicular hyperplasia. Florid PTGC refers to cases where PTGC is the dominant pattern. Florid cases occur more commonly in young men and are asymptomatic and solitary. Florid cases may show repeated recurrences but do not apparently progress to lymphoma (Chang et al., 2003; Hicks et al., 2002).

In PTGC there is a male predominance with a 3:1 male to female ratio. PTGC has a wide age distribution, ranging from 4 years to 82 years of age. The median age in children is 11 years and 28 years in adults. However, in Japan, PTGC is more common in patients in the fourth to sixth decades of life (Kojima et al., 2003). Adults are affected 4 times more often by PTGC than children. In children, PTGC is more likely to be florid and persistent with multiple recurrences (Osborne et al., 1992; Chang et al., 2003; Verma et al., 2002).

Involvement confined to one lymph node is more frequent than involvement of multiple lymph nodes. Peripheral lymph nodes are more commonly affected. Asymptomatic head and neck involvement occurs in approximately 75% of patients, with cervical lymph nodes affected in about half of the cases. Inguinal and axillary lymph nodes are affected less frequently (Kojima et al., 2010).

Rarely, extranodal PTGC occurs in the skin, subcutaneous soft tissues, the orbit, the gastrointestinal tract including the oral cavity, Waldeyer's ring, the stomach, and the large intestine (Ferry et al., 1992; Nguyen et al., 1999). The large intestine is the most commonly affected extranodal site. Extranodal cases have a female predominance with a male to female ratio of 1:3 and occur more frequently in an older age group in 60% of the cases. More frequently PTGC is florid in extranodal sites. The morphologic features are similar to that of nodal PTGC (Osborne et al., 1992).

PTGC may be seen in association with Hodgkin's lymphoma, particularly nodular lymphocyte predominant Hodgkin's lymphoma (NLPHL) in about 16 to 35% of the cases. PTGC may coexist, precede, or follow Hodgkin's lymphoma (Burns et al., 1984; Osborne et al., 1984). Nevertheless, the majority of lymph nodes with PTGC are not associated with Hodgkin's lymphoma. There is no increased risk of lymphoma in patients with PTGC or florid PTGC (Osborne et al. 1992).

Exceedingly rare cases of follicular lymphoma in situ concurrently occur with PTGC. Children and young adults with nodal and rarely extranodal marginal zone lymphomas may also present with follicles resembling PTGC. Rare cases of multiple myeloma have been reported to follow PTGC. PTGC can be also associated with localized chronic inflammation such as chronic sialoadenitis and chronic tonsillitis, infectious epidermal cyst, and/or autoimmune disorders such as hyperthyroidism and bronchial asthma (Chang et al., 2003; Verma et al., 2002).

Pathogenesis

The pathogenesis of PTGC remains unknown. The prospective associations among hyperplastic follicles, Hodgkin's lymphoma, and follicular lysis to PTGC are also unclear. Stimulated follicles are postulated to undergo a continuum of chronological phases, including follicular hyperplasia, follicular lysis, and PTGC (Chang et al., 2003). PTGC is postulated to possibly represent a spectrum in the progression of hyperplastic changes in follicles, occurring as the final end point over a period of time in response to the antigenic stimuli. PTGC may perhaps also represent an inherent developmental progression of reactive germinal centers (Schnitzer, 1995; Hansmann et al., 1990).

In PTGC, T cells enter into the germinal centers followed by entrance of mantle zone B cells. Ineffective B-cell proliferative response to antigens, homing mechanisms, and cell regulatory factors are postulated as possibly invoking overproduction of cytokines and growth factors resulting in PTGC (Burns et al., 1984). PTGC has been shown to contain disrupted follicular dendritic cell networks intermingled with mantle zone B cells that have entered into the germinal center (Guettier et al., 1986). There is an associated corresponding decrease of normal follicular center B cells. Helper T cells are increased while suppressor T cells are proportionally decreased in PTGC, implicating a possible role of T cell dysregulation in the formation of PTGC as well (Stein et al., 1982).

In one case of PTGC, a minor subpopulation of lymphoid cells is reported to harbor a translocation involving chromosome 3q27 presumably at the Bcl-6 gene locus, suggesting that perhaps PTGC and the nodular lymphocyte predominant Hodgkin's lymphoma (NLPHL) may be related. Bcl-6 expression present with follicles resembling is critical for germinal center formation. Bcl-6 is inactivated in post-germinal center B cells (Bouron-Dal Soglio et al., 2008). Although PTGC is associated with chronic inflammatory conditions, the role of infection in causing PTGC is unclear (Licup et al., 2006). Nonetheless, an Epstein–Barr virus (EBV) genome has been detected in a large number of PTGC cases (Weiss et al., 1991).

Approach to Diagnosis (Clinical Workup)

A complete history and physical examination are essential for the determination of the possible causes for enlarged lymph nodes. Laboratory data and lymph node biopsy may be necessary to rule out infections such as tuberculosis, toxoplasmosis, and infectious mononucleosis, as well as autoimmune disorders, and malignancies such as lymphoma and metastatic carcinoma.

Morphologic Aspects

Lymph nodes in PTGC are enlarged, and pale gray to tan with a nodular or lobulated surface. The normal lymph node architecture is maintained without effacement in PTGC. Large nodular follicles that are usually 2 to 5 times the size of reactive follicles are often present in a background of smaller hyperplastic lymphoid follicles (Figure 13.13). Follicles are round to oval, and either well delineated and/or ill-defined from the surrounding interfollicular areas. There may be one or multiple nodules of PTGC present within a single lymph node. Germinal centers in PTGC transform to ultimately become fragmented, disrupted, and replaced by abundant small lymphocytes (Figure 13.14). (Chang et al., 2003; Verma et al., 2002).

A progressive sequence of morphologic changes is evident in PTGC. Initially there is an inward migration of mantle zone small B and T lymphocytes into the germinal center (Figure 13.15). These mantle zone lymphocytes have round to slightly irregular nuclei without significant atypia (Figure 13.21). Predominantly B cells with only a minor population of T cells migrate into the follicles. This occurs in a continuous stepwise, multifocal manner in which there is a progressive accumulation, expansion, and disruption of the germinal center (Figure 13.17). This leads in the fragmentation and lysis of the germinal center cells into small aggregates of centrocytes and centroblasts (Figure 13.18). Some follicles in PTGC may also show

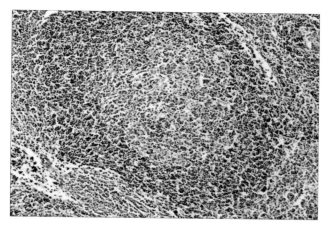

FIGURE 13.14 **Typical PTGC on medium power with residual germinal centers and peripheral mantle cell encroachment.**

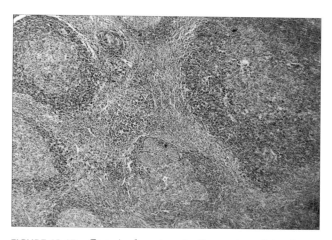

FIGURE 13.15 Germinal centers in the center of the figure and top are incompletely transformed. Small darker mantle zone lymphocytes are seen moving into and transforming the paler germinal centers in contrast to the completely transformed and larger germinal center on the right.

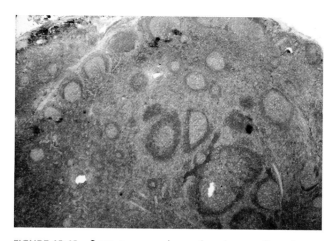

FIGURE 13.13 **Low-power view showing a few larger darker follicles with attenuated pale transformed germinal centers (center) and multiple normal follicles with pale germinal centers.** In contrast, a PTGC follicle has about 2 to 3× the diameter.

follicular lysis. The border between the mantle zones and the irregular germinal centers becomes obscure and indistinct due to the ingress of mantle zone cells into the follicle (Figure 13.19). Mantle zone lymphocytes also migrate into the adjacent interfollicular sinusoids (van den Oord et al., 1985; Hicks et al., 2002).

Subsequent progression leads to an enlarged transformed follicle that contains a preponderance of small B lymphocytes, and an irregular germinal center with only occasional remnants of follicular center cells and dendritic cells (Figure 13.20). Eventually mantle zones vanish and are no longer discernable. Infrequently germinal centers show

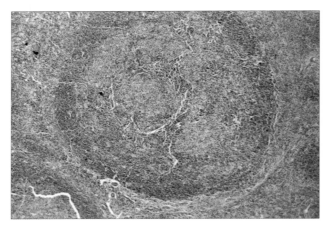

FIGURE 13.16   Incompletely transformed PTGC at medium-power view.

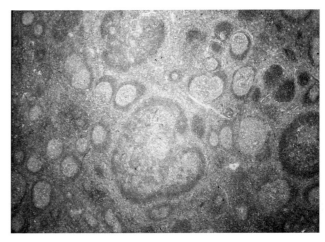

FIGURE 13.18   **Some irregular, scalloped, transformed centers that have undergone follicular fragmentation into several parts.**

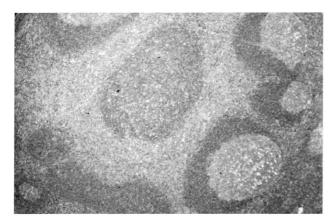

FIGURE 13.17   **PTGC (center) contrasted with the distinct polarized germinal centers (right).** Note the obscured germinal center and mantle zone that are no longer clear, unlike the clearly defined germinal centers and mantle zones of the hyperplastic follicles.

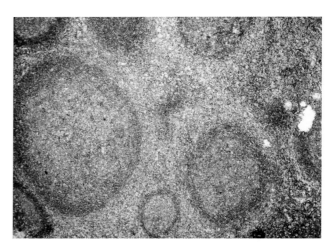

FIGURE 13.19   **Two progressively transformed follicles with smaller hyperplastic germinal centers below at edge.**

merged or shared mantle zones with adjacent follicles (Licup et al., 2006). Follicular dendritic cell networks are disrupted and expanded. Secondary germinal center components such as centrocytes, centroblasts, dendritic cells, and plasma cells become sparse (Figure 13.21). Residual centroblasts and immunoblasts may morphologically mimic mononuclear and polylobated L&H (lymphocytic and/or histiocytic) cells of nodular lymphocyte predominant Hodgkin's lymphoma (NLPHL). (Stein et al., 2001; Burns et al., 1984; Nguyen et al., 1999).

Residual germinal center elements such as tingible body macrophages and mitotic figures, although rare, are still evident in the transformed follicles of PTGC. Epithelioid granulomas occur occasionally

within the transformed germinal centers as well as surround it. Occasional HV-like germinal centers, reminiscent of the HV type of Castleman's disease are seen. Rare immunoblasts and eosinophils are also seen in the follicles. Aggregates of polyclonal plasma cells may be present at the periphery of PTGC. Secondary lymphoid follicles can also infrequently surround nodules of PTGC. Ultimately the transformed germinal center consists predominantly of numerous small lymphocytes with an obscured irregular germinal center without an obvious mantle zone (Kojima et al., 2005; Chang et al., 2003; Verma et al., 2002).

In PTGC the lymph node capsule may be thickened. There may be focal infiltration of lymphocytes

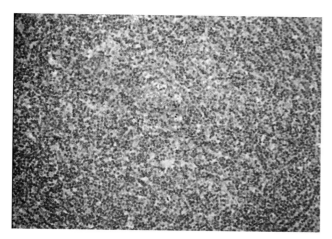

FIGURE 13.20   **Medium-power view of a transformed germinal center with almost total obliteration by smaller mantle zone B lymphocytes**. Remnants of residual larger centroblasts showing a paler pinkish appearance and centrocytes are scattered diffusely amongst occasional histiocytes and dendritic cells.

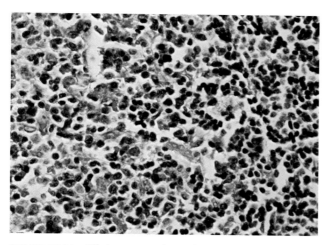

FIGURE 13.21   **High-power view showing benign mantle zone cells**. The mantle cells on the right migrating into and obliterating centroblasts and larger cells of the germinal center on the left.

and plasma cells into the capsule. Vasculature in the interfollicular areas is often prominent with occasional hyalinized vessels. There may be striking interfollicular sclerosis. Sinuses are slightly compressed but patent, containing small lymphocytes, plasma cells admixed with occasional immunoblasts, plasmacytoid lymphocytes, and histiocytes. Rare cases may also contain plasmacytoid monocytes. The paracortical zone seldom shows hyperplasia (Chang et al., 2003; Verma et al., 2002).

Marginal zone hyperplasia may be prominent in a minority of PTGC. This is characterized by expansion of the marginal zones mostly by monocytoid B cells and small lymphocytes. The monocytoid B cells show abundant pale and/or clear cytoplasm, medium size slightly indented or round nuclei with inconspicuous nucleoli. A variable number of admixed larger activated lymphocytes are also present in the marginal zones (Kojima et al., 2010).

Immunophenotyping/Cytochemistry

Lymphoid follicles in PTGC are composed of predominantly migrated mantle zone B cells expressing CD20, and a minor subpopulation of T cells expressing CD3, CD5, CD43, and CD45RO. Mantle zone B cells characteristically express Bcl-2, CD20, surface IgM, and surface IgD and are negative for CD3, CD43, and cyclin D1. A subset of mantle zone lymphocytes weakly express CD5. Moreover the expression of Bcl-2 is retained in mantle zone lymphocytes that have migrated into the transformed germinal centers in PTGC. The Bcl-2 protein regulates lymphocyte apoptosis and is typically expressed in mantle zone B cells as well as T cells. However, non-neoplastic follicle center B cells lack expression of Bcl-2 and CD3. These Bcl-2 positive mantle zone B lymphocytes along with migrating Bcl-2 positive T cells outline large expanded Bcl-2 positive nodules in a background of sparse Bcl-2 negative follicle center B cells in PTGC. This results in the characteristic diffuse Bcl-2 positive staining pattern in follicles of PTGC. (Kojima et al., 2005; Chang et al., 2003; Verma et al., 2002).

Remnants of residual follicular center B cells characteristically express CD20, focally express CD10 and Bcl-6, and lack expression of Bcl-2, IgD, and EMA (epithelial membrane antigen). Epstein–Barr virus (EBV) may also be expressed in residual follicle B cells of PTGC. Both L&H cells of nodular lymphocyte predominant Hodgkin's lymphoma (NLPDH) and residual follicular center B cells express CD20, Bcl-6, and CD45. In contrast, L&H cells classically express EMA, and are usually negative for CD10 and CD15.

T-cell-associated antigens (CD3, CD5, CD45RO) demonstrate randomly distributed T cells scattered singly or in small aggregates within the transformed follicles in PTGC. T cells in the normal germinal center are more frequent in the light zones and at the interface of the germinal center and mantle zone. The majority of T cells in PTGC are positive for CD57. In NLPHL, T cells that form rosettes around L&H cells are positive for CD3, CD57, and PD-1 (programmed death 1). PD-1, also known as PDCD1, is a member of the extended CD28/CTLA-4 family of T-cell receptors. It is expressed on the surface of activated T cells, B cells, and macrophages and serves as a negative regulator of immune responses. PD-1 (CD279) is also expressed by germinal center T cells. In PTGC there are no prominent CD57/CD3/PD-1 positive T-cell rosettes around large B cells. However, occasional cases of PTGC show focal CD3/CD57 positive T-cell rosettes around immunoblasts and/or centroblasts in a few follicles. Nonetheless, T-cell-forming rosettes in PTGC are significantly less prominent than those of NLPHL (Nguyen et al., 1999; Krishnan et al., 2010; Kojima et al., 2005; Chang et al., 2003; Verma et al., 2002).

Marginal zone B cells of PTGC classically express CD20, may express surface IgM, but lack expression of surface IgD, CD5, CD10, CD21, CD23, CD43, CD45RO, and EMA. Bcl-2 is typically positive on marginal zone B cells; however, a subpopulation of marginal zone cells can be Bcl-2 negative. B immunoblasts, scattered within the follicle and in the interfollicular areas, express CD30 and CD20 but are negative for CD15 and EMA. CD 30 reactivity is similar in both NLPHL and PTGC, since rare L&H cells can also be weakly positive for CD30. Kappa and lambda light chains are polyclonal. There is no clonal rearrangement of the immunoglobulin heavy chain (Kojima et al. 2005; Chang et al., 2003; Verma et al., 2002).

Dendritic cell markers, CD21, CD23, CD35, and CAN.42, outline tight concentric and/or disrupted and expanded dendritic cell networks in PTGC. In PTGC, dendritic networks commonly are entirely disrupted and separated into tight clusters. Follicular dendritic cell networks of PTGC show a similar staining pattern as the networks in follicular lysis and NLDHD, which are also disrupted (Guettier et al., 1986).

Differential Diagnosis

The pathologic features of PTGC can mimic nodular lymphocyte predominant Hodgkin's lymphoma (NLPHL), nodular variant of lymphocyte rich classic Hodgkin's lymphoma, Castleman's disease (CD) either of hyaline vascular or plasmablastic types, various low-grade B-cell non-Hodgkin's lymphomas, florid reactive follicular hyperplasia, florid follicular lysis, granulomatous disease, as well as infections including the early stage of human immunodeficiency virus (HIV) infection. There are similarities in the clinical features of PTGC, Hodgkin's lymphoma, and follicular lymphoma as well. Monoclonality and molecular studies may be crucial for the distinction of PTGC from the various lymphomas.

NLPHL can coexist in the same lymph node as PTGC. Moreover, florid cases of PTGC can mimic NLPHL morphologically because of its nodular pattern and presence of scattered large cells in the follicles. The number of L&H cells in NLPHL is variable, with some cases showing only a few L&H cells that may resemble immunoblasts and centroblasts of PTGC. The morphologic features are impressively similar between early involvement by NLPHL and PTGC when only a few L&H cells are present. In PTGC, the B cells in follicles are confluent and arranged in a sheet-like fashion with only few scattered T cells. There are no Hodgkin and/or Reed–Sternberg cells evident in PTGC. In contrast, in NLPHL there is effacement of nodal architecture with an irregular distribution of B cells intermingled with large aggregates of T cells imparting a moth-eaten appearance, as well as prominent T-cell rosettes around L&H cells. Indeed, in low-power view, the single most important distinction between PTGC and NLPHL is the mass or pushing effect by neoplastic NLPHL nodules against the surrounding normal tissue, often resulting in compressed normal lymphoid follicles seen on edge of the lymph node involved by lymphoma. Exceedingly rare cases of NLPHL are in extranodal sites including Waldeyer's ring, skin, soft tissue, and large intestine. Therefore the differential diagnosis of extranodal PTGC should also include NLPHL (Chang et al., 1995, Poppema et al., 2008).

A variety of low-grade non-Hodgkin's lymphomas can mimic PTGC and therefore are considered important in the differential diagnosis of PTGC. PTGC associated with prominent marginal zone hyperplasia should be distinguished from lymphomas distributed in a marginal zone pattern. These include marginal zone B-cell lymphoma, small lymphocytic B-cell lymphoma, mantle cell lymphoma with marginal zone differentiation, and follicular lymphoma with marginal zone differentiation. Furthermore disrupted germinal centers in PTGC may appear similar to follicular colonization of germinal centers by marginal zone B-cell lymphoma, or rarely follicular colonization by mantle cell lymphoma. A distinctive feature in PTGC is the clustering of small T cells around residual germinal center remnants, which is not characteristically seen in follicular colonization by lymphoma. Florid variant of follicular lymphoma, follicular lymphoma in situ and mantle zone lymphoma are included in the differential diagnosis. In mantle zone lymphoma, the nodular growth pattern may resemble florid PTGC. Generally, neoplastic lymphoid cells tend to egress from germinal centers; in contrast, non-neoplastic cells in PTGC ingress into the germinal centers. Mono-clonality and molecular studies may be crucial for the distinction of PTGC from the various lymphomas (Kojima et al., 2010).

The floral variant of follicular lymphoma and follicular lymphoma (FL) in situ may strongly mimic PTGC. FL in situ can coexist in the same lymph node with PTGC. Synchronous FL may be evident at other sites in these cases. Approximately 23% of de novo FL in situ eventually develop FL. In the floral variant of FL, the majority of neoplastic follicles are encircled by prominent mantle zones that invaginate into the centers in an irregular disorderly manner resulting in a floral pattern. This floral pattern can be confused with PTGC, since there are numerous mantle zone B cells and T cells intermingled with neoplastic B cells in the follicles (Sandhaus et al., 1988, Osborne et al., 1987). The floral variant of FL has a female predominance and occurs more commonly in the sixth decade of life, with only rare cases in patients younger than 40 years of age. Bcl-2 can be positive in both the neoplastic follicles of floral variant of FL and FL in situ as well as the follicles of PTGC. Therefore Bcl-2 positivity of follicles is not always indicative of lymphoma. In the floral variant of FL, the neoplastic nodules are often densely packed with effacement of nodal architecture. Neoplastic cells are seen not only in the follicles but also in the interfollicular areas and may show extranodal extension. PTGC, in contrast, is usually seen in the background of reactive follicular hyperplasia, and the cells may infiltrate into but not beyond the capsule. Bcl-6 and CD10 staining is confined to the follicles in PTGC. In FL, Bcl-6 and CD10-positive neoplastic B cells often are present in interfollicular areas. In PTGC, only sparse residual follicle center B cells are CD10 positive. In contrast, in FL, numerous CD10-positive cells may be present in the neoplastic follicles (Goates et al., 1994; Sandhaus et al., 1988; Osborne et al., 1987).

Florid PTGC may mimic nodular variant of lym-phocyte rich classic Hodgkin's lymphoma (LRHL). In PTGC, there is no effacement of nodal architec-ture and remnants of residual germinal centers are indistinct. In contrast, in the LRHL, there is efface-ment of the lymph node architecture and residual germinal center are small and distinct. Rarely, PTGC changes are seen in association with mixed cellularity and nodular sclerosing classic Hodgkin's lymphoma; however, these have unique pathologic features and do not morphologically mimic PTGC (Osborne et al., 1992; Hansmann et al., 1990).

PTGC may coexist with the hyaline vascular type of Castleman's disease in the same nodal site. Fur-thermore HV like germinal centers may be seen in cases of PTGC. It is essential to exclude PTGC prior to rendering a diagnosis of CD (Kojima et al., 2005). The plasmablastic variant of CD can be distinguished from PTGC by its characteristic expression of HHV-8 (human herpes virus-8) genome, IgM and lambda light chains, and lack of expression for CD138 (Dupin et al., 2000).

In children the presence of epithelioid granulo-mas in PTGC may possibly lead to the consideration of granulomatous disease and/or infection. In follicular lysis the germinal centers are distorted by numerous invading benign mantle zone cells similar to that seen in PTGC. However, in follicular lysis the proportion of mantle zone cells within follicles is significantly less than that of PTGC. In florid reactive follicular hyperplasia (FFH) the follicles are not expanded by mantle zone B cells, and the mantle zones are distinct and well demarcated. There are equal numbers of Bcl-2-positive and CD3-positive cells, indicating the presence of T cells and the virtual absence of Bcl-2 positive mantle zone cells. FFH is more common in younger patients and rare in individuals over the age of 50. In adults, FFH is often associated with rheuma-toid arthritis, early stage human immunodeficiency virus (HIV) infection, syphilis, and multicentric CD (Osborne et al., 1991; Kojima et al., 1998).

Treatment of Choice and Prognosis

PTGC does not have malignant potential and does not transform into lymphoma. However, it can pre-cede, coexist, or follow lymphoma. PTGC can recur multiple times after local surgical resection. Monitor-ing for recurrences and subsequent development of lymphoma, most commonly NLPHD, is warranted (Osborne et al., 1992; Chang et al., 2003; Verma et al., 2002).

MARGINAL ZONE HYPERPLASIA AND MANTLE CELL HYPERPLASIA

Mantle Cell Hyperplasia

Although uncommon, mantle cell hyperplasia may be seen in reactive lymph nodes as a solitary, enlarged lymph node in a young patient or an incidental find-ing with nonspecific etiology. A study of 35 cases with mantle cell/marginal zone hyperplasia pat-tern disclosed a low incidence of development of non-Hodgkin lymphoma over a long term follow-up (Hunt et al., 2001). The hyperplastic mantle is seen in lymph node adjacent to and involved with Castleman's disease or non-Hodgkin lymphoma. In

CD, interfollicular vascularity, lollipop follicles, and single follicle with expanded mantle zones and with multiple atrophic follicles are present. Hyperplastic mantle may be seen with two or more lollipop follicles. A hyperplastic mantle zone is one of the patterns of mantle cell lymphoma, the so-called mantle zone lymphoma subtype.

Morphologically mantle cell hyperplasia is characterized by an expanded mantle zone in relation to the relatively intact normal looking germinal center. Mantle cell hyperplasia has to be differentiated from clustered primary follicles or tangential sections of secondary follicles with small or early germinal centers. The primary follicle is identified in a lymph node in the cortex or medullary cords as dark small nodules composed of small lymphocytes. These are often smaller than most reactive germinal centers in diameter. Like secondary follicles, these cells mark with CD20, but unlike secondary follicles, the nodules are Bcl2 positive. The B cells present in primary follicles and mantle zones are described as often CD5+ and could be the putative origin of mantle cell lymphomas.

Distinction of primary follicle hyperplasia or mantle cell hyperplasia from mantle cell lymphoma is critically important. The presence expanded mantle zones in germinal center is abnormal and require ancillary investigation such as flow cytometry, immunohistochemistry, or molecular test to rule out a lymphoma (see Figure 13.22, which shows a unilaterally enlarged tonsil with mantle zone hyperplasia that was not clonal by flow cytometry on biopsy). On follow-up the patient developed nodal marginal zone lymphoma after 3 months. The

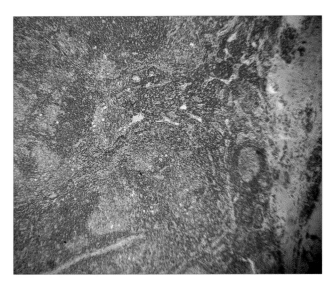

FIGURE 13.23 **Prominent medullary cords and primary follicles and early follicle with relative mantle zone hyperplasia, in a reactive lymph node**.

cells of mantle cell lymphoma morphologically show atypical round and irregular lymphocytes. Unlike most primary follicles or mantle cel hyperplasia, mantle cell lymphoma nodules overtake the lymph node, and show monotypic light chains with expression of CD20, CD43, CD5, and cyclin D1 but lacking CD23. On rare occasions the medullary areas show prominent nodules of primary follicles with few early secondary follicles (see Figure 13.23). High-power view reveals the cells to be composed of small lymphocytes typical of primary follicles, and although Bcl2 will be positive, other markers for mantle cell lymphoma will be negative.

A particular form of mantle cell lymphoma presents in the bowel in about a fifth of the cases. The bowel shows polyps mimicking colonic polyps. The polyps are, however, lymphoid rich and has been called lymphomatous polyposis (see Figure 13.24). A histologic section shows naked germinal centers with a sea of mantle zone lymphocytes around (see Figure 13.25).

Marginal Zone Pattern

Marginal zone B cells are normal components of lymph nodes, and splenic and gastrointestinal tissue, although they are easily more appreciated in normal spleen and mesenteric lymph nodes. The human lymph node, like the spleen, harbors a small number of normal marginal zone cells and is typically located adjacent to the outside facet of the mantle zones (van den Oord, de Wolf-Peeters, and Desmet, 1986).

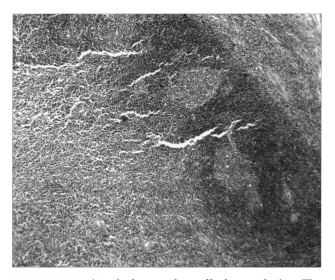

FIGURE 13.22 **Atypical mantle cell hyperplasia**. The patient on follow-up developed marginal zone lymphoma.

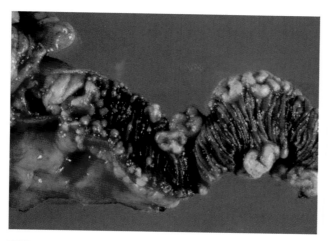

FIGURE 13.24 Mantle cell lymphomatous polyposis in bowel.

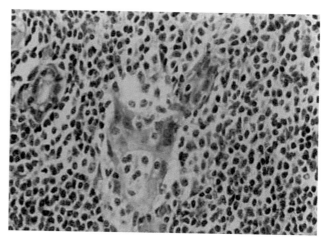

FIGURE 13.26 Marginal zone cells or centrocyte-like cells in MALTOMA.

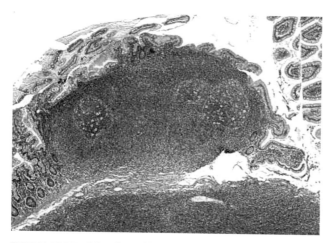

FIGURE 13.25 Mantle cell lymphoma surrounding reactive germinal centers in small bowel.

toxoplasmic lymphadenitis, HIV lymphadenopathy, CMV lymphadenitis, and lymphogranuloma venereum (Sheibani et al., 1990; Sohn et al., 1985). In addition monocytoid B cells are a prominent component in certain low-grade lymphomas, and can be seen in some autoimmune setting like Sjögren's syndrome or hepatitis viral infections.

Another type of cell similar to monocytoid B cells is the epithelial associated marginal zone B cell. This type of cell is particularly prominent in extranodal marginal zone of the MALT type where the mucosal and lymph nodes show these cells as principal tumor cells (Figure 13.26). Lymph nodes involved by MALTOMA show a perifollicular pattern with expanded marginal zones visible as pale bands around the mantle (Figure 13.27). Unlike marginal

In extranodal lymphoid tissue, the normal human Peyer's patch shows a mantle zone that is continuous with a population of slightly larger cells with more cytoplasm and irregular nuclear outlines, resembling centrocytes in the germinal center, corresponding to the marginal zone B cells (Spencer, Perry, and Dunn-Walters, 1998).

Monocytoid cell nuclei have about 2× the diameter of small lymphocytes. They are indistinguishable from marginal zone B cells but may differ in having more cytoplasm,or may be associated with neutrophilic collections or less plasmacytic differentiation. Monocytoid B cells can be seen in any number of reactive follicular hyperplasia and could be found in about 14% of reactive lymph nodes (Plank, Hansmann, and Fischer, 1993). The reaction, however, is particularly prominent in a few specific lymphadenitis that include cat-scratch disease,

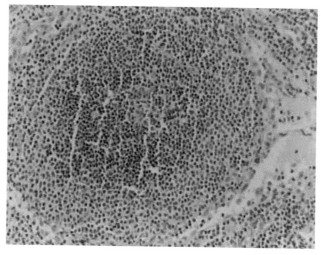

FIGURE 13.27 Marginal zone pattern in a gastric lymph node involved by MALTOMA.

zone cells of marginal zone lymphoma, which are Bcl2 and CD43 positive, reactive monocytoid cells are Bcl2 and CD43 negative (Kojima et al., 2006). The relationship of these cells to the splenic marginal zone cells and the nodal monocytoid B cells is not completely known, but recent studies show evidence of similar phenotypic antigen sets between each of these cells. It has been suggested that monocytoid cells are more immature marginal zone B cells, but the issue is still unclear (Camacho et al., 2001), and monocytoid B cells or MALT marginal zone B cells may be unrelated to marginal zone B cells (Johrens et al., 2005).

REACTIVE FOLLICULAR PATTERN, MIXED WITH OTHER PATTERNS, SPECIFIC ENTITIES

HIV-Persistent Generalized Lymphadenopathy and Involuted Phase of HIV-Related Lymphadenopathy

Although the most common cause of lymphadenopathy in HIV infection is secondary to the virus itself, the lymph node enlargement can be secondary to lymphoma, Kaposi sarcoma, multicentric Castleman disease, and a variety of infections.

ICD-10 Code B23.1

Definition

Persistent generalized lymphadenopathy is the term applied to the hyperplastic phase of HIV lymphadenopathy characterized by florid follicular hyperplasia, usually in a setting of homosexual risk activity, that persist for at least three months. Involuted lymphadenopathy is the terminal phase histology following the hyperplastic phase, characterized by depletion of follicles.

Synonym HIV Lymphadenitis

Epidemiology About 25 million people have already died of acquired immune deficiency syndrome since its discovery. HIV remains a major health problem in the world and in Western societies. It is a major cause of childhood mortality in Africa, and despite availability of medications, more than a million people had HIV infection in the United States. In the United States, 4 to 8% of those with HIV infection tested at STD clinics are acutely infected (antibody findings negative, antigen findings positive). Acute infection is associated with having a known HIV-positive partner within the past 12 months and a history of chlamydia, syphilis, and hepatitis B infection in the past 2 years (Truong et al., 2006; Pilcher et al., 2005).

Pathogenesis

Seroconversion to an acute infection is defined as a series of events between exposure to the virus and completion of the initial immune responses (when an antibody test becomes positive for HIV). The following is a simplified outline of events that occur during acute HIV infection (Zetola and Pilcher, 2007). After the individual is exposed to HIV, infection begins, and at day 8, the virus is detectable in blood using polymerase chain reaction (PCR) only since the antibody test are negative. HIV has tropism for CD4 membrane antigen gp 120 and infects CD4 helper T cells, monocytes, and dendritic cells. At weeks 2 to 4, after the infected CD4 cells nearly double every day, early antibodies to HIV may be detected using newer antibody assays that detect low-affinity antibodies. As the immune system reacts by generating antibodies and CD8 cytotoxic cells, the viral load begins to decline. Because the individual is asymptomatic, if untested and unaware of infection, this is a period of high communicability. At weeks 10 to 24, the HIV viral load drops to its lowest point. Antibodies at this point, have higher reactivity, and the routine antibody tests become positive for HIV, so seroconversion is now complete. At this point chronic HIV infection commences. The reservoir of the virus is found in follicle dendritic reticulum cells and contributes to its persistent disease. The depletion of immune response contributes to the development of a host of opportunistic infections and the emergence of immune deficiency associated malignancies.

Approach to Diagnosis

Lymph node biopsy is indicated in the HIV-infected patients with unexplained generalized symptoms or with atypical enlargement of the lymph nodes. Lymph node histopathology identifies secondary infections and neoplasms, which occur in about 10% of enlarged lymph nodes (Gerstoft et al., 1989).

Morphology

The morphology mirrors an overlapping histology spectrum that begins at an acute hyperplastic phase, followed by intermediate phase; then terminates in a depleted phase. The differential diagnosis depends on the phase. Overlapping findings from acute and depleted phases are seen in the intermediate phase. Presence of polykaryotes or Warthin–Finkeldey giant cells are better appreciated in the intermediate and atrophic phases. Since these giant

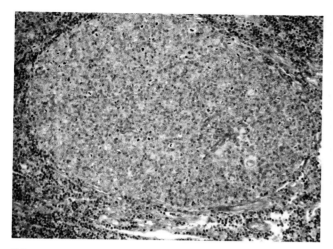

FIGURE 13.28 **Hyperplastic mishapen germinal centers with attenuated mantle zones.**

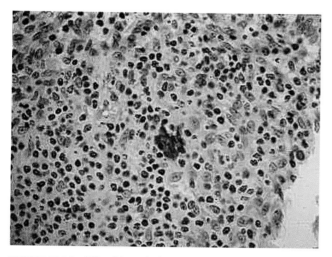

FIGURE 13.29 **Warthin–Finkeldey polykaryotes.**

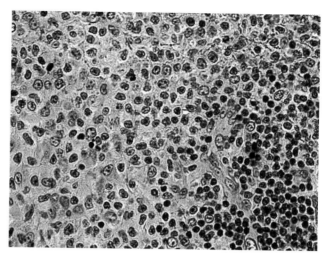

FIGURE 13.30 **Monocytoid hyperplasia.**

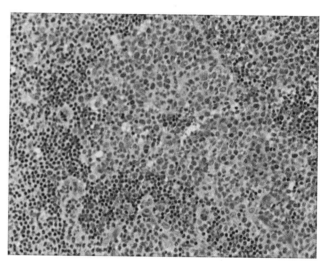

FIGURE 13.31 **Follicle lysis with disaggregated germinal center with hemorrhage, and follicular fragmentation.**

polykaryotes originate from follicular dendritic cells, they are much commonly seen during those phases (see Chapter 12); see Figures 13.28–13.31.

Characteristic features of hyperplastic phase include the following:

1. Florid follicular hyperplasia replacement of the lymph node with large, mishapen, naked, back-to-back germinal centers.
2. Germinal centers with an increase of large centroblasts, tingible body macrophages, and inconspicuous mantle zone.
3. Follicle lysis with invaginated mantle zones as well as follicles with hemorrhages.
4. Paracortex with increased HEVs vascularity, plasma cells, monocytoid cells, or granulomas.

Immunohistochemistry

CD8 T cytotoxic cells increase in the germinal centers in between sheets of the CD21 + follicular dendritic cell network, which is disrupted. The paracortex shows a decreased CD4:CD8 ratio and increased dendritic cells positive for S100. In the depleted stage there is virtual absence of CD4 in paracortex, which is completely replaced by CD8 T cells.

Regressed (Atrophic) Germinal Centers Pattern

For the involuted phase of HIV-related lymphadenopathy, see Figures 13.32 and 13.33. Characteristic

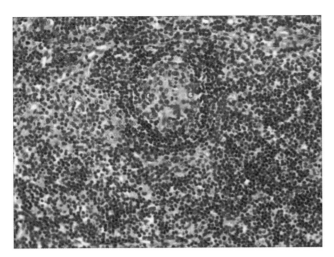

FIGURE 13.32 Involuted phase of AIDS lymphadenopathy with atrophic follicle with scant mantle and interfollicular vascularity.

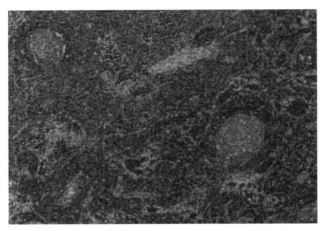

FIGURE 13.33 Atrophic follicle with cortical and paracortical sinuses filled with reactive lymphocytes displayed as dark round to elliptical cords.

features of the involuted or atrophic phase are as follows:

1. Small follicles with atrophic germinal centers with increased follicular dendritic cells, fibrosis, and attenuated mantle zones.
2. Paracortex with expansion, as well as prominent vascularity secondary to HEVs.
3. Fibrotic and depletion stage in the terminal phase with absence of follicles and increased histiocytes and plasma cells.

Differential Diagnosis

The hyperplastic phase raises concern for a nonspecific follicular hyperplasia or follicular large-cell

lymphoma. The lack of polarity, the attenuated mantle, and the highly prolliferative centers are features seen in some follicular large-cell lymphoma composed of centroblasts in sheets (i.e., follicular large cell lymphoma, grade IIIB). Ancillary tests include finding Bcl-2 negative follicles and the presence of a polyclonal population by flow cytometry or the absence of a molecular gene rearrangement. The differential diagnosis of the involuted phase include Castleman disease of the hyaline vascular type, angioimmunoblastic T-cell lymphoma, and in the fibrotic and highly vascular paracortex, Kaposi sarcoma, vascular tranformation, and infections such as *Mycobacterium avium intracellulare.*

MIXED PATTERN WITH FOLLICULAR HYPERPLASIA, MICROGRANULOMAS, MONOCYTOID HYPERPLASIA

Toxoplasmic Lymphadenopathy

The Greek word *Toxoplasma*, derives from "toxon" for "arc or bow-shaped" and the word *gondii* derives from a North African desert rodent *gundi* where *T. gondii* was originally found by Nicole and Manceaux in 1908 (Sima and Rasin, 1973). Toxoplasmosis is a common infection of which *T. gondii* is the causative agent, and is usually asymptomatic, and self-limiting but in certain clinical settings can develop grave or fatal course. The following section extends the discussion of toxoplasma on Chapter 6 regarding its blood manifestations and contributes the lymphadenopathy findings. (For the laboratory diagnosis and treatment of defined clinical forms of toxoplasmosis, see Chapter 6.)

Definition

Toxoplasmic lymphadenitis is a zoonotic infection caused by the parasite *T. gondii* with specific characteristics and pattern of lymph node reaction.

ICD-10 Code B58

Synonyms

Piringer–Kuchinka lymphadenitis, cat-poo disease.

Epidemiology

T. gondii is worldwide in distribution. It is estimated that over 50 million is infected, with clusters of infection in France, Central America, and Asia (Zimmer, 2000). In France and other European countries, infection has been associated with eating raw or undercooked meat (steak *tartare* or its variations), while in Central America and Asia, infection has been largely from zoonotic transmission from stray cats. The overall seroprevalence in the United States decreased (1999–2004 NHANES survey). The prevalence among the general population decreased from the previous decade to 9% which is in parallel with a drop in seroprevalence to 11% among women of childbearing age (15–44 years) (Jones et al., 2007).

Humans become infected with *Toxoplasma gondii* in five ways : (1) mainly by ingesting uncooked meat, fruits, or vegetables containing viable oocysts; (2) drinking contaminated water; (3) via transplacentally; (4) via blood transfusion, or (5) very rarely through allogeneic organ transplant. Until recently waterborne transmission of *T. gondii* was considered uncommon, but a large outbreak traced to contamination of a water reservoir in Canada by wild felids and human infection by marine mammals in the United States argues against this consideration (Dubey, 2004).

Etiology

Toxoplasma gondii are single-cell protozoa in the genus Toxoplasma. The organism has a nucleus, contains membrane bound organelles including *apical complexes*, which are used in host cell invasion and are structures characteristic of the phylum Apicomplexa. These are parasites of humans, companion mammals, wild animals, and birds with three infective forms: sporozoites, bradyzoites, and tachyzoites. Oocysts are passed between them through feces and transmission between a cat and the rodents to carry out its sexual life cycle (see Chapter 6 for the parasite life cycle). The life cycle of *Toxoplasma* begins as a noninfective oocyst that sporulates and makes infective cells called sporozoites. These sporozoites are found in the feces of infected cats or otherwise may contaminate water, garden soil, vegetables, or fruits. If ingested, they multiply, forming pseudocysts containing bradyzoites, which they use to hide in the host's tissues, and they burst later releasing tachyzoites sytemically (see Chapter 6 for figures of toxoplasma cysts in smears and in tissue.)

Pathophysiology

T. gondii has a sneaky way of surviving the host immune response by invading the parasitophorous vacuoles inside macrophages (see Figure 13.34). Since these sacs do not fuse with lyzosomes, they resist dissolution, parasites get nutrition, and they escape immune reaction allowing unimpeded multiplication

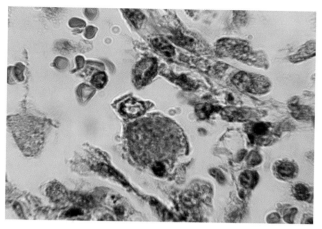

FIGURE 13.34 **Toxoplasmosis**. Toxoplasma bradyzoites inside a macrophage in lung tissue of an immunocompromised patient with disseminated disease.

until the cell ruptures and releases tachyzoites. These are the motile, bow shaped form of the parasite, that distribute via the blood stream, and are recognized by the host immune system. Similar to the mechanism used by some viruses, toxoplasma is also able to dysregulate the immune effector cells by secreting a factor that inhibits the cell cycle of nearby cells. Other factors secreted are implicated in behavioral changes seen in experimental animals and that are also postulated to be involved in altered human behaviors via the factors' dopaminergic effects in the brain (Zimmer, 2000).

Clinical Features

Sites of Involvement. Typical lymphadenopathy presentation is characterized as cervical neck lymph nodes enlargement associated with fever and malaise. Clinically most patients are young children with a history of exposure to domestic cat or kitten. The clinical syndrome simulates an infectious mononucleosis, but the Monospot test is negative. The acute stage lasts several days and then proceeds to the latent stage, which persists for months. In immunocompetent persons, the chronic phase is asymptomatic. In immunocompromised patients (infected HIV or transplant recipients on immunosuppressive therapy), the symptoms are dramatic and serious. The most dramatic manifestation is toxoplasmic encephalitis. Similarly, if transmitted transplacentally, severe congenital infection can be spontaneous abortion (miscarriage) or intrauterine death secondary to cerebral complications and, less severe, may later manifest as bilateral chorioretinitis.

Approach to Diagnosis. A combination of the following findings indicate acute toxoplasmosis:

characteristic lymphadenopathy, the presence of a high IgG IFA titer ($\geq$1:1000), and the detection of toxoplasma-specific IgM. In surgical pathology or microbiology laboratories, confirmation of the diagnosis include the following set of modalities. Serologic test for toxoplasma is the mainstay for immunocompetent persons, although serology may be negative in initial infection. Therefore an evaluation of the lymph node pathology should be made to document the diagnostic histologic triad, along with a confirmatory PCR test for presence of toxoplasma DNA material. If there is toxoplasma tissue or cytology material (especially in a clinical setting where the patient is immunosuppressed), isolation from blood or tissue by culture can be performed. Infection from the protozoal organism *Toxoplasma gondii* is common and involves lymph nodes either locally or in a generalized manner. The posterior cervical nodes are commonly involved.

Morphology. A histopathology and serologically confirmed study in Turkey noted a 15% incidence of toxoplasma when based on the classic histologic triad among 731 reactive lymph node biopsies (Tuzuner et al., 1996). The histologic triad correlates highly with positive serology. The component of the triad includes follicular hyperplasia, microgranulomas, and monocytoid hyperplasia. On sections, lymph nodes show prominent follicles and activated germinal centers with tingible bodies, small poorly formed microgranulomas or loose histiocytic clusters impinging on the germinal centers, and crescentic areas of monocytoid hyperplasia in the subcapsule, trabeculae, or perifollicular areas (see Figure 13.35). Taken individually, the findings are nonspecific but in combination, along with confirmed serology, are characteristic permitting a diagnosis of toxoplasmosis.

Microgranulomas (or loose aggregates of histiocytes) surrounding or abutting the mantle zones and germinal centers may be the single most important feature not seen in other lymphadenopathies. It is rare to find microorganisms in histologic sections or imprints, except in immunocompromised patients. Because the pale areas of monocytoid B cells are often subcapsular, these cells were thought to be histiocytes and initially called immature sinus histiocytosis. Other findings include presence of scattered immunoblasts, periadenitis, and plasmacytosis.

Immunohistochemistry/Cytochemistry

The morphologic triad correlates historically with the Sabin–Feldman dye test and the IgM immunofluorescent antibody test (Dorfman and Remington, 1973). PCR has a reported 91% specificity and 63% sensitivity when correlated with the classic triad (Weiss et al., 1992). An antitoxoplasma IgM ELIZA assay (Diagnostic Bioprobes, Milan, Italy) was reported to have 98% and 99% sensitivity and specificity, respectively. The caveat is that the ELIZA should performed within three months of infection. Investigators using the IgM assay as a standard suggested that the classic histologic triad be modified (with 100% sensitivity and 96.6% specificity of correct diagnosis) as follows (Eapen, Mathew, and Aravindan, 2005):

1. Presence of microgranulomas
2. Follicular hyperplasia
3. Absence of multinucleated giant cells

They described the microgranulomas to be composed of fewer than 25 epithelioid cells, with localization not only in mantle or germinal centers but also in interfollicular and paracortical areas and diffusely in the sinus pattern. Monocytoid hyperplasia may be an inconstant or a later finding based on this single study, in contrast with the classic findings.

Differential Diagnosis

Monocytoid cells, when present, are a useful positive finding because these are rarely seen in other lymphadenitis associated with granulomas, such as sarcoidosis, syphilis, brucellosis, and chlamydia infections. The presence of monocytoid cells is hence useful in the differential diagnosis. When epithelioid clusters and reactive follicles are seen, it is important to look for Interfollicular Hodgkin lymphoma or because of monocytoid hyperplasia, MALT lymphoma involving the lymph nodes. There is no necrosis or fibrosis and extremely unusual to find Langhan's giant cells. The clusters of epithelioid histiocytes appear to have more histiocyte cytoplasm than the epithelioid cells in sarcoidosis or tuberculosis, the letter conditions often showing spindle epithelioid cells. The monocytoid cells are often in trabecular spaces and in between follicles as elliptical or elongated collections in low-power view, sometimes with a sprinkle of neutrophils. Moreover monocytoid cells are seen in a variety of diseases including HIV, viral adenitis, MALT lymphoma, and types of suppurative granulomatous lymphadenitis including CSD. Cat-scratch lymphadenitis, if biopsied early, may only have monocytoid hyperplasia or few early clusters of epithelioid histiocytes. The presence of plasmacytoid monocytes in the paracortex around the high endothelial venules may be a clue to an early CSD. The presence of plasmacytoid dendritic cell

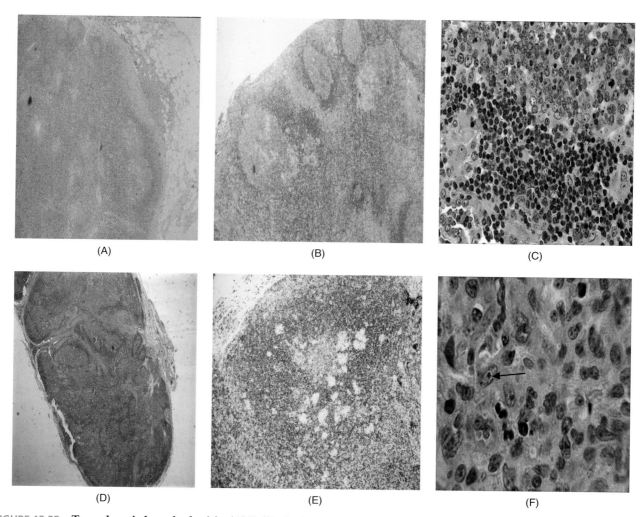

(A)   (B)   (C)

(D)   (E)   (F)

FIGURE 13.35   **Toxoplasmic lymphadenitis**. (**A**) Follicular hyperplasia, pale monocytoid cells in subcapsular and interfollicular areas, small clusters of epithelioid histiocytes encroaching on germinal centers are the minimal criteria for diagnosis. Monocytoid cells are also seen in *B. henselae lymphadenitis* but rarely if ever seen in sarcoid, brucellosis, or syphilis. (**B**) Microgranulomas impinging on germinal centers and interfollicular as well as in sinusoidal areas, adjacent sheets of pale monocytoid cells. No multinucleated cells or associated necrotic granulomas are seen. (**C**) Microgranulomas in mantle zone of germinal center. (**D**) Low-power view with florid follicular hyperplasia pushing medullary compartments and vessel outward, as well as pale monocytoid aeas in intertrabeculare sites. (**E**) The triad of microgranulomas, follicles, monocytoid cells. (**F**) Monocytoid B cells formerly called immature sinus histiocytosis. Unlike histiocytes, these cells show less cytoplasm, more pleomorphic, and the nuclei have thicker and more basophilic nuclear membranes, darker chromatin and many chromocenters. Larger histiocytes and endothelial cells on left show open cleared nuclei with a prominent central nucleolus (arrow) Two neturophils present.Immunoblasts with prominent nucleolus is also easily found (100×, H&E). Monocytoid B cells are different from marginal zone B cells; the latter appear around the mantle zoned especially in the spleen white pulp Peyer's patch and, mesenteric nodes, and in MALTOMAs. These are bcl-2 and CD43 positive, and the monocytoid cells are negative in both said markers.

clusters, which are associated with a high endothelial venule, is not a feature of toxoplasmic lymphadenitis. Paucity of the organism is a key finding that separates toxoplasmosis from leismaniasis, which often shows numerous intracellular amastigotes.

Other differential diagnosis commonly encountered in lymph nodes in North America include fungal and TB lymphadenitis, which have a more straightforward tissue workup. Tuberculosis (TB) is always a consideration in countries with high frequency of TB in population especially if biopsied early or after treatment. Classically TB shows fully formed, caseous granulomas, in association with Langhan's multinucleated giant cells, unlike the small epithelioid clusters in Toxoplasma. AFB stain is diagnostic but bacilli may be difficult to find.

Treatment of Choice and Prognosis

Recovery in a few months is the rule and treatment is seldom needed unless complications occur. In general, treatment is reserved for immunosuppressed individuals, congenital infections, ocular disease and infections during pregnancy. see Chapter 6 for recommendations on prevention of infection for the general population.

Additional Information

Washing vegetables thoroughly before eating them and cooking meat to recommended temperatures are just a few ways to reduce the risk of toxoplasmosis.

FOLLICULAR HYPERPLASIA WITH CAPSULAR FIBROSIS AND PLASMACYTOSIS-SYPHILIS

The name "syphilis" was coined by the Italian physician and poet Girolamo Fracastoro in his epic poem, written in Latin, titled *Syphilis sive morbus gallicus* (Latin for "Syphilis or the French Disease") in 1530. The origin of the name, however, is not faithful to the current understanding of the disease's near-worldwide distribution.

Definition

Syphilis is a bacterial disease caused by infection with the spirochete, *Treponema pallidum var pallidum*, almost always through sexual contact with an infected person.

ICD-10 Codes A50.0 - A53.0 and A53.9

Synonyms

The great imitator, the French pox, the Italian pox, lues, great pox, black lion.

Etiology

Syphilis is a sexually transmitted disease caused by the bacterial spirochete, *Treponema pallidum var pallidum*. There are several subspecies of *T. pallidum* that cause human disease, but syphilis is the most common. The disease arises from direct contact with an infected lesion, usually on the genitals.

Epidemiology

Syphilis is a relatively rare disease in the United States, but its incidence has been increasing since its decline in the latter part of the twentieth century.

The incidence is highest in large urban areas, and in 2006 there were about 10,000 cases of syphilis in Los Angeles, Chicago, and New York City. Transmission by infected prostitutes is still the most common route of *T. pallidum* infection worldwide, and infected women can pass congenital syphilis to their unborn children. An emerging association between asymptomatic syphilis and the transmission of HIV, especially among men who have sex with men, is causing concern and prompting reevaluation of screening programs for sexually transmitted diseases (Buchacz et al., 2008, Branger et al., 2009).

Pathogenesis

T. pallidum bacteria are motile, Gram-negative spirochaetes that are obligate human parasites. They die quickly outside the body and do not persist on surfaces as some organisms do. Within the human body the bacteria can move relatively quickly by means of their flagella and surface proteins facilitate cell adherence and penetration. Some virulent strains are able to acquire a coating of host fibronectin that renders them less likely to be phagocytosed. In pregnant women infected with syphilis, the bacteria are also able to enter the placenta and infect the fetus causing congenital syphilis.

Unless treated, primary syphilis will progress into secondary and tertiary disease. Tertiary disease occurs in 30 to 50% of cases. The primary chancre has a neutrophilic infiltrate early on and later shows a chronic inflammatory infiltrate of T and B lymphocytes. The secondary form follows an emergence of a new bacterial strain that is resistant to immune antibodies. Later the secondary syphilis manifestation may be immune complex mediated. As more anti-treponemal antibodies become reactive to this new strain and cell-mediated immunity is restored; a latent or quiescent phase emerges that ushers the tertiary phase.

Clinical Features

Site of Infection. The principal infection sites are the genitals, anus, and rectum, but transmission can also occur orally. Approximately 30% of exposed people contract the disease. The principal lesion, a hard chancre, develops following an incubation period of approximately 3 weeks. The hard chancre, a firm, painless sore, appears at the site of entry marking the primary stage of syphilis. Palpable lymphadenopathy usually does not occur until the secondary phase during which the person is most infectious. Some cases of cervical lymphadenitis in persons otherwise unsuspected of the presence of a sexually transmitted disease have been identified by examination of fine-needle aspirates from the enlarged nodes (Van CR et al., 2009).

Bacterial infection occurs from lesions on an infected individual through skin breaks or abrasions, usually during sexual activity. A hard chancre appears at the infection site on average about 3 weeks after contact, but during this period, the infected person is usually asymptomatic. Six to 8 weeks after the lesion appears, the disease has progressed to what is known as secondary syphilis characterized by lymphadenopathy, headache, malaise, and frequently a pale, reddish rash on the trunk and extremities, particularly the palms of the hands and the soles of the feet. Secondary stage syphilis can appear to resolve on its own, but the disease actually enters a state of latency that can last for years during which the infected person shows no symptoms but tests positive for *T. pallidum*. The final stage of syphilis is called the tertiary and occurs on average 1 to 10 years after the secondary stage, but may not become manifest for as long as 50 years. Tertiary syphilis, which may be fatal, can involve the brain, cardiovascular system, and other organs, and often produces large, nodular granulomas.

Approach to Diagnosis. Primary syphilis often goes undiagnosed because of the frequent lack of symptoms. The Rapid Plasma Reagin Test and the Venereal Disease Research Laboratory test are the principle tools for assessing syphilis infection through a blood or CSF sample. More sensitive and specific tests involve immunofluorescence, PCR, and enzyme immunoassay.

Immunohistochemistry/Cytochemistry. The *T. pallidum* bacteria cannot be cultured in the lab, but the organisms can be seen microscopically by using dark-field illumination. In skin biopsies of patients suspected of secondary syphilis, immunohistochemistry for *T. pallidum* may be a more sensitive method to detect spirochetes than silver stain (Hoang, High, and Molberg, 2004).

Morphology. Regional lymphadenopathy adjacent to the chancre may develop during all stages of syphilis. The nodes are firm and nonsuppurative. It may persist for months, despite healing of the chancre. The most prominent histologic features are vascular changes caused by endarteritis and periarteritis (perivascular cuffing). Although the histologic picture is not diagnostic and includes follicular hyperplasia (Figures 13.36, 13.37), along with plasmacytosis (Figure 3.36, inset), vasculitis (Figure 13.38), as well as capsular and trabecular fibrosis (Figure 13.39), the

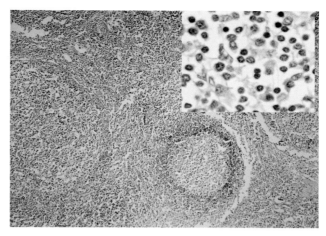

FIGURE 13.36 **Syphilis lymphadenopathy.** Follicular hyperplasia is seen at low-power view with attenuated mantle and interfollicular hypervascularity (inset). Abundant plasma cells in parenchyma are present.

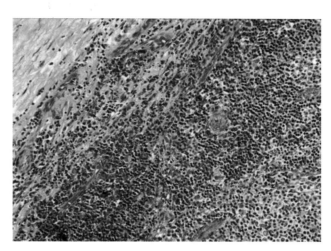

FIGURE 13.37 **Syphilis.** There is capsular fibrosis with many mature plasma cells and increased vessels.

constellation of findings would prompt consideration of syphilis. In tertiary syphilis, granulomatous involvement of lymph node may rarely be seen. The granulomas are non-caseating and may show Langhans giant cells. Progressive inflammation of the blood vessels can cause endarteritis. The organisms may or may not be observable.

Differential Diagnosis. Other subspecies of *T. pallidum* can cause human diseases such as yaws (*Treponema pallidum var pertenue*) and pinta (*Treponema pallidum var carateum*), and positive identification may require immunofluorescence or other molecular assays. Another disease to differentiate includes chancroid or soft chancre disease, which is an acute sexually transmitted disease characterized by genital

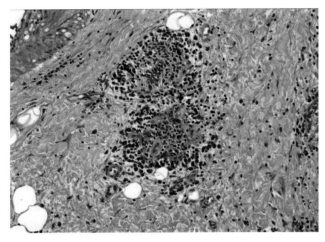

FIGURE 13.38 **Syphilis**. Vasculitis in the fibrosed capsule.

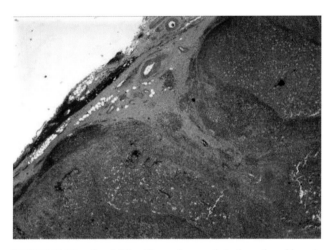

FIGURE 13.39 **Syphilis**. Capsular and trabecular fibrosis and follicular hyperplasia.

ulceration and suppuration caused by the organism *Haemophilus ducreyi*. Also genital herpes type 2 infection, lymphogranuloma venereum, granuloma inguinale, and trauma have to be considered for lesions found around the genitalia. Sometimes acute suppurative and necrotizing granulomas are prominent, and it is important to differentiate from other sexually transmitted infection such as gonococcal lymphadenitis or those secondary to *Yersinia* infections.

Treatment and Prognosis. The initial infection, known as primary syphilis, causes a sore called a chancre at the point of entry but few symptoms. The next stage, secondary syphilis, may result in palpable lymphadenopathy and is associated with a pale reddish rash on the palms of the hands, the soles of the feet and other parts of the body. If untreated, the disease can progress to the tertiary stage with formation of granulomas and involvement of the nervous system and other organs. Early treatment with antibiotics can effect a complete cure with no permanent damage (Kent and Romanelli, 2008).

A paradoxical course may follow treatment called Jarisch–Herxheimer reaction. It is an intensification of existing syphilitic lesions and/or exacerbation of old ones following administration of penicillin; the reaction subsides in 24 hours.

REFERENCES

Amin HM, Medeiros LJ, Manning JT, Jones D. 2003. Dissolution of the lymphoid follicle is a feature of the HHV8+ variant of plasma cell Castleman's disease. Am J Surg Pathol 27:91–100.

Androulaki A, Giaslakiotis K, Giaslakiotis K, Giakoumi X, Aessopos A, Lazaris AC. 2007. Localized Castleman's disease associated with systemic AA amyloidosis. Regression of amyloid deposits after tumor removal. Ann Hematol 86:55–7.

Azam M, Husen YA, Pervez S. 2009. Calcifying fibrous pseudotumor in association with hyaline vascular type Castleman's disease. Indian J Pathol Microbiol 52:527–9.

Barbounis V, Efremidis A. 1996. A plasma cell variant of Castleman's disease treated successfully with cimetidine: case report and review of the literature. Anticancer Res 16:545–7.

Baserga M, Rosin M, Schoen M, Young G. 2005. Multifocal Castleman disease in pediatrics: case report. J Pediatr Hematol Oncol 27:666–9.

Berek CA, Berger, Apel M. 1991. Maturation of the immune response in germinal centers. Cell 67:1121–9.

Bouron-Dal Soglio D, Truong F, Fetni R, Hazourli S, Champagne J, Oligny LL, Fournet JC. 2008. A B-cell lymphoma-associated chromosomal translocation in a progressive transformation of germinal center. Hum Pathol 39:292–7.

Bowne WB, Lewis JJ, Filippa DA, Niesvizky R, Brooks AD, Burt ME, Brennan MF. 1999. The management of unicentric and multicentric Castleman disease: a report of 16 cases and a review of the literature. Cancer 85:706–17.

Branger J, van der Meer JT, van Ketel RJ, Jurriaans S, Prins JM. 2009. High incidence of asymptomatic syphilis in HIV-infected MSM justifies routine screening. Sex Transm Dis 36:84–85.

Buchacz K, Klausner JD, Kerndt PR, Shouse RL, Onorato I, McElroy PD, Schwendemann J, Tambe PB, Allen M, Coye F, Kent C, Park MN, Hawkins K, Samoff E, Brooks JT. 2008. HIV incidence among men diagnosed with early syphilis in Atlanta, San Francisco, and Los Angeles, 2004 to 2005. J Acquir Immune Defic Syndr 47:234–40.

Buesing K, Perry D, Reyes C, Abdessalam S. 2009. Castleman disease: surgical cure in pediatric patients. J Pediatr Surg 44:e5–8.

BURNS BF, COLBY TV, DORFMAN RF. 1984. Differential diagnostic features of nodular L&H Hodgkin's disease, including progressive transformation of germinal centers. Am J Surg Pathol 8:253–61.

CAMPO E, MIQUEL R, KRENACS L, SORBARA L, RAFFELD M, JAFFE ES. 1999. Primary nodal marginal zone lymphoma of splenic and MALT type. Am J Surg Pathol 23:59–68.

CASPER C. 2005. The aetiology and management of Castleman disease at 50 years: translating pathophysiology to patient care. Br J Hematol 129:3–17.

CASTLEMAN B, IVERSON L, MENENDEZ VP. 1056. Localized mediastinal lymph node hyperplasia resembling thymoma. Cancer 9:822–30.

CHAN WC. 1999. Cellular origin of nodular lymphocyte-predominant Hodgkin's disease: immunophenotypic and molecular studies. Semin Hematol 36:242–52.

CHANG CC, OSIPOV V, WHEATON S, TRIPP S, PERKINS SL. 2003. Follicular hyperplasia, follicular lysis, and progressive transformation of germinal centers: a sequential spectrum of morphologic evolution in lymphoid hyperplasia. Am J Clin Pathol 102:322–6.

CHANG KL, KAMEL OW, ARBER DA, HORYD D, WEISS LM. 1995. Pathologic features of nodular lymphocyte predominance Hodgkin's disease in extranodal sites. Am J Surg Pathol 19:1323–4.

CHEN CH, LIU HC, HUNG TT, LIU TP. 2009. Possible roles of Epstein–Barr virus in Castleman disease. J Cardiothorac Surg 4:31.

CHEN WC, JONES D, HO CL, CHEUG CN, TSENG JY, TSAI HP, CHAUG KC. 2006. Cytogenetic anomalies in hyaline vascular Castleman disease: report of two cases with reappraisal of histogenesis. Cancer Genet Cytogenet 164:110–7.

CHOI JH, JO YJ, GONG SJ, HONG BW, LEE HJ, SON BK, JUN DW, KIM SH, PARK YS, SEOK JW. 2008. Unicentric Castleman disease is not clearly distinguished from multicentric type: a case report. Clin Lymphoma Myeloma 8:256–9.

COOPER MD, CHASE HP, LOWMAN JT, et al. 1966. Wiskott–Aldrich syndrome: an immunologic deficiency disease involving the afferent limb of immunity. Am J Med 44:499–513.

COTTER H, KRAFT R, MEISTER F. 1991. Primary immunodeficiency syndromes and their manifestations in lymph nodes. Curr Top Pathol 84(pt 2) 81–155.

DISPENZIERI A, GERTZ MA. 2004. Treatment of POEMS syndrome. Curr Treat Options Oncol 5:249–57.

DISPERIZIERI A, GERTZ MA. 2005. Treatment of Castleman's disease. Curr Treat Options Oncol 6:255–66.

DOGAN A, BAGDI E, MUNSON P, ISAACSON PG. 2000. CD10 and BCL-6 expression in paraffin sections of normal lymphoid tissue and B-cell lymphomas. Am J Surg Pathol 24:846–52.

DORFMAN RF, REMINGTON JS. 1973. Value of lymph-node biopsy in the diagnosis of acute aquired toxoplasmosis. New Engl J Med 289:878–81.

DORFMAN RF, WARNKE R. 1974. Lymphadenopathy simulating the malignant lymphoma. Hum Pathol 5:519–50.

DORFMAN RF, REMINGTON JS. 1973. Value of lymph-node biopsy in the diagnosis of acute acquired toxoplasmosis. N Engl J Med 289:878–81.

DUBEY JP 2004. Toxoplasmosis—a waterborne zoonosis. Vet Parasitol 126:57–72.

DUPIN N, DISS TL, KELLAM P, TULLIEZ M, DU M-Q, SICARD D, WEISS RA, ISAACSON PG, BOSHOFF C. 2000. HHV-8 is associated with a plasmablastic variant of Castleman disease that is linked to HHV-8-positive plasmablastic lymphoma. Blood 95:1406–12.

DUPIN N, DISS TL, KELLAM P, TULLIEZ M, DU M-Q, SICARD D, WEISS RA, ISAACSON PG, BOSHOFF C. 2000. HHV-8 is associated with a plasmablastic variant of Castleman disease that is linked to HHV-8–positive plasmablastic lymphoma. Blood 15(95):1406–12.

EAPEN M, MATHEW CF, ARAVINDAN KP. 2005. Evidence based criteria for the histopathological diagnosis of toxoplasmic lymphadenopathy. J Clin Pathol 58:1143–6.

EDVARD SMITH CI, BÄCKESJÖ CM, BERGLÖF A, BRANDÉN LJ, ISLAM T, MATTSSON PT, MOHAMED AJ, MÜLLER S, NORE B, VIHINEN M. 1998. X-linked agammaglobulinemia: lack of mature B lineage cells caused by mutations in the Btk kinase. Springer Sem Immunopathol 19(4):369–81.

EL-DALY H, BOWER M, NARESH KN. 2010. Follicular dendritic cells in multicentric Castleman disease present human herpes virus type 8 (HHV8)-latent nuclear antigen 1 (LANA1) in a proportion of cases and is associated with an enhanced T-cell response. Eur J Haematol 84:133–6.

FACCHETTI F, APPIIANAI C, SALVI L, et al. 1995. Immunohistologic analysis of ineffective CD40-CD40L ligand interactions in lymphoid tissue from patients with X-linked immunodeficiency with hyper-IgM. Abortive germinal center reaction and severe deletion of follicular dendritic cells. J Immunol 154:6624–33.

FACCHETTI F, BLANZUOLI L, UNGARI M, ALEBARDI O, VERMI W. 1998. Lymph node pathology in primary combined immunodeficiency diseases. Springer Seminars in Immunopathology 19(4):459–78.

FARHI DC, McGUIRE PW, LUCKEY CN. 1993. Monoclonality in reactive lymphadenopathy: gene rearrangement and multiparameter analysis. Hematol Pathol 7:143–52.

FAZAKAS A, CSIRE M, BERENCSI G, SZEPESI A, MATOLCSY A, JAKAB L, KARÁDI I, VÁRKONYI J. 2009. Multicentric plasmocytic Castleman's disease with polyneuropathy, organomegaly, endocrinopathy, M protein, skin changes syndrome and coexistent human herpes virus-6 infection—a possible relationship. Leuk Lymphoma 50:1661–5.

FERRY JA, ZUKERBERG LR, HARRIS NL. 1992. Florid progressive transformation of germinal centers: a syndrome affecting young men, without early progression to nodular lymphocyte predominant Hodgkin's disease. Am J Surg Pathol 16:252–8.

FLENDRIG JA, SCHILLINGS PM. 1969. Benign giant lymphoma: the clinical signs and symptoms. Folia Medica Neerlandica 12:119–20.

FRIZZERA G, MASSARELLI G, BANKS PM, ROSAI J. 1983. A systemic lymphoproliferative disorder with morphologic features of Castleman's disease: pathological findings in 15 patients. Am J Surg Pathol 7:211–31.

FRIZZERA G. 2001. Atypical lymphoproliferative disorders. In: Knowles DM, ed., Neoplastic Hematopathology. Lippincott Williams and Wilkins, Philadelphia, 569–622.

GERSTOFT J, PALLESEN G, MATHIESEN LR, PEDERSEN C, GAUB J, LINDHARDT BO. 1989. The value of lymph node histology in human immunodeficiency virus related persistent generalized lymphadenopathy. APMIS (suppl 8):24–27.

GHOSH A, PRADHAN SV, TALWAR OP. 2010. Castleman's disease-hyaline vascular type-clinical, cytological and histological features with review if literature. Indian J Pathol Microbiol 53:244–7.

GOATES JJ, KAMEL OW, LEBRUN DP, BENHARROCH D, DORFMAN RF. 1994. Floral variant of follicular lymphoma: immunological and molecular studies support a neoplastic process Am J Surg Pathol 18:37–47.

GOOD DJ, GASCOYNE RD. 2009. Atypical lymphoid hyperplasia mimicking lymphoma. Hematol Oncol Clin North Am 23:729–45.

GUETTIER C, GATTER KC, HERYET A, MASON DY. 1986. Dendritic reticulum cells in reactive lymph nodes and tonsils: an immunohistological study. Histopathology 10:15–24.

HANSMANN ML, FELLBAUM C, HUI PK, MOUBAYED P. 1990. Progressive transformation of germinal centers with and without association to Hodgkin's disease. Am J Clin Pathol 93:219–26.

HENRY K. 1972. Follicular hyperplasia. In: HENRY K, SYMMERS St. Claire W, eds. Thymus, Lymph Node, Spleen and Lymphatics. Systemic Pathology, vol. 7, 3rd ed. Churchill Livingstone, Edinburgh p 183–192.

HEYMER B, NIETHAMMER D, HAAS R, MEISTER H, HAFERKAMP O. 1976. Pathomorphologic findings in severe combined immunodeficiency and reticular dysgenesia. Virchows Arch A Pathol Anat Histol 370(2):151–62.

HICKS J, FLAITZ C. 2002. Progressive transformation of germinal centers: review of histopathologic and clinical features. Int J Pediatr Otorhinolaryngol 65:195–202.

HOANG MP, HIGH WA, MOLBERG KH. 2004. Secondary syphilis: a histologic and immunohistochemical evaluation. J Cutan Pathol 31:595–9.

HSIAO CJ, HSU MM, LEE JY, CHEN WC, HSIEH WC. 2001. Paraneoplastic pemphigus in association with a retroperitoneal Castleman's disease presenting with a lichen planus pemphigoides-like eruption: a case report and review of literature. Br J Dermatol 144:372–6.

HSU SM, COSSMAN J, JAFFE ES. 1983. Lymphocyte subsets in normal human lymphoid tissues. Am J Clin Pathol. 80:21–30.

HUANG J, WANG L, ZHOU W, JIN J. 2007. Hyaline vascular Castleman disease associated with POEMS syndrome and cerebral infraction. Ann Hematol 86:59–61.

HUBER J, ZEGERS BJM, SCHUURMAN HJ. 1992. Pathology of congenital immunodeficiencies. Semin Diagn Pathol 9:31.

HUNG IJ, LIN JJ, YANG CP, HSUEH C. 2006. Paraneoplastic syndrome and intrathoracic Castleman disease. Pediatr Blood Cancer 15:616–20.

HUNT JP, CHAN JA, SAMOSZUK M, BRYNES RK, HERNANDEZ AM, BASS R, WEISENBURGER DD, MÜLLER-HERMELINK K, NATHWANI BN. 2001. Hyperplasia of mantle/marginal zone B cells with clear cytoplasm in peripheral lymph nodes: a clinicopathologic study of 35 cases. Am J Clin Pathol 116:550–9.

IOACHIM HL, CRONIN W, ROY M, MAYA M. 1990. Persistent lymphadenopathies in people at high risk for HIV infection. Clinicopathologic correlations and longterm follow-up in 79 cases. Am J Clin Pathol 93:208–18.

ISAACSON PG. 2001. Gastrointestinal lymphoma and lymphoid hyperplasia. In: Knowles DM, ed., Neoplastic Hematopathology, 2nd ed. Lippincott Williams and Wilkins, New York, 1235–61.

JACKSON CE, PUCK JM. 1999. Autoimmune lymphoproliferative syndrome, a disorder of apopotosis. Curr Opin Pediatr 11:521–7.

JOHRENS K, SHIMIZU Y, ANAGNOSTOPOULOS I, SCHIFFMANN S, TIACCI E, FALINI B, STEIN H. 2005. T-β-positive and IRTA1-positive monocytoid B cells differ from marginal zone B cells and epithelial-associated B cells in their antigen profile and topographical distribution. Haematologica 90:1070–7.

JONES JL, KRUSZON-MORAN D, SANDERS-LEWIS K, WILSON M. 2007. *Toxoplasma gondii* infection in the United States, 1999–2004: decline from the prior decade. Am J Trop Med Hyg 77:405–10.

JONGSMA T, VERBURG R, GEELHOED-DUIJVESTIJN P. 2007. Castleman's disease: a rare lymphoproliferative disorder. Eur J Intern Med 8:87–9.

KARUBE K, OHSHIMA K, TSUCHIYA T, YAMAGUCHI T, KAWANO R, SUZUMIYA J, HARADA M, KIKUCHI M. 2005. A "floral" variant of nodal marginal zone lymphoma. Hum Pathol 36(2):202–6.

KATAYANAGI K, TERADA T, NAKANUMA Y, UENO T. 1994. A case of pseudolymphoma of the liver. Pathol Int 44:704–11.

KAVLI B, ANDERSEN S, OTTERLEI M, LIABAKK, NB, IMAI K, FISCHER A, DURANDY A, KROKAN HE, SLUPPHAUG G. 2005. B cells from hyper-IgM patients carrying UNG mutations lack ability to remove uracil from ssDNA and have elevated genomic uracil. J Exp Med 201(12):2011–21.

KELLER AR, HOCHHOLZER L, CASTLEMAN B. 1972. Hyaline-vascular and plasma-cell types of giant lymph node hyperplasia of the mediastinum and other locations. Cancer 29:670–83.

KENT ME, ROMANELLI F. 2008. Reexamining syphilis: an update on epidemiology, clinical manifestations, and management. Ann Pharmacother 42:226–36.

KOJIMA M, MURAYAMA K, HIGUCHI K, MATSUMOTO, M, TAMAKI Y, MASAWA N. 2006. Reactive lymphoid hyperplasia with giant follicles associated with post-therapeutic state of hematological malignancies: a report of six cases. Leuk Lymphoma 47:1404–6.

Kojima M, Nakamura S, Itoh H, Motoori T, Sugihara S, Shinkai H, Masawa N. 2001. Angioimmunoblastic T-cell lymphoma with hyperplastic germinal centers: a clinicopathological and immunohistochemical study of 10 cases APMIS. 109(10):699–706.

Kojima M, Nakamura S, Lijima M, Murayama K, Sakata N, Masawa N. 2005. Lymphoid variant of hyaline vascular Castleman's disease containing numerous mantle zone lymphocytes with clear cytoplasm. APMIS 113:75–80.

Kojima M, Nakamura S, Miyawaki S, Ohno Y, Sakata N, Masawa N. 2005. Progressive transformation of germinal center presenting with histological features of hyaline-vascular type of Castleman's disease. APMIS 113: 288–95.

Kojima M, Nakamura S, Motoori T, Itoh H, Shimizu K, Yamane N, Ohno Y, Ban S, Yoshida K, Hoshi K, Oyama T, Shimano S, Sugihara S, Sakara N, Masawa N. 2003. Progessive transformation of germinal centers: a clinicopathological study of 42 Japanese patients. Int J Srg Pathol 11: 101–7.

Kojima M, Nakamura S, Motoori T, Shimizu K, Ohno Y, Itoh H, Masawa N. 2002. Follicular hyperplasia presenting with a marginal zone pattern in a reactive lymph node lesion. Areport of six cases. APMIS 110:325–31.

Kojima M, Nakamura S, Nishikawa M, Miyawaki S, Massawa N. 2005. Idiopathic multicentric Castleman's disease. A clinicopathologic and immunohistochemical study of five cases. Pathol Res Pract 201:325–32.

Kojima M, Nakamura S, Shimizu K, Itoh H, Yoshida K, Hosomura Y, Yamane N, Ban S, Joshita T, Suchi T. 1998. Florid reactive follicular hyperplasia in elderly patients: a clinicopathological study of 23 cases. Pathol Res Pract 194:391–8.

Kojima M, Nakarmura N, Sakamoto K, Sakurai S, Tsukamoto N, Itoh H, Ikota H, Enomoto Y, Shimizu K, Motoori T, Hoshi K, Igarashi T, Masawa N, Nakamine H. 2010. Progressive transformation of the germinal center of extranodal organs: a clinicopathological, immunohistochemical, and genotypic study of 14 cases. Pathol Res Pract 206: 235–40.

Kojima M, Shimizu K, Okota H, Ohno Y, Motoori T, Itoh H, Masawa N, Nakamura S. 2008. "Follicular variant" of hyaline-vascular type of Castleman's disease: histopathological and immunohistochemical study of 11 cases. J Clin Exp Hematop 48:39–45.

Kojima M, Tanaka H, Matsuda H, Iijima M, Motoori T, Masawa N. 2005. Floral variant of follicular lymphoma containing marginal zone B-cell component: a report of two cases. APMIS 113:638–42.

Kop EN, MacKenzie MA. 2010. Clinical images: Castleman disease and paraneoplastic pemphigus. CMAJ 182:61.

Kreft A, Weber A, Springer E, Hess G, Kirkpatrick CJ. 2007. Bone marrow findings in multicentric Castleman disease in HIV-negative patients. Am J Surg Pathol 3:398–402.

Krishnan C, Warnke RA, Arber DA, Natkunam Y. 2010. PD-1 expression in T-cell lymphomas and reactive lymphoid entities: potential overlap in staining patterns between lymphoma and viral lymphadenitis. Am J Surg Pathol 34:178–89.

Lai R, Arber DA, Chang KL, Wilson CS, Weiss LM. 1998. Frequency of bcl-2 expression in non-Hodgkin's lymphoma: a study of 778 cases with comparison of marginal zone lymphoma and monocytoid B-cell hyperplasia. Mod Pathol 11:864–9.

Lee J, Ban JY, Won KY, Kim GY, Lin SJ, Lee S, Kim YW, Park YK, Lee SS. 2008. Expression of EGFR and follicular dendritic markers in lymphoid follicles from patients with Castleman's disease. Oncol Rep 20:851–6.

Leiti AC, Nascimento OJ, Lima MA, Andrada-Serpa MJ. 2007. POEMS (polyneuropathy, organomegaly, endocrinopathy, M protein, skin lesions) syndrome: a South America's report. Arg Neuropsiquiatr 65: 516–20.

Lennert K, Hansmann M. 1987. Progressive transformation of germinal centers: clinical significance and lymphocytic predominance Hodgkin's disease: the Kiel experience. Am J Surg Pathol 11:149–50.

Liang J, Newman JG, Frank DM, Chalian AA. 2009. Cervical unicentric Castleman disease presenting as a neck mass: case report and review of the literature. Ear Nose Throat J 88:E8.

Licup AT, Campisi P, Ngan BY, Forte V. 2006. Progressive transformation of germinal centers: an uncommon cause of pediatric cervical lymphadenopathy. Arch Otolaryngol Head Neck Surg 132:797–801.

Lim MS, Straus SE, Dale JK, Fleisher TA, Stetler-Stevenson M, Strober W, Sneller MC, Puck JM, Lenardo MJ, Elenitoba-Johnson KS, Lin AY, Raffeld M, Jaffe ES. 1998. Pathological findings in human autoimmune lymphoproliferative syndrome. Am J Pathol 153(5):1541–50.

Martin JV, Willoughby PB, Giusti V, Price G, Cerezo L. 1995. The lymph node pathology of Omenn's syndrome. Am J Surg Pathol 19(9):1082–7.

Martino G, Cariati S, Tintisona O, Veneroso S, De Villa F, Vergine M, Monti M. 2004. Atypical lymphoproliferative disorders: Castleman's disease. Case report and review of the literature. Tumori 90:352–5.

Mathew P, Hudnall SD, Elghetany MT, Payne DA. 2001. T-gamma gene rearrangement and CMV mononucleosis. Am J Hematol 66:64–66.

McCarty MJ, Vukelja SJ, Banka PM, Weiss RB. 1995. Angiofollicular lymph node hyperplasia (Castleman's disease). Cancer Treat Rev 21:219–310.

Menenakos C, Braumann C, Hartmann J, Jacobi CA. 2007. Retroperitoneal Castleman's tumor and paraneoplastic pemphigus: report of a case and review of the literature. World J Surg Oncol 5:45.

Müller-Hermelink HK, Lennert K. 1978. The cytologic, histologic, and functional bases for a modern classification of lymphomas. In: Lennert K, Mohri N, Stein H, Kaiserling E, Muller-Hermelink HK, eds., Malignant Lymphomas Other Than Hodgkin's Disease. Springer, Berlin, 1–71.

Mylona E, Baraboutis I, Lekakis L, Georgiou O, Papastamopoulos V, Skoutelis A. 2008. Multicentric

Castleman's disease in HIV infection: a systematic review of the literature. AIDS Rev 10:25–35.

NAM-CHA SH, SAN-MILLÁN B, MOLLEJO M, GARCIA-COSIO M, GARIJO G, GOMEZ M, WARNKE RA, JAFFE ES, PIRIS MA. 2008. Light-chain-restricted germinal centres in reactive lymphadenitis: report of eight cases. Histopathology 52(4):436–44.

NEWLON J, COUCH M, BRENNAN J. 2007. Castleman's disease: three case reports and a review of the literature. Ear Nose Throat J 86:414–18.

NGUYEN PL, FERRY JA, HARRIS NL. 1999. Progressive transformation of germinal centers and nodular lymphocyte predominant Hodgkin's disease: comparative immunohistochemical study. Am J Surg Pathol 23:27–33.

NOTARANGELO LD, LANZI G, TONIATI P, GILIANI S. 2007. Immunodeficiencies due to defects of class-switch recombination. Immunol Res 38(1–3):68–77.

OKSENHENDLER E, BOULANGER E, GALICIER L, DU M-Q, DUPIN N, DISS TC, HAMOUDI R, DANIEL M-T, AGBALIKA F, BOSHOFF C, CLAUVEL J-P, ISAACSON PG, MEIGNIN V. 2002. High incidence of Kaposi sarcoma-associated herpes virus-related non-Hodgkin lymphoma in patients with HIV infection and multicentric Castleman disease. Blood 99:2331–6.

OSBORNE BM, BUTLER JJ, GRESIK MV. 1992. Progressive transformation of germinal centers: comparison of 23 pediatric patients to the adult population. Mod Pathol 5:135–40.

OSBORNE BM, BUTLER JJ, VIRIAKOJIS D, KOTT M. 1982. Reactive lymph node hyperplasia with giant follicles. Am J Clin Pathol 78:493–9.

OSBORNE BM, BUTLER JJ. 1984. Clinical implications of progressive transformation of germinal centers. Am J Surg Pathol 8:725–33.

OSBORNE BM, BUTLER JJ. 1987. Follicular lymphoma mimicking progressive transformation of germinal centers. Am J Clin Pathol 88(3):264–9.

OSBORNE BM, BUTLER JJ. 1991. Clinical implications of nodal reactive follicular hyperplasia in the elderly patient with enlarged lymph nodes. Mod Pathol 4(1):24–30.

PAREZ N, BADER-MEUNIER B, ROY CC, DOMMERGUES JP. 1999. Paediatric Castleman disease: report of seven cases and review of the literature. Eur J Pediatr 158:631–7.

PAUWELS P, DAL CIN P, VIASSVELD LT, ALEVA RM, VAN ERP WF, JONES D. 2000. A chromosomal abnormality in hyaline vascular Castleman's disease: evidence for clonal proliferation of dysplastic stromal cells. Am J Surg Pathol 24:882–8.

PAYDAS S, ERGIN M, SIKGENC M, BICAKCI K, KIROGLU M. 2009. Castleman-like reaction due to toxic substance ingestion. Eur J Intern Med 20:328–30.

PEH SC, SHAMINIE J, POPPEMA S, KIN LH. 2003. The immunophenotypic patterns of follicle centre and mantle zone in Castleman's disease. Singapore Med 44:185–91.

PETERSON BA, FRIZZERA G. 1993. Multicentric Castleman's disease. Semi Oncol 20:636–47.

PETERSON RDA, et al. 1966. Lymphoid tissue abnormalities associated with Ataxia-telangiectasia. Am J Med 41:341–59.

PILCHER CD, FISCUS SA, NGUYEN TQ, FOUST E, WOLF L, WILLIAMS D, ASHBY R, O'DOWD JO, McPHERSON JT, STALZER B, HIGHTOW L, MILLER WC, ERON JJ Jr., COHEN MS, LEONE PA. 2005. Detection of acute infections during HIV testing in North Carolina. N Engl J Med 352:1873–83.

PLANK L, HANSMANN ML, FISCHER R. 1993. The cytological spectrum of the monocytoid B-cell reaction: recognition of its large cell type. Histopathology 23:425–31.

POPPEMA S, DELSOL G, PILERI S, STEIN H, SWERDLOW SH, WARNKE RA, JAFFE ES. 2008. Nodular lymphocyte predominant Hodgkin lymphoma. In: Swerdlow SH, Campo E, Harris NL, Jaffe ES, Pileri SA, Stein H, Thiele V, Vardiman JW (Eds.), WHO Classification of Tumours of Haematopoietic and Lymphoid Tissues. IARC Press, Lyon. p 323–325.

POPPEMA S. 1992. Lymphocyte-predominance Hodgkin's disease. Int Rev Exp Pathol 33:53–79.

PUCK JM, SNELLER MC. 1997. ALPS: an autoimmune human lymphoproliferative syndrome associated with abnormal lymphocyte apoptosis. Semin Immunol 9(1):77–84.

REVY P, MUTO T, LEVY Y, GEISSMANN F, PLEBANI A, SANAL O, CATALAN N, FORVEILLE M, DUFOURCQ-LABELOUSE R, GENNERY A, et al. 2000. Activation-induced cytidine deaminase (AID) deficiency causes the autosomal recessive form of the Hyper-IgM syndrome (HIGM2). Cell 2102(5):565–75.

ROCA B. 2009. Castleman's disease: a review. AIDS Rev 11:3–7.

RUSHIN JM, RIORDAN GP, HEATON RB, SHARPE RW, COTELINGAM JD, JAFFE ES. 1990. Cytomegalovirus-infected cells express Leu-M1 antigen: a potential source of diagnostic error. Am J Pathol 136(5):989–95.

SANDHAUS LM, VOELKERDING K, RASKA K Jr. 1988. Follicular lymphoma mimicking progressive transformation of germinal centers: immunologic analysis of a case. Am J Clin Pathol 90:518–9.

SATO Y, KOJIMA M, TAKATA K, MORITO T, ASSAOKU H, TAKEUCHI T, MIZOBUCHI K, FUJIHARA M, KURAOKA K, NAKAI T, ICHIMURA K, TANAKA T, TAMURA M, NISHIKAWA Y, YOSHINO T. 2009. Systemic IgG4-related lymphadenopathy: a clinical and pathologic comparison to multicentric Castleman's disease. Mod Pathol 22:589–99.

SCHNITZER B. 1995. Reactive lymphoid hyperplasias. In Jaffe ES, ed., Surgical Pathology of the Lymph Nodes and Related Organs, 2nd ed. Saunders, Philadelphia, 98–132.

SCHNITZER B. 2001. The reactive lymphadenopathies. In: Knowles DM, ed., Neoplastic Hematopathologym, 2nd ed. Lippincott Williams and Wilkins, Philadelphia, 537–568.

SEGAL GH, PERKINS SL, KJELDSBERG CR. 1995. Benign lymphadenopathies in children and adolescents. Semin Diagn Pathol 12:288–302.

SHEIBANI K, BEN-EZRA J, SWARTZ WG, ROSSI J, KEZIRIAN J, KOO CH, WINBERG CD. 1990. Monocytoid B-cell lymphoma in a patient with human immunodeficiency virus infection: demonstration of human immunodeficiency virus sequences in paraffin-embedded lymph node sections by polymerase chain reaction amplification. Arch Pathol Lab Med 114:1264–7.

Sima O, Rasin K. 1973. [*Toxoplasma gondii* Nicole et Manceaux 1909—Antibodies in domestic rabbits]. Vet Med (Praha) 18:633–40.

Snover DC, Filipovich AH, Dehner LP, Krivit W. 1981. Pseudolymphoma: a case associated with primary immunodeficiency disease and polyglandular failure syndrome. Arch Pathol Lab Med 105(1):46–9.

Sohn CC, Sheibani K, Winberg CD, Rappaport H. 1985. Monocytoid B lymphocytes: their relation to the patterns of the acquired immunodeficiency syndrome (AIDS) and AIDS-related lymphadenopathy. Hum Pathol 16:979–85.

Spencer J, Perry ME, Dunn-Walters DK. 1998. Human marginal zone B-cells. Immunol Today 19:421–6.

Stebbing J, Pantanowitz L, Dayyani F, Sullivan R, Bower M, Dezube B. 2008. HIV-associated multicentric Castleman's disease. Am J Hematol 83:498–503.

Stein H, Delsol G, Pileri S, Said J, Mann R, Poppema S, Swerdlow SH, Jaffe ES. 2001. Nodular lymphocyte predominant Hodgkin lymphoma. In: Jaffe ES, Harris NL, Stein H, Vardiman JW (eds): Pathology and genetics of tumours of haematopoietic and lymphoid tissues. IARC Press, Lyon. p 240–243.

Stein H, Gerdes J, Mason DY. 1982. The normal and malignant germinal center. Haematoll l:531–59.

Straus SE, Jaffe ES, Puck JM, Dale JK, Elkon KB, Rösen-Wolff A, Peters AM, Sneller MC, Hallahan CW, Wang J, et al. 2001. The development of lymphomas in families with autoimmune lymphoproliferative syndrome with germline Fas mutations and defective lymphocyte apoptosis. Blood 98(1):194–200.

Swerdlow SH. 2004. Pediatric follicular lymphomas, marginal zone lymphomas, and marginal zone hyperplasia. Am J Clin Pathol 122(suppl): S98–S109.

Tanizawa T, Eishi Y, Kamiyama R, Nakahara M, Abo Y, Sumita T, Kawano N. 1996. Reactive lymphoid hyperplasia of the liver characterized by an angiofollicular pattern mimicking Castleman's disease. Pathol Int 46:782–786.

Tomasini D, Zampatti C, Serio G. 2009. Castleman's disease with numerous mantle zone lymphocytes with clear cytoplasm involving the skin: case report. J Cutan Pathol 36:887–91.

Truong HM, Kellogg T, Klausner JD, Katz MH, Dilley J, Knapper K, Chen S, Prabhu R, Grant RM, Louie B, McFarland W. 2006. Increases in sexually transmitted infections and sexual risk behaviour without a concurrent increase in HIV incidence among men who have sex with men in San Francisco: a suggestion of HIV serosorting ? Sex Transm Infect 82:461–6.

Tuzuner N, Dogusoy G, Demirkesen C, Ozkan F, Altas K. 1996. Value of lymph node biopsy in the diagnosis of acquired toxoplasmosis. J Laryngol Otol 110:348–52.

Vakiani E, Nandula SV, Subramaniyam S, Keller CE, Alobeid B, Murty VV, Bhagat G. 2007. Cytogenetic analysis of B-cell posttransplant lymphoproliferations validates the World Health Organization classification and suggests inclusion of florid follicular hyperplasia as precursor lesion. Hum Pathol 38:315–25.

van CR, Grefte JM, van DD, Sturm P. 2009. Syphilis presenting as isolated cervical lymphadenopathy: two related cases. J Infect 58:76–8.

van den Berge M, Pauwels P, Jakimowicz JJ, Creemers GJ. 2002. Hyaline vascular Castleman's disease: a case report and brief review of the literature. Neth J Med 60:444–7.

van den Oord JJ, de Wolf-Peeters C, Desmet VJ. 1985. Immunohistochemical analysis of progressively transformed follicular centers. Am J Clin Pathol 83: 560–4.

Van den Ord JJ, de Wolf-Peeters C, Desmet VJ. 1986. The marginal zone in the human reactive lymph node. Am J Clin Pathol 86:475–9.

van Krieken JH, Lennert K. 1990. Proliferation of marginal zone cells mimicking malignant lymphoma. Pathol Res Pract 186:399–402.

van Krieken JH, von Schilling C, Kluin PM, Lennert K. 1989. Splenic marginal zone lymphocytes and related cells in the lymph node: a morphologic and immunohistochemical study. Hum Pathol 20:320–5.

Vassilios L, Raffaele B, Simona F, Alessandro P. 2005. Hyper immunoglobulin M syndrome due to CD40 deficiency: clinical, molecular, and immunological features. Immunol Rev 203(1):48–66.

Vasudev Rao T, Alkindi S, Pathare AV. 2007. Follicular dendritic cell hyperplasia in plasma cell variant of Castleman's disease with interfollicular Hodgkin's disease. Pathol Res Pract 203:479–84.

Verma A, Stock W, Norohna S, Shah R, Bradlow B, Platanias LC. 2002. Progressive transformation of germinal centers. Report of 2 cases and review of the literature. Acta Haematol 108:33–8.

Wang J, Ziu X, Li R, Tu P, Wang R, Zhang L, Li T, Chen X, Wang A, Yang S, Wu Y, Yang H, Ji S. 2005. Paraneoplastic pemphigus associated with Castleman tumor: a commonly reported subtype of paraneoplastic pemphigus in China. Arc Dermatol 141:1285–93.

Waterston A, Bower M. 2004. Fifty years of multicentric Castleman's disease. Acta Oncol 43:698–704.

Weiss LM, Chen YY, Berry GJ, Strickler JG, Dorfman RF, Warnke RA. 1992. Infrequent detection of *Toxoplasma gondii* genome in toxoplasmic lymphadenitis: a polymerase chain reaction study. Hum Pathol 23: 154–8.

Weiss LM, Chen YY, Liu XF, Shibata D. 1991. Epstein–Barr virus and Hodgkin's disease. A correlative in situ hybridization and polymerase chain reaction study. Am J Pathol 139:1259–65.

Wolff JA. 1967. Wiskott–Aldrich syndrome: clinical, immunologic, and pathologic observations. J Pediatr 70(2):221–32.

Yasuda N, Ohmori S, Usui T, Nanba K. 1996. Atypical follicular hyperplasia with clonal rearrangement for immunoglobulin and T-cell receptor genes: biclonal pro-liferation of B cell and T cell [letter]. Am J Hematol 51:177–8.

ZETOLA NM, PILCHER CD. 2007. Diagnosis and manage-ment of acute HIV infection. Infect Dis Clin North Am 21:19–48.

ZIMMER C. 2000. Evolution: parasites make scaredy-rats foolhardy. Science 289:525–7.

ZUTTER M, HOCKENBERY D, SILVERMAN GA, KORSMEYER S. 1991. Immunolocalization of the Bcl-2 protein within hematopoietic neoplasms. Blood 78:1062–8.

CHAPTER FOURTEEN

REACTIVE LYMPHADENOPATHY WITH PARACORTICAL PATTERN, NONINFECTIOUS ETIOLOGY

Ling Zhang and Jeremy W. Bowers

PARACORTICAL HYPERPLASIA

Lymph nodes are classically divided into four compartments: the cortex, paracortex, sinus, and medulla. B cells, T cells, and histiocytes home in to separate areas within these compartments. The lymphocytes interact with antigen-presenting cells and undergo clonal expansion (Willard-Mack, 2006). There are several reactive patterns that take place in a normal lymph node after an immune response and presentation of an antigen. Four reactive patterns are recognized in morphologic evaluation of the lymph node: (1) follicle (or germinal) center cell reaction, (2) paracortical reaction, (3) histiocytic reaction (van der Valk and Meijer, 1987; Willard-Mack, 2006), and (4) mixed pattern comprised of a combination of the reactions above and specialized patterns, such as granulomas or necrosis. The first three patterns are recognized as a predominant pattern or one among other patterns coexisting in one or more compartments.

Using histology and immunohistochemical stains, a trained histopathologist can easily identify the various compartments and the localization of B cells in the follicles and medullary cords, the T cells in the paracortex, and the histiocytes in the sinuses (van der Valk and Meijer, 1987). Follicular hyperplasia can be seen in infections, autoimmune disorders, and nonspecific reactions; paracortical hyperplasia is often found in viral infections, skin diseases, and nonspecific reactions; and sinus histiocytosis is frequently noted in lymph nodes draining limbs with inflammatory disorders and malignancies; and mixed reactions are often seen in infectious diseases. In this chapter our focus is mainly on the morphologic and phenotypic changes in the paracortex in response to noninfectious etiology such as drug-induced paracortical pattern, skin disorder associated dermatopathic lymphadenopathy, and the commonly seen paracortical hyperplasia of nonspecific etiology. We also discuss the differential diagnoses, which include infectious or malignant lymphadenopathy, that should be considered when evaluating paracortical hyperplasia. See Table 14.1 for a complete list of disease entities under the four patterns of reactive lymphadenopathy.

Definitions

Nodular paracortical hyperplasia, or nonspecific paracortical hyperplasia, is a nodular paracortical expansion composed of high endothelial venules (HEVs), small T cells, interdigitating reticulum cells,

TABLE 14.1 Differential Diagnosis of Interfollicular Pattern

Benign	Malignant
Dermatopathic lymphadeno-pathy	Mycosis fungoides
Paracortical T nodules	T zone lymphoma
Viral lymphadenitis	PTLD (post-transplant lymphoproliferative disorder)
Reactive immunoblastic proliferation	Peripheral T-cell lymphoma
Interfollicular infiltrate, NOS	Metastatic disease
	Granulocytic sarcoma
	Mast cell disease
	Anaplastic large-cell lymphoma
	Interfollicular Hodgkin lymphoma
	Langerhans cell histiocytosis
	Kaposi's sarcoma
	Monocytoid B-cell lymphoma
	Immunoblastic diffuse large B-cell lymphoma
	Plasmacytoma
	Lymphoplasmacytic lymphoma

histiocytes, and rare immunoblasts creating a mottled or "moth-eaten" nodular pattern.

Diffuse paracortical hyperplasia, or reactive immunoblastic proliferation, is a type of paracortical hyperplasia showing a diffuse expansion of the paracortex or interfollicular area of the entire cortex by a heterogeneous population of cells consisting of predominantly sheets of immunoblasts, plasma cells, small T lymphocytes, and histiocytes associated with increased HEVs and dendritic cells imparting a mottled diffuse pattern.

ICD-10 Codes

I88.8   Other nonspecific lymphadenitis
I88.9   Nonspecific lymphadenitis, unspecified

Synonyms

Paracortical hyperplasia: nonspecific paracortical reaction, nodular paracortical hyperplasia, T zone nodules, diffuse paracortical hyperplasia, reactive immunoblastic proliferation, florid immunoblastic proliferation, diffuse polymorphic hyperplasia.

Epidemiology

Paracortical hyperplasia is one of the most common reactions of a nonspecific or specific etiology under reactive lymphoid hyperplasia that is not otherwise specified; it is second only to follicular hyperplasia. This pattern may occur at any age and gender as a general reactive lymphoid hyperplasia, and it is a major subdivision of non-neoplastic lymphadenopathy. This pattern has generated some confusion and a myriad of terms, including interfollicular hyperplasia, diffuse paracortical hyperplasia, immunoblastic proliferation, T zone nodules, nodular alterations of the paracortex, T cell hyperplasia, and diffuse polymorphic hyperplasia. Whatever the terminology is used, however, there are generally two patterns of paracortical hyperplasia: nodular and diffuse.

The more common nodular pattern is seen as a component reaction in a nonspecific local immune reaction, a reaction to adjacent tumor, or as a predominant pattern in certain specific reactive lymph nodes. Nodular alterations of the paracortex comprise 42% of the cases of nonspecific chronic lymphadenitis or reactive hyperplasia studied by Ree (Ree and Fanger, 1975). Focal nodular paracortical hyperplasia comprise 47.6% of the more specific set of cases studied using immunohistochemistry by van den Oord (van den Oord et al., 1985a). About half of their cases include specific diagnosis such as toxoplasmosis or Castleman's disease. Paracortical hyperplasia, as the only diagnosis, comprise 13% in their series. The common location of nodular alteration in the paracortical area of lymph nodes include the axillary, cervical, and inguinal regions, and rarely in abdominal, mediastinal, and retroperitoneal groups (van den Oord et al., 1985a). The most recognized form of nodular paracortical hyperplasia is dermatopathic lymphadenopathy or lymphadenitis. In a series of 370 lymph node biopsies from India, a paracortical hyperplasia of the dermatopathic lymphadenitis type accounted for 9.2% of the cases, while sinus histiocytosis comprised 4% and the disease specific lymphadenitis accounted for 14%. The nonspecific reactive lymphoid hyperplasia, which includes predominantly follicular hyperplasia and sinus hyperplasia, was the most common pattern, comprising 75.6% of patients with noninfectious lymphadenopathy followed by dermatopathic lymphadenitis (Chhabra et al., 2006).

The other pattern is diffuse paracortical hyperplasia. Diffuse paracortical hyperplasia is often cited as synonymous with the term paracortical hyperplasia in the literature. This terminology has caused confusion. Namely the term diffuse paracortical hyperplasia, on one hand, is associated with viral and other specific lymphadenitis that mimic the diffuse pattern in lymphoma; on the other hand, a form of paracortical hyperplasia often associated with skin disorders is also sometimes called diffuse paracortical hyperplasia when most cases present as nodular alterations in the paracortex or dermatopathic lymphadenopathy. To avoid confusion, nodular paracortical hyperplasia and in its most florid form, dermatopathic lymphadenopathy, should be separately designated from the diffuse paracortical hyperplasia, a pattern associated with florid immunoblastic proliferation, and usually with atypical lymphoproliferation raising concern for lymphoma.

The incidence of diffuse form of paracortical hypeplasia is difficult to study because of its high association with more specific conditions. The diffuse form of paracortical hyperplasia has a large set of differential diagnoses (Abbondazo, Irey, and Frizzera, 1995; Abbondanzo SL, 2004, Kojima et al., 2006, Kojima et al., 2010) but is commonly seen in viral, drug, autoimmune, and postvaccinial reactions. It is also sometimes called florid or reactive immunoblastic reaction or even diffuse polymorphic hyperplasia, the latter term especially used in association with EBV infection or post-transplantation reactive lymphadenopathies.

Clinical Aspects

Etiology

There are a variety of diseases that elicit paracortical hyperplasia of either the nodular or diffuse category. Nodules of the paracortical hyperplasia underlie a dermatopathic lymphadenopathy reaction (Cooper and Dawson, 1967), and a diffuse paracortical hyperplasia can be secondary to an infection, such as the Epstein–Barr virus (EBV) (Gowing, 1975), HIV-positive lymphadenopathy (Baroni and Uccini, 1990), and other viral-induced lymphadenitis. It has also been reported as a reactive pattern in the lymph node of patients who have systemic lupus erythematosus (SLE) (Kojima et al., 2007) or can be a nodal reaction to malignancy (van den Oord et al., 1985a). More worrisome is the implication of nodular or diffuse paracortical hyperplasia: a pattern seen in both B-cell and T-cell lymphomas. In a retrospective analysis of 457 patients, it was noted that paracortical hyperplasia is a typical pattern noted in T-cell lymphomas and in Hodgkin lymphoma with prominent fibrosis (Melikian et al., 2007), and the diffuse immunoblastic reaction is the most easily confused benign pattern with large-cell lymphoma.

Sites of Involvement

The lymph node site of involvement of paracortical hyperplasia depends on specific disorders that evoke either mostly local or rarely generalized lymphadenopathy. In nonspecific nodular paracortical hyperplasia, the lymph nodes from axillary, cervical, and inguinal regions are more commonly involved by paracortical hyperplasia than that of the abdominal, mediastinal, and retroperitoneal areas (Ree and Fanger, 1975). In specific diseases, for example, in HIV-positive drug abusers and homosexual men, the neck and axillary lymph nodes are characteristically involved (Baroni and Uccini, 1990). Dermatopathic lymphadenopathy involves primarily axillary, neck and inguinal lymph nodes (Cooper and Dawson, 1967) and sites adjacent to an inflammatory or malignant skin disorder. In contrast, autoimmune disorders and other systemic diseases, including iatrogenic lymphadenopathy, typically present in a more generalized distribution.

Pathogenesis

The paracortical area is the lymphocyte-rich region located between the cortical lymphoid follicles and the medullar cords and sinuses (Cottier et al., 1972). There are two layers of nodal cortex: a superficial cortex and a deep cortex. Pathologists often refer to the deep cortex as the paracortex (Willard-Mack, 2006). The superficial cortex includes the follicles and the interfollicular (or diffuse) cortex. The paracortex, however, conventionally encompasses the area in between and deep to the follicles. High endothelial venules (HEVs) or postcapillary venules are recognized as structures typically associated with the paracortex. The term ''high'' refers to the plump or ''high'' cuboidal endothelial lining cells these vessels possess. T lymphocytes home in to the paracortex after entry into the lymph node via the HEVs, where they interact in the paracortex with dendritic cells (Willard-Mack, 2006) and promote a paracortical reaction. Thus the paracortex is rich with HEVs, T lymphocytes, and interdigitating type of dendritic cells (DCs) (van den Oord et al., 1985a).

Paracortical hyperplasia is an immune response to antigen stimulation (Stansfeld, 1985) with a preferential local stimulation of the parafollicular T cells. A majority of paracortical T cells are T helper/inducer subset and a minorirty are suppressor/cytotoxic subset (Poppema, 1981). T cells generate a peculiar nodular alteration (T zone nodule) upon stimulation (Ree and Fanger, 1975). In van den Oord's study, T zone nodules have been divided into three subtypes: primary, secondary, and tertiary, according to their location in paracortical region, and the arrangement of interdigitating dendritic cells (DCs) and high endothelial venules (HEV) (van den Oords et al., 1985a). Primary T zone nodules are usually located in interfollicular areas and composed of centrally located CD4 positive T helper cells and DCs and surrounded by concentrically located HEVs (van den

Oords et al., 1985a). The primary nodule shows a ring of HEVs surrounding the nodule. Secondary T zone nodules, however, show as nodules of "starry sky" mottled collection consisting of CD8+/CD4+ T lymphocytes, scattered DCs, and an increased number of HEVs in and around the nodule (van den Oords et al., 1985a). Tertiary T zone nodules include a large number of DCs forming pale sheets and few HEVs forming a nodular pattern characteristic of dermatopathic lymphadenopathy. The DCs presenting in all three types are composed of S100+ interdigitating reticulum cells. The tertiary T nodule is commonly seen with dermatopathic lymphadenopathy, as well as various kinds of reactive disorders (van den Oords et al., 1985a; O'Malley, 2009a; Cooper and Dawson, 1967; Hurwitt 1942). The pale nodules of dermatopathic lymphadenopathy are sometimes refered to as "alopecia-like" in pattern because of the stark contrast with the darker cells of the surrounding small lymphocytes.

The formation of T nodules plays an important role in the presentation of antigens to helper/inducer T cells and in proliferation of antigen-responsive T cells (van den Oord et al., 1985a; Gutman and Weissman, 1972; Poppema et al., 1981). Dendritic cells are potent antigen presenting cells (APC) that process antigens from tissues, home in to the paracortex and present them to T cells thereafter generating T-cell proliferation (Romani et al., 2001). After stimulation by its cognate antigen via interaction with DCs, the T cells seek help from their B-cell counterparts to eventually form a yet unstimulated primary follicle (van den Oord et al., 1985a). In the ensuing reaction T nodules and adjacent B-cell follicles form an ovoid, distinct nodular structure termed a "composite nodule" (van den Oord et al., 1986b) because of their mixed composition, and together play a key role in antigen triggering, B-cell maturation, and antibody production.

In the spleen T cells are mainly located in the red pulp and the periarteriolar lymphoid sheats (Cesta, 2006). T-cell hyperplasia is rarely seen in spleen but once it occurs, it presents with a selective white pulp expansion (O'Malley, 2009a). DCs have been found in splenic white pulp as in lymph node (Heusermann et al., 1974; Kaiserling and Lennert, 1974), and they are also key player in reactive hyperplasia of the spleen.

Approach to Diagnosis

Clinical and Laboratory Investigations

Reactive paracortical hyperplasia, nonspecific is a diagnosis based on histologic evaluation of a lymph node biopsy. However, the clinical history and laboratory result may present clues that indicate an etiology for paracortical hyperplasia. These may include viral infection, autoimmune disorder, drug or vaccine administration, and possible malignancy. A laboratory investigation including a routine chemistry profile, a serology for virus infections and autoimmune conditions, should be carried out for the purpose of determining a diagnosis that would not require a biopsy. If the results are nonconclusive, an excisional biopsy of an enlarged lymph node is preferred over needle core biopsy or fine needle aspirate (FNA) in order to clearly assess the histologic pattern of the lymph node. The biopsy would also provide additional materials needed for a lymphoma protocol, including specimen for flow cytometry and tissue for immunohistochemical stains or molecular tests to identify clonal B-cell proliferation, abnormal T-cell population with aberrant expression, and loss of any surface antigen. Immunohistochemical stains or nucleic acid in situ hybridization are also useful in detection of a viral infection.

Morphologic Aspects

Follicular hyperplasia can be seen together with nonspecific paracortical hyperplasia (Figure 14.1). (O'Malley et al., 2009a; Kojima et al., 2006a). The sinuses could be normal, but in a lymph node adjacent to a tumor, a dilated sinus with or without sinus histocytosis is commonly associated with paracortical hyperplasia (Melikian, 2007). Paracortical hyperplasia could also be a prominent pattern, which may present as nodular alterations or a diffuse pattern in a lymph node. Nodular paracortical hyperplasia can be divided into a primary, secondary, and tertiary nodular hyperplasia. As described in pathogenesis above, the three kinds of T nodules are all composed of lymphocytes and DCs in a background of prominent vessels lined by thick or enlarged endothelial cells (HEVs) with unique distribution patterns (Figure 14.1A, B). Cytologically T cells in paracortical hyperplasia are usually small with mild irregular contours. DCs contain a large pale convoluted nucleus with smooth nuclear membrane, clear cytoplasm, and cytoplasmic processes that impart a dendritic configuration. In low-power view, the presence of increased DCs impart a "mottled" or "starry sky" appearance (Crivellato et al., 1993; Willard-Mack, 2006). The primary T zone nodules usually are small and well defined, and comprised of a nodular collection of small mature appearing lymphocytes surrounded by DCs and circumferential HEVs (van den Oords et al., 1985a). The secondary T zone nodule is slightly loose without clear border, with increased DCs, and with HEVs scattered throughout the nodule intermingled with small lymphocytes exhibiting "starry sky" pattern (Figure 14.2)

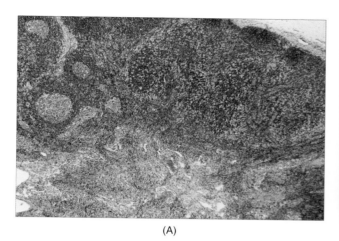

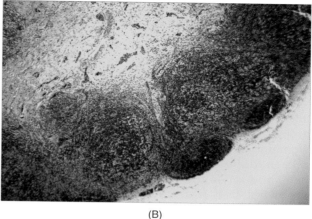

(A)

(B)

FIGURE 14.1 Paracortical hyperplasia. (A) Paracortical reaction dominated with nodular proliferation of reactive T cells admixed with pale stained dendritic cells and histiocytes adjacent to reactive germinal centers (secondary follicles); also associated with open sinusoidal spaces or increased vascular channels in medulla (H&E, 16×). **(B)** Pure paracortical reaction, nonspecific paracortical hyperplasia, two T zone nodules, and overlying primary follicles (H&E, 40×).

(van den Oords et al., 1985a). The tertiary T nodule is large with very large aggregates of DCs that show as pale areas under low-power view. Small lymphocytes and HEVs in tertiary T nodules are not as numerous as those in primary or secondary T nodules (van den Oords et al., 1985a; Cooper and Dawson, 1967). Paracortical hyperplasia that is nonspecific, with predominance of T nodules, shows fewer numbers of scattered immunoblasts.

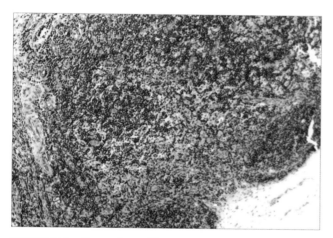

FIGURE 14.2 Secondary T zone nodule. Paracortical hyperplasia with admixed high endothelial venules is a secondary type of paracortical hyperplasia where discrete nodules comprised of T cells are easily seen under low-power view. Secondary T zone forms due to proliferation of T cells in the region in response to stimulation, where consist of predominantly T helper cells intermingled with interfollicular dendritic reticulum cells and high endothelial venules, forming a mottled or "starry sky" pattern (H&E, 400×).

In contrast, a diffuse pattern of paracortical hyperplasia is often found in viral lymphadenitis, in drug reactions, and in autoimmune diseases and shows as diffuse proliferation of reactive immunoblasts.

Immunophenotyping

Flow cytometric analysis frequently reveals no diagnostic immunophenotypic abnormalities in nonspecific paracortical hyperplasia. Immunohistochemistry, however, highlights the CD3 expressing T cells in the paracortex and the CD20 expressing B cells in the follicles, which are used as clues as to whether there is a normal or abnormal increased of one phenotype or aberrancy in distribution. The CD20-positive B cells, including immunoblasts, are scattered in the paracortex. Immunohistochemical stains highlight a predominance of T cells in a hyperplastic paracortex. CD3 stains predominantly small and mature appearing T lymphocytes, while the subset of CD4+ T helper cells is commonly increased in contrast to the CD8+ cytotoxic T cells (Poppema et al., 1981). S100-positive DCs, called interdigitating reticulum cells, are the antigen-presenting cells in the paracortex and they are increased in T zone nodules (Cocchia et al., 1983; Takahashi et al., 1981; Isobe and Okuyama, 1978). Langerin (CD207) positive, CD1a positive and S100 positive Langerhans cells (Cheong et al., 2007) are present even in tertiary T zone nodules. Staining with follicular dendritic cell markers (CD21 and CD35) outlines the germinal centers near the hyperplastic paracortex (Liu et al., 1997; Reynes et al., 1985).

Differential Diagnosis

The differential diagnosis of diffuse paracortical hyperplasia includes infection, autoimmune, drug, or postvaccine reactions, and other atypical immunoblastic proliferations.

Viral Infections. One of the common entities causing paracortical hyperplasia is lymphadenitis secondary to the herpes family of viruses, specifically EBV, CMV, HSV, and VZV (see Chapter 15). The clinical history should be investigated and laboratory studies are performed for the specific virus. Viral cytopathic effects may also be a morphologic clue to diagnosis. Immunohistochemical stains and/or in situ hybridization for specific viruses may be useful in equivocal cases (Ferry, 2007).

Viral lymphadenitis frequently presents as paracortical hyperplasia with increased histiocytes/macrophages in the lymph node (Ferry, 2007). Morphologically viral lymphadenitis does not exhibit a clear-appearance as dermatopathic lymphadenopathy by low-power view because DCs and histiocytes are not increased in a viral infection (Ioachim and Medeiros, 2009a). Instead, viral lymphadenitis shows increased polymorphic immunoblasts, plasma cells, and Reed–Sternberg-like cells (see Chapter 15), which should differentiate with reactive, diffuse immunoblastic hyperplasia that is noninfectious. Immunohistochemical stains, in situ hybridization, and the cytopathologic viral effect may be used to identify some types of viral infections (Ferry, 2007; Ioachim and Medeiros, 2009a). Other laboratory tests, including antivirus antibody titers, may be useful in cases of suspected viral lymphadenitis.

The differential diagnosis of nodular paracortical hyperplasia includes dermatopathic lymphadenopathy secondary to skin malignancy (especially mycosis fungoides), lymph node draining an adjacent carcinoma, non-Hodgkin lymphomas (T-cell lymphomas, B-cell lymphomas), Hodgkin lymphoma, and other lymphomas. When confronted with nonspecific paracortical hyperplasia, other malignancies, both extrinsic and intrinsic to the lymph node, have to be considered. These include adjacent carcinoma, non-Hodgkin lymphoma, and Hodgkin lymphoma.

Adjacent Carcinomas. Carcinoma metastases to lymph nodes will cause an enlargement of the node. Prominent paracortical hyperplasia, along with open sinusoids and sinus histiocytosis, is often seen with metastatic disease, which can mask the foci of carcinoma cells. Small-cell carcinoma of the lung or other primary site is considered the most critical due to the morphologic similarity and the degree of crush artifact. However, a detailed examination of the small-cell carcinoma cells will reveal ''salt–pepper'' granular chromatin rather than the clumped chromatin pattern typically seen in mature T lymphocytes. Tumor cell molding, angulated nuclei, and a cohesive arrangement are additional features favoring metastatic small-cell carcinoma (Batsakis et al., 1981). Pan-cytokeratin staining, especially low-molecular-weight cytokeratin (Cam5.2) is able to detect a majority of small-cell carcinoma, with the exception of some undifferentiated cases. Synaptophysin, chromogranin, and/or CD56 may highlight neoplasms with neuroendocrine differentiation. Organ-specific markers such as TTF1 are helpful in identification of lung as the primary site (Kargi et al., 2007). The sinusoidal space may harbor individual or small collections of mestastic tumor cells. Breast carcinoma, especially lobular variant, can be picked up by IHCs with cytokeratins (Cohen et al., 2002). Worthy of mention is undifferentiated nasopharyngeal carcinoma, since it presents with unique morphologic features including syncytial appearance, indistinct cell margins, prominent inflammatory infiltrate (plasma cells, eosinophils), and many lymphocytes (Batsakis et al., 1981; Micheau, 1986). The etiology of nasophargeal carcinoma is multifactorial with differences in risk attributed to race, genetics, (EBV) infection, and other environmental factors. It is more prevalent in Southeast Asia than other areas. In situ hybridization for EBV and additional immunohistochemical stain with cytokeratin are useful in detecting carcinoma cells intermixed with similar appearing lymphocytes (Liebowitz, 1994; Lopategui et al., 1994).

Hodgkin Lymphoma. Interfollicular Hodgkin lymphoma is considered a morphologic variant of the classical Hodgkin lymphoma. Although paracortical hyperplasia may be one of the features associated with this disease, the presence of large atypical Hodgkin cells that coexpress CD30 and CD15 is characteristic. In contrast, in reactive hyperplasia the increased DCs are usually negative for CD30 or CD15. Furthermore these DCs are highlighted by S100, and Langerhans cells are positive for S100, CD1a and langerin (Gould et al., 1988; Asano et al., 1987; Shamoto et al., 1995, Cheong et al., 2007).

Non-Hodgkin Lymphoma. Marginal zone lymphoma (MZL) can shows paracortex expansion, especially in the early phase (Nathwani et al., 1999). These cells are intermingled with paracortical histiocytes and mature T cells that may resemble paracortical hyperplasia, NOS. Immunohistochemical stains and flow cytometry studies reveal these cells to be of B-cell origin with a light chain restriction, expressing CD20 but often lacking coexpression of CD5, CD10, or CD23. Paracortical nodular hyperplasia composed of benign mantle or monocytoid B cells with a clear cytoplasm but without dendritic cells (DCs), is present in this setting (Hunt et al., 2001, Kojima et al., 2006b). Confirmation of the B-cell origin is achieved by immunohistochemical stains (CD3, CD5, CD43, CD20, PAX-5, and light chains) and/or by flow cytometry. The reactive B cells do not show coexpression of CD5 and CD43 (Hunt et al., 2001). If no definitive clonal population is detected by flow cytometry but there is clinical suspicion of lymphoma, a clonality assay by PCR may be performed to further clarify the disease entity.

CLL/SLL can have unusual patterns of involvement, including marginal zone, perifollicular, and interfollicular patterns that can be difficult to separate from paracortical hyperplasia, NOS, histologically (Gupta et al., 2000). These might or might not have vaguely recognizable pseudoproliferation centers consisting of prolymphocytes and paraimmunoblasts. Importantly, the interfollicular spaces are packed with B cells, instead of T cells, which express CD19, CD20, CD23, and CD5.

A striking mantle zone expansion is noted in the earlier phase of mantle cell lymphoma or in situ mantle cell lymphoma (Richard et al., 2006; Bassarova et al., 2008), which is also easily misinterpreted as paracortical hyperplasia, NOS. A lymphoid infiltrate expands out into the paracortex forming a diffuse or vaguely nodular proliferation of neoplastic B cells with positivity for CD20, BCL-1, and CD5 by immunohistochemistry. A FISH study probing with immunoglobulin (IgH) and cyclin D1 should demonstrate a fusion-signal pattern.

Peripheral T-cell lymphoma can present in a pattern of paracortical hyperplasia (Melikian et al., 2007). The T-cell lymphoma, especially the T zone variant, shows a morphology similar to that of reactive paracortical hyperplasia, which is characterized by paracortical or perifollicular proliferation of T cells throughout the lymph node with minimal cytologic atypia (Rudiger et al., 2000). The T nodules may be vague or easily discernible and cause minimal to partial architectural distortion (Macon et al., 1995). However, T zone lymphomas usually demonstrate a surface antigen loss of CD5 and CD7 (Warnke et al., 2007), a finding not associated with reactive paracortical T-cell hyperplasia. Paracortical hyperplasia has also been observed in anaplastic T-cell lymphoma (Melikian et al., 2007). In general, anaplastic T-cell lymphoma is characterized by large atypical CD30+ and ALK-1 +/− lymphoid cells with C-shaped or "horseshoe-shaped" nuclei

(Benharroch et al., 1998). These features distinguish the lymphoma from reactive paracortical hyperplasia.

Mycosis fungoides (MF) can show lymph node involvement that is typical of dermatopathic lymphadenopathy or florid paracortical hyperplasia (Burke and Colby, 1981; Burke et al., 1986). The lymph node affected by MF shows dermatopathic lymphadenopathy and is characterized by medium or large atypical lymphoid cells exhibiting irregular to pleomorphic nuclei and an increased mitotic rate with downregulated expressions of CD5 and CD7. A molecular study for clonal TCR gene rearrangement is helpful in detection of the clonal T cells. A complete clinical history is, in particular, crucial for a differential diagnosis. In fact in lymph node grading, dermatopathic lymphadenopathy is used as a hallmark in grading of involvement of MF.

DERMATOPATHIC LYMPHADENOPATHY

Definition

Dermatopathic lymphadenopathy is characterized as a reactive paracortical hyperplasia in response to skin antigen stimulation, composed of mainly T-cell proliferation, increased pale-appearing interdigitating reticulum cells (DCs), Langerhans cells, and histiocytes containing lipid or melanin (Cooper and Dawson, 1967). This entity occurs in the regional or adjacent lymph node of skin lesions, including various forms of generalized dermatitis or long-standing skin irritations, including neoplastic or non-neoplastic processes.

ICD-10 Codes   WHO 2007

R59.1   Generalized enlarged lymph nodes
I88.1   Chronic lymphadenitis, except mesenteric

Synonyms

Dermatopathic lymphadenitis, lipomelanotic reticulosis, lipomelanosis reticularis of Pautrier.

Epidemiology

Dermatopathic lymphadenopathy is primarily seen in adults aged 20 to 60 years old. It is found in lymph nodes draining an inflammatory dermatitis or neoplastic entities such as mycosis fungoides (MF) (Colby et al., 1981; Weiss, 1985a, 2008a; Ioachim and Medeiros, 2009a). However, 12% of patients do not have concurrent clinical evidence of skin lesions; therefore changes present in the lymph node should indicate a remote history of dermatitis (Gould et al., 1988). A study from 960 consecutive lymph node biopsies found 40 cases with dermatopathic lymphadenopathy, comprising 4.8% of total biopsies (Cooper and Dawson, 1967). In a retrospective histological evaluation of 250 cases of non-neoplastic superficial lymphadenopathy, dermatopathic lymphadenopathy was seen in 15 patients (6%) (Chhabra et al., 2006). Dermatopathic lymphadenopathy is more common in males than in females (2:1) (Cooper and Dawson, 1967).

Clinical Aspects

Etiology

There are many benign and malignant skin disorders that can trigger dermatopathic lymphadenopathy. Benign entities include psoriasis, pemphigus, neurodermatitis, eczema, atrophic senilis, and toxic shock syndrome (Hurwitt, 1942; Gould et al., 1988; Cooper and Dawson, 1967). Dermatopathic lymphadenopathy has also been reported in uremic pruritis (Westhoff et al., 2006). It also often accompanies cutaneous malignancies such as mycosis fungoides (MF) with or without Sezary syndrome (SS). There are approximately 75% of these patients have palpable lymphadenopathy at the time of diagnosis identified as dermatopathic lymphadenopathy, MF, or both (Bunn et al., 1980). The duration for dermatopathic lymphadenopathy to develop in patients with skin irritation is variable and can range from months to years (Hurwitt, 1942; Steffen, 2004). Some dermatopathic lymphadenopathy may be linked to a remote history of skin dermatitis (Gould et al., 1988).

Sites of Involvement

The most common sites include axillary and inguinal lymph nodes with rare involvement of deep-seated intra-abdominal or mediastinal lymph nodes (Hurwitt, 1942; Gould et al., 1988; Cooper and Dawson, 1967).

Pathogenesis

Dermatopathic changes in the lymph node are, in general, associated with inflammatory dermatoses or neoplastic disease, with rare occurrences in the absence of skin diseases (Gould et al., 1988). The pathogenesis of the lymph node changes in dermatopathic lymphadenopathy remains obscure but is considered an immune response (Cooper and Dawson, 1967). It likely represents a lymph node reaction

to the drainage of melanin and various skin antigens (Ioachim and Medeiros, 2009a).

In skin dermis, langerin/CD207-positive Langerhans cells (LCs) constitute a predominant population of immature dendritic cells (DCs) (Banchereau and Steinman, 1998; Sallusto and Lanzavecchia, 1999). During development of dermatopathic lymphadenopathy, inflammatory stimuli in the skin increase the migration of Langerhans cells to the lymph node (Geissmann et al., 2002). These immature Langerhans cells in the lymph node communicate with other mature dendritic cells and T cells to regulate immune responses (Geissmann et al., 2002; O'Malley et al., 2009a). Maturation of DCs is therefore a crucial step in the initiation of specific immune responses (Sallusto and Lanzavecchia, 1999). Recent studies have demonstrated that plasmacytoid DCs are also increased within reactive nodular T-cell areas and sinuses in lymph node (Sozzani et al., 2006, Yoneyama et al., 2004). The role of plasmacytoid DCs in dermatopathic lymphadenopathy is not yet well studied and considered to be related to type-specific immune responses (Sallusto and Lanzavecchia, 1999; O'Malley et al., 2009a).

Approach to Diagnosis

Clinical and Laboratory Investigations

Dermatopathic lymphadenopathy is usually secondary to generalized dermatitis, including inflammatory dermatoses (e.g., psoriasis) and neoplastic diseases (e.g., MF) (Ioachim and Medeiros, 2009a; Colby et al., 1981; Weiss, 2008a). It is rarely seen in the absence of clinical skin disease (Gould et al., 1988). Clinically skin lesions are commonly exfoliative or eczematoid, both associated with itching and irritation (Hurwitt, 1942; Gould et al., 1988; Cooper and Dawson, 1967). Presentations could include scales, plaques, pigmentation, nodules, and masses (Cooper and Dawson, 1967). Reactive eosinophilia in peripheral blood has been noted in patients with dermatopathic lymphadenopathy (Weiss, 2008a). Clinical examination of the involved lymph nodes reveals firm, rubbery, and mobile nodules with a majority exhibiting enlarged size.

Morphologic Aspects

Grossly, the lymph node is enlarged with a bulging cut surface and is pale yellow in color. If florid dermatopathic lymphadenopathy is present, the lymph node often shows black linear areas in the periphery, representing clumps of melanin simulating metastatic melanoma.

The most common microscopic lymph node findings can be divided into three stages. (1). Early dermatopathic lymphadenopathy exhibits cortical sinuses just deep to a germinal follicle containing small aggregates of pale histiocytes. Massive expansion of the paracortical region results in a wide pale area between the capsule and the lymphoid follicles (Figure 14.3A). A high-power view of the paracortical region shows numerous cells with oval vesicular nuclei, which correspond to an admixture of interdigitating dendritic cells (DCs) and Langerhans cells (Figure 14.3B). Pigment is present in cortical sinuses within germinal center histiocytes, intracellular histiocytes, and extracellular spaces. Reactive small and mature T cells are highlighted by BCL-2 and CD4 immunostains (Figure 14.3C, D). (2). Dermatopathic lymphadenopathy, an intermediate stage, shows replacement of the central portion of tertiary cortical nodules with an accumulation of CD68 positive histiocytes (Figure 14.4A). Abundant melanin pigment is present at the borders of the nodule (3). Dermatopathic lymphadenopathy, advanced

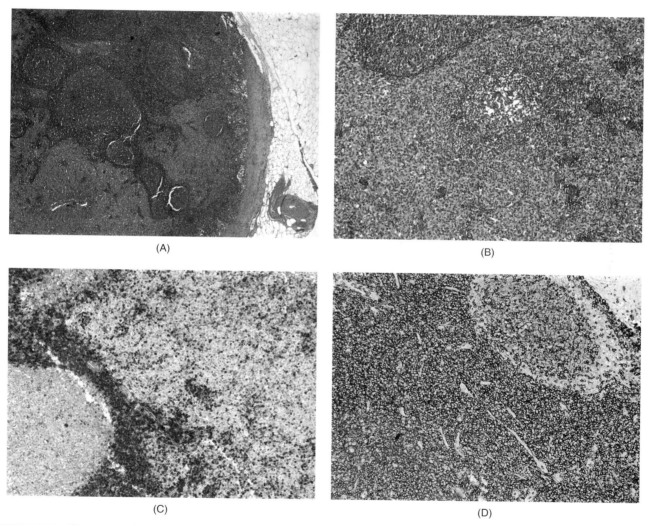

(A)

(B)

(C)

(D)

FIGURE 14.3 **Dermatopathic lymphadenopathy. (A)** Low-power view of lymph node section shows several pale nodules with reactive germinal centers and intact, slightly thickened capsule. The lymphoid follicles are variable in size with adjacent expansion of paracortical zone filled increased histiocytes with eosinophilic cytoplasm, dendritic cells with clear cytoplasm, brownish pigmentation intracellularly or extracellularly, and small reactive T lymphocytes. **(B)** Medium-power view of paracortical hyperplasia shows numerous interdigitating dendritic reticulum cells, histiocytes, and small lymphocytes present (H&E, ×200). **(C)** BCL-2 stain demonstrates no immunoreactivity in the T zone area in dermatopathic changes and in reactive germinal center as expected, but is positive in scattered T cells. **(D)** Immunohistochemical stain with CD4 highlights increased CD4 T helper cells in expanded interfollicular area; CD4 stain also shows cross reaction to monocytes and histiocytes.

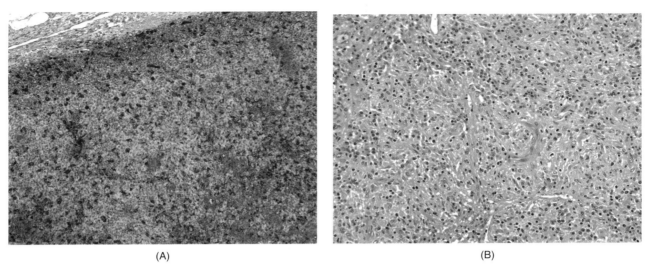

(A)   (B)

FIGURE 14.4 **CD68 macrophage staining pattern in dermatopathic lymphadenopathy. (A)** CD68 stains the increased histiocytes or plasmacytoid T cells (of monocytic origin) in the reactive interfollicular area. **(B)** In the paucicellular area in dermatopathic lymphadenopathy, there are increased collagen bundles and vasculatures.

stage, is present when the tertiary cortical nodule is extensively replaced by histiocytes with only a rim of small lymphocytes remaining (Figure 14.4*B*). The circumscribed character of the histiocytic infiltrate end at the medulla and is a form of tertiary T zone nodule (van den Oord, 1985a; Ree and Fanger, 1975; Asano et al., 1987; Rausch et al., 1977; Cooper and Dawson, 1967).

In summary, the involved lymph node retains it nodal architecture and shows a pale widened paracortical zone that is occupied by large nonlymphoid cells thought to be of three types: histiocytes containing phagocytosed melanin and neutral fat, Langerhans cells, and interdigitating dendritic cells (Asano et al., 1987; Rausch et al., 1977). In the background, plasma cell infiltration, sinus histiocytosis, and follicular hyperplasia are present with scattered eosinophils (O'Malley et al., 2009a).

Immunohistochemistry/Cytochemistry

In lymph nodes with dermatopathic changes, brownish pigmentations are highlighted by Fontana–Masson (melanin) stain and negative for Prussian-blue (iron) stain (Ioachim and Medeiros, 2009a). If melanocyte-specific markers (e.g., Melan A, tryrosinase, HMB-45) are selected for staining, the pigmented cells should be negative. A study elucidated that the majority of DCs in dermatopathic lymphadenopathy were Langerhans cells, which are positive for S100 and CD1a (Gould et al., 1988; Asano et al., 1987; Shamoto et al., 1995). Histocytes or macrophages, in contrast to interdigitating dendritic cells or Langerhans cells, stain positive

for histocytic markers such as CD68, lysozyme, and CD163, with cross reaction with T helper marker CD4 (Ioachim and Medeiros, 2009a; Weiss, 2008a). CD123 (interleukin-3 receptor alpha chain), which is expressed at high levels only in plasmacytoid dendritic cells (or type 2 DCs) and basophils, would be useful in characterizing these cells located the periphery of T nodule (Sozzani et al., 2006).

Differential Diagnosis

Differential diagnosis includes MF, Hodgkin lymphoma, viral infections, and Langerhans cell histiocytosis.

Mycosis Fungoides (MF). Dermatopathic lymphadenopathy is often noted in lymph nodes adjacent to skin irritations caused by MF (Rausch et al., 1977; Colby et al., 1981; Burke and Colby, 1981; Scheffer et al., 2000). A study of 76 patients with MF showed that dermatopathopic lymphadenopathy was the most common change found in biopsies of palpable lymph nodes (Colby et al., 1981). There are more than one histopathological staging systems for abnormal lymph node in MF (Sausville et al., 1985; Scheffer et al., 2000; Olsen et al., 2007). According to the Sausville's study or NCI classification, MF involving the lymph nodes demonstrates four different infiltration patterns: LN1 has single infrequent atypical lymphocytes in the paracortical T-cell region, LN2 has small clusters of paracortical atypical cells, LN3 has large clusters of atypical cells, and LN4 shows partially or totally effaced architecture by atypical lymphocytes (Sausville et al., 1985). Involvement histologically manifests either as a presence of cerebriform cells or as large anaplastic cells that mimic Hodgkin cells. Paracortical expansion of histiocytes with elongated, folded, and delicate nuclei is a characteristic lymph node finding in MF, although it can be misinterpreted as simply dermatopathic lymphadenopathy by morphology without additional studies. It is a diagnostic challenge in the earlier phase of MF in a lymph node, such as LN1 and LN2, by convention indicating no MF involvement because of the coexistence of dermatopathic lymphadenopathy. Many studies have indicated that minimal involvement by MF is subtle using only histologic criteria and show no evidence of immunophenotypic abnormalities (Colby et al., 1981; Burke and Colby, 1981; Weiss, 1985a,b). In this situation, PCR study for T-cell gene rearrangement is a useful strategy. Positive results suggest the presence of clonal T cells and possible involvement by MF. However, the clinical significance is uncertain if there is no overt evidence of histologic findings (Fraser-Andrews et al., 2006; Weiss, 1985b). When partial or full effacement of lymph node is noted in later phase of MF, as in LN3 or LN4, respectively, immunohistochemical stains help reveal the common immunophenotypic features for MF: CD2+, CD3+, CD4+, CD5+, and CD8−, CD7−. Interpretation of lymph node involvement by MF should be cautious when encountered a phenotypic variant of MF e.g. CD8+. Flow cytometry and PCR for TCR gene rearrangements are useful modalities for a workup of lymph node involvement (Assaf et al., 2005; Fraser-Andrews et al., 2006; Weiss, 1985b). Cytogenetic studies may also help identify cytogenetic aberrations in T-cell lymphoma.

Hodgkin Lymphoma. The classical Hodgkin lymphoma often shows a partial effacement of the nodal architecture, sometimes exhibiting pale staining paracortical areas due to increased macrophages and histiocytes. The findings could mimic dermatopathic lymphadenitis (Ioachim and Medeiros, 2009a). Of note, there is no increase in interdigitating dendritic cells or Langerhans cells. CD30+/CD15+ cells highlighted by immunohistochemical stains help make a diagnosis of the classical Hodgkin lymphoma.

Langerhans Cell Histiocytosis. Reactive proliferations with a major dendritic cell component include dermatopathic lymphadenopathy and Langerhans cell histiocytosis (Jaffe, 1988). Langerhans cell histiocytosis shows dilation of the sinuses with cells characterized by elongated nuclei and nuclear grooves (Jaffe, 1988; Weiss, 2008b). Increased histiocytes in paracortical areas might resemble

dermatopathic lymphadenopathy. Proliferative Langerhans cells are typically positive for S100 and CD1a (Gould et al., 1988; Asano et al., 1987; Shamoto et al., 1995). In addition they are positive for CD68, CD163, langerin (CD207), BCL-2, and p53 (Cheong et al., 2007; O'Malley et al., 2009a). Subtle involvement by Langerhans cell histiocytosis requires careful morphologic assessments in conjunction with results of other diagnostic reports, such as electron microscopic findings with Birbeck granules in Langerhans cell histiocytes (Weiss, 2008b).

Treatment is focused on the underlying cutaneous disease. Systemic management is necessary for lymph node involvement by cutaneous lymphoma or other neoplastic entities.

REACTIVE IMMUNOBLASTIC PROLIFERATION

Definition

Reactive immunoblastic proliferation is characterized by diffuse interfollicular expansion in the lymph nodes, or splenic periarteriolar involvement, by large transformed lymphocytes/immunoblasts with immunologic features (O'Malley et al., 2009a). Interfollicular Hodgkinoid lymphadenopathy is a reactive immunoblastic proliferation featuring interfollicular proliferation of lymphocytes, immunoblasts, plasma cells, eosinophils, and epithelioid histiocytes, which may mimic Hodgkin lymphoma (Fletcher, 2007).

ICD-10 Codes   WHO 2007

R59.1 Generalized enlarged lymph nodes
I88.1 Chronic lymphadenitis, except mesenteric
I88.8 Other nonspecific lymphadenitis
I88.9 Nonspecific lymphadenitis, unspecified

Synonyms

Reactive immunoblastic hyperplasia; reactive immunoblastic proliferation, nonspecific; plasmacytoid immunoblastic proliferation; diffuse immunoblastic reaction; Diffuse polymorphic hyperplasia

Epidemiology

Reactive immunoblastic proliferation is associated with various clinical situations. It is encountered more frequently in patients with a history of infectious mononucleosis, other viral infections, vaccination, some autoimmune disorders, or drug reactions. Age or gender prevalence varies based on related disease categories. Infectious mononucleosis or vaccine reaction occurs more commonly in age under 20 and uncommonly in adult and elderly (see Chapter 15 and the section on postvaccinal lymphadenitis). In advanced rheumatoid arthritis (RA), immunoblastic proliferation is associated with the elderly, with a female predominance, reflecting the age distribution and sex ratio of RA (Kojima et al., 2006a). The majority of the RA patients with immunoblastic proliferation have the B-cell phenotype and exhibit an increased frequency of large-cell lymphoma of the diffuse large B-cell type (Kojima et al., 2006a).

Clinical Aspects

Etiology

The etiology of a reactive, non-neoplastic plasmacytic-immunoblastic infiltrate is related to viral infection, drug use (e.g., phenytoin, methotrexate), postvaccinal reactions, and various kinds of autoimmune disorders (Gowing, 1975; Abbondanzo et al., 1995; Hartsock, 1968; Lim et al., 1998; Kojima et al., 2010). The common autoimmune diseases that result in lymphoplasmacytic infiltration, immunoblastic proliferation, or interstitial Hodgkinoid reaction include RA, systemic lupus erythemates (SLE), Still disease and Sjögren syndrome have been well documented (Jeon et al., 2004, Kojima et al., 2006a, 2007, 2010).

Interstitial Hodgkinoid lymphadenopathy has also been observed in noninfectious or non–drug-related reactive processes besides viral lymphadenitis including infectious mononucleosis (Gowing, 1975), CMV (Shimojima et al., 2010), immunodeficiency lymphoproliferative disorder (Slatter et al., 2010), senile Epstein–Barr virus+ B-cell lymphoproliferative disorder (Said, 2007) as well as methothrexate induced lymphoproliferative disorders (Kamel et al., 1996; Kikuchi et al., 2010; Gaulard et al., 2008).

Sites of Involvement

No specific site has been determined. Immunoblastic proliferation is related to various disease categories that could be localized or systemic, nodal or extranodal location.

Pathogenesis

Immunoblasts play a critical role in immune response. Immunoblastic proliferation could be seen in either malignant or non-neoplastic disorders. Due to various etiologies that could induce reactive immunoblastic proliferations, the pathogenesis is complex and thought to be antigen related. Peterson's group reported 4 cases of extensive reactive polyclonal immunoblastic proliferation with uncertain pathogenesis (Peterson et al., 1988) although 3 of 4 presented with some degree of acute immune disorders. One study determined that the pathogenesis of atypical lymphoplasmacytic and immunoblastic proliferation in lymph nodes of patients with autoimmune disease is probably related to a deficiency in suppressor T-cell function, which results in an unopposed proliferation of B cells with autoantibody formation and polyclonal gammopathy (Koo et al., 1984; Strelkauskas et al. 1978). Post-viral infection, postvaccine administration, and drug use may alter the immune response pathway resulting in reactive atypical immunoblastic hyperplasia. The pathogenesis regarding the alterations will be discussed in the corresponding sections.

Approach to Diagnosis

Clinical and Laboratory Investigations

Clinical presentations are related to underlying disorders. Detailed clinical history helps identify the etiology. Patients with autoimmune disorders often initially present with constitutional symptoms, such as fever, sweats, weight loss, and skin rashes, and then progress to having generalized lymphadenopathy, hepatosplenomegaly, and, in some cases, pulmonary infiltrates (Koo et al., 1984). Viral infection, such as infectious mononucleosis, is associated with "flu-like" symptoms in the earlier phase and is asymptomatic or induces mild fatigue in the chronic phase (Frizzera, 1987) (also see Chapter 15). Lymphadenopathy induced by vaccine administration might present with localized symptoms at the injection site, with or without accompany systemic symptoms or signs (see postvaccinal lymphadenopathy). Laboratory investigation is necessary, including autoantibodies in different autoimmune disorders, serum titer of anti-virus antibodies if virus infection is suspected, as well as routine CBCs and chemical profile. Biopsy of the enlarged lymph node is performed in conjunction with ancillary studies, including flow cytometry, immunohistochemical stains, and in situ hybridization in order to exclude lymphoma. PCR for T- and B-cell gene rearrangement is further performed as necessary.

Morphologic Aspects

Microscopic examination of the sectioned lymph node typically shows an essentially intact architecture or partially effaced with a mild to moderate expansion of interfollicular spaces filled with increased number of immunoblasts in the background of small mature lymphocytes, variable number of plasma cells, histiocytes, and vasculature (Figure 14.5A–C, low-power to high-power view) (O'Malley et al.,

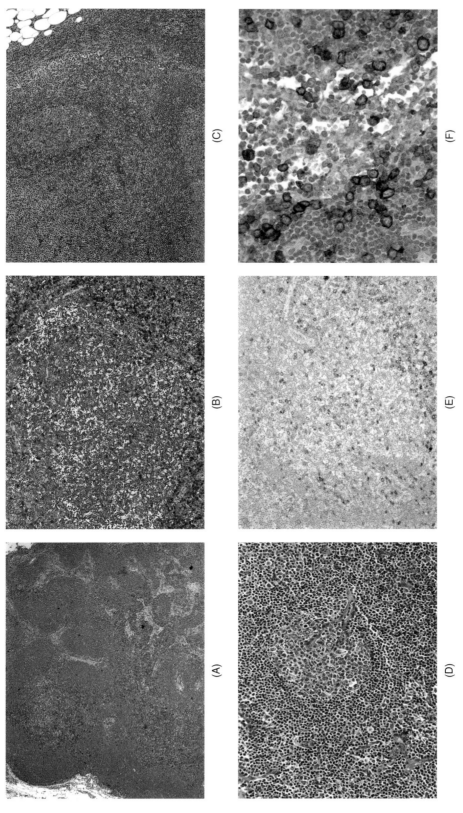

FIGURE 14.5 Reactive immunoblastic proliferation. (A) Interfollicular immunoblastic proliferation seen at low power with nodules of reactive follicles (immunoblasts highlighted in dark blue by this RNA stain with hematoxylin counterstain). **(B)** Atypical immunoblastic reaction with mottled pattern showing large dendritic cells (clear cytoplasm) and immunoblasts (dark blue cytoplasm, Hematoxylin and RNA stain). **(C)** Reactive germinal centers in between diffuse paracortical immunoblastic proliferation. **(D)** Reactive follicle with capillary and interfollicular large cells (immunoblasts highlighted by CD30 stain). **(E)** Interfollicular large cells, CD30 +, F. CD30 + immunoblasts, are increased raising differential diagnoses of lymphomas, especially Hodgkin lymphoma.

2009a). Follicular hyperplasia could coexist and some reactive germinal centers could contain prominent vasculature (Figure 14.5 C–D). Immunoblasts are large in size, often with large nuclei, a vesicular chromatin pattern, prominent nucleolus, distinct paranuclear hallo (clear zone), and dark-blue cytoplasm (Hoppe et al., 2007). Plasmacytosis is typically marked. Pynoninophilia could be shown by methyl green pyronin stain (MGP) or RNA stain (Figure 14.5). In both stains the immunoblasts are highlighted by coloration of the cytoplasm in purple pink or dark blue, respectively (Figure 14.5A, B). These immunoblasts may be of the B- or the T-cell type, and they may be mononuclear, binucleated, or multinucleated (Nathwani and Brynes, 1988).

Occasionally immunoblasts are multinucleated, resembling Reed–Sternberg cells and are therefore called Hodgkinoid cells (Hoppe et al., 2007). In interfollicular Hodgkinoid lymphadenitits the immunoblasts are not as large as true Reed–Sternberg cells. Their nucleoli tend to be basophilic compared to the "cherry-red" or eosinophilic typically seen in Hodgkin lymphoma. Cytoplasm is basophilic/amphophilic rather than eosinophilic. In this setting, scattered immunoblasts or sheets of immunoblasts are present in the paracortical regions, either with or without hyperplastic follicles (Figure 14.6A, B, low- a and high-power view). When follicles are absent, the appearance can be easily misinterpreted as a classic Hodgkin lymphoma, mixed-cellularity subtype; when follicles are present, it could mimic interfollicular Hodgkin lymphoma (Hoppe et al., 2007. Figure 14.5C, D).

In some autoimmune disorders immunoblastic proliferation displays a histological diversity that can be useful in distinguishing it from the other diseases (Koo, 1984, O'Malley 2009a; Kojima et al., 2010). For example, immunoblastic proliferation is one of the most common pathologic patterns noted in patients with RA (Kojima et al., 2006a), along with follicular and paracortical hyperplasia. Patients with SLE may sometimes present with atypical lymphoplasmacytic and immunoblastic proliferation, but most often these patients present follicular hyperplasia with giant follicles, histologic findings resembling Castleman's disease, atypical paracortical hyperplasia with lymphoid follicles or a combination of above these findings (Kojima et al., 2007). Still's disease with lymphadenopathy shows a dynamic histological spectrum. An exuberant immunoblastic reaction may occur, frequently with accompanying lymphadenopathy (Jeon et al., 2004). In this setting the patchy/diffuse infiltration of large T immunoblasts shows high mitotic activity that could be misinterpreted as malignant lymphoma (Jeon et al., 2004); therefore, consideration of clinical history with additional laboratory tests is warranted.

As reported, reactive immunoblastic proliferation could be a part of neoplastic lymphadenopathy with dysproteinemia (AILD) (Frizzera et al., 1974), which currently is regarded as an entity that is overlapping with AILD/angioimmunoblastic T-cell lymphoma (AILT) (Dogan et al., 2008). Immunoblastic proliferation is also seen in other B-cell lymphomas. So benign and neoplastic immunoblastic proliferations are difficult to distinguish if examined only on the basis of their cytologic features. Careful assessment

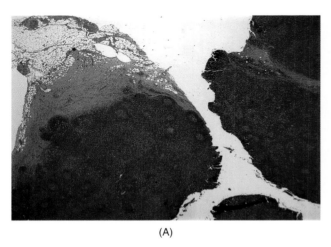

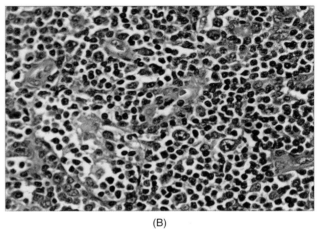

(A) (B)

FIGURE 14.6 Interfollicular Hodgkinoid cells. (A) Very low magnification view of section of lymph node with several reactive lymphoid follicles. In between increased large cells are noted (H&E, 16×). **(B)** Medium-power view of the large atypical cells exhibiting big, round to oval nucleus with prominent nucleoli and clear cytoplasm associated with increased vasculature (H&E, 200×).

of all histologic parameters such as the architectural arrangement, the cellular composition of the proliferation, the relationships among the different cell types, and the cytologic features of the immunoblasts is needed (Nathwani and Brynes, 1988).

*Immunohistochemistry/Cytochemistry/*In situ *Hybridization*

In situ hybridization with EBV-encoded RNA probe (EBER) could play a critical role in identifying EBV-associated reactive lymphadenitis or neoplastic lymphoproliferative disorders (e.g., infectious mononucleosis, Hodgkin lymphoma) and separating them from non-infectious, reactive immunoblastic proliferation, NOS, and an interfollicular Hodgkinoid reaction. EBER is rarely positive in autoimmune disorders (Kojima et al., 2006a; Jeon et al., 2004).

Immunohistochemical stains demonstrate a T- or B-cell origin of reactive immunoblasts, with diffuse, strong positivity for CD30 (Figure 14.5*E, F*). Immunoblasts do not express CD15 (Fletcher, 2007), which can be used to distinguish this entity from Hodgkin lymphoma. The B immunoblast shows a polyclonal light chain expression, which distinguishes it from clonal B-cell lymphoproliferative disorders or lymphoma. Since CD30 positive cells can be seen in both neoplastic and reactive processes (Hartsock, 1968; Segal et al., 1994; Abbondanzo et al., 1995; Kojima et al., 2010); the distinction between reactive and neoplastic lymphoid infiltrates is a common challenge in clinical and pathology practice. Appropriate clinical correlation and ancillary laboratory data are necessary to assist in differentiating CD30+ immunoblastic reactive disorders from similar-appearing malignant lymphomas.

Differential Diagnosis

Angioimmunoblastic T-Cell Lymphoma (AITL). AITL is a rare peripheral T-cell lymphoma characterized by diffuse lymphadenopathy, fever, hepatosplenomegaly, hemolytic anemia, and polyclonal hypergammaglobulinemia (Frizzera et al., 1974; Sallah and Gagnon, 1998, Dogan et al., 2008). The involved lymph nodes demonstrate complete architectural effacement, prominent neovascularization, and infiltration by immunoblasts and plasma cells. Immunologic and molecular studies have demonstrated that the majority of AITL cases are T-cell clonal disorders by abnormal proliferation of CD4+ follicular helper T-cells. AITL is found mostly in the elderly and has an aggressive clinical course (Dogan et al., 2008). In contrast to drug- or autoimmune-induced reactive immunoblastic proliferation with hyperplastic follicles, AITL has

infrequent or absent follicles (Dogan et al., 2008; de Leval and Gaulard, 2008). Importantly, the pathognomonic feature of AITL is the presence of multiple clusters of immunoblasts, transformed cells, or clear cells of varying size and number (Ree et al., 1998). Immunohistochemical stains highlight neoplastic T cells in AITL. These T cells are frequently CD4+, with only rare loss of pan-T markers (CD2, CD3, CD5, or CD7). There is also a background of increased reactive cytotoxic T-cells (CD8+, TIA+, perforin+ and granzyme B+) (Dogan et al., 2008). Typically proliferation of follicular T helper cells shows immunoreactivity to CD10, CXCL13, and PD1 (Dorfman et al., 2006; Rodriguez-Justo et al., 2009). Clonal T-cell gene rearrangements with strong, distinct oligoclonal bands favor AITL over reactive angioimmunoblastic proliferation (Dogan et al., 2008).

Peripheral T-Cell Lymphoma. Peripheral T-cell lymphoma with features of increased angiogenesis and expansion of paracortical spaces with T lymphocytes mimics reactive angioimmunoblastic proliferation in lymph nodes. There is a spectrum of architectural or cytologic changes in peripheral T-cell lymphoma including paracortical or diffuse effacement and composed of numerous medium sized, and/or some large, atypical lymphoid cells (Jaffe, 2006). Therefore, an important feature distinguishing reactive immunoblastic proliferation from peripheral T-cell lymphoma of the mixed cell type is the absence of atypia in the small to medium sized lymphocytes and lack of T-cell clonality.

Kaposi Sarcoma. Reactive angioimmunoblastic proliferation shows increased capillaries and abundant infiltrate of plasma cells that may resemble Kaposi sarcoma; however, the classical Kaposi sarcoma features of spindle cells proliferation, cleft-like vascular spaces, and extavasated erythrocytes are absent. Since HHV8 is present in peripheral blood mononuclear cells and endothelial cells in a majority of Kaposi sarcomas, immunohistochemical stains or molecular studies for viral detection are useful for diagnosis (Dictor et al., 1996; Schwartz et al., 2003; Whitby et al., 1995).

Hodgkin lymphoma. Reactive immunoblastic proliferations may be confused with Hodgkin lymphoma when relying only on histopathology (Fletcher, 2007; Segal et al., 1994). It is critical to distinguish Hodgkin lymphoma from interfollicular Hodgkinoid lymphadenitis. Morphologically, in interfollicular Hodgkinoid lymphadenitits, the immunoblasts are not as large as mononuclear

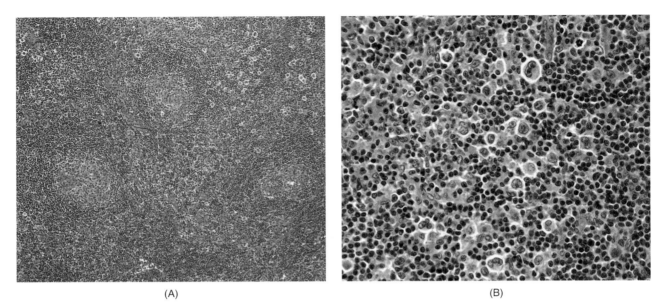

(A)   (B)

FIGURE 14.7 **Interfollicular Hodgkin lymphoma.** **(A)** Low magnification view of a lymph node section shows numerous large cells with clear cytoplasm in between several reactive lymphoid follicles (H&E, 200×). **(B)** These large atypical cells exhibit big, round to oval nucleus with prominent nucleoli and abundant clear cytoplasm. Binucleation or multinucleation is also present (H&E, 400×).

Reed–Sternberg cells. Additionally nucleoli tend to be basophilic, instead of "cherry-red" or eosinophilic, and the cytoplasm is basophilic/amphophilic rather than eosinophilic (Fletcher, 2007). Reactive immunoblasts are more evenly dispersed, while Reed–Sternberg cells in Hodgkin lymphoma are more irregularly clustered (Hoppe et al., 2007). Interstitial Hodgkin lymphoma (Figure 14.7) has morphologic similarity to the interstitial Hodgkinoid reaction. It is difficult to distinguish them without additional studies. In contrast to classical Hodgkin lymphoma (CD45−/CD30+/CD15+), reactive Hodgkinoid cells are usually CD45+ and they react with B- or T-cell antibodies but not with CD15 (Fletcher, 2007; Hoppe et al., 2007; O'Malley et al., 2009a). Some variants of classical Hodgkin lymphoma present with increased large Hodgkin cells that only show diffuse CD30 surface and cytoplasmic expression with lack of coexpression of CD15. The morphologic and phenotypic findings could resemble reactive immunoblastic proliferation, CD45 expression on the large cells is crucial in identifying true CD45 positive immunoblasts from CD45 negative Hodgkin cells/Reed–Sternberg cells in classical Hodgkin lymphoma (Stein, 2008).

Lymphocyte predominant Hodgkin lymphoma is characterized with L&H cells ("popcorn cells") surrounded by small reactive T cells (CD4+, and/or

CD57+) arranged in a rosette pattern, whereas reactive immunoblastic proliferation does not have these features. In addition "popcorn cells" are positive for CD20 and negative for CD30, which is useful in differentiating LP-Hodgkin from immunoblastic proliferation (Poppema et al., 2008).

T-Cell/Histiocyte-Rich B-Cell Lymphoma. An immunoblastic variant of T-cell/histiocyte-rich B-cell lymphoma may share similar morphologic changes noted in reactive immunoblastic proliferation. The clinical features favoring reactive immunoblastic proliferation include young age, partial nodal involvement, and a polymorphous morphology of mixed T and B phenotypes. History or clinical evidence of infectious mononucleosis, other viral infections, vaccination, and drug use should be investigated. Ancillary studies are necessary to exclude malignant lymphoma if no distinct morphologic pattern or clinical evidence suggestive of a benign reactive process is identified. In general, EBV infection is uncommon in DLBCL (approximately 10%) except in immunosuppressed patients (Park et al., 2007). Benign entities do not have clonal light chain restriction detected by flow cytometry, immunohistochemical stains, or molecular studies. Gene rearrangement studies may be requested in difficult cases. Immunoblastic proliferation is often characterized by clinically spontaneous regression (Isaacson et al., 1988).

Treatment of Choice and Prognosis

There is no specific treatment for reactive immunoblastic proliferation other than treatment of the underlying etiology.

POSTVACCINAL LYMPHADENITIS

Localized lymphadenopathy typically occurs adjacent to the vaccine injection site. An enlarged lymph node shows paracortical hyperplasia (nodular proliferation) with mottling, accompanied by interstitial proliferation of immunoblasts and occasional multinucleated or Hodgkin-like large atypical cells (Hartsock, 1968). Lymph nodes show active, hyperplastic changes after the administration of a variety of vaccines, for example, Bacillus Calmette-Guérin (BCG), varicella-zoster, measles-mumps-rubella, and smallpox (O'Malley et al., 2009b).

Definition

Postvaccinal lymphadenitis is a reactive process in local lymph node adjacent to vaccine injection site, demonstrating paracortical hyperplasia with moth-eaten appearing by interstitial proliferation of immunoblasts or Hodgkinoid cells.

ICD-10 Codes   WHO 2007

L04.9. suppurative (see also Lymphadenitis, acute)
T88.1   vaccination, reaction (allergic)
R59.1   Generalized enlarged lymph nodes
I88.   Chronic or subacute lymphadenitis.

Synonyms

Vaccinia lymphadenitis (smallpox vaccination adenitis), postvaccinal lymphadenopathy, postvaccinal reaction.

Epidemiology

Vaccination is the administration of antigenic material to humans or animals to produce immunity to a disease. The age for vaccination varies from newborn to the elderly and includes those with and without immunocompromised status. Vaccines are, in particular, given to young children or school students whose naïve immune systems have not been exposed to susceptible antigens. Thus postvaccinal reaction commonly occurs in this population. Immunization has enabled the global eradication of smallpox; however, reconstitution of vaccination for smallpox would increase the prevalence of postvaccinal lymphadenitis (O'Malley et al., 2009b).

Incidence of postvaccinal lymphadenitis is not well documented, with a single study showing the incidence of postvaccinal lymphadenitis in 5.8% of patients (26 of 480) who received BCG vaccination in Iran. Of those, 84.6% cases had simple or nonsuppurative lymphadenitis while 15.4% had suppurative lymphadenitis (Behjati and Ayatollahi, 2008).

Clinical Aspects

Etiology

Vaccines can be live or weakened forms of pathogens (bacteria, virus) and can be killed, inactivated, or purified material (e.g., protein). Smallpox was the first disease that people tried to prevent from by purposely inoculating themselves with other types of infections, with smallpox inoculation first occurring in China or India circa 200 BC (Lombard et al., 2007). Vaccines developed against infectious diseases-for example, influenza, hepatitis A and B, chickenpox, meningitis, peneumonia, human papilloma virus (HPV), measles-mumps-rubella (MMR and H1N1)-are now widely used (Fiore et al., 2009; Offit, 2007; Chang et al., 2009; Freeman et al., 1993; Rodriguez-Rieiro et al., 2010). Besides the use against infectious diseases, vaccines have gained their use in other areas, such as for antitumor therapy (Jones et al., 2004; Frazer et al., 2011; Madan and Gulley, 2011). Dendritic cell vaccination with anti-CD25 monoclonal antibody is implicated in phase I/II trial in patients with melanoma (Jacobs et al., 2010). BCG vaccine is currently in use for bladder cancer treatment (Takeuchi et al., 2011). Postvaccinal reaction in patients undergoing cancer therapy, with or without lymphadenitis/lymphadenopathy, is a new entity with more investigations warranted.

Site of Involvement

Lymphadenitis, when present, is in the lymph nodes draining the injection site, commonly supracervical or axillary (Ioachim and Medeiros, 2009b).

Pathogenesis

Vaccines appear to have more side effects than previously realized. Information is limited regarding pathophysiology despite postvaccinal reactions having been reported since the 1960s (Hartsock, 1968). For example, for smallpox vaccine, the vaccinia is a poxvirus, considerably less virulent and with a broader host range than smallpox (Ginsberg, 1990). The vaccinia virus and smallpox virus, both being DNA poxviruses, share similar antigenicities, but the former is used to vaccinate for smallpox.

After administration, circulating viral antigens have been reported to activate the complex T- and B-cell response, resulting in smallpox vaccination adenitis and its characteristic early histologic appearance in lymph nodes (O'Malley et al., 2009b). The BCG vaccine may also induce a delayed type of hypersensitivity reaction and cell-mediated immunity in the host 4 to 8 weeks after vaccination. There are many studies regarding post–BCG lymphadenitis; however, the pathogenesis is not well documented and could also be related to its delayed immune response (Merry and Fitzgerald, 1996; Sadeghi and Kumar, 1990; Aggarwal et al., 1990).

Cancer vaccines are designed and developed for specific types of cancer. For cancer vaccines, the general mechanism is to induce the body's primary immune response. For example, tumor-antigen-loaded DC vaccination is an important tool for tumor-antigen-specific immunotherapy in the treatment of cancer, since DCs are antigen-presenting cells in the immune system that are able to induce primary T-cell responses (Mitchell and Abbot, 1965; Tuettenberg et al., 2007, Aguzzi and Krautler, 2010).

Approach to Diagnosis

Clinical and Laboratory Investigations

The first step in diagnosis is verifying the clinical history of vaccine administration followed by an examination for unilateral or bilateral lymphadenopathy. Routine CBCs, metabolic panels, and liver function tests may not be required if a recent vaccination history is documented. The latent period from vaccination to enlargement of lymph node is variable but generally, postvaccinal lymphadenitis occurs 1 to 3 weeks after smallpox vaccination (Hartsock, 1968), whereas lymph node enlargement occurs 12 weeks after BCG vaccination (Lehmann et al., 1978). Lymphadenitis can also occur after measles-mumps-rubella (MMR) vaccination (Freeman et al., 1993). Nasal discharge or rash may also be present. The BCG vaccine could be complicated by ulceration and regional lymphadenitis (Milstien and Gibson, 1990; Sadeghi and Kumar, 1990; Kroger et al., 1994). Lymphadenitis occurs usually 2 to 8 weeks after vaccination, although an interval delay of up to 8 or more months can happen (Milstien and Gibson, 1990; Aggarwal et al., 1990; Merry and Fitzgerald, 1996; Nazir and Qazi, 2005). The involved nodes are usually ipsilateral to the vaccination site. A number of factors such as age, technique of vaccination, BCG strain, dose, potency, viability and immunogenicity of the vaccine, and prior exposure to mycobacterial antigens are implicated in the pathogenesis of lymphadenitis (Milstien and Gibson, 1990; Aggarwal

et al., 1990; Merry and Fitzgerald, 1996; Behjati and Ayatollahi, 2008). BCG is also used as a vaccine in bladder or prostate antitumor therapy (Madan and Gulley, 2011), but lymphadenitis with this form of vaccination has not been reported.

Morphologic Aspects

Postvaccinial lymph node findings could be a reactive immunoblastic proliferation, follicular hyperplasia, or suppurative, based on the type and duration. Typically viral vaccination elicits the former followed by follicular hyperplasia. After smallpox vaccination, morphologic changes can occur as early as 8 to as late as 15 days later. In the earlier setting (8 days postvaccine), changes include diffusely hyperplastic changes in the regional lymph nodes. A typical "moth-eaten" appearance or mottling is present due to profound proliferation of immunoblasts, which are present throughout the entire parenchyma. After day 15, follicular hyperplasia is dominant (Hartsock, 1968; Ioachim and Medeiros, 2009b; O'Malley et al., 2009b). Plasma cells, eosinophils, and mast cells are present in the later biopsy (Hartsock, 1968).

Morphologic examination of biopsied lymph nodes in patients who receive measles vaccination reveals features similar to those occurring with smallpox vaccination; however, plasmacytosis with Warthin–Finkeldey-type giant cells is typical (Nozawa et al., 1994; O'Malley et al., 2009b). In contrast, BCG vaccination complication is primarily characterized by suppurative lymphadenitis (Nazir and Qazi, 2005).

Immunohistochemistry/Cytochemistry

Immunohistochemistry could be used to determine an infectious etiology, but the critical application is to differentiate between reactive immunoblastic hyperplasia versus Hodgkin or non-Hodgkin lymphoma. Immunoblasts or reactive Hodgkin-like cells express CD30 but not CD15 (Fletcher, 2007).

Differential Diagnosis

Vaccine-induced lymphadenitis could mimic some infections that cause diffuse paracortical hyperplasia with immunoblast proliferation, and in some cases with granulomas and necrosis. These include viral lymphadenitis, Hodgkin lymphoma, non-Hodgkin lymphoma, and drug-induced lymphadenitis.

Viral lymphadenitis is morphologically indistinguishable from postvaccinial lymphadenitis, but serology and in situ hybrididization for viral etiology could delineate the two etiologies (refer to Chapter 15). The presence of Hodgkin-like cells, eosinophils, plasma cells, with or without fibrosis in postvaccinial lymphadenitis, could resemble the pathohistological features of classical Hodgkin lymphoma (Hartsock, 1968). Appropriate immuno-histochemical stains and in situ hybridization help to distinguish these two entities. Postvaccinal lymphadenitis with marked immunoblastic proliferation is the classic example of a large-cell lymphoma mimicker because of the presence of sheets of large immunoblasts, necrosis, and variable nuclear atypia. B-cell clonality by flow cytometry, immunostains, and PCR study should be performed to separate a reactive versus a neoplastic process. Phenytoin or methotrexate drug induced lymphadenopathy demonstrates paracortical hyperplasia presenting with immunoblasts or Hodgkin-like cells. A history of drug administration and regression of lymphadenopathy after drug withdrawal or vaccine administration would point to the etiology.

Treatment of Choice and Prognosis

Postvaccinial lymphadenitis is a reactive process that usually resolves spontaneously within weeks or months requiring no treatment. A sustained lymphadenopathy or progressive enlargement of a lymph node should be followed with excisional biopsy if clinically suspicious for lymphoma or persistent mass exceeding many months. Post–BCG or antitumor vaccinal reactions may behave differently with a delayed or prolonged reaction (Aggarwal et al., 1990; Merry and Fitzgerald, 1996; Nazir and Qazi, 2005).

DRUG-INDUCED LYMPHADENOPATHY

Many drugs may induce generalized lymphadenopathy-mimicking malignancies, especially those used for long-term therapy in chronic inflammatory disorders, autoimmune disorders, connective tissue disorders, epilepsy, infections and for some malignancies. More commonly implicated drugs include methotrexate, phenytoin, phenobarbitital, sulfasalazine, antithymocytes globulin, and gold salts (Ioachim and Medeiros, 2009c) with phenytoin and methotrexate being the most commonly encountered agent in reactive lymphadenopathy (Abbondazo, 1995; Ioachim and Medeiros, 2009c). Phenytoin can cause a pseudolymphoma syndrome with generalized lymphadenopathy, fever, skin rashes, eosinophilia, and hepatosplenomegaly with a slightly increased risk of lymphoma (Abbondazo, 1995; Choi

et al., 2003). Therefore it could be misdiagnosed as systemic lymphoma or cutaneous lymphoma such as MF (Choi et al., 2003). Lymphadenopathy in the setting of methotrexate (MTX) therapy is frequently granulomatous in nature and may represent a form of drug-induced sarcoidosis (Verdich and Christensen, 1979; Sybert and Butler, 1978). In addition MTX-related lymphoproliferative disorders are well studied (Hoshida et al., 2007; Gaulard et al., 2008; Hasserjian et al., 2009). Since MTX is widely used in the treatment of malignancy, it is also possible to mistake methotrexate-induced lymphadenopathy for metastatic disease or secondary lymphoproliferative disorder. The drug-induced lymphoproliferative disorders can be divided into nonneoplastic tumors (also called pseudolymphoma) and lymphoma. For the latter, it has been listed in the 2008 World Health Organization classification of lymphoid neoplasms under the subcategory "iatrogenic immunodeficiency-associated lymphoproliferative disorders," which include both Hodgkin and non-Hodgkin lymphomas (Gaulard et al., 2008). Treatment includes discontinuation of the offending drug, monitoring for organ involvement, or the use of systemic steroids (Ang et al., 2010).

ANTICONVULSANT (PHENYTOIN)-RELATED LYMPHOPROLIFERATIVE DISORDER

Definition

ICD-10 Codes   WHO 2007

R59.1   Generalized enlarged lymph nodes
I88.1   Chronic lymphadenitis, except mesenteric
I88.8   Other nonspecific lymphadenitis
I88.9   Nonspecific lymphadenitis, unspecified

Synonyms

Anticonvulsant hypersensitivity syndrome; phenytoin (Dilantin) lymphadenopathy; phenytoin (Dilantin) induced hypersensitivity; anticonvulant-associated hypersensitivity; anticonvulant-associated lymphadenopathy; anticonvulsant-induced pseudolymphoma syndrome; iatrogenic immuno-deficiency-associated lymphoproliferative disorders.

Epidemiology

Although there are a number of studies on phenytoin-related lymphoproliferative disorders (Abbondanzo et al., 1995, Choi et al., 2003; Scheinfeld, 2003, Weedon, 1975), the incidence is not known. There are no differences in age or gender as any patient with long-term exposure to the drug may be affected. In a small series of 25 lymph node lesions from 1965 to 1991 that were suspected to be related to phenytoin, six were coded as probable phenytoin associated, 17 as possible and 2 as coincidental. The male-to-female ratio was 11:14, and patient ages ranged from 24 to 81 years (median of 53 years). Documented lymphadenopathy developed 1 week to 30 years (median of 5 years) after the start of phenyotoin (Abbondazo, 1995).

Clinical Aspects

Etiology

The drugs commonly used to treat epilepsy are carbamazepine, phenytoin (diphenylhydantoin, Dilatin), phenobarbital, and valproic acid. Phenytoin acts to suppress the abnormal brain activity seen in seizures by reducing electrical conductance among brain cells by stabilizing the inactive intracellular state of voltage-dependent sodium channels (Chao and Alzheimer, 1995; Segal and Douglas, 1997). Aside from seizures, it is an option in the treatment of trigeminal neuralgia in the event that carbamazepine or other first-line treatment is deemed inappropriate (Cheshire, 2007). Phenytoin is the most common cause of the anticonvulsant hypersensitivity syndrome (Moss et al., 1999; Scheinfeld, 2003). A number of hypersensitivity reactions have been reported in association with phenytoin use. These reactions frequently involve generalized rashes, eosinophilia, fever, lymphadenopathy, and hepatic disease and despite the ominous presentation, lymphadenopathy is also called "pseudolymphoma," because of its benign self-limited nature with rare exceptions (Choi et al., 2003; Scheinfeld, 2003). Newell et al. reported that atypical lymphocytosis and eosinophilia were observed in 72% and 56% of 32 pediatric patients with anticonvulsant hypersensitivity syndrome, respectively (Newell et al., 2009).

Sites of Involvement

Most case reports have indicated a high frequency of extranodal involvement in phenytoin-related hypersensitivity, namely for cutaneous reactions (Scheinfeld, 2003). Lymph nodes, spleen, and liver are also commonly involved (Ioachim and Medeiros, 2009c). Hilar or mediastinal lymphadenopathy has also been noted as a common presentation for a few drug-induced lymphoproliferative disorders including anticonvulsants (Abbonadazo SL et al., 1995).

Pathogenesis

Prolonged administration of phenytoin has been implicated as a possible etiologic factor in alteration of immune function with subsequent development of a lymphoproliferative disorder; however, the mechanism is not entirely clear. Phenytoin has complex effects on the immune system, including suppression of cytotoxic activities of natural killer (NK) cells and cytotoxic T lymphocytes (CTL) but not lymphokine-activated killer (LAK) cells (Okamoto et al., 1989). Phenytoin also significantly depresses interferon augmentation of NK cell cytotoxicity in a dose-dependent manner (Margaretten et al., 1987). Phenytoin suppresses the level of cortisol specifically by inducing the liver cytochrome P450 enzyme system to stimulate steroid clearance and by directly suppressing adrenal production (Putignano et al., 1998). These effects may partially explain the ability of phenytoin to cause lymphoproliferative disorder.

Approach to Diagnosis

Clinical and Laboratory Investigations

A detailed clinical and medication history is helpful in establishing the diagnosis of anticonvulsant lymphoproliferative disorder. The duration from anticonvulsant use to the onset of a lymphoproliferative disorder or lymphadenopathy varies based on the type of drug use, the nature of the underlying disorder, and the genetic background of the patient. Laboratory monitoring of serum anticonvulsant levels is routinely used in clinical setting. Skin eruption may occur 3 to 24 weeks (mean 7 weeks) from the start of anticonvulsant therapy (Choi et al., 2003). The skin lesions manifest as generalized maculopapular eruptions (Choi et al., 2003). Other clinical presentations include facial edema, fever, and gingival hyperplasia due to folate deficiency (Lafzi et al., 2007). Lymphadenopathy is present in 63% of patients, while hepatomegaly is present in 25% of patients (Choi et al., 2003). The anticonvulansant-induced pseudolymphoma syndrome can rarely be fatal if there are extensive skin lesions, severe hepatitis, agranulocytosis, and neutropenia (Choi et al., 2003). Pseudomononucleosis induced by phenytoin use has been reported with occurrence typically 3 to 7 weeks after starting therapy (Weedon, 1975). Laboratory investigation reveals leukocytosis, atypical lymphocytes, eosinophilia, monocytosis, neutrophilia, lymphocytosis, and abnormal liver function tests (Choi et al., 2003).

Molecular tests for clonality are helpful since rare cases show monoclonality. A negative T-cell or B-cell receptor gene rearrangement will favor pseudolymphoma, since presence of T-cell receptor–gamma gene rearrangement has been reported in one of eight cases (Choi et al., 2003). It is critical to determine the presence of a clonal population in an enlarged lymph node to aid in ruling out a lymphoma or a development of one on a background of pseudolymphoma.

Morphologic Aspects

Phenytoin-related lymphoproliferative disorder has a wide spectrum of heterogeneous clinical behaviors from benign to malignant. In one study, 15 of 25 cases (60%) of suspected anticonvulsant-related pseuolymphoma showed a benign histology, which was classified according to the presence or absence of immunoblastic hyperplasia. The remaining 10 cases showed 7 (28%) with non-Hodgkin lymphoma and 3 (12%) with Hodgkin lymphoma (Abbondazo, 1995). A progression from reactive hyperplasia to malignant lymphoma was observed in 2 of 5 sequential biopsies (Abbondazo, 1995). MF-like skin lesions are also reported to be associated with phenytoin and other anticonvulsants (Rijlaarsdam et al., 1991; Choi et al., 2003). Some patients may develop generalized lymph node hyperplasia together with MF-like lesions (Wolf et al., 1985). Angioimmunoblastic proliferation in enlarged lymph nodes from patients who has received phenytoin has also been frequently documented (Choi et al., 2003; Tsung and Lin, 1981; Abbondazo, 1995). Proliferation and infiltration by Langerhans cell histiocytes in enlarged lymph nodes, along with eosinophilia, skin eruption, and hepatosplenomegaly was observed in a 2-year-old girl during phenobarbital prophylaxis for convulsion (Nagata et al., 1992). Pseudolymphoma in a phenytoin-related disorder is difficult to separate from malignant lymphoma by morphology alone. A diagnosis of anticonvulsant hypersensitivity syndrome/pseudolymphoma could be made if clinical signs and symptoms improve after anticonvulsant therapy is discontinued (Nathan and Belsiito, 1998; Gaulard et al., 2008).

Differential Diagnosis

Mycosis Fungoides. Phenytoin-related drug hypersentitivity exhibits similar morphologic features with MF, for example, epidermotropism of atypical lymphocytes and Pautrier's microabcess-like structures (38%) (Choi et al., 2003). But, in contrast to MF, phenytoin-related drug sensitivity reveals moderate to marked spongiosis (75%), necrotic keratinocytes (63%), and infiltration of eosinophils (25%) in the epidermis and, in the dermis, papillary dermal edema (100%). Other inflammatory cells including neutrophils are also present in subset of cases (50%) (Choi et al., 2003). MF involving lymph nodes reveals variable patterns (Sausville et al., 1985). Besides atypical lymphocytes, paracortical expansion of histiocytes and dermatopathic lymphadenopathy are characteristic findings that contrast with the immunoblastic proliferation findings in phenytoin. In patients suspected of MF, T-cell gene rearrangement should be routinely ordered, since clonal T cells are associated with MF and rarely seen with phenytoin-related lymphadenopathy.

Infectious Mononucleosis (IM). Phenytoin could cause pseudomononucleosis similar to IM (Weedon, 1975). Appropriate tests for EBV lympadenitis should be performed if IM is suspected. (Detailed diagnostic tools for EBV-related mononucleosis are described in Chapter 15.)

Hodgkin and Non-Hodgkin Lymphoma. Phenytonin induced lymphadenopathy including benign lymph node hyperplasia, pseudolymphoma, lymphoma, and Hodgkin disease have been reported (Choi et al., 2003; Gaulard et al., 2008). Distinguishing reactive or hypersensitive processes (pseudolymphoma syndrome) from true neoplastic processes could be difficult (Choi et al., 2003). All CD30-positive lymphomas should be considered in the differential diagnosis. Immunohistochemical staining is a useful because some lymphoproliferative disorders with Hodgkinoid features are positive for CD20 and CD30 but negative for CD15 (Gaulard et al., 2008). Classical Hodgkin lymphoma is CD30+, CD15+, and CD45 negative (Stein, 2008). Anaplastic large T-cell lymphoma often displays a sinusoidal infiltrate with large cells having C-shaped or "horseshoe-shaped" anaplastic nuclei characteristic of "hallmark cells" (Benharroch et al., 1998). ALK stain is positive (Ioachim and Medeiros 2009c). Angioimmunoblastic T-cell lymphoma (AILT) is abnormal proliferation of follicular T helper cells, admixed with immunoblasts or sometimes Hodgkin-like cells with angioimmunoblastic-like pattern of arborizing vessels. Unlke anticonvulsant-related lymphadenopathy with focal immunoblastic proliferation and follicular hyperplasia, AILT shows a complete effacement of nodal architecture (Dogan et al., 2008). If a T- or B-cell non-Hodgkin lymphoma is suspected, but without definite evidence to prove malignancy by flow cytometry or molecular study, cessation of phenytoin would be the initial step with subsequent close follow-up. Resolution of signs and symptoms would favor phenytoin-induced lymphadenopathy instead of malignancy.

Treatment and Prognosis

Patients with anticonvulsant hypersensitivity syndrome should avoid all traditional anticonvulsants. Benzodiazepines, valproic acid, or one of the newer anticonvulsants may be used for seizure control in such cases (Knowles et al., 1999). In addition family counseling is a vital component of patient management (Knowles et al., 1999). In general, treatment includes discontinuation of the offending drug, monitoring for organ involvement, and using topical or systemic steroids for cutaneous reactions (Ang et al., 2010), especially for benign reactive lymphoid hyperplasia. Since anticonvulsant-induced pseudolymphoma syndrome has a prolonged course even after the cessation of causative agents, close follow-up and additional biopsies are needed for early detection of malignant lymphoma transformation (Choi et al., 2003).

METHOTREXATE-RELATED LYMPHOPROLIFERATIVE DISORDER

Definition

Methotrexate-associated lymphoproliferative disorders (MTX-LPD) are a heterogeneous group of lymphoid proliferation or lymphoma that develop in patients with autoimmune diseases treated with MTX. MTX-LPDs are often associated with EBV infection and could regress after cessation of MTX therapy.

ICD-10 Codes   WHO 2007

R59.1   Generalized enlarged lymph nodes
I88.1   Chronic lymphadenitis, except mesenteric
I88.8   Other nonspecific lymphadenitis
I88.9   Nonspecific lymphadenitis, unspecified

Epidemiology

MTX is widely used in the treatment of autoimmune disorders, predominantly in patients with rheumatoid arthritis (RA) (Wolfe and Michaud, 2007; Rizzi et al., 2009; Isomaki et al., 1978; Kinlen, 1985a; Gridley et al., 1994; Matteson et al., 1991). Long-term

of use of MTX has caused many patients to develop lymphoproliferative disorders (LPD) that could be transient, a long-standing reactive process, or malignant. Clinically, a study showed that when compared with sporadic LPD, late onset with female predominance was observed in 76 patients with rheumatoid arthritis-lymphoproliferative disorder (RA-LPD) when compared with sporadic LPD, of those, 48 patients were diagnosed as MTX-LPD and 28 were non-MTX-LPD (Hoshida et al., 2007). The study also showed that the interval between the diagnosis of RA and LPD in MTX-LPD was significantly shorter than that in non–MTX-LPN (132 months versus 240 months) (Hoshida et al., 2007).

Clinical Aspects

Etiology

MTX is an antimetabolite and antifolate drug used in the treatment of neoplasms and autoimmune diseases (e.g., rheumatoid arthritis, psoriasis, connective disorders) alone or combined with other immunomodulator or anti-inflammatory agents. It is well known that patients with RA, treated or untreated, have a high risk of developing lymphoproliferative disorders as well as other autoimmune disorders such as Sjögren's or Felty's syndromes (Isomaki et al., 1978; Gridley et al., 1994; Masaki and Sugai, 2004). EBV, a ubiquitous herpes virus, has been etiologically linked to lymphoma in MTX-treated patients and over-represented in these patients (Tosato et al., 1984; Dawson et al., 2001). Overall, about 40% of lymphoproliferative disorders/lymphoma in RA patients treated with MTX are EBV positive (Gaulard et al., 2008; Rizzi et al., 2009). A subpopulation of patients has detectable EBV-encoded small nonpolyadenylated RNA (EBER) (Dawson et al., 2001; Niitsu et al., 2010).

Sites of Involvement

In approximately 40% of the reported cases, the affected sites were extranodal and have included the gastrointestinal tract, skin, lung, kidney, and soft tissues (Hoshida et al., 2007; Sallum et al., 1996; Ioachim and Medeiros, 2009c). Hilar or mediastinal lymphadenopathy has also been reported in association with drug-induced lymphoproliferative disorder including MTX-LPD (Verdich J and Christensen AL, 1979; Zisman DA et al., 2001).

Pathogenesis

MTX is administered mostly to patients with autoimmune disorders. Thus, the hyperimmune state of disease itself and the immunosuppressive state induced by MTX treatment might contribute to the development of LPD (Hoshida et al., 2007). Studies have revealed abnormally increased frequency of EBV-induced atypical cells in the blood of patients with RA (Tosato et al., 1984). However, the frequency of EBV infection could be variable in MTX-LPD (Salloum et al., 1996; Gaulard et al., 2008). Several observations support the suggestion of an increased risk of EBV-associated lymphoproliferations in patients with arthritis receiving immunosuppressive drugs. T cells play a critical role in immune surveillance, and a potential pathologic link between RA and LPD was suggested based on the reduced ability of T cells to control EBV infection in these patients (Bardwick et al., 1980; Depper et al., 1981; Vaugham, 1985). The mechanisms of MTX related lymphoproliferative disorder are similar to those found in post transplant patients; both showed a high susceptibility to EBV infection and immunosuppression. The occurrence of MTX associated lymphoproliferative disorder usually takes a long period of the drug exposure. During the development of LPD, the role of T-cells in LPD in response to EBV infection cannot be ignored. A study indicated that a healing from posttransplant related lymphoproliferative disorder was due to a rapid increase of EBV specific T-cells concomitant to a decrease of viral load (Smets et al. 2002). Miceli-Richard et al's further study revealed that there was no significant alteration of EBV specific T-lymphocyte response or the EBV load after a short time exposure to MTX or anti-TNF therapy (Miceli-Richard et al., 2009). Non-EBV related mechanism of lymphomagenesis should also be considered in driving LPD and needs further exploration.

Approach to Diagnosis

Clinical and Laboratory Investigations

A wide spectrum of clinical presentations is observed in MTX-LPD. There are many subtypes of lymphomas in the category of MTX-LPD, including B cell–LPD/lymphoma (DLBC, polymorphilic/lymphoplasmacytic LPD, follicular lymphoma, Burkitt lymphoma, MZL, lymphoplasmacytic lymphoma, CLL/SLL), T cell–LPD/lymphomas (peripheral T-cell lymphoma, NOS, extranodal NH/T cell lymphoma, nasal type), Hodgkin-like lesions, and, classical Hodgkin lymphoma (Gaulard et al., 2008). Among MTX-LPD, DLBCL accounts for about half (Niitsu et al., 2010; Gaulard et al., 2008). Mantle cell lymphoma (Tran et al., 2008) and cutaneous T- and B-cell lymphomas (Huwait et al., 2010) were occasionally reported in MTX-treated patients. Increased awareness is needed on the possible

occurrence of LPD spontaneous remission following immunosuppressant discontinuation in regard to initiating cytotoxic therapy (Rizzi et al., 2009).

Laboratory study for antibodies against EBV and CMV infections and routine chemical profile is commonly applied to MTX-LPD. CBC and peripheral blood smear examination, in combination with flow cytometric profile, are used for detection of atypical lymphocytosis in peripheral blood samples. The initial management of patients who diagnosed LPD while on MTX therapy is to stop medication and put in observation.

Morphologic Aspects

The histologic features in MTX-related lymphadenopathy are variable, depending on the duration and the phase of therapy. These could range from atypical lymphoid hyperplasia to definitive lymphoma. Lymphoid proliferations may consist of nodular, interstitial, immunoblastic, or mixed patterns. However, the most common lymph node findings can be divided into two patterns: (1) polymorphous, consisting of various kinds of lymphocytes including small reactive lymphocytes, immunoblasts, centroblasts, Reed–Sternberg-like cells and plasmacytes, and (2) monomorphous, presenting with increase in monotonous population of immunoblasts or centroblasts resembling diffuse large B-cell lymphoma (Gaulard et al., 2008). For MTX-related lymphadenopathy, polymorphous lymphocytic or lymphoplasmacytic infiltrates have been described in 15% of the cases (Gaulard et al., 2008). In the polymorphous pattern the architecture of lymph node is only partially effaced with interfollicular hyperplasia, reactive germinal centers, and portions of demarcated T-cell zone. The monomorphous subtype is characterized by proliferating B cells resembling DLBCL (Gaulard et al., 2008; Ioachim and Medeiros, 2009c). Some Reed–Sternberg-like lymphocytes are also occasionally noted. A Hodgkin-like lesion, defined as a lesion containing Reed–Sternberg-like cells but not fulfilling the criteria for Hodgkin lymphoma, has been reported in patients receiving long-term low-dose MTX therapy (Kamel et al., 1996; Kikuchi et al., 2010; Gaulard et al., 2008). The infiltrating pattern in MTX-related lymphadenopathy could also mimic the nodular lymphocyte predominant Hodgkin lymphoma displaying progressive transformation of germinal centers and presence of "L&H" cells or "popcorn cells". On rare occasions MTX-LPD has shown similar morphologic features to angioimmunoblastic lymphoma (Hatanaka et al., 2010). True paniculitis-like T-cell lymphoma (Nemoto et al., 2010) and lymphomatoid granulomatosis (Schalk et al., 2009) have also been documented in MTX-LPD. A secondary infection with CMV has occurred in patients with RA treated with MTX and inflixmab (Shimojima et al., 2010) with morphologic changes in lymph nodes resembling infectious mononucleosis (IM)-like syndrome with viral inclusion and immunoblast proliferation.

Immunohistochemistry/Cytochemistry

For diagnosis of MTX-induced lymphadenopathy, excisional biopsy of the enlarged lymph node is needed for architectural pattern assessment. In addition flow cytometry and immunohistochemical stains are required to determine if B lymphocytosis is accompanied by light chain clonality. PCR for T- and B-cell gene rearrangement should be applied in the cases suspicious for lymphoma. CD30+/CD15−/CD45+ immunoblasts are different from classical Hodgkin lymphoma (CD30+/CD15+/CD45−) (Stein, 2008). EBV infection or reactivation can be detected by in situ hybridization, EBV-latent infection membrane protein-1(LMP-1) immunostain, and PCR for LMP-1 and EBNA-2 (Kikuchi et al., 2010).

Differential Diagnosis

MTX-induced lymphadenopathy covers a wide spectrum from reactive to neoplastic process. Distinguishing neoplastic from non-neoplastic lymphadenopathy largely depends on morphologic assessment, light chain clonality by flow cytometry, immunoperoxidase stains, and molecular studies by PCR for T-cell and/or B-cell gene rearrangement. A mixture of polymorphous, monomophous, and lymphoma stage disease could occur simultaneously when examining the same lymph node from the same patient (Ioachim and Medeiros, 2009c).

Diffuse Large B-Cell Lymphoma

It has been reported that DLBCL is frequently present in MTX-treated patients (Mariette et al. 2002; Hoshida et al., 2007). MTX-induced lymphoid hyperplasia could mimic DLBCL, especially if there is significant increase in transformed B cells with atypical features or arranged in monomorphic proliferative pattern (Ioachim and Medeiros, 2009c). Commonly MTX-related LPD, but not de novo DLBCL, is associated with EBV infection or reactivation (Salloum et al., 1996; Hoshida et al., 2007). Thus testing serum EBV titer and detecting EBV-positive cells in tissue section would be helpful. Many studies also show that when MTX therapy was interrupted, MTX-related lymphomas resolved, and chemotherapy was not necessary (Salloum et al., 1996; Hsiao et al., 2009).

Hodgkin Lymphoma

Hodgkin-like lesions, as well as MTX-induced Hodgkin lymphoma, have been reported in patients receiving long-term, low-dose MTX therapy (Kamel et al., 1996; Kikuchi et al., 2010; Khopkar and Bhor, 2009). Hodgkin-like lesions are usually CD30+, CD15−, by immunostaining and EBER+/− by in situ hybridization. MTX-related Hodgkin lymphoma often presents with extranodal involvement, in contrast to mostly nodal pattern of classical Hodgkin lymphoma (Salloum et al., 1996; Hoshida et al., 2007; Kojima et al. 2006).

Angioimmunoblstic T-Cell Lymphoma

There are some RA patients who developed MTX-associated LPDs resembling AITL (Hatanaka et al., 2010). A study demonstrated that the biopsies of lymph nodes from three patients showed polymorphous infiltrates, mainly T-cells, and arborizing HEVs with EBV-positive B-cells in two cases. The lymphadenopathy spontaneously regressed with cessation of MTX in all three cases, but one case recurred (Hatanaka et al., 2010). PCR for T-cell gene rearrangements might be helpful in distinguishing true AITL from MTX-AITL-like disorder.

EBV-Associated LPD

EBV-associated LPD/lymphomas can clinically present as infectious mononucleosis, Burkitt lymphoma, plasmablastic lymphoma, nasal type natural killer-cell/T-cell lymphoma, and HIV or immunodeficiency related LPDs and lymphomas (Maeda et al., 2009; Carbone et al., 2008). Infectious mononucleosis occurs primarily in young persons with recent flu-like symptoms and high IgM titer for EBV in serum. Burkitt lymphoma is characterized by relatively uniform proliferation of medium size B cells and tingible body macrophages, displaying a "starry sky" pattern under low-power view. Burkitt lymphoma is immunophenotypically CD5−, CD10+, CD20+, and BCL-2 and involves translocation of the c-MYC gene. Plasmablastic lymphoma is unique in its morphology with plasmacytoid or immunoblastoid differentiation that corresponds to the terminal phase of B-cell differentiation. Immunophenotypically, plasmablastic lymphoma is CD20−, CD38 cytoplasmic +, CD138+, MUM-1+, EBV +/− (Flaitz et al., 2002, Vega et al., 2005). Nasal type of NK/T-cell lymphoma is located in nasal-oral area, and shows a very aggressive clinical behavior. Morphologically it presents with a diffuse angiocentric and angioinvasive infiltration by medium to large atypical lymphoid cells, which are positive for CD2+, CD56+, cytoplasmic CD3 epsilon, and TIA by immunohistochemical stains

(Al-Hakeem et al., 2007; Chan et al. 1997). There is overlap between MTX-LPD and immunodeficiency-related LPD by histology and pathogenesis. Identification of etiology of diseases and correlation with clinical history and medication record are necessary for further differential diagnosis. In addition testing for HIV, if clinically indicated, aids in diagnosis of HIV-related LPD.

Treatment of Choice and Prognosis

Treatment for drug induced hypersensivity or lymphoproliferative disorder includes discontinuation of the offending drug, monitoring for organ involvement, and using systemic steroids (Ang et al., 2010). There are a number of intriguing reports of lymphoproliferative disorders diagnosed during immunosuppressive treatment for underlying autoimmune disease that spontaneously abated shortly after treatment discontinuation (Satoh et al., 2009; Rizzi et al., 2009). The same phenomenon is seen in MTX-LPD, which is even reversible in the lymphoma phase (Satoh et al., 2009; Rizzi et al., 2009). Complete remission usually occurs within 4 weeks after discontinuation of the drug and appears to be durable (Rizzi et al., 2009). In one study, 37 patients with RA treated with MTX developed lymphoproliferative disorder/lymphoma with 16 showing initial spontaneous regression without antitumor therapy and only 6 had no response to MTX withdrawal (Salloum et al., 1996). For the patients not responding to MTX withdrawal and presenting with high-grade or progressive clinical courses, chemotherapy should be considered. A study of 29 patients who developed DLBCL after receiving MTX for RA demonstrated that a majority of these patients achieved complete response after consequent chemotherapy (Niitsu et al., 2010).

REFERENCES

Abbondanzo SL, Irey NS, Frizzera G. 1995. Dilantin-associated lymphadenopathy. Spectrum of histopathologic patterns. Am J Surg Pathol 19:675–86.

Aggarwal NP, Kallan BM, Grover PS, Aggarwal M. 1990. Clinico-excisional study of lymphadenitis following BCG vaccination. Indian J Pediatr 57:585–6.

Aguzzi A and Krautler NJ. 2010. Characterizing follicular dendritic cells: a progress report. Eur J Immunol 40:2134–8.

Al-Hakeem DA, Fedele S, Carlos R, Porter S. 2007. Extranodal NK/T-cell lymphoma, nasal type. Oral Oncol 43:4–14.

Ang CC, Wang YS, Yoosuff EL, Tay YK. 2010. Retrospective analysis of drug-induced hypersensitivity syndrome: a study of 27 patients. J Am Acad Dermatol 63:219–27.

Asano S, Muramatsu T, Kanno H, Wakasa H. 1987. Dermatopathic lymphadenopathy. Electronmicroscopic, enzyme-histochemical and immunohistochemical study. Acta Pathol Jpn 37:887–900.

Assaf C, Hummel M, Steinhoff M, Geilen CC, Orawa H, Stein H, Orfanos CE. 2005. Early TCR-beta and TCR-gamma PCR detection of T-cell clonality indicates minimal tumor disease in lymph nodes of cutaneous T-cell lymphoma: diagnostic and prognostic implications. Blood 105:503–10.

Banchereau J, Steinman RM. 1998. Dendritic cells and the control of immunity. Nature 392:245–52.

Bardwick PA, Bluestein HG, Zvaifler NJ, Depper JM, Seegmiller JE. 1980. Altered regulation of Epstein–Barr virus induced lymphoblast proliferation in rheumatoid arthritis lymphoid cells. Arthritis Rheum 23:626–32.

Baroni CD, Uccini S. 1990. Lymph nodes in HIV-positive drug abusers with persistent generalized lymphadenopathy: histology, immunohistochemistry, and pathogenetic correlations. Prog AIDS Pathol. 2:33–50.

Bassarova A, Tierens A, Lauritzsen GF, FossAA A, Delabie J. 2008. Mantle cell lymphoma with partial involvement of the mantle zone: an early infiltration pattern of mantle cell lymphoma? Virchows Arch. 453:407–11.

Batsakis JG, Solomon AR, Rice DH. 1981. The pathology of head and neck tumors: carcinoma of the nasopharynx. Head Neck Surg 3:511–24.

Behjati M, Ayatollahi J. 2008. Post BCG lymphadenitis in vaccinated infants in Yazd, Iran. Iran J Pediatr 18:351–6

Benharroch D. Meguerlan-Bedoyan Z, Lamant L, Amin C, Brugieres L, Terrier-Lacombe MJ, Haralambieva E, Pulford K, Pileri S, Morris SW, Maason Dy, Delsci G. 1998. ALK-positive lymphoma: a single disease with a broad spectrum of morphology. Blood 91:2076–84.

Bunn PA Jr., Huberman MS, Whang-Peng J, Schechter GP, Guccion JG, Matthews MJ, Gazdar AF, Dunnick NR, Fischmann AB, Ihde DC, Cohen MH, Fossieck B, Minna JD. 1980. Prospective staging evaluation of patients with cutaneous T-cell lymphoma. Demonstration of a high frequency of extracuaneous dissemination. An Intern Med 93:223–30.

Burke JS, Colby TV. 1981. Dermatopathic lymphadenopathy: comparison of cases associated and unassociated with mycosis fungoides. Am J Surg Pathol 5:343–52.

Burke JS, Scheibani K, Kappaport H. 1986. Dermatopathic lymphadenopathy: an immunophenotypic comparison of cases associated with and unassociated with mycosis fungoides. Am J Surg Pathol 123:256–63.

Carbone A, Gloghini A, Dotti G. 2008. EBV-associated lymphoproliferative disorders: classification and treatment. Oncoloist 13:577–85.

Cesta MF. 2006. Normal structure, function, and histology of the spleen. Toxicol Pathol 34:455–65.

Chan JK, Sin VC, Wong KF, Ng CS, Tsang WY, Chan CH, Cheung MM, Lau WH. 1997. Nonnasal lymphoma expressing the natural killer cell marker CD56: a clinico-pathologic study of 49 cases of an uncommon aggressive neoplasm. Blood 89:4501–13.

CHANG Y, BREWER NT, RINAS AC, SCHMITT K, SMITH JS. 2009. Evaluating the impact of human papillomavirus vaccines. Vaccine 27:4355–62.

CHAO TI, ALZHEIMER C. 1995. Effects of phenytoin on the persistent Na+ current of mammalian CNS neurones. Neuroreport 6:1778–80.

CHEONG C, IDOYAGA J, DO Y, PACK M, PARK SH, LEE H, KANG YS, CHOI JH, KIM JY, BONITO A, INABA K, YAMAZAKI S, STEINMAN RM, PARK CG. 2007. Production of monoclonal antibodies that recognize the extracellular domain of mouse langerin/CD207. J Immunol Methods 324:48–62.

CHESHIRE WP. 2007. Trigeminal neuralgia: for one nerve a multitude of treatments. Expert Rev Neurother 7:1565–79.

CHHABRA S, MOHAN H, BAL A. 2006. A retrospective histological evaluation of non-neoplastic superficial lymphadenopathy. Internet J Int Med 6(1).

CHOI TS, DOH KS, KIM RH, JANG MS, SUH KS, KIM ST. 2003. Clinicopathological and genotypic aspects of anticonvulsant-induced pseudolymphoma syndrome. Br J Dermatol 148:730–6.

COCCHIA D, TIBERIO G, SANTARELLI R, MICHETTI F. 1983. S-100 protein in "follicular dendritic" cells of rat lymphoid organs. Cell Tiss Res 230:95–103.

COHEN C, ALAZRAKI N, STYBLO T, WALDROP SM, GRANT SF, LARSEN T. 2002. Immunohistochemical evaluation of sentinel lymph nodes in breast carcinoma patients. Appl Immunohistochem Mol Morphol 10:296–303.

COLBY TV, BURKE JS, HOPPE RT. 1981. Lymph node biopsy in mycosis fungoides. Cancer 47:351–9

COOPER RA, DAWSON PJ. 1967. Dermatopathic lymphadenopathy: a clinicopathologic analysis of lymph node biopsy over a fifteen-year period. California Med 106:170–5.

COTTIER H, TURK J, SOBIN L. 1972. A proposal for a standardized system of reporting human lymph node morphology in relation to immunological fundtion. Bull WHO 47:375–406.

CRIVELLATO E, BALDINI G, BASA M, FUSAROLI P 1993. The three-dimensional structure of interdigitating cells. Ital J Anat Embryol 98:243–58.

DAWSON TM, STARKEBAUM G, WOOD BL, WILLKENS RF, GOWN AM. 2001. Epstein–Bar virus, methotrexate, and lymphoma in patients with rheumatoid arthritis and primary Sjoegren syndrome: case series. J Rheumatol 28:47–53.

DE LEVAL L, GAULARD P. 2008. Pathobiology and molecular profiling of peripheral T-cell lymphomas. Hematology Am Soc Hematol Educ Program. 2008:272–9.

DEPPER JM, BLUESTEIN HG, ZVAIFLER NJ. 1981. Impaired regulation f Epstein–Bar virus-induced lymphocyte proliferation in rheumatoid arthritis is due to T-cell defect. Arthritis Rheum 24:1899–1902.

DICTOR M, RAMBECH E, WAY D, et al. 1996. Human herpes virus 8 (Kaposi's sarcoma-associated herpevirus) DNA in Kaposi's sarcoma lesions, AIDS Kaposi's sarcoma cell lines, endothelial Kaposi's sarcoma simulators and the skin of immunosuppressed patients. Am J Path 148:2009–16.

DOGAN A, GAULAND P, JAFFE ES, RALFKIAER E, MUELLER-HERMEINK HK. 2008. Angioimmunoblastic T-cell lymphoma. In: Swerdlow SH, ed., WHO Classification of Tumors of Hematopoietic and Lymphoid Tissues. IARC, Lyon, 323–5.

DORFMAN DM, BROWN JA, SHAHSAFAEI A, FREEMAN GJ. 2006. Programmed death-1 (PD-1) is a marker of germinal center-associated T cells and angioimmunoblastic T-cell lymphoma. Am J Surg Pathol. 30:802–10.

FERRY JA. 2007. Reactive lymph nodes and atypical lymphoproliferative disorders. In: Hsi E, ed., Hematopatholgoy. Churchill Livingstone/Elsevier, Philadelphia, 113–56.

FIORE AE, BRIDGES CB, COX NJ. 2009. Seasonal influenza vaccines. Curr Top Microbiol Immunol 333:43–82.

FLAITZ CM, NICHOLS CM, WALLING DM, HICKS MJ. 2002. Plasmablastic lymphoma: an HIV-associated entity with primary oral manifestations. Oral Oncol 38:96–102.

FLETCHER CDM. 2007. Tumor of lymphoreticular system. In: Fletcher CDM, ed., Diagnostic Histopathology of Tumors, vol. 2, 3rd ed. Churchill Livingston/Elsevier, Philadelphia, 1165.

FRASER-ANDREWS EA, MITCHELL T, FERREIRA S, SEED PT, RUSSELL-JONES R, CALONJE E, WHITTAKER SJ. 2006. Molecular staging of lymph nodes from 60 patients with mycosis fungoides and Sézary syndrome: correlation with histopathology and outcome suggests prognostic relevance in mycosis fungoides. Br J Dermatol 155:756–62.

FRAZER IH, LEGGATT GR, MATTAROLLO SR. 2011. Prevention and treatment of papillomavirus-related cancers through immunization. Annu Rev Immunol. 2011 Apr 23;29:111–38.

FREEMAN TR, STEWART MA, TURNER L. 1993. Illness after measles-mumps-rubella vaccination. CMAJ 149:1669–74.

FRIZZERA G, MORAN EM, RAPPAPORT H. 1974. Angio-immunoblastic lymphadenopathy with dysproteinaemia. Lancet 1:1070–3.

FRIZZERA G. 1987. The clinio-pathologic expressions of Epstein–Barr virus infection in lymphoid tissues. Virchows Arch B Cell Pathol Incl Mol Pathol 53:1–12.

GAULARD P, SWERDLOW SH, HARRIS NL, JAFFE ES, SUNDSTRIOEM C. 2008. Other iatrogenic immunodeficiency-associated lymphoproliferative disorders. In: SWERDLOW SH, ed., WHO Classification of Tumours of Haematopoietic and Lymphoid Tissues. IARC, Lyon, 350–1.

GEISSMANN F, DIEU-NOSJEAN MC, DEZUTTER C, VALLADEAU J, KAYAL S, LEBORGNE M, BROUSSE N, SAELAND S, DAVOUST J. 2002. Accumulation of immature Langerhans cells in human lymph nodes draining chronically inflamed skin. J Exp Med 196:417–30.

GINSBERG HS. 1990. Poxviruses. In: DAVID BD, DULBECCO R, EISEN HN, and GINSBERG HS. eds. Microbiology, 4th ed. Lippincott, Philiadelphia, PA, pp. 947–959.

GOULD E, PORTO R, ALBORES-SAAVEDRA J, IBE MJ. 1988. Dermatopathic lymphadenitis: the spectrum and significance of its morphologic features. Arch Pathol Lab Med 112:1145–50.

GOWING NFC. 1975. Infectious mononucleosis: histopathologic aspects. Pathol An 10:1–20.

GRIDLEY G, KLIPPEL GH, HOOVER RN, FRAUMENI JF Jr. 1994. Incidence of cancer among men with the Felty syndrome. An Intern Med 120:35–9.

GUPTA D, LIM MS, MEDEIROS LJ, ELENITOBA-JOHNSON KSJ. 2000. Small lymphocytic lymphoma with perifollicular, marginal zone, or interfollicular distribution. Mod Pathol 13:1161–6.

GUTMAN GA, WEISSMAN IL. 1972. Lymphoid tissue architecture: experimental analysis of the origin and distribution of T-cells and B-cells. Immunology 23:465–79.

HARTSOCK RJ. 1968. Postvaccinial lymphadenitis: hyperplasia of lymphoid tissue that simulates malignant lymphomas. Cancer 21:632–49.

HASSERJIAN RP, CHEN S, PERKINS SL, de Leval, KINNEY MC, BARRY TS, SAID J, LIM MS, FINN WG, MEDERIOR LJ, HARRIS NL, O'MALLEY DP. 2009. Immunomodulator agent-related lymphoproliferative disorders. Mod Pathol 22:1532–40.

HATANAKA K, NAKAMURA N, KOJIMA M, ANDO K, IRIE S, BUNNO M, NAKAMINE H, UEKUSA T. 2010. Methotrexate-associated lymphoproliferative disorders mimicking angioimmunoblastic T-cell lymphoma. Pathol Res Pract 206:9–13.

HEUSERMANN U, STUTTE HJ, MUELLER-HERMELINK HK. 1974. Interdigitating cells in the white pulp of the human spleen. Cell Tiss Res 158:415–7.

HOPPE RT, MAUCH PT, ARMITAGE JO, DIEHL V, WEISS LM. 2007. Section II: biology and pathology. In: Hoppe R, et al., ed., Hodgkin lymphoma, 2nd ed. Wolters Kluwer/Lippincott Williams and Wilkins, Philadelphia, p41–54.

HOSHIDA Y, XU JX, FUJITA S, NAKAMICHI I, IKEDA J, TOMITA Y, NAKATSUKA S, TAMARU J, LIZUKA A, TAKEUCHI T, AOZASA K. 2007. Lymphoproliferative disorders in rheumatoid arthritis: clinicopathological analysis of 76 cases in relation to methotrexate medication. J Rheumatol 34: 322–31.

HSIAO SC, ICHINOHASAMA R, LIN SH, LIAO YL, CHANG ST, CHO CY, CHUANG SS. 2009. EBV-associated diffuse large B-cell lymphoma in a psoriatic treated with methotrexate. Pathol Res Pract 205:43–9.

HUNT JP, CHAN JA, SAMOSZUK M, BRYNES RK, HERNANDEZ AM, BASS R, WEISENBURGER DD, MÜLLER-HERMELINK K, NATHWANI BN. 2001. Hyperplasia of mantle/marginal zone B cells with clear cytoplasm in peripheral lymph nodes: a clinicopathologic study of 35 cases. Am J Clin Pathol 116:550–9.

HURWITT E. 1942. Dermatopathic lymphadenitis: focal granulomatous lymphadenitis associate with chronic generalized skin lesion. J Invest Dermatol 5:197–204.

HUWAIT H, WANG B, SHUSTIK C, MICHEL RP. 2010. Composite cutaneous lymphoma in a patient with rheumatoid arthritis treated with methotrexate. Am J Dermatopathol 32:65–70.

IOACHIM HL, MEDEIROS LJ. 2009a. Dermatopathic lymphadenopathy. In: Ioachim HL, ed., Lymph Node Pathology, 4th ed. Wolters Kluwer/Lippincott Williams and Wilkins, Philadelphia, 223–6.

IOACHIM HL, MEDEIROS LJ. 2009b. Vaccina lymphadenitis. In: Iochim HL, ed., Lymph Node Pathology, 4th ed. Wolters Kluwer/Lippincott Williams and Wilkins, Philadelphia, 95–6.

IOACHIM HL, MEDEIROS LJ. 2009c. Iatrogenic lymphadenopathies. In: IOACHIM HL, ed., Lymph Node Pathology, 4th ed. Wolters Kluwer/Lippincott Williams Wilkins, Philadelphia, 248–62.

ISOMAKI HA, MUTRU O, JOUTSENLAHTA U. 1978. Excess risks of lymphoma, leukemia and myeloma in patients with rheumatoid arthritis. J Chronic Dis 31:691–9.

ISAACSON PG, SPENCER J, WRIGHT DH. 1988. Classifying primary gut lymphoma. Lancet 2:1148–9.

ISOBE T, OKUYAMA T. 1978. The amino acid sequence of S100 protein (PAP-1b protein) and its relation to the calcium binding proteins. Eur J Biochem. 89:379–88.

JAFFE ES. 1988. Histiocytoses of lymph nodes: biopsy and differential diagnosis. Semin Diagn Pathol 5:376–90.

JAFFE ES. 2006. Pathobiology of peripheral T-cell lymphomas. Hematology Am Soc Hematol Educ Program 317–22.

JACOBS JF, PUNT CJ, LESTERHULIS WJ, SUTMULLER RP, BROUWER HM, SCHARENBORG NM, KLASEN IS, HIBRANDS LB, FIGDOR CG, de VRIES IJ, ADEMA GJ. 2010. Dendritic cell vaccination in combination with anti-CD25 monoclonal antibody treatment: a phase I/II study in metastatic melanoma patients. Clin Cancer Res 16:5067–78.

JEON YK, PAIK JH, PARK SS, PARK SO, KIM YA, KIM JE, SONG YW, KIM CW. 2004. Spectrum of lymph node pathology in adult onset Still's disease: analysis of 12 patients with one follow up biopsy. J Clin Pathol 57:1052–6.

JONES RL, CUMMINGHAM D, COOK G, ELL PJ. 2004. Tumour vaccine associated lymphadenopathy and false positive positron emission tomography scan changes. Br J Radiol 77:74–5.

KAISERLING E, LENNERT K. 1974. Interdigitating reticulum cell in the human lymph node: a specific cell of the thymus dependent region. Virchows Arch B Cell Pathol 16:51–61.

KAMEL OW, van de RM, WEISS LM, DEL ZOPPO GJ, HENCH PK, ROBBINS BA, MONTGOMERY PG, WARNKE RA, DORFMAN RF. 1993. Brief report: reversible lymphomas associated with Epstein–Barr virus occurring during methotrexate therapy for rheumatoid arthritis and dermatomyositis. N Engl J Med 328:1317–21.

KAMEL OW, WEISS LM, van de REJIN M, COLBY TV, KINGMA DW, JAFFE ES. 1996. Hodgkin disease and lymphoproliferations resembling Hodgkin's disease in patients receiving long term low-dose methotrexate therapy. Am J Surg Pathol 20:1279–87.

KAMEL OW. 1997. Iatrogenic lymphoproliferative disorders in nontransplantation settings. Semin Diagn Pathol 14:27–34.

KARGI A, GUREL D, TUNA B. 2007. The diagnostic value of TTF-1, CK 5/6, and p63 immunostaining in classification of lung carcinomas. Appl Immunohistochem Mol Morphol 15:415–20.

KHOPKAR U, BHOR U. 2008. Hodgkin's lymphoma in a patient of psoriasis treated with long-term, low-dose methotrexate therapy. Indian J Dermatol Venereol Leprol 74:379–82.

KIKUCHI K, MIYAZAKI Y, TANAKA A, SHIGEMATU H, KOJIMO M, SAKASHITA H, KUSAMA K. 2010. Methotrezate-related Epstein–Barr virus (EBV)-associated lymphoproliferative disorder: so-called "Hodgkin-like lesion" of the oral cavity in a patient with rheumatoid arthritis. Head Neck Pathol 4:305–11,

KINLEN LJ. 1985a. Incidence of cancer in rheumatoid arthritis: epidermiologic considerations. Am J Med 78(suppl 1A):15–21.

KNOWLES SR, SHAPIRO LE, SHEAR NH. 1999. Anticonvulsant hypersensitivity syndrome: incidence, prevention and management. Drug Safety 21:489–501.

KOJIMA M, ITOH H, HIRABAYASHI K, IGARASHI S, TAMAKI Y, MURAYAMA K, OGURA H, SAITOH R, KASHIWABARA K, TAKIMOTO J, MASAWA N, NAKAMURA S. 2006. Methtrexate-associated lymphoproliferative disorders: a clinicopathological study of 13 Japanese cases. Pathol Res Pract 202:679–85.

KOJIMA M, MOTOORI T, NAKAMURA S. 2006a. Benign, atypical and malignant lymphoproliferative disorders in rheumatoid arthritis patients. Biomed Pharmacother 60:663–72.

KOJIMA M, MOTOORI T, IIJIMA M, ONO T, YOSHIZUMI T, MATSUMOTO M, MASAWA N, NAKAMURA S. 2006b. Florid monocytoid B-cell hyperplasia resembling nodal marginal zone B-cell lymphoma of mucosa associated lymphoid tissue type. A histological and immunohistochemical study of four cases. Pathol Res Pract 202:877–82.

KOJIMA M, MOTOORI T, ASANO S, NAKAMURA S. 2007. Histological diversity of reactive and atypical proliferative lymph node lesions in systemic lupus erythematosus patients. Pathol Res Pract 203:423–31.

KOJIMA M, NAKAMURA N, TSUKAMOTO N, ITOH H, MATSUDA H, KOBAYASHI S, UEKI K, IRISAWA K, MURAYAMA K, IGARASHI T, MASAWA N, NAKAMURA S. 2010. Atypical lymphoplasmacytic and immunoblastic proliferation of autoimmune disease: clinicopathologic and immunohistochemical study of 9 cases. J Clin Exp Hematopath 50:113–9.

KOO CH, NATHWANI BN, WINBERG CD, HILL LR, RAPPAPORT H. 1984 Atypical lymphoplasmacytic and immunoblastic proliferation in lymph nodes of patients with autoimmune disease (autoimmune-disease-associated lymphadenopathy). Medicine (Baltimore). 63:274–90.

LAFZI A, FARAHANI RM, SHOJA MA. 2007. Phenobarbital-induced gingival hyperplasia. J Contemp Dent Pract 8:50–6.

LEHMANN HG, HENNESSEN W, ENGELHARDT H, FREUDENSTEIN H, WIDMARK R, WEBER-OLDECOP H, OEHME J,

SIEGLE-JOOS H, SINIOS A, SCHMIDT-DOHNA W, NEVERMANN L, BEUTNAGEL H, SCHUMANN K, SCHULZ R, KÜHL H, SCHMÖGER R. 1978. Investigations carried out to ascertain the dose-effect relationship of a BCG vaccine, strain 1331 Copenhagen, in neonates and young infants. Zentralbl Bakteriol Orig B 166:250–63. (Article in German)

LIEBOWITZ D. 1994. Nasopharyngeal carcinoma: the Epstein–Barr virus association. Semin Oncol 21:382–97.

LIM MS, STRAUS ES, DALE JK, FLEISHER TA, SNELLER MC, PUCK W, LENARDO MJ, ELENITOBA-JOHNSON KSJ, LIN AY, RAFFELD M, JAFFE S. 1998. Pathologcal findings in human autoimmune lymphoproliferative syndrome. Am J Pathol. 153:1541–50.

LIU J, DE BOUTEILLER O, PARHAM CL, DJOSSOU O, DE SAINT-VIS B, LEBECQUE S, BANCHEREAU J, MOORE KW. 1997. Follicular dendritic cells specifically express the long CR2/CD21 isoform. J Exp Med 185:165–70.

LOMBARD M, PASTORET PP, MOULIN AM. 2007. A brief history of vaccines and vaccination. Rev Off Int Epizoot 26:29–48.

LOPATEGUI JR, GAFFEY MJ, FRIERSON HF Jr, CHAN JK, MILLS SE, CHANG KL, CHEN YY, WEISS LM. 1994. Detection of Epstein–Barr viral RNA in sinonasal undifferentiated carcinoma from Western and Asian patients. Am J Surg Pathol 18:391–8.

MACON WR, WILLIAMS ME, GREER JP, COUSAR JB. 1995. Paracortical nodular T-cell lymphoma. Identification of an unusual variant of peripheral T-cell lymphoma. Am J Surg Pathol 19:297–303.

MADAN RA, GULLEY JL. 2011. Therapeutic cancer vaccine fulfills the promise of immunotherapy in prostate cancer. Immunotherapy 3:27–31.

MAEDA E, AKAHANE M, KIRYU S, KATO N, YOSHIKAWA T, HAYASHI N, AOKI S, MINAMI M, UOZAKI H, FUKAYAMA M, OHTOMO K. 2009. Spectrum of Epstein–Barr virus-related diseases: a pictorial review. Jpn J Radiol 27:4–19.

MARGARETTEN NC, HINCKS JR, WARREN RP, COULOMBE RA Jr. 1987. Effects of phenytoin and carbamazepine on human natural killer cell activity and genotoxicity in vitro. Toxicol Appl Pharmacol 87:10–17.

MARIETTE X, CAZALS-HATEM D, WARSZAWKI J, LIOTE F, BALANDRAUD N, SIBILIA J. 2002. Lymphomas in rheumatoid arthritis patients treated with methotrexate: a 3-year prospective study in France. Blood 99:3909–15.

MASAKI Y, SUGAI S. 2004. Lymphoproliferative disorders in Sjögren's syndrome. Autoimmun Rev 3:175–82.

MATTESON EL, HICKEY AR, MAGUIRE L, TILSON HH, UROWITZ MB. 1991. Occurrence of neoplasia in patients with rheumatoid arthritis enrolled in a DMARD registry. J Rheumatol 18:809–14.

MELIKIAN AL, NIKITIN EA, KAPLANSKAIA IB, FRANK GA. 2007. Paraneoplastic lymphadenopathy. Ter Arkh. 79:44–52. (Article in Russian)

MERRY C, FITZGERALD RJ. 1996. Regional lymphadenitis following BCG vaccination. Pediatr Surg Int 11:269–71.

MICELI-RICHARD C, GESTERMANN N, AMIEL C, SELLAM J, ITTAH M, PAVY S, URRUTIA A, GIRAULD I, CARCELAIN G, VENET A, MARIETTE X. 2009. Effect of methotrexate and anti-TNF on Epstein–Barr virus T-cell response and viral load in patients with rheumatoid arthritis or spondylarthropathies. Arthritis Res Ther 11:R77.

MICHEAU C. 1986. What's new in histological classification and recognition of nasopharyngeal carcinoma (NPC). Pathol Res Pract 181:249–53.

MILSTIEN JB, GIBSON JJ. 1990. Quality control of BCG vaccine by WHO: a review of factors that may influence vaccine effectiveness and safety. Bull WHO 68:93–108.

MITCHELL J., ABBOT A. 1965. Ultrastructure of the antigen-retaining reticulum of lymph node follicles as shown by high-resolution autoradiography. Nature 208:500–2.

MOSS DM, RUDIS M, HENDERSON SO. 1999. Cross-sensitivity and the anticonvulsant hypersensitivity syndrome. J Emerg Med 17:503–6.

NAGATA S, GOLSTEIN P. 1995. The Fas death factor. Science 267:1449–56.

NAGATA T, KAWAMURA N, MOTOYAMA T, MIYAKE M, YODEN A, YOSHIKAWA K, OGUNI T, YAMASIRO K, MINO M. 1992. A case of hypesensitivity syndrome resembling Langerhans cell histiocytosis during phenobarbital prophylaxis for convulsion. Jpn J Clin Oncol 22:421–7.

NATHAN DL, BELSIITO DV. 1998. Carbamazepine-induced pseudolymphoma with CD30 positive cells. J Am Acad Dermatol 38:806–9.

NATHWANI BN, BRYNES RK. 1988. Reactive immunoblastic proliferations. Semin Diagn Pathol 5:317–28.

NATHWANI BN, ANDERSON JR, ARMITAGE JO, CAVALI F, DIEBOLD J, DRACHENBERG MR, HARRIS NL, MacLENNAN KA, MULLER-HERMELINK HK, ULLRICH FA. WEISEN-BURGER DD. 1999. Margional zone-B-cell lymphoma: a clinical comparison of nodal and mucosa-associated lymphoid tissue type. Non-Hodgkin's lymphoma classification project. J Clin Oncol 17:2486–92.

NAZIR Z, QAZI SH. 2005. Bacillus Calmette-Guerin (CBG) lymphadenitis: changing trends and management. J Ayub Med Coll Abbottabad 17:16–18.

NEMOTO Y. TAIGUCHI A, KAMIOKA M, NAKAOKA Y, HIROI M, YOKOYAMA A, ENZAN H, DAIBATA M. 2010. Epstein–Barr virus-infected subcutaneous panniculitis-like T-cell lymphoma associated with methotrexate treatment. Int J Hematol 92:364–8.

NEWELL BD, MOINFAR M, MANCINI AJ, NOPPER AJ. 2009. Retrospective analysis of 32 pediatric patients with anticonvulsant hypersensitivity syndrome (ACHSS). Pediatr Dermatol. 26:536–46.

NIITSU N, OKAMOYO M, NAKAMINE H, HIRANO M. 2010. Clinicopathologic correlations of diffuse large B-cell lymphoma in rheumatoid arthritis patients treated with methotrexate. Cancer Sci 101:1309–13.

NOZAWA Y, ONO N, ABE M, SAKUMA H, WAKASA H. 1994. An immunohistochemical study of Warthin–Finkeldey cells in measles. Pathol Int 44:442–447.

OFFIT PA. 2007. Vaccinated: one man's quest to defeat the world's deadliest diseases. HarperCollins Publishers, New York, NY 10022 Smithsonian Book, p 107.

OKAMOTO Y, SHIMIZU K, TAMURA K, YAMADA M, MATSUI Y, HAYAKAWA T, MOGAMI H. 1989. Effects of anticonvulsants on cellular immunity. No To Shinkei 41:299–304. (article in Japanese)

OLSEN E, VONDERHEID E, PIMPINELLI N, WILLEMZE R, KIM Y, KNOBLER R, ZACKHEIM H, DUVIC M, ESTRACH T, LAMBERG S, WOOD G, DUMMER R, RANKI A, BURG G, HEALD P, PITTELKOW M, BERNENGO MG, STERRY W, LAROCHE L, TAUTINGER F, WHITTAKER S, ISCL/EORTC. 2007. Revisions to the staging and classification of mycosis fungoides and Sezary syndrome: a proposal of the International Society for Cutaneous Lymphoma (ISCL) and the cutaneous lymphoma task force of the European Organization of Research and Treatment of Cancer (EORTC). Blood 110:1713–22.

O'MALLEY DP, GERORGE TI, ORAZI A, ABBONDANZO S. 2009a. General reactive conditions in lymph node and spleen. Specific clinical entities. In: O'Malley DP, et al. eds., Atlas of Nontumor Pathology. First Series, Fascicle 7. Benign and Reactive Conditions of Lymph Node and Spleen. ARP Press, Washington, DC 20306-6000, 105–83.

O'MALLEY DP, GERORGE TI, ORAZI A, ABBONDANZO S. 2009b. Postvaccinal lymphadenitis. under viral lymphaenopathies. In: O'Malley DP, et al., eds., Atlas of Nontumor Pathology. First Series, Fascicle 7. Benign and reactive conditions of lymph node and spleen. ARP Press, Washington, DC 20306-6000, 320–2.

PARK S, LEE J, KO YH, HAN A, JUN HJ, LEE SC, HWANG IG, PARK YH, AHN JS, JUNG CW, KIM K, ANN YC, KANG WK, PARK K, KIM WS. 2007. The impact of Epstein–Barr virus status on clinical outcome in diffuse large B-cell lymphoma. Blood 110:972–8.

PATEL RM, GOLDBLUM JR, HSI ED. 2004. Immunohistochemical detection of human herpes virus-8 latent nuclear antigen-1 is useful in the diagnosis of Kaposi sarcoma. Mod Pathol 17:456–460.

PETERSON L, KEUCK B, ARTHUR DC, DEDEKER K, BRUNNING R. 1988. Systemic polyclonal immunoblastic proliferations. Cancer 61:1350–8.

POPPEMA S, BHAN AK, REINHERZ EL, McCLUSKY RT, SCHLOSSMAN SF. 1981. Distribution of T cell subsets in human lymph nodes. J Exp Med 153:30–41.

POPPEMA S, SWERDLOW SH, DELSOL G, WARNKE RA, PIERI SA, JAFFE ES, STEIN H. 2008 Nodular lymphocyte predominant Hodgkin lymphoma. In: SWERDLOW SH, ed., WHO Classification of Tumors of Hematopoietic and Lymphoid Tissues. IARC, Lyon, 323–5.

PUTIGNANO P, KALTSAS GA, SATTA MA, GROSSMAN AB. 1998. The effects of anti-convulsant drugs on adrenal function. Horm Metab Res 30:389–97.

RAUSCH E, KAISERLING E, GOOS M. 1977. Langerhans cells and interdigitating reticulum cells in the thymus-dependent region in human dermatopathic lymphadenitis. Virchows Arch 25:327–43.

REE H, FANGER H. 1975. Paracortical alteration in lymphadenopathic and tumor-draining lymph nodes: histologic study. Hum Pathol 6:363–72.

REE HJ, KADIN ME, KIKUCHI M, KO YH, GO JH, SUZU-MIYA J, KIM DS. 1998. Angioimmunoblastic lymphoma (AILD-type T-cell lymphoma) with hyperplastic germinal centers. Am J Surg Path 22:643–55.

REYNES M, AUBERT JP, COHEN JH, AUDOUIN J, TRICOTTET V, DIEBOLD J, KAZATCHKINE MD. 1985. Human follicular dendritic cells express CR1, CR2, and CR3 complement receptor antigens. J Immunol 135:2687–94.

RICHARD P, VASSALLO J, VALMARY S, MISSOURY R, DELSOL G, BROUSSET P. 2006. "In situ-like" mantle cell lymphoma: a report of two cases. J Clin Pathol. 59:995–996.

RIJLAARSDAM U, SCHEFFER E, MEIJER CJ, KRUYSWIJK MR, WILLEMZE R. 1991. Mycosis fungoides-like lesions associated with phenytoin nd carbamazepine therapy. J Am Acad Dermatol 24:216–20.

RIZZI R, CURCI P, DELIA M, RINALDI E, CHIEFA A, SPECCHIA G, LISO V. 2009. Spontaneous remission of "methotrexate-associated lymphoproliferative disorders" after discontinuation of immunosuppressive treatment for autoimmune disease: review of the literature. Med Oncol 26:1–9.

ROMANI N, RATZINGER G, PFALLER K, SALVENMONSER. W, STISSEL H., KOCH F, STOITZNER P. 2001. Migration of dendritic cells into lymphatics: the Langerhans cell example. Routes, regulation, and relevance. Int Rev Cytol 207:237–70.

RODRIGUEZ-JUSTO M, ATTYGALLE AD, MUNSON P, TONCADOR. G, MARAFIOTI T, PIRIS MA. 2009. Angioimmunoblastic T-cell lymphoma with hyperplastic germinal centres: a neoplasia with origin in the outer zone of the germinal centre? Clinicopathological and immunohistochemical study of 10 cases with follicular T-cell markers. Mod Pathol 22:753–61.

RODRIGUEZ-RIEIRO C, ESTEBAN-VASALLO MD, DOMINGUEZ-BERJON MF, ASTRAY-MOCHALES J, INIESTA-FORNIES D, BARRANCO-ORDONEZ D, CAMENO-HERAS M, JIMENEZ-GARCIA R. 2010. Coverage and predictors of vaccination against 2009 pandemic H1N1 influenza in Madrid, Spain. Vaccine. Rev Esp Salud Publica. 2010 Sep–Oct;84(5):609–21.

RUDIGER T, ICHINOHASAMA R, OTT MM, MULER-DEUBERT S, MIURA I, OTT G, MULLER-HERMELINK HK. 2000. Peripheral T-cell lymphoma with distinct perifollicular growth pattern: a distinct subtype of T-cell lymphoma ? Am J Surg Pathol 24:117–22.

SADEGHI E, KUMAR PV. 1990. Eczema vaccination and post BCG adenitis. Tuberculosis. 71:145–6.

SAID JW. 2007. Immunodeficiency-related Hodgkin lymphoma and its mimics. Adv Anat Pathol 14:189–94.

SALLAH S, GAGNON GA. 1998 Angioimmunoblastic lymphadenopathy with dysproteinemia: emphasis on pathogenesis and treatment. Acta Haematol 99:57–64.

SALLOUM E, COPPER DL, HOWE G, LACY J, TALLINI G, CROUCH J, SCHULTZ M. 1996. Spontaneous regression of lymphoproliferative disorders in patients treated with methotrxate for rheumatoid arthritis and other rheumatic diseases. J Clin Oncol 14:1943–9.

SALLUSTO F, LANZAVECCHIA A. 1999. Mobilizing dendritic-cells for tolerance, priming, and chronic inflammation. J Exp Med 189:611–4.

SATOH K, YOSHIDA N, IMAIZUMI K, YAJIMA M, WAKUI H, SAWADA K, KOMTSUDA. 2009. Reversible methotrexate-associated lymphoproliferative disorder resembling advanced gastric cancer in a patient with rheumatoid arthritis. Am J Med Sci 338:334–5.

SAUSVILLE EA. WORSHAM GF, MATTHEWS MJ, MAKUCH RW, FISHMANN AB, SCHECHTER GP, GAZDAR AF, BUNN PA Jr. 1985. Histologic assessment of lymph nodes in mycosis fungoides/Sezary syndrome (cutaneous T-cell lymphoma): clinical correlations and prognostic import of a new classification system. Hum Pathol 16:1098–1109.

SCHALK E, KROGEL E, SCHEINPFLUG K, MOHREN M. 2009. Lymphomatoid granulomatosis in a patient with rheumatoid arthritis receiving methotrexate: successful treatment with the anti-CD20 antibody mabthera. Onkologie 32:440–1.

SCHEFFER E, MEIJER CJLM, and VAN VLOTEN WA. 1980. Dermatopathic lymphadenopathy and lymph node involvement in mycosis fungoides. Cancer 45:137–48.

SCHEINFELD N. 2003. Phenytoin in cutaneous medicine: its uses, mechanisms and side effects. Dermatol Online J 9:6.

SEGAL GH, KJELDSBERG CR, SMITH GP, PERKINS SL. 1994. CD30 antigen expression in florid immunoblastic proliferations: a clinicopathologic study of 14 cases. Am J Clin Pathol 102:292–8.

SEGAL MM, DOUGLAS AF. 1997. Late sodium channel openings underlying epileptiform activity are preferentially diminished by the anticonvulsant phenytoin. J Neurophysiol 77:3021–34.

SHAMOTO M, OSADA A, SCHINZATO M, KANEKO C, SHIMIZU M. 1995. A comparative study on Langerhans cells in lymph nodes with dermatopathic lymphadenopathy and histiocytosis X cells. Adv Exp Med Biol 378:139–41.

SHIMOJIMA Y, ISHII W, MATSUDA M, NAKAZAWA H, IKEDA S. 2010. Cytomegalovirus-induced infectious mononucleosis-like syndrome in a rheumatoid arthritis patient treated with methotrexate and infliximab. Intern Med 49:937–40.

SLATTER MA, ANGUS B, WINDEBANK K, TAYLOR A, MEANEY C, LESTER T, NORBURY G, HAMBLETON S, ABINUN M, FLOOD TJ, CANT AJ, GENNERY AR. 2010. Polymorphous lymphoproliferative disorder with Hodgkin-like features in common gamma-chain-deficient severe combined immunodeficiency. J Allergy Clin Immunol 2011 Feb;127(2):533–35.

SMETS F, LATINNE D, BAZIN H, REDING R, OTTE JB, BUTS JP, SOKAL EM. 2002. Ratio between Epstein–Barr viral load and anti-Epstein–Barr virus specific T-cell response as a predictive marker of posttransplant lymphoproliferative disease. Transplantation 73:1603–10.

SOZZANI S, PRETE AD, OTEERMI W and FACCHETTI F. 2006. Migration of dendric cell subset. In: Badolato R, Sozzani S, eds., Lymphocye Trafficking in Health and Disease. Birkhaueyser Verlag Basel/Switzerland, 74–76

STANSFELD AG. 1985. Inflammatory and reactive disorders. In: Stansfeld AG, ed., Lymph Node Biopsy Interpretation. Churchill Livingstone, New York, 85–141.

STEFFEN C. 2004. Frédéric Woringer: Pautrier–Woringer disease (lipomelanotic reticulosis/dermatopathic lymphadenitis). Am J Dermatopathol 26:499–503.

STEIN H. 2008. Hodgkin lymphoma, In: Swerdlow SH, et al. eds., WHO Classification of Tumors of Hematopoietic and Lymphoid Tissues. IARC, Lyon, 322–34.

STRELKAUSKAS AJ, CALLERY RT, MCDOWEL J, BORE1 Y, SCHLOSSMAN SF. 1978. Direct evidence for loss of human suppressor cells during activeautoimmune diseases. Proc Nat Acad Sci USA 75:5150–4.

SCHWARTZ EJ, DORFMAN RF, KOHLER S. 2003. Human herpesvirus-8 latent nuclear antigen-1 expression in endemic Kaposi sarcoma: an immunohistochemical study of 16 cases. Am J Surg Pathol 27:1546–50.

SWERDLOW SH, ZUKERBERG LR, YANG W-I, HARRIS NL, WILLIAMS ME. 1996. The morphologic spectrum of non-Hodgkin lymphomas with BCL-1/cyclin D1 gene rearrangements. Am J Surg Pathol 20:627–40.

SYBERT A, BUTLER TP. 1978. Sarcoidosis following adjuvant high-dose methotrexate therapy for osterosarcoma. Arch Intern Med 138:488–9

TAKAHASHI K, YAMAGUCHI H, ISHIZEKI J, NAKAJIMA T, NAKAZATO Y. 1981. Immunohistochemical and immunoelectron microscopic localization of S-100 protein in the interdigitating reticulum cells of the human lymph node. Virchows Arch 37:125–35.

TAKEUCHI A, DEJIMA T, YAMADA H, SHIBATA K, NAKAMURA R, ETO M, NAKATANI T, NAITO S, YOSHIKAI Y. 2011. IL-17 production by γδ T cells is important for the antitumor effect of Mycobacterium bovis bacillus Calmette–Guérin treatment against bladder cancer. Eur J Immunol 41:246–51.

TOSATO G, STEINBERG AD, YARCHOAN R, HEILMAN CA, PIKE SE, DE SEAU V, BLAESE RM. 1984. Abnormally elevated frequency of Epstein–Barr virus-infected B-cells in the blood of patients with rheumatoid arthritis. J Clin Invest 73:1789–95.

TRAN H, CHEUNG C, GILL D, DUA U, NOURSE J, BOYLE R, GANDHI MK. 2008. Methotrexate-associated mantle-cell lymphoma in an elderly man with myasthenia gravis. Nat Clin Pract Oncol 5:234–8.

TSUNG SH and LIN JI. 1981. Angioimmunoblstic lymphadenopathy in a patient taking diphenylhydantoin. Ann Clin Lab Sci 11:542–5.

TUETTENBERG A, SCHMITT E, KNOP J, JONULEIT H. 2007. Dendritic cell-based immunotherapy of malignant melanoma: success and limitations. J Dtsch Dermatol Ges 5:190–6.

van den OORD JJ, de WOLF-PEETERS C, DESMET VJ, TAKAHASHI K, OHTSUKI Y, AKAGI T. 1985a. Nodular alteration of the paracortical area: an in situ immunohistochemical analysis of primary, secondary, and tertiary T-nodules. Am J Pathol 120:55–66.

van den OORD JJ, de WOLF-PEETERS C, DESMET VJ. 1986b. The composite nodule. A stuctural and functional unit of the reactive human lymph node. Am J Pathol 122:83–91.

van der VALK P, MEIJER CJ. 1987. The histology of reactive lymph nodes. Am J Surg Surg Pathol 11:866–82.

VAUGHAN JH. 1985. Immune system in rheumatoid arthritis: possible implications in neoplasms. Am J Med 78(suppl 1A):6–11.

VERDICH J, CHRISTENSEN AL. 1979. Pulmonary disease complicating intermittent methotrexate therapy of psoriasis. Acta Derm Venereol 59:471–3.

VEGA F, CHANG CC, MEDEIROS LJ, UDDEN MM, CHO-VEGA JH, LAU CC, FINCH CJ, VILCHEZ RA, MCGREGOR D, JORGENSEN JL. 2005. Plasmablastic lymphomas and plasmablastic plasma cell myelomas have nearly identical immunophenotypic profiles. Mod Pathol 18:806–15.

VERDICH J, CHRISTENSEN AL. 1979. Pulmonary disease complicating intermitter methotrexate therapy of psoridasis. Acta Derm Venereol 59:471–3.

WARMKE RA, JONES RD, HIS ED. 2007. Morphologic and immunophenotypic variants of nodal T-cell lymphoma. Am J Clin 127: 511–27.

WEEDON AP. Diphenylhydantoin sensitivity. 1975. A syndrome resembling infectious mononucleosis with a morbilliform rash and cholestatic hepatitis. Aust N Z J Med 5:561–3.

WEISS LM, WOOD GS, WARNKE RA. 1985a. Immunophenotypic differences between dermatopathic lymphadenopathy and lymph node involvement in mycosis fungoides. Am J Pathol 120:179–85.

WEISS LM, HU E, WOOD GS, MOULDS C, CLEARY ML, WARNKE R, SKLAR J. 1985b. Clonal rearrangements of T-cell receptor genes in mycosis fungoides and dermatopathic lymphadenopathy. N Engl J Med 313:539–44.

WEISS, L. 2008a. Dermatopathic lymphadenitis under Benign lymphadenopathy. In: WEISS L, ed., Lymph Node. Illustrated Surgical Pathology Series. Cambridge University Press, Cambridge, 45–51.

WEISS, L. 2008b. Langerhan's cell histiocytosis under Histiocytic and dendritic neoplasm. In: WEISS L, ed., Lymph Node. Illustrated Surgical Pathology Series. Cambridge University Press, Cambridge, 234–40.

WESTHOFF TH. LODDENKEMPER C, HOERL MP, SCHMIDT S. ANAGNOSTOPOULOS I, HUMMEL M, ZIDEK W, van der GIET M. 2006. Dermatopathic lymphadenopathy: a differential diagnosis of enlarged lymph nodes in uremic pruritus. Clin Nephrol 66:472–5.

WHITBY E. HOWARD MR, TENANT-FLOWERS M, et al. 1995. Detection of Kaposi sarcoma-associated herpesvirus in peripheral blood of HIV-infected individuals and progression to Kaposi's sarcoma. Lancet 346:799–802.

WILLARD-MACK CL. 2006. Normal structure, function, and histology of lymph nodes. Toxicologic Pathol 34:409–24.

WOLFE F, MICHAUD K. 2007. The effect of methotrexate and anti-tumor necrosis factor therapy on the risk of lymphoma in rheumatoid arthritis in 19,652 patients during 89,710 person-years of observation. Arthritis Rheumat 56:1433–39.

WOLF R, KHANE E, SANDBANK M. 1985. Mycosis-fungoides-like lesions associated with phenytoin therapy. Arch Dermatol 121:1181–2.

YONEYAMA H, MATSUNO K, ZHANG Y. 2004. Evidence for recruitment of plasmacytoid dendritic cell precursors to inflamed lymph nodes through high endothelial venules. Int Immunol 16:915–28.

ZISMAN DA, MCCUNE WJ, JINO G, LYNCH JP. 2001. 3rd. Drug-Induced pneumonitis: the role of methotrexate. Sarcoidosis Vasc Diffuse Lung Dis. 18:243–52.

CHAPTER FIFTEEN

REACTIVE LYMPHADENOPATHY WITH DIFFUSE PARACORTICAL PATTERN—INFECTIOUS ETIOLOGY

Jeremy W. Bowers and Ling Zhang

INTRODUCTION

Diffuse hyperplasia composed of reactive immunoblastic proliferation in lymph nodes is a nonspecific histopathologic finding that may be associated with benign or malignant processes. This pattern is a subset of paracortical hyperplasia and has to be distinguished from the relatively more common reactive paracortical hyperplasias, which are usually nodular and not diffuse. This diffuse pattern is most easily confused with non-Hodgkin lymphomas. In contrast, the nonspecific paracortical hyperplasia with "mottling" due to increased interdigitating reticulum cells and not immunoblastic proliferation is also called primary or secondary T zone reactive nodules and easily recognized as a benign process. In its most florid form, with formation of pale nodules with pigmented histiocytes, paracortical hyperplasia is called tertiary T zone paracortical reaction, also known as dermatopathic lymphadenopathy.

Histologically, diffuse hyperplasia in lymph nodes exhibits overall preservation of architecture with paracortical distortion rather than effacement. Low-power microscopic findings are typically described as "mottled" or "moth-eaten" due to immunoblastic hyperplasia. Residual or reactive germinal centers may be present (Figure 15.1). The distinguishing feature is diffuse paracortical hyperplasia with a heterogeneous population of cells, including, but not limited to, polymorphic immunoblasts, small lymphocytes, plasma cells, and histiocytes (Figure 15.2). The interfollicular infiltrate of reactive immunoblasts is CD30 positive (Figure 15.3). The differential diagnosis includes the viral lymphadenitides, drug-associated lymphadenitis, postvaccine lymphadenitis, and lymphomas, specifically diffuse large B-cell lymphoma, Hodgkin lymphoma, and CD30-positive anaplastic large-cell lymphoma (Table 15.1) (Abbondanzo, 2004). This chapter focuses on the main herpesvirus lymphadenitides with general information on the viruses themselves, lymph node histopathology, clinical features of disease, and differential diagnoses.

INFECTIOUS MONONUCLEOSIS LYMPHADENITIS

Definition

A clinical syndrome and lymphadentitis caused by Epstein–Barr virus (EBV).

Non-Neoplastic Hematopathology and Infections, First Edition. Edited by Hernani D. Cualing, Parul Bhargava, and Ramon L. Sandin.
© 2012 Wiley-Blackwell. Published 2012 by John Wiley & Sons, Inc.

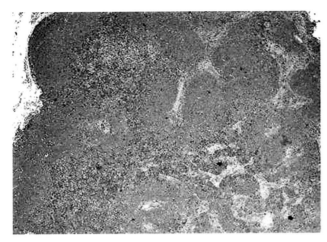

FIGURE 15.1 **Lymph node with pan-hyperplasia, especially paracortical hyperplasia comprised of reactive immunoblasts, and reactive germinal centers.** (Used with permission of Hernani Cualing, MD)

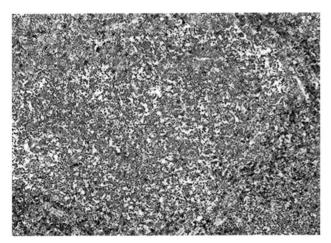

FIGURE 15.2 **"Mottled appearance" with numerous paracortical immunoblasts.** (Used with permission of Hernani Cualing, MD)

ICD-10 Codes

B27. Infectious mononucleosis
B27.0 gammaherpesviral mononucleosis [WHO, 2007].

Synonyms

Infectious mononucleosis, EBV lymphadenitis, "mono."

Epidemiology

EBV [human herpesvirus 4 (HHV-4)] is a cancer-causing virus and the etiologic agent of acute

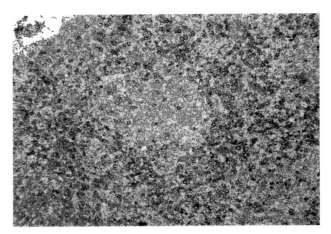

FIGURE 15.3 **CD30 rich interfollicular infiltrate of reactive immunoblastic proliferation.** (Used with permission of Hernani Cualing, MD)

TABLE 15.1 Differential Diagnosis of Diffuse Paracortical Hyperplasia, Nonspecific

Viral lympadenitides

- Acute infectious mononucleosis
- Cytomegalovirus lymphadenitis
- Herpes simplex lymphadenitis
- Varicella zoster lymphadenitis

Drug-related lymphadenitis
Postvaccine lymphadenitis
Lymphomas

infectious mononucleosis (IM). The clinical syndrome of IM was first described in 1920 (Sprunt and Evans, 1920). EBV was detected by electron microscopy in lymphoblasts from Burkitt lymphoma in 1964 (Epstein et al., 1964). Three years later, in an attempt to grow the virus in irradiated Burkitt lymphoma cells cultured with normal human lymphocytes, it was discovered that the virus stimulated proliferation of the B lymphocytes for an indefinite period (Henle et al., 1967). This immortalization phenomenon is a probable mechanism for the viral associated lymphoproliferative disorders and carcinomas. The etiologic association with IM was made in 1968 (Henle et al., 1968). Transmission of EBV via saliva was apparent shortly after its discovery with the presence of active virus shedding in the saliva of 50% of patients symptomatic for infectious mononucleosis and in up to 25% of asymptomatic carriers (Gerber et al., 1972). It was also discovered that EBV was etiologically associated with Burkitt lymphoma, nasopharyngeal carcinoma, Hodgkin lymphoma, and other lymphoproliferative diseases in the congenital and acquired immunosuppressed state (Henle et al., 1968; Cohen, 2000).

Early studies in the United States showed patients from 10 to 19 years old with the highest incidence of IM, while infections in patients younger than 10 or older than 30 was less than 1 in 1000 persons per year (Ebell, 2004; Fry, 1980; Henke et al., 1973). IM does occur in 2% of adults presenting with sore throat; however, when compared to younger patients, symptoms may be atypical with absence of pharyngitis and lymphadenopathy with negative heterophile antibodies (Aronson et al., 1982; Axelrod and Finestone, 1990; Horowitz et al., 1976). It is likely that IM may be underdiagnosed in the very young or older populations due to atypical presentations. Most persons in developing countries are infected at younger ages, with over 90% of 5- to 9-year-old children being infected. In contrast, approximately 50% of patients in the same age group are infected in Western countries. As predicted, infection rates are highest in populations where younger persons from different geographic backgrounds congregate, such as universities and the military, where incidence is as high as 48 cases per 1000 persons (Crawford et al., 2006; Hallee et al., 1974). The overall incidence currently in the United States is approximately 500 cases per 100,000 persons per year with highest incidences in the 15- to 24-year-old age group. Approximately 10 to 20% of susceptible persons become infected each year with IM developing in 30 to 50% of that subset. EBV infection has no racial predilection and no seasonal variation with males and females affected equally (Luzuriaga and Sullivan, 2010).

Clinical Aspects

Etiology

Epstein–Barr virus is a human herpes virus (HHV), specifically HHV-4. It is subclassified as a γ-1 herpesvirus, the lymphocryptoviruses. The double-stranded DNA genome with 172 kbp, encoding approximately 100 proteins, is contained within a nucleocapsid that is surrounded by a tegument and encased in a viral envelope derived from the host cell membrane (Cohen, 2000; Sanghavi et al., 2009). The γ-herpesviruses genome has conserved gene blocks separated by coincident divergent loci. Homologous genes within these divergent loci have a high degree of sequence divergence, suggesting that these viruses can acquire new functions resulting in speciation and occupation of unique biological roles. These genes have not been found in other viruses and may be responsible for the pathogenicity of neoplasms associated with the family (Nicholas, 2000).

Two strains of EBV have been identified, EBV-1 and EBV-2. The majority of isolates in IM infections in Western countries is EBV-1, while EBV-2 is more rare and classically attributed to central Africa and Southeast Asia (Abdel-Hamid et al., 1992; Arrand et al., 1989; Rowe et al., 1989; Sixbey et al., 1989; Young et al., 1987; Zimber et al., 1986). A small portion of persons, up to 10%, is doubly infected, shedding DNA from both strains. Likewise strains have been identified with both EBV-1 and EBV-2 polymorphisms, suggesting intertypic recombination (Sixbey et al., 1989). It is debatable whether viral strains contribute specifically to known associated malignancies or environmental factors, along with the locally prevalent strain, are providing impetus for malignant transformation. One study indicates that Burkitt lymphoma can be attributed to either EBV-1 or EBV-2 and that the incidence of lymphoma is dependent on prevalence of infection in the general population, with no increase in lymphomagenic risk attributed to either strain (Young et al., 1987). Another study suggests that strain difference may play a role in nasopharyngeal carcinoma, and that unusual rare strains with features of both EBV-1 and EBV-2 may play a role in pathogenesis in certain populations (Abdel-Hamid et al., 1992).

Sites of Involvement

A variety of organs, including lymph nodes, spleen, tonsils, bone marrow, appendix, liver, and central nervous system, show histopathologic changes associated with EBV infection (Gowing, 1975). Other cells that have more rarely been reported to be infected by EBV are T cells, natural killer cells, smooth muscle cells, and monocytes (Guerreiro-Cacais et al., 2004; Kawa, 2000; Savard et al., 2000). EBV gene expression has been described in diffuse large B-cell lymphoma, Burkitt lymphoma, Hodgkin lymphoma, plasmablastic lymphoma, T-cell lymphoma, HIV- or post-transplant lymphoproliferative disease, nasopharyngeal carcinoma, a subset of gastric carcinomas, and leiomyosarcoma (Ambinder and Mann, 1994; Carbone et al., 2008; McClain et al., 1995; Sunde et al., 2010).

EBV can infect both epithelial cells and B lymphocytes, as apparent by its association with upper respiratory disease, carcinoma, and lymphomas. The infected B cells become proliferating lymphoblasts eventually becoming memory B cells (Thorley-Lawson, 2001). Models of EBV persistence have been proposed and involve interactions between B cells and epithelial cells. Initially memory B cells sporadically release viruses that infect adjacent epithelial cells. The infection spreads exponentially until random termination by an immune response (natural killer and cytotoxic T cells), leaving behind infected plaques of epithelial cells that in turn shed viruses. The nature of the infection is cyclical but because of the nearly constant presence of epithelial plaques, the shedding of EBV in the saliva is continuous. In young persons, EBV is rapidly cleared from the blood but not the oropharynx (Balfour et al., 2005; Hadinoto et al., 2009).

Pathogenesis

The incubation after exposure to symptoms is approximately 30 to 50 days (Luzuriaga and Sullivan, 2010). Viral attachment to and penetration of B cells and epithelial cells has been studied extensively (Fingeroth et al., 1984; Hutt-Fletcher, 2007; Sanghavi et al., 2009). Viral transfer from B cells to epithelial cells also occurs and is a complex process (Hutt-Fletcher, 2007; Molesworth et al., 2000). Within hours of entry, the DNA is transferred to the nucleus where immortalization takes place, followed by DNA replication, transcription, translation, and eventual virion production (Sanghavi et al., 2009).

The host immune response involves cytotoxic (CD8+) T cells against infected B lymphocytes, resulting in enlarged atypical lymphocytes (Downey cells) (Hoagland, 1975). A brisk cellular response, involving both CD4+ and CD8+ T cells, is critical, controlling the primary EBV infection with subsequent suppression. The cellular immune response is also responsible for the signs and symptoms of IM as antigens are released by the destruction of infected cells (Hadinoto et al., 2009; Luzuriaga and Sullivan, 2010). Ineffective T-cell response may lead to B-cell proliferation and/or lymphoma (Cohen, 2000).

Virus latency is complex, involving numerous host and viral protein interactions, including Epstein–Barr virus-encoded RNA (EBER), an important target of in situ hybridization (ISH) probes (Strickler et al., 1993). Variable expressions of the genes will produce a specific pattern of latency that may be associated with certain EBV-induced malignancies (Niedobitek et al., 1997; Young et al., 2000). Latency could be life-long with circulating B cells serving as reservoirs (Hochberg et al., 2004; Souza et al., 2005).

Approach to Diagnosis

Clinical Workup and Laboratory Findings

Most patients (up to 98%) with IM will experience the classic symptoms/signs of fatigue, malaise, pharyngitis, lymphadenopathy, fever, and tonsillar enlargement (Hoagland, 1975). However, in adults, infection rarely occurs over age of 40, and in those patients there may be absent or atypical symptoms (Axelrod and Finestone, 1990). In most, the symptoms will resolve in 3 to 4 weeks. Rash, hepatomegaly, palatal petechiae, splenomegaly, splenic rupture, anemia, thrombocytopenia, myocarditis, hepatitis, genital ulcers, and neurological complications have also been rarely documented in IM (Cohen, 2000; Ebell, 2004).

Hoagland's criteria for diagnosis include the classic symptoms/signs described above with lymphocytosis comprising 50% of WBC count, at least 10% transformed lymphocytes (immunoblasts), and positive serological tests (Hoagland, 1975). The transformed lymphocytes (Downey cells) are predominantly T cells with abundant pale blue cytoplasm, large nuclei and prominent nucleoli (Sheldon et al., 1973). Only about 50% of all patients with IM meet all of the criteria (Ebell, 2004).

Paul and Bunnell made the first laboratory test for the diagnosis of IM in 1932 with the test bearing the discoverers' names. They observed that sera from patients with IM agglutinated red blood cells, with autoreactive heterophile antibodies (Ebell, 2004; Sanghavi, et al., 2009). Relatively specific sensitivity is problematic. The false-negative rate is 25% in the first week, 5 to 10% in the second, and 5% in the third (Hoagland, 1975). Improvements of the heterophile antibody test were made whereby horse erythrocytes were used instead of sheep, which became the basis for the modern Monospot test. The agglutinin titers are up to three times higher, conferring a greater sensitivity (Ebell, 2004; Lee et al., 1968). EBV-specific antibodies including VCA-IgM, which declines to undetectable levels in 8 to 10 weeks, and VCA-IgG, which appears early and persists for life, may be measured but are more properly utilized when disease is suspected and heterophile antibody tests are negative (Bruu et al., 2000; Ebell, 2004).

Lymph Node Histopathology

It is generally accepted that clinical evidence of IM does not warrant a lymph node biopsy, as it may be difficult to distinguish EBV lymphadenitis from lymphoma on histopathologic evaluation alone; however, peripheral blood changes and heterophile antibody testing are limited such that a lymph node biopsy may be performed (Fleisher et al., 1983; Henle et al., 1974). General lymphadenopathy is common including, but not limited to, cervical, axillary, epitrochlear, inguinal, mediastinal, and mesenteric nodes (Sanghavi et al., 2009).

Grossly, lymph nodes are soft in consistency with a uniform cut surface but may have foci of necrosis.

Enlargement is usually minimal with normal capsule thickness; however, the capsule may contain marked infiltrations of lymphocytes, plasma cells, and immunoblasts. Nodes are discreet without matting. Even enlarged nodes retain their reniform shape (Gowing, 1975).

The histology of lymph nodes has been described by numerous authors with similar findings (Childs et al., 1987; Dorfman and Warnke, 1974; Gowing, 1975; Strickler et al., 1993). The overall histology has a mottled appearance similar to other types of viral infections with distortion rather than effacement of architecture and occasional geographic necrosis (Figures 15.4–15.5). The primary microscopic feature is diffuse paracortical hyperplasia consisting of variably sized lymphocytes, polymorphic immunoblasts, histiocytes, and plasma cells (Figure 15.6). Other features include Reed–Sternberg-like cells, frequent mitoses, abundance of postcapillary venules, endothelial cell swelling, and focal necrosis (Figure 15.5). The transformed large lymphocytes have small peripherally located nucleoli and pale amphophilic cytoplasm. Occasionally these cells display large vesicular nuclei, prominent and central nucleoli, and abundant amphophilic or basophilic cytoplasm. The lymphoid follicles may be large in early infections, showing follicular hyperplasia with numerous mitoses and a starry sky pattern due to marked phagocytosis of debris by macrophages. The rim of the follicle will become blurred as interfollicular cells proliferate and lymphocytes transform into immunoblasts. As the infection progresses, nodules

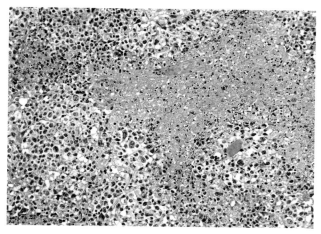

FIGURE 15.5 **Focal geographic necrosis**. (Used with permission of Hernani Cualing, MD)

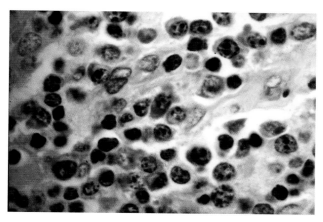

FIGURE 15.6 **Increased immunoblasts and plasma cells**. (Used with permission of Hernani Cualing, MD)

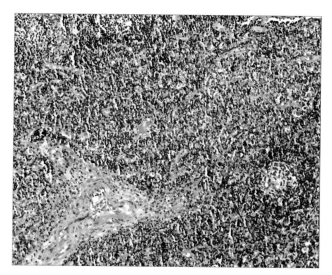

FIGURE 15.4 **Mottled-appearing histology with obscured germinal centers**. (Used with permission of Hernani Cualing, MD)

will lose their identity and will be easily missed on routinely stained sections. The preserved sinuses are frequently infiltrated with immunoblasts and proteinaceous fluid. The polymorphous nature of the hyperplasia is typically apparent but may be difficult to perceive in cases where immunoblasts are numerous and in large sheets.

Immunohistochemistry/In situ *Hybridization*

The immunoblasts in EBV lymphadenitis are positive for CD30 (a cell membrane protein of the tumor necrosis factor receptor family with both membranous and perinuclear staining) and CD 45 (common leukocyte antigen with membranous and cytoplasmic staining), and negative for CD15 (a carbohydrate adhesion molecule) (Niedobitek et al., 1997; Reynolds et al., 1995), a phenotype

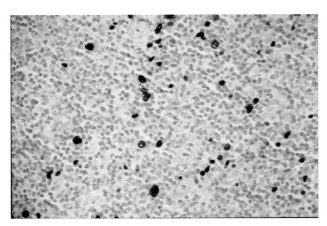

FIGURE 15.7 **Scattered EBER + immunoblasts (ISH).** (Used with permission of Hernani Cualing, MD)

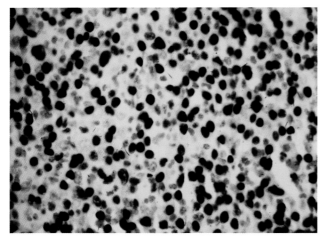

FIGURE 15.8 **Diffuse EBER + immunoblasts (ISH).** (Used with permission of Hernani Cualing, MD)

distinguishing EBV lymphadenitis from classical Hodgkin lymphoma. Immunohistochemistry (IHC) and in situ hybridization (ISH) are used to detect the EBV infection in formalin-fixed, paraffin-embedded tissue. IHC targets antibodies to latent membrane protein 1(LMP1) (Isaacson et al., 1992; Niedobitek et al., 1997). ISH uses EBV-encoded RNA (EBER) probes, and because of the sheer abundance of target, the technique is very sensitive and has been detected in malignant cells of EBV-associated tumors, with variation in staining depending on the tumor type (Ambinder and Mann, 1994). ISH signal may be variable from scattered to diffuse (Figures 15.7, 15.8). The use of IHC and ISH is extremely important in entities that can simulate EBV lymphadenitis (Strickler et al., 1993).

Differential Diagnosis

Diffuse paracortical hyperplasia is nonspecific; therefore the differential diagnosis in the absence of other clinical information is broad (Strickler et al., 1993). Other viruses, particularly other herpesviruses, commonly cause lymphadenitis virtually identical to IM; therefore clinical, serological, and ISH may be helpful (Abbondanzo, 2004). CMV infection could show some pathologic features similar to EBV lymphadenitis but lack autoreactive heterophile antibodies (herophile-negative mononucleosis syndrome). The specifics of CMV and other viral entities are discussed later in this chapter.

Drug-induced lymphadenopathy, most commonly caused by the anticonvulsant drug phenytoin, may show similar histopathologic changes to EBV lymphadenitis, including paracortical immunoblastic hyperplasia with disruption or atrophy of the germinal centers (Abbondanzo et al., 1995; Abbondanzo, 2004). Clinical history is paramount in cases involving drug-induced lymphadenopathy. Short exposure time will be characterized by classic hypersensitivity reactions including fever, rash, eosinophilia, and hepatosplenomegaly. Longer exposure times may not show hypersensitivity syndrome; therefore a drug history is important, as the disease will subside after cessation of the drug.

The difficulty in distinguishing EBV lymphadenitis from lymphomas in the absence of ancillary studies is well documented (Abbondanzo, 2004; Childs et al., 1987; Dorfman and Warnke, 1974; Gowing, 1975; Salvador et al., 1971; Strum et al., 1970; Tindle et al., 1972). Histologic changes outlined above in EBV lymphadenitis, especially paracortical hyperplasia, may be present in several lymphomas. It is critical to incorporate the traditional clinical and laboratory findings of IM when considering a diagnosis of lymphoma in a lymph node biopsy. In general, if lymph node architecture is preserved with only focal disruption and presence of a mottled appearance, a reactive process is favored over a malignant process. Cytologically, a polymorphic population of different type of cells composed of small lymphocytes, plasma cells, and immunoblasts favor a reactive process. Diffuse large B-cell lymphoma, with few exceptions, tends to be composed of a monomorphic population with nuclear contour irregularities and atypia. However, if there is architectural effacement with sheets of large transformed B cells, additional studies (i.e., flow cytometry, IHC, and molecular studies) should be performed to determine if a diffuse large B-cell lymphoma is present. Likewise prominent immunoblastic hyperplasia with sheets of large cells may be confused with CD30-expressing anaplastic large-cell lymphoma, especially since CD30 is also positive in EBV lymphadenitis. However, systemic anaplastic large-cell lymphoma is positive in a majority of cases for anaplastic large-cell lymphoma kinase (ALK), 84% in one study (Benharroch et al., 1998). In addition anaplastic large-cell lymphoma is epithelial membrane antigen (EMA) positive in addition to having T-cell receptor gene rearrangements and chromosomal translocations, the most common being t(2;5)(p23;q35). The presence of CD30+ large atypical Reed–Sternberg-like cells in EBV lymphadentitis may be mistaken for Hodgkin lymphoma. However, classical Hodgkin lymphoma will show effacement of nodal architecture with abnormal nodular proliferation or a mixed inflammatory infiltrate associated with CD30+/CD15+/CD45 negative Reed–Sternberg (RS) cells (EBV Reed–Sternberg-like cells will be CD15– and CD45+). Classical Hodgkin lymphoma, nodular sclerosis subtype, will show capsular thickening and collagen bands that create nodules enclosing lacunar RS cells, features that are not present in acute EBV lymphadenitis. Caution should be exercised in diagnosing EBV lymphadenitis based on immunohistochemical staining for EBV because the virus has been detected in Hodgkin lymphoma and even has been implicated in contributing to its development (Flavell and Murray, 2000; Reynolds et al., 1995).

Treatment of Choice and Prognosis

Supportive care is recommended for patients with IM. Appropriate medications, such as acetaminophen or ibuprofen, are recommended for symptoms of fever and pain. Corticosteroids can also be considered in patients with significant pharyngeal edema that threatens airway obstruction; however, steroids have not been shown to be efficacious in symptom relief (Ebell, 2004; Luzuriaga and Sullivan, 2010). A possible complication is splenic rupture, which typically occurs within three weeks of diagnosis but has been reported as late as seven weeks. Avoidance of sports is recommended for at least three weeks with uncertainty as the appropriate time to resume contact sports (Putukian et al., 2008).

Antiviral treatments show mixed results. Acyclovir reduces viral shedding in the saliva but only during treatment without decreasing duration or severity of symptoms (Jenson, 2004). A valacyclovir study in a small group of young adults demonstrated a decrease in salivary viral shedding and reduction in severity of symptoms but without decreasing viral load (Balfour et al., 2007). Valacyclovir, however, reduced frequencies of EBV-infected memory B cells in peripheral circulation in patients treated for one year (Hoshino et al., 2009). This study demonstrates that the EBV reservoir relies on continuous lytic replication and infection of new B cells. Theoretically the infection could be cleared with sustained treatment of valacyclovir; however, this process would take many years.

An EBV vaccine is currently under study. Early results show recipients are not protected against infection but are less likely to develop symptoms during primary infection (Sokal et al., 2007).

The symptoms of IM can cause substantial functional impairment; however, most cases resolve spontaneously. Signs and symptoms such as fever and splenomegaly, as well as many laboratory tests, return to normal within one month. Fatigue, cervical lymphadenopathy, pharyngitis, and general health status improve more slowly, and may be quite protracted in some cases (Rea et al., 2001). Prolonged fatigue or chronic fatigue syndrome has been reported with a separate and smaller risk of post-IM depression (Katz et al., 2009; Petersen et al., 2006). Although most cases resolve, there is a very small subset of patients with immunodeficiency disorders, such as X-linked lymphoproliferative syndrome, which may develop fatal IM (Wick et al., 2002).

CYTOMEGALOVIRUS LYMPHADENITIS

Definition

Lymphadenitis caused by cytomegalovirus (CMV).

ICD-10 Codes

B25   Cytomegaloviral disease.
B35.2 Congential cytomegalovirus infection.
B27.1 Cytomegaloviral mononucleosis [WHO, 2007].

Synonyms

CMV lymphadenitis, CMV mononucleosis.

Epidemiology

Cytomegalovirus (CMV), also known as human herpesvirus 5 (HHV-5) is a β-herpesvirus that only naturally occurs in humans. Infected lymph nodes contain large atypical lymphoid cells with visible or prominent intranuclear inclusions. These histologic findings, thought initially to be protozoal in origin, were first identified in the early twentieth century (Sanghavi et al., 2009). A viral etiology was confirmed in 1926 (Kuttner and Cole, 1926). CMV was first isolated from human tissue culture in 1956 (Rowe et al., 1956; Smith, 1956). At first thought to be a purely congenital infection, the virus is now recognized as an opportunistic infection in immunodeficient persons and organ-transplant patients (Brown and Abernathy, 1998; Colugnati et al., 2007). The pathogen is prevalent with at least 40% of the population showing exposure by serology. Numerous sites may be primarily infected (Taylor, 2003). CMV is not highly contagious and is contracted from close person-to-person contact. It is shed directly from the throat and uterine cervix and is found in various body fluids including saliva, urine, breast milk, semen, and blood (Taylor, 2003).

CMV has a worldwide distribution and is prevalent in all populations depending on location. Areas with low socioeconomic conditions, such as India, have serologic prevalence greater than 90% with no statistical differences between age groups (Kothari et al., 2002). In the United States the prevalence of CMV is approximately 60% in persons six years and older. The seroprevalence increases with age with 36% in 6- to 11-year-olds to over 90% in persons 80 and older. There are significant racial differences with seroprevalence of 51% in non-Hispanic white persons, 76% in non-Hispanic black persons, and 82% in Mexican-Americans (Staras et al., 2006). Ethnic differences between women of childbearing age are most dramatic. When comparing 10- to 14-year-olds with 20- to 24-year-olds, seroprevalence increased 38% for non-Hispanic black persons, 7% for non-Hispanic white persons, and <1% for Mexican-Americans. These differences are still present when controlling for social and geographic factors from data generated from 1988 to 1994 (Staras et al., 2006).

A 2007 study determined that approximately 27,000 new CMV infections occur each year in the United States among seronegative pregnant women (Colugnati et al., 2007). CMV can be transferred transplacentally or passed to the infant as it passes through the birth canal, as well as being transmitted in breast milk and on fomites (Brown and Abernathy, 1998). The overall prevalence of congenital CMV is under 1%, but this varies depending on racial and socioeconomic factors. Only about 11% of infants with congenital CMV infections are symptomatic. Rates of transmission to newborns is 32% in mothers with primary infections and under 2% in mothers with recurrent infections. Mothers with CMV IgM, likely representing both primary and recurrent infections, transmit congenital CMV approximately 20% of the time (Kenneso and Cannon, 2007). Because of the potential disabilities (e.g., hearing loss, mental

retardation, and cerebral palsy) of congenital CMV infections, and given its ubiquitous nature worldwide, effective treatments and preventive care such as a vaccine are crucial.

CMV continues to cause significant morbidity and mortality in immunocompromised persons, especially AIDS and post-transplant patients. A study of patients with AIDS showed that approximately 50% had evidence of CMV at autopsy with 20% of those dying from organ failure related to CMV. Interestingly, therapy for CMV prolonged course of the disease but ultimately did not prevent death from CMV (Klatt and Shibata, 1988).

Transplant patients also experience significant morbidity and mortality associated with CMV infection. In transplant patients, both solid-organ and hematopoietic stem cell recipients, CVM may cause a febrile syndrome associated with myelosuppression, hepatitis, pneumonitis, gastroenteritis, and encephalitis with increased propensity for development of life-threatening opportunistic infections (Razonable, 2005). New strategies such as frequent use of newer antiviral drugs have decreased incidence of CMV in transplant patients (Razonable and Emery, 2004). However, late-onset infection in the year following transplantation is a growing problem. Additionally the emergence of subsequent antiviral drug resistant strains has been associated with higher morbidity and mortality (Razonable, 2005).

Clinical Aspects

Etiology

CMV is a β-herpesvirus, specifically human herpesvirus 5 (HHV-5). It has an icosahedral nucleocapsid approximately 150 to 200 nm in diameter. The nucleocapsid is surrounded by an amorphous tegument and lipid envelope. Glycoproteins of the lipid envelope are genetically homologous with herpes simplex virus (Sanghavi et al., 2009). The virus is a linear, double-stranded DNA virus and contains the largest genome of the eight human herpesviruses with approximately 165 genes (Davison et al., 2003; Dolan et al., 2004). The study of CMV strains is difficult due to the size of the genome and the differences between in vitro and wild type CMV isolates; however, it has been proposed that polymorphisms could be related to differing clinical manifestations of CMV infection (Pignatelli et al., 2004).

Sites of Involvement

Cytomegalovirus (CMV) has been reported from numerous sites infecting different types of cells, including endothelial cells and reticular cells. Sites of involvement of disseminated CMV include cardiac myocytes, hepatocytes, GI tract, spleen, lymph nodes, endometrial stromal and glandular cells, breast stromal cells, renal glomeruli, tubules and interstitia, adrenal cortex and medulla, fallopian tube submucosa, myometrium, CNS, eyes, and anterior pituitary (Klatt and Shibata, 1988; Myerson et al., 1984).

In lymph nodes, it has been determined that CMV also infects both CD4+ and CD8+ T cells but not B cells (Younes et al., 1991). Other blood cells infected are polymorphonuclear leukocytes and monocytes, especially in immunocompromised patients (Gerna et al., 1992).

Pathogenesis

CMV exhibits a typical herpesvirus replication cycle with initial attachment to membrane receptors, fusion of viral envelope with the cell membrane, entrance of the nucleocapsid with subsequent travel to the nucleus, viral DNA entrance into the nucleus, and DNA replication, transcription, and translation into progeny virions with eventual release from the cell membrane. Infection results in lifelong latency with the genome persisting intracellularly without replication until reactivated by a variety of triggers (Sanghavi et al., 2009).

The dissemination of CMV seems to be an interplay between endothelial cell and leukocyte replication, which provides the pathogenesis of disease as well as transmission of the virus (Gerna et al., 2004). The first is infection of endothelial cells with subsequent giant cells formation. These cells then break off and enter the blood stream to spread CMV to distant sites (Percivalle et al., 1993). In addition studies have supported the replication of CMV in polymorphonuclear leukocytes, monocytes, and macrophages, with subsequent dissemination to other organs via these cells (Gerna et al., 1992, 2004).

CMV may cause disease in immunocompetent persons, but usually the disease is held in check by the patient's immune response; therefore, it is usually considered a disease of the immunocompromised (Vancikova and Dvorak, 2001). Direct effects of CMV may be IM-like symptoms that are indistinguishable from EBV (Taylor, 2003). Indirect effects of CMV include end-organ damage, acute or chronic graft rejection, accelerated transplant vasculopathy, and opportunistic superinfection, commonly noted in patients post-organ transplantation (Rubin, 1989). It has been shown that infected T cells lack expressions of HLA-DR and IL-2R, suggesting a probable mechanism for CMV-induced immunosuppression (Younes et al., 1991).

Approach to Diagnosis

Clinical Workup and Laboratory Findings

Nonspecific signs and symptoms of primary CMV infection include, but are not limited to, fever, chills, malaise, fatigue, pharyngitis with erythema, headache, lymphadenopathy, splenomegaly, rash, increased liver transaminases, and, less frequently, encephalitis, myocarditis, fulminant hepatitis, and Guillain–Barré syndrome (Taylor, 2003). CMV is a differential diagnosis in patients with febrile illness and more than 10% reactive lymphocytes in the peripheral circulation; however, other infectious causes, particularly EBV, are more likely (Tsaparas et al., 2000). If heterophile-antibodies for EBV are negative, CMV should be considered. CMV IgM antibodies should be present in all symptomatic patients but may be present for up to a year following infection, in which case CMV may not be the cause of the fever. IgG antibodies should increase up to fourfold during the acute infection; therefore monitoring of IgG should be used to determine if the febrile illness is truly due to CMV (Taylor, 2003). CMV PCR quantitation is an increasingly common method for detecting CMV, but it is not useful in diagnosing primary infection because a positive test may be due to viral shedding from reactivation in a latent state (Taylor, 2003). However, CMV DNA levels as measured by PCR quantitation are important in the immunocompromised when determining prognosis, for initiating pre-emptive therapy, and for assessing therapy response (Razonable and Emery, 2004).

Lymph Node Histopathology

CMV causes lymphadenopathy less commonly than EBV, histologically but clinically and histopathologically, both share similar features (Abbondanzo, 2004; Betts, 1980; Klemola and Kaariainen, 1965; Ramsay, 2004; Swerdlow, 1993). Overall lymph node architecture is retained. Nonspecific findings of diffuse paracortical hyperplasia resulting in a mottled appearance, composed of tingible body macrophages, monocytoid cells, small lymphocytes, Reed–Sternberg-like cells, and larger immunoblasts are common (Figure 15.9). CMV-infected cells may be very large with eosinophilic intranuclear inclusions surrounded by a clear halo, prominent nucleoli, and smaller basophilic cytoplasmic inclusions (Figure 15.10). The nuclear inclusion is often referred to as an "owl's eye" due to its large striking appearance. The presence of the unique intranuclear inclusion is pathognomonic for CMV infection (Mattes et al., 2000). In addition to the obviously infected cells, many normal appearing cells are also

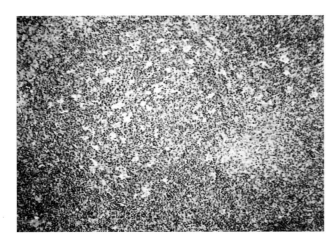

FIGURE 15.9 **Parafollicular B-cells with tingible body macrophages.** (Used with permission of Steven H. Swerdlow, MD)

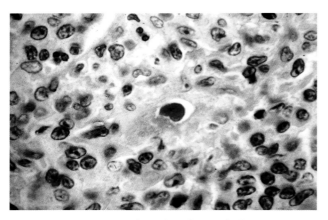

FIGURE 15.10 **CMV infected cells with large intranuclear inclusions and multiple intracytoplasmic inclusions.** (Used with permission of Steven H. Swerdlow, MD)

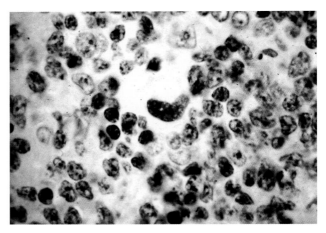

FIGURE 15.11 **CMV infected cell stained with anti-CMV monoclonal antibody (E-13, Chemicon, Temecula, CA).** (Used with permission of Steven H. Swerdlow, MD)

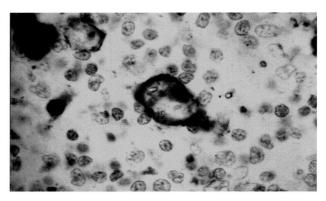

FIGURE 15.12 **Large cells with CD-15 positive membranous and Golgi staining patterns.** (Used with permission of Steven H. Swerdlow, MD)

infected, located primarily in the medulla of lymph node (Myerson et al., 1984).

Immunohistochemistry/In situ Hybridization

CMV can be detected in formalin-fixed, paraffin-embedded tissue by either IHC using anti-CMV antibodies or by ISH with biotinylated DNA probes (Figure 15.11) (Eizuru et al., 1991; Lu et al., 2009; Strickler et al., 1990; Swerdlow, 1993). These techniques have moderate sensitivities with high specificities and high positive predictive values. Both techniques have been shown to be more sensitive than H&E alone or classical viral culture (Andrade et al., 2004; Eizuru et al., 1991; Chemaly et al., 2004). CMV cells may also stain with CD15 (Leu-M1) (Figure 15.12) but not with CD30, necessitating additional stains to rule out Hodgkin lymphoma (Rushin

et al., 1990). The smaller, basophilic cytoplasmic inclusions contain DNA and polysaccharides and as a result will stain with Feulgen and Periodic-Acid-Schiff (PAS) (Abbondanzo, 2004).

Differential Diagnosis

Other viral lymphadenopathies, particularly those caused by other herpesviruses, can show similar histomorphology with CMV lymphadenitis. If the pathognomonic owl's eye inclusions are present, a diagnosis of CMV can be readily made. Immunohistochemical staining and ISH are of great utility in cases lacking characteristic CMV cytopathologic changes (Abbondanzo, 2004, Eizuru et al., 1991; Mattes et al., 2000; Ramsay, 2004; Strickler et al., 1990).

CMV lymphadenitis may also simulate some types of lymphoma. In particular, Hodgkin lymphoma is part of the differential diagnosis due to the large cells with large nuclei and inclusions simulating Reed–Sternberg cells. The infected cells also frequently have perinuclear cytoplasmic staining for CD15, potentially mimicking Reed–Sternberg cells (Rushin et al., 1990). In such cases immunohistochemical staining and ISH for both CMV and Hodgkin lymphoma (CD45−, CD15+, CD30+) should be performed to prevent an inappropriate diagnosis. Other lymphomas may also simulate CMV lymphadenitis but will lack the characteristic intranuclear inclusions. If lymphoma is considered, ancillary studies should be considered in the clinical workup. An interesting finding is that CMV may cause a clonal expansion of T large granular lymphocytes, apparently a reactive process and not one associated with neoplasia; therefore caution should be exercised if a T-LGL clonal population is identified in the setting of suspected CMV infection (Delobel et al., 2005).

As seen with EBV, phenytoin-associated lymphadenitis may display the same histopathology as CMV lymphadentitis; therefore clinical history of phenytoin therapy may be helpful (Abbondanzo et al., 1995; Abbondanzo, 2004). IHC and/or ISH should be performed in cases of suspected phenytoin-associated lymphadenopathy with concurrent clinical suspicion of viral lymphadentitis to make a definitive diagnosis.

Treatment of Choice and Prognosis

Drugs targeting CMV DNA polymerase are commonly used and include acyclovir, ganciclovir, valganciclovir, foscarnet, and cidofovir (Sanghavi et al., 2009). Ganciclovir, both oral and intravenous administrations, is the drug of choice for prophylaxis in immunosuppressed organ transplant patients, but the oral formulation has poor bioavailability while the intravenous formulation is plagued with side effects such as neutropenia. Oral valganciclovir has higher bioavailability and has shown effectiveness similar to intravenous ganciclovir with fewer side effects (Razonable and Emery, 2004). Prophylaxis for three months post-transplant may be used in high-risk organ recipients; however, once therapy is discontinued, late-onset CMV disease as well as development of drug-resistant strains continues to be problematic (Limaye et al., 2004). Preemptive therapy is also given to prevent progression of asymptomatic to symptomatic disease and commonly employs ganciclovir in solid-organ transplants and foscarnet in bone marrow transplants as it has less hematotoxicity (Razonable and Emery, 2004). Symptomatic congenital CMV benefits from intravenous ganciclovir but may be limited by neutropenia (Tanaka-Kitajima et al., 2005). Prenatal therapy in women with CMV DNA in amniotic fluid diminishes CMV DNA with

no symptomatic disease in the newborn (Puliyanda et al., 2005). CMV-Ig has been shown to be effective as an adjunct treatment in prevention of disease in organ transplant patients and in pregnant women with CMV DNA in amniotic fluid (Snydman et al., 2001; Nigro et al., 2005). Prevention of CMV by way of vaccine is currently in development (Schleiss, 2005).

HERPES SIMPLEX VIRUS LYMPHADENITIS

Definition

Lymphadenitis is caused by herpes simplex viruses 1 or 2 (HSV-1 and HSV-2, respectively).

ICD-10 Code

B00   Herpes viral [herpes simplex] infections [WHO, 2007].

Synonym

HSV lymphadenitis.

Epidemiology

Herpes, from the Greek for creeping or crawling, has been recognized for millennia. Hippocrates may have been the first to describe the disease now known to be caused by herpes simplex (Roizman and Whitley, 2001). It was not until the late nineteenth century when researchers discovered that herpes simplex is passed from human to human by the fluid of vesicular lesions. HSV-1, HSV-2, and varicella-zoster virus (VZV) are related in that they are neurotropic with latency in ganglia. HSV typically causes asymptomatic or mild uncomplicated mucocutaneous infections, most often orolabial or anogenital. Though not receiving the medical urgency afforded other herpesviruses such as CMV, HSV continues to be important in its ability to cause severe systemic disease, especially in the immunocompromised (Fatahzadeh and Schwartz, 2007; Whitley and Roizman, 2001).

Epidemiology differs for HSV-1 and HSV-2 with the former accounting for the majority of infections in humans (Fatahzadeh and Schwartz, 2007). In less developed countries, seroconversion occurs earlier in life with about a third of five-year-olds affected and approximately 80% of adolescence. In more developed countries those numbers drop to 20% of five-year-olds and 40 to 60% by 20 to 40 years (Whitley and Roizman, 2001). In one large study conducted in the United States, in persons 12 years old and older, approximately 27% were seronegative for HSV-1 and HSV-2, 51% were seropositive for HSV-1 only, 5% were positive for HSV-2 only, and 16% were positive for both HSV-1 and HSV-2 (Xu et al., 2002). Interestingly in this study, 16% of persons with HSV-2 only reported a history of symptoms compared to 6% if coinfected with HSV-1, indicating that seroprevalence of HSV-1 may influence epidemiology of clinical genital herpes. Race also affects HSV-1 epidemiology in the United States with approximately 35% of African-American versus 18% of white children affected by age 5 (Whitley and Roizman, 2001).

HSV-2 infections are usually transmitted sexually, with most genital infections attributed to that virus; however, HSV-1 is increasingly the cause of genital herpes. Genital herpes caused by HSV-1 are more mild and less likely to recur than those caused by HSV-2 (Whitley and Roizman, 2001). A study in the United States in the 1990s compared seroprevalence of HSV-2 to those of the 1970s, showing a 30% increase with the greatest gains among white teenagers and whites in their twenties (Fleming et al., 1997). This study shows over 20% of the population to be seropositive but less than 10% of those reporting a history of genital herpes infection. Risk factors include female gender, older age, lower socioeconomic status, illicit drug use, and greater number of sexual partners. A more recent study from 2005 to 2008 shows a decrease in seroprevalence to 16% with more than 80% of those persons being unaware of infection (CDC, 2010). Socioeconomic factors also significantly affect the rate of being undiagnosed (Pouget, 2010).

There are approximately 1500 annual cases of neonatal HSV disease in the United States with that number expected to rise. Approximately one-third of cases are encephalitis with disseminated cases accounting for one-half to two-thirds. The small remainder of cases is confined to the eyes, skin, and/or mouth (Kimberlin, 2007).

Clinical Aspects

Etiology

HSV, an α-herpesvirus, is approximately 150 to 200 nm in diameter with the typical double-stranded DNA genome, capsid, tegument, and envelope (Aurelian, 2009). The glycoproteins of the envelope are unique for HSV-1 and HSV-2, providing antigens for host immune response (Steiner et al., 2007). The HSV genome contains over 150 kbp coding for more than 80 different proteins (Whitley et al., 1998). HSV-1 and HSV-2 share 70% homology and can be distinguished by both DNA composition and antigen expression (Steiner et al., 2007). Genetic differences suggest the

two viruses have evolved different regulatory functions (Aurelian, 2009).

Sites of Involvement

In general, HSV infects mucocutaneous sites with HSV-1 primarily associated with orolabial infections while HSV-2 is primarily associated with anogenital disease. Primary and recrudescent lesions are indistinguishable clinically (Xu et al., 2002). HSV can also cause encephalitis, other skin infections such as herpetic whitlow, visceral infections, keratoconjunctivitis, Kaposi's varicella-like eruption, and association with erythema-multiforme (Nahamias, 1970; Whitley et al., 1998). Neonatal HSV encephalitis and disseminated disease particularly have significant morbidity and mortality, creating the need for rapid diagnosis and effective treatment strategies (Kimberlin, 2007). Despite the high prevalence of HSV, lymphadenitis is rare with only a few cases reported in the literature, most involving patients with immunodeficiency or underlying malignancy (Robertson et al., 2007).

Pathogenesis

The HSV replication cycle begins at the site of inoculation, typically mucocutaneous epithelial cells that have been exposed to the virus from another individual, either by vesicular fluid or by direct epithelial shedding of virions. The replication cycle in the epithelial cells is similar to the replication cycle of other herpesviruses. The HSV attaches to the host cell membrane via several classes of receptors. The nucleocapsid is transported to the nucleus and releases its DNA into the nucleus. HSV then replicates through three cycles using alpha, beta, and gamma proteins for viral replication, synthesis and packaging of DNA, and structural virion particles, respectively (Whitley and Roizman, 2001). This replicative cycle causes vesicle formation with virion release in the resulting clear liquid. Viruses also travel retrograde through the periaxonal sheath of sensory nerves to the trigeminal, lumbosacral, or autonomic ganglia where they either destroy the neuron or establish life-long latency (Fatahzadeh and Schwartz, 2007; Stevens, 1989). During reactivation, viruses travel anterograde in axons, cross into epithelial cells, and cause infection with the production of lesions. It is not uncommon for primary infection or reactivations to be asymptomatic (Stevens, 1989). Reactivation producing clinical disease is classically called a recrudescence while asymptomatic reactivation is called a recurrence (Fatahzadeh and Schwartz, 2007). After primary infection, antibodies are produced that do not prevent reactivation but typically cause recrudescent outbreaks to be less severe and may confer a degree of partial protection against the other serotype. HSV-2 has been shown to recur six times more frequently than HSV-1 (Beauman, 2005). HSV-2 is also considered a cocarcinogen causing neoplastic transformation of immortalized cells under conditions that interfere with viral replication (Aurelian, 2009).

Approach to Diagnosis

Clinical Workup and Laboratory Findings

The classic signs and symptoms of HSV often establish the diagnosis; however, diagnosis is difficult when symptoms are atypical. Commonly utilized laboratory tests include Tzanck smear, tissue biopsy, tissue culture of the virus, DNA detection by PCR, and serology (Fatahzadeh and Schwartz, 2007). The Tzanck smear is a rapid and inexpensive cytopathologic method of examining the cells from the base of freshly opened vesicles for viral cytopathologic changes; however, the changes, when present, cannot differentiate between HSV-1, HSV-2 or VZV (Oranje and Folkers, 1988). Likewise skin biopsy of the ulcers may be utilized to search for cytopathologic effect and IHC for viral typing (Cohen, 1994). Using vesicle fluid for viral isolation in tissue culture is the gold standard as it has relatively high sensitivity and specificity, and is the preferred method of virus detection. DNA detection by PCR, by traditional methods or more rapid real-time methods, is even more sensitive than viral culture and is suggested for rapid diagnosis of herpes encephalitis eliminating the need for brain biopsy (Kimberlin, 2006, 2007; Shi, 2010; Weidmann et al., 2003). Serology is used when other techniques are impractical or in patients with recrudescent lesions, healing lesions, or no lesions (Ashley and Wald, 1999). As there is evidence that some populations are experiencing an increase in HSV-1 prevalence of genital herpes, serology may be of benefit in patients with clinical disease (Lafferty, 2002). Due to delayed humoral response, HSV antibodies are absent in acute serum specimens but appearance of HSV-specific IgM and/or fourfold increase in anti-HSV IgG is specific for primary infection. A recurrent infection has IgG antibodies in acute serum specimens with the subsequent appearance of IgM antibodies and then increasing IgG antibodies. Enzyme-linked immunofluorescent assays can also be used discriminate between HSV-1 and HSV-2 (Fatahzadeh and Schwartz, 2007; Ohana et al., 2000).

Lymph Node Histopathology

Although HSV lymphadenitis is considered rare and lymph node biopsy is not indicated in viral infections, several case reports have been published likely because HSV lymphadenitis is often associated with hematopoietic malignancy or other causes of immunodeficiency increasing the likelihood of lymph node biopsy (Audouin et al., 1985; Banks, 2004; Epstein et al., 1986; Finberg and Mattia, 1994; Gaffey et al., 1991; Higgins and Warnke, 1999; Joseph et al., 2001; Lapsley et al., 1984; Mariette et al., 1999; Miliauskas and Leong, 1991; Pilichowska et al., 2006; Robertson et al., 2007; Tamaru et al., 1990; Taxy et al., 1985; Wat et al., 1994; Witt et al., 2002). The histopathology of HSV-infected lymph nodes is very similar, if not identical, to those described for EBV and CMV above. Published cases to date show nonspecific features by morphology in the biopsied lymph node, the most prominent is nodal architectural distortion, rather than effacement, with expansion of the paracortical regions (Figure 15.13). The interfollicular areas are infiltrated primarily with immunoblasts, but also with lymphocytes, plasmacytoid cells, eosinophils, macrophages, and Reed–Sternberg-like cells (large atypical immunoblasts) (Figure 15.14). Atrophic germinal centers may remain around the periphery of the node. Endothelial cells of the epithelioid venules are prominent. Medullary sinuses are preserved and may show sinus histiocytosis. Necrosis, less commonly seen in EBV or CMV lymphadenitis, is common in HSV lymphadenitis and is surrounded at the periphery by virally infected cells. Distinctly HSV-infected cells may be present showing a number of characteristics, including delicate chromatin clearing (Cowdry type A changes), degeneration with dark inclusions (Cowdry type B changes), enlarged cells with multinucleation and molding of adjacent

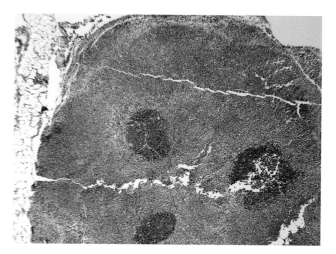

FIGURE 15.13 **Distinct follicular structures with cellular interfollicular expansion.** (Used with permission of Peter Banks, MD)

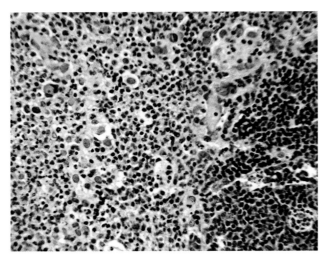

FIGURE 15.14 **Interfollicular mixed cellularity with large atypical cells and single degenerating cells.** (Used with permission of Peter Banks, MD)

nuclei; amphophilic to eosinophilic nuclear inclusions; and margination of chromatin with halo formation (Figure 15.14). In some cases, however, HSV-infected cells may resemble CMV infected cells or may show none of the classic features.

Immunohistochemistry/In situ Hybridization

HSV-1 and HSV-2 specific IHC and ISH may be used to identify virally infected cells in paraffin-embedded tissue (Figure 15.15). In addition, if lymphoma is also suspected, the appropriate IHC and ISH for those entities should be utilized. As HSV may be associated with hematologic malignancies, a broad panel of studies for both HSV and lymphoma is prudent for accurate diagnosis, treatment, and prognosis.

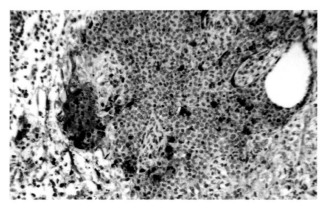

FIGURE 15.15 **Immunohistochemistry stain for HSV 1 and 2.** (Used with permission of Peter Banks, MD)

Differential Diagnosis

Other viral lymphadenitites show similar histopathology to HSV lymphadenitis. In cases of suspected viral lymphadenitis, clear cytopathologic changes of a specific entity obviate the need for ancillary studies. If viral etiology is suspected with unknown etiology, IHC and/or ISH are readily available to distinguish EBV, CMV, HSV, and VZV (Abbondanzo, 2004).

As HSV lymphadenitis is routinely characterized by necrosis, etiologies of necrotic lymphadenopathy should be considered in the differential diagnosis (Gaffey et al., 1991; Wat et al., 1994). Infectious entities that may mimic HSV lymphadenitis by causing necrotic lymphadenopathy are tuberculosis, *Bartonella hensalae*, fungi, and other bacteria. Tuberculosis will typically show caseating granulomas with acid-fast organisms. *Bartonella hensalae* will have paracortical microabscesses and necrotizing chronic granulomas with bacilli staining with various silver stains. Fungi and other bacteria may also be associated with necrosis and granulomas whereby special stains may be utilized to see the causative organisms. Kikuchi–Fujimoto lymphadenitis and systemic lupus erythematosus also typically have necrotic lymphadenopathy and with overlapping but not identical features (Helal et al., 2001; Khana et al., 2010). They may be differentiated from HSV lymphadenitis by the absence of viral cytopathologic changes and by the presence of a paracortical infiltrate composed primarily of histiocytes, lymphocytes, abundant extra- and intracellular karyorrhectic debris, and paucity of neutrophils and plasma cells.

HSV lymphadenitis can simulate several types of lymphomas and may be present concurrently with lymphoma. Several cases of patients with chronic lymphocytic leukemia (CLL) and subsequent or recurrent HSV lymphadenitis have been reported (Epstein et al., 1986; Gaffey et al., 1991; Higgins and Warnke, 1999; Joseph et al., 2001; Mariette et al., 1999). The immunocompromised states of CLL patients likely lead to susceptibility to HSV lymphadenitis. It has also been shown that neoplastic B cells express higher levels of herpes viral entry protein and are resistant to the cytopathologic effects of the virus, likely due to expression of bcl-2 (Robertson et al., 2007). Mantle cell lymphoma with concurrent HSV lymphadenitis has been reported (Pilichowska et al., 2006). A case of HSV lymphadenitis in a patient in remission for Hodgkin lymphoma has also been reported (Audouin et al., 1985). In cases of suspected HSV infection, or lymphoma with concurrent HSV infection, ancillary tests such as flow cytometry,

IHC, and ISH are crucial, especially to rule out lymphoma.

Treatments of Choice and Prognosis

Treatment of HSV relies on DNA polymerase inhibitors, including acyclovir, valacyclovir, and famciclovir. For uncomplicated orolabial or genital infections including primary infections and recrudescence, or for suppressive therapy, oral antiviral drugs are appropriate (Aurelian, 2009; Brady and Bernstein, 2004; Tyring et al., 2002). Suppressive therapy is safe but concerns include reactivation after cessation of treatment, drug resistance, and that nonreplicating HSV is potentially oncogenic (Aurelian, 2009). Treatment of choice for HSV encephalitis and/or disseminated disease, especially in neonates, is intravenous acyclovir, which has decreased mortality at 1 year of age from 85% of patients with disseminated disease and 50% of patients with CNS disease to 29% and 4%, respectively (Kimberlin et al., 2001; Kimberlin, 2007).

VARICELLA ZOSTER LYMPHADENITIS

Definition

Lymphadenitis is caused by varicella zoster virus (VZV).

ICD-10 Codes

B01   Varicella [chickenpox].
B02   Zoster [herpes zoster] [WHO, 2007].

Synonyms

VZV lymphadenitis, herpes zoster (HZ) lymphadenitis, chickenpox lymphadenitis, shingles lymphadenitis.

Epidemiology

VZV is the etiologic agent of chickenpox, establishes life-long latency, and may recur manifesting as a number of conditions. The earliest reports of rashes due to the herpesviruses, including VZV, date to antiquity while the relationship between chickenpox and herpes zoster was not identified until the 1880s (Wood, 2000). In the 1950s it was determined conclusively that varicella infection is caused by a virus, causing cytopathologic changes in tissue culture, and that it is highly specific for human hosts (Weller and Stoddard, 1952). Since the discovery of the virus much

has been accomplished from sequencing of the entire VZV genome to production of a clinically available vaccine (Wood, 2000).

VZV is a cosmopolitan virus, with infections occurring in all populations, even those with historical isolation (Grose, 2006). Transmitted by aerosol droplets, a cyclical pattern of infections is noted with most occurring in winter and spring in temperate countries, due to higher contact rates of children attending school (Gershon et al., 2010). The incidence of HZ prior to vaccinations is age dependent with 20 per 100,000 person-years in children aged 5 years to more than 1000 per 100,000 person-years for those older than 75 years. The estimated lifetime risk of HZ is 30% (Donahue et al., 1995; Guess et al., 1985). Epidemiology has changed as millions of people have been vaccinated since 1995. Before vaccination, most children, up to 90%, were infected by age 10 years with the susceptibility to VZV infection dropping dramatically to 4% of 20- to 29-year-olds (Finger et al., 1994; Wharton, 1996). The overall incidence of primary varicella has been reduced by 76 to 87% (Gershon et al., 2010). Nevertheless, incidence of HZ remains high as the patient population typically affected is older persons who have latent VZV infections from childhood. The current incidence at age 50 is approximately 300 per 100,000 person-years and by age 80 reaches 1000 per 100,000 patient-years, similar to the incidence before vaccination (Gershon et al., 2010). Females have a significantly higher incidence than males with differences increasing with age (Toyama et al., 2009). Patients with immunodeficiency diseases, such as HIV and certain malignancies, are at greater risk for severe varicella complications or serious to life-threatening HZ with increased incidence (Gershon et al., 1997; Gnann, 2002).

Clinical Aspects

Etiology

VZV, an α-herpesvirus, is related to HSV, with indistinguishable morphology between the viruses (Mueller et al., 2008; Sanghavi et al., 2009). VZV has the typical herpesvirus morphology of nucleocapsid surrounded by a tegument enclosed by a lipid envelope derived from the host cell membrane. The virions are 150 to 200 nm in diameter. The double-stranded DNA genome of VZV is approximately 125 kbp encoding roughly 70 proteins (Davison and Scott, 1986). VZV is closely related to HSV with similar gene layout and homology suggesting evolution from an ancestral genome.

VZV is the most stable herpesvirus; however, variances have been identified. A polymorphism in glycoprotein gE is associated with a strain capable of an accelerated cell spread phenotype (Grose et al., 2004; Tyler et al., 2007). In addition four to five clades of VZV have been identified and have geographical significance, possibly affecting epidemiology in their native environments (Quinlivan and Breuer, 2006; Sengupta et al., 2007).

Sites of Involvement

The primary site of involvement of VZV, occurring most commonly in children, is a diffuse rash on the skin and rarely mucosa, with latency in various ganglia of sensory nerves (Mueller et al., 2008). CNS and vasculature infections are rare complication of primary VZV infection in children and may cause significant morbidity and mortality in those affected (Askalan et al., 2001; Guess et al., 1986). Adults with primary infections usually have more severe disease, which may be systemic, the most significant being varicella pneumonia, a frequent cause of adult hospitalization. HZ, the reactivation of latent VZV, typically occurs as a prodrome of neuralgia followed by painful vesicular dermatosis in a dermatomal pattern but may just be present as a prodrome with no rash (zoster sine herpete). Reactivation also less commonly causes vasculopathy, myelopathy, cerebellitis, or retinal necrosis, most of these without accompanying rash (Mueller et al., 2008). Cervical lymphadenopathy is common and often a heralding event of VZV infection (Dwyer and Cunningham, 2002); however, these nodes are not typically biopsied as concurrent fever signals an infectious etiology.

Pathogenesis

VZV, a highly contagious virus, is transmitted by direct contact with skin lesions or by respiratory aerosols from infected individuals, a unique mode of transmission for herpesviruses (Mueller et al., 2008). The incubation period is 10 to 21 days, during which time the virus infects respiratory epithelial cells eventually spreading to T cells in the tonsils (Ku et al., 2004). VZV preferentially infects T cells with skin homing capabilities and indeed are transferred to skin by T cells where epithelial infection takes place. The skin epithelium mounts a potent antiviral response by up-regulating interferon-α. It is likely the prolonged incubation period is due to the time required for VZV to overcome this response. After replication cycles similar to those of other herpesviruses, virions may either be released from the superficial skin cells or be transferred from cell to cell. Spread of VZV to other organs occurs but is typically inconsequential in

the immunocompetent host; however, immunocompromised individuals are at great risk for hepatitis, pneumonia, or encephalitis (Gershon et al., 2010).

Latency is established when VZV infects sensory ganglia. Two hypotheses have been proposed to explain VZV infection of ganglia cells. One is that VZV infects epidermal projections of sensory neurons then travels retrograde to sensory ganglia. The other is that circulating T cells directly infect ganglia cell bodies but do not complete the proliferation cycle, preventing neuron death (Gershon et al., 2010; Kennedy, 2002). Viral antigens are not present on the surface of infected neurons during latency, thereby protecting them from the host's immune system.

During latency, 6 VZV genes are regularly expressed with their products limited to the cytoplasm, whereas 71 genes are expressed in lytic infections (Gershon et al., 2008, 2010). Reactivation to produce HZ occurs when VZV ORF61p, a nonstructural protein, is expressed in latently infected neurons, switching from a latent to lytic state. Inflammatory mediators have also been implicated in the reactivation of VZV. During reactivation, VZV travels along sensory axons to infect epithelial cells, causing the typical dermatomal pattern of HZ dermatosis. Trigeminal, cervical, and thoracic dermatomes are most commonly the sites of reactivation and viremia is usually not present (Gershon et al., 2010). Reactivation is a result of decline in cell-mediated immunity due to either normal senescence or immunocompromised states (Burke et al., 1982).

Approach to Diagnosis

Clinical Workup and Laboratory Findings

Classic, uncomplicated varicella zoster or HZ infections, which are apparent clinically, require no additional workup or laboratory testing. Circumstances when VZV testing is appropriate include immunocompromised patients, suspected neonatal infections, presumed immune or vaccinated persons, HZ in a young person, complicated infections, atypical lesions that mimic HSV, and suspected small pox lesions in cases of bioterrorism (Sanghavi et al., 2009).

Several methods are available for VZV detection. A simple Tzanck smear can be performed on scrapings from fresh vesicles of either varicella or HZ. Typical microscopic findings include large cells with multinucleation, molding of nuclei, margination of chromatin, and possibly a central dense nuclear inclusion surrounded by a clear zone (Figure 15.16). These characteristics are identical to and indistinguishable from the cytopathologic changes of HSV (Oranje and Folkers, 1988; Woods and Walker, 1996).

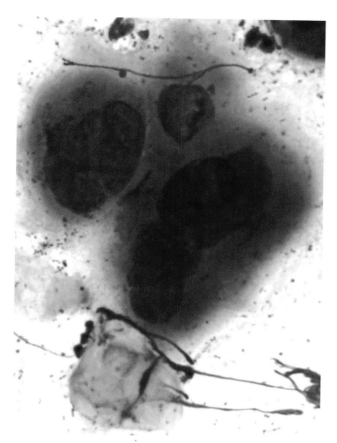

FIGURE 15.16 Tzanck smear of herpes zoster showing giant cells with multinucleation, molding of nuclei, and margination of chromatin.

Cytologic preparations from fresh vesicles and other tissues may also be used for direct immunofluorescence with conjugated monoclonal antibodies specific for VZV, distinguishing it from HSV, with higher specificity compared to tube cell culture (Coffin and Hodinka, 1995; Schmidt et al., 1980). Culturing of virus on fibroblasts grown on glass coverslips is now standard in most laboratories. After 3 to 6 days the cells are stained with fluorescent monoclonal antibodies to VZV. Positive cells will fluoresce, providing a more sensitive and rapid technique compared to older tube cultures (West et al., 1988). Viral DNA detection by PCR, in both vesicular fluid and CSF, has become an important and rapid tool for detection with 100% sensitivity and specificity for VZV allowing for the differentiation between VZV, HSV-1, and HSV-2 (Beards et al., 1998; Weidmann et al., 2003). Serologic methods are still employed but are of limited value because of false-positive results and lack of sensitivity and specificity (Arvin, 1996). However, serology may be used to assess the immune status of immunocompromised patients or to ascertain immune status postvaccination (Sanghavi et al., 2009).

Lymph Node Histopathology

Lymphadenopathy is a common sign and symptom of primary VZV infection but may be lacking in HZ due to lack of disseminated disease. In either situation, lymph node biopsy is rarely performed because the infectious etiology is clinically apparent or there is no lymph node enlargement. Nevertheless, there are a small number of reports of VZV lymphadenitis in the literature (Dorfman and Warnke, 1974; Patterson et al., 1980). Lymph nodes infected with VZV show diffuse cellular proliferation distorting the capsule and normal lymph node architecture, thereby creating a mottled appearance. The infiltrate is composed primarily of immunoblasts, small lymphocytes, prominent histiocytes engulfing debris, occasional plasma cells, and eosinophils, resulting in diffuse paracortical hyperplasia. An earlier review states that HZ lymphadenitis is histologically identical to postvaccinia vaccination lymphadenitis, with prominent histiocytes (Butler, 1969). These findings are similar to the other herpesvirus lymphadenitites described elsewhere in this chapter. Likewise the nonspecific nature of findings simulates other entities such as lymphoma.

Immunohistochemistry/In situ Hybridization

IHC specific for VZV IE63 and gE compounds may be performed on smears and biopsies where the etiology, specificially distinguishing between HSV and VZV, is not obvious (Nikkels et al., 1993; Nikkels and Pierard, 2009). Additional IHC or ISH may be performed to distinguish VZV lymphadenitis from various lymphomas that may be simulated due to lymph node architectural distortion and expansion of paracortical areas.

Differential Diagnosis

Other viral lymphadenitides may mimic VZV lymphadenitis. In cases where clear cytopathologic changes are not evident, IHC may be performed to distinguish etiologies. In particular, HSV lymphadenitis with the absence of the characteristic necrosis, may show cytopathologic changes of large cells with multinucleation, molding of nuclei, margination of chromatin, and/or presence of intranuclear inclusions with halos. In addition atypical clinical presentations of any VZV, HZ, or HSV lesions may make diagnosis unclear, warranting the use of IHC or ISH on surgical pathology specimens (Nikkels et al., 2009). Lymphadenitis caused by small pox vaccination, though rare, is identical to herpesvirus lymphadenitis and may also be confused with lymphoma; therefore vaccination history is important when nonspecific histologic features of paracortical hyperplasia with a mixed cellular response is present (Harstock, 1968).

VZV lymphadenitis, with its paracortical expansions of immunoblasts and Reed–Sternberg-like cells, may simulate various lymphomas, especially if the lymph node is biopsied in the absence of clear clinical features of varicella or HZ (Butler, 1969; Dorfman and Warnke, 1974; Patterson et al., 1980). A histopathologic feature that may favor a benign process would be distortion rather than complete effacement of the lymph node. Appropriate ancillary tests such as flow cytometry, IHC, ISH, and molecular studies should be performed in any cases where lymphoma is suspected. There have also been a few cases of cutaneous pseudolymphoma caused by VZV and mimicking malignancies such as CD30+ anaplastic large-cell lymphoma, indicating a need for careful clinical and pathologic correlation (Shiohara et al., 2009).

Treatment of Choice and Prognosis

Several anti-viral drugs are now approved for use in treating both primary varicella and HZ infections (Dworkin et al., 2007). Oral acyclovir administered in the first 24 hours after appearance of dermatosis in immunocompetent children and adults with primary varicella decreases severity and longevity of symptoms; however, latency is not affected nor is the acquisition of long-term immunity (Arvin, 1996; Dunkle et al., 1991). Alternative oral drugs include famciclovir and valacyclovir, the prodrugs of penciclovir and acyclovir respectively, both with increased bioavailability. Foscarnet may be used for acyclovir-resistant VZV; however, resistance has been reported (Sanghavi et al., 2009). Immunocompromised patients or immunocompetent patients with high-risk comorbidities, such as pneumonia or encephalitis, are at greater risk for developing life-threatening complications; therefore treatment is crucial and intravenous acyclovir is recommended. It has been shown that treatment within the first 72 hours dramatically reduces mortality in immunocompromised children from approximately 7 to 0% (Arvin, 1996; Balfour, 1988). Recommendations are similar for HZ cutaneous lesions and ophthalmic disease, with acyclovir, valacyclovir, and famciclovir as first-line treatment administered within 72 hours after onset. All drugs have shown efficacy in reducing complications and further pain (Arvin, 1996; Dworkin et al., 2007; Shaikh and Ta, 2002). Acyclovir has also been shown to reduce incidence of reactivation in high-risk persons, such as post-allogeneic bone marrow transplant patients; however, incidence is not affected once prophylaxis is discontinued (Thomson et al., 2005).

A live attenuated vaccine, containing the Oka strain, was developed in Japan in the 1970s and was approved for use in the United States in 1995 (Arvin, 1996; Nguyen et al., 2005). The universal childhood vaccination program has resulted in a sharp decline in mortality in the United States from 0.37 per 1 million whites and 0.66 per 1 million for all other races to 0.15 per million averaged for all races (Nguyen et al., 2005). As this is a live vaccine, it is capable of causing disease, especially in immunocompromised patients, and may not fully protect against breakthrough infections with wild-type strains (LaRussa et al., 2000).

The morbidity of HZ, specifically the prolonged often debilitating neuralgia, is significant and increases with age. Anti-viral medications may reduce the severity and duration of HZ, but the neuralgia may persist indefinitely. To alleviate this morbidity, a HZ vaccine, which is a version of the Oka vaccine with 14 times more potency, was developed in the 2000s and approved for use in the United States in 2006 (Oxman et al., 2005; Sanghavi et al., 2009). In clinical trials, the vaccine was shown to reduce the burden of illness due to HZ by 61%, reduce the incidence of post-herpetic neuralgia by 67%, and reduce the incidence of HZ by 51% (Oxman et al., 2005).

REFERENCES

ABBONDANZO SL. 2004. Epstein-Barr virus-associated lymphadenitis: the differential diagnosis of diffuse paracortical lymphoid hyperplasia. Pathol Case Rev 9:192–8.

ABBONDANZO SL, IREY NS, FRIZZERA G. 1995. Dilantin-associated lymphadenopathy: spectrum of histopathologic patterns. Am J Surg Pathol 19:675–86.

ABDEL-HAMID M, CHEN JJ, CONSTANINE N, MASSOUD M, RAAB-TRAUB N. 1992. EBV strain variation: geographical distribution and relation to disease state. Virology 190:168–75.

AMBINDER RF, MANN RB. 1994. Detection and characterization of Epstein–Barr virus in clinical specimens. Am J Pathol 145:239–52.

ANDRADE ZR, GARIPPO AL, SALDIVA PHN, CAPELOZZI VL. 2004. Immunohistochemical and in situ detection of cytomegalovirus in lung autopsies of children immunocompromised by secondary interstitial pneumonia. Pathol Res Pract 200:25–32.

ARONSON MD, KOMAROFF AL, PASS TM, ERVIN CT, BRANCH WT. 1982. Heterophil antibody in adults with sore throat: frequency and clinical presentation. An Int Med 96:505–8.

ARRAND JR, YOUNG LS, TUGWOOD JD. 1989. Two families of sequences in the small RNA-encoding region of Epstein–Barr virus (EBV) correlate with EBV types A and B. J Virol 63:983–6.

ARVIN AM. 1996. Varicella-zoster virus. Clin Microbiol Rev 9:361–81.

ASHLEY RL, WALD A. 1999. Genital herpes: review of the epidemic and potential use of type-specific serology. Clin Microbiol Rev 12:1–8.

ASKALAN R, LAUGHLIN S, MAYANK S, CHAN A, MACGREGOR D, ANDREW M, CURTIS R, MEANEY B, DE VEBER G. 2001. Chickenpox and stroke in children: a study of frequency and causation. Stroke 32:1257–62.

AUDUOIN J, LE TOURNEAU A, AUBERT JP, DIEBOLD J. 1985. Herpes simplex virus lymphadenitis mimicking tumoral relapse in a patient with Hodgkin's disease in remission. Virchows Arch 408:313–21.

AURELIAN L. 2009. Herpes simplex viruses. In: Specter S, Hodinka RL, Young SA, Wiedbrauk DL, ed., Clinical Virology Manual, 4th ed. ASM Press, Washington, DC, pp. 424–53.

AXELROD P, FINESTONE AJ. 1990. Infectious mononucleosis in older adults. Am Fam Phys 42:1599–1606.

BALFOUR HH. 1988. Varicella zoster virus infections in immunocompromised hosts: a review of the natural history and management. Am J Med 85(2A): 68–73.

BALFOUR HH, HOKANSON KM, SCHACHERER RM, FIETZER CM, SCHMELING DO, HOLMAN CJ, VEZINA HE, BRUNDAGE RC. 2007. A virologic pilot study of valacyclovir in infectious mononucleosis. J Clin Virol 39:16–21.

BALFOUR HH, HOLMAN CJ, HOKANSON KM, LELONEK MM, GIESBRECHT JE, WHITE DR, SCHMELING DO, WEBB CH, CAVERT W, WANG DH, BRUNDAGE RC. 2005. A prospective clinical study of Epstein–Barr virus and host interactions during acute infectious mononucleosis. J Infect Dis 192:1505–12.

BANKS PM. 2004. Herpes lymphadenitis: case of the month, February 2004. http://drpeterbanks.com/CaseOfTheMonth.cfm?mo=Feb04&Year=2004&idx=2 (Accessed 26 December 2010.)

BEARDS G, GRAHAM C, PILLAY D. 1998. Investigation of vesicular rashes for HSV and VZV by PCR. J Med Virol 54:155–7.

BEAUMAN JG. 2005. Genital herpes: a review. Am Fam Phys 72:1527–34.

BENHARROCH D, MEGUERIAN-BEDOYAN Z, LAMANT L, AMIN C, BRUGIERES L, TERRIER-LACOMBE MJ, HARALAMBIEVA E, PULFORD K, PILERI S, MORRIS SW, MASON DY, DELSOL G. 1998. ALK-positive lymphoma: a single disease with a broad spectrum of morphology. Blood 91:2076–84.

BETTS RF. 1980. Syndromes of cytomegalovirus infection. Adv Intern Med 26:447–66.

BRADY RC, BERNSTEIN DI. 2004. Treatment of herpes simplex virus infections. Antiviral Res 61:73–81.

BROWN HL, ABERNATHY MP. 1998. Cytomegalovirus infection. Sem Perinatol 22:260–6.

BRUU, AL, HJETLAND R, HOLTER E, MORTENSEN L, NATAS O, PETTERSON W, SKAR AG, SKARPAAS T, TJADE T, ASJO B.

2000. Evaluation of 12 commercial tests for detection of Epstein–Barr virus-specific and heterophile antibodies. Clin Diagn Lab Immunol 7:451–6.

BURKE BL, STEELE RW, BEARD OW, WOOD JS, CAIN TD, MARMER DJ. 1982. Immune responses to varicella-zoster in the aged. Arch Intern Med 142:291–3.

BUTLER JJ. 1969. Non-neoplastic lesions of lymph nodes of man to be differentiated from lymphomas. Nat Cancer Inst Monograph 32:233–55.

CARBONE A, GLOGHINI A, DOTTI G. 2008. EBV-associated lymphoproliferative disorders: classification and treatment. Oncologist 13:577–85.

Centers for Disease Control and Prevention (CDC). 2010. Seroprevalence of herpes virus type 2 among persons aged 14–49 years—United States, 2005–2008. Morb Mortal Wkly Rep 59:456–9.

CHEMALY RF, YEN-LIEBERMAN B, CASTILLA EA, REILLY A, ARRIGAIN S, FARVER C, AVERY RK, GORDON SM, PROCOP GW. 2004. Correlation between viral loads of cytomegalovirus in blood and bronchoalveolar lavage specimens from lung transplant recipients determined by histology and immunohistochemistry. J Clin Microbiol 42:2168–72.

CHILDS CC, PARHAM DM, BERARD CW. 1987. Infectious mononucleosis: the spectrum of morphologic changes simulating lymphoma in lymph nodes and tonsils. Am J Surg Path 11:22–132.

COFFIN SE, HODINKA RL. 1995. Utility of direct immunofluorescence and virus culture for detection of varicella-zoster virus in skin lesions. J Clin Microbiol 33:2792–95.

COHEN, JI. 2000. Epstein–Barr virus infection. NEJM 343:481–92.

COHEN, PR. 1994. Tests for detecting herpes simplex virus and varicella-zoster infections. Dermatol Clin 12:51–68.

COLUGNATI FAB, STARAS SAS, DOLLARD SC, CANNON MJ. 2007. Indicence of cytomegalovirus infection among the general population and pregnant women in the United States. BMC Infect Dis 7:71.

CRAWFORD DH, MACSWEEN KF, HIGGINS CD, THOMAS R, MCAULAY K, WILLIAMS H, HARRISON N, REID S, CONACHER M, DOUGLAS J, SWERDLOW AJ. 2006. A cohort study among university students: identification of risk factors for Epstein–Barr virus seroconversion and infectious mononucleosis. Clin Infect Dis 43:276–82.

DAVISON AJ, DOLAN A, AKTER P, ADDISON C, DARGAN DJ, ALCENDOR DJ, MCGEOCH DJ, HAYWARD GS. 2003. The human cytomegalovirus genome revisited: comparison with the chimpanzee cytomegalovirus genome. J Gen Virol 84:17–28.

DAVISON AJ, SCOTT JE. 1986. The complete DNA sequence of varicella-zoster virus. J Gen Virol 67:1759–1816.

DELOBEL P, GODEL A, THEBAULT S, ALRIC L, DUFFAUT M. 2005. Transiet clonal expansion of T-large granular lymphocytes during primary cytomegalovirus infection. J Infect 53:e65–67.

DOLAN A, CUNNINGHAM C, HECTOR RD, HASSAN-WALKER AF, LEE L, ADDISON C, DARGAN DJ, MCGEOCH DJ, GATHERER D, EMERY VC, GRIFFITHS PD, SINZGER C, MCSHARRY

BP, WILKINSON GWG, DAVISON AJ. 2004. Genetic content of wild-type human cytomegalovirus. J Gen Virol 85:1301–12.

DONAHUE JG, CHOO PW, MANSON JE, PLATT R. 1995. The incidence of herpes zoster. Arch Intern Med 155:1605–09.

DORFMAN RF, WARNKE R. 1974. Lymphadenopathy simulating the malignant lymphomas. Hum Pathol 5:519–50.

DUNKLE LM, ARVIN AM, WHITLEY RJ, ROTBART HA, FEDER HM, FELDMAN S, GERSHON AA, LEVY ML, HAYDEN GF, McGUIRT PV, HARRIS MA, BALFOUR HH. 1991. A controlled trial of acyclovir for chickenpox in normal children. NEJM 325:1539–44.

DWORKIN RH, JOHSNON RW, BREUER J, GNANN JW, LEVIN MJ, BACKONJA M, BETTS RF, GERSHON AA, HAANPAA ML, McKENDRICK MW, NURMIKKO TJ, OAKLANDER AL, OXMAN MN, PAVAN-LANGSTON D, PETERSEN KL, ROWBOTHAM MC, SCHMADER KE, STACEY BR, TYRING SK, VAN WIJCK AJM, WALLACE MS, WASSILEW SW, WHITLEY RJ. 2007. Recommendations for management of herpes zoster. Clin Infect Dis 44:S1–S26.

DWYER DE, CUNNINGHAM AL. 2002. Herpes simplex and varicella-zoster infections. Med J Australia 177:267–73.

EBELL MH. 2004. Epstein-Barr virus infectious mononucleosis. Am Fam Phys 70:1279–87.

EIZURU Y, MINEMATSU T, MINAMISHIMA Y, EBIHARA K, TAKAHASHI K, TAMURA K, HOSODA K, MASUHO Y. 1991. Rapid diagnosis of cytomegalovirus infections by direct immunoperoxidase staining with human monoclonal antibody against an immediate-early antigen. Microbiol Immunol 35:1015–22.

EPSTEIN MA, ACHONG BG, BARR YM. 1964. Virus particles in cultured lymphoblasts from Burkitt's lymphoma. Lancet 1:702–3.

EPSTEIN JI, AMBINDER RF, KUHAJDA FP, PEARLMAN SH, REUTER VE, MANN RB. 1986. Localized herpes simplex lymphadenitis. Am J Clin Pathol 86:444–8.

FATAHZADEH M, SCHWARTZ RA. 2007. Human herpes simplex virus infections: epidemiology, pathogenesis, symptomatology, diagnosis, and management. J Am Acad Dermatol 57:737–63.

FINBERG RW, MATTIA AR. 1994. [Case records of the Massachusetts General Hospital] weekly clinicopathological exercises: case 45–1994: a 47-year-old man with inguinal lymphadenopathy and fever during preparation for a bone marrow transplant. NEJM 331:1703–10.

FINGER R, HUGHES JP, MEADE BJ, PELLETIER AR, PALMER CT. 1994. Age-specific incidence of chickenpox. Pub Health Rep 109:750–5.

FINGEROTH JD, WEIS JJ, TEDDER TF, STROMINGER JL, BIRO PA, FEARON DT. 1984. Epstein-Barr virus receptor of human B lymphocytes is the C3d receptor CR2. Proc Natl Acad Sci 81:4510–4.

FLAVELL KJ, MURRAY PG. 2000. Hodgkin's disease and the Epstein–Barr virus. J Clin Pathol: Mol Pathol 53:262–9.

FLEISHER GR, COLLINS M, FAGER S. 1983. Limitations of available tests for diagnosis of infectious mononucleosis. J Clin Microbiol 17:619–24.

FLEMING DT, McQUILLAN GM, JOHNSON RE, NAHMIAS AJ, ARAL SO, LEE FK, ST. LOUIS ME. 1997. Herpes simplex virus type 2 in the United States, 1976–1994. NEJM 337:1105–11.

FRY J. 1980. Infectious mononucleosis: some new observations from a 15-year study. J Fam Prac 10:1087–9.

GAFFEY MJ, BEN-EZRA JM, WEISS LM. 1991. Herpes simplex lymphadenitis. Am J Clin Pathol 95:709–14.

GERBER P, NONOYAMA M, LUCAS S, PERLIN E, GOLDSTEIN LI. 1972. Oral excretion of Epstein–Barr virus by healthy subjects and patients with infectious mononucleosis. Lancet ii:988–9.

GERNA G, BALDANTI F, REVELLO MG. 2004. Pathogenesis of human cytomegalovirus infection and cellular targets. Hum Immunol 65:381–6.

GERNA G, ZIPETO D, PERCIVALLE E, PAREA M, REVELLO MG, MACCARIO R, PERI G, MILANESI G. 1992. Human cytomegalovirus infection of the major leukocyte subpopulations and evidence for initial viral replication in polymorphonuclear leukocytes from viremic patients. J Infect Dis 6:1236–44.

GERSHON AA, CHEN J, GERSHON MD. 2008. A model of lytic, latent, and reactivating varicella-zoster virus infections in isolated enteric neurons. J Infect Dis 197:S61–5.

GERSHON AA, GERSHON MD, BREUER J, LEVIN MJ, OAKLANDER AL, GRIFFITHS PD. 2010. Advances in the understanding of the pathogenesis and epidemiology of herpes zoster. J Clin Virol 48:S2–7.

GERSHON AA, MERVISH N, LaRUSSA P, STEINBERG S, LO SH, HODES D, FIKRIG S, BONAGURA V, BAKSHI S. 1997. Varicella-zoster virus infection in children with underlying human immunodeficiency virus infection. J Infect Dis 176:1496–1500.

GNANN JW. 2002. Varicella-zoster virus: atypical presentations and unusual complications. J Infect Dis 186:S91–8.

GOWING NFC. 1975. Infectious mononucleosis: histopathologic aspects. Pathol Annu 10:1–20.

GROSE C. 2006. Varicella zoster virus: out of Africa and into the research laboratory. Herpes 13:32–6.

GROSE C, TYLER S, PETERS G, HIEBERT J, STEPHENS GM, RUYECHAN WT, JACKSON W, STORLIE J, TIPPLES GA. 2004. Complete DNA sequence analyses of the first two varicella-zoster virus glycoprotein E (D150N) mutant viruses found in North America: evolution of genotypes with an accelerated cell spread phenotype. J Virol 78:6799–6807.

GUERREIRO-CACAIS AO, LI LQ, DONATI DD, BEJARANO MT, MORGAN A, MASUCCI MG, HUTT-FLETCHER L, LEVITSKY V. 2004. Capacity of Epstein–Barr virus to infect monocytes and inhibit their development into dendritic cells is affected by the cell type supporting virus replication. J Gen Virol 85:2767–78.

GUESS HA, BROUGHTON DD, MELTON LJ, KURLAND LT. 1985. Epidemiology of herpes zoster in children and adolescents: a population-based study. Pediatrics 76:512–7.

GUESS HA, BROUGHTON DD, MELTON LJ, KURLAND LT. 1986. Population-based studies of varicella complications. Pediatrics 78:723–7.

HADINOTO V, SHAPIRO M, SUN CC, THORLEY-LAWSON DA. 2009. The dynamics of EBV shedding implicate a central role for epithelial cells in amplifying viral output. PLoS Pathogens 5:e1000496.

HALLEE TJ, EVANS AS, NIEDERMAN JC, BROOKS CM, VOEGTLY JH. 1974. Infectious mononucleosis at the United States Military Academy: a prospective study of a single class over four years. Yale J Biol Med 47:182–95.

HARSTOCK RJ. 1968. Postvaccinial lymphadenitis: hyperplasia of lymphoid tissue that simulates malignant lymphoma. Cancer 21:632–49.

HELAL TA, TALAAT W, DANIAL MF. 2001. Kikuchi histiocytic necrotizing lymphadenitis: clinicopathological immunohistochemical study. Eastern Mediterranean Health J 7:153–62.

HENKE CE, KURLAND LT, ELVEBACK LR. 1973. Infectious mononucleosis in Rochester, Minnesota, 1950 through 1969. Am J Epidemiol 98:483–90.

HENLE G, HENLE W, DIEHL V. 1968. Relation of Burkitt's tumor-associated herpes-type virus to infectious mononucleosis. Proc Nat Acad Sci 59:94–101.

HENLE W, DIEHL V, KOHN G, ZUR HAUSEN H, HENLE G. 1967. Herpes-type virus and chromosome maker in normal leukocytes after growth with irradiated Burkitt cells. Science 157:1064–5.

HENLE W, HENLE GE, HOROWITZ CA. 1974. Epstein-Barr virus specific diagnostic tests in infectious mononucleosis. Hum Pathol 5:551–65.

HIGGINS JPT, WARNKE RA. 1999. Herpes lymphadenitis in association with chronic lymphocytic leukemia. Cancer 86:1210–5.

HOAGLAND RJ. 1975. Infectious mononucleosis. Prim Care 2:295–307.

HOCHBERG D, SOUZA T, CATALINA M, SULLIVAN JL, LUZURIAGA K, THORLEY-LAWSON DA. 2004. Acute infection with Epstein–Barr virus targets and overwhelms the peripheral memory B-cell compartment with resting, latently infected cells. J Virol 78:5194–5204.

HOROWITZ CA, HENLE W, HENLE G, SEGAL M, ARNOLD T, LEWIS FB, ZANICK D, WARD PCJ. 1976. Clinical and laboratory evaluation of elderly patients with heterophil-antibody positive infectious mononucleosis. Am J Med 61:333–9.

HOSHINO Y, KATANO H, ZOU P, HOHMAN P, MARQUES A, TYRING SK, FOLLMANN D, COHEN JI. 2009. Long-term administration of valacyclovir reduces the number of Epstein–Barr virus (EBV)-infected B cells but not the number of EBV DNA copies per B cell in healthy volunteers. J Virol 83:11857–61.

HUTT-FLETCHER LM. 2007. Epstein–Barr virus entry. J Virol 81:7825–32.

ISAACSON PG, SCHMID C, PAN LX, WOTHERSPOON AC, WRIGHT DH. 1992. Epstein-Barr virus latent membrane protein expression by Hodgkin and Reed–Sternberg-like cells in acute infectious mononucleosis. J Pathol 167:267–271.

JENSON HB. 2004. Virologic diagnosis, viral monitoring, and treatment of Epstein–Barr virus infectious mononucleosis. Curr Infect Dis Rep 6:200–7.

JOSEPH L, SCOTT MA, SCHICHMAN SA, ZENT CS. 2001. Localized herpes simplex lymphadenitis mimicking large-cell (Richter's) transformation of chronic lymphocytic leukemia/small lymphocytic lymphoma. Am J Hematol 68:287–91.

KATZ BZ, SHIRAISHI Y, MEARS CJ, BINNS HJ, TAYLOR R. 2009. Chronic fatigue syndrome after infectious mononucleosis in adolescents. Pediatrics 124:189–93.

KAWA K. 2000. Epstein–Barr virus–associated diseases in humans. Int J Hematol 71:108–17.

KENNEDY PGE. 2002. Varicella-zoster virus latency in human ganglia. Rev Med Virol 12:327–34.

KENNESON A, CANNON MJ. 2007. Review and meta-analysis of epidemiology of congenital cytomegalovirus (CMV) infection. Rev Med Virol 17:253–76.

KHANA D, SHRIVASTAVA A, MALUR PR, KANGLE R. 2010. Necrotizing lymphadenitis in systemic lupus erythematosus: is it Kikuchi-Fujimoto disease ? J Clin Rheumatol 16:123–4.

KIMBERLIN DW, LIN CY, JACOBS RF, POWELL DA, COREY L, GRUBER WC, RATHORE M, BRADLEY JS, DIAZ PS, KUMAR M, ARVIN AM, GUTIERREZ K, SHELTON M, WEINER LB, SLEASMAN JW, DE SIERRA TM, WELLER S, SOONG SJ, KIELL J, LAKEMAN FD, WHITLEY RJ, National Institute of Allergy and Infecious Diseases Collaborative Antiviral Study Group. 2001. Safety and efficacy of high-dose intravenous acyclovir in management of neonatal herpes simplex virus infections. Pediatrics 108:230–8.

KIMBERLIN DW. 2006. Diagnosis of herpes simplex virus in the era of polymerase chain reaction. Pediatr Infect Dis J 25:841–2.

KIMBERLIN DW. 2007. Herpes simplex virus infections of the newborn. Sem Perinatol 31:19–25.

KLATT EC, SHIBATA D. 1988. Cytomegalovirus infection in the acquired immunodeficiency syndrome. Clinical and autopsy findings. Arch Pathol Lab Med 112:540–4.

KLEMOLA E, KAARIAINEN L. 1965. Cytomegalovirus as a possible cause of a disease resembling infectious mononucleosis. Brit Med J 5470:1099–1102.

KOTHARI A, RAMACHANDRAN VG, GUPTA P, SINGH B, TALWAR V. 2002. Seroprevalence of cytomegalovirus among voluntary blood donors in Delhi, India. J Health Popul Nutr 20:348–51.

KU CC, ZERBONI L, ITO H, GRAHAM BS, WALLACE M, ARVIN AM. 2004. Varicella-zoster virus transfer to skin by T cells and modulation of viral replication by epidermal cell interferon-α. J Exp Med 200:917–25.

KUTTNER AG, COLE R. 1926. Further evidence concerning the significance of nuclear inclusions as indicator of transmissible agents. Proc Soc Exp Biol Med 23:49–62.

LAFFERTY WE. 2002. The changing epidemiology of HSV-1 and HSV-2 and implications for serological testing. Herpes 9:51–55.

LAPSLEY M, KETTLE P, SLOAN JM. 1984. Herpes simplex lymphadenitis: a case report and review of the published work. J Clin Pathol 37:1119–22.

LARUSSA P, STEINBERG SP, SHAPIRO E, VAZQUEZ M, GERSHON AA. 2000. Viral strain identification in varicella vaccinees with disseminated rashes. Pediatr Infect Dis J 19:1037–9.

Lee CL, Davidsohn I, Panczyszyn O. 1968. Horse agglutinins in infectious mononucleosis. II. The spot test. Am J Clin Pathol 49:12–18.

Limaye AP, Bakthavatsalam R, Kim HW, Kuhr CS, Halldorson JB, Healey PJ, Boeckh M. 2004. Late-onset cytomegalovirus disease in liver transplant recipients despite antiviral prophylaxis. Transplantation 78:1390–6.

Lu DY, Qian J, Easley KA, Waldrop SM, Cohen C. 2009. Automated in situ hybridization and immunohistochemistry for cytomegalovirus detection in paraffin-embedded tissue sections. Appl Imunohistochem Mol Morphol 1717:158–64.

Luzuriaga K, Sullivan JL. 2010. Infectious mononucleosis. NEJM 362:1993–2000.

Mariette X, Molina JM, Asli B, Brouet JC. 1999. A patient with chronic lymphoid leukemia and recurrent necrotic herpetic lymphadenitis. Am J Med 107:403–4.

Mattes FM, McLaughlin JE, Emery VC, Clark DA, Griffiths PD. 2000. Histopathological detection of owl's eye inclusions is still specific for cytomegalovirus in the era of human herpesviruses 6 and 7. J Clin Pathol 53:612–4.

McClain KL, Leach CT, Jenson HB, Joshi VV, Pollock BH, Parmley RT, DiCarlo FJ, Chadwick EG, Murphy SB. 1995. Association of Epstein-Barr virus with leiomyosarcoma in children with AIDS. NEJM 332:12–8.

Miliauskas JR, Leong ASY. 1991. Localized herpes simplex lymphadenitis: report of three cases and review of the literature. Histopathology 19:355–60.

Molesworth SJ, Lake CM, Borza CM, Turk SM, Hutt-Fletcher LM. 2000. Epstein–Barr virus gH is essential for penetration of B cells but also plays a role in attachment of virus to epithelial cells. J Virol 74:6324–32.

Mueller NH, Gilden DH, Cohrs RJ, Mahalingam R, Nagel MA. 2008. Varicella zoster virus infection: clinical features, molecular pathogenesis of disease, and latency. Neurol Clin 26:675–97.

Myerson D, Hackman RC, Nelson JA, Ward DC, McDougall JK. 1984. Widespread presence of histologically occult cytomegalovirus. Hum Pathol 15:430–9.

Nahamias A. 1970. Disseminated herpes-simplex virus infections. NEJM 282:684–5.

Nguyen HQ, Jumaan AO, Seward JF. 2005. Decline in mortality due to varicella after implementation of varicella vaccination in the United States. NEJM 352:450–8.

Nicholas J. 2000. Evolutionary aspects of oncogenic herpesviruses. J Clin Pathol:Mol Pathol 53:222–37.

Niedobitek G, Agathanggelou A, Herbst H, Whitehead L, Wright DH, Young LS. 1997. Epstein–Barr virus (EBV) infection in infectious mononucleosis: virus latency, replication and phenotype of EBV-infected cells. J Pathol 182:151–9.

Nigro G, Adler SP, La Torre R, Best AM. 2005. Passive immunization during pregnancy for congenital cytomegalovirus infection. NEJM 353:1350–62.

Nikkels AF, Debrus S, Sadzot-Delvaux C, Piette J, Delvenne P, Rentier B, Pierard GE. 1993. Comparative immunohistochemical study of herpes simplex and varicella-zoster infections. Virchows Arch A 422:121–6.

Nikkels AF, Pierard GE. 2009. Occult varicella. Ped Infect Dis J 28:1073–5.

Ohana B, Lipson M, Vered N, Srugo I, Ahdut M, Morag A. 2000. Novel approach for specific detection of herpes simplex virus type 1 and 2 antibodies and immunoglobulin G and M antibodies. Clin Diagn Lab Immunol 7:904–8.

Oranje AP, Folkers E. 1988. The Tzanck smear: old, but still of inestimable value. Pediatr Dermatol 5:127–9.

Oxman MN, Levin MJ, Johnson GR, Schmader KE, Straus SE, Gelb LD, Arbeit RD, Simberkoff MS, Gershon AA, Davis LE, Weinberg A, Boardman KD, Williams HM, Zhang JH, Peduzzi PN, Beisel CE, Morrison VA, Guatelli JC, Brooks PA, Kauffman CA, Pachucki CT, Neuzil KM, Betts RF, Wright PF, Griffin MR, Brunell P, Soto NE, Marques AR, Keay SK, Goodman RP, Cotton DJ, Gnann JW, Loutit J, Holodniy M, Keitel WA, Crawford GE, Yeh SS, Lobo Z, Toney JF, Greenberg RN, Keller PM, Harbecke R, Hayward AR, Irwin MR, Kyriakides TC, Chan CY, Chan ISF, Wang WWB, Annunziato PW, Silber JL. 2005. A vaccine to prevent herpes zoster and postherpetic neuralgia in older adults. NEJM 352:2271–84.

Patterson SD, Larson EB, Corey L. 1980. Atypical generalized zoster with lymphadenitis mimicking lymphoma. NEJM 302:848–51.

Percivalle E, Revello MG, Vago L, Morini F, Gerna G. 1993. Circulating endothelial giant cells permissive for human cytomegalovirus (HCMV) are detected in disseminated HCMV infections with organ involvement. J Clin Invest 92:663–70.

Petersen I, Thomas JM, Hamilton WT, White PD. 2006. Risk and predictors of fatigue after infectious mononucleosis in a large primary-care cohort. Q J Med 99:49–55.

Pignatelli S, Dal Monte P, Rossini G, Landini MP. 2004. Genetic polymorphisms among human cytomegalovirus (HCMV) wild-type strains. Rev Med Virol 14:383–410.

Pilichowska ME, Smouse JH, Dorfman DM. 2006. Concurrent herpes simplex viral lymphadenitis and mantle cell lymphoma: a case report and review of the literature. Arch Pathol Lab Med 130:536–9.

Pouget ER. 2010. Racial/ethnic disparities in undiagnosed infection with herpes simplex virus type 2. Sex Transm Dis 37:538–43.

Puliyanda DP, Silverman NS, Lehman D, Vo A, Bunnapradist S, Radha RK, Toyoda M, Jordan SC. 2005. Successful use of oral ganciclovir for the treament of intrauterine cytomegalovirus infection in a renal allograft recipient. Transpl Infec Dis 7:71–4.

Putukian M, O'Connor FG, Stricker PR, McGrew C, Hosey RG, Gordon SM, Kinderknecht J, Kriss VM, Landry GL. 2008. Mononucleosis and athletic participation: an evidence-based subject review. Clin J Sport Med 18:309–15.

Quinlivan M, Breuer J. 2006. Molecular studies of varicella zoster virus. Rev Med Virol 16:225–50.

Ramsay AD. 2004. Reactive lymph nodes in pediatric practice. Am J Clin Pathol 122(S1):S87–97.

Razonable RR. 2005. Epidemiology of cytomegalovirus disease in solid organ and hematopoietic stem cell transplant recipients. Am J Health Syst Pharm 62S1:S7–13.

Razonable RR, Emery VC. 2004. Management of CMV infection and disease in transplant patients. Herpes 11:77–86.

Rea TD, Russo JE, Katon W, Ashley RL, Buchwald DS. 2001. Prospective study of the natural history of infectious mononucleosis caused by Epstein–Barr virus. J Am Board Fam Pract 14:234–42.

Reynolds DJ, Banks PM and Gulley ML. 1995. New characterization of infectious mononucleosis and a phenotypic comparison with Hodgkin's disease. Am J Pathol 146:379–88.

Robertson JL, Cebe K, Landrum ML. 2007. Herpes simplex lymphadenitis: 2 cases and review of the literature. Infect Dis Clin Pract 15:154–9.

Roizman B, Whitley RJ. 2001. The nine ages of herpes simplex virus. Herpes 8:23–7.

Rowe M, Young LS, Cadwallader K, Petti L, Kieff E, Rickinson AB. 1989. Distinction between Epstein-Barr virus type A (EBNA 2A) and type B (EBNA 2B) isolates extend to the EBNA 3 family of nuclear proteins. J Virol 63:1031–9.

Rowe WP, Hartley JW, Waterman S, Turner HC, Huebner RJ. 1956. Cytopathogenic agent resembling human salivary gland virus recovered from tissue cultures of human adenoids. Proc Soc Exp Biol Med 92:418–24.

Rubin RH. 1989. The indirect effects of cytomegalovirus infection on the outcome of organ transplantation. JAMA 261:3607–9.

Rushin JM, Riordan GP, Heaton RB, Sharpe RW, Cotelingam JD, Jaffe ES. 1990. Cytomegalovirus-infected cells express Leu-M1 antigen: a potential source of diagnostic error. Am J Pathol 136:989–95.

Salvador AH, Harrison EG, Kyle RA. 1971. Lymphadenopathy due to infectious mononucleosis: its confusion with malignant lymphoma. Cancer 27:1029–40.

Sanghavi SK, Rowe DT, Rinaldo CR. 2009. Cytomegalovirus, varicella-zoster virus, and Epstein–Barr virus. In: Specter S, Hodinka RL, Young SA, Wiedbrauk DL, ed., Clinical Virology Manual, 4th ed. ASM Press, Washington, DC, pp. 454–93.

Savard M, Balanger C, Tardif M, Gourde P, Flamand L, Gosselin J. 2000. Infection of primary human monocytes by Epstein–Barr virus. J Virol 74:2612–9.

Schleiss M. 2005. Progress in cytomegalovirus vaccine development. Herpes 12:66–75.

Schmidt NJ, Gallo D, Devlin V, Woodie JD, Emmons RW. 1980. Direct immunofluorescence staining for detection of herpes simplex and varicella-zoster virus antigens in vesicular lesions and certain tissue specimens. J Clin Microbiol 12:651–5.

Sengupta N, Taha Y, Scott FT, Leedham-Green ME, Quinlivan M, Breuer J. 2007. Varicella-zoster-virus genotypes in east London: a prospective study in patients with herpes zoster. J Infect Dis 196:1014–20.

Shaikh S, Ta CN. 2002. Evaluation and management of herpes zoster ophthalmicus. Am Fam Phys 66:1723–30.

Sheldon PJ, Hemsted EH, Papamichail M, Holborrow EJ. 1973. Thymic origin of atypical lymphoid cells in infectious mononucleosis. Lancet 301:1153–1155.

Shi J. 2010. Rapid diagnosis of herpetic encephalitis in children by PCR-microarray technology for simultaneous detection of sever human herpes viruses. Eur J Pediatr 169:421–5.

Shiohara J, Koga H, Uhara H, Takata M, Saida T, Uehara T. 2009. Herpes zoster histopathologically mimicking CD30-postive anaplastic large cell lymphoma. J Eur Acad Dermatol and Venereol 23:618–9.

Sixbey JW, Shirley P, Chesney PJ, Buntin DM, Resnick L. 1989. Detection of a second widespread strain of Epstein–Barr virus. Lancet ii:761–5.

Smith MG. 1956. Propagation in tissue cultures of a cytopathogenic virus from human salivary gland virus (SGV) disease. Proc Soc Exp Biol Med 92:424–30.

Snydman DR, Falagas ME, Avery R, Perlino C, Ruthazer R, Freeman R, Rohrer R, Fairchild R, O'Rourke E, Hibberd P, Werner BG. 2001. Use of combination cytomegalovirus immune globulin plus ganciclovir for prophylaxis in CMV-seronegative liver transplant recipients of a CMV-seropositive donor organ: a multicenter, open-label study. Transplant Proc 33:2571–5.

Sokal EM, Hoppenbrouwers K, Vandermeulen C, Moutschen M, Leonard P, Moreels A, Haumont M, Bollen A, Smets F, Denis M. 2007. Recombinant gp350 vaccine for infectious mononucleosis: a phase 2, randomized, double-blind, placebo-controlled trial to evaluate the safety, immunogenicity, and efficacy of an Epstein–Barr virus vaccine in healty young adults. J Infect Dis 196:1749–53.

Souza T, Stollar BD, Sullivan JL, Luzuriaga K, Thorley-Lawson DA. 2005. Periperhal B-cells latently infected with Epstein–Barr virus display molecular hallmarks of classical antigen-selected memory B cells. Proc Natl Acad Sci 102:18093–8.

Sprunt IP, Evans FA. 1920. Mononuclear leukocytosis in reaction to acute infection (infectious mononucleosis). Bull Johns Hopkins Hosp 31:410–7.

Staras SAS, Dollard SC, Radford KW, Falnders WD, Pass RF, Cannon MJ. 2006. Seroprevalence of cytomegalovirus infection in the United States, 1988–1994. Clin Infect Dis 43:1143–51.

Steiner I, Kennedy PGE, Pachner AR. 2007. The neurotropic viruses: herpes simplex and varicella-zoster. Lancet Neurol 6:1015–28.

Stevens JG. 1989. Human herpesviruses: a consideration of the latent state. Microbiol Rev 53:318–32.

Strickler JG, Fedeli F, Horwitz CA, Copenhaver CM, Frizzera G. 1993. Infectious mononucleosis in lymphoid tissue: histopathology, in situ hybridization, and differential diagnosis. Arch Pathol Lab Med 117:269–78.

STRICKLER JG, MANIVEL JC, COPENHAVER CM, KUBIC VL. 1990. Comparison of in situ hybridization and immuno-histochemistry for detection of cytomegalovirus and herpes simplex virus. Hum Pathol 21:443–8.

STRUM SB, PARK JK, RAPPAPORT H. 1970. Observation of cells resembling Sternberg–Reed cells in conditions other than Hodgkin's disease. Cancer 26:176–90.

SUNDE J, CHETTY-JOHN S, SHLOBIN OA, BOICE CR. 2010. Epstein-Barr virus-associated uterine leiomyosarcoma in an adult lung transplant patient. Obstet Gynecol 115:434–6.

SWERDLOW SH. 1993. Society of Hematopathology, Case of the Quarter, August. 5 pp.

TAMARU J, MILKATA A, HORIE H, ITOH K, ASAI T, HONDO R, MORI S. 1990. Herpes simplex lymphadenitis: report of two cases with review of the literature. Am J Surg Pathol 14:571–7.

TANAKA-KITAJIMA N, SUGAYA N, FUTATANI T, KANEGANE H, SUZUKI C, OSHIOR M, HAYAKAWA M, FUTAMURA M, MORISHIMA T, KIMURA H. 2005. Ganciclovir therapy for congenital cytomegalovirus infection in six infants. Pediat Infect Dis J 24:782–5.

TAXY JB, TILLAWI I, GOLDMAN PM. 1985. Herpes simplex lymphadenitis: an unusual presentation with necrosis and viral particles. Arch Pathol Lab Med 109:1043–4.

TAYLOR GH. 2003. Cytomegalovirus. Am Fam Phys 67:519–24.

THOMSON KJ, HART DP, BANERJEE L, WARD KN, PEGGS KS, MACKINNON S. 2005. The effect of low-dose aciclovir on reactivation of varicella zoster virus after allogeneic hemopoietic stem cell transplantation. Bone Marrow Trans 35:1065–9.

THORLEY-LAWSON DA. 2001. Epstein–Barr virus: exploiting the immune system. Nat Rev Immunol 1:75–82.

TINDLE BH, PARKER JW, LUKES RJ. 1972. "Reed-Sternberg cells" in infectious mononucleosis ? Am J Clin Pathol 58:607–17.

TOYAMA N, SHIRAKI K, Members of the Society of the Miyazaki Prefecture Dermatologists. 2009. Epidemiol-ogy of herpes zoster and its relationship to varicella in Japan: a 10-year survey of 48,388 herpes zoster cases in Miyazaki Prefecture. J Med Virol 81:2053–55.

TSAPARAS YF, BRIDGEN ML, MATHIAS R, THOMAS E, RABOUD J, DOYLE PW. 2000. Proportion of positive for Epstein–Barr virus, cytomegalovirus, human her-pesvirus 6, Toxoplasma, and human immunodeficiency virus types 1 and 2 in heterophile-negative patients with an absolute lymphocytosis or an instrument-generated atypical lymphocyte flag. Arch Pathol Lab Med 124:1324–30.

TYLER SD, PETERS GA, GROSE C, SEVERINI A, GRAY MJ, UPTON C, TIPPLES GA. 2007. Genomic cartography of varicella-zoster virus: a complete genome-based analysis of strain variability with implications for attenuation and phenotypic differences. Virology 359:447–58.

TYRING SK, BAKER D, SNOWDEN W. 2002. Valacyclovir for herpes simplex virus infection: long-term safety and sus-tained efficacy after 20 years' experience with acyclovir. J Infect Dis 186:S40–6.

VANCIKOVA Z, DVORAK P. 2001. Cytomegalovirus infec-tion in immunocompetent and immunocompromised individuals—a review. Curr Drug Targets Immune Endocr Metabol Disord 1:179–87.

WAT PJ, STRICKLER JG, MYERS JL, NORDSTROM MR. 1994. Herpes simplex infection causing acute necrotizing ton-sillitis. Mayo Clin Proc 69:269–71.

WEIDMANN M, MEYER-KONIG U, HUFERT FT. 2003. Rapid detection of herpes simplex virus and varicella-zoster virus infections by real-time PCR. J Clin Microbiol 41:1565–8.

WELLER TH, STODDARD MB. 1952. Intranuclear inclusion bodies in cultures of human tissue inoculated with var-ciella vesicle fluid. J Immunol 68:311–9.

WEST PG, ALDRICH B, HARTWIG R, HALLER GJ. 1988. Increased detection rate for varicella-zoster virus with combination of two techniques. J Clin Microbiol 26:2680–81.

WHARTON M. 1996. The epidemiology of varicella-zoster virus infections. Infect Dis Clin North Am 10:571–81.

WHITLEY RJ, KIMBERLIN DW, ROIZMAN B. 1998. Herpes simplex viruses. Clin Infect Dis 26:541–55.

WHITLEY RJ, ROIZMAN B. 2001. Herpes simplex virus infec-tions. Lancet 357:1513–8.

WITT MD, TORNO MS, SUN N, STEIN T. 2002. Herpes sim-plex virus lymphadenitis: case report and review of the literature. Clin Infect Dis 34:1–6.

WICK MJ, WORONZOFF-DASHKOFF KP, MCGLENNEN RC. 2002. The molecular characterization of fatal infectious mononucleosis. Am J Clin Pathol 117:582–8.

WOOD MJ. 2000. History of varicella zoster virus. Herpes 7:60–5.

WOODS GL, WALKER DH. 1996. Detection of infection or infectious agents by use of cytologic and histologic stains. Clin Microbiol Rev 9:382–405.

World Health Organization (WHO). ICD Version 2007. http://apps.who.int/classifications/apps/icd/icd10 online (accessed 24 October 2010).

XU F, SCHILLINGER JA, STERNBERG MR, JOHNSON RE, LEE FK, NAHMIAS AJ, MARKOWITZ LE. 2002. Seroprevalence and coinfection with herpes simplex virus type 1 and type 2 in the United States 1988–1994. J Infect Dis 185:1019–24.

YOUNES, M, PODESTA A, HELIE M, BUCKLEY P. 1991. Infection of T but not B lymphocytes by cytomegalovirus in lymph node: an immunophenotypic study. Am J Surg Pathol 15:75–80.

YOUNG LS, DAWSON CW, ELIOPOULOS AG. 2000. The expres-sion and function of Epstein-Barr virus encoded latent genes. J Clin Pathol: Mol Pathol 53:238–47.

YOUNG LS, YAO QY, ROONEY CM, SCULLEY TB, MOSS DJ, RUPANI H, LAUX G, BORNKAMM GW, RICKINSON AB. 1987. New type B isolates of Epstein–Barr virus from Burkitt's lymphoma and from normal individuals in endemic areas. J Gen Virol 68:2853–62.

ZIMBER U, ADLDINGER HK, LENOIR GM, VUILLAUME M, KNEBEL-DOEBERITZ MV, LAUX G, DESGRANGES C, WITTMANN P, FREESE UK, SCHNEIDER U, BORNKAMM GW. 1986. Geographical prevalence of two types of Epstein–Barr virus. Virology 154:56–66.

CHAPTER SIXTEEN

REACTIVE LYMPHADENOPATHY WITH SINUS PATTERN

Hernani D. Cualing

SINUSES AND VASCULAR SUPPLY

The lymph node sinuses comprise structures and functions that can be identified histologically as well as functionally. Sinuses support monocytic immune activity and filtration of lymphatics. Sinuses are relatively open spaces bounded by sinus lining cells where fluid and cells flow through the node. Unlike the lymph node parenchyma, sinuses show relatively few lymphocytes, so that lymphatic fluid can readily pass through and flow from afferent lymphatic vessels in the capsule to the efferent vessel in the hilum. Subcapsular sinuses lie immediately below the capsule to received the afferent flow. The subcapsular sinuses are continuous with intermediate sinus channels, located in the paratrabeculae and hence also called trabecular sinuses. Trabecular sinuses are also continuous with medullary sinuses. Flattened fibroblastic reticular cells (FRCs) line the sinuses. These specialized lining cells express fibronectin, which facilitates lymphocyte adhesion and ameboid movements, and other specific receptors that control passages of lymphocytes into the pulp. Macrophages, referred to as sinus histiocytes, reside in between a tethered fibroblastic reticular meshwork in the sinuses, and akin to an intricate web, capture bacteria, cancer cells, and foreign particulate as it flows through the sinuses (Willard-Mack, 2006).

This structure is easily seen in low-power histology. The sinuses appear as pale pink structures surrounded by a sea of dark blue lymphocytes in low-power view. It is good practice to first examine the sinuses when evaluating a lymph node. This approach allows the pathologist a starting point to survey the sinus for metastatic disease, reactive cells such as monocytoid cells, histiocytes, and infections such as lymph-borne parasites. Sinuses may show reactive sinus histiocytosis, metastatic tumor cells, and even early involvement of Hodgkin lymphoma as well as a number of reactive lymphadenopathy with a sinus pattern.

When the sinuses are prominent, dilated, and filled with cells, we have a sinus pattern of reaction. Focal sinus histiocytosis is a common reaction identified by presence of reactive histiocytes. Sometimes other cells including red blood cells, neutrophils, eosinophils, and plasma cells may be additionally present, especially during abnormal immune conditions.

SINUS HISTIOCYTOSIS, NONSPECIFIC

Reactive sinus histiocytosis (SH) or hyperplasia often occurs together with reactive paracortical or follicular

TABLE 16.1 Sinus Pattern, Noninfectious and Infectious

Sinus histiocytosis, nonspecific
Sinus histiocytosis, secondary to adjacent tumor drainage
Signet ring histiocytosis
Sinus histiocytosis with massive lymphadenopathy
Pigmented sinus histiocytic pattern
Histiocytic reactions to foreign materials
Lymphangiography lymphadenopathy
Mucicarminophilic histiocytosis (PVP Lymphadenopathy)
Histiocytosis postmetallic joint prosthesis
Sinus histiocytosis pattern of Extramedullary hematopoieisis
Immature "sinus histiocytosis" or Monocytoid B-cell hyperplasia
Histiocytic hemophagocytic syndromes
Vascular transformation of sinuses
Whipple (*T. whipelli*) lymphadenopathy

hyperplasia as a nonspecific finding and is seldom the only finding. Florid sinus histiocytosis or SH-like pattern is found in a number of specific conditions summarized in Table 16.1

Definition

Sinus histiocytosis is a benign disorder of lymph nodes showing distended sinuses filled by syncytial sheets of benign sinus histiocytes. The sinus pattern mimics the appearance of sinus histiocytosis but has features and cytologic components brought about by a variety of nonneoplastic and neoplastic-specific conditions.

ICD-10 Code CM 180–189

Diseases of veins, lymphatic vessels and lymph nodes, not elsewhere classified

ICD-10 Code CM 189.9

Noninfective disorder of lymphatic vessels and lymph nodes, unspecified

Synonym

Sinus catarrh.

Incidence

As an isolated primary finding in an otherwise unremarkable lymph node, sinus histiocytosis comprises an incidence of 4 to 6% of surgically excised specimen (Black and Speer, 1958, Chhabra, 2006).

Normal Histology and Function

The lymphatic sinuses vary in size and shape. They can be thin or dilated, irregular in shape, and filled with histiocytes and other cells (Figure 16.1). The sinuses contain a variable number of pale staining nucleated histiocytes—readily recognized as different from lymphocytes, which contain dark staining nuclei (see Figure 16.2). The sinuses are lined with flattened sinus lining cells, providing an envelope that separates the sinus from other compartments of the lymph node. Penetrating the sinus lining

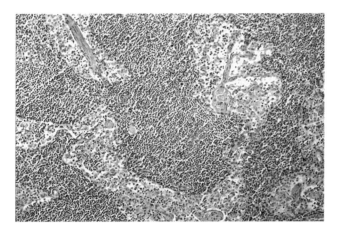

FIGURE 16.1 **Normal sinuses as readily seen in reactive lymph nodes.** These sinuses have a normal serpiginous anastomosing appearance with or without expansion by sinus histiocytosis. Trabecular fibrous tissue could, at times, be identified in the center of these sinuses identifying these as trabecular sinuses.

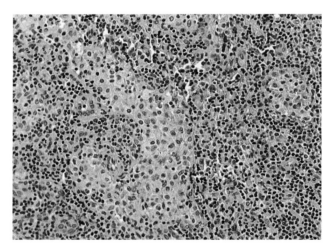

FIGURE 16.2 **Sinus histiocytosis, intermediate to marked, surrounding small lymphocytes.** Normal sinus histiocytes distictly identified and differentiated from lymphocytes.

cells are thin anastomosing fluid conduits forming a web.

The lymph from the subcapsular sinus reaches the lymph node cellularity and parenchyma via a relatively closed system of conduits made up of fibroblastic reticular cells (FRCs) network, which also compose the sinus lining. FRCs, at least in lower mammals, have some characteristics of epithelial cell, fibroblasts, and endothelium. They express cytokeratins 8 and 18 and secrete matrix known as reticular fibers. Reticular fibers are composed of a core of collagen fibrils enveloped in a layer of basement membrane and express collagen types I, III, and IV, elastin, entactin, fibronectin, laminin-1, tenascin, vitronectin, and heparan sulfate (Sainte-Marie and Peng, 1986). These thin fibers can sometimes be seen on routine stains inside sinuses (see Figure 16.3). These conduits are easily seen in reticulin stained or anti–type I collagen immunostained lymph node. When stained with reticulin, this network is visible in parenchyma as well as in the sinuses. These tubular hollow pipes show as thin anastomosing conduits conducting lymph fluid (Gretz, Anderson, and Shaw, 1997; Roozendaal et al., 2009) The lymph fluid bathes both B-cell and T-cell areas as these tubular channels or conduits extend into the follicles to deliver small antigens (less than 70 kD) to follicular dendritic cells and interdigitating reticulum cells (Roozendaal et al., 2009). The conduits are pathways intimately in contact with antigen-processing dendritic cells. This arrangement provides a direct interface of lymph-borne antigens with the follicular cortex and the paracortex. The lymphatic fluid that bypass the conduit system goes directly into paracortical sinuses and intermediate sinuses.

The sinus lymphatic fluid carries cells, fluid, and macromolecules into the lymph node sinuses and parenchyma. Unwelcome traffickers may include trapped tumor cells, parasites, or other infectious agents, all of which are best appreciated in subcapsular or in intermediate sinuses. These lymph channels inside the lymph node start as subcapsular sinus, then meander inside the pulp as intermediate or trabecular sinuses (also called marginal sinuses), and end in the hilum as medullary sinuses (see Figure 16.4). The anastomosing subcapsular sinuses are continuous with the medullary sinuses. Eventually the lymph fluid with its passenger cells exit the lymph node via an efferent lymphatic vessel into other nodes in the chain and end up in the systemic circulation. In this way the effluent of antigen-rich fluid that carries solutes and lymphocytes permits a dynamic matrix for antigen and cellular interaction. In addition the constant movement of naïve lymphocytes in the lymph nodes maximizes the chance that a cell encounters its cognate antigen, an encounter that triggers events that contribute to the lymphocyte becoming functional and fully competent.

Relation to Cancer and Sinus Histiocytosis Grading

Sinus histiocytosis is common in lymph nodes in reaction to adjacent cancer or to other inflammatory or

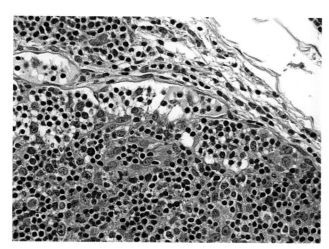

FIGURE 16.3 Thin conduits visible inside sinuses in H & E stain but poorly visualized in the pulp without additional reticulin or type I collagen staining.

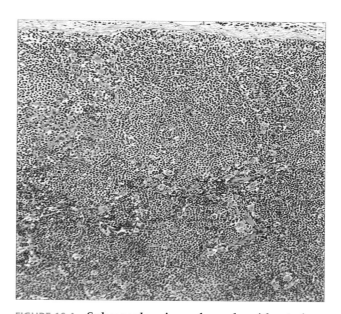

FIGURE 16.4 **Subcapsular sinus channels without sinus histiocytosis.** The subcapsular channels are continuous with the cortical and paracortical sinuses.

infectious causes. Many of the lymph nodes obtained for staging of cancer show sinus histiocytosis. A grading system popular in surgical pathology is used for prognosis. An intermediate grade of sinus histiocytosis is defined as histiocytes three to four layers thick, mild sinus histiocytosis is below three layers, and marked grade is above four layers (see Figure 16.2). Though the literature is not conclusive if there is an enhanced survival advantage in patients with carcinoma and sinus histiocytosis reaction, it is generally believed that sinus histiocytosis is a positive response against tumor (Silverberg et al., 1970) (Silverberg, Frable, and Brooks, 1973). Failure to find a relationship is believed to be due to the differences in timing of surgery, the inconsistent grading used for sinus histiocytosis, and observer variabillity.

Immunohistochemistry

Sinus histiocytes reveal sheets of CD68+ macrophages that characteristically do not co-express S100 or CD1a proteins. This pattern of staining contrasts with that of other histiocytic-like cells such as Langerhans cells, which additionally express S100 and CD1a and lack Fascin, or paracortical interdigitating reticulum cells (IDRC), which express S100, CD1a, CD68 weakly, and Fascin. (Nishikawa et al., 2009) (Facchetti et al., 1988) or Rosai–Dorfman sinus cells, expressing CD68, CD163, and S100 as well as fascin, but, which lacks CD1a staining (Jaffe, DeVaughn, and Langhoff, 1998). Three types of histiocytes are found in dermatopathic lymphadenitis: interdigitating reticulum cells (IDRC), Langerhans cells, and macrophages (van der Oord et al., 1984).

Special Types of Sinus Reaction

The dynamic appearance of sinuses gives clues to either a normal physiology or abnormal reaction. In addition to the nonspecific sinus histiocytosis, five special types of sinus pattern are described:

1. Inflammatory sinus histiocytosis. Blood or lymphocytes are not normally present in the sinus unless there is recent surgery, local trauma, or a reaction to florid immune response. In some sinuses, admixed lymphocytes and detached histiocytes are present along with prominent plump lining cells. The presence of blood and lymphocytes in sinuses could sometimes be seen in postsurgical lymphadenectomy—and is also called inflammatory sinus histiocytosis (see Figure 16.5).

2. Immature "sinus histiocytosis" or monocytoid hyperplasia. This is not a true sinus histiocytosis

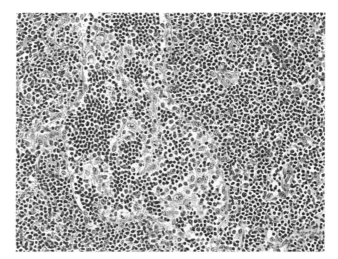

FIGURE 16.5 **Sinuses with lymphocytes admixed with histiocytes**. The sinuses are sometimes called inflammatory sinus histiocytosis. Notice the flat sinus lining cells on the boundaries of the sinuses.

because the cells are mostly composed of monocytoid B lymphocytes with admixed histiocytes. This pattern is generated as follows. Since the sinuses drain fluid carried by afferent vessels, lymphocytes and monocytes are carried along with other cells. Lymphocytes migrate from the sinuses and settle inside the lymph node pulp. In the early immune response characterized by IgM secretion and IgM-complex formation, monocytoid hyperplasia may be prominent. Similarly the marginal zone cells of the spleen are postulated to be carriers of immune complexes into the splenic white pulp, specifically depositing complexes on the membrane receptors of follicle dendritic cells (Ferguson, Youd, and Corley, 2004). Since monocytoid B cells become prominent inside paratrabecular and subcapsular sinuses and also form parafollicular bands, which mimic marginal zone pattern seen in the spleen, monocytoid B cells may arguably assume a similar role in human lymph nodes (Camacho et al., 2001) These cells were once called "immature sinus histiocytosis," a historical misnomer, since we now know these to be B cells and not histiocytes. These cells, when present, are seen in low-power view as pale crescentic bands inside and around sinuses and follicles. High-power view reveals their lymphoid nature, albeit with generous amount of cytoplasm akin to the appearance of monocytes (see Chapter 13, Figure 13.35, for monocytoid cells.)

3. Lactation sinus histiocytosis. The sinus fluid may also carry endogenous or exogenous materials such as hemosiderin, antharacotic pigments, metals, polyesters, or lipids. Lactation sinus histiocytosis is

a condition that manifests in lymph nodes sinuses when there is accumulation of lipid globules, from an adjacent lactating breast, inciting sinus hyperplasia with foamy histiocytes.

4. Sinus catarrh. In mesenteric or abdominal lymph nodes, the sinuses may normally be filled with pink proteinaceous fluid with few histiocytes—a situation refered to as sinus catarrh. This finding is nonspecific and regarded a physiologic reaction to the richly laden fluid from the gut.

5. Signet ring histiocytosis. A rare type with morphology of signet ring histiocytes that is concerning for metastatic signet ring cancer is discussed further below (see Figure 16.11 and 16.12).

Occasionally, in between medullary sinuses, there may be prominent plasma cells collections forming medullary cords (see Figure 16.6). The medullary cords are bounded by medullary sinus lining cells. The cords are formed by reactive lymphocytes and plasma cells. Rarely, medullary cords may be so prominent and concerning for nodular lymphoma (see Figure 16.7). These findings are seen in association with an exuberant immune response as in florid reactive follicular hyperplasia, in some autoimmune disorders, or in Castleman's disease.

Differential Diagnosis of Sinus Histiocytosis

Several histologic features set some diseases apart from the nonspecific sinus histiocytosis (see Table 16.2). These include intedigitating reticulum cell tumor, signet ring histiocytosis, sinus histiocytosis with massive lymphadenopathy (SHML),

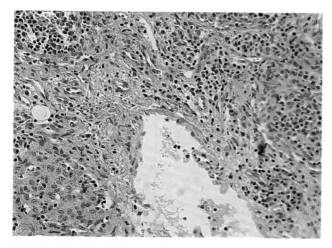

FIGURE 16.6 **Medullary cords and sinus**. Sheets of reactive plasma cells inside medullary cords.

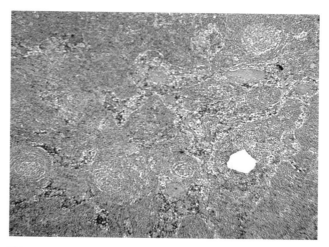

FIGURE 16.7 **Prominent medullary cords in florid hyperplasia**. Some cords have inconspicuous follicle centers that may be concerning for nodular lymphoma. These are also Bcl2 and IgD positive, and on high power they will show primary follicles composed of small lymphocytes lacking markers for both mantle cell or follicular lymphoma.

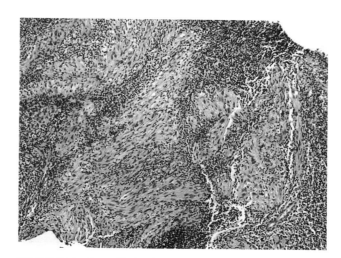

FIGURE 16.8 **Interdigitating reticulum tumor in a lymph node**. Low power sinusoidal pattern of IRCT.

Langerhans cell histiocytosis, reactive or neoplastic hemophagocytic syndrome, and lymphomas with a high content of histiocytes.

The intedigitating reticulum cell tumor mimics a sinus pattern in low power (Figure 16.8), although the spindle-shaped histiocyte is a clue as to the correct diagnosis. The interdigitating reticulum tumor or interdigitating reticulum cell sarcoma (IDRCS) are neoplastic cells mixed with reactive lymphoplasmacytes. Although rare, they often present with solitary lymphadenopathy that clinically may be innocuous and be mistaken for a benign process. However,

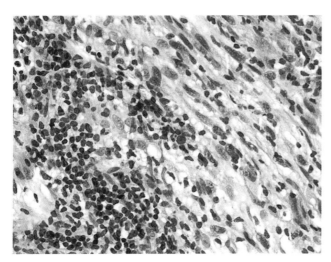

FIGURE 16.9 **Spindle cell nuclear and pleomorphic cellular appearance of the interdigitating reticulum tumor in the lymph node.** Shown are the occasional tumor giant cells. The nuclei are hyperchromatic and positive for CD68+ and vimentin but lack a follicular dendritic marker CD21 or CD35.

they do metastasize to viscera and other lymph nodes. Histologically they present in the paracortex mimicking a sinus pattern in low power. Although most tumor cells are spindly, some are epithelioid and rounded and on high power may be bland-looking with rare cytologic atypia (Figure 16.9). By electron microscopy, they lack well-formed desmosomes, unlike those in follicular dendritic cells, and they are devoid of Birbeck granules, unlike Langerhans cells. Although their immunostain is rather nondescript, they are invariably S100 positive with variable CD45, vimentin, CD68, and lysozyme expression (Figure 16.10). They lack the histiocyte marker CD163, follicular dendritic markers CD21, CD23, and

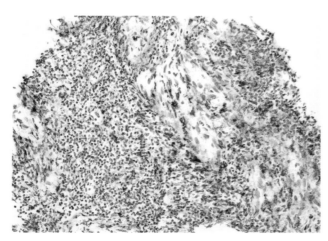

FIGURE 16.10 **Interdigitating reticulum tumor in lymph node CD68-positive spindle histiocytes.**

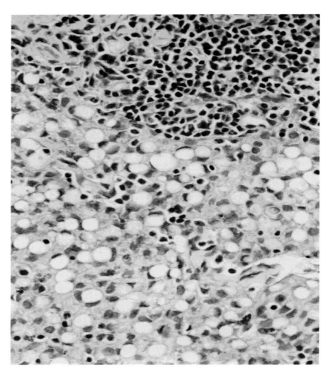

FIGURE 16.11 **Signet ring histiocytosis of pelvic lymph node sinuses with signet ring morphology H&E.** (From Guerrero-Medrano et al., 2000. Copyright Am Cancer Soc. Reprinted with permission from John Wiley and Sons, Inc.)

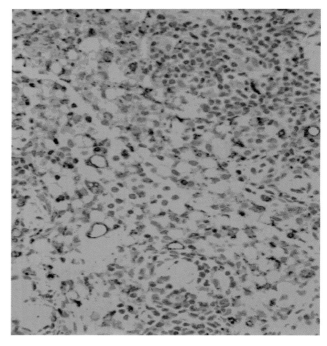

FIGURE 16.12 **Signet ring histiocytosis, CD68+, pankeratin negative.** (From Guerrero-Medrano et al., 2000. Copyright Am Cancer Soc. Reprinted with permission from John Wiley and Sons, Inc.)

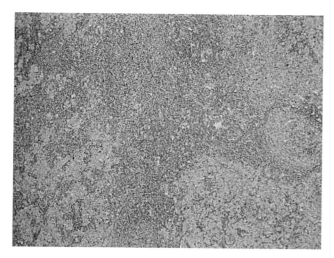

FIGURE 16.13 **Anaplastic large-cell lymphoma in sinusoidal pattern of infiltration in low-power view**.

CD35, as well as CD30, T and B markers, pankeratin, and EMA. Variable Ki67 in low percentage is seen. Although reactive cells are often of the T-cell type, tumors lack the T-cell gene rearrangement. Unlike melanoma, HMB45 and melan A are negative. The other differential diagnosis is signet ring histiocytosis (see Figure 16.11, 16.12). The following texts discuss the entities in more detail.

In patients suspected of lymphoma, the sinusoidal pattern is one of the features of CD30+ anaplastic large-cell lymphoma (ALCL) (see Figure 16.13). A prominent sinusoidal pattern in ALCL is seen in Figure 16.13. Although at low power ALCL appear to mimic sinus histiocytes, on higher power examination, they have a bland appearance only in rare cases. Mostly these cells show nuclear atypia, with the "hallmark cells" appearing multinucleated, fetaloid, or wreath-like. CD30 stains are invariably positive with variable expression of ALK-1, CD43, cytotoxic marker granzyme or TIA-1.

The most frequently found differential diagnosis in the electronic media is sinus histiocytosis with massive lymphadenopathy (SHML) (see Figure 16.14), characterized as a sinus pattern with abnormal large histiocytes with emperipolesis or lymphophagocytosis (see Figure 16.15–16.17). Emperipolesis is rare in sinus histiocytosis.

Langerhans cell histiocytosis (LCH) shows expanded lymph node sinuses by a histiocytic proliferation of langerhans histiocytes, with markers S100 and CD1a as well as CD68 (see Figure 16.18, 16.19). However, unlike SHML, Langerhans cells have smaller, oval grooved nuclei and are associated with eosinophils clusters.

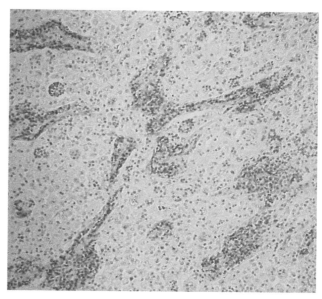

FIGURE 16.14 **Sinus pattern of Rosai–Dorfman disease**. Note the islands of lymphocytes in between the lymphophagocytic cells.

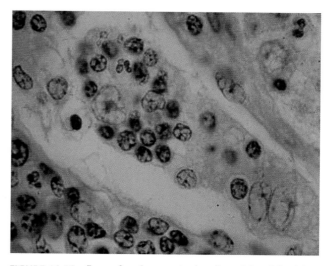

FIGURE 16.15 **Lymphophagocytosis by bland-looking macrophages in Rosai–Dorfman disease**. The detailed view shows reactive macrophages with lymphocytes, neutrophil, and plasma cell's emperopolesis. The lymphoplasmacytes and plasma cells are shown in the adjacent lower field and in the islets.

The other challenge is distinguishing the hemophagocytic syndrome, for which erythrophagocytosis or hemophagocytosis is commonly seen, displayed by a variety of reactive and neoplastic histiocytic proliferations (see Figure 16.31). Nonspecific sinus histiocytes display rare cytophagic bodies and, when present, should suggest either an infectious or autoimmune

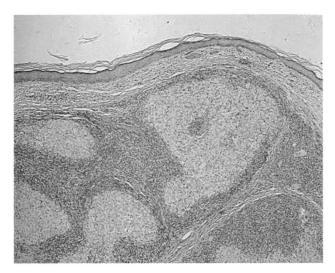

FIGURE 16.16 **Skin involved by RDD with similar sinus pattern surrounded by reactive lymphocytes**.

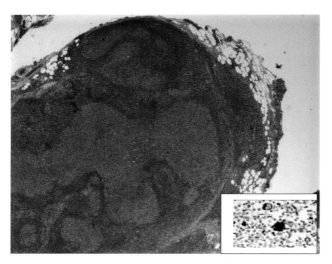

FIGURE 16.17 **CD68 (inset) in an atypical lymph node with florid follicular hyperplasia**. Note the scattered parenchymal histiocytes with lymphophagocytosis and the pericapsular extension of a recurrent RDD as CD163+ S100+ CD68+ histiocytes.

etiology. (See Table 16.2 for the neoplastic and nonreactive differential diagnosis of the sinus pattern.)

SIGNET RING HISTIOCYTOSIS

Definition

Sinus histiocytes that morphologically show a signet ring appearance.

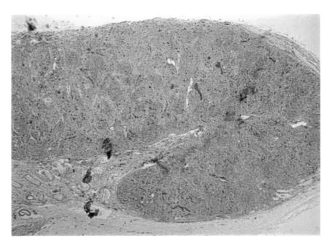

FIGURE 16.18 **Sinus pattern in low-power view in Langerhans cell histiocytosis**. The lymph node was excised from 2-year-old patient.

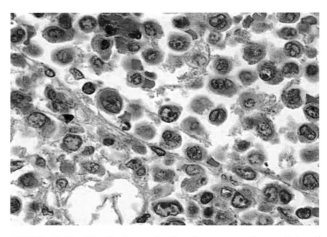

FIGURE 16.19 **Typical and classic grooved nuclei of Langerhans cell histiocytosis** (H&E 1000×).

ICD-10 Code 189.9 Noninfective disorder of lymphatic vessels and lymph nodes, unspecified

Incidence

Of 9741 lymph nodes reviewed by Guerrero-Medrano (Guerrero-Medrano, Delgado, and Bores-Saavedra, 1997), 37 (24 pelvic and 13 axillary lymph nodes) had signet-ring sinus histiocytosis, for an incidence of 0.38%.

Histology

Microscopically, distended sinuses show numerous histiocytes with clear cytoplasm and nuclei that appear as signet ring flat surface. Pale granular

TABLE 16.2 **Table Differential Diagnosis of Sinus Pattern**

Non-neoplastic	Neoplastic or Nonreactive
Sinus histiocytosis (SH) nonspecific or from tumor drainage	Metastatic disease
	Langerhans cell histiocytosis(LCH)
	Interdigitating reticulum cell sarcoma (IDRCS)
	Lymphomas
Signet ring histiocytosis	Carcinoma, lymphoma, melanoma
Pigmented sinus histiocytosis	Hemochromatosis
	Metastatic melanoma
Histiocytic reaction to foreign matter	Metastatic disease
	storage diseases
Extramedullary hematopoieisis	Granulocytic sarcoma
Sinus Histiocytosis with massive lymphadeno-pathy (or RDD)	Lymphoma with hemophagocytosis
	Malignant histiocytosis
	LCH (Langerhans cell histiocytosis)
Monocytoid hyperplasia	Marginal zone B-cell lymphomas
	MALT lymphomas
Hemophagocytic histiocytes	Lymphoma with hemophagocytosis T-cell lymphomas
Vascular transformation	Kaposi's sarcoma
	Vascular neoplasm
Whipple's disease	Enteropathy T-cell lymphoma
	T-cell lymphomas
	Storage diseases

or foamy cytoplasm is invariably present on some histiocytes. The signet ring histiocyte shows a bland dark nucleus without a nucleolus.

Cytochemistry/Immunohistochemistry

The histiocytes show with diastase-resistant, PAS positive cytoplasmic globules. These cells are immunoreactive for histiocytic markers CD68 and were pancytokeratin and lymphoid markers negative (see Figures 16.11, 16.12).

Differential Diagnosis

Metastatic carcinoma (Guerrero-Medrano, Delgado, and Bores-Saavedra, 1997; Gould et al., 1989), Frost, Shek, and Lack 1992) or signet ring lymphoma (Cross, Eyden, and Harris, 1989; Eyden, 2000; Eyden and Banerjee, 1990; Eyden, Cross, and Harris, 1990; Harris, Eyden, and Read 1981) are the foremost considerations. Signet ring histiocytes can be differentitated

from carcinoma because they usually lack nuclear atypia. These are also mucin negative.

Rarely signet ring melanoma (Sheibani and Battifora, 1988) Eckert et al., 1992) may arise. Immunostain markers for lymphoid or melanoma lineages are key to delineate these cases from signet ring histiocytosis.

SINUS HISTIOCYTOSIS WITH MASSIVE LYMPHADENOPATHY (OR ROSAI–DORFMAN DISEASE)

Since its original description in 1969 (Rosai and Dorfman, 1969), SHML has remained a disorder arising from cells of histiocytic and dendritic derivation of unknown etiology. Pathologists Rosai and Dorfman defined the entity (Rosai and Dorfman, 1972) that now bears the eponymic title Rosai–Dorfman disease (RDD).

Definition

Sinus histiocytosis with massive lymphadenopathy (SHML) is a rare disorder characterized by a non-neoplastic proliferation of cytophagocytic histiocytic cells in sinuses of lymph node and in some extranodal sites.

ICD-10 Code D76.3 D76.360

Synonyms

Destombes–Rosai–Dorfman syndrome, Rosai-Dorfman disease.

Epidemiology

SHML has worldwide distribution, with equal incidence in Caucasian and African origin, but the disorder is less seen in people of Asian descent (Foucar, Rosai, & Dorfman 1990). It is primarily a disease of children and young adults.

Etiology

Pathognomonic cells in SHML are activated phagocytic macrophages distinct from Langerhans cells, follicular dendritic cells, or interdigiting reticulum dendritic cells.

Pathogenesis

The study of pathogenesis is hampered by lack of markers specific to histiocytes, the absence of standard means for detection of monoclonality, and the clinicopathologic overlap with reactive infectious and neoplastic proliferations hinder insight into their pathogenesis. Many different infectious agents have been implicated in its pathogenesis including parvovirus B19 (Mehraein et al., 2006), HHV6 (Willman et al., 1994), but causal relationship is not established. HPV-DNA and EBV-mRNA are known to be not positive with RDD.

Recent findings suggest SHML may represent an acquired disorder of deregulation of apoptotic and other signaling pathways. Autoimmune lymphoproliferative syndrome (ALPS) has specific mutations of Fas and Fas ligand and RDD may share some of these mutations (Maric et al., 2005). Familial genetic studies disclose a cell mutation in the familial form of RDD and shares with other familial histiocytosis a nucleoside transporter mutation: belonging to SLC29 protein family (Morgan et al. 2010). Similar familial syndromes include the Faisalabad histiocytosis syndrome described in a family in Pakistan that also carry the said mutation, and these kindreds similarly show lymphadenopathy.

Clinical Aspects

The typical patient presents with fever, neutrophilic leukocytosis, elevated erythrocyte sedimentation rate, and hypergammaglobulinemia along with bilateral cervical adenopathy.

Sites of Involvement

Lymphadenopathy is the most frequent presenting finding and involves the cervical region in up to 90% of patients. Extranodal disease is documented in 43% of patients, some without lymphadenopathy or this may develop later on (Foucar, Rosai, and Dorfman, 1990). The most common extranodal sites include skin, soft tissues, upper respiratory tract, and bone. Also seen are tumors in kidneys, lower respiratory tract, and the oral cavity. Simultaneous involvement of multiple extranodal sites is not uncommon.

Morphology

Excised lymph nodes look yellow-white with capsular fibrosis. A normal lymph node architecture is often preserved and effacement indicates a longstanding lymphadenopathy. Classically, the lymph node sinuses are expanded by a proliferation of large histiocytes exhibiting round or oval vesicular nuclei with fine nuclear membranes and prominent nucleolus (Rosai and Dorfman, 1972) (see Figure 16.14). Nuclear atypia and mitoses are rare. The histiocytes show enlarged eosinophilic cytoplasm; occasionally with foamy vacuolated appearance. Associated with

the histiocytic proliferation are many reactive looking plasma cells often seen around postcapillary venules. Eosinophils are not a feature and when present raise a differential diagnosis of Langerhans histiocytosis (LCH), Hodgkin, or peripheral T-cell lymphoma. Lymphophagocytosis or emperopolesis is present with intracellular collections of lymphocytes inside the histiocytes (see Figure 16.15).

Extranodal Rosai–Dorfman disease (RDD) shows similar features to its nodal counterpart, although more fibrosis and fewer histiocytes with emperipolesis are encountered (Figure 16.16). Cutaneous RDD, without lymphadenopathy, is relatively commonly seen in dermatopathology practice usually in a setting of either old or young patient, some initially presenting with CBC abnormality of neutrophilic leucocytosis.

In RDD most of the cases show regression of enlarged lymph nodes, but in a few cases the clinical course is characterized by prolonged periods of remission and exacerbation and required therapy. In those cases surgical debulking and administration of alpha-interferon or steroids/chemotherapy were given, but usually applied in cases with organ compression or extranodal masses. Recurrence of lymphadenopathy may also prompt for excision of the lymph node given the rare association with lymphoma. Because of the rarity, histologic findings of treated RDD are not completely characterized although one such case showed a reactive lymph node follicular hyperplasia with focal residual disease characterized by parenchymal nonsinusoidal emperopolesis in histiocytes. Typical sinus histiocytosis pattern is not present (see Figure 16.17).

Immunohistochemistry/Cytochemistry.

Rosai–Dorfman histiocytes mark with CD68 (KP1 or PGM1) S100, fascin, CD31, and CD163 and negative for CD21, CD35, CD23, and CD1a (Lau, Chu, and Weiss, 2004). Other markers include pan-macrophage antigens HAM 56, CD14, CD15, as well as CD64 antigen, which is associated with phagocytosis, and a classic lysosomal marker such as lysozyme. CD31 is also positive, especially seen in our experience, in extranodal cases.

The most useful immunohistologic marker for SHML histiocytes is the expression of the S100 protein, CD163, and the lack of expression of CD1a, CD21, CD23, or CD35 (markers of dendritic differentiation). The overlap in morphologic and immunophenotypic features among histiocytic proliferation, especially in the young, requires a thorough panel to sort out the diagnosis (see Table 16.3).

TABLE 16.3 Histiocytosis and Immunophenotypic Markers

Histiocytic Disorders by Cell Type	Immunophenotypic Features					
	CD45	CD1a	S100	CD21	CD35	FactorXIII
Macrophage	+	−	±	−	−	−
Langerhans cell	+	+	+	−	−	−
Follicular dendritic cell	−	−	±	+	+	−
Interdigitating reticulum	+	−	+	−	−	−
Dendrocyte (dermal)	+	−	−	−	−	+
Indeterminate dendritic	+	±	+	−	−	−

Source: Adapted from Onciu (2004).

Differential Diagnosis

Perhaps the most frequently initial response is that of distinguishing SHML from reactive sinus histiocytic proliferations that occur as a nonspecific response to a variety of instigating agents. Emperipolesis is rare or absent in reactive histiocytic proliferations where the histiocytes are relatively small, and lymphophagocytosis absent. Although erythrophagocytosis is seen in reactive and neoplastic histiocytic proliferations, including LCH, emperipolesis of histiocytes that are not of SHML is extremely rare. Langerhans cells have frequently folded or grooved nuclei and are associated with eosinophilic microabscesses (Figures 16.18, 16.19). Bone marrow megakaryocytes may show emperopolesis, but the engulfed cells are often erythroid in lineage. Other malignancies that manifest with cytophagocytic morphology also should be considered including lymphomas, carcinomas, melanomas, and sarcomas.

Treatment of Choice and Prognosis

SHML lymphadenopathy tends to spontaneously resolve especially when presenting with a localized form. Persistence of lymphadenopathy or progression to widespread dissemination may occur, and with SHML involvement of the kidney, lower respiratory tract, or liver, the prognosis is worse. Of the 423 cases in the SHML registry, 17 patients died of persistent disease (Komp, 1990).

Treatment is not necessary in the majority of patients, but in a minority of patients showing massive nodal or extranodal tumor that is associated with organ dysfunction, treatment is needed. Steroid therapy often decreased lymphadenopathy and associated fevers. The ideal treatment for SHML is as yet undefined, and asymptomatic patient often require watchful observation.

The most frequent immune dysfunction is autoimmune hemolytic anemia, which leads to severe hemolysis or even fatality in a subset of patients. Involvement of the kidney, lower respiratory tract, and liver are associated with a worse clinical outcome. Liver and spleen involvement is uncommon.

PIGMENTED SINUS HISTIOCYTIC PATTERN SECONDARY TO IRON OVERLOAD FROM HEMOCHROMATOSIS, TRANSFUSION, OR HEMOLYSIS

ICD-10 Codes   E83.111   Iron overload due to repeated red blood cell transfusions
          E83.119   hemochromatosis

Definition

Pigmented sinus histiocytic pattern is a rare observation, usually as a complication of hemolytic anemia, blood transfusion, or a sign of hereditary disease that results in a surplus of iron deposits throughout the body manifested as pigmented sinus histiocytosis in excised lymph nodes.

Epidemiology

Although generally rare, hereditary hemochromatosis is one of the most common genetic disorders in the United States. Iron overload diseases afflict as many as 1.5 million persons in the United States. Men and women are equally affected by hemochromatosis, but women are diagnosed later in life. The disease manifest at ages of 40 to 60 years because it takes a long time to accumulate excessive iron.

Blood transfusion is common in patients with ineffective erythropoieisis such as myelodysplasia. Almost a three fold odds ratio for iron overload is seen in patients who have had frequently transfused red blood cells. (Delea, Hagiwara, and Phatak, 2009). The long-term effect of treatment of hematologic malignancies, along with transfusion, also result in secondary iron overload (Lichtman et al., 1999). In addition treatment of anemia of renal failure with parenteral iron dextran appears to be a major factor in causing iron overload in haemodialysis patients (Murray et al. 1984).

Pathogenesis

The hemochromatosis gene is called HFE and is on chromosome 6. The gene product interacts with the cell receptor for transferrin that binds and transports iron in the blood. Approximately one in nine Caucasian individuals have one abnormal hemochromatosis gene or 11% of the population. They are called carriers since they only carry one abnormal allele. About 1/200 to 1/400 persons have two abnormal genes for hemochromatosis and are homozygous and manifest the disease. Hemochromatosis is so common, however, that families and generations are seen with both diseased and carrier members. It is autosomal recessive in transmission. The disorder causes increased absorption of intestinal iron, well beyond that required to replace the normal loss of iron. In other instances secondary to administration of blood or iron products, the pathogenesis is the inability to excrete excess iron, which gets to be deposited in tissues as well as in lymph nodes.

Clinical Features

In hemochromatosis, the symptoms are commonly connected with heart failure, diabetes, or cirrhosis of the liver and includes fatigue, dyspnea, or symptoms of hyperglycemia. Pigmentation of the skin may appear bronze or a tanned or yellow (jaundice) appearance and, when combined with diabetes, has earned the alternative name "bronze diabetics."

Lymphadenopathy is also seen in iron overload secondary to hemolysis of thalassemia. Abdominal lymphadenopathy is seen in about a third of patients with thalassemia hemolytic disease (Papakonstantinou et al., 2005). Up to 32% of patients show a lymph node diameter greater than 0.8 cm with both perihepatic and periaortic lymph nodes showing lymph nodes with mean diameters of 2.2 to 2.5 cm, respectively.

Laboratory

A laboratory clue to presence of iron overload is given by testing for ferritin. The serum ferritin assay parallel the size of iron stores during normal development as well as in iron deficiency and iron overload (Siimes, Addiego Jr., and Dallman, 1974).

Morphology

Perihepatic lymphadenopathy could also be used for diagnosis of hemochromatosis and other hepatic diseases (Braden et al., 2008). Lymph node is mildly to moderately enlarged with the predominant source of expansion attributed to sinus histiocytosis. The coalescing sinuses impart a golden greenish color on low-power view. On high-power view, the hemosiderin tend to be refractile unlike many other similar brown pigments.

Although liver biopsy remains the gold standard in diagnosis, the occasional lymph node biopsied for suspicion of neoplasm may reveal a brown lymph node on cut section and histologically show sinus histiocytosis with iron deposits. Sinuses are dilated with presence of golden brown hemosiderin deposits in sinus histiocytes visible in low power magnification (see Figure. 16.20).

Differential Diagnosis

There are a multitude of pigments that cause sinus histiocytosis. These include melanin, hemosiderin, lipofuscin, anthracosis, carbon particles, metals, tatoo,

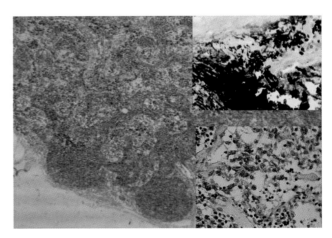

FIGURE 16.20 Hemochromatosis. Low-power view shows prominent pigmented sinus histiocytosis and generally preserved architecture. (Inset, right bottom) High-power view shows dense and interspersed refractile golden pigment laden macrophages. (Inset, right top). The granular golden pigments stained with Prussian blue, consistent with iron laden hemosiderin pigments, Pearls Iron stain.

as well as malaria pigments. Appropriate cytochemical stains are available in most places to determine the type of deposits. Pigmented melanoma has to be ruled out with morphologic exam and immunohistostains.

Treatment

Treatment is reserved for underlying conditions as well treatment with iron chelating regimen. In patients younger than 40 years who have a serum ferritin concentration of less than 750 ng/ml and normal liver enzyme levels, phlebotomy therapy may preceed any biopsy. In all other cases, biopsy is recommended for diagnosis and optimal management.

HISTIOCYTIC REACTION TO FOREIGN MATTER

Definition

Histiocytic reaction to foreign matter is predominantly a histiocytic reaction to injected or adsorbed substances such as lipodiol, polyvinylpyrrolidone (PVP) plasma cell expander, as well as hip replacement materials including metals (gold, cobalt/chromium/titanium) or plastic-like polyesters, polyethylene, or polyformaldehyde.

Lymphangiographic Effect

Lymphangiography was in common use for staging lymphomas about five decades ago. The side effects include lipodiol lymphangiographic lymphadenopathy (Ravel 1966). Although this modality has since been replaced by newer techniques (Armitage 2010), this pattern of lymphadenopathy has many mimics and may not just be a manifestation of lipodiol injections.

Lipid deposition from radio-opaque lipid-based dye has similar features with other lipid deposition lymphadenopathy. These include lipid lymphadenopathy from parenteral hyperalimentation, exogenous administration of lipid-based vitamin supplements, mineral oil enema, and fatty skin emolients. Gallbladder disease may also contribute to cholelipodystrophic lipogranulomatous findings in lymph nodes draining the biliary duct system. However, the most dramatic changes are those from direct injection of lipid contrast dyes to map out the visceral extent of Hodgkin lymphoma. An exuberant classic reaction to lipid characterizes this type of lymphadenopathy.

Morphology

The specimen is often an abdominal lymph node sampled during a staging laparotomy. The dominant pattern is the presence of sinusoidal expansion and prominent vacuoles of clear fatty appearance. The oily substance is not visible in the paraffin-processed section but only in fresh frozen materials. Histologically, the vacuoles are surrounded by reactive phagocytic cells and many confluent clusters of epithelioid histiocytes. There are multinucleated foreign body giant cells, some with oval or rounded intracellular materials. Scalloped vacuolated contours and partially digested small fat vacuoles can be seen inside and outside the giant cells. The appearance may be related to the duration of reaction so that early changes may consists mostly of sinus histiocytosis with numerous histiocytes with rare giant cells (see Figure 16.21). With longer duration, numerous foreign body giant cells are characteristic (see Figure 16.22).

Differential Diagnosis

Unlike Whipple's disease, which it resembles, postlymphangiogram finding does not include of PAS+ granular intracellular materials. Storage diseases may show expanded foamy or textured histiocytes: tissue paper texture for Gaucher's disease (Figure 16.23) and foamy PAS+ granules in Nieman–Pick diseases (Figure 16.24).

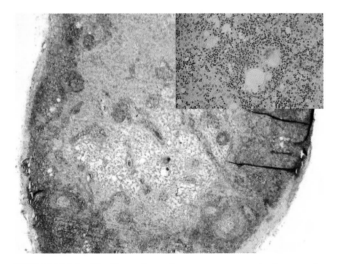

FIGURE 16.21 **Postlymphangiogram mesenteric node post-Hodgkin staging with a prominent pale sinusoidal pattern and visible clear vacuoles in low-power view**. (Inset). Giant cells with scalloped edges engulfing oily material. Background small lymphocytes, plasma cells, and eosinophils and epithelioid sarcoidal granuloma are present.

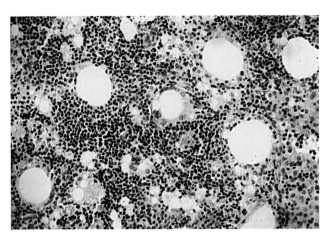

FIGURE 16.22　Clusters of epitheloid histiocytes in sinuses and few multinucleated foreign body giant cell reactions.

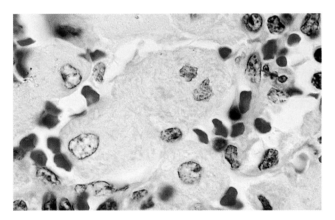

FIGURE 16.23　Gaucher's "crumpled tissue paper" cytoplasm.

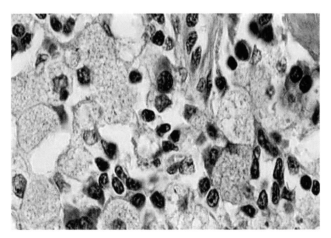

FIGURE 16.24　Foamy pink granular PAS macrophages in Nieman–Pick disease.

Cholegranulomatous Lymphadenitis

The location of lymphadenopathy overlaps with that of lymphangiography lymphadenopathy. Often the patient has gallbladder complaint and cholecystitis. The cystic and hepatic nodes are usually affected.

Histology. Characteristic lesions are foamy macrophage collections in sinuses. Vacuoles from fatty endogenous materials are present in both subcapsular and intermediate sinuses, sometimes with prominent foreign body giant cell reaction and lymphoid reactive nodules. Bile can sometimes be seen inside the phagocytic macrophages. Sarcoidal noncaseating granulomas may also be seen.

Hyperlipidemia

In both exogenous and endogenous origin, hyperlipidemia induces lipid granulomas. The lipid granulomas contain foamy macrophages, and faintly pigmented macrophages, which are Sudanophilic and stain faintly with PAS, given their lipoid origin. Touton-type giant cells are more common than the foreign body giant cell type.

Hip Replacement Adenopathy

There are many foreign body materials that are included with hip replacement surgery, and each component such as polyesters or metals may incite a histiocytic reaction (Benz et al., 1996, Gray et al., 1989).

Lymphadenopathy from Polyesters/Polyethylene

By light microscopy, the lymph nodes from patients show dilated nodal sinuses filled with macrophages with eosinophilic, PAS-positive, granular material. Polarization microscopy shows needle-like particles within the cytoplasm. This is a florid foreign body reaction to fragments of polyester or polyethylene derived from the articulating surfaces of the joint prostheses. Routine stain show expanded sinus macrophages with adjacent normal lymphocytes. Polyethylene particles are identified by their characteristic needle-like shape and bright birefringence under polarized light, within macrophages and multinucleated giant cells.

Lymphadenopathy Secondary to Metals

Usually after hip replacement, the pelvic lymph nodes becomes enlarged with a black brown cut surface. Histologically, there is florid sinus histiocytosis by polygonal pink large histiocytes filling the sinuses and interfollicular regions. The histiocytes are foamy and the cytoplasm contains cobalt-chromium and titanium microparticles elucidated using ultrastructure and X- ray microanalysis (Albores-Saavedra et al., 1994). The lymph nodes uninvolved by the histiocytic reaction lack the heavy metal microparticles. Polyethylene particles are also present, inciting the histiocytic response. By immunohistochemistry, the foamy cells display immunoreactivity for macrophage-associated markers such as CD68 and lysozyme.

Polyvinylpyrrolidone (PVP) or Mucicarminophilic Lymphadenopathy

After a mammaplasty with associated silicone injection, histiocytes become mucicarmine-positive secondary to a silicone lymphadenopathy. Signet ring, foamy, or globule-filed histiocytes are present. Some contain small globules of electron dense, granular material similar to that seen in the histiocytes with giant lysosomes or lipofuscin granules. Mucicarminophilic histiocytosis is secondary to the histiocytes containing PVP (Kuo and Hsueh, 1984).

SINUS PATTERN FROM EXTRAMEDULLARY HEMATOPOIESIS

Definition

Extramedullary hematopoiesis (EMH) is the presence of hematopoietic tissue outside of the bone marrow.

ICD-10 Codes   C92.3 myeloid sarcoma;
C94 Other leukemias;
D75 Other diseases of blood, unspecified

Epidemiology

In an adult, EMH should engender confirmatory studies to determine a benign or malignant cause. EMH in liver, spleen, and lymph nodes is normal in infants and young children.

EMH of varied etiology can localize in lymph nodes in only 15% of a reported series (Koch et al., 2003). However, findings at autopsy of patients with myelofibrosis, lymph nodes followed by kidneys are the most common sites of EMH (Pitcock et al., 1962).

Etiology

Any disorder that cause displacement of marrow elements by restricting the marrow space can cause EMH. These include bone trabeculae anomalies such as osteoid fibrosis, uremic osteitis, Paget's disease, as well as tumors or fibrosises such as myeloma and myeloproliferative disorders. In adults, myeloproliferative syndromes and treatment with myeloproliferative cytokines have also been associated with extramedullary hematopoiesis (see Tables 16.4, 16.5). In children, any hereditary disorders of red cells and anemia can cause EMH.

The disorder can be due to any of the following pathogeneses:

1. Damage to marrow microenvironment.
2. Clonal expansion secondary to malignant myeloid proliferation.
3. Hyperplasia of benign marrow elements secondary to extrinsic stimuli such as drugs or myeloid stimulating cytokine factors.
4. Incidental presence of marrow elements as these are trapped passing through the microvasculature of any organ, namely lungs and, lymph nodes.

TABLE 16.4 Conditions Associated with Extramedullary Hematopoieisis

Primary myelofibrosis
Thalassemia
Hereditary spherocytosis
Sickle cell anemia
Congenital dyserythropoietic anemia
Immune thrombocytopenic purpura
Chronic myeloid leukemia
Polycythemia vera
Myelodysplastic syndrome
Paget disease
Osteopetrosis
Gaucher disease
Treatment with myeloid growth factors
Acute leukemia
Idiopathic

TABLE 16.5 Locations of EMH

Organs Involved by EMH	Frequency
Spinal/thoracic tissue	26%
Lymph nodes	15%
Retroperitoneum	15%
Lungs pleura	11%
Genitourinary	7%
Cutaneous	7%
Others	19%

Source: Adapted from Koch et al. (2003).

Approach to Diagnosis

Clinical history, hematopoietic status including bone marrow or peripheral blood findings, and heme molecular testing are required to resolve the benign or malignant nature of the infiltrate especially when atypical cell precursors are identified.

Morphology

Lymph nodes with EMH are often normal to mildly enlarged. There is sparing of the residual follicles and paracortex even by extensive extramedullary hematopoiesis. Incidental megakaryocytes trapped in sinuses or pulp may be seen in patients without a hematologic disease (see Figure 16.25).

The pattern, as visualized on low-power view showing as pale areas, is generally of sinus or interfollicular appearance. The pale areas on high-power view often show a mixture of elements in benign or nonleukemic conditions: the most striking cells at low power are the megakaryocytes appearing dark multilobated and larger than surrounding cells. Other cells may be erythroid or myeloid lineage. Sheets of red cell precursors may also be prominent and obvious on low power as perfectly rounded dark nuclei with evenly distributed internuclear spaces (see Figure 16.26). This pattern is from the abundant red cell cytoplasm in nucleated red cell precursors. When sheets of cells are composed of more immature cells, erythroblasts may be difficult to differentiate from myeloblasts. Short of using stem cell immunostains, PAS stain may help the distinction by coloring myeloid precursors pink, erythroid

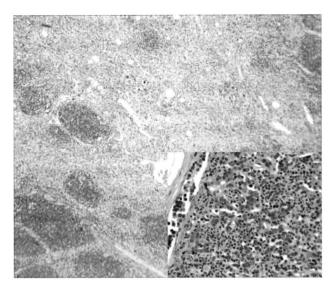

FIGURE 16.26 **Sinusoidal or interfollicular pattern of mature extramedullary hematopoieisis.** (40×inset). Medium power of expanded sinus spaces and pulp infiltrated by many nucleated red cell precursors as well as pronormoblasts.

precursors gray or clear, and megakaryocytes fuschia red.

Often benign EMH are focal and does not form a mass. The most common situation is an incidental single or few megarkaryocytes seen in a surgical specimen such as tissue from lung, liver, spleen or lymph node (see Figure 16.25).

Neoplastic infiltrate may be multifocal, sinusoidal or may obliterate the lymph node architecture with immature extramedullary hematopoiesis. In this situation, megakaryocytes usually form clusters and may be dysplastic (see Figure 16.27).

Differential Diagnosis

The differential diagnosis of EMH include immature extramedullary hematopoieisis and granulocytic sarcoma. Morphologically, the distinction may be difficult and ancillary immunostain is key: seeing CD34 and CD117 markers are positive in cluster of blasts. Lack of sheets of blasts suggest an immature extramedullary hematopoieisis, a finding that may be seen associated in majority with myelodysplasia or myeloproliferative diseases. In certain organs, like the uterus, there has been found nevertheless no association of a multilineage EMH with hematopoeietic neoplasm except for presence of anemia in many of these patients (Gru et al. 2010).

The most important disease in the differentiation is myeloid sarcoma. In differentiating benign

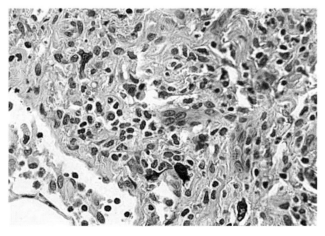

FIGURE 16.25 **High-power view of incidental presence of entrapped mature megakaryocytes in the lymph node sinuses and parenchyma.** The dark mishapen nuclei of megakarycytes are visible in between reactive lymphocytes.

TABLE 16.6 Morphologic Features of Benign and Neoplastic Extramedullary Proliferations

Non-neoplastic	Neoplastic
Megakaryocytes common	Megakaryocytes present dysplastic
Erythroid cells identifiable	Immature left-shifted multilineage proliferation with clusters of immature myeloid cells (CD34+ CD117+ blasts most often seen)
Multilineage proliferation of mature forms	
May be normal in infants	
Abnormal in adults: Marrow hyperplasia Marrow fibrosis Myelophtysis Metastasis Osteitis Drugs/cytokine treatment	Clinically with concurrent myeloproliferative or myelodysplastic diseases

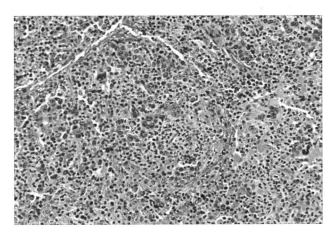

FIGURE 16.27 **Immature EMH spilled into the nodal pulp with sheets of dysplastic megakaryocytes and mononuclear cell infiltrate in the sinuses**. The patient has primary myelofibrosis and lymphadenopathy with transformation to acute leukemia.

and malignant EMH, clinical history is important (see Table 16.6). Although morphologic clues are not infallible, they may be useful in deciding whether to perform additional studies. The presence of sheets or clusters of immature myeloid or blast cells, and dysplastic megakaryocytes, would be in favor of neoplasm especially if clusters of CD117, CD34, or TdT staining cells are present.

Immunohistochemistry

Rare or no expression of CD34, CD117, or TdT favor mature nonneoplastic EMH or a immature

differentiated extramedullary hematopoieisis. Chronic myeloproliferative disorders may also display mature or immature extramedullary hematopoiesis, and diagnosis may need direct bone marrow evaluation. Diffuse positivity for stem cell markers supports diagnosis of myeloid sarcoma. In extramedullary sites like the skin, a CD3-negative CD43-positive phenotype supports a myelomonocytic infiltrate. In those cases co-expression with CD68, CD45 on blasts arrayed in linear pattern is supportive. Expression of many cells with CD34 or CD117, or in their absence, typical blasts cluster, may signal leukemic change of chronic myeloid neoplasm or myelodysplasia to an acute myeloid leukemia. Molecular or cytogenetic abnormalities are confirmatory. Presence of cytogenetic abnormalities by conventional karyotype or FISH support a diagnosis of neoplastic proliferation. Specific defects like t(9;22) or JAK2 (Hsieh et al., 2007) mutation can confirm diagnosis.

Treatment

For incidental findings treatment may not be required, but for symptomatic patients with neoplastic underlying diseases, treatment is directed to the specific disease. In symptomatic patients secondary to mass effect of reactive ectopic hematopoietic tissue, low doses of radiation may be useful (Koch, et al., 2003).

IMMATURE "SINUS HISTIOCYTOSIS" OR MONOCYTOID B-CELL HYPERPLASIA

Marginal zone B cells and monocytoid B cells (MBC) are morphologically similar, and because these cells are found in similar locations, the prevailing understanding seems to equate the two as similar if not identical (Camacho, et al., 2001).

Location of Marginal Zone Cells

Careful examination of the cytology of the cells between the sinus and the mantle lymphocytes will show an inconspicuous collection of lymphocytes with a larger amount of pale-staining cytoplasm characteristic of marginal zone lymphocytes. These cells are not prominent except in certain reactive conditions, in splenic white pulp, and in mesenteric and abdominal lymph nodes.

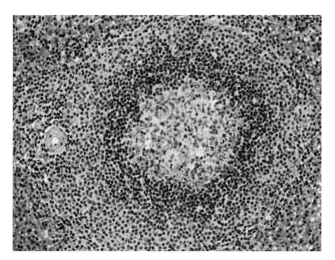

FIGURE 16.28 **Marginal zone B cells in spleen**.

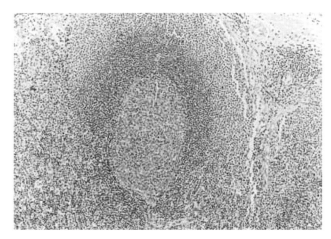

FIGURE 16.29 **Marginal zone B cell in mesenteric lymph node**.

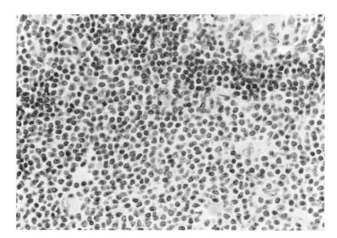

FIGURE 16.30 **High-power view of marginal zone cells in relation to mantle cells (top)**.

Plasma cells and plasmacytic differentiation may be present.

Marginal zone B cells are associated with normal histology in spleen, in mesenteric lymph nodes, and in Peyer's patch centers. These marginal zone lymphocytes are often prominent in the reactive white pulp in splenic follicles (see Figure 16.28), in mesenteric lymph nodes, as well as underneath the surface of the mucosal membrane of the intestinal tract as normal Peyer'patches. Marginal zone B cells, localized in the marginal sinus of the spleen, are functionally associated with immune complex transport to the follicular dendritic cells in mice, and it remains to be seen if these cells' function is similar to those in humans (Ferguson, Youd, and Corley, 2004). These cells may also form a prominent marginal zone in lymph nodes adjacent to a MALT lymphoma (see Figure 16.29, 16.30).

Location of Monocytoid B Cells (MBCs)

Subcapsular and peritrabecular sinuses may contain an arc or band of monocytoid cells with clear cytoplasm. In some nodes these cells also encompass the perifollicular location akin to the location of marginal zone B cells. Cytological features of MBCs are the presence of abundant pale to clear cytoplasm, medium size, and bland-looking irregular nuclei with inconspicuous nucleoli. Segmented neutrophils are often seen in these aggregates.

Monocytoid B cells can also be seen in perifollicular locations in reactive conditions, although marginal zone lymphocytes typically comprise these areas. The monocytoid B cells often have associated neutrophils, often within their centers, but marginal zone B cells tend to have plasmacytic differentiation.

Differential Diagnosis

Monocytoid B cells (MBCs) are a subset of B cells that may be recognized in several reactive and tumoral lymph node conditions, including toxoplasmic lymphadenitis, (Stansfeld 1961), infectious mononucleosis, and Hodgkin lymphoma (Ohsawa et al. 1994).

Relationship of MBCs and Marginal Zone Hyperplasia

A relationship of MBCs with marginal zone (MZ) B lymphocytes has been claimed for this B-cell subpopulation, based mainly on architectural localization and cytology. Although a clear relationship may be established between splenic MZ cells and Peyer's patches MZ lymphocytes, based on the presence of an immunophenotype of IgM1, IgD2 (Spencer et al., 1985; Spencer and Dogan, 2009), the immunophenotype of MZ cells in mesenteric lymph nodes or spleens differs strongly from that which is observed in MBCs. Thus MZ cells show distinct immunoglobulin staining (IgM), bcl-2 expression, with a low growth fraction. Monocytoid cells are often Bcl-2 and CD43 negative while marginal zone B cells origin of marginal zone lymphoma are Bcl2 and CD43 positive. All reactive monocytoid cells are basically bcl-2-negative cells. In contrast, nodal MZ lymphoma, and splenic MZ lymphoma show a distinct expression of IgM and bcl-2 (Camacho et al., 2001).

These features could be used to separate reactive monocytoid hyperplasia from marginal zone B cell lymphoma. Nodal MZ lymphoma cases display an immunophenotype different from the one observed in MBCs, and similar to that of MZ B cells. Most tumoral cells in all cases showed bcl-2 positivity.

REACTIVE HEMOPHAGOCYTIC SYNDROMES

Definition

Hemophagocytic syndrome (HS) is a rare hematologic disorder that typically manifests as fever, splenomegaly, and jaundice and has the pathologic finding of hemophagocytic lymphohistiocytosis (HLH).

ICD-10 Codes D76.1, D76.2

Synonyms

Histiocytic medullary reticulosis, reactive hemophagocytic lymphohistiocytosis.

Etiology

HS has been associated with the following disorders (Risdall 1984):

1. Malignancies.
2. Genetic mutations (i.e., familial hemophagocytic lymphohistiocytosis).
3. Infections (e.g., EBV, HIV).
4. Autoimmune diseases (e.g., connective tissue disease).

Morphology

Hemophagocytic lymphohistiocytosis describes the pathologic finding of activated macrophages, engulfing erythrocytes, leukocytes, platelets, and their precursor cells seen in bone marrow, liver, or lymph nodes (see Figure 16.31). These cells appear to be "stuffed" with other blood cells and has been sometimes called "bean-bag" cells.

Pathogenesis

Hemophagocytosis is a hallmark of overstimulated macrophages. Most studies of the pathogenesis of HLH favor a defect in the regulatory and effector lymphocyte pathways, resulting in a dysregulated immune response.

Pediatric Hemophagocytic Syndrome

Genetic mutations in the inherited form, or "familial hemophagocytic lymphohistiocytosis," an autosomal recessive disorder, is invariably fatal when untreated. It is the main subset of pediatric hemophagocytic syndrome. Typically patients become acutely ill with high and unremitting fever. Splenomegaly is the second most common clinical finding and can be associated with hepatomegaly, lymphadenopathy, jaundice, and CNS symptoms. These clinical findings are suggestive of acute viral infections such as the Epstein–Barr virus (EBV) infection, cytomegalovirus infection, or viral hepatitis, and the diagnosis is further complicated by the association of these infections with HLH.

Activated T cells and macrophages infiltrate multiple organs, and histopathologically, hemophagocytosis is seen in bone marrow, spleen, liver, lymph

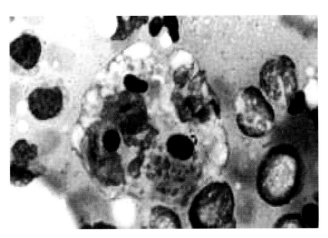

FIGURE 16.31 **Cytophagic histiocytes with nucleated red cells, platelets, and neutrophils engulfed inside the cytoplasm.**

nodes, and occasionally the CNS and skin. In the brain, the inflammatory cells form perivascular foci, suggesting a blood-derived tissue infiltration.

Familial Hemophagocytic Lymphohistiocytosis (FHL)

This syndrome was first described by Farquhar (Farquhar, Macgregor, and Richmond, 1958) as familial erythrophagocytic lymphohistiocytosis. The incidence of FHL has been estimated to be 1 in 50,000 births. FHL is invariably lethal unless treatment with allogeneic stemcell transplantation is performed.

Molecular defects underlying FHL include perforin and munc 13–4 deficiencies, and these features account for two-thirds of patients with FHL. Patients whose disease is associated with FHL3 locus present typical features of FHL and are indistinguishable from patients with a perforin (i.e., FHL2) defect (Morgan NV et al, 2010).

Primary hemophagocytosis is a hallmark of overstimulated macrophages. Genetic defects in perforin-mediated cytotoxicity have been identified in HLH. Perforin is a pore-forming protein secreted by activated cytotoxic T lymphocytes and natural killer (NK) cells that is critical for inducing the apoptosis of infected target cells. Patients with defective cell-mediated cytotoxicity, but normal expression of perforin and other proteins involved in cytotoxicity, can also manifest HLH.

Acquired Hemophagocytic Lymphohistiocytosis

Autoimmune-associated hemophagocytic syndrome is associated with rheumatoid diseases. In the early 1980s several reports described patients with systemic onset juvenile rheumatoid arthritis (JRA). Several recent observations have demonstrated that RA patients appear to be deficient in their ability to regulate EBV infection and that B cells in the blood of patients with RA are frequently infected by EB viruses.

Although HS has also been observed in a small number of patients with polyarticular JRA and in those with collagen diseases (including lupus, vasculitis, Kawasaki disease, dermatomyositis, and panniculitis), it is most commonly seen in patients with the systemic form of JRA.

A hemophagocytic syndrome associated with SLE has been reported in Hong Kong as acute lupus hemophagocytic syndrome (ALHS) (Wong et al., 1991). ALHS was described as SLE with febrile illness, fulminant pancytopenia, and bone marrow proliferation of reactive histiocytes that phagocytize hemopoietic cells.

VASCULAR TRANSFORMATION OF SINUSES (VTS)

Definition

Reactive replacement of the lymph node sinuses into capillary-like vascular channels, often accompanied by fibrosis.

ICD-10 Code D18.0

Synonyms

Angiomyomatous hamartoma hemangiomatoid transformation, nodal angiomatosis, stasis lymphadenopathy.

Epidemiology

VTS has sex predilection and occurs at any age. It is worldwide in distribution.

Etiology

Venous obstruction occurs, as well as lymphatic vessel obstruction derived from any etiology including tumoral masses, thrombosis, congestive cardiac disorders, or even the presence of an angiogenic paraneoplastic effect from cancer (Catalano et al., 2002; Meysman et al., 1997).

Pathophysiology

Venous or lymphatic obstruction is thought to be the underlying mechanism, and contributing factors include adjacent tumor, thrombosis, congestive heart failure, previous surgery, or radiotherapy (Samet et al. 2001).

Clinical Aspects

The at-risk population includes postsurgical patients, patients with heart or lung conditions that increase pulmonary vascular pressure and patients with local radiotherapy. In addition the presence of tumor that caused the vascular stasis is associated with development of VTS.

Sites of Involvement

Most cases involve the abdominal areas. Rarely, the head and neck lymph nodes are involved.

Approach to Diagnosis

Most cases are incidental findings associated with a workup for lymph node metastasis in a patient with known carcinoma.

Morphologic Aspects

The lymph node may be normal or enlarged with fatty or fibrous consistency. The cut section often shows a thickening of the hilum with no capsular fibrosis. On histology, the architecture is generally preserved (Figures 16.32, 16.33) with a conspicuous nodularity and dilated or ectatic vessels, most appreciated in the medulla (see Figure 16.32). The lymph node is compartmentalized and each compartment is bounded by pale looking band of fine vessels without intraluminal blood (see Figure 16.33). These bands are secondary to a vasoproliferative expansion of the subcapsular, intermediate, and medullary sinuses of the lymph nodes that have transformed to a hemangiomatoid histopathology (Chan, Warnke, and Dorfman, 1991). Single or multiple lymph nodes in a chain may show the same findings. On high-power view, there is an anastomosing of narrow-clefted channels. A sieve-like or solid appearance may be seen, some with rounded lumina, some with flat or plump endothelial lining, and often associated with variable degrees of sclerosis (see Figure 16.34, 16.35). The vascular spaces may be empty or filled with lymph-like fluid, and the larger rounded vessels may be with some blood or occasionally thrombosed. Extravasation of red cells

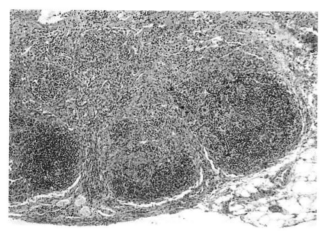

FIGURE 16.32 **VTS**. A sparing of the lymph node parenchyma is seen in low power view. Note the disproportionate lack of capsular thickened sclerosis.

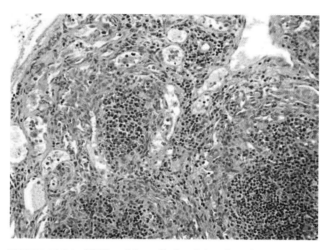

FIGURE 16.34 **VTS with cellular islands admixed with solid sheets of spindly pink endothelial cells and dilated channels with scant cells**.

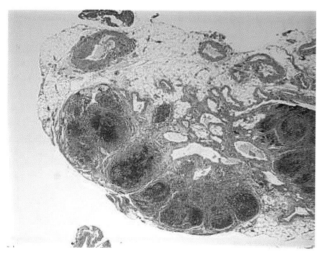

FIGURE 16.33 **VTS with capsule spared**. The capsule was not thickened with nodular comparmentalized composite nodules of lymphoid cells. The architecture is mostly preserved but with dilated thick-walled vessels and vascularized subcapsular, intermediate, and medullary sinuses as seen in low power.

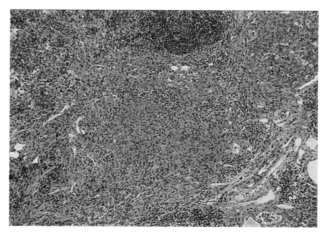

FIGURE 16.35 **VTS with solid and diffuse pattern in the subcapsular and intermediate sinuses obliterated by solid sheets of spindled cells**.

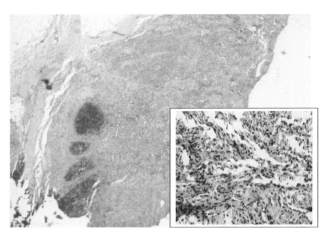

FIGURE 16.36 **Kaposi sarcoma with solid areas from the hilum to the capsules**. (Inset) Atypical distinct spindles cells.

is common. A nodular spindle cell variant that is worrisome for Kaposi sarcoma (KS) is described (see Figure 16.36) (Cook et al., 1995).

Immunohistochemistry/Cytochemistry

The endothelial nature of the vessels is characterized by factor VIII (Scherrer and Maurer 1985) with admixed myofibroblasts and actin filaments (Michal, Koza, and Fakan, 1992).

Differential Diagnosis

The solid form of the vascular transformation may resemble Kaposi's sarcoma. Morphologically, the subtle difference in VTS may include a pure sinusoidal instead of parenchymal distribution, the absence of distinct spindle cellularity in the fascicles, and the lack of associated capsular fibrosis as is frequently seen in Kaposi's sarcoma. On high-power view, areas with well-formed vascular channels, arrayed in nodular compartments, and lack of nuclear atypia favor VTS more than KS.

The bacillary angiomatosis may show a nodular vascular proliferation with blood-filled lumina in the nodal parenchyma. Special stains for *Bartonella spp.* can be used to sort out difficult cases. Inflammatory pseudotumor tends to have a prominent capsular fibrosis with extensive involvement of the nodal framework, and fibroblastic as well as plasmacytic infiltration. Other parenchymal vascular tumors include the vascular hamartomas and angiomas, which tend to have prominent vessels instead of spindled elements.

Hemangiomas of capillary/cavernous types show compact aggregates of blood-filled vessels, variable in size, that replace the nodal architecture partly or almost completely with associated acute or chronic inflammatory cells, and those associated with the hilum may be difficult to separate from the VTS. These are often inside the parenchyma instead of inside the sinuses. Likewise the parenchymal epithelioid hemangioendothelioma variant, with the spindle and epithelioid cells and hemangioendothelioma, may be difficult to distinguish from VTS except for its localization. Lymphangiomas of lymph nodes usually show simultaneous multifocal and extranodal involvement and are characterized by cystic endothelium-lined spaces filled predominantly with lymph fluid.

Treatment of Choice and Prognosis

Surgically excised VTS, unlike the similar looking but treatable neoplasms, may require no treatment.

WHIPPLE'S DISEASE (WD) LYMPHADENOPATHY

First described by American pathologist George Whipple in 1903, it was only in 1961 that a bacterial etiology was considered for Whipple's disease based on ultrastructural and light microscopy. *T. whippelii* was partially characterized at the molecular level by PCR in 1991, which contributed to its improved diagnosis. Despite these improvements, the disease presents with variable manifestations and is still a diagnostic challenge, if not considered in a differential diagnosis. Relman et al. (1992) proposed the new genus and species designation "*Tropheryma whippelii*." This name derives from the Greek words "trophe" meaning nourishment, "eryma" meaning barrier in reference to the malabsorption syndrome, and "*whippelii*" to honor George H. Whipple.

Definition

WD is a disease caused by bacterial *Tropheryma whippelii*.

ICD-10 Code K90.8

Synonyms

Intestinal lipodystrophy.

Epidemiology and Geolocation

Whipple's disease (WD) is considered a rare pathology, with less than 1000 cases having been reported.

In postmortem studies, the frequency of the disease is quoted as being less than 0.1%.

WD predominantly affects Caucasian males, with a male-to-female ratio of approximately 8:1 and a mean age of onset around 50 years. Some studies have shown a statistically significantly higher prevalence of Whipple's disease in farmers than in persons with other occupations (Dobbins, III 1995).

Etiology

The organism belongs to the Gram-positive actinomycetes. Members of this class are present in a wide range of habitats including the soil, where they are active in the decomposition of organic materials.

Pathogenesis

Certain genetic factors influencing the body's immune system may accelerate the disease. This theory is supported by the existence of a relatively high number of asymptomatic carriers. A specific genetic susceptibility to the illness is suggested by the fact that about 30% of people with Whipple disease have a specific abnormality in their T cells.

Tropheryma whippellii infection can cause intestinal villi lesions, take on an abnormal, club-like appearance. The damaged intestinal lining fails to properly absorb nutrients, causing diarrhea and malnutrition. Anemia is caused by vitamin B_{12} malabsorption, intestinal blood loss, and iron deficiency. Hypoalbuminemia is frequent and is largely due to malabsorption.

Clinical Aspects

Initial symptoms of the disease include fever, muscle pain, heart murmur, pedal edema, and lymphadenopathy. Long-term infection leads to joint pains, weight loss, anemia in up to 90% and diarrhea in up to 85% of cases. Whipple disease can be chronic, fall into a relapse, and persist in the body of the host after treatment. Infection of the heart can lead to endocarditis. It can also lead to myocarditis and/or pericarditis. Rare involvement of the central nervous system can lead to severe illness with loss of memory, seizures, dementia, and death.

Sites of Involvement

Systemic symptoms like fever, night sweats, and lymphadenopathy are quite frequent in Whipple's disease. Lymphadenopathy comprise 40 to 60% of cases (Dutly and Altwegg, 2001).

Approach to Diagnosis

Culture has not been successful. False-positive PCR has been found in gastric fluid and/or duodenal biopsy specimens in at least 10% of persons without clinical manifestations typical of Whipple's disease (Ehrbar et al., 1999) and in the saliva of at least 30% of healthy individuals (Street, Donoghue, and Neild, 1999).

In the absence of clinical clues or radiological evidence (i.e., thickening of bowel wall seen in CT scan), in order to confirm Whipple's disease, laboratory tests play a pivotal role. These include biopsy for histology with microbiology and PAS staining, including PCR on tissue specimens, as well as using joints fluid or cerebrospinal fluid specimen.

Pathognomonic PAS-positive macrophages may also be present in the peripheral and mesenteric lymph nodes and various other organs. PAS-positive macrophages may be found in liver, spleen, joints, bone marrow, heart, lungs, CNS, eyes, and mediatinal lymph nodes underlining the systemic nature of the disease. Gastric or rectal biopsy specimens are not recommended to diagnose Whipple's disease, since faintly PAS-positive lipid-containing macrophages in the stomach and strongly PAS-positive macrophages in the rectum have been observed in patients with other diseases. In addition a finding of granulomas does not rule out WD. Whipple's granulomas similar to sarcoid has been reported, and up to 40% of sarcoidal granulomas in Whipple's are PAS negative.

Morphologic Aspects

The confirmation of Whipple's disease is based on the demonstration of PAS-positive inclusions in macrophages detected mainly in the lamina propria of duodenal biopsy specimens or in excised lymph node (see Figure 16.37, 16.38). In intestinal biopsies there is villous atrophy and bulbous distension of the normal villous architecture by an infiltrate of foamy macrophages with a coarsely granular cytoplasm, which stain a magenta color with PAS. The nodes are easily palpable and are clinically indistinguishable from lymphadenopathy due to other infectious diseases, sarcoidosis, or lymphomas. Lymphomas associated with Whipple's disease are also reported (Fest et al., 1996, Gillen et al., 1993). A few cases with mediastinal lymphadenopathy have been described (Kubaska et al., 1998).

Ultrastructure by Electron Microscopy

Although this modality was used in the recent past, this approach may still be used if all other findings are not forthcoming. The bacteria are free

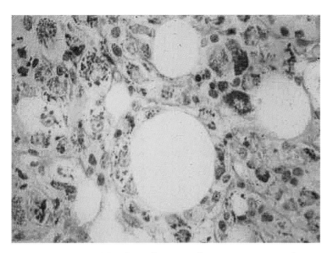

FIGURE 16.37 **Whipple's disease.** The sinus patterns shows medullary sinuses packed with PAS-positive particles phagocytosed by macrophages.

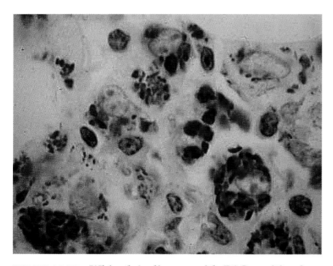

FIGURE 16.38 **Whipple's disease with PAS positive bacterial in macrophages.** In this view, the appearance of these bacteria is described as taking a "sickle form."

dense bodies with a diameter of 0.25 microns and a trilaminar cell wall. Whipple's disease bacteria can be found inside or outside the cells. WD can also be found inside the cytoplasm of peripheral blood mononuclear cells and CSF macrophages.

Immunohistochemistry/Cytochemistry

The PAS-positive material remaining in the foamy macrophages corresponds to the mucopolysaccharide-containing capsule of the bacteria. The Gram-positive staining and the staining with Giemsa support the view that these structure's are bacteria.

Differential Diagnosis

PAS-positive macrophages can be seen in association with other infectious agents (e.g., *M. avium-intracellulare*). To distinguish Whipple's disease from infections due to *M. avium* and *M. intracellulare* in AIDS patients, an acid-fast stain of the biopsy specimen is required. Whipple's disease bacilli are not acid fast. However, granulomas related to Whipple's disease may be PAS negative. Therefore, electron microscopy or PCR may be required to confirm the diagnosis (Wilcox et al., 1987). Malignant diseases that mimics Whipple's disease include lymphomas in the bowel that cause villous atrophy such as enteropathy-associated T-cell lymphoma. Appropriate immunostains and molecular clonality studies may help in sorting these conditions.

Treatment of Choice and Prognosis

Whipple's disease is treated with antibiotics for extended periods of time, but there are no randomized, controlled trials of different antibiotic regimens upon which to base recommendations. Based on observational studies, the treatment with the most success in improving symptoms and preventing recurrences is initial therapy with penicillin given by vein plus streptomycin given by injection into the muscle for two weeks, followed by trimethoprim-sulfamethoxazole given orally for one year. Ceftriaxone can be substituted for the initial penicillin and streptomycin. A combination oral antibiotic that can enter the cerebrospinal fluid and brain is commonly used to treat Whipple's disease.

Generally, antibiotic treatment to destroy the bacteria that caused the disease results in relief of symptoms. However, the disorder may be persistent despite sustained treatment with antibiotics. Relapses are frequent. With treatment, the disorder can be cured. Untreated, Whipple's disease is fatal.

People with neurologic Whipple's disease who relapse tend to have much poorer health outcomes, including serious neurologic symptoms and even death. Therefore some scientists argue that all cases of Whipple's disease should be considered neurologic. Relapsing neurologic Whipple's disease is sometimes treated with a combination of antibiotics and weekly injections of interferon gamma.

REFERENCES

Albores-Saavedra J, Vuitch F, Delgado R, Wiley E, Hagler H. 1994. Sinus histiocytosis of pelvic lymph nodes after hip replacement: a histiocytic proliferation induced by cobalt-chromium and titanium. Am J Surg Pathol 18:83–90.

ARMITAGE JO 2010. Early-stage hodgkin's lymphoma. N Engl J Med 363:653–62.

BENZ EB, SHERBURNE B, HAYEK JE, FALCHUK KH, SLEDGE CB, SPECTOR M. 1996. Lymphadenopathy associated with total joint prostheses: a report of two cases and a review of the Literature. J Bone Joint Surg Am 78:588–93.

BLACK M, SPEER F. 1958. Sinus histiocytosis of lymph nodes in cancer. Surg Gynecol Obstet 106:163–75.

BRADEN B, FAUST D, IGNEE A, SCHREIBER D, HIRCHE T, DIETRICH CF. 2008. Clinical relevance of perihepatic lymphadenopathy in acute and chronic liver disease. J Clin Gastroenterol 42:931–36.

CAMACHO FI, GARCIA JF, SANCHEZ-VERDE L, SAEZ AI, SANCHEZ-BEATO M, MOLLEJO M, PIRIS MA. 2001. Unique phenotypic profile of monocytoid B cells: differences in comparison with the phenotypic profile observed in marginal zone B cells and so-called monocytoid B cell lymphoma. Am J Pathol 158:1363–369.

CATALANO C, BALBI T, COCCO P, FABBIAN F, DAVI L, CONZ PA, FARRUGGIO A. 2002. [Thoracic lymphadenopathy due to vascular transformation of lymph node sinuses associated with upper limb edema in a chronic hemodialysis patient with congestive heart failure]. G Ital Nefrol 19:60–73. (in Italian)

CHAN JK, WARNKE RA, DORFMAN R. 1991. Vascular transformation of sinuses in lymph nodes: a study of its morphological spectrum and distinction from Kaposi's sarcoma. Am J Surg Pathol 15:732–43.

CHHABRA S, MOHAN H, BAL A. 2006 A retrospective histological evaluation of non-neoplastic superficial lymphadenopathy. Internet Int Med 6(1).

COOK PD, CZERNIAK B, CHAN JK, MACKAY B, ORDONEZ NG, AYALA AG, ROSAI J. 1995. Nodular spindle-cell vascular transformation of lymph nodes: a benign process occurring predominantly in retroperitoneal lymph nodes draining carcinomas that can simulate Kaposi's sarcoma or metastatic tumor. Am J Surg Pathol 19:1010–20.

CROSS PA, EYDEN BP, HARRIS M. 1989. Signet ring cell lymphoma of T cell type. J Clin Pathol 42:239–45.

DELEA TE, HAGIWARA M, PHATAK PD. 2009. Retrospective study of the association between transfusion frequency and potential complications of iron overload in patients with myelodysplastic syndrome and other acquired hematopoietic disorders. Curr Med Res Opin 25:139–47.

DESTOMBES P. 1965. Adhites avec surcharge lipidiqne, de l'enfant ou de l'adulte jeune, observkes aux Antilles et au Mali (Quatre observations). Bull Sac Pathol Exot 58:1169–75.

DOBBINS WO, III 1995. The diagnosis of Whipple's disease. N Engl J Med 332:390–2.

DUTLY F, ALTWEGG M. 2001. Whipple's disease and "Tropheryma Whippelii." Clin Microbiol Rev 14:561–83.

ECKERT F, BARICEVIC B, LANDTHALER M, SCHMID U. 1992. Metastatic signet-ring cell melanoma in a patient with an unknown primary tumor: histologic, immunohistochemical, and ultrastructural findings. J Am Acad Dermatol 26:870–75.

EHRBAR HU, BAUERFEIND P, DUTLY F, KOELZ HR, ALTWEGG M. 1999. PCR-positive tests for *Tropheryma Whippelii* in patients without whipple's disease. Lancet 353:2214.

EYDEN BP 2000. Filiform and signet-ring cells in large B-cell lymphoma: ultrastructural interpretation. Histopathology 36:186–7.

EYDEN BP, CROSS PA, HARRIS M. 1990. The ultrastructure of signet-ring cell non-Hodgkin's lymphoma. Virchows Arch A Pathol Anat Histopathol 417:395–404.

EYDEN BP, BANERJEE SS. 1990. Multiple myeloma showing signet-ring cell change. Histopathology 17:170–2.

FACCHETTI F, DE WOLF-PEETERS C, MASON DY, PULFORD K, VAN DEN OORD JJ, DESMET VJ. 1988. Plasmacytoid T cells: immunohistochemical evidence for their monocyte/macrophage origin. Am J Pathol 133:15–21.

FARQUHAR JW, MACGREGOR AR, RICHMOND J. 1958. Familial haemophagocytic Reticulosis. Br Med J 2:1561–64.

FERGUSON AR, YOUD ME, CORLEY RB. 2004. Marginal zone B cells transport and deposit IgM-containing immune complexes onto follicular dendritic cells. Int Immunol 16:1411–22.

FEST T, PRON B, LEFRANC MP, PIERRE C, ANGONIN R, DE WB, SOUA Z, DUPOND JL. 1996. Detection of a clonal BCL2 gene rearrangement in tissues from a patient with Whipple disease. An Intern Med 124:738–40.

FOUCAR E, ROSAI J, DORFMAN R. 1990. Sinus histiocytosis with massive lymphadenopathy (Rosai–Dorfman disease): review of the entity. Semin Diagn Pathol 7:19–73.

FROST AR, SHEK YH, LACK EE. 1992. "Signet ring" sinus histiocytosis mimicking metastatic adenocarcinoma: report of two cases with immunohistochemical and ultrastructural study. Mod Pathol 5:497–500.

GALL EA. 1964. The enlarged lymph node: differential diagnosis. In: Pack G. T, Ariel I. M, eds., Treatment of Cancer and Allied Diseases, Harper and Row, New York, vol. 9, 31.

GILLEN CD, CODDINGTON R, MONTEITH PG, TAYLOR RH. 1993. Extraintestinal lymphoma in association with Whipple's disease. Gut 34:1627–29.

GLEW RH, HAESE WH, MCINTYRE PA. 1973. Myeloid metaplasia with myelofibrosis: the clinical spectrum of extramedullary hematopoiesis and tumor formation. Johns Hopkins Med J 132:253–70.

GOULD E, PEREZ J, BORES-SAAVEDRA J, LEGASPI A. 1989. Signet ring cell sinus histiocytosis: a previously unrecognized histologic condition mimicking metastatic adenocarcinoma in lymph nodes. Am J Clin Pathol 92:509–12.

GRAY MH, TALBERT ML, TALBERT WM, BANSAL M, HSU A. 1989. Changes seen in lymph nodes draining the sites of large joint prostheses. Am J Surg Pathol 13:1050–56.

GRETZ JE, ANDERSON AO, SHAW S. 1997. Cords, channels, corridors and conduits: critical architectural elements facilitating cell interactions in the lymph node cortex. Immunol Rev 156:11–24.

GRU AA, HASSAN A, PFEIFER JD, HUETTNER PC. 2010. Uterine extramedullary hematopoiesis: what is the clinical significance? Int J Gynecol Pathol 29:366–73.

GUERRERO-MEDRANO J, DELGADO R, ALBORES-SAAVEDRA J. 1997. Signet-ring sinus histiocytosis: a reactive disorder that mimics metastatic adenocarcinoma. Cancer 80:277–85.

HARRIS M, EYDEN B, READ G. 1981. Signet ring cell lymphoma: a rare variant of follicular lymphoma. J Clin Pathol 34:884–91.

HSIEH PP, OLSEN RJ, O'MALLEY DP, KONOPLEV SN, HUSSONG JW, DUNPHY CH, PERKINS SL, CHENG L, LIN P, CHANG CC. 2007. The role of Janus Kinase 2V617F mutation in extramedullary hematopoiesis of the spleen in neoplastic myeloid disorders. Mod Pathol 20:929–35.

JAFFE R, DEVAUGHN D, LANGHOFF E. 1998. Fascin and the differential diagnosis of childhood histiocytic lesions. Pediatr Dev Pathol 1:216–21.

KIM H, DORFMAN RF, RAPPAPORT H. 1978. Signet ring cell lymphoma. Am J Surg Pathol 2:119–32.

KIM SH, KIM DH, LEE KG. 2007. Prominent Langerhans' cell migration in the arthropod bite reactions simulating Langerhans' cell histiocytosis. J Cutan Pathol 34(12):899–902.

KOCH CA, LI CY, MESA RA, TEFFERI A. 2003. Non-hepatosplenic extramedullary hematopoiesis: associated diseases, pathology, clinical course, and treatment. Mayo Clin Proc 78:1223–33.

KOMP DM 1990. The treatment of sinus histiocytosis with massive lymphadenopathy (Rosai–Dorfman disease). Semin Diagn Pathol 7:83–86.

KORSTEN J, GROSSMAN H, WINCHESTER PH, CANALE VC. 1970. Extramedullary hematopoiesis in patients with thalassemia anemia. Radiology 95:257–63.

KUBASKA SM, SHEPARD JA, CHEW FS, KEEL SB. 1998. Whipple's disease involving the mediastinum. AJR Am J Roentgenol 171:364.

KUO TT, HSUEH S. 1984. Mucicarminophilic Histiocytosis. A polyvinylpyrrolidone (PVP) storage disease simulating signet-ring cell carcinoma. Am J Surg Pathol 8:419–28.

LAU SK, CHU PG, WEISS LM. 2004. CD163: a specific marker of macrophages in paraffin-embedded tissue samples. Am J Clin Pathol 122:794–801.

LICHTMAN SM, ATTIVISSIMO L, GOLDMAN IS, SCHUSTER MW, BUCHBINDER A. 1999. Secondary hemochromatosis as a long-term complication of the treatment of hematologic malignancies. Am J Hematol 61:262–64.

MARIC I, PITTALUGA S, DALE JK, NIEMELA JE, DELSOL G, DIMENT J, ROSAI J, RAFFELD M, PUCK JM, STRAUS SE, JAFFE ES. 2005. Histologic features of sinus histiocytosis with massive lymphadenopathy in patients with autoimmune lymphoproliferative syndrome. Am J Surg Pathol 29:903–11.

MEHRAEIN Y, WAGNER M, REMBERGER K, FAZESI L, MIDDEL P, KAPTUR S, SCHMITT K, MEESE E. 2006. Parvovirus B19 detected in Rosai–Dorfman disease in nodal and extranodal manifestations. J Clin Pathol 59:1320–6.

MEYSMAN M, DILTOER M, RAEVE HD, MONSIEUR I, HUYGHENS L. 1997. Chronic thromboembolic pulmonary hypertension and vascular transformation of the lymph node sinuses. Eur Respir J 10:1191–3.

MICHAL M, KOZA V, FAKAN F. 1992. Myoid differentiation in vascular transformation of lymph node sinuses due to venous obstruction. Immunohistochemical and ultrastructural studies. Zentralbl Pathol 138:27–33.

MORGAN NV, MORRIS MR, CANGUL H, GLEESON D, STRAATMAN-IWANOWSKA A, DAVIES N, KEENAN S, PASHA S, RAHMAN F, GENTLE D, VREESWIJK MP, DEVILEE P, KNOWLES MA, CEYLANER S, TREMBATH RC, DALENCE C, KISMET E, KOSEOGLU V, ROSSBACH HC, GISSEN P, TANNAHILL D, MAHER ER. 2010. Mutations in SLC29A3, encoding an equilibrative nucleoside transporter ENT3, cause a familial histiocytosis syndrome (Faisalabad histiocytosis) and familial Rosai–Dorfman disease. PLoS Genet 6:e1000833.

MURRAY JA, SLATER DN, PARSONS MA, FOX M, SMITH S, PLATTS MM. 1984. Splenic siderosis and parenteral iron dextran in maintenance haemodialysis patients. J Clin Pathol 37:59–64.

NISHIKAWA Y, SATO H, OKA T, YOSHINO T, TAKAHASHI K. 2009. Immunohistochemical discrimination of plasmacytoid dendritic cells from myeloid dendritic cells in human pathological tissues. J Clin Exp Hematop 49:23–31.

O'MALLEY DP. 2007. Benign extramedullary myeloid proliferations Mod Pathol 20, 405–41.

OHSAWA M, KANNO H, NAKA N, AOZASA K. 1994. Occurrence of monocytoid B-lymphocytes in Hodgkin's disease. Mod Pathol 7:540–3.

ONCIU M 2004. Histiocytic Proliferations in Childhood. Am J Clin Pathol 122 (Suppl): S128–36.

PAPAKONSTANTINOU O, MARIS TG, KOSTARIDOU S, LADIS V, VASILIADOU A, GOURTSOYIANNIS NC. 2005. Abdominal lymphadenopathy in beta-thalassemia: MRI features and correlation with liver iron overload and posttransfusion chronic hepatitis C. AJR Am J Roentgenol 185:219–24.

PITCOCK J, REINHARD E, JUSTUS B, MENDELSOHN R. 1962. A clinical and pathological study of seventy cases of myelofibrosis. An Intern Med 57:73–84.

PITTALUGA M I, DALE JK, NIEMELA JE, DELSOL G, DIMENT J, ROSAI J, RAFFELD M, PUCK JM, STRAUS SE, JAFFE ES. 2005. Histologic features of sinus histiocytosis with massive lymphadenopathy in patients with autoimmune lymphoproliferative syndrome. Am J Surg Pathol 29:903–11.

RAVEL R 1966. Histopathology of lymph nodes after lymphangiography. Am J Clin Pathol 46:335–40.

REDMOND J III, KANTOR RS, AUERBACH HE, SPIRITOS MD, MOORE JT. 1994. Extramedullary hematopoiesis during therapy with granulocyte colony-stimulating factor. Arch Pathol Lab Med 118:1014–5.

RELMAN DA, SCHMIDT TM, MACDERMOTT RP, FALKOW S. 1992. Identification of the uncultured bacillus of Whipple's disease. N Engl J Med 327:293–301.

RISDALL RJ, BRUNNING RD, HERNANDEZ JJ. 1984. Bacteria associated hemophagic syndrome. Cancer 54:2968–72.

ROOZENDAAL R, MEMPEL TR, PITCHER LA, GONZALEZ SF, VERSCHOOR A, MEBIUS RE, VON ANDRIAN UH, CARROLL MC. 2009. Conduits mediate transport of low-molecular-weight antigen to lymph node follicles. Immunity 30:264–76.

ROSAI J, DORFMAN RF. 1969. Sinus histiocytosis with massive lymphadenopathy: a newly recognized benign clinicopathological entity. Arch Pathol 87:63–70.

ROSAI J, DORFMAN RF. 1972. Sinus histiocytosis with massive lymphadenopathy: a pseudolymphomatous benign disorder. Analysis of 34 cases. Cancer 30: 1174–88.

ROTH MJ, MEDEIROS LJ, ELENITOBA-JOHNSON K, et al. 1995. Extramedullary myeloid cell tumors: an immunohistochemical study of 29 cases using routinely fixed and processed paraffin-embedded tissue sections. Arch Pathol Lab Med 119:790–8.

SAINTE-MARIE G, PENG FS. 1986. Diffusion of a lymph-carried antigen in the fiber network of the lymph node of the rat. Cell Tissue Res 245:481–6.

SAMET A, GILBEY P, TALMON Y, COHEN H. 2001. Vascular transformation of lymph node sinuses. J Laryngol Otol 115:760–2.

SCHERRER C, MAURER R. 1985. [Vascular sinus transformation of the lymph nodes. morphological and immunohistochemical analysis of 6 cases]. An Pathol 5:231–8.

SHEIBANI K, BATTIFORA H. 1988. Signet-ring cell melanoma: a rare morphologic variant of malignant melanoma. Am J Surg Pathol 12:28–34.

SIIMES MA, ADDIEGO JE JR., DALLMAN PR. 1974. Ferritin in serum: diagnosis of iron deficiency and iron overload in infants and children. Blood 43:581–90.

SILVERBERG SG, CHITALE AR, HIND AD, FRAZIER AB, LEVITT SH. 1970. Sinus histiocytosis and mammary carcinoma: study of 366 radical mastectomies and an historical review. Cancer 26:1177–85.

SILVERBERG SG, FRABLE WJ, BROOKS JW. 1973. Sinus histiocytosis in non-diagnostic scalene lymph node biopsies. Cancer 32:177–80.

SPENCER J, FINN T, PULFORD KA, MASON DY, ISAACSON PG. 1985. The human gut contains a novel population of B lymphocytes which resemble marginal zone cells. Clin Exp Immunol 62:607–12.

SPENCER J, DOGAN A. 2009. A common migratory highway between human spleen and mucosa-associated lymphoid tissues: data from nature's own experiments. Mucosal Immunol 2:380–2.

STANSFELD AG 1961. The histological diagnosis of toxoplasmic lymphadenitis. J Clin Pathol 14:565–73.

STREET S, DONOGHUE HD, NEILD GH. 1999. *Tropheryma Whippelii* DNA in saliva of healthy people. Lancet 354:1178–9.

TRUONG L, CARTWRIGHT J, GOODMAN D, WOZNICKI D. 1988. Silicone lymphadenopathy associated with augmentation mammoplasty: morphologic features of nine cases. Am J Surg Pathol 12:484–91.

VAN DER OORD JJ, DE WOLF-PEETERS C, DE VR, DESMET VJ. 1984. The paracortical area in dermatopathic lymphadenitis and other reactive conditions of the lymph node. Virchows Arch B Cell Pathol Incl Mol Pathol 45:289–99.

WEISS LM, WOOD GS, DORFMAN RF. 1985. T-cell signet-ring cell lymphoma: a histologic, ultrastructural, and immunohistochemical study of two cases. Am J Surg Pathol 9:273–80.

WILCOX GM, TRONIC BS, SCHECTER DJ, ARRON MJ, RIGHI DF, WEINER NJ. 1987. Periodic acid-Schiff-negative granulomatous lymphadenopathy in patients with Whipple's disease: localization of the Whipple bacillus to non-caseating granulomas by electron microscopy. Am J Med 83:165–70.

WILLMAN CL, BUSQUE L, GRIFFITH BB, FAVARA BE, McCLAIN KL, DUNCAN MH, GILLILAND DG. 1994. Langerhans'-cell histiocytosis (histiocytosis X)—a clonal proliferative disease. N Engl J Med 331:154–60.

WOLF BC, NEIMAN RS. 1987. Hypothesis: splenic filtration and the pathogenesis of extramedullary hematopoiesis in agnogenic myeloid metaplasia. Hematol Pathol 1:77–80.

WONG KF, HUI PK, CHAN JK, CHAN YW, HA SY. 1991. The acute lupus hemophagocytic syndrome. An Intern Med 114:387–90.

CHAPTER SEVENTEEN

MIXED LYMPH NODE PATTERNS: STROMAL AND HISTIOCYTIC REACTIONS, NONINFECTIOUS

Hernani D. Cualing

PROTEINACEOUS LYMPHADENOPATHY INCLUDING IMMUNOGLOBULIN DEPOSITION LYMPHADENOPATHY

The histopathologist should be familiar with the morphological appearance of proteinaceous lymphadenopathy, which can be confused with amyloidosis. A number of diseases may contribute to proteinaceous deposits and enlargement of lymph nodes, but this term should not be applied to deposits secondary to amyloidosis. The proteinaceous lymphadenopathy includes immunoglobulin (Ig) and nonimmunoglobulin deposition diseases, deposits secondary to hemodialysis, and deposits in association with chronic diseases like rheumatoid arthritis (RA) (Hazenberg et al., 1999).

Definition

Proteinaceous lymphadenopathy is a rare disorder that shows nonamyloid hyaline deposition in lymph nodes and tissues that are congo red negative (Michaeli et al., 1995).

Synonyms

Angiocentric sclerosing lymphadenopathy, nonimmunoglobulin deposition disease, immunoglobulin-related deposition diseases, nonamyloid proteinaceous deposition disease.

ICD-10 Code R59.9 Enlarged lymph node, unspecified.

Etiology

Two types are described based on the proteinaceous material deposited: a nonimmunoglobulin sclerotic type (Osborne, Butler, and Mackay, 1979, Michaeli et al., 1995) and an immunoglobulin-related type (Banerjee et al., 1990a; Buxbaum and Gallo, 1999a).

Morphology

The nonimmunoglobulin, sclerotic type of deposition disease shows polyclonal hypergammaglobulinemia with organomegaly and lymphadenopathy. The lymph node histopathology shows lymphoid depletion. The normal architecture is replaced by a hyaline sclerosis that is also congo red negative and lacks electron microscopic evidence of an

Non-Neoplastic Hematopathology and Infections, First Edition. Edited by Hernani D. Cualing, Parul Bhargava, and Ramon L. Sandin.
© 2012 Wiley-Blackwell. Published 2012 by John Wiley & Sons, Inc.

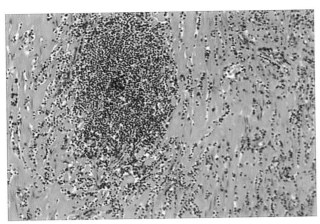

FIGURE 17.1 **Light chain deposition disease with mesenteric lymph node showing pink amorphous proteinaceous deposits around a lymphoid aggregate** (H&E).

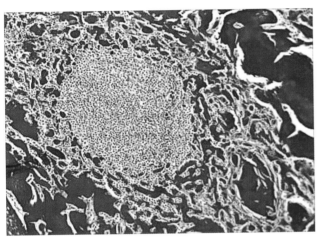

FIGURE 17.2 **Light chain deposition disease with PAS-positive deposits between lymphoid cells surrounding a kappa monoclonal small lymphoplasmacytic lymphoid aggregate.**

amyloid. Prominent sclerosis around blood vessels is a key feature, and hence the process has been also called "angiocentric sclerosing lymphadenopathy" (Michaeli et al., 1995). Immunoglobulin deposition disease shows amorphous hyaline deposits (see Figure 17.1) that are PAS positive (see Figure 17.2). These are also congo red negative (see Figure 17.3) proteinaceous deposits.

Immunohistochemistry/Cytochemistry

Antibody to heavy or light chains as well as substance P are helpful in classifying the type of deposits. Congo red cytochemical stain or thiamine red immunofluorescent stain are standard tests for amyloid in lieu of electron microscopy.

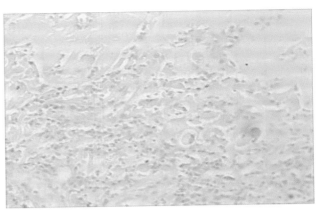

FIGURE 17.3 **Light chain deposition disease with negative congo red stain.**

Differential Diagnosis

A congo red or fluorescent thiamine red stain will highlight amyloidotic deposits in the lymph node or tissue. The congo red stain will distinguish amyloid deposits from the noncongophilic, proteinaceous, and immunoglobulin light and heavy chain deposition diseases. A positive congo red in brightfield microscopy appears orange or orangeophilic, (see Figure 17.4), and crystalline apple-green or pale green birefringent in polarization microscopy (see Figure 17.5). In addition to plasma cell dyscrasia, congo red is positive in chronic debilitating disease or in patients undergoing hemodialysis. Rheumatoid arthritis should be included in the differential diagnosis of patients with deposition lymphadenopathy. Since congophilic deposits can be as a sequelae to a neoplasm, a positive stain requires exclusion of an underlying monoclonal B cell lymphoma or plasma cell dyscrasia (see Table 17.4). If the tissue with proteinaceous amyloid-looking depositi is congo red negative, a number of noncongophilic deposition diseases, in addition to the sclerosing nonimmunoglobuling angiocentric adenopathy, should be considered as described below.

The heavy or light chain immunoglobulin deposition disease is also called "Randall disease" and is noncongophilic. It is a plasma cell dyscrasia characterized by amorphous, extensive, diffuse, or patchy deposits that are congo red negative, nonbirefringent by polarized microscopy, and do not stain with the amyloid P antibody. In addition some laboratory results may be misleading especially the serum paraprotein. This monoclonal lymphoproliferative disorder may be missed since the serum monoclonal paraprotein may be absent in 15% (Buxbaum et al.,

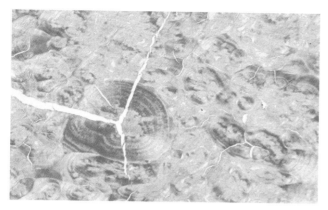

FIGURE 17.4 **Amyloidosis expressed by congo red positive amyloidoma crystal with refractile congophilic crystalline material taken under brighfield light microscopy** (congo red).

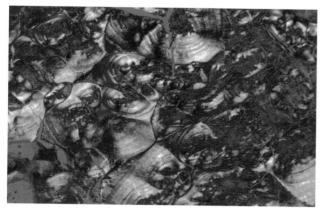

FIGURE 17.5 **Amyloidosis expressed by polarized birefringent green and gold polarization spectra of congophilic crystals.**

1990). These deposits are composed of incomplete or unstructured immunoglobulins and differ in characteristics from AL fibrillar amyloid deposits (see Table 17.1).

Monoclonal heavy or light chain deposition diseases are rare diseases that should be also considered when evaluating a congo red negative proteinaceous lymphadenopathy. A wide spectrum of organ compromise, including renal disease, is seen in light chain and heavy chain depositiion diseases. Their tissue biopsy shows a monoclonal staining with anti–light or heavy chain, bright pink amorphous deposits in tissues including the glomeruli by PAS staining (LIN et al., 2001, Aucouturier et al., 1993) Entrapped clonal lymphoid aggregates of lymphocytes or lympho-plasmacytes may be seen

(see Figure 17.2). A monoclonal disease of either a lymphoplasmacytic lymphoma or a plasma cell neoplasm may be the underlying disorder (Banerjee et al., 1990b; Buxbaum and Gallo, 1999b).

Heavy chain disease is extremely rare as the sole primary manifestation. Hence a search for an underlying low-grade B-cell lymphomas such as lymphoplasmacytic or marginal zone B-cell type has to be done to determine if this is a primary or a secondary monoclonal immunoglobulin deposition disease.

Treatment

Corresponding therapy for the underlying disease is necessary. RA-associated proteinaceous lymphadenopathy regress following successful treatment of arthritis. (Al Rikabi et al., 1995). Treatment for the other conditions depends on the underlying etiology.

LYMPH NODE FIBROSIS OR FIBROTIC CHANGES, NONSPECIFIC

Definition

Fibrosis of lymph node is a reactive process characterized by a diffuse distribution of collagenous sclerosis in the parenchyma, usually associated with lymphatic or vascular obstruction.

Fibrotic changes are focal sclerosis not involving the entire lymph node.

ICD-10 Code R59.9 Enlarged lymph node, unspecified.

Clinical Aspects

Lower leg lymphedema is the classic associated clinical finding that leads to fibrosis of lymph nodes (Kinmonth and Wolfe, 1980). Milroy's disease (familial congenital lymphedema) or late onset lymphedema are associated with a lymph node pathology of fibrosis. Surgical procedures that lead to stasis of lymphatic drainage can also cause fibrosis of lymph nodes. In these cases the lymph nodes are small and fibrosed. Lymph nodes from mediastinal region of coal miners often show fibrosis in addition to dust particles (Leigh and Wiles, 1987).

Pathogenesis

An initial vascularization of the lymph node that begins at the medullary region is seen. As the lesion

TABLE 17.1 Characteristics of Amyloidosis and Amyloid-like Deposition Diseases

Congophilic Amyloid (AL)	Congophilic Non-AL Amyloid (AA)	Congophilic FamilialAmyloid (AF)	Non-congophilic Proteinaceous Hemodialysis Associated (β2) Deposits	Non-congophilic Light/Heavy Chain Deposition Disease
No monoclonal paraprotein (M) in 80% (usually lambda)	No M component	No M component	No M component	M component often present (usually kappa)
Clonal plasma cells	Non-clonal	Non-clonal	Non-clonal	Clonal plasma cells may be demonstrable in marrow
Clonal light chain in deposits may be demonstrable	No clonal light chain deposits	No clonal light chain deposits	No clonal light chain deposits	Clonal light/heavy chain deposits may be demonstrable
Congo red positive	Congo red positive	Congo red positive	Congo red negative	Congo red negative

progresses, the vascularity is replaced by collagenized bands of fibrosis going toward the capsule. The medullary sinuses are obliterated with recanalization and dilatation of the lymphatics. The histologic findings are not easily distinguised from vascular transformation of the sinuses, and in some cases these two may be identical in origin.

Morphology

A focal fibrosis limited to the medullary region is a normal finding in many lymph nodes. Extension of fibrosis from medullary sinuses to the paracortex and cortex and into the subcapsular region is seen in long-standing fibrosis (see Figure 17.6). In the cortex and paracortex, the residual lymphoid tissues are often seen as vague nodules infiltrated by dense knots of fibrosclerosis. Dense serpiginous pattern of sclerosis may be accentuated in the pulp (see Figure 17.7). Admixed histiocytic and fibroblastic infiltrate can be seen, and sinuses may be obliterated and fused. The medullary arterioles, and in severe cases capsular arterioles, display markedly thickened walls while the venule walls appear normal. Efferent and afferent lymphatic vessels also show thickened luminal walls (see Figure 17.8).

Differential Diagnosis

Vascular transformation of the sinuses as well as inflammatory pseudotumors resemble some of the findings of lymph node fibrosis in low-power histologic view. However, in vascular transformation, although there is sclerosis of the hilum, there is more prominent small and medium vessel hyperplasia

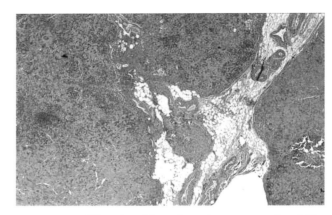

FIGURE 17.6 **Fibrosis of lymph nodes expressed as hilar sclerosis and thickened arteriolar walls with extension into paracortex.** Note the decreasing degree of fibrosis from the hilum to the pulp.

displaying round to elliptical vascular lumina associated with lymphoid tissue. In an inflammatory pseudotumor the fibrosis is seen in both the hilum and the capsule with intervening widened but fibrous trabeculae distinctly framing the nodal framework. In addition varying degrees of follicular and paracortical reactions along with mixed inflammatory infiltrates of plasma cells and inflammatory venulitis are seen. In contrast, there are minimal chronic inflammatory plasma cells and no prominent vasculitis in the lymph node with fibrosis.

Treatment

Treatment is directed at relieving the lymphedema or the cause of vascular obstruction.

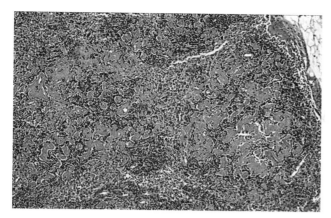

FIGURE 17.7 **Fibrosis of lymph nodes expressed as knots of collagenous bundles in serpiginous pattern in and around reactive residual lymphoid tissue.** The patient had a long-standing lymphedema from breast surgery.

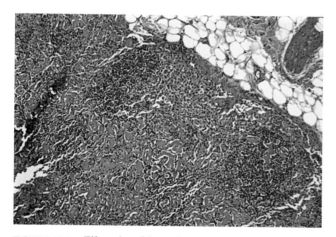

FIGURE 17.8 **Fibrosis of lymph nodes expressed as sclerosis of the cortex and residual lymphoid tissue with obliteration of sinuses.** A histiocytic reaction in subcapsular area with fibrosis is seen. Capsular fibrosis extends to the pulp. Afferent lymphatic wall is thickened at the right upper corner.

INFLAMMATORY PSEUDOTUMOR OF LYMPH NODES

The inflammatory pseudotumor is likely a heterogeneous disease; it presents in a wide age range and occurs in almost all organs. The inflammatory pseudotumor of the lymph nodes and the spleen may be a nonneoplastic process distinct from the inflammatory myofibroblastic tumors (IMT) that may arise at other sites, which may be neoplastic.

Although the original description pointed to a morphologic similarity of the pseudotumor arising in nodal and extranodal sites, IMTs arising at extranodal organs are now largely regarded to be different from the inflammatory pseudotumor of the lymph node and spleen. Recent evidence shows that extranodal IMTs are in fact neoplastic processes that often harbor balanced chromosomal translocations involving the ALK kinase gene, with an overexpression of ALK kinase being detectable by immunostaining. The lung IMT had a reported a 20% ALK positivity (Tavora et al., 2007) and in all other nonlymphatic organs IMT showed a 21.7% ALK positivity rate, especially noted in patients 40 years or younger in a series of 61 cases (Chan, Cheuk, and Shimizu, 2001).

The nonlymphatic inflammatory myofibroblastic tumors that have been described in almost all organs seem to have a clonal proliferation and may be associated with chromosomal rearrangements in 2p23, ALK translocation, or an EBV-induced transformation. The neoplastic nature of this subset of IMT, characterized as tumor with aneuploidy and ALK abnormalities, with a more aggressive clinical behavior, imply that we should separate these cases from the true inflammatory pseudotumor (Coffin et al., 1995; Coffin, Dehner, and Meis-Kindblom, 1998; Coffin, Humphrey, and Dehner, 1998; Hussong et al., 1999; Alaggio et al., 2010; Kutok et al., 2001).

Definition

An inflammatory pseudotumor of lymph nodes is a rare reactive lymphadenopathy arising from the lymph node stromal framework. It is composed of fibrous and spindle cell proliferation, with variable inflammatory component, and an absence of chromosomal rearrangement, ALK translocation, or EBV infection.

ICD-10 Code R59.9 Enlarged lymph node, unspecified.

Synonyms

Inflammatory pseudotumor, plasma cell granuloma.

Etiology

The inflammatory pseudotumor of lymph nodes was first described by Perrone as a distinct pattern of lymph node reactions in young adults associated with systemic symptoms (Perrone, de Wolf-Peeters, and Frizzera, 1988).

The inflammatory pseudotumor of lymph nodes presents predominantly in young male adults with a median age of 40 years, in either single or multiple lymph node sites, with or without splenomegaly (Kutok et al., 2001). Lymphatic pseudotumors have no positive staining for ALK kinase.

Laboratory Findings

There is often anemia, hypergammaglobulinemia, and an elevated erythrocyte sedimentation rate in patients with inflammatory pseudotumor of lymph nodes.

Sites of Involvement

Lymph node, spleen, and occasionally liver are the sites.

Approach to Diagnosis

Since the disease shares morphologic features, clinical and immunohistochemical workup will be necessary to separate true inflammatory from the neoplastic types. Inflammatory myofibroblastic tumor of childhood may deserve special consideration and treatment. IMT of childhood may affect all organs with many reported in lungs, abdominal areas, and CNS. In children the lung and thorax are the most common IMT sites.

Morphologic Aspects

Inflammatory pseudotumors of the lymph nodes are composed of spindle cells admixed with variable amounts of extracellular collagen, lymphocytes, and plasma cells. At least three patterns have been described: a myxoid vascular pattern, a compact spindle cell pattern, and/or a hypocellular fibrous pattern.

In low-power view, the lymph node may show thickened capsule with residual lymphoid nodules (see Figure 17.9). Residual lymphoplasmacytic aggregates are typically separated by interlacing and thick fibrous bands extending from the hilum to trabeculae (see Figure 17.10). Occasionally, in solid areas, the fibroblastic networks are arranged in poorly formed fascicles and in a storiform pattern with admixed plasma cells (see Figure 17.11). At higher magnification, the pseudotumor nodules contained numerous mature plasma cells mixed with few immunoblasts, myofibroblasts, lymphocytes, and histiocytes (see Figure 17.12). There is no sharp demarcation between the inflammatory and fibroblastic areas (see Figure 17.13). Small and large venulitis could be seen in the hilum and in the parenchyma mixed with interlacing cords of fibroblastic stroma (see Figure 17.14).

IMT, in contrast, may affect all organs with many reported in lungs, abdominal areas, and CNS. The IMT tumors also occur in adults and morphologically show a wide histologic spectrum typical of inflammatory pseudotumors/myofibroblastic tumors, but there are variable or focal nuclear atypia (Chan,

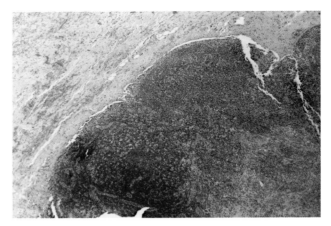

FIGURE 17.9 **Inflammatory pseudotumor of lymph node expressed as a perinodal extension of spindle cells admixed with sclerosis and edema overlying vaguely nodular residual cortical and paracortical tissue**.

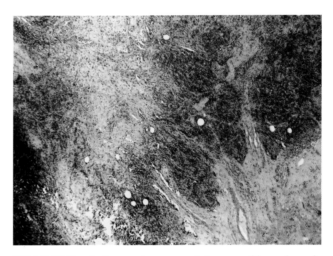

FIGURE 17.10 **Inflammatory pseudotumor of lymph node expressed as prominent hilar sclerosis with extension into trabeculae and into the pulp with vaguely nodular residual paracortical lymphoid tissue**.

Cheuk, and Shimizu, 2001). In IMT of childhood, cytologic atypia, low inflammatory infiltrate, and a rich myxoid pattern are characteristics in patients who have recurrent disease or a poor prognosis (Alaggio et al., 2010).

Immunohistochemistry/Cytochemistry

In a benign inflammatory pseudotumor of lymph nodes, the lesional spindle cells are negative for anaplastic lymphoma kinase-1 (ALK). Immunohistochemically, the fibroblastic or myofibroblastic spindle cells are positive for vimentin, human smooth muscle actin, and muscle actin but negative for desmin, CD8,

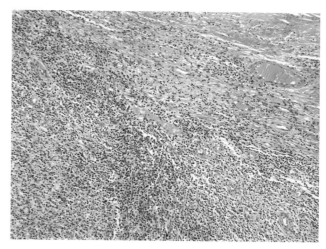

FIGURE 17.11   Inflammatory pseudotumor of lymph node with sheets of reactive plasma cells and admixed fibroblastic spindled cells and dense hyaline sclerosis.

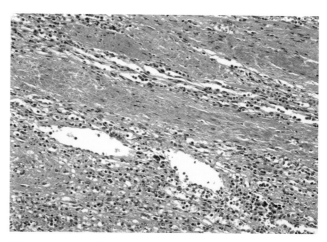

FIGURE 17.13   Inflammatory pseudotumor of lymph node with increased vascularity. Note the overlapping fibroblastic vascular area with dense inflammatory area.

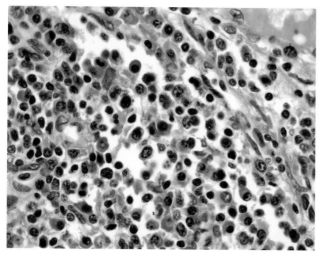

FIGURE 17.12   Inflammatory pseudotumor of lymph node with immunoblasts and mature plasma cells admixed with lymphocytes, histiocytes, and eosinophils.

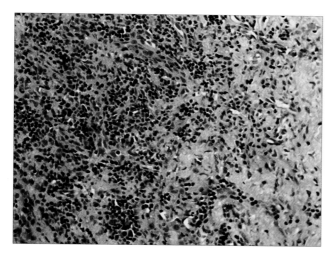

FIGURE 17.14   Inflammatory pseudotumor of lymph node with venulitis and interlacing cords of fibroblastic stroma.

CD21, CD23, CD34, CD35, p80, S-100, Epstein–Barr virus LMP, and human herpesvirus type 8. In contrast, positivity for CD21 or CD35 coupled with EBV staining are characteristic of follicular dendritic cell-like inflammatory pseudotumors that has been described in the spleen, liver, or CNS.

In IMT, immunostaining for ALK typically shows a granular cytoplasmic staining in the neoplastic cells, with occasional cell membrane highlight. In childhood IMT, ALK is positive in 33%. In some series ALK immunohistochemistry positivity was up to 36% with a higher rate observed using fluorescence in situ

hybridization. ALK rearrangements is seen in up to 47% of cases (Coffin et al., 1995; Coffin, Dehner, and Meis-Kindblom, 1998; Coffin, Humphrey, and Dehner, 1998). Background plasma cells are polyclonal and a variable increased CD45RO memory T cells and scattered B cells are present.

Differential Diagnosis

One needs to distinguish the type of inflammatory pseudotumor and use clinical cytogenetics and immunohistochemical tests for characterizing a lesion that is morphologically compatible with inflammatory pseudotumor.

The nonlymphatic IMT tumor presents in a wide age range, and has been described in persons as young an infant to an octogenarian, who often presents with fever of unknown origin or other vague, nonspecific symptoms such as malaise and night sweats (Chan, Cheuk, and Shimizu, 2001). Inflammatory myofibroblastic tumors of childhood have a median age of presentation at 5 years and presents predominantly in the lung–bronchus, abdominal, and thoracic wall (Alaggio et al., 2010). Evaluation of ALK-1 staining would be useful, since abnormalities of ALK and evidence of chromosomal rearrangements of 2p23 occur in a significant proportion of IMTs.

In addition a subset of EBV positive follicular dendritic-like tumor has been described in the spleen and in the lymph nodes. Both lesions show similarity with inflammatory pseudotumors and have also been called inflammatory pseudotumor-like follicular dendritic tumor in those lesions that expressed CD21 and CD35 (Lewis et al., 2003). Myxoid stroma with prominent interlacing spindle cells apposed to inflammatory elements may be found (see Figure 17.15). In those instances follicular dendritic markers CD21 (see Figure 17.16) and CD35 would be positive in the spindle cells, and in situ hybridization for EBV would be positive as well (see Figure 17.17) (Horiguchi et al., 2004; Lewis et al., 2003).

Vascular transformation of sinuses show similarity with an increased spindle cells and vessels, but typically, unlike inflammatory psedotumor of lymph nodes, increased vascularity and fibrosis is prominent in the hilum with sparing of the capsular fibrous tissue in vascular transformation (see Figure 17.18). Typically a thickened capsule, hilum, and trabecular nodal framework is the low-power appearance

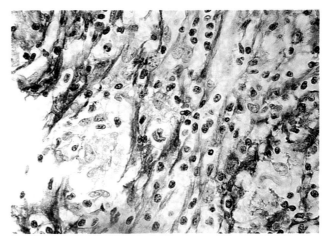

FIGURE 17.16 **Follicle dendritic-like inflammatory pseudotumor of lymph node showing CD21 + spindle cells.**

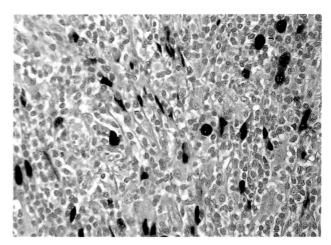

FIGURE 17.17 **Follicle dendritic-like inflammatory pseudotumor of lymph node showing EBER + spindle cells.**

of inflammatory pseudotumors. These findings also contrast with idiopathic fibrosis of lymph nodes, which shows discrete serpiginous knotty hyaline sclerosis (see Figure 17.19).

Lymphomatoid granulomatosis (LYG) is a differential diagnosis because inflammatory pseudotumors may show vasculitis and intravascular infiltrate similar to LYG, but unlike LYG, the infiltrate in inflammatory pseudotumor of lymph nodes is typically EBV negative. A caveat in this scheme is a subset of neoplastic inflammatory pseudotumors that have been described to be different and show clonal EBV integration that are neither LYG or follicular dendritic neoplasms based on a postulated mesenchymal differentiation of inflammatory pseudotumors in spleen and liver (Lewis et al., 2003).

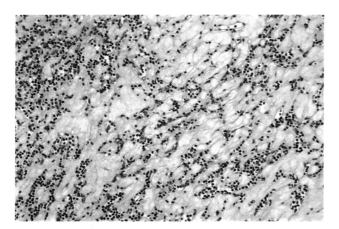

FIGURE 17.15 **Inflammatory pseudotumor-like follicular dendritic tumor or follicular dendritic-like inflammatory pseudotumor of lymph node.** Note the myxoid interlacing chicken-wire distribution of spindle cells and inflammatory cells.

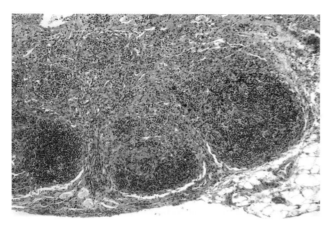

FIGURE 17.18 **Vascular transformation of sinuses**. Note the different pattern from the inflammatory pseudotumor of the lymph node, showing sparing of capsule and hilar vascularity.

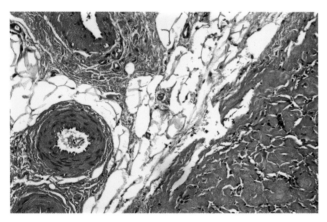

FIGURE 17.19 **Fibrosis of lymph nodes with sclerosed lymph node hilar arterioles without venulitis**.

Last, tumors in immunocompromised individuals such as Kaposi sarcoma (KS) and spindled mycobacterial pseudotumor could be confused with IMT or inflammatory pseudotumor. In addition to the Ziehl–Neelsen acid-fast bacteria, immunostaining for HHV-8 in atypical spindled MTB and KS, respectively would be useful in those cases. Furthermore the spindle cells in mycobacterial pseudotumor are positive for S-100 and CD68 protein, whereas those of Kaposi sarcoma are CD31 and CD34 positive.

Treatment of Choice and Prognosis

This is dictated by the type of inflammatory pseudotumor subset. IMTs of childhood are locally aggressive lesions with a local recurrence rate of 23%, and the 5-year and 10-year event-free survival rates were 87.4

and 72.8%, respectively. The treatment of choice is a complete excision with option for chemotherapy in residual disease (Alaggio et al., 2010). Inflammatory myofibroblastic tumor is a neoplasm of intermediate biological potential that may recur (Marino-Enriquez et al., 2011). The inflammatory pseudotumor in lymph nodes appears nevertheless to have a benign behavior on clinical follow-up (Kojima et al., 2001).

FATTY REPLACEMENT OR FATTY CHANGES, NONSPECIFIC

Fatty change is a pattern seen in normal lymph nodes, commonly along the axillary chain.

Definition

The lymph node is replaced almost totally by a centrally located fatty tissue leaving a rim of normal lymphoid tissue and sinuses.

Synonyms

Fatty replacement or fatty changes, nonspecific.

ICD-10 Code R59.9 Enlarged lymph node, unspecified.

Etiology

A small section of fatty tissue in a lymph node appears to be a normal pattern, if found close to or adjacent to the medullary areas. A fatty tissue inside a small lymph node may also be a transient early finding seen in a developing lymph node, a relatively common incidental finding in mesenteric and omental specimen. In addition lymphoid tissue involutes with age and involution with fatty change or fibrosis are features of some lymph nodes taken from older patients.

Sites of Involvement

These fatty changes are often incidental findings in lymph nodes, commonly seen in axillary and mesenteric nodal areas. It is not a common finding in inguinal or pelvic lymph nodes where we usually see focal fibrosis.

Morphologic Aspects

This is a diagnosis on low-power magnification, characterized as discrete continuous mature fibroadipose tissue inside subcortical areas. Small areas of fat characteristic of fatty change may also be seen in lieu of subtotal replacement (see Figure 17.20). Fatty replacement shows as a rim of lymphoid tissue comprised of normal follicles and nodules of paracortex that appear to have been replaced by extensive mature adipose tissue centrally (see Figs 17.20, 17.21, 17.22, 17.23).

Differential Diagnosis

Unlike findings in lipoid replacement or lipid foreign body reactions in lymph nodes, also called lipogranulomas or lipophagic granulomas (Weiss, 2008), there is well-demarcated normal fat without any associated histiocytic or inflammatory response. Lipogranulomas also manifest histiocytes with foamy vacuoles often associated with multinucleated giant cells. No treatment is needed unless the node is involved by metastatic disease or lymphoma.

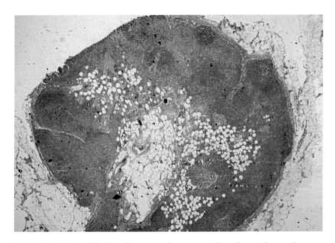

FIGURE 17.20 **Fatty changes in a reactive lymph node**.

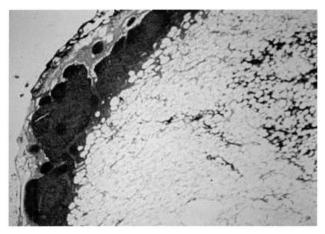

FIGURE 17.21 **Fatty replacement**.

TUMOR REACTIVE GRANULOMATAS

Malignant neoplasms associated with granulomas may be a pitfall in differential diagnosis when granulomas are so pervasive that the neoplasm is obscured.

Tumor cells with epithelioid histiocytes may be difficult to diagnose accurately, especially when florid granulomas overlay the neoplasm or when in the setting of limited presenting materials such as some aspirates or cytologic preparations. Hence, in favor of caution, a differential diagnosis of a "granulomatous" process in a tissue core biopsy and aspirate cytology should include malignant neoplasms of either Hodgkin, non-Hodgkin, or even epithelial and other malignancies (Khurana et al., 1998).

Definition

Epithelioid granulomas is tissue or lymph nodes that are associated with malignant neoplasms.

ICD-10 Code R59.9 Enlarged lymph node, unspecified.

Synonym

Sarcoid-like tumor reactions.

Epidemiology

Sarcoid-like granulomatous reactions occur in 4.4% of carcinomas, in 13.8% of patients with Hodgkin's disease, and in 7.3% of cases of non-Hodgkin lymphomas (Brincker, 1986).

Clinical Associations

Although the most recognized malignancy associated with epithelioid granulomas is Hodgkin lymphoma (Sacks et al., 1978), a variety of non-Hodgkin lymphomas (Hollingsworth, Longo, and Jaffe, 1993, Braylan et al., 1977) and cutaneous lymphomas (Bessis et al., 1996), solid tumors, including keratinizing squamous cell carcinoma (Carneiro et al., 1989) and seminomas (Richter and Leder, 1979) can present with obscuring or admixed granulomatous reactions.

Morphology

The sarcoid-like granulomas often show noncaseating epithelioid histiocytes with or without Langhans-type or foreign body-type giant cells. Lymphoid-rich granuloma should prompt caution, since this type of granuloma can coexist with sarcoidal granulomas with

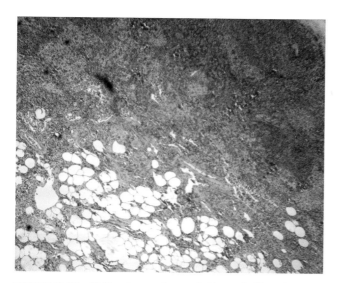

FIGURE 17.22   Fatty change in medulla with fibrosis.

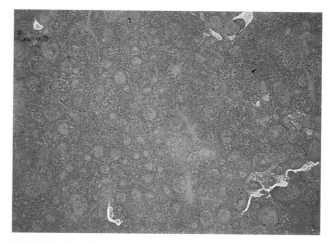

FIGURE 17.24   **Tumor reactive granulomatas with mantle cell lymphoma obscured the neoplastic proliferation in the spleens and abdominal lymph nodes.**

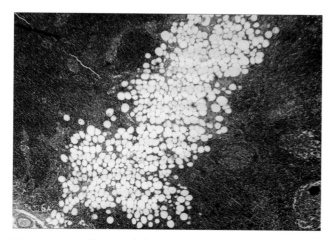

FIGURE 17.23   **Tangential section through medulla highlighting the medullary fatty change.**

FIGURE 17.25   **Tumor reactive granulomatas with epithelioid granulomas showing cuffs of mantle cell small lymphocytes in spleen involved with mantle cell lymphoma with sarcoidal reaction.**

prominent epithelioid histiocytes in some low-grade lymphomas or mantle cell lymphomas "obscured by granulmatous reaction" (see Figures 17.24–17.27).

Differential Diagnosis

Sarcoidosis can be a diagnostic dilemma. Occasionally serologic and histologic clues of sarcoidosis may mask a lymphoma especially when lymphocytes are small, bland, and mature looking. In addition sarcoidosis may present independent of and concurrent with non-Hodgkin lymphoma (Karakantza et al., 1996). More confusing is presence of extensive sarcoid-like granulomas in juxtaposed coexistence with low-grade lymphomas. Further confusion from sarcoidosis may arise because an elevated serum calcium level

and increased serum angiotensin converting enzyme activity may be seen in patients with non-Hodgkin lymphoma (Dunphy, Panella, and Grosso, 2000). In the skin, cutaneous granulomatous infiltration looking like sarcoidosis may turn out to be a rare form of granulomatous mycosis fungoides or part of granulomatous slack skin disease (Bessis et al., 1996).

Careful adherence to a lymph node protocol, including the performance of ancillary tests, including flow cytometry and molecular clonality tests, will help in determining the presence or absence of non-Hodgkin lymphoma. Immunohistochemical battery

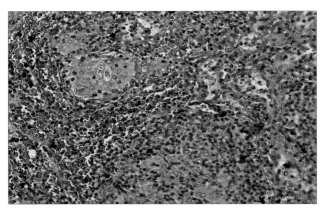

FIGURE 17.26 **Tumor reactive granulomatas with epithelioid sarcoidal-type granulomas adjacent with lymphoid rich granuloma**.

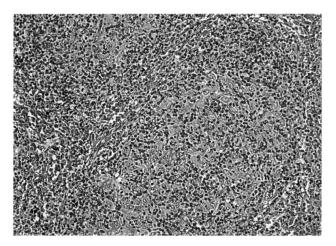

FIGURE 17.27 **Tumor reactive granulomatas with lymphoid rich granuloma in mantle cell lymphoma obscured by granulomas**.

of tests to rule out Hodgkin lymphoma, undifferentiated carcinoma, melanoma, myeloma, and seminoma may be performed to avoid misdiagnosis and missing a malignant neoplasm.

Treatment

Treatment should be geared toward a regimen directed to the reactive diagnosis or an underlying neoplasm.

REFERENCES

ANSARI-LARI MA, ALI SZ Fine-needle aspiration of abdominal fat pad for amyloid detection: a clinically useful test? 2004 Diagn Cytopathol 30:178–81.

AL RIKABI AC, NADDAF HO, AL BALLA SR, AL SOHAIBANI MO. 1995. Proteinaceous lymphadenopathy in a Patient with known rheumatoid arthritis: report and review of literature. Rheumatology 34:1087–9.

ALAGGIO R, CECCHETTO G, BISOGNO G, GAMBINI C, CALABRO ML, INSERRA A, BOLDRINI R, DE SALVO GL, DALL'IGNA P. 2010. Inflammatory myofibroblastic tumors in childhood: a report from the Italian cooperative group studies. Cancer 116:216–26.

AUCOUTURIER P, KHAMLICHI AA, TOUCHARD G, JUSTRABO E, COGNE M, CHAUFFERT B, MARTIN F, PREUD'HOMME JL. 1993. Heavy-chain deposition disease. N Eng J Med 329:1389–93.

BANERJEE D, MILLS DM, HEARN SA, MEEK M, TURNER KL. 1990a. Proteinaceous lymphadenopathy due to monoclonal nonamyloid immunoglobulin deposit disease. Arch Pathol Lab Med 114:34–9.

BESSIS D, SOTTO A, FARCET JP, BARNEON G, GUILHOU JJ. 1996. Granulomatous mycosis fungoides presenting as sarcoidosis. Dermatology 193:330–2.

BRAYLAN RC, LONG JC, JAFFE ES, GRECO FA, ORR SL, BERARD CW. 1977. Malignant lymphoma obscured by concomitant extensive epithelioid granulomas: report of three cases with similar clinicopathologic features. Cancer 39:1146–55.

BRINCKER H 1986. Sarcoid reactions in malignant tumours. Cancer Treat Rev 13:147–56.

BUXBAUM J, GALLO G. 1999a. Nonamyloidotic monoclonal immunoglobulin deposition disease: light-chain, heavy-chain, and light- and heavy-chain deposition diseases. Hematol Oncol Clin North Am 13:1235–48.

BUXBAUM JN, CHUBA JV, HELLMAN GC, SOLOMON A, GALLO GR. 1990. Monoclonal Immunoglobulin deposition disease: light chain and light and heavy chain deposition diseases and their relation to light chain amyloidosis. An Int Med 112:455–64.

CARNEIRO PC, GRAUDENZ MS, ZERBINI MC, DE MY, DOS SANTOS LR, FERRAZ AR. 1989. [Granulomatous reaction associated with metastatic epidermoid carcinoma: the importance of the use of multiple methods in diagnostic pathology]. Rev Hosp Clin Fac Med Sao Paulo 44:29–32. (in Portugese)

CHAN JK, CHEUK W, SHIMIZU M. 2001. Anaplastic lymphoma kinase expression in inflammatory pseudotumors. Am J Surg Pathol 25:761–8.

COFFIN CM, DEHNER LP, MEIS-KINDBLOM JM. 1998. Inflammatory myofibroblastic tumor, inflammatory fibrosarcoma, and related lesions: an historical review with differential diagnostic considerations. Semin Diag Pathol 15:102–10.

COFFIN CM, HUMPHREY PA, DEHNER LP. 1998. Extrapulmonary inflammatory myofibroblastic tumor: a clinical and pathological survey. Semin Diag Pathol 15:85–101.

COFFIN CM, WATTERSON J, PRIEST JR, DEHNER LP. 1995. Extrapulmonary inflammatory myofibroblastic tumor (inflammatory pseudotumor): a clinicopathologic and immunohistochemical study of 84 cases. Am J Surg Pathol 19:859–72.

DUNPHY CH, PANELLA MJ, GROSSO LE. 2000. Low-grade B-cell lymphoma and concomitant extensive sarcoidlike granulomas: a case report and review of the literature. Arch Pathol Lab Med 124:152–6.

GIORGADZE TA, SHIINA N, BALOCH ZW, TOMASZEWSKI JE, GUPTA PK. 2004. Improved detection of amyloid in fat pad aspiration: an evaluation of congo red stain by fluorescent microscopy. Diagn Cytopathol 31: 300–6.

HALLOUSH RA, LAVROVSKAYA E, MODY DR, LAGER D, TRUONG L. 2010. Diagnosis and typing of systemic amylo idosis: The role of abdominal fat pad fine needle aspiration biopsy. Cytojournal 15(6): 24.

HAZENBERG BP, LIMBURG PC, BIJZET J, VAN RIJSWIJK MH. 1999. A quantitative method for detecting deposits of amyloid A protein in aspirated fat tissue of patients with arthritis. An Rheum Dis 58:96–102.

HOLLINGSWORTH HC, LONGO DL, JAFFE ES. 1993. Small non-cleaved cell lymphoma associated with florid epithelioid granulomatous response: a clinicopathologic study of seven patients. Am J Surg Pathol 17:51–59.

HORIGUCHI H, MATSUI-HORIGUCHI M, SAKATA H, ICHINOSE M, YAMAMOTO T, FUJIWARA M, OHSE H. 2004. Inflammatory pseudotumor-like follicular dendritic cell tumor of the spleen. Pathol Int 54:124–31.

HUSSONG JW, BROWN M, PERKINS SL, DEHNER LP, COFFIN CM. 1999. Comparison of DNA ploidy, histologic, and immunohistochemical findings with clinical outcome in inflammatory myofibroblastic tumors. Mod Pathol 12:279–86.

KARAKANTZA M, MATUTES E, MACLENNAN K, O'CONNOR NT, SRIVASTAVA PC, CATOVSKY D. 1996. Association between sarcoidosis and lymphoma revisited. J Clin Pathol 49:208–12.

KHURANA KK, STANLEY MW, POWERS CN, PITMAN MB. 1998. Aspiration cytology of malignant neoplasms associated with granulomas and granuloma-like features: diagnostic dilemmas. Cancer 84:84–91.

KINMONTH JB, WOLFE JH. 1980. Fibrosis in the lymph nodes in primary lymphoedema: histological and clinical studies in 74 patients with lower-limb oedema. An R Coll Surg Engl 62:344–54.

KOJIMA M, NAKAMURA S, SHIMIZU K, HOSOMURA Y, OHNO Y, ITOH H, YAMANE N, YOSHIDA K, MASAWA N. 2001. Inflammatory pseudotumor of lymph nodes: clinicopathologic and immunohistological study of 11 Japanese cases. Int J Surg Pathol 9:207–14.

KUTOK JL, PINKUS GS, DORFMAN DM, FLETCHER CD. 2001. Inflammatory pseudotumor of lymph node and spleen: an entity biologically distinct from inflammatory myofibroblastic tumor. Hum Pathol 32:1382–7.

LEIGH J, WILES AN. 1987. Central lymph node changes and progressive massive fibrosis in coalworkers. Thorax 42:559–60.

LEWIS JT, GAFFNEY RL, CASEY MB, FARRELL MA, MORICE WG, MACON WR. 2003. Inflammatory pseudotumor of the spleen associated with a clonal Epstein–Barr virus genome: case report and review of the literature. Am J Clin Pathol 120:56–61.

LIN J, MARKOWITZ GS, VALERI AM, KAMBHAM NR, SHERMAN WH, APPEL GB, D'AGATI VD. 2001. Renal monoclonal immunoglobulin deposition disease: the disease spectrum. J Am Soc Nephrol 12:1482–92.

MARINO-ENRIQUEZ A, WANG WL, ROY A, LOPEZ-TERRADA D, LAZAR AJ, FLETCHER CD, COFFIN CM, HORNICK JL. 2011. Epithelioid inflammatory myofibroblastic sarcoma: an aggressive intra-abdominal variant of inflammatory myofibroblastic tumor with nuclear membrane or perinuclear ALK. Am J Surg Pathol 35:135–44.

MICHAELI J, NIESVIZKY R, SIEGEL D, LADANYI M, LIEBERMAN PH, FILIPPA DA. 1995. Proteinaceous (angiocentric sclerosing) lymphadenopathy: a polyclonal systemic, nonamyloid deposition disorder. Blood 86:1159–62.

OSBORNE BM, BUTLER JJ, MACKAY B. 1979. Proteinaceous lymphadenopathy with hypergammaglobulinemia. Am J Surg Pathol 3:137–45.

PERRONE T, DE WOLF-PEETERS C, FRIZZERA G. 1988. Inflammatory pseudotumor of lymph nodes: a distinctive pattern of nodal reaction. Am J Surg Pathol 12:351–61.

RICHTER HJ, LEDER LD. 1979. Lymph node metastases with PAS-positive tumor cells and massive epithelioid granulomatous reaction as diagnostic clue to occult seminoma. Cancer 44:245–9.

SACKS EL, DONALDSON SS, GORDON J, DORFMAN RF. 1978. Epithelioid granulomas associated with Hodgkin's disease: clinical correlations in 55 previously untreated patients. Cancer 41:562–7.

SWERDLOW SH, CAMPO E, HARRIS NL, JAFFE ES, PILERI SA, STEIN H, THIELE J, VARDIMAN JW. 2008. WHO Classification of Tumours of Haematopoietic and Lymphoid Tissues. International Agency for Research on Cancer, Lyon.

TAVORA F, SHILO K, OZBUDAK IH, PRZYBOCKI JM, WANG G, TRAVIS WD, FRANKS TJ. 2007. Absence of human herpesvirus-8 in pulmonary inflammatory myofibroblastic tumor: immunohistochemical and molecular analysis of 20 cases. Mod Pathol 20:995–9.

WARNKE RA, WEISS LM, CHAN JKC, CLEARY ML, DORFMAN RF. 1995. Tumors of the lymph nodes and spleen. Atlas of Tumor Pathology, AFIP Third Series.

WEISS L. 2008. Lymph Nodes. Cambridge University Press, New York.

CHAPTER EIGHTEEN

MIXED LYMPH NODE PATTERNS: INCLUDING GRANULOMATOUS LYMPHADENOPATHY, NONINFECTIOUS

Xiaohui Zhang and Hernani D. Cualing

MIXED PATTERN WITH FOLLICULAR HYPERPLASIA AND EOSINOPHILIA

Kimura's Disease

The first report of Kimura's disease was in 1937 by Kim and Szeto in the Chinese literature (Kung and Chan, 1988), in which they described seven cases of a condition they termed "eosinophilic hyperplastic lymphogranuloma." It received its current name after a report by Kimura et al. in 1948 in a Japanese journal (Kimura, 1948). There has been confusion between Kimura's disease and angiolymphoid hyperplasia with eosinophilia (ALHE), but now they are considered to be different entities.

Definition

Kimura's disease is a benign rare chronic inflammatory disorder of unknown etiology, predominantly involving the lymph nodes and subcutaneous tissue of the head and neck region, and is characterized by angiolymphoid proliferation and eosinophilia.

ICD-10 Code I89

Synonyms

Kimura disease, Kimura lymphadenopathy, eosinophilic granuloma.

Epidemiology

Kimura's disease is rare and is predominantly seen in young males of Asian descent. The reported range of age is as big as 2.5 to 61 years with a median age from 25 to 32 years (Wang et al., 2009; Sun et al., 2008; Chen et al., 2004; Takeishi et al., 2007). Male to female ratio is roughly 3 to 19:1. There have been only a few hundred cases reported all worldwide and most cases are in East and Southeast Asia. However, a small number of cases have been reported in Europe and the United States in all races (Sun et al., 2008; Chen et al., 2004). The exact prevalence of Kimura's disease is unknown.

Clinical Aspects

Etiology. The exact etiology of Kimura's disease is unknown. An aberrant immune reaction, namely autoimmunity, allergic reaction, or an alteration of

Non-Neoplastic Hematopathology and Infections, First Edition. Edited by Hernani D. Cualing, Parul Bhargava, and Ramon L. Sandin.
© 2012 Wiley-Blackwell. Published 2012 by John Wiley & Sons, Inc.

immune regulation, has been suspected (Thomas et al., 2008; Abuel-Haija and Hurford, 2007).

Sites of Involvement. Kimura's disease usually affects deep subcutaneous tissue and regional lymph nodes of the head and neck, with or without salivary gland involvement (Chen et al., 2004). Uncommon sites of involvement have been described, including axilla, groin, popliteal region, limbs, oral cavity, and trunk (Abuel-Haija and Hurford, 2007; Chung et al., 2010). It is associated with renal disease, with various forms of renal pathology such as membranous nephropathy, minimal change disease, and mesangial proliferative glomerulonephritis in 15 to 18% of adult patients (Wang et al., 2009).

Pathogenesis

The pathogenesis of Kimura's disease is unclear. Allergic reaction, autoimmune reaction, and association with an infectious process including parasite, virus, fungi, or toxin have been suggested in different studies (Chen et al., 2004; Thomas et al., 2008).

Approach to Diagnosis

Incisional biopsy is recommended to obtain the diagnosis of Kimura's disease.

Clinical Workup

CBC count with differential almost always shows peripheral eosinophilia. Serum IgE levels are often elevated. BUN, creatinine should be obtained to assess the renal function. Imaging studies, particularly ultrasonography and magnetic resonance imaging (MRI), may help determine the extent of the disease.

Morphology

The enlarged lymph node can be very large in size simulating a tumor. The key morphological features of Kimura's disease are summarized in Table 18.1. Generally, the nodal architecture is largely preserved. There may be capsular fibrosis, subcapsular sinusoid obliteration, and perinodal soft tissue involvement. Florid germinal centers are surrounded by well-defined mantle zones that may invaginate or intrude inside germinal centers. Marked eosinophilic infiltrates are present in the paracortex and sinuses. Eosinophil microabscesses may or may not be present, and eosinophils in germinal centers are often present. Eosinophilic folliculolysis is a helpful feature. Polykaryocytes (Warthin–Finkeldey-type giant cells) are often seen in the germinal centers. Vascular proliferation of high endothelial venules is seen mostly in the paracortex, at times so prominent that these venules impinges on into the mantle zones.

TABLE 18.1 Kimura's Disease

Key Morphologic Features
Florid reactive hyperplasia
Germinal center hyperplasia well-defined mantle zone lymphocytes invaginating into the germinal centers (Figure 18.1)
Polykaryotes in germinal centers (Figure 18.2)
Germinal center eosinophils (Figure 18.3)
Vascularization of germinal centers (Figure 18.4)
Proteinaceous precipitate bodies in germinal centers (Figure 18.5)
Cortical and paracortical eosinophilia
Paracortex with eosinophils with or without paracortical eosinophilic abscess (Figure 18.6, 18.7)
Paracortical hypervascularity (Figure 18.6)
Patchy sclerosis of arteriolar vessels with onion-skinning pattern (Figure 18.8)

As delineated by Hui, there are constant, frequent, and rare features (Hui et al., 1989; Chen et al., 2004). Constant features include a preserved nodal architecture, florid germinal centers' hyperplasia, eosinophilic infiltration in the paracortex, and proliferation of postcapillary venules. Frequent features include sclerosis of the paracortex and blood vessels, polykaryocytes in germinal centers, vascularization of germinal centers and the paracortex, proteinaceous precipitate bodies in germinal centers, necrosis of germinal centers, eosinophil abscess, and atrophic venules in sclerotic areas (Figures 18.1–18.8).

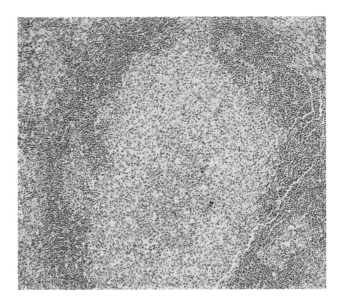

FIGURE 18.1 Germinal centers surrounded by well-defined mantle with dark zone invagination into the pale centers (250×).

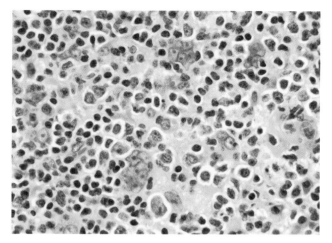

FIGURE 18.2   Polykaryocytes   (Warthin–Finkeldey-type giant cells) in the germinal centers.

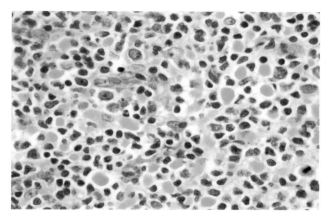

FIGURE 18.5   Proteinaceous precipitate bodies in germinal centers.

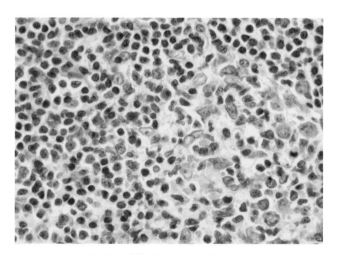

FIGURE 18.3   Eosinophils in germinal centers.

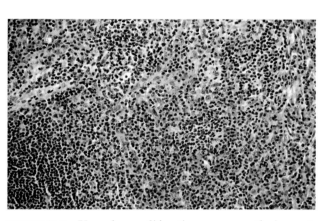

FIGURE 18.6   Vascular proliferation seen mostly in post-capillary venules in mantle zone and interfollicular eosinophilia.

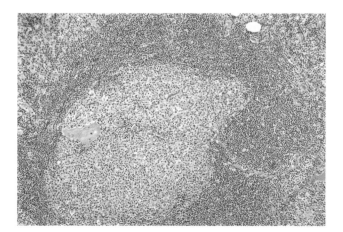

FIGURE 18.4   Hypervascularity of the germinal center.

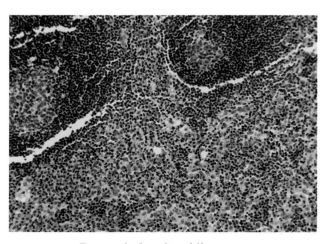

FIGURE 18.7   Paracortical eosinophila.

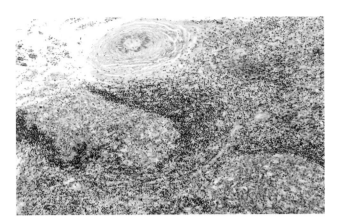

FIGURE 18.8 **Patchy sclerosis of vessels and onion-skinning around sclerosed arterioles**.

Rare feature includes progressive transformation of germinal centers.

Immunophenotyping/Cytochemistry

Immunohistochemical stains with IgE show a characteristic reticular staining pattern of the germinal centers (Hui et al., 1989). These stainings may correspond to the pink proteinaceous precipitates inside the germinal centers.

Differential Diagnosis

Kimura's disease has been confused with ALHE (Angiolymphoid Hyperplasia with Eosinophilia) both clinically and microscopically. Although it was assumed that the diseases represent two ends of the same spectrum, it is now accepted that Kimura's disease is a separate entity from ALHE. In contrast to Kimura's disease, ALHE occurs in all racial groups, typically middle-aged females in the

TABLE 18.2 **Angiolymphoid Hyperplasia with Eosinophilia**

Key Morphologic Features
Presence of arteriovenous malformation or damaged muscular artery or vein adjacent to mass in many cases (Figure 18.9)
Proliferation of blood vessels with plump or hobnailed high endothelial venules, surrounded by eosinophils (Figure 18.10)
Reactive small lymphoid aggregates with minimal or absent germinal centers and predominance of eosinophils (Figure 18.11)
Prominent arteriolar sclerosis and eosinophilic arteriolitis (Figure 18.12)
Discrete paucicellular pale edematous stroma, with eosinophilic matrix, on a sea of eosinophils (Figure 18.13)
Focal ischemic necrosis (Figure 18.14)

Western population. Regional lymphadenopathy, serum eosinophilia, and elevated IgE levels are rare. There are three major components in ALHE: branching vessels (malformed or damaged large vessels) with protuberant epithelioid endothelial cells, a lymphocytic infiltrate, and fairly numerous eosinophils. The vascular proliferation with epithelioid endothelial cells is more prominent. Some other features of ALHE are summarized in Table 18.2 (Figures 18.9–18.14).

Other differential diagnoses include Hodgkin disease, angioimmunoblastic T-cell lymphoma, Langerhans cell histiocytosis, florid follicular hyperplasia, Castleman's disease, dermatopathic lymphadenopathy, allergic granulomatosis/Churg–Strauss syndrome, lymphadenopathy of drug reactions, and parasitic lymphadenitis. A lymphoma workup including molecular and phenotypic analysis would

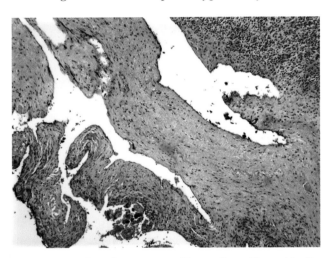

FIGURE 18.9 **Arteriovenous malformation adjacent to the mass**.

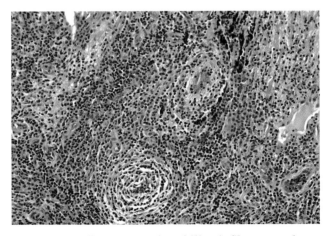

FIGURE 18.10 **Intense eosinophilic infiltrates, plump endothelial venules with onion skinning**.

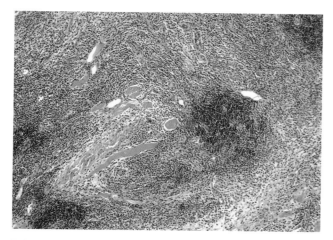

FIGURE 18.11 **Residual lymphoid aggregates with entrapped degenerated skeletal muscle, edema**.

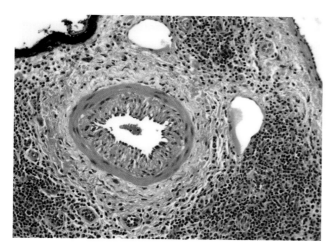

FIGURE 18.12 **Arteriolar sclerosis and eosinophilic arteriolitis**.

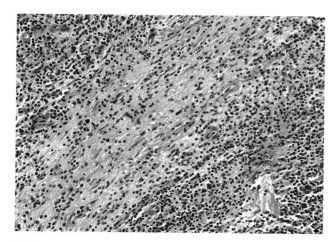

FIGURE 18.13 **Paucicelluar edematous stroma with eosinophils**.

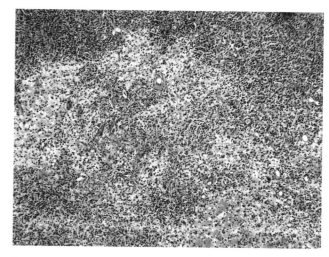

FIGURE 18.14 **Focal ischemic necrosis (right bottom) with proliferation of vessels and admixed eosinophils**.

be essential to exclude neoplastic hematologic diseases. The other entities have insinuating morphologic signatures.

Treatment of Choice and Prognosis

The primary treatment is surgical resection. Immunosuppressants, steroid, cytotoxic agents, and radiation are used to reduce morbidity and to prevent complications. The course is chronic and frequently waxes and wanes over time. The prognosis is good, with no potential for malignant transformation.

Allergic Granulomatosis/Churg–Strauss Syndrome

Also known as Churg–Strauss syndrome, allergic granulomatosis was first described by Churg and Strauss in 1951 (Churg and Strauss, 1951). It is a rare, systemic necrotizing vasculitis that involves multiple organs or systems.

Definition

As defined by the Chapel Hill Consensus Conference on the classification of vasculitis in 1994 (Jennette et al., 1994b), Churg–Strauss syndrome is an eosinophil-rich and granulomatous inflammation involving the respiratory tract, necrotizing vasculitis affecting small- to medium-size vessels, and associated with asthma and eosinophilia.

ICD-10 Code M30.1

Synonyms

Churg–Strauss syndrome, Churg–Strauss vasculitis, allergic granulomatosis, allergic angiitis and granulomatosis, allergic granulomatosis and angiitis, eosinophilic granulomatous vasculitis.

Epidemiology

Churg–Strauss syndrome is rare with an annual incidence between 0.05 and 0.68 cases per 100,000 patients (Pagnoux, 2010), while among asthma patients, an average of 3.4 cases per 100,000 patients has been reported (Pagnoux et al., 2007). Gender predilection varies according to different sources, and it is believed there is no sex predominance (Pagnoux, 2010). The range of age is between 4 and 75 years with a median age around 50 years (Abril et al., 2003). There is no strong evidence of racial predilection and a differential geographic distribution pattern.

Clinical Aspects

Etiology. The exact cause of Churg–Strauss syndrome is unknown. Several triggering factors have been suspected, including allergen inhalation, vaccinations, desensitization, and drugs. Some drugs linked to this disease are macrolides, carbamazepine, quinine, anti-asthma medications such as leukotriene antagonists or modifiers (montelukast, zafirlukast, etc.), and more recently omalizumab (Pagnoux, 2010; Jaworsky, 2008; Bibby et al., 2010; Wechsler et al., 2009). However, no conclusion of causal effects has been drawn. Although association with asthma is typical, cases without history of asthma have been described (Abril et al., 2003).

Sites of Involvement. Three clinical phases of the disease have been characterized. Phase 1, or the prodromal phase, is characterized by adult-onset asthma with or without allergic rhinitis. Phase 2, or the eosinophilic phase, is marked by peripheral eosinophilia and tissue eosinophilic infiltration involving lungs, gastrointestinal tract, and skin. Phase 3, or the vasculitic phase, has manifestations of systemic vasculitis that may occur in lung, skin, peripheral nerves, heart, kidney, liver, muscle, central nervous system, and lymph node (Gross, 2002). The most frequent involved organs are lungs (Figure 18.15), skin, peripheral nerves, gastrointestinal tract, and heart (Sinico and Bottero, 2009; Cualing et al., 2001). In pediatric patients, pulmonary and cardiac involvement is predominant (Zwerina et al., 2009c). A restricted indolent form with involvement limited to specific organs, including the eyes, the skin, the gastrointestinal tract, or the lymph node, has been recognized and is labeled as the limited form of Churg–Strauss syndrome (Cualing et al., 2001).

Pathogenesis

The pathogenetic mechanism for Churg–Strauss syndrome remains unclear, but it is believed to be

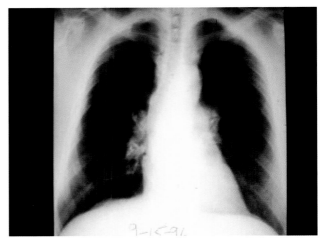

FIGURE 18.15 **Prominent hilar vessels and nodes.**

an autoimmune process, supported by the presence of immune complexes, heightened T-cell immunity, and altered humoral immunity. A strong Th2-type immune response are postulated to play a role in the prodromal phase (Zwerina et al., 2009a). Eosinophils are activated in the progression of the disease, and eosinophilic cationic protein, eosinophil-derived neurotoxin, and eosinophil peroxidase are released by eosinophils that directly cause tissue and endothelial damage and trigger the oxidative stress cascade (Guilpain et al., 2007; Pagnoux, 2010). The formation of immunoglobulin (Ig) E-containing complexes and their interactions with eosinophils is also suggested to play a role (Ishii et al., 2009). In addition an antineutrophil cytoplasm autoantibody (ANCA) participates in the development of vasculitic lesions (Zwerina et al., 2009b). Hereditary factors, like the HLA-DRB1*04 and HLA-DR1*07 alleles and the HLA-DRB4 gene, are also risk factors (Wieczorek et al., 2010).

Approach to Diagnosis

An algorithm was developed and validated for the clinical diagnosis of Churg–Strauss syndrome (Sinico and Bottero, 2009; Watts et al., 2007). In a patient with either histological proof of vasculitis or surrogate markers for vasculitis, the Lanham or the American College of Rheumatology (ACR) criteria can be applied to make the diagnosis (Watts et al., 2007). Lanham criteria require the following: (1) a history of asthma, (2) eosinophilia higher than 1500 cell mm^3, and (3) clinical/histological vasculitis involving two or more extrapulmonary organs (Lanham et al., 1984). The ACR criteria need at least four of the following six: (1) asthma, (2) eosinophilia greater than 10% on differential white blood cell count, (3) mononeuropathy (including multiplex) or polyneuropathy, (4) migratory or transient pulmonary infiltrates detected radiographically, (5) paranasal sinus abnormality, and (6) biopsy containing a blood vessel with extravascular eosinophils (Masi et al., 1990). The sensitivity and specificity of the ACR criteria are 85 and 99.7% respectively.

Clinical Workup

CBC count, erythrocyte sedimentation rate (ESR), and ANCA testing should be performed. Systemic vasculitis screening including cryoglobulins, antiphospholipid antibodies, immunoglobulins (Igs), especially IgE, and complement levels may be included in the initial workup. Multiple system functional tests are helpful to evaluate the systemic involvement of the disease. European League Against Rheumatism (EULAR) recommends that tissue biopsy should be obtained whenever possible (Mukhtyar et al., 2008).

Morphology

Regardless of the organs involved, two pathological findings are confirmatory of Churg–Strauss syndrome: necrotizing vasculitis and extravascular necrotizing granulomas, associated with eosinophilic infiltrates (Lie, 1990; Churg and Strauss, 1951). The granulomas are composed of a center of necrotic eosinophils debris and surrounded by eosinophils, palisading histiocytes, and few multinucleated giant cells. However, the granulomas are not pathognomonic because they are also present in Wegener granulomatosis, polyarteritis nodosa, systemic lupus erythematosus, rheumatoid arthritis, lymphoproliferative disorders, and other immunoreactive disorders.

In the involved lymph node, a benign lymph node architecture is preserved but is distorted by the eosinophilic granuloma (Figure 18.16). Arterioles and venules are thickened with prominent sclerosis and eosinophilic angiitis (Figure 18.18). The interfollicular areas contain eosinophils, transformed lymphocytes, histiocytes, and proliferation of endothelial venules (Figure 18.19) (Cualing et al., 2001). Charcot–Leyden crystals may also be present (Casey et al., 2000). Well-formed epithelioid granulomas, surrounding germinal centers, are C-shaped and ring-shaped, some centrally necrotic with eosinophilic abscess (Figure 18.19). Key morphological features are summarized in Table 18.3.

Immunophenotyping/Cytochemistry

The immunophenotype of the lymph node involved by Churg–Strauss syndrome is typical of a reactive process with preserved B-cells as well as T-cell areas. Flow cytometric results of immunoglobulin

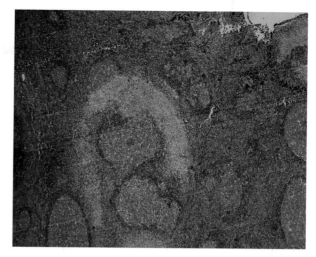

FIGURE 18.16 **Low-power view of the benign lymph node architecture distorted by a ring-shaped granuloma encircling germinal centers**.

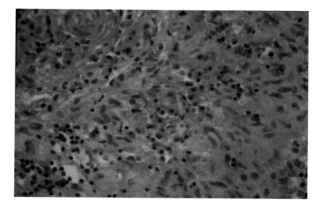

FIGURE 18.17 **High-power view of an eosinophilic granulomatous inflammation**. The epithelioid histiocytes are admixed with an inner central collection of eosinophils resembling eosinophilic microabscess.

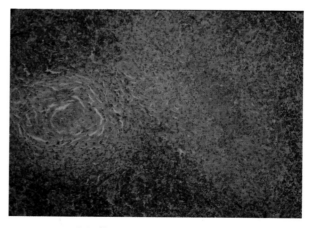

FIGURE 18.18 **Medium-power view of periarteriolar granulomatous focus with palisading histiocytes and eosinophilic collection**.

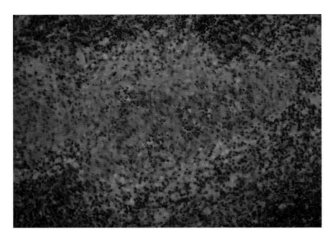

FIGURE 18.19 **Medium-power view showing dispersed eosinophils, lymphocytes, immunoblasts, clusters of histiocytes, and allergic eosinophilic granuloma.**

TABLE 18.3 **Churg–Strauss Syndrome/Allergic Granulomatosis**

Key Morphologic Features
Prominent vessels with sclerosis, eosinophilic vasculitis
Necrotizing and nonnecrotizing confluent epithelioid granulomas
Follicular hyperplasia with progressive transformation of germinal centers
Interfollicular area contained numerous eosinophils and clusters of plasma cells, immunoblasts, and mummified cells and Warthin–Finkeldey giant cells

light chains (kappa and lambda) should be polyclonal. CD15, CD30, and S100 immunostaining may be helpful to differentiate from Hodgkin lymphoma and Langerhans cell histiocytosis/eosinophilic granuloma.

Approach to Diagnosis

Eosinophilia is the hallmark laboratory finding. However, workup is needed to exclude the other causes of eosinophilia and to establish the presence of a vasculitic process. Anemia, leukocytosis, thrombocytosis, and an elevated ESR are usually found in the vasculitic phase in CBC. Rheumatoid factor (RF) and antinuclear antibody (ANA) may be weakly positive. Perinuclear ANCA (P-ANCA)/myeloperoxidase ANCA (MPO-ANCA) was initially reported in as many as 75 to 80% of patients, but more recent studies have shown much lower frequency of positivity (Sinico and Bottero, 2009).

Differential Diagnosis

The eosinophilic granuloma type of Langerhans cell histiocytosis needs to be ruled out based on the absence of infiltrate of characteristic S100-positive Langerhans cell histiocytes in a diffuse sinusoidal pattern. In addition sheets of Langerhans cells with grooved nuclei are present in eosinophilic granuloma, but these cells are rare and scattered in allergic granulomas. Although granulomas may frequently be seen in Hodgkin disease, the absence of Reed–Sternberg cells or the variant "popcorn" cells of the lymphocyte-predominant type and the absence of typical immunoreactivity for Hodgkin lymphoma would rule it out. Peripheral T-cell lymphomas can be associated with eosinophilia, which would show atypical pleomorphic small to large T cells and show aberrant flow cytometry T-cell reactivities. Tissue eosinophilia may be observed in diffuse large B-cell non-Hodgkin lymphomas with eosinophilia, but it does not typically show granulomatous changes (Navarro-Roman et al., 1994).

Among the reactive conditions, Kimura's disease tends to have a triad of follicular hyperplasia, infiltration by eosinophils, and proliferation of postcapillary venules (Kuo et al., 1988). Sarcoidosis does not have eosinophilic abscesses. Other systemic vasculitides may involve the same organs as the Churg–Strauss syndrome, and may also be ANCA positive, but the presence of asthma and eosinophilia is uncommon. In Wegener granulomatosis the eosinophils are usually absent or in a small number. Polyarteritis nodosa has less intense eosinophilic infiltration and intravascular granulomas are rarely seen. A drug effect is commonly associated with a cutaneous and mucosal allergic reaction with a particular medication history.

Treatment of Choice and Prognosis

Corticosteroids are the first-line therapy. Immunosuppressive medications such as cyclophosphamide, azathioprine, and mycophenolate mofetil may be initiated in unresponsive patients. Tumor necrosis factor (TNF) blockers, infliximab, and etanercept may be used for severe cases. The majority of patients usually achieve a full recovery but relapses and fatalities may occur. Coronary arteritis and myocarditis are the main causes of morbidity and mortality (Sinico and Bottero, 2009).

MIXED NONNECROTIZING "DRY" GRANULOMAS

Sarcoidosis

Sarcoidosis is well known to affect the lungs and intrathoracic lymph nodes primarily, while virtually almost every organ can be involved. Extrathoracic lymphadenopathy is estimated to occur in 15% of the patients. Although it has been described since 1875, causes and pathogenesis still remain mysterious.

Definition

Sarcoidosis is a multisystem inflammatory disease of unknown etiology that predominantly affects the young adults, and it is characterized by the presence of noncaseating granulomas in affected organs.

ICD-10 Code D86

Synonyms

Sarcoid, Besnier–Boeck disease, Besnier–Boeck–Schaumann disease.

Epidemiology

Sarcoidosis is seen throughout the world with an incidence ranging from 5 to 40 per 100,000 population per year. The prevalence among African-Americans are 10 times higher than among the Caucasians. It commonly affects people younger than 50 with a peak of incidence between ages 20 and 40 (Lazarus, 2009). A second peak of incidence in females older than 50 years of age has been reported (Tachibana et al., 2010). Male to female ratio is 2:1.

Clinical Aspects

The lungs are the most common site involved followed by skin and lymph nodes. A third of patients have skin involvement and peripheral lymph nodes are involved in one-sixth or 15% of patients (Yanardag et al., 2007). Significant liver pathology could be seen as granulomatous hepatic involvement (Devaney et al., 1993). The bone marrow is also involved with noncaseating granulomas in 10% of sarcoidosis (Yanardag et al., 2007).

Pathogenesis

No definite etiologic agent has been identified. Possible causing agents are infection, irritants, chemical agents, and occupational exposures. T cells play a central role in the development of sarcoidosis, as they likely present an excessive immune response. Several cytokines are also critical in the pathogenesis. Th1 cytokines (IFN-gamma and interleukin-2) production is increased while Th2 cytokines (interleukin-4 and interleukin-5) are low. In addition the tumor necrosis factor (TNF) and TNF receptors are increased [Lazarus, 2009].

Approach to Diagnosis

Biopsy is the approach to diagnose sarcoidosis in most cases. Noncaseating epithelioid granulomas shoud be present in at least two organs, commonly lung or mediastinum, followed by cervical/axillary lymph nodes with unusual sparing of small and large intestinal organs and mesenteric nodes. Spleen may be massively involved in 20% of cases. Infectious and noninfectious etiologies have to be ruled out before diagnosing sarcoidosis.

Clinical Workup

Serum angiotensin converting enzyme (ACE) levels are elevated in 60% of patients at the time of diagnosis, but the sensitivity and specificity of this test is limited (60 and 80%, respectively) (Ainslie and Benatar, 1985). Besides imaging studies, fiberoptic bronchoscopy with mucosal and transbronchial biopsy and bronchoalveolar lavage (BAL), will establish a histological diagnosis. Notably BAL with CD4+/CD8+ lymphocyte ratio greater than 3.5 shows a high specificity of 94 to 96%, while the sensitivity is 52 to 59% (Costabel et al., 2008). Peripheral blood counts, serum calcium levels, liver enzymes, and creatinine may be helpful for the evaluation of the disease status. There may be hypercalcemia or hypercalciuria. An elevated alkaline phosphatase level suggests hepatic involvement.

Morphology

Morphological features are summarized in Table 18.4. In full-blown sarcoidosis, the lymph node histology is characteristic with an extensive architectural replacement by rounded, discrete, sometimes coalescing epithelioid cell granulomas (Figures 18.20–18.22). Occasional central areas of the granuloma show pink necrotic acellular appearance (Figure 18.23). Giant cells are present in many foci (Figure 18.24). Early sarcoid in lymph nodes may show scattered granulomas composed of loose macrophages with few epithelioid or spindle forms usually found adjacent to B-cell follicles (Figure 18.20). More advanced sarcoid show back to back (Figure 18.27), almost confluent, granulomas diffusely present in the cortex to medulla (Figure 18.21), and progressive disease may show replacement of epithelioid islands with mature fibrous or collagenous tissue. Uninvolved lymph node show dilated sinuses with reticulin tethers (Figure 18.25), and prominent high endothelial or postcapillary venules in the paracortex.

In some granulomas, within giant cells or non-granulomatous areas, some or all of the following inclusion bodies may be present: birefringent amorphous crystalline inclusion bodies, concentric calcified basophilic conchoid, or Schaumann bodies (Figure 18.26). These may take on a birefringent

TABLE 18.4 Sarcoidosis

Common Morphologic Features

Noncaseating epithelioid granulomas, showing compact fully developed rounded collection of epithelioid macrophages, multinucleated giant cells, and scant lymphocytes (not specific, need to rule out infectious and noninfectious eitologies)

Mostly discrete granulomas with few confluent forms displacing reticulin or collagen fibers around the granulomas

Giant cells may be foreign body or Langhan's type, rarely numerous unlike in tuberculosis or fungal infections

Caseation is characteristically absent; rare focal fibrinoid central necrosis could be present

Minimal or nonexistent suppurative abscess

Presence of inclusion bodies: crystalline inclusion bodies, concoid bodies, Schaumann bodies, asteroid bodies, or Hamazaki–Wesenberg (HW, or rice) bodies

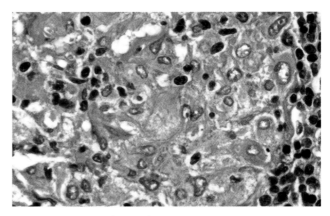

FIGURE 18.22 Epithelioid granuloma in routine stains with compact arrangement. Reticulin stain often show dense fibrous scaffolding in the granulomas.

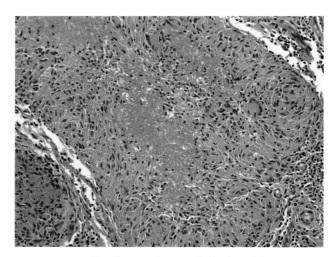

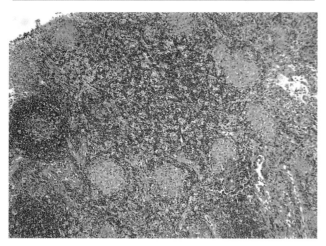

FIGURE 18.20 Ring of granulomas around a paracortex nodule and a germinal center.

FIGURE 18.23 Focal central necrosis in sarcoid.

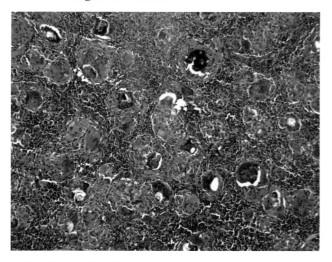

FIGURE 18.21 Confluent epithelioid granulomas in sarcoidosis.

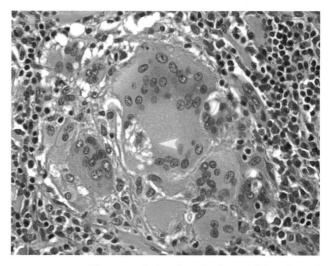

FIGURE 18.24 Cluster of foreign body multinucleated giant cells.

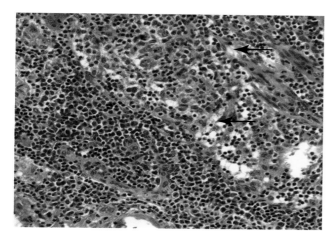

FIGURE 18.25 **Uninvolved lymph node area showing increase in vascularity, and presence of intense sinus histiocytosis with prominent sinus fibroblastic reticular scaffolding (arrow).**

could be seen inside or outside of macrophages of reactive lymph nodes—often those showing sinus reactions. They are not easily seen unless a high-power magnification is used. In routine H & E, they appear as ovoid, round, or spindle shaped—the latter resembling a rice seed in shape—but colored brownish-yellow, dark or gray brown. They are easily masked by the eosinophilia of the cytoplasm of surrounding cells. When seen in high-power magnification, they impart a sharp relief with the center of these bodies, appearing denser in color than the edges. The bodies often are seen in collection where other parts of the node appear devoid of them. These collections are often in sinuses, in medullary spaces, adjacent to venules, and rarely in and around germinal centers. Special stains for both AFB and Grocott for fungal microorganisms reveal these bodies to be

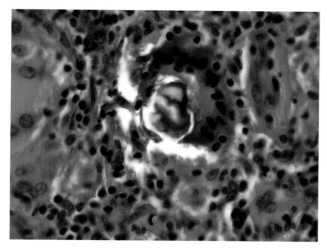

FIGURE 18.26 **Crystalline conchoid bodies in multinucleate giant cell.**

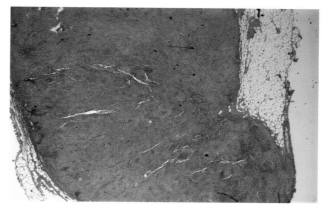

FIGURE 18.27 **Lymph node totally replaced by sarcoidosis.**

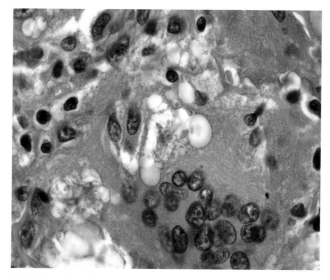

FIGURE 18.28 **Double asteroid bodies.**

polarized appearance. Asteroid bodies are also seen as a discrete stellate spiculated eosinophilic body with a clear background (Figure 18.28). Although none are specific to sarcoidosis, their presence and the corresponding absence of other findings of TB, fungal, Crohn's disease, or berylliosis may indicate sarcoidosis. Rice bodies or Hamazaki–Wesenberg (HW) bodies also belong to these inclusions that could be seen in sarcoidosis (Figures 18.29, 18.30).

HW bodies are sometimes called ceroid bodies owing to their fatty osmiophilic electron microscopy appearance. Although not specific for sarcoidosis, these spindle or ovoid bodies need to be recognized because of their resemblance to fungal bodies. These

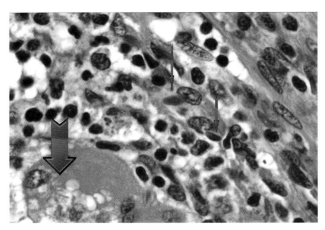

FIGURE 18.29 **Hamazaki–Wesenberg bodies or rice bodies adjacent to sinus lining cells.** HW bodies—thin arrows; asteroid body in giant cell—thick arrow.

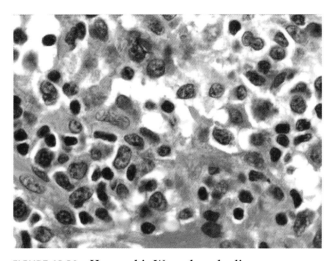

FIGURE 18.30 **Hamazaki–Wesenberg bodies.**

AFB staining in an intense blue color (Figure 18.31). PAS stain them dark pink. Gram stain and Giemsa impart Gram positive and greenish hue. Methyl green pyronin stains, owing to their light staining appearance, accentuate their brownish color. Silver or melanin stains impart a variable coloration results (Henry and Farrer-Brown, 1981).

Differential Diagnosis

Infectious granulomas, namely mycobacteria tuberculosis and fungal infections, are often the primary differential diagnosis, especially when the initial findings involve the lungs and mediastinum. Exposure to exogenous inorganic substance such as beryllium is also high in the differential since the reaction is typically a sarcoidal type with epithelioid

rounded granulomas. When seen in mesenteric or abdominal lymph nodes, Crohn's regional enteritis granulomatous lymphadenitis should be considered and appropriate mucosal biopsies should be performed. The most common side effects of recombinant IFN recombinant interferon-alpha (IFN-alpha) treatment of chronic hepatitis C is the development of sarcoidosis that is histologically similar to de novo sarcoidosis (Butnor, 2005; Ravenel et al., 2001). The presence of noncaseating granulomas in bone marrow is secondary to the following differential diagnosi: infectious disease (30%), hematologic disorders (25%), sarcoidosis (11%), nonhematologic malignancies (10%), drug reaction (5%), other diseases (6%), and no final diagnosis (6%) (Bhargava and Farhi, 1988).

Crohn's lymphadenitis manifest as regional abdominal lymph node enlargement as part of the intestinal pathology findings in a number of cases. The morphologic changes vary from a nonspecific follicular and paracortical hyperplasia to discrete presence of epithelioid granulomas that are noncaseating. Necrosis is rare and progression of disease show a tendency for the granulomas to undergo fibrosis.

Berylliosis may manifest as hilar pulmonary lymphadenopathy in response to exposure to beryllium salts in certain occupation and can be detected using specialized X-ray microscopic techniques (Butnor et al., 2003). Sarcoidal-type granulomas with inclusions seen in sarcoidosis are the typical appearance in histology. Beryllium salt spectrography may also be used to identify the etiology.

Treatment of Choice and Prognosis

Although the clinical course is variable, about two-thirds of the patients may recover with minimal

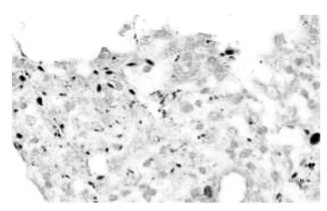

FIGURE 18.31 **AFB stain dark blue positive for HW bodies.**

residual changes. Lung function may be compromised in one-fifth, and a tenth of patients die of complications: progressive pulmonary fibrosis, central nervous system disease, or myocardial disease. Treatment is usually with steroids.

Berylliosis

Berylliosis is a hypersensitivity disorder that develops as a result of exposure to beryllium. It is similar to sarcoidosis clinically, radiologically and histopathologically, except that the cause, beryllium, is known.

Definition

Berylliosis is an occupationally acquired granulomatosis disease caused by beryllium exposure, affecting lungs and may also present with lymphadenopathy.

ICD-10 Code J63.2

Synonym

Chronic beryllium disease.

Epidemiology

It is estimated that at least 134,000 current workers and up to 1 million individuals have been exposed to beryllium in the United States (Samuel and Maier, 2008). A small percentage (1–10%) of those exposed people develop beryllium hypersensitivity, and some further develop berylliosis.

Clinical Aspects

Etiology. Beryllium is the inciting agent. The exposure is primarily by inhalation or contact through broken skin, which occurs in many industries, such as metal mining and processing, nuclear energy, defense industries, aerospace and aeronautics, computer manufacturing and other electronic industries (Santo Tomas, 2009). Secondary exposure from beryllium workers has also been reported to cause berylliosis.

Site of Involvement. The granuloma formation can be throughout the body, but lungs, intrathoracic lymph nodes and skin are the predominant sites.

Pathogenesis

The disease develops due to a cell-mediated delayed-type hypersensitivity in response to beryllium. The beryllium most likely functions as a hapten. Large number of CD4+ T cells accumulate in tissues with disease activity. The CD4+ T cells interact with human leukocyte antigen (HLA) class II on antigen presenting cells. HLA-DPB1 with glutamic acid at amino acid position 69 (HLA-DPB1-Glu69) is a marker associated with increased susceptibility to berylliosis (Amicosante et al., 2005).

Approach to Diagnosis

The diagnosis is based on demonstration of granulomatous changes and positive lung proliferative response to beryllium (BeLPT), which is done on blood or BAL cells. BeLPT test involves exposing peripheral blood mononuclear cells in vitro to beryllium salts, and cell proliferation in the presence of beryllium indicates a positive result. It is a highly specific and sensitive test, helping distinguish berylliosis from sarcoidosis (Rossman, 1996).

Clinical Workup

Blood or BAL BeLPT test, imaging studies, pulmonary function test are helpful to make the diagnosis.

Morphology

Characteristic finding is noncaseating granuloma, which is identical to the granulomas found in sarcoidosis and other noninfectious granulomatous diseases. The granulomas are primarily found along the bronchovascular bundle in the bronchial submucosa and in the pulmonary interstitium, and occasionally in regional lymph nodes (Maier, 2002). Varying degree of interstitial fibrosis may be evident. While beryllium can be detected within granulomas by specialized techniques, such as microscopic X ray, these techniques are not readily available (Rossman, 1996).

Differential Diagnosis

To distinguish berylliosis from sarcoidosis and other noncaseating granulomatous diseases including tuberculosis, blood BeLPT is the choice to identify beryllium workers who develop beryllium sensitization.

Treatment of Choice and Prognosis

Berylliosis is treated with corticosteroids. Methotrexate may be considered if corticosteroid therapy fails. Prognosis is usually excellent, but progression to loss of lung function and further respiratory failure occurs.

Crohn's Disease

Categorized under inflammatory bowel disease (IBD), Crohn's disease is a chronic inflammatory process of the gastrointestinal system. Enlarged reactive mesenteric lymphadenopathy can be found in as many as 60% of Crohn's disease patients (Maconi et al., 2005).

Definition

Crohn's disease is an idiopathic, chronic inflammatory disease that may involve any area of the gastrointestinal tract and is typically transmural. Mesenteric and regional lymph nodes can also be involved.

ICD-10 Code K50

Synonyms

Crohn disease, regional enteritis.

Epidemiology

Crohn's disease is found worldwide. The prevalence is estimated at 3.6 to 15.6 cases per 100,000 population in North America. It affects more women than men, and most individuals are diagnosed in their 20s to 30s.

Clinical Aspects

Etiology. Among a lot of factors implicated in the pathogenesis of Crohn's disease, the key factors are the environment, genetic makeup, commensal flora, and immune response (Scaldaferri and Fiocchi, 2007). How these factors interact and cause the disease is still under investigation.

Site of Involvement. Crohn's disease may occur in any area of the gastrointestinal tract. Both small intestine and colon can be involved. The most common sites are the terminal ileum, ileocecal valve and cecum (Kumar et al., 2010a). During the course, strictures, fistula, and abscesses tend to develop. Accompanying mesenteric lymphadenopathy is a common finding, with a prevalence of 50 to 60% of regional lymph nodes (Maconi et al., 2005). Extraintestinal involvement includes joints, skin, eyes, and other organs.

Pathogenesis

The exact pathogenesis is still not clear. It is believed that a combination of defects in host interactions with intestinal microbiota, intestinal epithelial dysfunction, and aberrant mucosal immune responses lead to the disease (Kumar et al., 2010a; Scaldaferri and Fiocchi, 2007). Genetics also plays a role, and it had been shown that mutation of NOD2 gene confers susceptibility to Crohn's disease (Thoreson and Cullen, 2007).

Approach to Diagnosis

There is no single gold standard for diagnosing Crohn's disease. A diagnosis is based on clinical findings, combined with endoscopic, radiologic, and pathologic findings, and exclusion of other pathologies (Stange et al., 2006; Panes et al., 2007).

Clinical Workup

Routine laboratory tests, serologic tests, imaging studies may be performed. A positive perinuclear antineutrophil cytoplasmic antibody (p-ANCA) and negative anti–Saccharomyces cerevisiae (ASCA) would favor Crohn's disease over other form of IBD, ulcerative colitis (Nikolaus and Schreiber, 2007). Endoscopic and histologic examinations can provide characteristic findings.

Morphology

The microscopic features of active Crohn's disease in bowel has been described (Kleer and Appelman, 2001). Noncaseating granuloma is a hallmark of Crohn's disease and can be found in approximately 35% of the cases. The enlarged mesenteric lymph nodes show characteristic noncaseating granulomas, increased lymphocytic aggregates, plasma cells, and reticuloendothelial proliferation (Guillou et al., 1973). Granulomatous lymph nodes were found in 20 to 38% of cases with Crohn's disease (Cook, 1972; Williams, 1964).

Differential Diagnosis

Lymphadenopathy in cases with Crohn's disease needs to be differentiated from other infectious or noninfectious noncaseating granulomatous process like tuberculosis and sarcoidosis. As mentioned, there is sparing of small and large intestinal organs and mesenteric lymph nodes in sarcoidosis.

Treatment of Choice and Prognosis

The goal of the therapy is to reduce morbidity, to prevent complications, and to maintain nutritious status. Anti-inflammatory agents such as mesalamine and sulfasalazine, immunosuppressants including infliximab, azathioprine, and methotrexate, and corticosteroids can be used. Crohn's disease is a chronic process with recurrent episodes, however, appropriate medical and surgical therapy may help patients maintain a reasonable quality of life. Complications and the mortality rates increase with the duration of the disease.

Primary Biliary Cirrhosis

Primary biliary cirrhosis (PBC) is an inflammatory disease affecting bile ducts of the liver. Besides the liver, the characteristic granulomatous changes can also involve the regional lymph nodes.

Definition

PBC is a chronic inflammatory autoimmune liver disease characterized by progressive destruction of intrahepatic bile ducts with cholestasis, portal inflammation, and fibrosis, which may lead to cirrhosis and other complications.

ICD-10 Code K74.3

Synonym PBC

Epidemiology

Variable prevalence of PBC has been noted worldwide (Gross and Odin, 2008). The overall prevalence is estimated at 40.2 per 100,000 population. It preferentially affects women than men, with a female to male ratio of 9:1, and most patients are between the age of 40s and 60s.

Clinical Aspects

Etiology. PBC is a result from a combination of multiple factors including genetic factors and superimposed environmental triggers. These factors may affect the immune system; thus this disease is believed to be an autoimmune disorder (Poupon, 2010). The exact etiology is unknown.

Site of Involvement. The liver is the primary affected organ. Lymphadenopathy is often seen in the porta hepatis, along the common bile duct, and less often in unexpected sites such as the mesentery and supradiaphragmatic paracardiac areas (Kaplan, 1996).

Pathogenesis

It is generally considered an autoimmune disease, supported by the presence of autoantibodies. Although several different pathogenetic models have been proposed, the exact mechanism is still unknown (Hohenester et al., 2009; Jones, 2008).

Approach to Diagnosis

The hallmark of PBC is the presence of serum antimitochondrial antibodies (AMAs). In the clinical setting the diagnosis should be based on the following three criteria: (1) abnormal tests with elevation of serum alkaline phosphatase (ALP) and gammaglutamyltranspeptidase (GGTP), and (2) presence of AMAs, or (3) histology of nonsuppurative destructive cholangitis. Both criteria (2) and (3) have high specificity (Poupon, 2010).

Clinical Workup

Laboratory tests will show abnormal liver function test, with significant elevations of ALP and GGTP. Besides the serum AMA test, histology examination of the liver is mandatory. Imaging studies including ultrasound, computed tomography (CT) scanning, or magnetic resonance imaging (MRI) are important to exclude biliary obstruction.

Morphology

In liver, chronic, nonsuppurative, destructive cholangitis of the small interlobular bile ducts is characteristic. There is also lymphocytic and plasma cell infiltration in portal areas. Epithelioid aggregates or noncaseating granulomas may be found around the bile ducts. In involved lymph node, there is nonspecific reactive follicular hyperplasia (Aisaka et al., 2006; Cassani et al., 1990). Granulomatous changes are commonly found in the portal lymph nodes (Hubscher and Harrison, 1989) (Figure 18.32). Deposits of lipofuscin in sinus histiocytes are observed, but they are also present in other chronic cholestatic liver diseases.

Differential Diagnosis

Other infectious or noninfectious noncaseating granulomatous process should be included in the differential diagnosis.

Treatment of Choice and Prognosis

Ursodeoxycholic acid (UCDA) is the mainstay of therapy. Adjuvant therapies include glucocorticoids and methotrexate. Liver transplantation is considered for selected cases (Silveira and Lindor, 2008). For asymptomatic patients the progress is slow. However, PBC can progress to symptomatic and further to end-stage liver cirrhosis. The median survival duration for symptomatic patients is between 5 and 12 years.

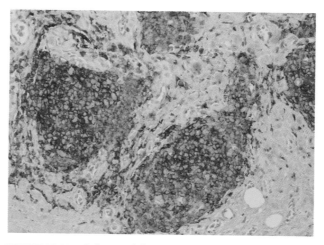

FIGURE 18.32 **Sclerosed lymph node adjacent the common bile duct with epithelioid granulomas admixed with lymphocytes and plasma cells** (40×). Double immunostain for CD68 (brown) and CD3 (red).

MIXED PATTERN WITH HEMORRHAGE AND INFARCTION

Fine Needle Associated Changes

Lymph node biopsy following a fine needle aspiration (a few days to more than a month) previously may have certain histological changes induced by the needle puncture.

ICD-10 Code Not applicable.

Morphology

Several patterns of histopathological changes can be caused by fine needle aspiration (Tsang and Chan, 1992; Davies and Webb, 1982): the presence of focal hemorrhage associated with granulation and variable degrees of tissue reorganization, wedge-shaped segmental infarction with marked depletion of lymphocytes associated with hemorrhage (Figure 18.33), or total infarction of the lymph node. A distinct linear hemorrhagic needle tract may be identifiable, with proliferation of fibroblasts. In the case of total infarction, only "ghost" cellular outlines may be remained and the diagnosis becomes difficult due to the lack of viable cells. Fibrosis can be present as early as six days (Behm et al., 1984) (Figure 18.34), and prior to that, acute phase of reaction usually includes infiltrates of neutrophils, lymphocytes, and histiocytes within the needle tract.

Pathogenesis

Segmental infarction could be caused by thrombosed hilar veins associated with the procedure (Davies and Webb, 1982). The total infarction of lymph node most likely represents an exaggerated host response to fine needle aspiration procedure (Nasuti et al., 2001).

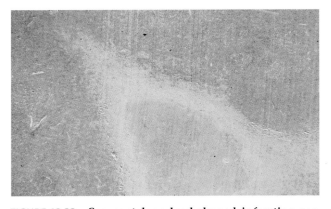

FIGURE 18.33 **Segmental wedged-shaped infarction secondary to arteriopathy or thrombus.**

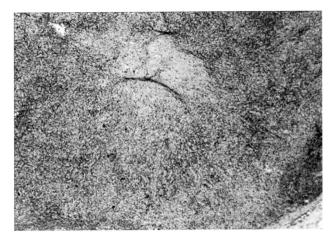

FIGURE 18.34 **Needle tract with fibrosis and surrounding lymphoid depleted reaction post FNA.**

Immunophenotyping/Cytochemistry

Immunohistochemical stains are shown to be helpful in identifying the original pathology in the totally infarcted lymph node obtained after a fine needle aspiration (Nasuti et al., 2001). In these cases metastatic carcinoma or melanoma, the "ghost" tumor cells, may be stained with particular tumor markers. Although morphologically it would be difficult to identify the tumor per se, findings are suggestive of the underlying diagnosis.

Differential Diagnosis

There may be a wedge-shaped segmental infarction, with marked depletion of lymphocytes associated with hemorrhage. A total infarction of the lymph node may rarely be seen. A distinct linear hemorrhagic needle tract may be identifiable, associated with proliferation of fibroblasts. In cases of total infarction, only "ghost" cellular outlines may remain, and the diagnosis becomes difficult sometimes due to the lack of viable cells. Subtotal or total infarction usually occurs in lymph nodes involved by malignant lymphoma (Tsang and Chan, 1992), and therefore these findings require additional investigation such as molecular gene rearrangement clonality assay to determine the presence of lymphoma.

The spindle fibroblasts proliferation raises a concern of sarcoma, such as angiosarcoma, or liposarcoma in cases with fat necrosis (Tabbara et al., 1991). The occurrence of total infarction makes it impossible to render a definitive diagnosis and to confirm the previous fine needle aspiration diagnosis, which may necessitate further biopsies.

Lymph nodes irradiated directly by radioactive colloidal materials induce varying degree of depletion and necrosis in experimental animals

(Christopherson and Berg, 1955) and in lymph nodes of patients treated with radiation for Hodgkin lymphoma (Congdon, 1966) (Figures 18.35, 18.36).

Lymph Node Infarction

Because lymph nodes have abundant vascularity, lymph node infarction is rare. However, associations between lymph node infarction and various non-neoplastic and neoplastic processes, most importantly lymphoma, make it an important condition that the pathologists and clinicians need to recognize.

Definition

Spontaneous lymph node infarction is characterized by extensive coagulation necrosis of medullary and cortical region with preservation of a subcapsular rim of viable lymphoid tissue [Davies and Stansfeld, 1972, Pietrafitta et al., 1983]. Infarction caused by

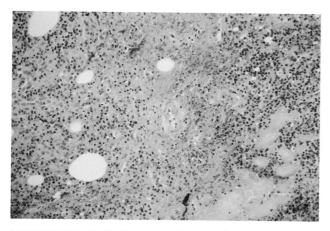

FIGURE 18.35 **Radiation necrosis in pelvic lymph nodes in a patient with intrapelvic radiotherapy for gonadal carcinoma.**

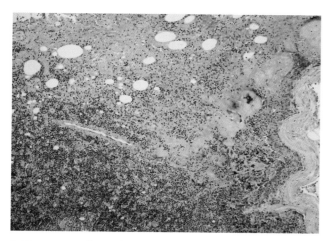

FIGURE 18.36 **Lymphoid depletion and geographic necrosis in irradiated lymph node.**

vascular occlusion ranges from subtotal necrosis to partial necrosis [Mahy and Davies, 1984].

ICD-10 Code R59.9 Enlarged lymph node, unspecified.

Synonym
None.

Epidemiology/Occurrence Rate
It has been estimated that lymph node infarction occurs in one of 13,000 tissue biopsies (Toriumi et al., 1988), and one of 450 lymph node biopsies in head and neck region (0.2%) (Maurer et al., 1986). In one recent study (Punia et al., 2009), six cases of lymph node infarction were retrieved in 3938 lymph node biopsies (0.15%) during a 10-year period. Notably, it has been reported that lymph node infarction can occur in as high as 25% of non-Hodgkin lymphoma patients, and this is not surprising because there is a frequent association between lymph node infarction and lymphoma (Yonemori et al., 2006).

Clinical Aspects
Etiology. Lymph node infarction was described as an idiopathic process with no identifiable etiology (Watts et al., 1980). Lymph node infarction has been reported in association with various processes, including non-neoplastic and neoplastic conditions. Possible associated non-neoplastic conditions include vascular thrombosis or obstruction, vasculitis, viral infections, gold injections for the treatment of rheumatoid arthritis, disseminated intravascular coagulation (DIC), and HIV infection (Punia et al., 2009; Kojima et al., 2002; Roberts et al., 2001; Rothschild and Marshall, 1986; Mahy and Davies, 1984; Rao et al., 2005; Wannakrairot et al., 2007). Neoplastic conditions are most commonly lymphoma (Cleary et al., 1982; Toriumi et al., 1988; Yonemori et al., 2006; Strauchen and Miller, 2003; Punia et al., 2009), with rare reports of other malignancies including myeloid sarcoma and metastatic tumors (Kojima et al., 2003; Kojima et al., 2005c; Nasuti et al., 2001). Varying types of lymphoma include Hodgkin lymphoma, follicular lymphoma, diffuse large B-cell lymphoma, and high-grade peripheral T-cell lymphoma. The reported incidence of lymphoma in patients with infarcted lymph node ranges from 32 to 89% (Cleary et al., 1982; Maurer et al., 1986; Strauchen and Miller, 2003). In one study (Maurer et al., 1986), lymphoma developed in 20 of 51 (39%) cases of lymph node infarction either concurrently (14 cases) or within a 2-year follow-up (6 cases). Thus pathologists should be alert about the possibility of an underlying lymphoma when examining an infarcted lymph node.

Sites of involvement. Both superficial and deep lymph nodes can be involved (DeFrance et al., 1976; Watts et al., 1980; Pietrafitta et al., 1983; Mahy and Davies, 1984).

Pathogenesis

Lymph node infarction presumably results from vascular compromise. Extranodal vascular lesions or vascular occlusion was observed in different conditions, such as polyarteritis nodosum and vovulus (Mahy and Davies, 1984). It should be pointed out that lymph nodes have dual circulation of blood and lymphatics, and experiments demonstrated that subcapsular areas of the lymph node remained intact with necrosis of the other areas when blood vessels were ligated. The morphology of the infarcts due to vascular occlusion thus may differ from those with underlying lymphoma (Mahy and Davies, 1984). Frank lymph node infarction is most likely due to occlusion of both blood and lymphatic vessels, which may be the results of the rapidly growing tumor cells in the case of lymphoma (Cleary et al., 1982).

Morphology

There is extensively coagulative necrosis with ghost cells that may be identifiable (Figure 18.37). A rim of subcapsular cortical tissue may be spared in peripheral lymph nodes. The capsule is thickened with occasional preserved subcapsular sinuses. The reticulum architecture of the lymph node is preserved, which may be shown by reticulin stain (Watts et al., 1980; Toriumi et al., 1988). In old lesion, granulation tissue and fibrosis form.

Lymph node infarction caused by ischemia was studied in mesenteric lymph nodes as well as in animal experiments (Mahy and Davies, 1984; Steinmann

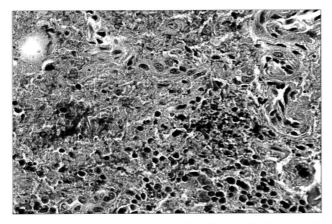

FIGURE 18.37 **Lymph node infarction with lymphoid depletion, "ghost" nuclei, hypervascularity, necrosis, nuclear smudge and dusts, and dystrophic stroma H & E, (400×).**

et al., 1982). Three lesions were observed: frank infarction, lymphoid depletion, and capsular hypervascularity. The necrosis more often only affects the central part, or there may be viable areas around the trabeculae.

Immunophenotyping

Against the common belief that necrotic tissue is suboptimal for immunophenotypic analysis, many studies have shown that antigens are frequently preserved in lymph node infarction and that immunohistochemistry sometimes is useful to render diagnosis (Yonemori et al., 2006; Kojima et al., 2005c; Kojima et al., 2004; Strauchen and Miller, 2003; Polski et al., 2003; Norton et al., 1988). CD20, CD79a, CD3, CD45RO, CD43, and CD10 were reported to be well preserved according to different reports (Strauchen and Miller, 2003; Polski et al., 2003), while some antigens such as CD45, bcl-2, and bcl-6 were undetecable (Yonemori et al., 2006; Kojima et al., 2004). Cytokeratin (AE1/AE3 and CAM5.2), and carcinoembronic antigen were also well-preserved (Kojima et al., 2005c). However, it is suggested that the interpretation should be cautious because there is occasional false-negative and false-positive results.

Differential Diagnosis

Benign lymphadenopathies should be considered in the differential diagnosis. Lymphadenitis secondary to bacterial agents may result in fibrinoid necrosis with many neutrophils. Infectious agents may cause necrotic region surrounded by histiocytes, which is not seen in lymph node infarction. Kikuchi–Fujimoto lymphadenopathy has distinct histologic features as described in this chapter. Lymphadenopathy in systemic lupus erythematosus may show areas of focal lymph node infarction, but there is numerous plasma cells and basophilic deposits in the vessel walls and paracortex (Toriumi et al., 1988).

Additional Newer Information

Gene rearrangement analysis using DNA extracts from the infarcted lymph node was demonstrated to be useful in addition to the immunopenotypic studies to evaluate the nature of the infarction (Laszewski et al., 1991).

MIXED NECROTIZING PATTERN WITH NO OR MINIMAL GRANULOMAS

Lupus Erythematosus

Localized or generalized lymphadenopathy is a frequent finding in patients with systemic lupus erythematosus (SLE). The prevalence of lymphadenopathy among SLE patients ranges from a third to half (Shapira et al., 1996).

Definition

SLE is an autoimmune disorder characterized by a chronic, often febrile illness characterized by injury to the skin, joints, kidney, serosal membranes, and virtually every other organs in the body (Kumar et al., 2010b). Lupus lymphadenopathy, also known as lupus lymphadenitis, is the lymph node reactive changes associated with SLE.

ICD-10 Code M32

Synonyms

Lupus lymphadenopathy, lupus lymphadenitis.

Epidemiology

The prevalence of SLE varies by race and ethnicity, with higher rates among black and Hispanic people. In North America the overall prevalence is 15 to 50 per 100,000 people. SLE affects females more frequently than males, at a rate of almost 9 to 1 (Danchenko et al., 2006).

Clinical Aspects

Site of Involvement. The SLE-associated lymphadenopathy may be localized or generalized, involving the superficial and deep lymph nodes mostly in cervical, mesenteric, axillary, or inguinal regions (Fox and Rosahn, 1943). Generalized lymphadenopathy was reported to be 12% of 140 cases in this review. Other locations reported include retroperitoneal, supraclavicular and infraclavicular, submaxillary, pelvic, epitrochlear, para-aortic, mediastinal and submental regions (Fox and Rosahn, 1943; Kassan et al., 1976).

Etiology. The causes of SLE remain unclear. Autoantibodies and genetic and environmental factors play roles (Kumar et al., 2010b). Multiple immune disturbances may predispose to SLE, and immune complex and immune system disregulation are the suspected causes (Rahman and Isenberg, 2008). More than 10 gene loci have been known to increase the risk of SLE. HLA-A1, B8, and DR3 are more common in patients with SLE than in the general population. As to lymphadenopathy, studies demonstrated that Epstein–Barr virus (EBV) might be the cause in some of the cases (Kojima et al., 2005b).

Pathogenesis

SLE is an organ-nonspecific autoimmune disorder characterized by various autoantibodies production, immune complex deposition, and hyperglobulinemia.

Approach to Diagnosis

The presentation and course of SLE are highly variable, and include constitutional, musculoskeletal, dermatological, renal, neuropsychiatric, pulmonary, gastrointestinal, cardiac, and hematologic symptoms and features. The diagnosis of SLE is based on a constellation of clinical findings and laboratory evidence. Diagnostic criteria was proposed by the 1982 American College of Rheumatology (ACR) (Tan et al., 1982, Hochberg, 1997). Most often the patient's age, clinical findings, and laboratory studies are characteristic. Lymph node biopsy is occasionally performed to exclude the possibility of malignant process, which has also been associated with SLE (Bernatsky et al., 2005; Landgren et al., 2006; Xu and Wiernik, 2001).

Clinical Workup

Laboratory studies to diagnose SLE include CBC, serum creatinine, urinalysis, and autoantibody tests (ANA, anti-dsDNA, anti-Sm, anti-SSA (Ro) or anti-SSB (La), antiribosomal P, anti-RNP, anticardiolipin, lupus anticoagulant, Coombs test, antihistone). Complement (C3 and C4) levels are also tested. The specificity and sensitivity of these tests are discussed in the literature.

Morphology

Generally, small-vessel vasculitis with necrosis of vascular walls is present in multiple systems and also in lymph node. The SLE-associated lymphadenopathy is characterized by irregularly shaped, focal or extensive, necrosis sometimes accompanied by LE bodies or hematoxylin bodies (Kojima et al., 2001; Fox and Rosahn, 1943) (Figure 18.38). Hematoxylin bodies, which are heavily hematoxylin-stained homogeneous nuclear remnant of cells reacted with ANAs, are strongly indicative of SLE (Bowerfind et al., 1956) (Figure 18.39). An Azzopardi phenomenon, which is basophilic outlining of blood vessels, can also be found. Surrounding the necrosis, there may be, though not always, macrophages and small lymphocytes, and scattered neutrophils, plasmacytoid monocytes, and immunoblasts (Figure 18.40, 18.41).

Besides the necrosis, other lymph node changes are generally nonspecific. The lymph node architecture is preserved. Subcapsular and medullary sinuses

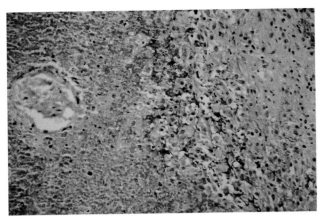

FIGURE 18.38 Geographic necrosis with hematoxylin bodies.

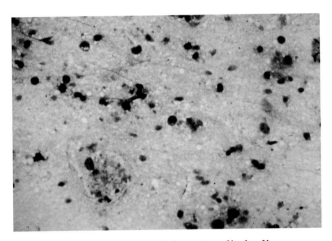

FIGURE 18.39 Dark and pink hematoxylin bodies.

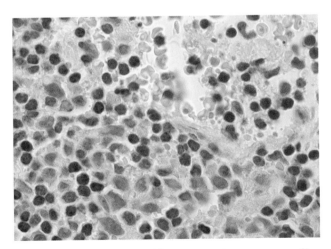

FIGURE 18.40 Plasmacytoid monocytes surrounding necrosed blood vessel, pink hematoxyphilic boides, and paracortical necrosis with karyorrhectic debris and inflammatory cells.

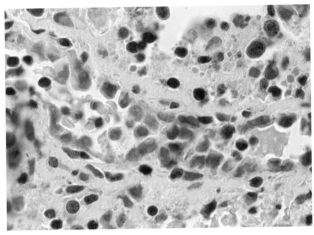

FIGURE 18.41 Plasma cells and single-cell necrosis.

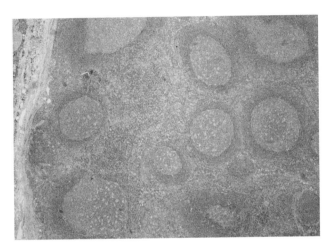

FIGURE 18.42 Follicular hyperplasia.

are patent. There are usually large follicles with reactive, usually enlarged, germinal centers (Figure 18.42). The follicular hyperplasia is often associated with increased vascularity and scattered immunoblasts and plasma cells (Kojima et al., 2005a). Occasionally lymph node changes are similar to those in the hyaline vascular or intermediate types of Castleman's disease, T-zone dysplasia with hyperplastic follicles (Kojima et al., 2000). Prominent lymphoplasmacytic infiltration with immunoblastic proliferation may be similar to angioimmunoblastic T-cell lymphoma.

Immunophenotyping/Cytochemistry

Immunohistochemistry would demonstrate the lymphoid follicles are a mixture of small and medium-size lymphocytes and immunoblasts that are positive for B-cell or T-cell markers. CD4 and CD8 stains would show a mixed nature of the interfollicular T lymphocytes. CD4-positive T cells may outnumber the CD-8 positive T cells in interfollicular region

(Kojima et al., 2001). Germinal centers B cells are Bcl-2 negative. Hematoxylin bodies are positive for the periodic acid-Schiff (PAS) and Feulgen stains.

Differential diagnosis

Kikuchi–Fujimoto's lymphadenitis can present similar clinicopathological features including a similar histological findings. Differential diagnosis of these two entities is discussed under Kikuchi–Fujimoto's lymphadenitis. Other differential considerations may include lymph node infarcts that may be associated with lymphoma. Infectious lymphadenitis caused by mycobacterium, HIV, and so on, may be diagnosed by special stains or serological tests.

Treatment of Choice and Prognosis

The treatment is usually supportive. Nonsteroidal anti-inflammatory drugs (NSAIDs) and corticosteroids are used. The prognosis is favorable, as this is generally a self-limited disease. Lymphadenopathy usually resolves within 1 to 6 months.

Kawasaki's Disease

Kawasaki's disease, also known as mucocutaneous lymph node syndrome, was first described in Japan in 1967, and the disease is now known as the number one cause of acquired heart disease in children in the developed countries (Yeung, 2010). It is a potentially fatal disease due to the complications in cardiovascular system.

Definition

Kawasaki's disease is an acute vasculitis that predominantly affects young children, manifested by a massive systemic symptoms, including prolonged fever, nonpurulent conjunctivitis, oral mucosal inflammation, cervical lymphadenopathy, induration and erythema of the hands and feet, and a diffuse polymorphous skin rash.

ICD-10 Code M30.3

Synonym

Mucocutaneous lymph node syndrome.

Epidemiology

Kawasaki's disease has been reported in children of all races and ethnicities. The incidence rate is estimated at 32.5, 16.9, 11.1, and 9.1 per 100,000 children under age 5 years in Asians and Pacific Islanders, non-Hispanic African-Americans, Hispanics, and Caucasians, respectively (Holman et al., 2003;

Newburger and Fulton, 2004). The highest rates are reported in Japan, at about 184 per 100,000 children under 5 years (Harnden et al., 2009). Boys outnumber girls at a ratio of 1.5:1 (Newburger and Fulton, 2004). Rare adult cases have been reported (Gomard-Mennesson et al., 2010).

Clinical Aspects

Etiology. The etiology remains unknown. Infectious etiology such as viruses and bacteria has been suspected, but no definite causative agents have been demonstrated. It is believed many factors, including viral or bacterial superantigen, can trigger immune activation and lead to a self-directed immune response (Pinna et al., 2008).

Sites of Involvement. Cervical lymphadenopathy, often unilateral, is found in as many as 40% of the patients. The lymph node is usually greater than 1.5 cm. Mediastinal lymphadenopathy as a variant of incomplete Kawasaki's disease was reported (Bosch Marcet et al., 1998). Lymphadenopathy can be the sole manifestation (Kubota et al., 2008).

Pathogenesis

Genetic predisposition to Kawasaki's disease is proposed based on the observation of the increased frequency among Asians and Asian-Americans. ITPKC, 1,4,5-triphosphate 3-kinase C, a negative regulator of T-cell activation, is identified as an Kawasaki's disease associated gene. Independent studies using animal model also identified that regulation of T-cell activation plays critical roles on susceptibility and severity of the disease (Yeung, 2010; Rowley and Shulman, 2010).

Approach to Diagnosis

The diagnosis is based on clinical criteria, which is published by the American Heart Association and American Academy of Pediatrics (Freeman and Shulman, 2006; Newburger et al., 2004). Incomplete cases in which the clinical features are not present in the required numbers can occur.

Clinical Workup

There is no specific laboratory test for Kawasaki's disease. A mild-to-moderate anemia, platelet elevation, and liver function abnormalities may be present. Very rarely, the lymph node is biopsied to rule out lymphadenitis or abscess.

Morphology

Focal areas of necrosis with adjacent microthrombosis of small vessels are the most common pathologic changes. The necrosis can be accompanied by intense polymorphonuclear infiltration within the necrotic foci. Other cases may have little polymorphonuclear or histiocytic infiltrate (Giesker et al., 1982; Marsh et al., 1980). The vasculitic changes is most common in large arteries, not in microvasculature. Varied nonspecific changes have been described in the literatures before 1990s (Marsh et al., 1980; Amano et al., 1980; Keim and Geltner, 1985). Those findings include swollen endothelial cells of postcapillary venules, acute lymphadenitis and histiocytosis, nonspecific lymphoid hyperplasia.

Differential Diagnosis

Differential diagnoses include the diseases with necrotic changes in lymph node, like cat-scratch disease, SLE-associated lymphadenopathy, tuberculosis, and Kikuchi–Fujimoto's lymphadenitis. The diagnostic value of the lymph node biopsy in Kawasaki's disease is minimal.

Treatment of Choice and Prognosis

Gamma globulin (IVIG) and aspirin is the standard therapy. Corticosteroids can be added according to some studies (Athappan et al., 2009). If coronary artery aneurysm is not developed, generally the patient is fully recovered.

NECROTIZING NONSUPPURATIVE GRANULOMATAS

Kikuchi–Fujimoto's Lymphadenitis/Kikuchi Disease

Also known as Kikuchi disease or histiocytic necrotizing lymphadenitis, Kikuchi–Fujimoto's lymphadenitis is an uncommon benign lymphadenitis, with or without systemic signs and symptoms. Clinically and histologically it can be confused with lymphoma or systemic lupus erythematosus (SLE).

Definition

Kikuchi–Fujimoto's lymphadenitis is a benign, self-limited disorder characterized by regional lymphadenopathy with focal proliferation of histiocytes and abundant karyorrhectic debris.

ICD-10 Code D76.3

Synonyms

Histiocytic necrotizing lymphadenitis, HNL, Kikuchi's histiocytic necrotizing lymphadenitis, Kikuchi–Fujimoto disease, necrotizing lymphadenitis, Kikuchi's disease, Kikuchi disease.

Epidemiology

Kikuchi–Fujimoto's lymphadenitis is a rare disease with a worldwide distribution, but a higher prevalence among Japanese and other Asian population has been reported (Bosch and Guilabert, 2006). Patients are predominantly under 30 years of age, although it can occur in a wide age range (2–75 years of age). It was reported that there was a female preponderance with a female to male ratio of 4:1, but recent studies have shown a female to male ratio of 1.25:1 (Bosch et al., 2004).

Clinical Aspects

Etiology. The cause is unknown. Infectious and autoimmune causes have been suggested. Viral infection, like Epstein-Barr virus (EBV), has been shown by some authors to be linked to the disease, but the studies are not conclusive (Hudnall, 2000).

Sites of Involvement. The disease typically manifests as cervical lymphadenopathy. Less commonly affected nodes include those in axillary, inguinal, and mesenteric region. Unusual cases have generalized adenopathy. Extranodal involvement is uncommon, but cutaneous lesions, hepatomegaly, and splenomegaly have been described (Hutchinson and Wang, 2010).

Pathogenesis

The pathogenesis remains unclear. Infectious and autoimmune causes have been hypothesized. Numerous triggering agents have been proposed, including EBV, human herpes virus 6, human immunodeficiency virus (HIV), herpes simplex virus, hepatitis B, and so on. An exuberant T-cell mediated hyperresponse to certain antigen in genetically susceptible might be induced. CD8+ cytotoxic T cells may proliferate and induce target cell apoptosis, accounting for the characteristic necrosis and cell debris (Kuo, 1995).

Approach to Diagnosis

The diagnosis is based on lymph node histology evaluation. Immunohistochemical analysis and flow cytometry can be used to rule out lymphoma.

Clinical Workup

Laboratory tests and imaging studies are nonspecific. The diagnosis is confirmed by excisional lymph node biopsy.

Morphology

The classic Kikuchi–Fujimoto's lymphadenitis in lymph nodes is characterized by irregular paracortical coagulative necrosis with abundant karyorrhectic debris, and large numbers of histiocytes, but no neutrophils and eosinophils present.

The lymph node capsule is usually intact but may be focally thickened in the areas overlying necrosis (Figure 18.43). The normal architecture of the lymph nodes is partially effaced, with inconspicuous germinal centers (Figure 18.44), by a paracortical expansion that is composed of circumscribed foci of apoptotic necrosis with abundant karyorrhectic debris (Figures 18.45, 18.46). A mixture in variable proportions of histiocytes, immunoblasts, plasmacytoid monocytes, and small lymphocytes is surrounding the necrotic foci (Figures 18.47–18.50). Neutrophils and eosinophils are absent. Plasma cells are absent or rare. In some cases large transformed lymphocytes with immunoblast morphology are markedly increased in a background of karyorrhectic debris and scattered tingible-body macrophages, which may resemble lymphoma (Figure 18.51). Kuo proposed to classify Kikuchi–Fujimoto's lymphadenitis into three phases: proliferative, necrotizing, and xanthomatous phases (Kuo, 1995). The proliferative phase features an expanded paracortex with increases in various histiocytes and plasmacytoid dendritic cells. The necrotizing phase has any degree of necrosis. The xanthomatous phase is predominated by foamy histiocytes, with or without necrosis (Figure 18.52). Table 18.5 summarizes the key morphological features of Kikuchi–Fujimoto's lymphadenitis.

Immunophenotyping/Cytochemistry

Immunohistochemistry is mainly used to rule out malignant lymphoma. The histiocytes stain positively for histiocyte-associated antigens such as lysozyme, myeloperoxidase (MPO), CD68, and CD4 (Pileri et al., 2001). The lymphocytes in Kikuchi–Fujimoto's lymphadenitis typically consist of a predominance of CD8+ T cells, with very few B cells. Immunoblasts in affected areas have T-cytotoxic phenotypes (Kucukardali et al., 2007; Tsang et al., 1994; Hutchinson and Wang, 2010). Plasmacytoid monocytes express neither histiocytic markers nor myeloperoxidase (Marafioti et al., 2008), but some studies showed that the cells were positive for CD68 (Bosch et al., 2004). These are also the so-called plasmacytoid dendritic cells that express CD123 (Facchetti and Vermi, 2002) (Figure 18.51).

Approach to Diagnosis

Lymph node biopsy and morphological assessment is the only way to render a definite diagnosis. So far no specific laboratory test is available. Flow cytometry is helpful to exclude the possibility of non-Hodgkin lymphoma. As mentioned above, the T

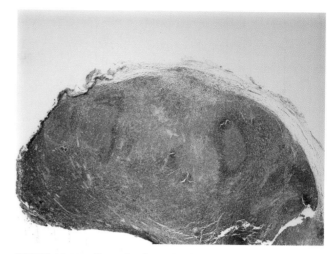

FIGURE 18.43 **Capsular lymphadenitis.**

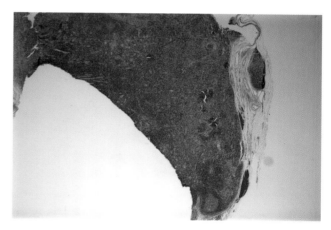

FIGURE 18.44 **Inconspicuous germinal centers.**

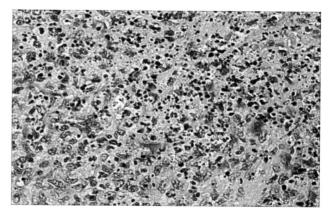

FIGURE 18.45 **Necrosis, karryorrhectic nuclear debris, and histiocytes without neutrophilic infiltrate- characteristic of Kikuchi–Fujimoto's lymphadenitis.**

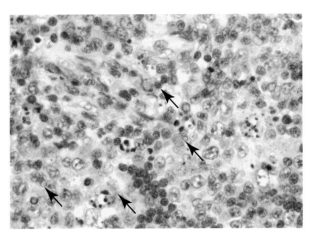

FIGURE 18.46 **Wall of necrotizing histiocytes with admixed epithelioid cells, immunoblasts, apoptotic cells, lymphocytes, histiocytes, and dendritic cells with crescentic or twisted nuclei (arrows) with wreath-shaped tingible-bodies and apoptotic beads.**

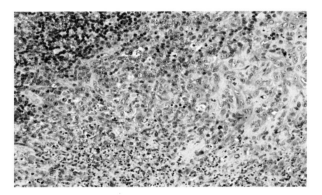

FIGURE 18.47 **Zonation with central karyorrhectic debris.** Note the intermediate area with less debris, and the intercellular matrix, epithelioid cells, and outer layer with plasmacytoid monocytes, histiocytes, immunoblasts, and small lymphocytes.

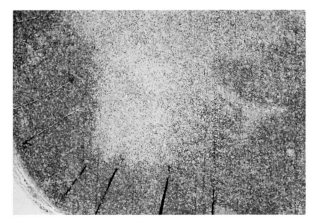

FIGURE 18.48 **Pale areas with mottling in subcapsular areas extending to paracortex.**

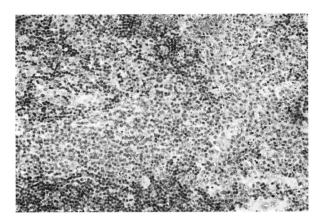

FIGURE 18.49 **Pale areas comprised of plasmacytoid monocytes.**

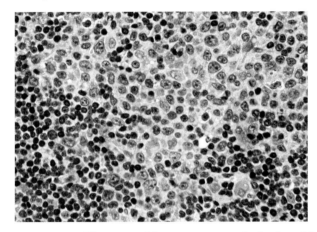

FIGURE 18.50 **Plasmacytoid monocytes admixed with many immunoblasts.** Note the large cells with dark chromatin, prominent nucleoli, darker cytoplasm.

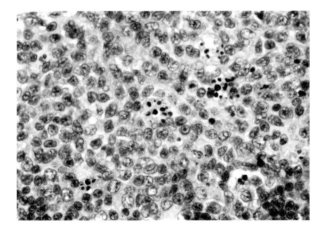

FIGURE 18.51 **Dense collection of plasmacytoid monocytes as a morphologic mimic of large-cell lymphoma with karyorrhectic debris.** Immunohistochemical studies typically show a CD4/CD3 + T small-cell infiltrate, admixed with CD123+ plasmacytoid monocytes (plasmacytoid dendritic cells), and rare CD20+ B cells.

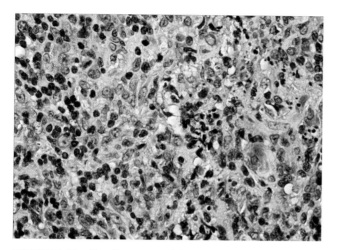

FIGURE 18.52 Xanthomatous histiocytes with foamy cytoplasm in focal areas of Kikuchi–Fujimoto lymphadenitis.

TABLE 18.5 Kikuchi–Fujimoto's Lymphadenitis

Morphologic Features
Necrosis of histiocytes without neutrophilic infiltrate
Crescentic or twisted nuclei in histiocytes with intracellular apoptotic beads
Capsular lymphadenitis
Inconspicuous germinal centers
Pale areas composed of plasmacytoid monocytes

cells are mainly phenotypically CD8+ cells. The other laboratory results are usually normal. However, some patients may have anemia, leukopenia or leukocytosis, elevated lactate dehydrogenase levels, elevated liver enzymes, and elevated erythrocyte sedimentation rates. Atypical lymphocytes are seen in peripheral blood in up to one-third of patients (Lin et al., 2003).

Differential Diagnosis

Differential diagnoses include lymphoproliferative disorders, reactive lymphadenitis associated with infectious etiologies, autoimmune diseases like Kawasaki disease and systemic lupus erythematosus (SLE), myeloid neoplasms, and metastatic adenocarcinoma (Hutchinson and Wang, 2010; Onciu and Medeiros, 2003; Chen et al., 2010; Bosch and Guilabert, 2006) (Table 18.6).

Kikuchi–Fujimoto's lymphadenitis may be confused with lymphoma because of the necrotizing process and the blastic lymphoid cells (Menasce et al., 1998). Both non-Hodgkin lymphoma and Hodgkin disease share some clinical and histologic features. Hodgkin disease has characteristic Reed–Sternberg cells or variants, which are stained with CD30 or CD15, with numerous eosinophils. A proliferation of

blastic cells may raise a concern of peripheral T-cell lymphoma. In difficult cases, flow cytometry analysis may be helpful.

Infectious agents, especially viruses like the herpes simplex virus, cytomegalovirus, and Epstein–Barr virus (EBV), as well as other agents like *toxoplasma gondii, Yersinia enterocolitica*, and *Bartonella henselae* may cause infectious lymphadenitis with histiocytic infiltrates and necrotic debris. Generally, the histiocytic infiltrates is usually less prominent and neutrophils are often present. Viral inclusions are very helpful. Immunohistochemical stains for the specific antigen if available will be extremely useful. In addition histiocytes from viral lymphadenitis and other lymphadenopathies are myeloperoxidase negative, whereas the histiocytes in Kikuchi–Fujimoto's disease are myeloperoxidase positive (Pileri et al., 2001).

SLE-associated lymphadenopathy may have identical histologic features with Kikuchi–Fujimoto's lymphadenitis. Hematoxylin bodies, which are aggregates of degenerated nuclear debris, an Azzopardi phenomenon, which is the presence of aggregates of degenerated nuclear material in the walls of blood vessels, sparse CD8+ T cells, abundant plasma cells, and capsular or pericapsular inflammation would favor a diagnosis of SLE. Careful evaluation of the clinical history and serological markers (antinuclear antibodies and complement CH50, C3, and C4 levels) will be helpful.

Treatment of Choice and Prognosis

Kikuchi–Fjimoto's lymphadenitis is a self-limiting condition that generally resolves spontaneously within 1 to 4 months, but persistent or recurrent cases have been reported, and rare fatal cases have also been documented (Onciu and Medeiros, 2003; Hutchinson and Wang, 2010). Therapy is generally symptomatic using analgesics and antipyretics. In patients with severe generalized or extranodal manifestation, steroids or nonsteroidal anti-inflammatory therapy may be considered.

NECROTIZING SUPPURATIVE GRANULOMATAS

Chronic Granulomatous Disease of Children

First described in 1950s, chronic granulomatous disease (CGD) is a rare primary immunodeficiency disorder characterized by recurrent bacterial and fungal infections involving reticuloendothelial system.

TABLE 18.6 Differential Diagnosis of Kikuchi–Fujimoto's Lymphadenitis

Lymphadenopathy Clinical Features	Histology	Immunohistology/Genetic
SLE Lymphadenopathy	Discrete pulp necrosis; nuclear basophilic smearing of vessels, Hematoxylin bodies; Plasmacytoid monocytes around HEVs preserved; plasma cells or neutrophils may be present	CD8 T cells increased
Herpes simplex	Viral inclusions, neutrophils, absent sheets of polymphorphic cells	Anti-HSV antibody
Infectious lymphadenitis	Granulomas; neutrophils; microorganisms may show on special stains	Specific antibody or molecular test positive
Non-Hodgkin lymphoma	Atypical lymphocytes; polymorphous histiocytes not prominent	CD20 for B-cell lymphoma; mostly CD4 for T-cell lymphoma; CD30 for anaplastic large cell lymphoma
Granulocytic sarcoma	Eosinophils, immature granulocytes may be seen;necrosis not prominent	CD34+, MPO or Lysozyme+, CD43+, maybe CD123+ if plasmacytoid blastic dendritic cell in origin
Kawasaki's disease	Extensive ischemic fibrinoid necrosis; microthrombi and hemorrhages; no prominent histoctyes or plasmacytosis	
Metastatic carcinoma	May not be obvious especially if morphology of small round blue cell tumor; signet ring or vacuolated cytoplasm; nuclear atypia Pankeratin or CK subset	

Definition

CGD is an inherited disease of the nicotinamide adenine dinucleotide phosphate (NADPH) oxidase system in phagocytic cells that leads to defective production of toxic oxygen metabolites and impaired killing of certain microbial pathogens. Patients with CGD develop recurrent life-threatening infections with catalase-producing organisms as well as tissue granuloma formation [Greenberg et al., 2006].

ICD-10 Code D71

Synonyms

CGD, chronic dysphagocytosis, chronic familial granulomatosis, septic progressive granulomatosis, fatal granulomatous disease of childhood, impotent neutrophil syndrome, congenital dysphagocytosis.

Epidemiology

The incidence of CGD in the United States is about 1 per 200,000 to 250,000 live births (Towbin and Chaves, 2010), with no apparent racial predilection. More than two-thirds of the cases are born with X-linked defects, and the remaining cases are autosomal recessive disease.

Clinical Aspects

Etiology. CGD is caused by a defect in NADPH oxidase. The defects prevents phagocytic cells from producing a respiratory burst, which is an event where oxygen is reduced and oxygen radicals are generated. The oxygen radicals are needed to kill catalase positive bacteria and fungi.

Sites of Involvement. CGD can affect every organ system. The most common involved organs include skin, lymph node, lungs, gastrointestinal tract, liver, spleen, bones, and joints. Lymphadenopathy is present in almost all CGD patients. The cervical nodal chain is most frequently affected, and other sites can also be involved (Mahomed et al., 2001).

Pathogenesis

The NADPH oxidase defect can be caused by mutations of any one of the four genes encoded the enzyme subunits. The X-linked recessive patients have a mutation of the CYBB gene, which encodes the gp91-phox subunit. The remaining cases are autosomal recessive and have mutations of CYBA, NCF-1, and NCF-2 genes, which encode p22-phox, p47-phox, and p67-phox, respectively. About 95%

of these mutations result in a complete absence or greatly diminished level of the affected protein, and the remaining mutations lead to a normal level of defective protein (Heyworth et al., 2003). The NADPH oxidase is needed to generate oxygen radicals such as the hydroxyl radical (OH−), hydrogen peroxide, peroxynitrite anion, and oxyhalides, for killing catalase-positive microorganisms. The catalase breaks down the endogenous hydrogen peroxide, thus a normally functioning phagocytic system is necessary. Some other microorganisms can still be killed because the phagocytes may use the endogenously produced hydrogen peroxide against the pathogens. The common pathogenetic bacteria and fungi in CGD include *Staphylococcus aureus, Serratia marcescens, Burkholderia cepacia, Nocardia*, and *Aspergillus* species (Greenberg et al., 2006).

Approach to Diagnosis

The diagnosis of CGD is usually made by a nitroblue tetrazolium (NBT) test or dihydrorhodamine (DHR) test. These tests measure the NADPH oxidase activity. The DHR test is considered the preferred screening and diagnostic test.

Clinical Workup

Laboratory screening and diagnostic tests include the above-mentioned NBT and DHR tests. Genetic testing to detect the specific gene mutation is useful to determine the inheritance pattern. Prenatal diagnosis using molecular testing is also available. The immunoblot may show an absence of corresponding protein products in the autosomal recessive mutations. Imaging is used to identify the involved sites.

Morphology

Histologic examination typically shows infection or postinfectious granuloma. In the lymph nodes the characteristic changes are necrotizing granulomas and pigmented histiocytes (Symchych et al., 1968; Levine et al., 2005). Numerous pigmented histiocytes are present around and between the granulomas, and there is also marked sinus histiocytosis. The pigment in histiocytes is yellow-brown, texture is granular, and ceroid-like, and it is typically stained greenish-blue with Giemsa (D'Amelio et al., 1984). The granulomas often resemble tuberculosis, with central necrosis and giant cells, although nonsuppurative infection can also occur (Towbin and Chaves, 2010). The calcified lymph node may be a consequence of the infection and granuloma.

Differential Diagnosis

Other granulomatous lesions in lymph node, including tuberculosis, cat-scratch disease and Kikuchi–Fujimoto's lymphadenitis, should be considered in lymph node biopsy.

Treatment of Choice and Prognosis

Antimicrobial prophylaxis, treatment of infections, and interferon-gamma are the current therapy for CGD. Hematopoietic stem cell transplantation is an attractive therapeutic approach. However, a substantial number of patients died in their 20s or 30s. The most common causes of death have been pneumonia, pulmonary abscess, septicemia, and brain abscess (van den Berg et al., 2009).

GRANULOMATOUS CHANGE WITHIN GERMINAL CENTERS

Henoch–Schönlein Purpura

First described in 1800s, and named after Johann Schönlein and Eduard Heinrich Henoch (Jennette, 2006), Henoch–Schönlein purpura (HSP) is a rare, self-limited small-vessel vasculitis, and is one of the most common forms of vasculitis in children, although it affects adults as well.

Definition

HSP is a systemic vasculitis characterized by "IgA-dominant immune deposits affecting small vessels and typically involving skin, gut, and glomeruli and associated with arthralgia or arthritis" (Jennette et al., 1994a). Only skin is involved in 100% of cases.

ICD-10 Code D69.0

Synonyms

Anaphylactoid purpura, Schönlein–Henoch purpura, allergic purpura, hemorrhagic capillary toxicosis, nonthrombocytopenic idiopathic purpura, peliosis rheumatica, rheumatic purpura, allergic vasculitis, Leukocytoclastic vasculitis.

Epidemiology

HSP typically occurs in children between 3 and 10 years of age, with 50% of the cases under 5 years of age, although adult cases have been described (Eleftheriou and Brogan, 2009). Gender preference is reportedly different in different studies (Gonzalez et al., 2009). There is no racial predominance, but a lower incidence in black children is noted comparing with white or Asian. The annual incidence is reported as between 10.5 and 20.4 per 100,000 children (McCarthy and Tizard, 2010).

Clinical Aspects

Etiology. The exact etiology of HSP is undetermined. It is noted that most HSP cases occur during the winter and fall months (Gonzalez et al., 2009), and it is often preceded by an upper respiratory tract infection (Saulsbury, 1999; Allen et al., 1960). Various bacterial and viral pathogens, parvovirus B19, hepatitis C virus, and streptococcus, have been postulated to be the etiologic agents. Drug-induced HSP is common in adults, which is most commonly associated with angiotensin-converting enzyme (ACE) inhibitors, antibiotics, or nonsteroidal anti-inflammatory drugs (NSAIDs). Genetic predisposition is supported by evidences of family clustering, and it has been reported that HLA DRB1*01 and *11 are positively associated with HSP while HLA DRB1*07 is negatively associated with HSP (Monach and Merkel, 2010).

Sites of Involvement. Typical symptoms of HSP include palpable purpura, arthralgia, abdominal pain, and proteinuria/hematuria. Characteristic palpable purpura is usually found on the lower extremeties and buttock. Joints involved typically are ankles, feet, and knees (Peru et al., 2008). In a web-based statistical study conducted by European League Against Rheumatism (EULAR)/Pediatric Rheumatology International Trials Organization (PRINTO)/Pediatric Rheumatology European Society (PRES), 827 pediatric patients were analyzed and 100% patients had purpura with lower limb predominance. Diffuse abdominal pain was present in 60% of the patients. Arthritis/arthalgia was present in 78%, and proteinuria/hematuria was in 33% of the patients (Ozen et al., 2010). Renal involvement often presents as glomerulonephritis, and renal failure is the most common cause of death in patients who succumb to HSP. Less frequently, HSP involves brain, testis, ureter, and lungs manifesting as cerebral vasculitis, orchitis, ureteritis, or pulmonary hemorrhage (Eleftheriou and Brogan, 2009). Lymphadenopathy has been noted in HSP patients (Veraldi et al., 1999; Akosa and Ali, 1989).

Pathogenesis

IgA deposition is the key factor in the pathogenesis of HSP. Deposition of IgA is demonstrated in the wall of lesional vascular tissue, such as dermal capillaries and postcapillary venules and mesangium (Yang et al., 2008). An aberrant glycosylation of IgA1 has been proposed as one possible mechanism (Lau et al., 2007). These altered glycosylated IgA1 proteins may form immune complex deposits. Recent studies suggested that nonspecific inflammatory mediators,

including tumor necrosis factor (TNF)-α, interleukin-1, and interleukin-6, may play roles (Yang et al., 2008; O'Neil, 2009). In lymph nodes it is hypothesized that the changes are due to ischemia caused by small-vessel vasculitis of the end arterioles of the germinal centers (Howat, 1990).

Approach to Diagnosis

The clinical features of HSP is usually classical. Palpable purpura and a positive direct immunofluorescence are sufficient to diagnose HSP. In 2006 EULAR/PRES published a new classification of childhood vasculitis, and Table 18.7 given the diagnostic criteria for HSP (Ozen et al., 2006). No laboratory test is specific for HSP.

Clinical Workup

Initial investigation for HSP may include CBC, erythrocyte sedimentation rate, clotting, biochemical profile, antistreptolysin O titer and antideoxyribonuclease B, urine dipstick, and protein/creatinine ratio. Hematuria and/or proteinuria, an altered renal function with increased creatinine and low albumin, and a preceding streptococcal infection may be present. A biopsy of the skin or the kidney may be warranted. Autoantibodies, complements, and immunoglobulins may be helpful to differentiate from other vasculitis.

Morphology

The lymphadenopathy is nonspecific. Histologically, the enlarged lymph node may show follicular granulomas, follicular microabscesses, and leukocytoclastic vasculitis (Akosa and Ali, 1989). The majority of germinal centers are replaced by histiocytes and dendritic cells, and the germinal centers usually contain aggregates of neutrophils. Leukocytoclastic vasculitis is characterized by vessel wall fibrinoid necrosis and perivascular accumulation of inflammatory cells, mostly polymorphonuclear leukocytes and mononuclear cells, surrounding the capillaries and postcapillary venules (Davin, 2006). Endothelial swelling and nuclear fragmentation of the infiltrating neutrophils are usually evident (Howat and Variend,

TABLE 18.7 Diagnostic Criteria for Henoch–Schönlein purpura

Palpable purpura (mandatory criterion) in the presence of at least one of the following four features:
Diffuse abdominal pain
Any biopsy showing predominant IgA deposition
Arthritis[a] or arthralgia
Renal involvement (any hematuria and/or proteinuria)

Source: Ozen et al., (2006).
[a] Acute, any joint.

1986). Biopsy of the skin shows changes of leukocytoclastic vasculitis, and typical renal lesion is a focal and segmental proliferative glomerulonephirits, in which glomeruli show segmental proliferation and increased numbers of infiltrating neutrophils or mononuclear cells (Asherson, 2001).

Immunophenotyping

Direct immunofluorescence (DIF) studies may reveal deposition of IgA, IgG, and C3 in the vessel walls, which are supportive findings for the diagnosis of HSP.

Laboratory Diagnosis

There is no specific laboratory diagnosis. Tests specific for antinuclear antibodies, double-stranded DNA, and the antineutrophil cytoplasmic antibody (ANCA) may be used to differentiate from systemic lupus erythematosus or other ANCA positive vasculitis. C3 and C4 are usually normal or low occasionally. IgG and IgM are normal but IgA may be increased (McCarthy and Tizard, 2010).

Differential Diagnosis

The vasculitis may be associated with lymphoproliferative disorder (Wooten and Jasin, 1996). Leukocytoclastic vasculitis can be accompanying lymphoma, such as cutaneous T-cell lymphoma, Hodgkin disease, and angioimmunoblastic lymphadenopathy, although they are unusual (Fox et al., 2008; Mor et al., 1987; Ng et al., 1988; Wooten and Jasin, 1996). Clinically, in patients whose presentation is atypical, the considerations may include juvenile rheumatoid arthritis, hemolytic uremic syndrome, and other forms of vasculitis.

Treatment of Choice and Prognosis

The natural course of HSP is most often self-resolving. The treatment is generally symptomatic and supportive. Renal manifestations in HSP are usually mild and transient. However, renal failure may develop and cause fatality in around 2% of the patients (Eleftheriou and Brogan, 2009). Steroids may be used but its efficacy is inconclusive (McCarthy and Tizard, 2010; Chartapisak et al., 2009).

Children with Shock or Bacteremia

Epithelioid granulomas in germinal centers are found in infants and children with various severe, fatal infections (Severson et al., 1988), or other circumstances like shock (Howat and Variend, 1986). Although it has been noted as early as in 1886 (Waschkwitsch, 1900; Klone, 1940–1; Councilman, 1900; Stilling, 1886), this entity is poorly understood and its significance is largely unknown.

Definition

In children with fatal infections or shock, germinal centers are replaced and expanded by a mixture of epithelioid histiocytes and follicular dendritic cells, with occasional central necrosis.

ICD-10 Code I89

Synonyms

Epithelioid germinal centers, follicular necrosis, toxische follikelalteration/toxic follicle alteration.

Epidemiology

Epithelioid germinal centers in infants and children are most commonly found in deaths of infants and young children, particularly ranging between ages of 1 and 3 years in one study (Howat and Variend, 1986), by postmortem examination.

Clinical Aspects

Etiology. Various infectious diseases, including bacterial meningitis, enterocolitis, laryngotracheobronchitis, bronchiolitis, pneumonia, myocarditis, and bacterial sepsis (Millikin, 1970, 1977), are the most often causes of death. Infections of viral origin have been reported as well (Millikin, 1970; Poscharisky, 1912). Other diseases such as Reye's syndrome, sudden infant death syndrome, have also been described (Millikin, 1977). Most cases have very short clinical courses of less than one week and all the reported cases have been fatal.

Sites of Involvement. The changes tend to affect all lymphoid tissue such as lymph nodes, spleen, tonsils, Peyer's patches, and appendix.

Pathogenesis

Pathogenesis is unknown. Systemic infections may cause cytolytic attack against germinal centers (Jones, 2002), and it is argued that circulatory, toxic, and hypovolemic shock may play roles in the pathogenesis (Howat and Variend, 1986, 1989).

Morphology

The germinal centers of the lymph node, spleen, or Peyer's patches show replacement and expansion by large, epithelioid-appearing cells with round to oval, centrally located nuclei and abundant eosinophilic cytoplasm (Severson et al., 1988). Occasional germinal centers contain necrotic cellular debris and lymphocytic infiltrates. Surrounding mantle zones are intact.

Immunophenotyping/Cytochemistry

The epithelioid cells are positive for follicular dendritic cell markers (S-100), and negative for monocyte/macrophage markers.

Differential Diagnosis

The progressive transformation of germinal centers (PTGC) is typically morphologically distinct with mantle zone lymphocytes replacing the focally expanded germinal centers. When there are increased follicular dendritic cells inside the germinal centers, PTGC may occasionally be difficult to distinguish from this entity. PTGC is associated with gradual expansion and homogenization of the outlines of the follicular dendritic cells, however, immunophenotypically, the majority of infiltrating cells in PTGC are small B cells and activated CD4+, often CD57+, T cells. Well-formed granulomas within germinal centers are also rarely seen in response to infectious agents.

MIXED PATTERN WITH PLASMACYTOSIS

Rheumatoid Arthritis Lymphadenopathy

Because of an increased risk of development of non-Hodgkin lymphomas, patients with rheumatoid arthritis (RA) lymphadenopathy often get biopsies to rule out atypical lymphoproliferative disorders and lymphomas.

Definition

Rheumatoid arthritis (RA) lymphadenopathy is a distinctive reactive lymphadenopathy seen in 50 to 75% of patients with RA.

Epidemiology

RA affects about 1% of the world's population (Gabriel et al., 1999).

Pathogenesis

There is a 2 to 20-fold increased risk of spontaneous lymphomas (Isomaki, Hakulinen, and Joutsenlahti, 1978; Symmons, 1985) and atypical lymphoproliferative disorders (Kamel et al., 1995b; Kamel, 1997) in rheumatoid arthritis. Immunosuppressive therapy especially low-dose methotrexate (MTX) therapy, as well as Epstein–Barr virus (EBV) infection may contribute to the development of these LPDs (Kamel et al. 1995a; Kamel 1997). In particular, an increased incidence of large B-cell lymphomas is described (Baecklund et al., 2003).

Morphology

Histologically, reactive lymphoproliferative disorders (LPDs) associated with RA usually demonstrate reactive follicular hyperplasia and polyclonal plasma cell infiltration in the interfollicular area (Figures 18.53, 18.54). Plasma cells tend to crowd in on the germinal centers (Nosanchuk and Schnitzer, 1969) (Figure 18.55). Although low proliferative activity, decreased tingible-body macrophages, and increased of cleaved cells in germinal centers of RA have been described (Kondratowicz et al., 1990), many rheumatoid lymph node germinal centers have hyperplasia with demarcated mantle zones filled with either a predominance of large centroblasts or a mixture of centrocytes or centroblasts, tingible-body macrophages, and polarized appearance (Nosanchuk and Schnitzer, 1969). Similar morphologic findings are seen in other autoimmune diseases like Felty's and Sjogren's syndrome (Talal, 1988; Talal and Flescher, 1988).

Atypical lymphadenopathy include mixed or multicentric Castleman's disease, atypical paracortical hyperplasia with lymphoid follicles (Kojima et al., 2001), and atypical immunoblastic proliferations

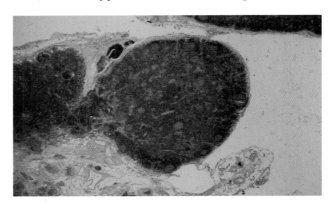

FIGURE 18.53 **Follicle center hyperplasia.**

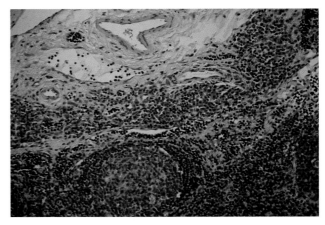

FIGURE 18.54 **Interfollicular and stromal reactive plasmacytosis in RA.**

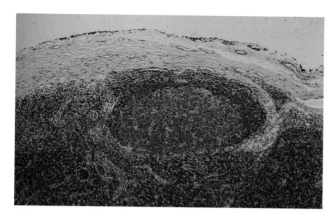

FIGURE 18.55 **Germinal center with interfollicular plasmacytosis in RA and crowding into the germinal center.**

(Kojima et al., 2010). Atypical lymphoplasmacytic immunoblastic proliferation in lymph nodes (Koo, 1984) has been seen in RA. Paracortical diffuse immunoblastic proliferation similar to EBV lymphadenopathy is described, although no EBV association is seen (Costenbader and Karlson, 2006).

Differential Diagnosis

Atypical paracortical hyperplasia with prominent vascular proliferation and many lymphoid follicles with germinal centers may simulate angioimmunoblastic T-cell lymphoma (AITL) pattern. The differences include atypical "clear" cells, atrophic germinal centers, and EBV EBER in situ positivity in AITL, whereas absent atypical cells, germinal center hyperplasia and absent EBV characterize RA.

Treatment with methotrexate may also give rise to Hodgkin-like atypical lymphoproliferative histology. Like Hodgkin cells, the large cells may be EBER+. In cases labeled as Hodgkin-like, the large cells are CD20+, CD30+, but CD15 negative.

Treatment

Methotrexate treatment may contribute to EBV+ lymphoproliferative disorders in RA. Withdrawal of methotrexate appear to cause partial regression of lymphomas or full regression of Hodgkin-like atypical lymphoproliferion, especially if EBV associated (Kamel et al., 1994).

Plasma Cell (Mott Cell) Granuloma

Definition

Mott cell granuloma is a type of plasma cell granuloma in which plasma cells show numerous intracytoplasmic globules referred to as Mott cells. Mott cells are abnormal plasma cells with multiple Russell bodies, or globular cytoplasmic inclusions.

Epidemiology

This is a rare reactive condition that has been described as either plasma cell granuloma, inflammatory pseudotumor, or myofibroblastic tumors, and it occurs in nodal and extranodal sites.

Sites

Lymph nodes (Kutok et al., 2001; Goldman et al., 2003), head and neck (Albizzati, Ramesar, and Davis 1988), lungs (Mohsenifar et al., 1979), spleen (Neuhauser et al., 2001), and stomach (Fujiyoshi et al., 2001).

Morphology

The Mott cell type of plasma cell granuloma shows a significant presence of Mott-type plasma cells in the cellular infiltrate (Goldman et al., 2003). The histology is characterized by increased sheets of Mott cells, the presence of intracytoplasmic hyaline globules, reactive multifocal necrotizing noncaseating granulomas, and epithelioid histiocytes with fibrotic areas (Table 18.8). Diagnosis relies on a triad of proliferation of Mott cells with polytypic immunoglobulin hyaline globules (Figure 18.56), reactive epithelioid multifocal necrotizing granulomas (Figure 18.57), and capsular and pulp fibrosis.

Approach to Diagnosis

A diagnosis of Mott cell granuloma can be made with histologic examination, immunohistochemical or immunoflorescence, or molecular genetic confirmation of polyclonality of plasma cells.

Ancillary Tests

Immunohistochemistry, flow cytometry, and immunofluorescence microscopy are crucial in differentiating between this benign lymphadenopathy and monoclonal extramedullary plasmacytoma.

TABLE 18.8 Plasma Cell Granuloma (Mott Cell Granuloma)

Morphologic Features
• Scattered epithelioid granulomas with no central necrosis, palisaded epithelioid histiocytes, and sheets of Mott cells (plasma cells laden with pink-orange hyaline globules)
• Lymph node capsule thickened and sclerosed trabeculae without vasculitis.
• Regressed follicles and interfollicular areas with fibroblastic as well as cellular proliferation composed of immunoblasts and plasma cells

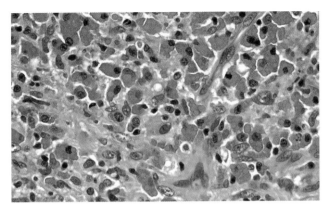

FIGURE 18.56 **Mott cells with intracytoplasmic globules of immunoglobulins.**

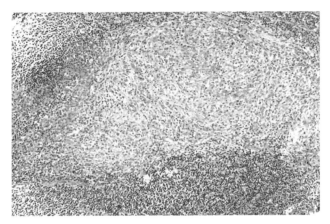

FIGURE 18.57 **Pale nodule of epithelioid granulomas.** Note the intense plasmacytosis with no necrosis and no multinucleated giant cells.

Pathogenesis

The etiology in this type of granulomata with a predominance of Mott cells implies an immunorelated process, while presence of necrosis and mixture with other inflammatory cells points to an infectious or postinflamatory process. In extranodal Mott cell granulomas, *H. pylori* infection may induce the reaction (Fujiyoshi et al., 2001).

Differential Diagnosis

The main differential diagnosis include plasmacytoma and lymphoplasmacytic disorders (Table 18.9). Polyclonality of the plasma cells by an immunologic and molecular test would support a reactive process. Specific infectious granulomas need to be excluded on the basis of histology, fungal and acid-fast stains, as well as viral serologies.

TABLE 18.9 Reactive Lymph Node with Plasmacytosis

Early immune normal reaction
Castleman's disease
Rheumatoid arthritis
Syphilis
SLE
Other autoimmune diseases
Plasma cell granuloma

REFERENCES

ABRIL A, CALAMIA KT, COHEN MD. 2003. The Churg–Strauss syndrome (allergic granulomatous angiitis): review and update. Semin Arthritis Rheum 33:106–14

ABUEL-HAIJA M, HURFORD MT. 2007. Kimura disease. Arch Pathol Lab Med 131:650–1

AINSLIE GM, BENATAR SR. 1985. Serum angiotensin converting enzyme in sarcoidosis: sensitivity and specificity in diagnosis. Correlations with disease activity, duration, extra-thoracic involvement, radiographic type and therapy. Q J Med 55:253–70

AISAKA Y, URABE A, YAMASAKI T, KOHNO H, AIMITSU S, FUJIHARA M. 2006. A case of primary biliary cirrhosis with systemic lymph node enlargement. Kanzo 47:392–7

AKOSA AB, ALI MH. 1989. Lymph node pathology in Henoch–Schonlein purpura. Histopathology 15:297–301

ALBIZZATI C, RAMESAR KC, DAVIS BC. 1988. Plasma cell granuloma of the larynx (case report and review of the literature). J Laryngol Otol 102:187–9. Analysis of nine cases. Pathol Res Pract 197:237–44

ALLEN DM, DIAMOND LK, HOWELL DA. 1960. Anaphylactoid purpura in children (Schonlein–Henoch syndrome): review with a follow-up of the renal complications. AMA J Dis Child 99:833–54

AMANO S, HAZAMA F, KUBAGAWA H, TASAKA K, HAEBARA H, HAMASHIMA Y. 1980. General pathology of Kawasaki disease: on the morphological alterations corresponding to the clinical manifestations. Acta Pathol Jpn 30:681–94

AMICOSANTE M, BERRETTA F, ROSSMAN M, BUTLER RH, ROGLIANI P, VAN DEN BERG-LOONEN E, SALTINI C. 2005. Identification of hla-drphebeta47 as the susceptibility marker of hypersensitivity to beryllium in individuals lacking the berylliosis-associated supratypic marker hla-dpglubeta69. Respir Res 6:94.

ASHERSON RA, CERVERA R, TRIPLETT DA, ABRAMSON SB. 2001. Vascular manifestations of systemic autoimmune diseases. CRC Press, West Palm Beach, FL.

ATHAPPAN G, GALE S, PONNIAH T. 2009. Corticosteroid therapy for primary treatment of Kawasaki disease–weight of evidence: a meta-analysis and systematic review of the literature. Cardiovasc J Afr 20:233–6.

BAECKLUND E, SUNDSTRÖM C, EKBONM A, CATRINA AI, BIBERFELD P, FELTELIUS N, et al. 2003. Lymphoma subtypes in patients with rheumatoid arthritis. Increased proportion of diffuse large B cell lymphoma. Arthritis Rheum 48:1543–50.

Behm FG, O'Dowd GJ, Frable WJ. 1984. Fine-needle aspiration effects on benign lymph node histology. Am J Clin Pathol 82:195–8.

Bernatsky S, Ramsey-Goldman R, Rajan R, Boivin JF, Joseph L, Lachance S, Cournoyer D, Zoma A, Manzi S, Ginzler E, Urowitz M, Gladman D, Fortin PR, Edworthy S, Barr S, Gordon C, Bae SC, Sibley J, Steinsson K, Nived O, Sturfelt G, St Pierre Y, Clarke A. 2005. Non-Hodgkin's lymphoma in systemic lupus erythematosus. An Rheum Dis 64:1507–9.

Ben-Chetrit E, Flusser D, Okon E, Ackerman Z, Rubinow A. 1989. Multicentric Castleman's disease assocoiated with rheumatoid arthritis: a possible role of hepatitis B antigen. An Rheum Dis 48:326–30.

Bhargava V, Farhi DC. 1988. Bone marrow granulomas: clinicopathologic findings in 72 cases and review of the literature. Hematol Pathol 2:43–50.

Bibby S, Healy B, Steele R, Kumareswaran K, Nelson H, Beasley R. 2010. Association between leukotriene receptor antagonist therapy and Churg–Strauss syndrome: an analysis of the fda aers database. Thorax 65:132–8.

Bosch Marcet J, Serres Creixams X, Penas Boira M, Inaraja Martinez L. 1998. Mediastinal lymphadenopathy: a variant of incomplete Kawasaki disease. Acta Paediatr 87:1200–2.

Bosch X, Guilabert A. 2006. Kikuchi–Fujimoto disease. Orphanet J Rare Dis 1:18.

Bosch X, Guilabert A, Miquel R, Campo E. 2004. Enigmatic Kikuchi–Fujimoto disease: A comprehensive review. Am J Clin Pathol 122:141–152.

Bowerfind ES Jr., Moore RD, Weisberger AS. 1956. Histochemical studies of lymph nodes in disseminated lupus erythematosus. AMA Arch Pathol 62:472–478.

Butnor KJ. 2005. Pulmonary sarcoidosis induced by interferon-alpha therapy. Am J Surg Pathol 29:976–9.

Butnor KJ, Sporn TA, Ingram P, Gunasegaram S, Pinto JF, Roggli VL. 2003. Beryllium detection in human lung tissue using electron probe X-ray microanalysis. Mod Pathol 16:1171–7.

Casey M, Radel E, Ratech H. 2000. Lymph node manifestations of limited Churg–Strauss syndrome. J Pediatr Hematol Oncol 22:468–71.

Cassani F, Zoli M, Baffoni L, Cordiani MR, Brunori A, Bianchi FB, Pisi E. 1990. Prevalence and significance of abdominal lymphadenopathy in patients with chronic liver disease: an ultrasound study. J Clin Gastroenterol 12:42–6.

Chartapisak W, Opastiraku S, Willis NS, Craig JC, Hodson EM. 2009. Prevention and treatment of renal disease in Henoch–Schonlein purpura: a systematic review. Arch Dis Child 94:132–7.

Chen H, Thompson LD, Aguilera NS, Abbondanzo SL. 2004. Kimura disease: a clinicopathologic study of 21 cases. Am J Surg Pathol 28:505–13.

Chen PH, Huang YF, Tang CW, Wann SR, Chang HT. 2010. Kikuchi–Fujimoto disease: an amazing response to hydroxychloroquine. Eur J Pediatr 169(12):1557–9.

Christopherson WM, Berg HF. 1955. A histopathological study of lymph nodes irradiated with colloidal au198. Cancer 8:1261–69.

Chung YG, Jee WH, Kang YK, Jung CK, Park GS, Lee AH, Bahk WJ, Cho HM, Park JW. 2010. Kimura's disease involving a long bone. Skeletal Radiol 39:495–500.

Churg J, Strauss L. 1951. Allergic granulomatosis, allergic angiitis, and periarteritis nodosa. Am J Pathol 27:277–301.

Cleary KR, Osborne BM, Butler JJ. 1982. Lymph node infarction foreshadowing malignant lymphoma. Am J Surg Pathol 6:435–42.

Congdon CC. 1966. The destructive effect of radiation on lymphatic tissue. Cancer Res 26:1211–20.

Cook MG. 1972. The size and histological appearances of mesenteric lymph nodes in Crohn's disease. Gut 13:970–2.

Costabel U, Ohshimo S, Guzman J. 2008. Diagnosis of sarcoidosis. Curr Opin Pulm Med 14:455–61.

Councilman WT, Mallory, F. B., Pearce, R. M. 1900. A study of the bacteriology and pathology of 220 fatal cases of diphtheria. J Boston Soc Med Sci 5:139–319.

Cualing H, Schroder L, Perme C. 2001. Allergic granulomatosis secondary to a limited form of Churg–Strauss syndrome. Arch Pathol Lab Med 125:954–7.

D'Amelio R, Bellavite P, Bianco P, de Sole P, Le Moli S, Lippa S, Seminara R, Vercelli B, Rossi F, Rocchi G, et al. 1984. Chronic granulomatous disease in two sisters. J Clin Immunol 4:220–7.

Danchenko N, Satia JA, Anthony MS. 2006. Epidemiology of systemic lupus erythematosus: a comparison of worldwide disease burden. Lupus 15:308–18.

Davies JD, Stansfeld AG. 1972. Spontaneous infarction of superficial lymph nodes. J Clin Pathol 25:689–96.

Davies JD, Webb AJ. 1982. Segmental lymph-node infarction after fine-needle aspiration. J Clin Pathol 35:855–7.

Davin JC, Sarzi-Puttini P, Doria A, Kuhn A. 2006. Henoch–Schonlein purpura. In: The Skin in Systemic Autoimmune Diseases. Elsevier, Amsterdam; 249–59.

DeFrance JH, Harriman BB, Azizkhan RG. 1976. Superficial lymph node infarction. Am J Surg 132:112–3.

Devaney K, Goodman ZD, Epstein MS, Zimmerman HJ, Ishak KG. 1993. Hepatic sarcoidosis: clinicopathologic features in 100 patients. Am J Surg Pathol 17:1272–80.

Eleftheriou D, Brogan PA. 2009. Vasculitis in children. Best Pract Res Clin Rheumatol 23:309–23.

Facchetti F, Vermi W. 2002. [Plasmacytoid monocytes and plasmacytoid dendritic cells. Immune system cells linking innate and acquired immunity]. Pathologica 94:163–75. [In Italian]

Fox MC, Carter S, Khouri IF, Giralt SA, Prieto VG, Nash JW, Hymes SR. 2008. Adult Henoch–Schonlein purpura in a patient with myelodysplastic syndrome and a history of follicular lymphoma. Cutis 81:131–7.

Fox RA, Rosahn PD. 1943. The lymph nodes in disseminated lupus erythematosus. Am J Pathol 19:73–99.

Freeman AF, Shulman ST. 2006. Kawasaki disease: summary of the American Heart Association guidelines. Am Fam Phys 74:1141–8.

GIESKER DW, PASTUSZAK WT, FOROUHAR FA, KRAUSE PJ, HINE P. 1982. Lymph node biopsy for early diagnosis in Kawasaki disease. Am J Surg Pathol 6:493–501.

GOMARD-MENNESSON E, LANDRON C, DAUPHIN C, EPAULARD O, PETIT C, GREEN L, ROBLOT P, LUSSON JR, BROUSSOLLE C, SEVE P. 2010. Kawasaki disease in adults: report of 10 cases. Medicine (Baltimore) 89:149–58.

GONZALEZ LM, JANNIGER CK, SCHWARTZ RA. 2009. Pediatric Henoch–Schonlein purpura. Int J Dermatol 48:1157–65.

GREENBERG DE, DING L, ZELAZNY AM, STOCK F, WONG A, ANDERSON VL, MILLER G, KLEINER DE, TENORIO AR, BRINSTER L, DORWARD DW, MURRAY PR, HOLLAND SM. 2006. A novel bacterium associated with lymphadenitis in a patient with chronic granulomatous disease. PLoS Pathol 2:e28.

GROSS RG, ODIN JA. 2008. Recent advances in the epidemiology of primary biliary cirrhosis. Clin Liver Dis 12:289–303.

GROSS WL. 2002. Churg–Strauss syndrome: Update on recent developments. Curr Opin Rheumatol 14:11–14.

GUILLOU PJ, BRENNAN TG, GILES GR. 1973. Lymphocyte transformation in the mesenteric lymph nodes of patients with Crohn's disease. Gut 14:20–24.

GUILPAIN P, AUCLAIR JF, TAMBY MC, SERVETTAZ A, MAHR A, WEILL B, GUILLEVIN L, MOUTHON L. 2007. Serum eosinophil cationic protein: a marker of disease activity in Churg–Strauss syndrome. An NY Acad Sci 1107:392–9.

HARNDEN A, TAKAHASHI M, BURGNER D. 2009. Kawasaki disease. BMJ 338:b1514.

HENRY K, FARRER-BROWN G. 1981. A Colour Atlas of Thymus and Lymph Node Histopathology. Wolf Medical Publications, London.

HEYWORTH PG, CROSS AR, CURNUTTE JT. 2003. Chronic granulomatous disease. Curr Opin Immunol 15:578–84.

HOCHBERG MC. 1997. Updating the American College of Rheumatology revised criteria for the classification of systemic lupus erythematosus. Arthritis Rheum 40:1725.

HOHENESTER S, OUDE-ELFERINK RP, BEUERS U. 2009. Primary biliary cirrhosis. Semin Immunopathol 31:283–307.

HOLMAN RC, CURNS AT, BELAY ED, STEINER CA, SCHONBERGER LB. 2003. Kawasaki syndrome hospitalizations in the United States, 1997 and 2000. Pediatrics 112:495–501.

HOWAT AJ. 1990. Lymph nodes in Henoch–Schonlein purpura. Histopathology 16:514–5.

HOWAT AJ, VARIEND S. 1986. Nuclear fragmentation and epithelioid change of germinal centers in the lymphoid tissue of child deaths. Pediatr Pathol 5:125–34.

HOWAT AJ, VARIEND S. 1989. Epithelioid germinal centers. Arch Pathol Lab Med 113:451.

HUBSCHER SG, HARRISON RF. 1989. Portal lymphadenopathy associated with lipofuscin in chronic cholestatic liver disease. J Clin Pathol 42:1160–5.

HUDNALL SD. 2000. Kikuchi–Fujimoto disease: is Epstein–Barr virus the culprit? Am J Clin Pathol 113:761–4.

HUI PK, CHAN JK, NG CS, KUNG IT, GWI E. 1989. Lymphadenopathy of Kimura's disease. Am J Surg Pathol 13:177–86.

HUTCHINSON CB, WANG E. 2010. Kikuchi–Fujimoto disease. Arch Pathol Lab Med 134:289–93.

ISHII T, FUJITA T, MATSUSHITA T, YANABA K, HASEGAWA M, NAKASHIMA H, OGAWA F, SHIMIZU K, TAKEHARA K, TEDDER TF, SATO S, FUJIMOTO M. 2009. Establishment of experimental eosinophilic vasculitis by ige-mediated cutaneous reverse passive arthus reaction. Am J Pathol 174:2225–33.

ISOMÄKI HA, HAKULINEN T, JOUTSENLAHTI U. 1978. Excess risk of lymphomas, leukemia and myeloma in patients with rheumatoid arthritis. J Chronic Dis 31:691–6.

JAWORSKY C. 2008. Leukotriene receptor antagonists and Churg–Strauss syndrome: an association with relevance to dermatopathology? J Cutan Pathol 35:611–3.

JENNETTE JC, FALK RJ, ANDRASSY K, BACON PA, CHURG J, GROSS WL, HAGEN EC, HOFFMAN GS, HUNDER GG, KALLENBERG CG, et al. 1994a. Nomenclature of systemic vasculitides: proposal of an international consensus conference. Arthritis Rheum 37:187–192.

JENNETTE JC, FALK RJ, ANDRASSY K, BACON PA, CHURG J, GROSS WL, HAGEN EC, HOFFMAN GS, HUNDER GG, KALLENBERG CG, et al. 1994b. Nomenclature of systemic vasculitides: proposal of an international consensus conference. Arthritis Rheum 37:187–92.

JENNETTE JC, OLSON, JL, SCHWARTZ MM, SILVA FG. 2006. Heptinstall's pathology of the kidney. Lippincott Williams and Wilkins, Philadelphia.

JONES D. 2002. Dismantling the germinal center: comparing the processes of transformation, regression, and fragmentation of the lymphoid follicle. Adv Anat Pathol 9:129–38.

JONES DE. 2008. Pathogenesis of primary biliary cirrhosis. Postgrad Med J 84:23–33.

KAMEL OW, WEISS LM, VAN DE RIJIN M, COLVY TV, KINGMA DW, JAFFE ES. 1996. Hodgkin's disease and lymphoproliferations resembling Hodgkin's disease in patients receiving long-term low-dose methotrexate therapy. Am J Surg Pathol 20:1279–87.

KAMEL OW. Iatrogenic lymphoproliferative disorders in nontransplantation settings. 1997. Semin Diag Pathol 14:27–34.

KAPLAN MM. 1996. Primary biliary cirrhosis. N Engl J Med 335:1570–80.

KASSAN SS, MOSS ML, REDDICK RL. 1976. Progressive hilar and mediastinal lymphadenopathy in systemic lupus erythematosus on corticosteroid therapy. N Engl J Med 294:1382–3.

KEIM DE, GELTNER JW. 1985. Mucocutaneous lymph node syndrome in an adult, with lymph node biopsy correlation. South Med J 78:872–4.

KIMURA T, YOSHIMURA, S., ISHIKAWA, E. 1948. On the unusual granulation combined with hyperplastic changes of lymphatic tissue. Trans Soc Pathol Jpn 37:179–80.

KLEER CG, APPELMAN HD. 2001. Surgical pathology of crohn's disease. Surg Clin North Am 81:13–30.

KLONE W. 1940–1. Die milz im ablauf der diphtherie. Beitr Pathol 105:73–90.

KOJIMA M, MOTOORI T, HOSOMURA Y, TANAKA H, SAKATA N, MASAWA N. 2006. Atypical lymphoplasmacytic and immunoblastic proliferation from rheumatoid arthritis: a case report. Pathol Res Pract 202:51–4.

KOJIMA M, NAKAMURA S, OYMA T, MOTOORI T, ITOH H, YOSHIDA K, et al. 2001. Autoimmune disease-associated lymphadenopathy with histological appearance of T-zone dysplasia with hyperplastic follicles. A clinicopathological analysis of nine cases. Pathol Res Pract 197(4):237–44.

KOJIMA M, MATSUDA H, IIJIMA M, YOSHIDA K, MASAWA N, NAKAMURA S. 2005a. Reactive hyperplasia with giant follicles in lymph node lesions from systemic lupus erythematosus patients: report of three cases. Apmis 113:558–63.

KOJIMA M, MOTOORI T, ITOH H, SHIMIZU K, IIJIMA M, TAMAKI Y, MURAYAMA K, OHNO Y, YOSHIDA K, MASAWA N, NAKAMURA S. 2005b. Distribution of Epstein–Barr virus in systemic rheumatic disease (rheumatoid arthritis, systemic lupus erythematosus, dermatomyositis) with associated lymphadenopathy: a study of 49 cases. Int J Surg Pathol 13:273–8.

KOJIMA M, NAKAMURA S, ITOH H, YOSHIDA K, SUCHI T, MASAWA N. 2001. Lymph node necrosis in systemic lupus erythematosus: a histopathological and immunohistochemical study of four cases. Apmis 109:141–6.

KOJIMA M, NAKAMURA S, MORISHITA Y, ITOH H, YOSHIDA K, OHNO Y, OYAMA T, ASANO S, JOSHITA T, MORI S, SUCHI T, MASAWA N. 2000. Reactive follicular hyperplasia in the lymph node lesions from systemic lupus erythematosus patients: a clinicopathological and immunohistological study of 21 cases. Pathol Int 50:304–12.

KOJIMA M, NAKAMURA S, SHIMIZU K, IIJIMA M, SARUKI N, SAKATA N, MASAWA N. 2005c. Usefulness of immunohistochemistry for recognizing metastatic colorectal adenocarcinoma in infarcted lymph nodes. Pathol Res Pract 200:771–4.

KOJIMA M, NAKAMURA S, SHIMIZU K, YAMANE Y, ITOH H, MASAWA N. 2003. Granulocytic sarcoma presenting with lymph node infarction at disease onset. Apmis 111:1133–6.

KOJIMA M, NAKAMURA S, SUGIHARA S, SAKATA N, MASAWA N. 2002. Lymph node infarction associated with infectious mononucleosis: report of a case resembling lymph node infarction associated with malignant lymphoma. Int J Surg Pathol 10:223–6.

KOJIMA M, NAKAMURA S, YAMANE Y, NISHIKAWA M, MURAYAMA K, SHIMIZU K, ITOH H, MASAWA N. 2004. Antigen preservation in infarcted nodal B-cell lymphoma, with special reference to follicular center cell markers. Int J Surg Pathol 12:251–5.

KOO CH, NATHWANI BN, WINBERG CD, HILL LR, RAPPAPORT H. 1984. Atypical lymphoplasmacytic and immunoblastic proliferation in lymph nodes of patients with autoimmune disease (autoimmune-disease associatedlymphadenopathy). Medicine (Baltimore) 63:274–90.

KUTOK JL, PINKUS GS, DORFMAN DM, FLETCHER CD. 2001. Inflammatory pseudotumor of lymph node and spleen: an entity biologically distinct from inflammatory myofibroblastic tumor. Hum Pathol. 32:1382–7.

KUBOTA M, USAMI I, YAMAKAWA M, TOMITA Y, HARUTA T. 2008. Kawasaki disease with lymphadenopathy and fever as sole initial manifestations. J Paediatr Child Health 44:359–62.

KUCUKARDALI Y, SOLMAZGUL E, KUNTER E, ONCUL O, YILDIRIM S, KAPLAN M. 2007. Kikuchi–Fujimoto disease: analysis of 244 cases. Clin Rheumatol 26:50–4.

KUMAR V, ABBAS AK, FAUSTO N, C. AJ. 2010a. Robbins S and Cotran R, Eds. Pathologic Basis of Disease. In: 8th ed. Saunders, Philadelphia, 807–11.

KUMAR V, ABBAS AK, FAUSTO NC. AJ. 2010b. Robbins S and Cotran R, Eds. Pathologic Basis of Disease. In: 8th ed. Saunders, Philadelphia, 213–21.

KUNG IT, CHAN JK. 1988. Kimura's disease or Kim's disease? Am J Surg Pathol 12:804–5.

KUO TT. 1995. Kikuchi's disease (histiocytic necrotizing lymphadenitis): a clinicopathologic study of 79 cases with an analysis of histologic subtypes, immunohistology, and DNA ploidy. Am J Surg Pathol 19:798–809.

KUO TT, SHIH LY, CHAN HL. 1988. Kimura's disease: involvement of regional lymph nodes and distinction from angiolymphoid hyperplasia with eosinophilia. Am J Surg Pathol 12:843–854.

LANDGREN O, ENGELS EA, PFEIFFER RM, GRIDLEY G, MELLEMKJAER L, OLSEN JH, KERSTANN KF, WHEELER W, HEMMINKI K, LINET MS, GOLDIN LR. 2006. Autoimmunity and susceptibility to Hodgkin lymphoma: a population-based case-control study in scandinavia. J Nat Cancer Inst 98:1321–1330.

LANHAM JG, ELKON KB, PUSEY CD, HUGHES GR. 1984. Systemic vasculitis with asthma and eosinophilia: a clinical approach to the churg-strauss syndrome. Medicine (Baltimore) 63:65–81.

LASZEWSKI MJ, BELDING PJ, FEDDERSEN RM, LUTZ CT, GOEKEN JA, KEMP JD, DICK FR. 1991. Clonal immunoglobulin gene rearrangement in the infarcted lymph node syndrome. Am J Clin Pathol 96:116–20.

LAU KK, WYATT RJ, MOLDOVEANU Z, TOMANA M, JULIAN BA, HOGG RJ, LEE JY, HUANG WQ, MESTECKY J, NOVAK J. 2007. Serum levels of galactose-deficient iga in children with iga nephropathy and Henoch–Schonlein purpura. Pediatr Nephrol 22:2067–2072.

LAZARUS A. 2009. Sarcoidosis: epidemiology, etiology, pathogenesis, and genetics. Dis Mon 55:649–60.

LEVINE S, SMITH VV, MALONE M, SEBIRE NJ. 2005. Histopathological features of chronic granulomatous disease (cgd) in childhood. Histopathology 47:508–16.

LIE JT. 1990. Illustrated histopathologic classification criteria for selected vasculitis syndromes. American College of Rheumatology Subcommittee on Classification of Vasculitis. Arthritis Rheum 33:1074–87.

LIN HC, SU CY, HUANG CC, HWANG CF, CHIEN CY. 2003. Kikuchi's disease: a review and analysis of 61 cases. Otolaryngol Head Neck Surg 128:650–3.

MACONI G, DI SABATINO A, ARDIZZONE S, GRECO S, COLOMBO E, RUSSO A, CASSINOTTI A, CASINI V, CORAZZA GR, BIANCHI PORRO G. 2005. Prevalence and clinical significance of sonographic detection of enlarged regional lymph nodes in crohn's disease. Scand J Gastroenterol 40:1328–33.

MAHOMED AA, BACHOO P, KING D, YOUNGSON GG. 2001. Recurrent cervical abscess: life-threatening presentation of chronic granulomatous disease in twin infants. Pediatr Surg Int 17:478–80.

MAHY NJ, DAVIES JD. 1984. Ischaemic changes in human mesenteric lymph nodes. J Pathol 144:257–67.

MAIER LA. 2002. Clinical approach to chronic beryllium disease and other nonpneumoconiotic interstitial lung diseases. J Thorac Imaging 17:273–84.

MARAFIOTI T, PATERSON JC, BALLABIO E, REICHARD KK, TEDOLDI S, HOLLOWOOD K, DICTOR M, HANSMANN ML, PILERI SA, DYER MJ, SOZZANI S, DIKIC I, SHAW AS, PETRELLA T, STEIN H, ISAACSON PG, FACCHETTI F, MASON DY. 2008. Novel markers of normal and neoplastic human plasmacytoid dendritic cells. Blood 111:3778–92.

MARSH WL, JR., BISHOP JW, KOENIG HM. 1980. Bone marrow and lymph node findings in a fatal case of Kawasaki's disease. Arch Pathol Lab Med 104:563–7.

MASI AT, HUNDER GG, LIE JT, MICHEL BA, BLOCH DA, AREND WP, CALABRESE LH, EDWORTHY SM, FAUCI AS, LEAVITT RY, et al. 1990. The American College of Rheumatology 1990 criteria for the classification of Churg–Strauss syndrome (allergic granulomatosis and angiitis). Arthritis Rheum 33:1094–1100.

MAURER R, SCHMID U, DAVIES JD, MAHY NJ, STANSFELD AG, LUKES RJ. 1986. Lymph-node infarction and malignant lymphoma: a multicentre survey of European, English and American cases. Histopathology 10:571–88.

MCCARTHY HJ, TIZARD EJ. 2010. Clinical practice: diagnosis and management of Henoch–Schonlein purpura. Eur J Pediatr 169:643–650.

MENASCE LP, BANERJEE SS, EDMONDSON D, HARRIS M. 1998. Histiocytic necrotizing lymphadenitis (Kikuchi–Fujimoto disease): continuing diagnostic difficulties. Histopathology 33:248–54.

MILLIKIN PD. 1970. Epitheloid germinal centers in the human spleen. Arch Pathol 89:314–20.

MILLIKIN PD. 1977. Epitheloid germinal centers: an acquired immunologic deficit? Am J Clin Pathol 67:545–9.

MOHSENIFAR Z, BEIN ME, MOTT LJ, TASHKIN DP. 1979. Cystic organizing pneumonia with elements of plasma cell granuloma. Arch Pathol Lab Med. 103:600–1.

MONACH PA, MERKEL PA. 2010. Genetics of vasculitis. Curr Opin Rheumatol 22:157–63.

MOR F, LEIBOVICI L, WYSENBEEK AJ. 1987. Leukocytoclastic vasculitis in malignant lymphoma: case report and review of the literature. Isr J Med Sci 23:829–32.

MOSUNJAC MB, FELICIANO DV, MAJMUDAR B. 2001. Pathologic quiz case: a mass of the spleen. Inflammatory myofibroblastic tumor of the spleen. Arch Pathol Lab Med. 125:1607–8.

MUKHTYAR C, FLOSSMANN O, HELLMICH B, BACON P, CID M, COHEN-TERVAERT JW, GROSS WL, GUILLEVIN L, JAYNE D, MAHR A, MERKEL PA, RASPE H, SCOTT D, WITTER J,

YAZICI H, LUQMANI RA. 2008. Outcomes from studies of antineutrophil cytoplasm antibody associated vasculitis: a systematic review by the european league against rheumatism systemic vasculitis task force. An Rheum Dis 67:1004–10.

NAM BH, RHA KS, YOO JY, PARK CI. 1994. Plasma cell granuloma of the temporal bone: a case report. Head Neck 16:457–459.

NASUTI JF, GUPTA PK, BALOCH ZW. 2001. Clinical implications and value of immunohistochemical staining in the evaluation of lymph node infarction after fine-needle aspiration. Diagn Cytopathol 25:104–7.

NAVARRO-ROMAN L, MEDEIROS LJ, KINGMA DW, ZARATE-OSORNO A, NGUYEN V, SAMOSZUK M, JAFFE ES. 1994. Malignant lymphomas of B-cell lineage with marked tissue eosinophilia: a report of five cases. Am J Surg Pathol 18:347–56.

NEUHAUSER TS, DERRINGER GA, THOMPSON LD, FANBURG-SMITH JC, AGUILERA NS, ANDRIKO J, CHU WS, ABBONDANZO SL. 2001. Splenic inflammatory myofibroblastic tumor (inflammatory pseudotumor): a clinicopathologic and immunophenotypic study of 12 cases. Arch Pathol Lab Med. 125:379–85.

NEWBURGER JW, FULTON DR. 2004. Kawasaki disease. Curr Opin Pediatr 16:508–14.

NEWBURGER JW, TAKAHASHI M, GERBER MA, GEWITZ MH, TANI LY, BURNS JC, SHULMAN ST, BOLGER AF, FERRIERI P, BALTIMORE RS, WILSON WR, BADDOUR LM, LEVISON ME, PALLASCH TJ, FALACE DA, TAUBERT KA. 2004. Diagnosis, treatment, and long-term management of Kawasaki disease: a statement for health professionals from the committee on rheumatic fever, endocarditis and Kawasaki disease, council on cardiovascular disease in the young, American Heart Association. Circulation 110:2747–71.

NG JP, MURPHY J, CHALMERS EM, HOGG RB, CUMMING RL, PEEBLES S. 1988. Henoch–Schonlein purpura and Hodgkin's disease. Postgrad Med J 64:881–2.

NIKOLAUS S, SCHREIBER S. 2007. Diagnostics of inflammatory bowel disease. Gastroenterology 133:1670–1689.

NORTON AJ, RAMSAY AD, ISAACSON PG. 1988. Antigen preservation in infarcted lymphoid tissue: a novel approach to the infarcted lymph node using monoclonal antibodies effective in routinely processed tissues. Am J Surg Pathol 12:759–67.

NOSANCHUK JS, SCHNITZER B. 1969. Follicular hyperplasia in lymph nodes from patients with rheumatoid arthritis: a clinicopathologic study. Cancer 24:343–54.

OHTSUKI Y, AKAGI T, MORIWAKI S, HATANO M. 1983. Plasma cell granuloma of the stomach combined with gastric cancer. Acta Pathol Jpn. 33:1251–7.

O'NEIL KM. 2009. Progress in pediatric vasculitis. Curr Opin Rheumatol 21:538–46.

ONCIU M, MEDEIROS LJ. 2003. Kikuchi–Fujimoto lymphadenitis. Adv Anat Pathol 10:204–11.

OZEN S, PISTORIO A, IUSAN SM, BAKKALOGLU A, HERLIN T, BRIK R, BUONCOMPAGNI A, LAZAR C, BILGE I, UZIEL Y, RIGANTE D, CANTARINI L, HILARIO MO, SILVA CA, ALEGRIA M, NORAMBUENA X, BELOT A, BERKUN

Y, Estrella AI, Olivieri AN, Alpigiani MG, Rumba I, Sztajnbok F, Tambic-Bukovac L, Breda L, Al-Mayouf S, Mihaylova D, Chasnyk V, Sengler C, Klein-Gitelman M, Djeddi D, Nuno L, Pruunsild C, Brunner J, Kondi A, Pagava K, Pederzoli S, Martini A, Ruperto N. 2010. Eular/printo/pres criteria for Henoch–Schonlein purpura, childhood polyarteritis nodosa, childhood Wegener granulomatosis and childhood Takayasu arteritis: Ankara 2008. Part II: Final classification criteria. An Rheum Dis 69:798–806.

Ozen S, Ruperto N, Dillon MJ, Bagga A, Barron K, Davin JC, Kawasaki T, Lindsley C, Petty RE, Prieur AM, Ravelli A, Woo P. 2006. Eular/pres endorsed consensus criteria for the classification of childhood vasculitides. Ann Rheum Dis 65:936–41.

Pagnoux C. 2010. Churg-strauss syndrome: Evolving concepts. Discov Med 9:243–52.

Pagnoux C, Guilpain P, Guillevin L. 2007. Churg–Strauss syndrome. Curr Opin Rheumatol 19:25–32.

Panes J, Gomollon F, Taxonera C, Hinojosa J, Clofent J, Nos P. 2007. Crohn's disease: a review of current treatment with a focus on biologics. Drugs 67: 2511–37.

Peru H, Soylemezoglu O, Bakkaloglu SA, Elmas S, Bozkaya D, Elmaci AM, Kara F, Buyan N, Hasanoglu E. 2008. Henoch–Schonlein purpura in childhood: clinical analysis of 254 cases over a 3-year period. Clin Rheumatol 27:1087–92.

Pietrafitta JJ, Grasberger RC, Deckers PJ, Giampaolo CM, Kondi ES. 1983. Superficial lymph node infarction. J Surg Oncol 24:212–4.

Pileri SA, Facchetti F, Ascani S, Sabattini E, Poggi S, Piccioli M, Rondelli D, Vergoni F, Zinzani PL, Piccaluga PP, Falini B, Isaacson PG. 2001. Myeloperoxidase expression by histiocytes in Kikuchi's and Kikuchi-like lymphadenopathy. Am J Pathol 159: 915–24.

Pinna GS, Kafetzis DA, Tselkas OI, Skevaki CL. 2008. Kawasaki disease: an overview. Curr Opin Infect Dis 21:263–70.

Polski JM, Dunphy CH, Evans HL, Brink DS. 2003. Lymph node infarction. Arch Pathol Lab Med 127:922.

Poscharisky JF. 1912. Zur frage des fettgehaltes der milz. Beitr Path Anat 54:369–84.

Poupon R. 2010. Primary biliary cirrhosis: a 2010 update. J Hepatol 52:745–58.

Punia RS, Dhingra N, Chopra R, Mohan H, Chauhan S. 2009. Lymph node infarction and its association with lymphoma: a short series and literature review. NZ Med J 122:40–4.

Rahman A, Isenberg DA. 2008. Systemic lupus erythematosus. N Engl J Med 358:929–39.

Rao IS, Loya AC, Ratnakar KS, Srinivasan VR. 2005. Lymph node infarction—a rare complication associated with disseminated intra vascular coagulation in a case of dengue fever. BMC Clin Pathol 5:11.

Ravenel JG, McAdams HP, Plankeel JF, Butnor KJ, Sporn TA. 2001. Sarcoidosis induced by interferon therapy. AJR Am J Roentgenol 177:199–201.

Roberts C, Batstone PJ, Goodlad Jr. 2001. Lymphadenopathy and lymph node infarction as a result of gold injections. J Clin Pathol 54:562–4.

Rossman MD. 1996. Chronic beryllium disease: diagnosis and management. Environ Health Perspect 104 (suppl 5): 945–7.

Rothschild B, Marshall H. 1986. Lymphadenopathy and lymph node infarction in the course of gold therapy. Am J Med 80:537–40.

Rowley AH, Shulman ST. 2010. Pathogenesis and management of Kawasaki disease. Expert Rev Anti Infect Ther 8:197–203.

Samuel G, Maier LA. 2008. Immunology of chronic beryllium disease. Curr Opin Allergy Clin Immunol 8:126–34.

Santo Tomas LH. 2009. Beryllium hypersensitivity and chronic beryllium lung disease. Curr Opin Pulm Med 15:165–9.

Saulsbury FT. 1999. Henoch–Schonlein purpura in children: report of 100 patients and review of the literature. Medicine (Baltimore) 78:395–409.

Scaldaferri F, Fiocchi C. 2007. Inflammatory bowel disease: progress and current concepts of etiopathogenesis. J Dig Dis 8:171–8.

Schnitzer B. 2001. The reactive lymphadenopathies: neoplastic hematopathology. Williams and Wilkins, Philadelphia, 537–68.

Severson GS, Harrington DS, Johansson SL, McManus BM. 1988. Epithelioid germinal centers in overwhelming childhood infections: the aftermath of nonspecific destruction of follicular b cells by natural killer cells. Arch Pathol Lab Med 112:917–21.

Shapira Y, Weinberger A, Wysenbeek AJ. 1996. Lymphadenopathy in systemic lupus erythematosus: prevalence and relation to disease manifestations. Clin Rheumatol 15:335–8.

Silveira MG, Lindor KD. 2008. Treatment of primary biliary cirrhosis: therapy with choleretic and immunosuppressive agents. Clin Liver Dis 12:425–43.

Sinico RA, Bottero P. 2009. Churg–Strauss angiitis. Best Pract Res Clin Rheumatol 23:355–66.

Stange EF, Travis SP, Vermeire S, Beglinger C, Kupcinkas L, Geboes K, Barakauskiene A, Villanacci V, Von Herbay A, Warren BF, Gasche C, Tilg H, Schreiber SW, Scholmerich J, Reinisch W. 2006. European evidence based consensus on the diagnosis and management of Crohn's disease: definitions and diagnosis. Gut 55 (suppl 1): 11–5.

Steinmann G, Foldi E, Foldi M, Racz P, Lennert K. 1982. Morphologic findings in lymph nodes after occlusion of their efferent lymphatic vessels and veins. Lab Invest 47:43–50.

Stilling M. 1886. Ueber progressive und regressive metamorphosen der milzfollikel. Virchows Arch A 103:15–31.

Strauchen JA, Miller LK. 2003. Lymph node infarction: an immunohistochemical study of 11 cases. Arch Pathol Lab Med 127:60–3.

Sun QF, Xu DZ, Pan SH, Ding JG, Xue ZQ, Miao CS, Cao GJ, Jin DJ. 2008. Kimura disease: review of the literature. Intern Med J 38:668–72.

SYMCHYCH PS, WANSTRUP J, ANDERSEN V. 1968. Chronic granulomatous disease of childhood: a morphologic study. Acta Pathol Microbiol Scand 74:179–88.

SYMMONS DPM. 1985. Neoplasms of the immune system in rheumatoid arthritis. Am J Med 78(suppl IA): 22–8.

TABBARA SO, FRIERSON HF JR., FECHNER RE. 1991. Diagnostic problems in tissues previously sampled by fine-needle aspiration. Am J Clin Pathol 96:76–80.

TACHIBANA T, IWAI K, TAKEMURA T. 2010. Sarcoidosis in the aged: review and management. Curr Opin Pulm Med 16:465–71.

TAKEISHI M, MAKINO Y, NISHIOKA H, MIYAWAKI T, KURIHARA K. 2007. Kimura disease: diagnostic imaging findings and surgical treatment. J Craniofac Surg 18:1062–67.

TAN EM, COHEN AS, FRIES JF, MASI AT, MCSHANE DJ, ROTHFIELD NF, SCHALLER JG, TALAL N, WINCHESTER RJ. 1982. The 1982 revised criteria for the classification of systemic lupus erythematosus. Arthritis Rheum 25:1271–7.

THOMAS J, JAYACHANDRAN NV, CHANDRASEKHARA PK, RAJASEKHAR L, NARSIMULU G. 2008. Kimura's disease—an unusual cause of lymphadenopathy in children. Clin Rheumatol 27:675–7.

THOMAS E, BREWSTER DH, BLACK RJ, MACFARLANE GJ. 2000. Risk of malignancy among patients with rheumatic conditions. Int J Cancer 88:497–502.

THORESON R, CULLEN JJ. 2007. Pathophysiology of inflammatory bowel disease: an overview. Surg Clin North Am 87:575–85.

TORIUMI DM, GOLDSCHMIDT RA, WOLFF AP. 1988. Lymph node infarction and malignant lymphoma: a case report. J Otolaryngol 17:128–30.

TOWBIN AJ, CHAVES I. 2010. Chronic granulomatous disease. Pediatr Radiol 40:657–68.

TSANG WY, CHAN JK. 1992. Spectrum of morphologic changes in lymph nodes attributable to fine needle aspiration. Hum Pathol 23:562–5.

TSANG WY, CHAN JK, NG CS. 1994. Kikuchi's lymphadenitis: a morphologic analysis of 75 cases with special reference to unusual features. Am J Surg Pathol 18:219–231.

VAN DEN BERG JM, VAN KOPPEN E, AHLIN A, BELOHRADSKY BH, BERNATOWSKA E, CORBEEL L, ESPANOL T, FISCHER A, KURENKO-DEPTUCH M, MOUY R, PETROPOULOU T, ROESLER J, SEGER R, STASIA MJ, VALERIUS NH, WEENING RS, WOLACH B, ROOS D, KUIJPERS TW. 2009. Chronic granulomatous disease: the European experience. PLoS One 4:e5234.

VERALDI S, MANCUSO R, RIZZITELLI G, GIANOTTI R, FERRANTE P. 1999. Henoch–Schonlein syndrome associated with human parvovirus b19 primary infection. Eur J Dermatol 9:232–3.

WANG DY, MAO JH, ZHANG Y, GU WZ, ZHAO SA, CHEN YF, LIU AM. 2009. Kimura disease: a case report and review of the chinese literature. Nephron Clin Pract 111: c55–61.

WANNAKRAIROT P, LEONG TY, LEONG AS. 2007. The morphological spectrum of lymphadenopathy in HIV infected patients. Pathology 39:223–7.

WASCHKWITSCH T. 1900. Ueber grosszellige heerde in den milz follikeln bei diphtheritis und anderen affectionen. Virchow Ach A 159:137–51.

WATTS JC, SEBEK BA, MCHENRY MC, ESSELSTYN CB, JR. 1980. Idiopathic infarction of intraabdominal lymph nodes: a case of fever of unknown origin. Am J Clin Pathol 74:687–90.

WATTS R, LANE S, HANSLIK T, HAUSER T, HELLMICH B, KOLDINGSNES W, MAHR A, SEGELMARK M, COHEN-TERVAERT JW, SCOTT D. 2007. Development and validation of a consensus methodology for the classification of the anca-associated vasculitides and polyarteritis nodosa for epidemiological studies. Ann Rheum Dis 66:222–7.

WECHSLER ME, WONG DA, MILLER MK, LAWRENCE-MIYASAKI L. 2009. Churg–Strauss syndrome in patients treated with omalizumab. Chest 136:507–18.

WIECZOREK S, HOLLE JU, EPPLEN JT. 2010. Recent progress in the genetics of Wegener's granulomatosis and Churg–Strauss syndrome. Curr Opin Rheumatol 22:8–14.

WILLIAMS WJ. 1964. Histology of Crohn's syndrome. Gut 5:510–6.

WOOTEN MD, JASIN HE. 1996. Vasculitis and lymphoproliferative diseases. Semin Arthritis Rheum 26:564–74.

XU Y, WIERNIK PH. 2001. Systemic lupus erythematosus and B-cell hematologic neoplasm. Lupus 10:841–50.

YANARDAG H, CANER M, PAPILA I, UYGUN S, DEMIRCI S, KARAYEL T. 2007. Diagnostic value of peripheral lymph node biopsy in sarcoidosis: a report of 67 cases. Can Respir J 14:209–11.

YANG YH, CHUANG YH, WANG LC, HUANG HY, GERSHWIN ME, CHIANG BL. 2008. The immunobiology of Henoch–Schonlein purpura. Autoimmun Rev 7:179–84.

YEUNG RS. 2010. Kawasaki disease: update on pathogenesis. Curr Opin Rheumatol 22:551–60.

YONEMORI K, KUSUMOTO M, MATSUNO Y, TATEISHI U, WATANABE S, WATANABE T, MORIYAMA N. 2006. Diffuse large B-cell lymphoma presenting as a unilateral solitary round pulmonary hilar node infarction. Respirology 11:224–6.

ZWERINA J, AXMANN R, JATZWAUK M, SAHINBEGOVIC E, POLZER K, SCHETT G. 2009a. Pathogenesis of Churg–Strauss syndrome: recent insights. Autoimmunity 42:376–9.

ZWERINA J, AXMANN R, MANGER B, SCHETT G. 2009b. The emergence of antineutrophil cytoplasmic antibodies may precede the clinical onset of Churg–Strauss syndrome. Arthritis Rheum 60:626–7.

ZWERINA J, EGER G, ENGLBRECHT M, MANGER B, SCHETT G. 2009c. Churg–Strauss syndrome in childhood: a systematic literature review and clinical comparison with adult patients. Semin Arthritis Rheum 39:108–15.

CHAPTER NINETEEN

MIXED PATTERNS IN LYMPH NODE, SUPPURATIVE NECROTIZING GRANULOMATOUS INFECTIOUS LYMPHADENOPATHY

Hernani D. Cualing and Gary Hellerman

CAT-SCRATCH DISEASE

Cat-Scratch disease was first described as part of the *Parinaud syndrome* (fever, conjunctivitis, lymphadenitis) by Henri Parinaud in 1889, but it was only in the 1950s that Dr. Debre recognized that the cat was the natural reservoir—hence the appellation "cat-scratch disease." The primary pathogen was not identified until 43 years later. It was initially ascribed to *Afipia felis* and formerly designated in the genus Rochalimaea, but is now classified as *B. henselae*. The bacteria are nonadherent to human erythrocytes but do stick to feline erythrocytes; thus cats may act as a reservoir for *B. henselae* (Hammoud 2008).

Definition

Gram-negative proteobacterium in the family *Bartonellaceae* is the most common cause of a suppurative granulomatous lymphadenitis known as cat-scratch disease (CSD).

ICD-10 Code A28.1

Synonyms

Cat-scratch disease, cat-scratch fever, inoculation lymphoreticulosis, subacute regional lymphadenitis, cat-scratch oculoglandular syndrome, Debre's syndrome.

Epidemiology

B. henselae is found worldwide in domestic and feral cats, and may be transmitted from one animal to another directly or through the bite of an infected cat flea. In Greece, about 20% of the healthy population were seropositive for *B. henselae* IgG antibody. The prevalence of infection varies considerably among cat populations with an increase from nil in cold climates (0% in Norway) to high in warm and humid climates (68% in the Philippines) (Boulouis et al., 2005). The incidence of CSD is about 1 in 10,000 persons and is the most common type of bartonellosis (Hammoud 2008).

Non-Neoplastic Hematopathology and Infections, First Edition. Edited by Hernani D. Cualing, Parul Bhargava, and Ramon L. Sandin.
© 2012 Wiley-Blackwell. Published 2012 by John Wiley & Sons, Inc.

Etiology

The causative agent of CSD is usually the Gram-negative proteobacterium, *Bartonella henselae*, but rarely may result from *Bartonella clarridgeiae*.

Pathophysiology

B. henselae is not known to adhere to human erythrocytes, but the bacteria are able to enter endothelial cells and cause vasoproliferative lesions in the skin and other organs (Scheidegger et al., 2009, McCord, Cuevas, and Anderson 2007). Bacterial infection induces the production of factors such as interleukin 8 that stimulate endothelial cell growth, block apoptosis, and promote angiogenesis (McCord, Resto-Ruiz, and Anderson, 2006). Disseminated bacteremia may occur in some infected persons, but is rare.

Sites of Involvement

CSD causes lymphadenitis, with the most common location being axillary followed by cervical and inguinal nodes (Hansmann et al., 2005). The infection is normally self-limiting, but there may be rare complications including encephalopathy. Endocarditis associated with *B. henselae* infection has been reported, but responded well to treatment (Dreier et al. 2008). Granulomas may occur on the conjunctiva but are more commonly found on the liver where they can cause a condition known as bacterial peliosis. *B. henselae* neuroretinitis has been reported with sudden loss of eyesight preceded by flu-like symptoms, but the illness resolved with antibiotic treatment (Curi et al. 2006).

When *B. henselae* infect an AIDS patient or a person undergoing immunosuppressive treatments, they can cause skin lesions associated with a condition known as bacillary angiomatosis. This is the second most commonly seen skin lesion in AIDS patients. The patient usually presents with multiple reddish or purplish papular or nodular areas that are frequently tender and show discharge and crusting. Bacteria may also cause angiomatosis in the mucosa or viscera and more rarely in the bone. Localized lymphadenopathy is common.

Diagnosis

Painful, swollen lymph nodes are the usual presenting symptom, but some 15 to 20% of infected persons may show little lymphadenopathy. They may have had a low-grade fever of unknown origin lasting for several days sometimes with muscle and joint pain. Questioning of the patient about exposure to cats and

a thorough examination, including the eyes, for the primary infection site is necessary. Elevated titer of antibodies against *B. henselae* is a characteristic sign of the disease. In bacillary angiomatosis, visceral infection may occur without any cutaneous lesions, but it is usually accompanied by fever.

In recent years the diagnosis of CSD using Bergmans criteria required three of the following four symptoms: (1) a history of contact with or a scratch from a cat and the presence of skin, eye, or mucous membrane lesions, (2) a positive cat-scratch skin test reaction, (3) negative laboratory testing for other causes of lymphadenopathy, and (4) characteristic histopathological lymph node biopsy findings or pathology at site of systemic involvement (Bergmans et al., 1997) (see Figures 19.1–19.3). Since the skin test is no longer used, the modified Hansmann criteria requires two of the following three symptoms: (1) close contact with cats or a scratch or bite from a cat, (2) a typical CSD histology, namely granuloma with a central pyogenic abscess (lymphoid hyperplasia not being sufficiently specific to establish a diagnosis of CSD), and (3) positive serology by an immunofluorescence assay for antibodies against *B. henselae* (Hansmann et al., 2005).

Laboratory Findings

Culturing *B. henselae* is difficult, so the majority of identification tests rely on PCR of lymph node or tissue specimens. The sensitivity is 76% and specificity is 100%, but a range is reported (Hansmann et al., 2005). Other tests include lymph node immunofluorescence assay (Rolain et al., 2003), or immunohistochemistry on tissue with varying sensitivity from high to a low of 25% (Caponetti et al., 2009). A negative serology for antibodies to *B. henselae* does not exclude the disease (Herremans et al., 2009). The indirect fluorescent antibody assay (using of antigen derived from *B. henselae*) of patient's serum has a 95% sensitivity and is probably the most useful test for primary clinics (Dalton et al., 1995) There is one caveat, however: serious neoplastic causes of lymphadenopathy may masquerade as CSD, and these may be missed unless histopathology is done (Rolain et al., 2006).

Morphology

CSD is the most significant cause of suppurative necrotizing granulomas (see Table 19.1 and Table 19.6). The usual histopathology in the progression includes an early nonspecific lymphoid hyperplasia with increased vascularity, followed by formation of monocytoid clusters with follicular hyperplasia, and terminating in the classic geographic suppurative

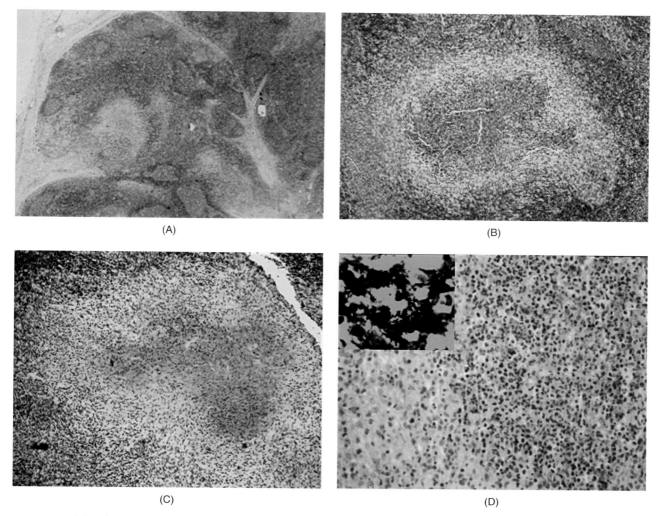

(A)

(B)

(C)

(D)

FIGURE 19.1 **Morphologic features of cat-scratch disease**. (**A**) Low-power view showing capsular and trabecular fibrosis, pale abscesses, and reactive follicle center hyperplasia. (**B**) Granuloma typical of CSD with central suppurative oval and branching abscess, pale wall of epithelioid histiocytes. (**C**) A granuloma with more necrotic center and better organized wall. (**D**) High-power view with dense neutrophils on right and wall of reactive histiocytes on left. (Inset) Warthin–Starry positive L-shaped and branching *B. henselae* inside macrophages and endothelia.

granulomatous lymphadenitis (Kojima et al., 1991; Facchetti et al., 1992). Like suppurative granulomas associated with B cells and monocytoid clusters, an increasing degree of suppuration may seen in the centers of monocytoid clusters as the disease progresses. At its peak the classic geographic, stellate, or confluent suppurative necrotizing pattern is seen (see Table 19.2).

Immunohistochemistry/Cytochemistry

Silver stain-positive pleomorphic bacilli can be seen in about 60% of the cases of acute suppurative lymphadenitis (Kojima et al., 1991; Kudo et al., 1988; Korbi et al., 1986). The Warthin–Starry or Steiner silver stains is the most common cytochemical test

used to diagnose CSD. In about 87% of the cases, the organism is detectable in the early phase, and in about 40% during the suppurative phase (Wear et al., 1983). These organisms appear as pleomorphic coccobacilli that display L-forms or branching chains. Endothelial cells and macrophages and vessels surrounding the monocytoid clusters usually harbor the organisms. When there are frank suppurative granulomas, or after antibiotic therapy, it is not uncommon to find Warthin–Starry-negative CSD lymphadenopathy.

Differential Diagnosis

Microbiologic analysis of 786 lymph node biopsy specimens from patients clinically suspected of having CSD yielded various neoplasms in 26%, an

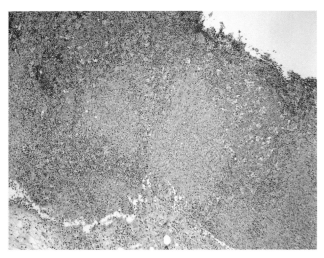

FIGURE 19.2 **Typical B cell associated granuloma is characteristic of CSD**. The monocytoid cluster is on the left; the central frank suppurative granuloma is surrounded by reactive follicles. Courtesy Dr. Wun-Ju Shieh and Dr. Sherif Zaki (Infectious Diseases Pathology Branch, Centers for Disease Control and Prevention).

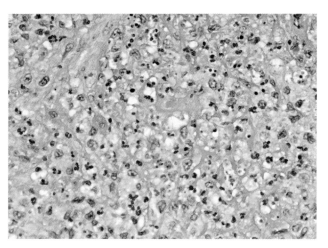

FIGURE 19.3 **Neutrophilic infiltrate with necrotic histiocytes**. Courtesy Dr. Wun-Ju Shieh and Dr. Sherif Zaki (Infectious Diseases Pathology Branch, Centers for Disease Control and Prevention).

infectious etiology in 50%, with CSD accounting for 31%, mycobacteria for 7%, and staph/streptococci as the third most frequently isolated agents. Q fever, tularemia, *B. quintana*, or *T. whipplei* are rare causes (Rolain et al., 2006).

During early infection the classic morphology of CSD may not be present. Instead, clusters of monocytoid cells with few or no neutrophils may be seen, which can resemble a viral infection like CMV

TABLE 19.1 Suppurative Necrotizing Granulomas

Suppurative Granulomatous Agents
1. Cat scratch (*Bartonella henselae bacilli*)
2. Tularemia *Francisella tularensis*
3. Lymphogranuloma venereum
4. Chancroid *H. ducreyi*
5. Yersinia enterocolitica/pseudotuberculosis
6. Brucellosis lymphadenitis
7. Melioidosis
8. Typhoid lymphadenitis
9. Fungal infections
10. Mycobacterial infections
11. Others

TABLE 19.2 Cat-Scratch Disease

Key Diagnostic Features of Cat-Scratch Disease
Etiology: *Bartonella henselae*
Regions: worldwide, with domestic cats in hot and humid climates but is the most common zoonosis in US
Transmission: cat, esp. kittens, and flea
Population at risk: cat owners
Organs involved: skin lymph nodes
Lymph node pathology: histiocytic suppurative lymphadenitis
Differential diagnosis: suppurative granulomatous lymphadenitis secondary to tularemia, LGV, MTB
Diagnosis: immunofluorescence assay, histology, Warthin–Starry silver stain
Unsual feature: self-limiting in normal individuals but can disseminate, cause peliosis, endocarditis, and hepatitis in immunocompromized persons and require antimicrobial treatment; Henoch–Schönlein purpura is associated with *B. henselae* positive serology

or toxoplasmosis. However, unlike toxoplasmosis, microgranulomas are not found, and unlike CMV, there is suppuration. In the necrotizing phase with few neutrophils, Kikuchi's disease is a differential diagnosis. However, Kikuchi's disease (KD) is characterized by histiocytic necrotizing lymphadenitis with neutrophils being absent. Unlike Kikuchi's disease, neutrophils are an essential component in CSD. In both KD and CSD, plasmacytoid monocytes and monocytoid lymphocytes can be seen with suppurative clusters (Kojima et al., 2006). Plasmacytoid monocytes are CD4+, CD68+, and CD123+ and negative for B cell associated markers but monocytoid cell marks with CD20 and other B cell markers. Acid-fast bacilli could be seen by using cytochemical stains in tissue when mycobacteria is highly suspected.

Course and Prognosis

A primary lesion in the form of pustules is usually seen at the site of infection some 5 to 10 days after a scratch or bite by a cat. Enlargement of the lymph nodes occurs within 1 month with swelling and tenderness, and this may be accompanied by fatigue and fever. Recovery within 2 to 4 months—even without treatment—usually occurs.

TULAREMIA

Tularemia disease was discovered in 1911 during an outbreak of rabbit fever around Tulare lake and is named after Tulare County, California (Petersen and Schriefer, 2005). The cause is a Gram-negative coccobacillus *Francisella tularensis*, named after Edward Francis, an American bacteriologist who first described the disease. Although most outbreaks occur in the south-central and western United States, from the bites of flies or ticks, other exposures may occur from infected rabbits, deer, or lemmings as well as infections from aerosols released in laboratory mishaps.

Definition

Tularemia is a serious zoonotic infectious disease caused by the bacterium *Francisella tularensis* and its subspecies.

ICD-10 Code A21

Synonyms

Pahvant Valley plague, rabbit fever, deer fly fever, Ohara disease, Japan "Yato-byo," and lemming fever.

Epidemiology

The disease is endemic in North America, Europe, the former Soviet republics, and Japan. Sporadic outbreaks occur all over the world. About 200 human tularemia infections are reported each year in the United States. Cats, dogs, cattle, primates, and some species of birds, fish, and amphibians are incidental hosts. *F. tularensis* can persist in the soil or in decaying leaves, and people can be exposed via inhaled dust while mowing the lawn, weed-whacking, or using a power blower.

Etiology

Francisella tularensis and its subtypes, the cause of tularemia, are Gram-negative, nonmotile, nonsporulating coccobacilli. The most virulent is *F. tularensis* *tularensis* (type A) infecting rabbits and humans. *F. tularensis palaearctica* (type B) occurs mainly in beavers and muskrats in North America and in hares and small rodents in northern Eurasia. It is less virulent for humans and rabbits. The primary vectors are ticks and deer flies, but the disease can also be spread by other arthropods.

Pathogenesis

F. tularensis is a facultative intracellular pathogen that multiplies predominantly within macrophages. The organisms initially enter macrophages through phagocytosis (Clemens, Lee, and Horwitz, 2004). The degree of *F. tularensis* virulence is determined, in part, by the ability of the organisms to replicate within macrophages. Bacteria are released from the macrophages following cell death by apoptosis.

Clinical Aspects

The incubation period for tularemia is 1 to 14 days, but symptoms usually appear 3 to 5 days after infection. The face and eyes redden and become inflamed and lymph node involvement is accompanied by high fever. Depending on the site of infection, tularemia has six characteristic clinical syndromes (Dennis et al., 2001):

Ulceroglandular tularemia (45–85% of naturally occurring cases)

Glandular tularemia (10–25% of naturally occurring cases)

Pneumonic tularemia (<5% of naturally occurring cases)

Oculoglandular tularemia (<5%)

Oropharyngeal tularemia (<5%)

Typhoidal tularemia (<5%, although this percentage may be much higher in outbreaks caused by aerosol exposure)

In the ulceroglandular form, the initial nidus forms a tender ulcerated lesion at the site of the papule. The ulcer is typically 2 to 4 cm in diameter and has an irregular raised border. A dark scab (akin to an eschar of anthrax) may occur over the area of ulceration. Organisms may spread hematogenously, and this can progress to septic syndrome or infection of multiple organs. In glandular tularemia, regional lymph node involvement occurs, but ulceration at the site of inoculation is not apparent.

Approach to Diagnosis

The integration of geographic location with risk history as well as clinical symptoms helps in arriving at a working diagnosis. The presence of skin ulcers, respiratory symptoms, and lymphadenopathy is indicative that skin, sputum, or blood samples should be taken for culture or PCR assay. The organism can be isolated from ulcer or lymph node aspirates.

Laboratory Findings

The agglutination serologic test may be useful, but many patients are seronegative. PCR has about 70% sensitivity in seropositive tularemia. Organisms can be cultured directly from lesions.

Morphologic Aspects

The painful cutaneous lesion at the inoculation site can lead to an ulcer and eschar. Organisms spread from the site of inoculation to regional lymph nodes, where they cause necrotizing lymphadenitis with a neutrophilic and granulomatous inflammatory infiltrate. Granulomas may eventually coalesce to form microabscesses. Affected lymph nodes may rupture and lead to draining cutaneous sinus tracts. In the very early stages of tularemia, only follicular hyperplasia is seen with some reactive changes but without necrosis. Pure necrotic abscess with or without epithelioid cell reaction may be seen during the second week and the caseous type of necrosis during the fourth week (Sutinen and Syrjala, 1986). Geographic necrosis with a necrotizing center, variable amounts of suppuration, and pink palisaded granulomatous walls characterize the morphology typical of lymphadenitis, but this is not strictly specific for tularemia (see Figures 19.4–19.6).

FIGURE 19.5 **Tularemia lymphadenitis with onset of suppurative necrotizing granuloma with pink palisaded wall** (10×). Courtesy Dr. Wun-Ju Shieh and Dr. Sherif Zaki (Infectious Diseases Pathology Branch, Centers for Disease Control and Prevention).

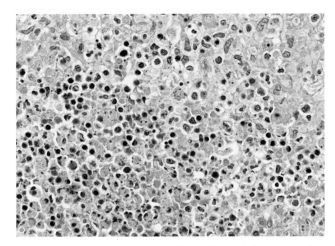

FIGURE 19.6 **Tularemia lymphadenitis with necrotizing granuloma**. Note the many necrotic cells and debris, few neutrophils and, at the top, the wall of epithelioid histiocytes (40×). Courtesy Dr. Wun-Ju Shieh and Dr. Sherif Zaki (Infectious Diseases Pathology Branch, Centers for Disease Control and Prevention).

Differential Diagnosis

In most cases tularemia in the lymph nodes cannot be histologically differentiated from cat-scratch disease and other causes of suppurative necrotizing lymphadenitis including tuberculosis (Sutinen and Syrjala, 1986). In the skin, the diseases requiring differential diagnosis include anthrax, plague, tick-bite, or rat-bite fever. In the pulmonary form, atypical pneumonia secondary to Q fever, mycoplasma, psittacosis, or legionella are considerations.

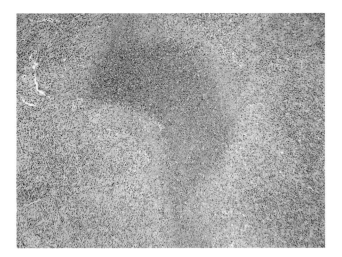

FIGURE 19.4 **Tularemia lymphadenitis**. Suppurative stellate or geographic granulomas, 5×. Courtesy Dr. Wun-Ju Shieh and Dr. Sherif Zaki (Infectious Diseases Pathology Branch, Centers for Disease Control and Prevention).

Treatment of Choice and Prognosis

Most patients respond rapidly to appropriate antibiotic therapy, with fever and generalized symptoms improving in 24 to 48 hours. Tularemia can be fatal if the person is not treated with appropriate antibiotics, but if therapy is initiated promptly, death occurs in fewer than 1% of cases. The drug of choice is streptomycin, but the disease will also respond to gentamycin, tetracycline, or chloramphenicol. An attenuated vaccine is available, but its use is restricted to high-risk groups. Before antibiotic therapy was available, the overall case-fatality rate was approximately 7%, although rates as high as 50% were seen with pneumonia and other forms of severe infection. [Dennis, Inglesby, Henderson, Bartlett, Ascher, Eitzen, Fine, Friedlander, Hauer, Layton, Lillibridge, McDade, Osterholm, O'Toole, Parker, Perl, Russell, & Tonat 2001].

LYMPHOGRANULOMA VENEREUM

Lymphogranuloma venereum (LGV) is a sexually transmitted disease caused by infection with *Chlamydia trachomatis* bacteria, which gain entry through breaks in the skin or the epithelial layer of the mucosal membranes. The disease was first described in 1913 (Durand, 1913), and historically the bacteria were transmitted during unprotected sexual intercourse. Recent outbreaks in Europe and the United States have been linked to male homosexuals (Spaargaren et al., 2005). Symptoms and outcomes depend on the site of introduction. The initial lesion may not even be noticed if it is internal and the infection may be passed on before symptoms appear. Coinfection with HIV is common.

Definition

Lymphogranuloma venereum (LGV) is a bacterial disease caused by infection with *Chlamydia trachomatis* and commonly introduced through unprotected sex.

ICD-10 Code A55

Synonyms

Climatic bubo, Durand–Nicolas–Favre disease, lymphogranuloma inguinale, poradenitis inguinale, strumous bubo.

Epidemiology

LGV has a worldwide distribution, but most of the cases of disease involve the L1, L2, or L3 serotypes. Incidence statistics had been quite low until the 2000s, when the number of cases increased substantially in Europe and North America due to a rise in the number of men having unprotected sex with men (Pathela, Blank, and Schillinger, 2007; Nieuwenhuis et al., 2004). The actual number of infections worldwide is unknown because the disease is often undiagnosed or misdiagnosed.

Etiology

Bacteria of the family Chlamydiae are obligate intracellular parasites that cause human ocular disease as well as lymphadenitis. There are at least fifteen pathogenic strains of *C. trachomatis*, but only three—L1, L2, and L3—are associated with LGV and severe lymphadenitis.

Pathogenesis

C. trachomatis L1, L2, or L3 gain entry to the lymphatic system through the genital or rectal mucosa and quickly establish an intracellular infection within lymph node monocytes. The immune system mounts an aggressive response against the bacteria causing swelling, pain, and purulent discharge. The chronic inflammation causes tissue necrosis and remodeling that may open fistulas to the surface of the skin or from the vagina into the rectum.

Sites of Infection

The *C. trachomatis* bacteria enter primarily through the vagina, penis, or rectum of individuals during unprotected sex with infected partners. There is usually an ulcer or abscess at the entry point, but this may go unnoticed if the site is internal. The entry point determines the nature of the disease with genital entry causing formation of inguinal buboes or abscesses while entry through the rectal mucosa may be associated with proctitis. Infection via the lung by fomites or aerosols is rare but has been documented.

Signs of LGV can be seen or felt from a few days after infection to as long as a month thereafter. The secondary stage occurs two to three weeks after the initial genital or rectal lesion and typically is signaled by lymphadenitis localized according to the route of infection. The lymph nodes become swollen and granulomatous and join together as the infection progresses. The surface skin over the area becomes indurated and roughened and may eventually ulcerate. In the case of anal infection, rectal symptoms may include bleeding, cramps, and painful bowel movements. If LGV continues without treatment, permanent damage to the lymphatic system with lymphedema and fibrosis can occur.

Since the primary lesion is often overlooked, especially in women, the patient may first present with painful, swollen unilateral lymph nodes in the groin or rectal area, red and swollen labia, and ulcerated areas on the skin or bloody stools. The disease may take up to a month to reach this stage and the patient may by then have forgotten the sexual encounter that caused the infection, although a history of promiscuity or men having sex with men constitute strong indicators of LGV. The exam may reveal vaginal or rectal fistulas or draining through the skin above the lymph nodes.

Approach to Diagnosis

The organism can be isolated from ulcers or lymph node aspirates.

Laboratory Findings

Cultures of fluid from discharges or lymph node biopsies can be done to test for *C. trachomatis* and assays for LGV can be performed on blood samples. Real time PCR is also useful (Chen et al., 2007). The tests are necessary to distinguish *C. trachomatis* infections from those of *Haemophilus ducreyi*, which causes soft chancre or chancroid.

Morphology

The lymph node histopathology is similar to an acute suppurative necrotizing granulomatous lymphadenitis (Martin et al., 2006) and may be difficult to differentiate from its many causes (see Table 19.1). One characteristic feature is the presence of vacuolated histiocytes around suppurative granulomas, which contain intracellular microorganisms, especially seen with cytochemical stains. In addition monocytoid B-cell clusters are features of LGV, similar to cat-scratch disease. Perilymphadenitis may also be seen.

Immunohistochemistry

Monocytoid B-cell clusters are a feature of LGV, and as in cat-scratch disease, the foci of suppuration may begin in the monocytoid clusters. These observations have resulted in this type of granuloma being referred to as a B cell associated granulomas.

Cytochemistry.

Warthin–Starry silver stain of infected tissues will show fine sand-like organisms inside vacuolated macrophages.

Treatment

Antibiotic treatment for LGV is nearly always successful, and the patient recovers with no long-term adverse effects provided that the disease is treated early.

CHANCROID, *H. DUCREYI*

Chancroid or soft chancre (to distinguish it from the "hard" chancre of syphilis) is a sexually transmitted infection first described by August Ducrey in 1889 (Ducrey, 1889).

Definition

Chancroid is a genital ulcer disease caused by infection with *Haemophilus ducreyi*, usually through unprotected sexual contact.

ICD-10 Code A57

Synonyms

Soft chancre.

Epidemiology

Infections are common among sex workers and purulent discharge from the painful ulcers can rapidly transmit the bacteria to others. While chancroid is relatively rare in the developed countries of Europe and North America, there is still a threat from imported disease or for those individuals engaging in sex with multiple partners. The global incidence of chancroid is only poorly known because of a lack of readily available tests for positively identifying the bacteria and inadequate record keeping in impoverished areas. The greater incidence of chancroid among sex workers and their clients in resource-limited countries correlates with the higher incidence of HIV infection and underscores its role as a major factor in the transmission of HIV (Mohammed, 2008).

Etiology

The infection is caused by *Haemophilus ducreyi*, a Gram-negative coccobacillus in the *Pasturellaceae* family (Morse, 1989).

Pathophysiology

As in other venereal diseases, *H. ducreyi* gains entry to the lymphatic system through small breaks in the mucosal barrier of the genitals or rectum. The incubation period is 4 to 7 days and results in soft-edged lesions with necrosis and purulent discharge. The entry of *H. ducreyi* into the body triggers an innate immune response, but the bacterium has evolved a number of virulence factors to evade destruction by macrophages. Antiphagocytic proteins are produced that blunt the attack and allow the bacteria to proliferate (Janowicz, 2010). The recruitment of numerous lymphocytes to the infection site can increase the likelihood of an HIV coinfection because these cells carry elevated levels of the HIV coreceptors, CCR5 and CXCR4.

Site of Infection

H. ducreyi enters the body during unprotected sex through small breaks in the vaginal or rectal mucosa. Entry of the bacteria is followed by lymphadenopathy and the formation of painful, erythematous papules three to seven days later. The papules progress to ulcers with purulent discharge and necrosis that eventually causes permanent scarring. Males are much more likely to evince symptoms than females, and infected female sex workers thus serve as a key reservoir of the disease.

Approach to Diagnosis

Positive identification of the organism *H. ducreyi* from ulcer exudate is the definitive test. It is advisable to test for other sexually transmitted diseases at the same time because multiple infections are common. There are several kinds of bacterial infection that produce genital ulcers, and distinguishing one from the other requires careful examination, history taking, and ordering and evaluation of lab tests. Chancroid ulcers commonly occur on the genitals, but may also be found on the legs or even orally. The accompanying inguinal lymphadenopathy may result in the formation of painful buboes.

Laboratory Findings

H. ducreyi is difficult to culture, and polymerase chain reaction-based methods applied to blood or exudates have become the standard for identification of chancroid and to distinguish it from other diseases causing venereal ulcers.

Morphology

Lymphadenopathy is seen in 87% of culture-proven chancroid (Ortiz-Zepeda, Hernandez-Perez, and Marroquin-Burgos, 1994), although the incidence averages 50%. Biopsies of skin show nonspecific features with edema, lymphohistiocytic inflammation, and fibrinoid vasculitis, as well as the presence of numerous eosinophils and Russell bodies (Ortiz-Zepeda, Hernandez-Perez, and Marroquin-Burgos 1994). Granulomatous lymphadenitis with coalescing microabscesses is also commonly present (Woods, 1993), although the definitive literature is scant.

Differential Diagnosis

In clinical practice, it is often not possible to distinguish LGV from chancroid. Another very similar clinical picture results from granuloma inguinale. This disease is also called donovanosis after the Donovan bodies discovered by Charles Donovan that are intracellular bacterial inclusions seen in macrophages infected with *Klebsiella granulomatis* (Velho, 2008). This is an ulcerative bacterial disease caused by infection with the pleomorphic Gram-negative bacillus, *K. granulomatis*, and is usually a result of sexual contact with an infected partner. The initial sign of infection is a small painless papule or nodule appearing 10 to 40 days after transmission. Continued growth of the bacteria results in large red, suppurating ulcers. The ulcers show characteristic serpiginous margins with the older, trailing edge undergoing healing while the leading edge is freshly ulcerated. The ulcers can form thickened nodular, granulomatous areas called pseudobuboes that resemble the lymph node buboes of other genital infections such as chancroid (Freinkel, 1988). Like chancroid, the infection is rare in developed countries in temperate climates, but is widespread in the tropics where it occurs under conditions of poor sanitation and limited access to health care (Rashid, 2006). Culture of *K. granulomatis* is difficult under resource-limited conditions, and identification can best be accomplished by staining of smears of purulent material with Giemsa or Wright–Giemsa and examination of the cells for the presence of Donovan bodies, which are the rod-shaped encapsulated forms of the bacilli (O'Farrell, 1993). *Treponema pallidum* infection may usually be ruled out by microscopic examination of exudates for the typical spirochaete forms of syphilis.

Treatment

Erythromycin as well as doxycycline are effective against chancroid, donovanosis, and LGV.

YERSINIA ENTEROCOLITICA/ PSEUDOTUBERCULOSIS LYMPHADENITIS

Yersinia enterocolitica infection, which primarily affects children 5 to 15 years of age was first described in 1939 (Pinninti, 2009). *Y. pseudotuberculosis* is a related strain that usually infects animals but can be transmitted to humans. Both species are Gram-negative enterobacteria that infect the intestine causing abdominal pain, fever, and, at least with *Y. enterocolitica*, bloody diarrhea (Long, 2010). Fever and right-side abdominal pain may mimic appendicitis. Persistent infections may spread to the liver, spleen, and lymph nodes resulting in granulomas and necrosis.

Definition

Infection with the zoonotic enteric coccobacilli *Yersinia enterocolitica or Yersinia pseudotuberculosis.*

ICD-10 Code (intestinal A04.6, extraintestinal yersiniosis A28.2)

Synonyms

Izumi fever, yersiniosis, Masshoff's disease.

Epidemiology

Animals, especially pigs, can be reservoirs for the disease and transmission can occur through unsanitary handling of raw meat products or drinking unpasteurized milk or contaminated water (Lieberman, 2009). Person-to-person transmission can occur by the fecal–oral route. In the United States, yersiniosis is uncommon with an average of one case per 100,000 persons being reported annually. The Centers of Disease Control and Prevention (CDC) estimates that about 17,000 cases of yersiniosis (including both *Y. enterocolitica* and *Y. pseudotuberculosis* infections) occur annually in the United States. Europe has from 5 to 7 cases per 100,000 per year (Rosner, 2010). The incidence can be locally much higher, especially in children less than 5 years old and in impoverished or resource-limited areas. Infection with *Y. enterocolitica* occurs most often in young children.

Etiology

Y. enterocolitica, a small rod-shaped, Gram-negative bacterium, is often isolated from clinical specimens such as wounds, feces, sputum, and mesenteric lymph nodes. However, it is not part of the normal human flora. *Y. pseudotuberculosis* has been isolated from the diseased human appendix or mesenteric lymph nodes.

Pathophysiology

Y. enterocolitica and *Y. pseudotuberculosis* possess a number of virulence factors that help generate and maintain infection in the host. They are encoded on the plasmid for yersinia virulence, pYV, and deletion of this plasmid abolishes bacterial infectivity. Some of the factors block neutrophil activation and macrophage attack, while others promote adhesion to the intestinal epithelium and penetration (Fahlgren, 2009).

Site of Infection

The incubation period is typically from three days to one week. The bacteria usually enter by the oral route into the intestine, but cases of infection through wounds have been reported. The majority of yersiniosis infections result in intestinal symptoms but sometimes the skin of an infected person shows areas of nodular erythema associated with the bacteria (Labbé, 1996). Systemic infection can also occur, especially in immunocompromised persons.

Yersiniosis is frequently characterized by gastroenteritis with diarrhea and/or vomiting; however, fever and abdominal pain are the hallmark symptoms. Yersinia infections mimic appendicitis and cause mesenteric lymphadenitis, but the bacteria may also cause infections of other sites such as wounds, joints, and the urinary tract.

Approach to Diagnosis

The above-mentioned intestinal symptoms are characteristic of infection by a number of different enteric bacteria, and positive identification requires culturing the organism from stool samples, blood, or lymph node aspirates. Molecular methods such as Taqman assay PCR can also be used on blood specimens (Sen, 2000).

Laboratory Findings

Culturing the bacteria from fecal samples, blood or other bodily fluids is the usual method of identifying *Y. enterocolitica*, or *Y. pseudotuberculosis*, but PCR assays can provide specific and sensitive data from relatively small amounts of material.

Morphology

Lymph nodes show granulomas with central necrosis (see Figure 19.7). Microabscesses or suppurative necrotizing granulomas are seen in the terminal phase preceded by nonspecific morphological findings (El-Maraghi and Mair, 1979). In addition nonsuppurative epithelioid granulomas without associated monocytoid cells are seen in the appendix as well as in the lymph nodes (Kojima et al., 2007). Lymph node capsules show a thickened edematous appearance overlying hyperplastic follicles with

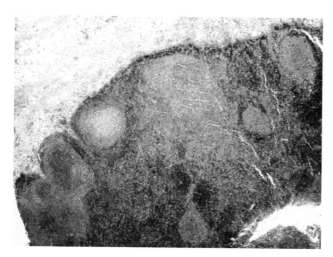

FIGURE 19.7 **Yersiniosis lymphadenitis.** Within the edematous capsule, hyperplastic follicles with granulomas are seen in low-power view.

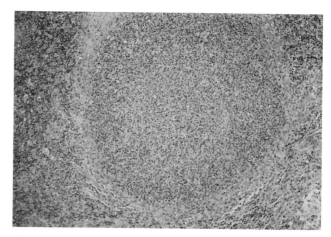

FIGURE 19.8 **Necrotizing abscess, surrounded by a pale epithelioid histiocyte wall.** Occasionally the microabsesses are in the germinal centers.

focal abscesses (Schapers et al., 1981). Colon and small bowel mucosa may show ulcerations, lymphoid hyperplasia, or granulomas. Also seen is a karyorrhexis of the neutrophils, with very rare or absent multinucleated giant cells (Mikhaleva, Zhavoronkov, and Kranchev, 1995). Chronic mesenteric adenitis, like other chronic infections, may lead to lymph node fibrosis as well.

Immunohistochemistry

Antibodies to *Yersinia pseudotuberculosis* antigen suitable for immunoassays have been described (Jain, Tuteja, and Batra, 2003), but immunostaining of paraffin sections has not been well documented.

Differential Diagnosis

The histological findings in *Yersinia enterocolitica* lymphadenitis appear similar to those of cat-scratch disease (CSD), but unlike CSD, there are no monocytoid B-cell clusters. Epithelioid granulomas with or without abscesses may be seen (Figure 19.8). Germinal centers may show microabscesses in yersiniosis, but these are rarely seen in CSD and other forms of suppurative granulomatous lymphadenitis. Clinically, other viral infections, *Campylobacter jejuni, Strep spp., salmonella spp.,* and mycobacteria could cause signs and symptoms of mesenteric adenitis.

Treatment and Prognosis

In severe or complicated infections, antibiotics such as aminoglycosides, doxycycline, trimethoprim-sulfamethoxazole, or fluoroquinolones may be useful. Infections usually resolve within a few weeks

with no lasting consequences, although some cases of persistent joint pain associated with bacteremia have been documented. Those most susceptible to post-enteritis arthritis are individuals with the antigen HLA-B27 (or related antigens such as B7). Both *Y. enterocolitica* and *Y. pseudotuberculosis* have been associated with reactive arthritis, which may occur even in the absence of obvious symptoms. The frequency of such post-enteritis arthritic conditions is 2 to 3% (Townes, 2008).

BRUCELLOSIS

Brucellosis disease was first described in 1850 in Malta during the Crimean War, but it was Dr. David Bruce who in 1887 established the bacterial etiology of the disease that now bears his name. Bernhard Bang, a Danish veterinarian, noted the association with unpasteurized milk soon thereafter. Infected persons who are not treated show a characteristic undulating fever that rises and falls in waves.

Definition

Brucellosis is a systemic disease caused by the Gram-negative coccobacilli, *Brucella abortus, B. melitensis, B. suis,* or *B. canis.* The necrotizing suppurative bacterial infections affect the lymph nodes and other organs.

Synonyms

Undulant fever, Malta fever, milk sickness, Bang's disease.

ICD-10 Code A22

Epidemiology

Since the discovery that marine mammals can be a reservoir for the agent of Malta fever, brucellosis is now regarded as an emergent zoonosis (Marcotty et al., 2009). Brucellosis is a rare disease in the United States, with an annual incidence of only 0.07 cases per 100,000. (Nadler et al., 1982). There are 100 to 200 cases of brucellosis seen annually in the United States, and *B. suis* is endemic in the swine population in 35 states. The worldwide incidence of all biovars is substantially larger than in the United States (Murray et al., 2000). Brucellosis is largely an occupational disease of those working with infected animals or their tissues. Sporadic cases and outbreaks occur among consumers of raw milk and milk products (especially unpasteurized soft cheese) from cows, sheep, and goats. In Texas and California, cases are seen within ethnic population known to be consumers of unpasteurized goat milk products ("queso fresco"). Isolated cases of infection with *B. canis* occur in animal handlers from contact with infected dogs. Infection may rarely occur in bison, elk, caribou, and some species of deer, and *B. canis* is an occasional problem in laboratory dog colonies and kennels. Coyotes have been found to be infected with *B. canis*. Marine mammals harboring *Brucella spp.* can cause human neurological granulomatous infection (Sohn et al., 2003, Whatmore et al., 2008). Marine mammal brucellosis due to the two new proposed *Brucella* species, *B. cetaceae* and *B. pinnipediae*, represents a potentially new zoonotic threat (Cloeckaert et al., 2003).

TABLE 19.3 Signs and Symptoms in Brucellosis (*B. melitensis*)

Signs/Symptoms	Frequency %
Fever	91
Chills	40
Sweats	39
Gastrointestinal symptoms	30
Headache	23
Respiratory symptoms	23
Musculoskeletal	22
Osteoarticular	37
Hepatomegaly	27 to 46.2% (Malik, 1997)
Splenomegaly	43.3% (Malik, 1997)
Lymphadenopathy	9% (Mousa et al., 1988b), 19.2% mainly cervical (Malik, 1997) to 32% (Madkour, 2009)

Etiology

Brucella abortus, biovars 1–6 and 9; *B. melitensis*, biovars 1–3; *B. suis*, biovars 1–5; and *B. canis* cause disease. The disease is acquired via direct contact, ingestion or through inhalation of airborne particles.

Pathogenesis

The dissemination and growth of Brucella systemically in lymph nodes, spleen, liver, bone marrow, mammary glands, and sex organs is facilitated by macrophages. The ability of Brucella to survive within macrophages is responsible for its persistence in chronic infections. Following ingestion or inhalation of contaminated aerosols, or through exposure of abraded skin or the mucosae, macrophages ingest the bacteria and transport them to the regional lymph nodes. Here they cause acute lymphadenitis with granulomas and/or microabscesses as in other extranodal organs. Brucella impairs the antibacterial myeloperoxidase–H_2O_2–halide systems in neutrophils preventing degranulation. In the macrophage, Brucella prevents phagosome-lysosome fusion, allowing the bacteria to multiply virulently. Brucella species do not elaborate exotoxin. Since the organisms often survive inside immune cells, acute disease may progress into chronic illness with recurrent episodes of exacerbation characterized by chills, malaise, and undulant fever. The clinical spectrum of the disease depends on the infecting Brucella species with milder symptoms caused by *B. abortus* and *B. canis* and more severe protracted disease as a result of infection with *B. melitensis* and suis (see Table 19.4).

Clinical Aspects

Signs and Symptoms

The frequency of various symptoms is given in Table 19.3 for *B. melitensis* in Kuwait in 379 patients (Mousa et al., 1988) and for 104 patients in Saudi Arabia (Malik, 1997).

Sites of Involvement

Lymphadenopathy, hepatomegaly, and splenomegaly occur at high frequency in most patients (Mousa et al., 1988; Malik, 1997). Osteoarticular complications with sacroiliitis are the most frequent joint manifestation. Genitourinary involvement is seen with orchitis and epididymitis as common symptoms. Erythematous, macular, desquamating skin lesions may show up on the arms and hands of farmers who hand-milk cows.

TABLE 19.4 **Brucella Types and Diseases**

Organism	Animal Reservoir	Human Disease	Complications
B. abortus	Cattle	Mild suppurative febrile infection	Rare
B. canis	Dogs	Mild suppurative febrile infection	Rare
B. suis	Swine	Prolonged disease that may lead to the formation of destructive lesions of the lymphoreticular organs and kidney	
B. melitensis	Goats/sheep	Severe and recurring disease	High incidence of serious complications

Incubation Period

Usually it takes 5 to 60 days from infection to onset of symptoms. There is no evidence of person-to-person communicability.

Approach to Diagnosis

Diagnosis starts with a strong suspicion based on a clinical presentation of myalgia, undulant fever, arthralgia, organomegaly, and occurrence in an endemic locale with a history of exposure. Laboratory diagnosis is through isolation of the infectious agent from discharges, blood, bone marrow, or other tissues. Even though the organisms are fastidious, definitive diagnosis can be made by culture. A fourfold rise in serum agglutination test (SAT) titer between the acute and convalescent phase sample is indicative of infection. Current serological tests allow a precise diagnosis in over 95% of cases. These methods do not apply for *B. canis*, where diagnosis requires tests detecting antibodies to rough-lipopolysaccharide antigens.

Morphology

Discrete yellow nodules may be seen in the spleen and other organs with rare caseation. Histologically, the granulomas are characterized by numerous multinucleated giant cells and palisaded histiocytes, with amorphous and stellate necrosis. Suppurative necrotizing granulomas are variably found in lymph nodes and other organs. Bone marrow shows round epithelioid granulomas, rarely necrotizing, with a variable number of neutrophils, many multinucleated giant cells and occasional surrounding eosinophils (Sundberg and Spink, 1947). Festooned macrophages around pink necrotic centers can produce the so-called Splendore–Hoeple effect (see Figure 19.9).

Differential Diagnosis

Chronic localized brucellosis is difficult to diagnose due to its rare occurrence and to the usually negative cultures and serological tests (Kerr et al., 1966). Tuberculosis is likely to be a diagnosis given when bone lesions are seen but the noncaseating appearance of brucellosis is useful. Histologic mimics include agents causing granulomatous necrotizing lymphadenitis with or without suppurative abscess.

Treatment and Prognosis

With treatment, a full recovery usually occurs, but rare complications can cause severe disability. The fatality rate of untreated brucellosis is 2% or less and usually results from complicating endocarditis associated with *Brucella melitensis* infections. Treatment with a combination of doxycycline, tetracycline, or trimethoprimsulfamethoxazole and gentamicin or rifampin for at least six weeks is usual to prevent recurrent infections. Animal vaccination and avoidance of infected material are effective control measures.

MELIOIDOSIS

Melioidosis was originally described in Burma in 1911, but is now considered a reemerging and under-diagnosed disease. Melioidosis is derived from the Greek *melis* meaning "a distemper of asses" because the bacteria is related to the cause of "glanders," a disease of horses, asses, and mules. The manifestations tend to be protean and easily mistaken for other diseases like tuberculosis.

Definition

Melioidosis is a systemic bacterial infection caused by *Burkholderia pseudomallei*.

ICD-10 Code A24.1 to A24.4

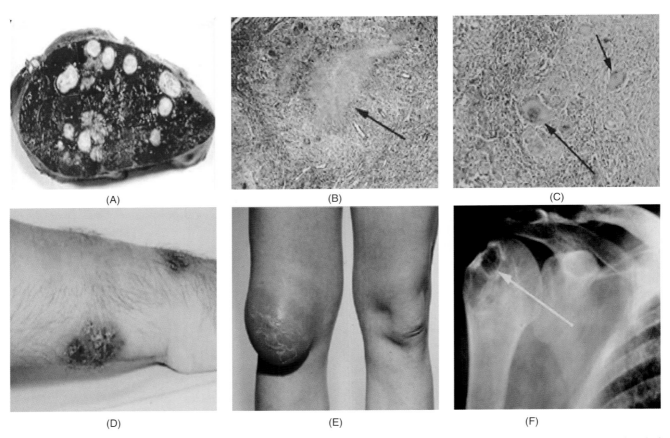

FIGURE 19.9　**Brucellosis**. (**A**) Splenic discrete yellow nodules. (**B**) Histology showing necrotizing granulomas and palisaded histiocytes (arrow), amorphous stellate necrosis festooned by macrophages—the so-called Splendore–Hoeple effect. (**C**) Numerous multinucleated giant cells (arrows). (**D**) Red macular desquamating lesions on arms caused by direct exposure, possibly from milking cows. (**E**) Joint lesions may or may not be obvious. (**F**) Bone X ray reveals deeper articular surfaces with erosion (yellow arrow). (Images courtesy of Dr. E. Koneman of Univ. of Colorado Pathology Department.)

Synonyms

Whitmore disease, Nightcliff gardener's disease, Vietnamese tuberculosis, paddy-field disease, Thai time bomb.

Epidemiology

The majority of disease occurs in southeast Asia, especially in Thailand, and northern Australia. Northeast Thailand has the highest incidence of melioidosis in the world (12.7 cases per 100,000 people per year) (Limmathurotsakul et al., 2010b).

The high-risk groups include rice paddy farmers, laborers, indigenous groups, and travelers. The risk of acute melioidosis is also increased in persons with chronic diseases and is highest in diabetics. Other risk factors include underlying medical conditions such as chronic renal failure, liver disease, respiratory diseases, and thalassemia (Suputtamongkol et al., 1999). Melioidosis is also a travel-related disease

affecting people who visit disease-endemic locations for pleasure, business, or military reasons (Inglis et al., 1999). Most cases of melioidosis in the United States have been in veterans of the Vietnam conflict (see Table 19.5).

Etiology

Melioidosis is caused by a Gram-negative bacillus from the beta-proteobacteria group known as *Burkholderia pseudomallei*. The species was previously known as *Pseudomonas pseudomallei*. It is not directly transmissible from human to human and therefore does not pose a serious epidemic threat although its high rate of mortality is a concern for potential use in bioterrorism.

Pathogenesis

The organism's production of membrane glycocalyx and survival within phagocytic cells are related to

TABLE 19.5 Melioidosis

Key Diagnostic Features of Melioidosis
Etiology: *Burkholderia pseudomallei* formerly *Pseudomonas pseudomallei*
Regions: Southeast Asia and Thailand, China, northern Australia, Brazil
Transmission: Inhalation and percutaneous inoculation presenting as community acquired septicemia in rice paddy communities; also occurs after atsunami and during rainy seasons
Population: Travelers, farmers, veterans, especially those with underlying chronic diseases such as renal failure or diabetes and other immunosuppressed states but paradoxically not HIV.
Organs: Lung, liver, spleen, skeletal muscle, lymph nodes, parotid gland, prostate, brain
Lymph node pathology: necrotizing suppurative granulomas in chronic melioidosis and suppurative abscesses in any organ in the acute form. Multinucleated giant cells with globi of bacteria are pathognomonic features.
Differential diagnosis: necrotizing suppurative granulomas: cat-scratch disease, tularemia, lymphogranuloma venereum. Caseation granulomas: mycobacterium tuberculosis
Diagnosis: culture from abscess; serology not helpful in endemic areas
Unsual feature: reactivation after decades of latent infection with the moniker "Vietnamese time bomb"

its pathogenicity and ability to relapse (Limmath-urotsakul et al., 2009). The bacterial capsule and a type III protein secretion apparatus enable *B. pseu-domallei* to survive intracellular killing and facilitate intercellular spread (Leelarasamee, 2004, Adler et al., 2009). In addition *B. pseudomallei* actively evades the autophagic pathway of the innate defense system (Cullinane et al., 2008). The bacterium can remain latent in the body for long periods of time (Gan, 2005) and also possesses mechanisms to evade the host immune response by inhibiting *NF-kappaB* and type I IFN pathway activation, thereby downregu-lating host inflammatory responses (Tan et al., 2010). Upregulation of toll-like receptors (TLRs), especially TLR-2, on peripheral blood leukocytes is observed in septic patients with melioidosis. (Wiersinga et al., 2007).

Clinical Aspects

Melioidosis has a wide range of disease presenta-tions, varying from septicemia with pneumonia and rapid deterioration to multiple organ failure. Infection results from inhalation, percutaneous inoculation, and possibly ingestion of this organism (Currie et al., 2000). Melioidosis also occurs as a self-limited febrile disease lacking specific features.

Sites of Involvement

Although infection of almost all organs has been described, lung involvement occurs in around half of all cases (Currie, 2003). Acute septicemic melioidosis causes discrete abscesses throughout the body. These occur most frequently in the lungs, liver, spleen, lymph nodes, and bone marrow, but any organ may be involved.

Approach to Diagnosis

Serologic testing has low diagnostic specificity for melioidosis in the disease-endemic setting, where the rate of background seropositivity in the healthy population is high (Cheng et al., 2006). Throat swabs can be used to identify active infection in children (Kanaphun et al., 1993). Blood culture remains the standard when compared with serology or molecular detection methods (Limmathurotsakul et al., 2010a).

Morphology

Suppurative lymphadenitis is evidenced by histopathologic appearance of *B. pseudomallei* in lymph nodes. Small, firm, yellowish lesions are sharply delimited from surrounding normal tissue and are often bounded by a narrow hemorrhagic and necrotic margin. The small foci may coalesce into larger abscesses. Microscopically, the centers of the abscesses are necrotic and contain neutrophils in a fibrin mesh (Maciej and Ban, 2006). Necrosis is a prominent feature of even the very early lesions, a finding that probably reflects toxin production by *B. pseudomallei*. Large numbers of bacteria are seen in the abscesses, but seldom in the surrounding tissue. There are numerous Gram-negative, non–acid-fast, intra- and extracellular bacilli, occurring either singly or in chains. Intracellular bacteria within macrophages and "giant cells" are so numerous as to resemble globi but are not easy to see in Gram-stained tissue (Wong, Puthucheary, and Vadivelu, 1995.) (see Table 19.5).

Immunohistochemistry

If the Gram stain does not reveal the bacteria, melioidosis in paraffin-embedded tissue sections may be detected by immunohistochemistry with poly-clonal antibody against *B. pseudomallei* (Wong et al., 1996).

Differential Diagnosis

Subacute melioidosis mimics tuberculosis and is characterized by fever, cough, and pneumonia.

TABLE 19.6 Infectious Causes of Granulomatous Reactions

Bacteria (actinomycosis, brucellosis, granuloma inguinale, listeriosis, meloidosis, nocardiosis, *R. Henselae* cat-scratch disease and bacillary angiomatosis, *Tropheryma whippeli* Whipple's disease), tularemia)

Mycobacteria (fish tank granuloma, Buruli ulcer, leprosy, tuberculosis)

Chlamydia (lymphogranuloma venereum, trachoma)

Cestodes (cryptococcosis, echiococcosis, sparganosis)

Fungi (aspergillus, candidiasis, coccidiomycosis, chromoblastomycosis, cryptococcosis, fusarium, histoplasmosis, mycetoma, sporotrichosis)

Nematodes (ascariasis, dirofilariasis, toxocariasis)

Protozoa (amoeboma, leishmaniasis, toxoplasmosis)

Rickettsia (Q fever)

Spirochetes (pinta, syphilis, yaws)

Trematodes (chronochiasis, fascioliasis, paragonimiasis, opisthorchiasis, schistosomiasis)

Viruses (cytomegalovirus, infectious mononucleosis, measles, mumps)

Source: Adapted from Gutierrez (1990).

Chronic disease may clinically and radiologically mimic pulmonary tuberculosis. Cutaneous melioidosis can present as persistent ulcer and mimics many diseases causing chronic skin ulcers (Thng et al., 2003). The melioidosis lymphadenitis mimics cat-scratch disease and other suppurative necrotizing granulomatous lymphadenitis.

Treatment of Choice and Prognosis

Burkholderia pseudomallei is oxidase positive, resistant to a wide range of antibiotics including gentamicin, polymyxin, and the second-generation cephalosporins, and can survive for long periods in a wide range of environments including distilled water, moist soil, and inside mammalian or plant (tomato) cells. Mortality rates range from 20 to 50%. Approximately one-fourth of septicemic patients will relapse at 10 to 14 days after onset of acute infection despite receiving intravenous antibiotics. Those at highest risk of fatal infection are patients with *B. pseudomallei* meningo-encephalitis. The overall in-hospital mortality was 48%, over half of which occurred in the first 72 hours after presentation (Veld et al., 2005). In Thailand, untreated septic melioidosis is usually fatal. Even with antibiotic therapy, half the people die.

The first-line treatment is an intravenous intensive course of ceftazidime or a carbapenem followed by a prolonged oral eradication course of cotrimoxazole or cotrimoxazole with doxycycline for 2 to 4 weeks (Cheng et al., 2008). This first line may be followed by a second eradication phase with a combination of oral agents such as cotrimoxazole and doxycycline for at least 12 weeks to mitigate relapse.

TYPHOID LYMPHADENITIS (*SALMONELLA TYPHI*)

Salmonella typhi was first described in 1880 by Karl Joseph Eberth who found the bacteria in the spleen and mesenteric lymph nodes of a patient who died of typhoid fever. The infamous "Typhoid Mary" was Mary Mallon, an asymptomatic carrier of *S. typhi*, who in 1907 unknowingly infected many people while working as a cook and baker for several families. Both in the past and in recent times, typhoid has been used intentionally as a biologic weapon by the military, extremists, and cult members.

Definition

Typhoid lymphadenitis is an infection of the lymph nodes, usually mesenteric, by *S. typhi* occurring secondary to typhoid fever.

ICD-10 Code A01.0

Synonyms

Typhoid, enteric fever.

Epidemiology

Typhoid fever is uncommon in developed countries where vaccination is practiced and food and water supplies are produced and distributed under clean conditions. Only about 400 cases per year are reported in the United States, and many of those are acquired during travel to countries where typhoid is endemic.

In Asia, the annual typhoid incidence (per 100,000 persons per year) varied from 24.2 in Vietnam and 29.3 China, to 180.3 in Indonesia, 412.9 in Pakistan, and 493.5 in India (Ochiai et al., 2008). In the Philippines, it is a major health issue with a reported increasing incidence of 29.6 per 100,000 person years in 1989 (Dr. M. Dayrit, PSMID scientific forum lecture, 1992) to more recent frequent regional outbreaks (Kawano, Leano, and Agdamag, 2007).

Etiology

S. typhi is the most common cause of typhoid fever. Areas of the world where sanitation is poor and vaccination and medical services are scarce can have a high incidence of typhoid fever. The disease is spread by fecal or other material from an infected person or sewage coming in contact with food or water that is ingested by others.

Pathogenesis

S. typhi is a colonizer of the intestine and thus may be expected to affect the mesenteric lymph nodes early in the disease, but later involvement of the inguinal nodes can occur. The earliest changes include colonization of the mucosa and hypertrophy of the lymphoid follicles of the Peyer's patches. The lymph nodes may become enlarged due to the influx of immune cells and production of inflammatory cytokines and reactive oxygen species that cause tissue damage and vascular leakiness, and this may set the stage for typhoid lymphadenitis.

Clinical Aspects

Site of Infection

Ingestion of food or water contaminated with *S. typhi* allows the bacteria to colonize the gut where they can multiply rapidly causing diarrhea or constipation, cramps, malaise, and high fever. From the intestine, the bacteria enter the blood where they can cause generalized lymphadenopathy, but *S. typhi* is considered one of the less common infectious agents. Infection of the lymph nodes by typhoid bacteria has been reported, but is uncommon (Faber, Simoons-Smith, and Razenberg, 1990). The presence of typhoid fever with abdominal pain, high fever, chills, and headache would likely be an indication of comorbid lymphadenitis.

Typhoid, like other food-borne bacterial diseases, is spread by food or water handled by persons infected with the disease that is later ingested by others. Infection with *S. typhi* results in a high fever (103–104°F, 39–40°C), fatigue, diarrhea or constipation, abdominal pain, and sometimes a rash of rose-colored areas on the lower chest or abdomen that lasts for only a few days. If the disease is not treated, the fever will continue and diarrhea or constipation will become severe leading to rapid weight loss. Death may follow if treatment is not begun.

Approach to Diagnosis

Symptoms of high fever combined with abdominal distress are indicators of typhoid fever. Identification of *S. typhi* in the feces is positive. Lymphadenitis causes swelling and tenderness of the lymph nodes, typically the mesenteric. Fine needle aspirates from swollen LNs will be positive for *S. typhi* (Lee et al., 1997).

Laboratory Findings

Blood and stool tests for *S. typhi* can be done to identify the causative agent. Fine needle aspirates from LNs can be examined for bacteria associated with lymphadenitis. Serology for *S. typhi* using Poly H and Vi antigens may be used. Blood culture as well as Vitek II and API 20 laboratory tests are complementary.

Morphology

The morphologic findings mainly show intestinal and lymph node pathology, but the disease can spread to the visceral organs. There is diffuse mucosal inflammation of the terminal small bowel and colonic mucosa followed by necrosis. Loosely formed focal granulomas or well-formed granulomas manifest as nodules containing "typhoid cells," histiocytic aggregates of macrophages that phagocytose red cells, bacteria, and lymphocytes along with plasma cells and lymphocytes with little suppurative component. Typhoid cells are large macrophages with abundant eosinophilic cytoplasm, ingested nuclear debris, bacteria, and other cells. They are noted in the lymph node sinuses as well as in foci of necrotizing granulomas.

Granulomas may also appear as foci of necrotic neutrophilic abscesses. They may also contain walls of histiocytes with giant cells and focally preserved lymphoid architecture (Bharadwaj et al., 2009). Sometimes large foci of bacterial clumps are seen in necrotic lymphadenitis. Although the most common sites of typhoid granulomas are the intestine and mesenteric lymph nodes (Lee et al., 1997), the spleen, liver, and bone marrow can are also be involved. Bone marrow, liver, and spleen may show well-formed necrotizing or non-necrotizing granulomas, some with hemophagocytosis (Shin, Paik, and Cho, 1994, Shin et al., 1995).

Cytochemistry

A modified Gram's stain (using Brown and Hopp) may show many Gram-negative bacilli, both within the histiocytes of typhoid cells and extracellularly especially in necrotic areas.

Differential Diagnosis

Yersinia enterocolitica lymphadenitis causes similar histological findings but can be differentiated by serology and culture. It uncommon, however, to find typical cytophagic typhoid cells in yersiniosis. Crohn's disease with epithelioid granulomas and secondary bacterial infection should be considered based on the location. Other causes of mesenteric lymphadenitis such as viral infections, *Campylobacter jejuni, Strep spp.*, other *salmonella spp.*, and mycobacteria should be included in the microbiologic workup for differential diagnosis.

Treatment

Administration of a combination of antibiotics has reduced the mortality rate to 1 to 2% from an untreated fatality rate of 20%. The prevention of overwhelming infections and complications such as pneumonia and intestinal perforation has been the primary reason for the reduced mortality. From 3 to 5% of patients become carriers of *S. typhi* after recovering from acute illness.

REFERENCES

ACHTMAN M, ZURTH K, MORELLI G, TORREA G, GUIYOULE A, CARNIEL E, 1999. *Yersinia pestis*, the cause of plague, is a recently emerged clone of *Yersinia pseudotuberculosis*. Proc Nat Acad Sci USA 96:14043–8.

ADLER NR, GOVAN B, CULLINANE M, HARPER M, ADLER B, BOYCE JD. 2009. The molecular and cellular basis of pathogenesis in melioidosis: how does *Burkholderia pseudomallei* cause disease? FEMS Microbiol Rev 33:1079–99.

ARIAS-STELLA J. Jr., ARIAS-STELLA J. 1997. Warthin–Starry stain identifies *Bartonella bacilliformis* in verruga peruana. Mod Pathol 10:41a.

BLANK S, SCHILLINGER JA, HARBATKIN D. 2005. Lymphogranuloma venereum in the industrialised world. Lancet 365:1607.

BORGES MC, COLARES JK, LIMA DM, FONSECA BA. 2009. *Haemophilus ducreyi* detection by polymerase chain reaction in oesophageal lesions of HIV patients. Int J STD AIDS 20:238–40.

BRANGER J, VAN DER MEER JT, VAN KETEL RJ, JURRIAANS S, PRINS JM. 2009. High incidence of asymptomatic syphilis in HIV-infected MSM justifies routine screening. Sex Transm Dis 36:84–5.

BUCHACZ K, KLAUSNER JD, KERNDT PR, SHOUSE RL, ONORATO I, MCELROY PD, SCHWENDEMANN J, TAMBE PB, ALLEN M, COYE F, KENT C, PARK MN, HAWKINS K, SAMOFF E, BROOKS JT. 2008. HIV incidence among men diagnosed with early syphilis in Atlanta, San Francisco, and Los Angeles, 2004 to 2005. J Acquir Immune Defic Syndr 47:234–40.

CHAMBERLIN J, LAUGHLIN LW, ROMERO S, SOLÓRZANO N, GORDON S, ANDRE RG, PACHAS P, FRIEDMAN H, PONCE C, WATTS D. 2002. Epidemiology of endemic *Bartonella bacilliformis*: a prospective cohort study in a Peruvian mountain valley community. J Infect Dis 186:983–90.

CHANG GJ. 1997. Molecular biology of dengue viruses. In: Gubler DJ, Kuno G, eds., Dengue and Dengue Hemorrhagic Fever. CAB International, London, 175–98.

CHANTRATITA N, MEUMANN E, THANWISAI A, LIMMATHUROTSAKUL D, WUTHIEKANUN V, WANNAPASNI S, TUMAPA S, DAY NP, PEACOCK SJ. 2008. Loop-mediated isothermal amplification method targeting the TTS1 gene cluster for detection of *Burkholderia pseudomallei* and diagnosis of melioidosis. J Clin Microbiol 46:568–73.

CHAPPUIS F, SUNDAR S, HAILU A, GHALIB H, RIJAL S, et al. 2007. Visceral leishmaniasis: what are the needs for diagnosis, treatment and control? Nature Rev Microbiol 5:873–82.

CHENG AC, CHIERAKUL W, CHAOWAGUL W, CHETCHOTISAKD P, LIMMATHUROTSAKUL D, DANCE DAB, PEACOCK SJ, CURRIE BJ. 2008. Consensus guidelines for dosing of amoxicillin-clavulanate in melioidosis. Am J Trop Med Hyg 78:208–9.

CHENG AC, CURRIE BJ. 2005. Melioidosis: epidemiology, pathophysiology, and management. Clin Micro Rev 18:383–416.

CHENG AC, PEACOCK SJ, LIMMATHUROTSAKUL D, WONGSUVAN G, CHIERAKUL W, AMORNCHAI P, GETCHALARAT N, CHAOWAGUL W, WHITE NJ, DAY NP, WUTHIEKANUN V. 2006. Prospective evaluation of a rapid immunochromogenic cassette test for the diagnosis of melioidosis in northeast Thailand. Trans R Soc Trop Med Hyg 100:64–7.

CHLEBICKI MP, TAN BH. 2006. Six cases of suppurative lymphadenitis caused by *Burkholderia pseudomallei* infection. Trans R Soc Trop Med Hyg 100:798–801.

CULLINANE M, GONG L, LI X, LAZAR-ADLER N, TRA T, WOLVETANG E, PRESCOTT M, BOYCE JD, DEVENISH RJ, ADLER B. 2008. Stimulation of autophagy suppresses the intracellular survival of *Burkholderia pseudomallei* in mammalian cell lines. Autophagy 4:744–53.

CURI AL, MACHADO D, HERINGER G, CAMPOS WR, LAMAS C, ROZENTAL T, GUTIERRES A, OREFICE F, LEMOS E. Cat-scratch disease: ocular manifestations and visual outcome. Int Ophthalmol 30(5):553–8. epub 2010 Jul 30.

CURRIE BJ 2003. Melioidosis: an important cause of pneumonia in residents of and travellers returned from endemic regions. Eur Respir J 22:542–50.

CURRIE BJ, FISHER DA, HOWARD DM, BURROW JN, LO D, SELVA-NAYAGAM S, ANSTEY NM, HUFFAM SE, SNELLING PL, MARKS PJ, STEPHENS DP, LUM GD, JACUPS SP, KRAUSE VL. 2000. Endemic melioidosis in tropical northern Australia: a 10-year prospective study and review of the literature. Clin Infect Dis 31:981–6.

FABER LM, SIMOONS-SMITH AM, RAZENBERG PP. 1990. An unusual late manifestation of a *Salmonella typhi* infection. Am J Gastroenterol 85:81–3.

FREIJ B. And J. SEVER. 1991. Toxoplasmosis. Pediatr Rev 12(8):227–236.

GAN YH 2005. Interaction between *Burkholderia pseudomallei* and the host immune response: sleeping with the enemy? J Infect Dis 192:1845–50.

GODFROID J, CLOECKAERT A, LIAUTARD JP, KOHLER S, FRETIN D, WALRAVENS K, GARIN–BASTUJ B, LETESSON

JJ. 2005. From the discovery of the Malta fever's agent to the discovery of a marine mammal reservoir, brucellosis has continuously been a re-emerging zoonosis. Vet Res 36(3):313–26.

Gutierrez Y. 1990. Diagnostic Pathology of Parasitic Infections with Clinical Correlations. Lea and Febiger, Pheladelphia.

Nadler H, Dolan C, Forgacs P, George H. 1982. *Brucella suis*: an unusual cause of suppurative lymphadenitis in an outpatient. JClin Microbiol 16(3):575–6.

Hoang MP, High WA, Molberg KH. 2004. Secondary syphilis: a histologic and immunohistochemical evaluation. J Cutan Pathol 31:595–9.

Inglis TJJ, Rolim DB, De Queiroz Sousa A. 2006. Melioidosis in the Americas. Am J Trop Med Hyg 75:947–54.

Kanaphun P, Thirawattanasuk N, Suputtamongkol Y, Naigowit P, Dance DA, Smith MD, White NJ. 1993. Serology and carriage of *Pseudomonas pseudomallei*: a prospective study in 1000 hospitalized children in northeast Thailand. J Infect Dis 167:230–3.

Kaufmann AF. 1976. Epidemiologic trends of leptospirosis in the United States, 1965–1974. In: Johnson RC, ed., The Biology of Parasitic Spirochetes. Academic Press, New York, 177–89.

Kent ME, Romanelli F. 2008. Reexamining syphilis: an update on epidemiology, clinical manifestations, and management. An Pharmacother 42:226–36.

Leelarasamee A. 2004. Recent development in melioidosis. Curr Opin Infect Dis 17:131–6.

Limmathurotsakul D, Chaowagul W, Day NP, Peacock SJ. 2009. Patterns of organ involvement in recurrent melioidosis. Am J Trop Med Hyg 81:335–7.

Limmathurotsakul D, Wongratanacheewin S, Teerawattanasook N, Wongsuvan G, Chaisuksant S, Chetchotisakd P, Chaowagul W, Day NP, Peacock SJ. 2010. Increasing incidence of human melioidosis in northeast Thailand. Am J Trop Med Hyg 82:1113–7.

Loulergue P, Bastides F, Baudouin V, Chandenier J, Mariani-Kurkdjian P, Dupont B, Viard JP, Dromer F, Lortholary O. 2007. Literature review and case histories of *Histoplasma capsulatum var. duboisii* infections in HIV-infected patients. Emerg Infect Dis 13(11):1647–52.

Madkour M. 2009. Brucellosis. In: Cook G, Zumla A, eds., Manson's Tropical Diseases. Saunders Elsevier, Hong Kong. 1075.

Maguiña C, Garcia P, Gotuzzo E, Cordero L, Spach D. 2001. Bartonellosis (carrion's disease in the modern era. Clin Infect Di 33:772–9.

Maguiña C, Gotuzzo E. 2000. Bartonellosis—new and old. Infect Dis Clin North Am 14:1–22.

Mccord AM, Cuevas J, Anderson BE. 2007. Bartonella-induced endothelial cell proliferation is mediated by release of calcium from intracellular stores. DNA Cell Biol 26:657–63.

Monack DM, Mecsas J, Ghori N, Falkow S. 1997. Yersinia signals macrophages to undergo apoptosis and Yopj is necessary for this cell death. Proc Nat Acad Sci USA 94:10385–90.

Nieuwenhuis RF, Ossewaarde JM, Gotz HM, Dees J, Thio HB, Thomeer MG, Den Hollander JC, Neumann MH, Van Der Meijden WI. 2004. Resurgence of *Lymphogranuloma venereum* in western Europe: an outbreak of *Chlamydia trachomatis serovar L2 proctitis* in the Netherlands among men who have sex with men. Clin Infect Dis 39(7):996–1003. epub 2004 Sep 8.

Rao PR, Banerjea S, Raju VP, Devi KI. 1969. Filarial lymphadenitis–a histopathological study. Indian J Pathol Bacteriol 12:154–7.

Raoult D, Roux V. 1997. Rickettsioses as paradigms of new or emerging infectious diseases. Clin Microbiol Rev 10(4):694–719.

Rapini, Ronald P.; Bolognia, Jean L.; Jorizzo, Joseph L. 2007. Dermatology: 2-Volume Set. St. Louis: Mosby.

Rean VM. 1962. The pathologic anatomy and pathogenesis of fatal human leptospirosis (Weil's disease). Am J Pathol 40:393–423.

Richens J. 2006. Donovanosis (granuloma inguinale). Sex Transm Infect 82(suppl 4):Iv21–2.

Ruckdeschel K, Roggenkamp A, Lafont V, Mangeat P, Heesemann J, Rouot B. 1997. Interaction of *Yersinia enterocolitica* with macrophages leads to macrophage cell death through apoptosis. Infect Immun 65:4813–21.

Scheidegger F, Ellner Y, Guye P, Rhomberg TA, Weber H, Augustin HG, Dehio C. 2009. Distinct activities of *Bartonella henselae* type IV secretion effector proteins modulate capillary-like sprout formation. Cell Microbiol 11:1088–101. epub 2009 Mar 12.

Spaargaren J, Schachter J, Moncada J, De Vries HJ, Fennema HS, Peña AS, Coutinho RA, Morré SA. 2005. Slow epidemic of *Lymphogranuloma venereum* L2b strain. Emerg Infect Dis 11:1787–8.

Suputtamongkol Y, Chaowagul W, Chetchotisakd P, Lertpatanasuwun N, Intaranongpai S, Ruchutrakool T, Budhsarawong D, Mootsikapun P, Wuthiekanun V, Teerawatasook N, Lulitanond A. 1999. Risk factors for melioidosis and bacteremic melioidosis. Clin Infect Dis 29:408–13.

Tan KS, Chen Y, Lim YC, Tan GY, Liu Y, Lim YT, Macary P, Gan YH. 2010. Suppression of host innate immune response by *Burkholderia pseudomallei* through the virulence factor TssM. J Immunol 184:5160–71.

Thng TG, Seow CS, Tan HH, Yosipovitch G. 2003. A case of nonfatal cutaneous melioidosis. Cutis 72:310–312.

Torrea G, Chenal-Francisque V, Leclercq A, Carniel E. 2006. Efficient tracing of global isolates of *Yersinia pestis* by restriction fragment length polymorphism analysis using three insertion sequences as probes. J Clin Microbiol 44:2084–92.

van CR, Grefte JM, van DD, Sturm P. 2009. Syphilis presenting as isolated cervical lymphadenopathy: two related cases. J Infect 58:76–8.

Veld D, Wuthiekanun V, Cheng AC, Chierakul W, Chaowagul W, Brouwer AE, White NJ, Day NJ, Peacock SJ. 2005. The role and significance of sputum cultures in the diagnosis of melioidosis. Am J Trop Med Hyg 73:657–61.

WIERSINGA WJ, WIELAND CW, DESSING MC, CHANTRATITA N, CHENG AC, LIMMATHUROTSAKUL D, CHIERAKUL W, LEENDERTSE M, FLORQUIN S, DE VOS AF, WHITE N, DONDORP AM, DAY NP, PEACOCK SJ, VAN DER PT. 2007. Toll-like receptor 2 impairs host defense in Gram-negative sepsis caused by *Burkholderia pseudomallei (melioidosis)*. PLoS Med 4:e248.

WONG KT, PUTHUCHEARY SD, VADIVELU J. 1995. The histopathology of human melioidosis. Histopathology 26:51–5.

WONG KT, VADIVELU J, PUTHUCHEARY SD, TAN KL. 1996. An immunohistochemical method for the diagnosis of melioidosis. Pathology 28:188–91.

WOODS GL, GUTIERREZ Y. 1993. Lea and Febiger, Philadelphia.

ZIMMER C. 2000. Parasite rex: Inside the bizarre world of nature's most dangerous creatures. Free Press, New York.

CHAPTER TWENTY

MIXED PATTERNS: EMERGENT/TROPICAL INFECTIONS WITH CHARACTERIZED LYMPHADENOPATHY

Hernani D. Cualing

MIXED PATTERN WITH GRANULOMATAS AND DIAGNOSTIC MICROORGANISMS

Filariasis

Wuchereria bancrofti was named in honor of the first two authors that described the disease that bears their name. Microfilaria was first found in chylous urine by O. Wucherer in 1866. The adult worm was described by J. Bancroft in 1876. Later Sir P. Manson described its biology and mosquito transmission from host blood. *Wuchereria bancrofti*, and the related *Mansona spp.* and *Brugia spp.* affect millions of people in tropical climates and developing countries. They cause severe disability and impose a great socioeconomic burden (Cuellar-Rodriguez et al., 2009). Their estimated encumbrance is almost 3.5-fold higher than that of schistosomiasis and approximately one-seventh of that of malaria (WHO, 2004).

Definition

Filariasis results from infection with the mosquito-borne filarial nematode manifesting a wide range of organ involvement, including lymphadenopathy. Lymphatic filariasis primarily affects the lymphatic vessels causing obstructive lymphedema.

ICD-10 Codes

Filariasis NOS	B74.0
Dirofilariasis	B74.9
Brugia malayi	B74.2
Brugia timori	B74.0
W. bancrofti	B74.9
Loa loa	B74.4
Mansoni perstans	B74.8

Synonyms

Calabar swelling, eyeworm disease, loasis, bancroftian filariasis, Brugian filariasis, dirofilariasis.

Non-Neoplastic Hematopathology and Infections, First Edition. Edited by Hernani D. Cualing, Parul Bhargava, and Ramon L. Sandin.

Epidemiology

Most filariasis infection is confined to warm climates but some are in temperate regions. Filariasis is endemic in tropical regions of Asia, Africa, Central and South America, and sporadic in the United States. *W. bancrofti* is the cause of 90% of human filariasis, altogether affecting about 128 million people in 80 countries. *Culex* is the predominant mosquito vector in most areas; in Africa, it is the *Anopheles* (Zagaria and Savioli, 2002). Although most filariasis of tropical countries are systemic and produce lymphangitic lymphedema, some of the Western filariasis are localized.

These worms are not present in the United States and Canada with the exception of cases from immigrants and travelers. However, *Dirofilaria spp.* and *Brugia spp.* are autochthonous infections in the Americas. Localized presentation is the rule in *Dirofilaria spp.* in contrast with the majority of world's filariasis. In North America and Europe, *Dirofilaria immitis, D. tenuis,* and *D. repens* are the infections associated with domesticated companion animals. *D. ursi and D. striata,* from bears and wild cats, respectively, are associated with sylvatic animals of the Americas. In Europe, *D. repens* is the common infection transmitted by household dogs (Kramer et al., 2007). Most infections in the United States are seen in immigrants from endemic countries with a few autochthonous native cases. Travelers who visit endemic areas for extended periods of time (generally longer than 3 months) and who are intensively exposed to infected mosquitoes are at greater risk of infection. Short-term travelers to endemic areas are at low risk for infection.

W. bancrofti is prevalent in Central Africa, coastal South Americas, India, Indonesia, some islands of northern Philippines while *Brugia spp.* are in Indonesia, Borneo, the Celebes, and Mindanao and Palawan of the Philippines (Tubangi, 1948). Risk locales previously cited in the Philippines include prevalence at sites of abaca plant cultivation (source of Manila hemp) and at towns with nearby swamps, where 8% of the population were positive by blood smear (Grove et al., 1977).

Etiology

Lymphatic filariasis is caused by infections with nematodes of the superfamily Filarioidea: *Wuchereria bancrofti, Brugia malayi,* and *Brugia timori.* Greater than 60% of infections are concentrated in Asia and the Pacific region while the rest are in Africa. Localized and subcutaneous filariasis is caused by *Dirofilaria spp* and *Brugia spp.*

Pathogenesis

In lymphatic filariasis, the larvae (microfilariae) circulate in the blood to become adults. Adult worms may be productive for more than 20 years. Mosquitoes pick up the larvae during a blood meal and transmit infection to and from the human hosts. The adult filarial worms lodge in the lymphatic system and induce debilitating disease. The presence of living worms in the body is mainly asymptomatic, but the death of adult worms leads to granulomatous inflammation and fibrosis leading to blockade of the lymphatic flow. Lymphedema can cause massive legs and genitalia called elephantiasis.

There is evidence of variation in susceptibility based on expressed human genes. Mannose-binding lectin (MBL) binds to bancroftian parasites. An association between expression of a gene encoding for production of MBL and immunity has been postulated (Meyrowitsch et al., 2010). The MBL is known to activate complement and augment opsonization and phagocytosis. Hence low-expressing MBL genotype individuals were three times more likely to present with filarial infection compared with high-expressing individuals.

Unlike the infections of tropical microfilaria, there is a striking absence of demonstrable microfilaremia in patients infected with Dirofilaria, Brugia, or other forms autochthonously acquired in the United States. In localized filariasis, such as *Dirofilaria spp.,* subcutaneous infection is the usual route. Lymphatic and systemic spread lead to localized subcutaneous nodules and lymphadenopathy. Systemic manifestation usually show in the lungs as radiographically visible nodules mimicking malignacy.

Clinical Aspects

Sites of Involvement. Most infected people are asymptomatic and will never develop clinical symptoms. Depending on the *Filaria spp.* filariasis may affect the lymphatics, lymph nodes, blood vessels, skin, or lungs. The most common acute clinical manifestations is acute dermato-lymphangio-adenitis (ADLA) attacks. They are usually associated with fever, chills, headache, and enlarged painful lymph nodes. The draining lymph nodes are swollen and tender with associated lymphangitis, lymphadenitis, or abscess formation.

Morphology. These parasites are very similar in their morphologic features, but in general *Wuchereria spp.* is much larger at a comparable stage of development than is *Brugia spp.* Both have a thin, smooth cuticle without external longitudinal ridges. (See Table 20.1 for cuticle and ridge characteristics.)

TABLE 20.1 **Comparison of External Longitudinal Ridges (Cuticle) between Filaria Species**

Species	External Longitudinal Ridges
W. bancrofti	None, smooth cuticle
Brugia spp.	None
D. immitis	None
D. striata	None
D. tenuis	Yes, beaded, blunt
D. repens	Yes, beaded
D. ursi	Yes, sharp crest
Oncocerca spp.	Yes, infrequent

Approach to Diagnosis

In lymphatic filariasis the standard for diagnosis is microscopic detection of microfilariae on a thick blood film. In most endemic areas the highest concentration of microfilariae in the peripheral blood occurs at night; therefore blood specimens should be collected between 10 pm and 2 am. Capillary finger-prick or venous blood is used for thick blood films. Microfilariae may also be observed in chylous urine and hydrocele fluid. Examination of the urine for chyluria followed by concentration can be used for microfilariae microscopy.

Microfilariae, however, may be absent in adenolymphangitis (ADL) or late chronic lymphatic disease with lymphadenopathy. Lymph node biopsy has been useful in diagnosis of these cases. Identification of characteristic features of the cross section of the worms is key to diagnosis. Mazzotti test can be used for cutaneous filariasis. In endemic filariasis, biopsy is only recommended in localized or cutaneous disease. Adult worms of *O volvulus, L loa, and Dirofilaria spp.* can be found in the nodules and fibrotic tissue of the skin.

The presence of circulating filarial antigen and serum immunoglobulin G4 (IgG4) or IgE antibodies in the peripheral blood are also considered diagnostic of filarial infection and is used to monitor the effectiveness of therapy. Commercial kits are available to test venous blood (Weil and Ramzy, 2007; Weil, Lammie, and Weiss, 1997). A urine ELISA (*Wb*-SXP-1ELISA) showed a sensitivity of 95.6% with *W. bancrofti*-infected subjects in Sri Lanka, and specificity of 99.0% (Itoh et al., 2007). Determination of serum antifilarial immunoglobulin (IgG) is also a diagnostically useful test (Parasitic Diseases Laboratory at the National Institutes of Health (NIH) or through CDC's Division of Parasitic Diseases).

Differential Diagnosis

Congenital lymphedema (Milroy syndrome), nonfilarial elephantiasis (in highlands of East Africa), and congenital hydrocele are some of the diseases under consideration when diagnosing lymphatic filariasis. In localized forms, the coin nodules seen in *Dirofilaria immitis* mimic metastatic disease. The differential diagnosis, when presenting other than a subcutaneous nodule, could be worrisome and in those cases that present as lung masses, ELISAs and PCR probes can usefully differentiate between pulmonary dirofilariasis and lung cancer. Lymphadenopathy may mimic fungal lymphadenitis, acute and/or streptococcal lymphadenitis, because of the painful presentation.

Treatment of Choice and Prognosis

Diethylcarbazine (DEC) kills circulating microfilariae and is partially effective against the adult worms. Although ivermectin kills microfilariae, it does not kill the adult worms. Many patients with lymphedema do not benefit from antifilarial drug treatment.

Newer diagnostic modalities have proved useful in developed and developing countries. Rapid diagnosis of filariasis serologically uses affordable test cards. *Binax Filariasis Now* is sensitive and specific for *W. bancrofti*. *Brugia timori* or *malayi* still relies on IgG4 dipstick test for verifying infection.

LYMPHADENOPATHY SECONDARY TO LOCALIZED FILARIASIS

Dirofilaria *spp.* in Subcutaneous Lymph Node

Unlike the more prevalent lymphatic filariasis, where in a lymph node biopsy is not advised because of exacerbation of lymphedema, biopsy of subcutaneous localized filariasis is diagnostic. Patients with lymphadenopathy or advance disease may benefit from examination of blood film for filariasis.

Because human infections of filarial parasites are found often in tissue section, identification depends on familiarity with characteristic microscopic features of the parasite wall, external longitudinal ridges, and internal organs allowing differentiation of species and sex, respectively (Gutierrez, 1984; Orihel, 1998). Although subcutaneous nodules as a presentation of *Dirofilaria spp.* is frequently reported, granulomatous lymphadenitis secondary to this zoonotic infection is rarely reported (Orihel, 1989; Cualing and Sandin, 2010).

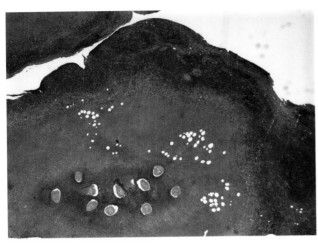

FIGURE 20.1 *Dirofilaria immitis* **and Hoeppli-splendore effect**. An epitrochlear lymph node with granulomatous lymphadenitis: pink necrotic center, palisaded histiocytic layer, and transverse worm sections. The lymph node shows a necrotizing granuloma and an outermost layer of eosinophils, plasma cells, and lymphocytes.

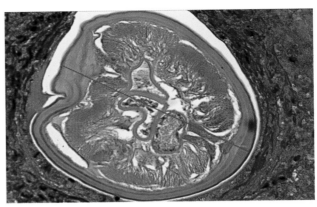

FIGURE 20.2 *Dirofilaria immitis.* A transverse section through a mature adult male shows cuticle of 11 to 14 μm in thickness, with smooth outer lining and pink wall with distinct multilamination, at least 4 layers. Note the even thickness of the cuticles without external longitudinal ridges, the pathognomonic internal cuticular wedged-shaped ridges with small lateral cords, a muscular layer, and reproductive and intestinal tubules. Note the tall coelomyarian muscles and the centrally located intestine and reproductive tubes. Worms are 165 μm in diameter, at this level (red line), indicating a small adult (100–350 μm in diameter for mature worms). (H&E, 200×) A Lovins micrometer and a digital amscope micrometer were used for the diameter sizing.

Human infection of dirofilarial worm is unusual in the United States. Two clinical forms are recognized: those that manifest in subcutaneous location and those with pulmonary involvement. Pulmonary dirofilarisis is usually caused by *D. immitis*, also called dog heartworm (Figures 20.1, 20.2). The adult worm inhabits the right ventricle of dogs, but in human only immature worms have been found, in both lungs and subcutaneous areas. Worms are 100 to 350 μm in diameter evenly with thick layered cuticles projecting into the central worm cavity as internal longitudinal ridges. *D. tenuis and D. repens* can also infect humans. Infection in humans presents as lesions of the skin, conjunctivae, arms, or legs but rarely in the lymph node (Figures 20.3–20.6). This location contrasts with the more frequent involvement of the lymph node in *Brugia spp.* infection in the Americas (Orihel and Beaver, 1989).

Dirofilaria tenuis is the species most frequently encountered infecting humans in the southeastern United States. Unlike *D. immitis*, the *D. tenuis* cuticle is relatively unevenly and irregularly thick and shows prominent external ridges. A subcutaneous route instead of the blood route is a likely route of infection. Subcutaneous tissue, localized or regional lymph nodes are the usual presenting sites.

Similarly *D. repens* shows thick multilayered cuticles, spiked longitudinal ridges, and internal cuticular ridges, averaging 450 to 650 μm in transverse diameter and 7 to 17 cm in length. *D. striata*, a parasite of wild cats, from bobcats and panther in United States, is distinguished from other *Dirofilaria spp.*

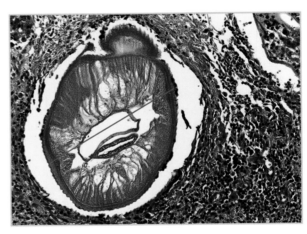

FIGURE 20.3 *D. tenuis*. Unlike *D. immitis*, the cuticle shows prominent external cuticular longitudinal rounded or beaded ridges and spaced about 10 μm apart, with up to 3 layers of transverse ridges, 5 to 8 μm thick. Under the cuticle and above the muscles is a thin layer of hypodermis that expands to parallel bilateral thick lateral cords (red line). The diameter is 265 μm (0.26 mm) at this level but ranges from 150 to 295 μm (H&E, 150×).

with a pathognomonic cuticular appearance: a larger transverse diameter than others, with weak irregular longitudinal ridges, a paired small lateral ala, and a weakly developed transverse striations. *D. ursi*, a

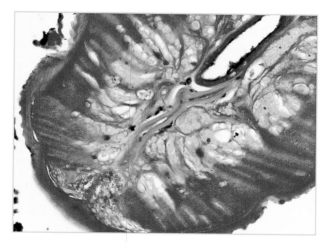

FIGURE 20.4 *D. tenuis* in **high-power view**. Note the cuticles with transverse ridges, thick muscles, and intestinal tubule (H&E).

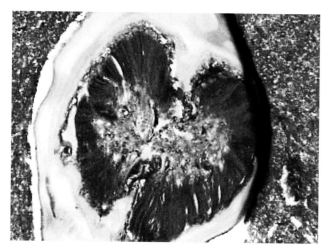

FIGURE 20.6 *D. immitis* **showing necrotic and degenerated worm**. The worms found in lungs are necrotic, poorly preserved, and sometimes calcified.

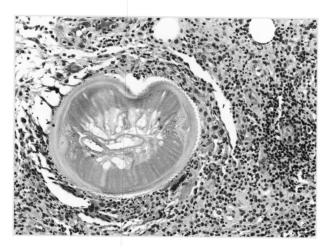

FIGURE 20.5 *D. tenuis* **preserved sections**. Apparent are intense granulomatous lymphadentis and eosinophilic and neutrophilic reactions (H&E).

parasite of bears, show very large diameters and prominent sharp spikes (see Table 20.1).

Bancroftian spp. Lymphadenopathy

The incidence of lymphadenopathy cases with identified worms has ranged from 20 to 28% (Rao et al., 1969, Rifkin, 1945, Wartman, 1944).

Bacroftian lymphadenopathy was characterized in 58 cases in which worms were identified in microscopic sections of lymph nodes (Jungmann, Figueredo-Silva, and Dreyer, 1991). Most of the patients were younger than 20 years, with involvement of inguinal nodes (74.1%), epitrochlear (15.5%), axillary nodes (8.6%), and cervical (1.7%) lymph nodes. Pain, inflammation, and mass were the

presenting findings. Blood smears were negative in patients suspected to be infected. None had elephantiasis or signs of lymphedema. Duration of symptoms ranged from a week to 15 years. Lymph nodes averaged 2.5 cm with largest about 4 cm.

Histologically, filarial worms were found in both efferent and afferent vessels and sinuses, sometimes without eliciting reactions except dilated vessels. Capsular, trabecular, or hilar fibrosis were variably noted. The granulomas show sheets of eosinophils, collections of macrophages, and sometimes Hoeppli–Splendore phenomena. Spent or quiescent granulomas with fibrosis and calcified worm were seen in about 20% of the cases. Similar incidence of mild lymphangitis without granulomas sometimes associated with lymphatic dilatation, with thickened wall or with inflammatory reactive intralumenal collection were seen. Epithelioid granulomas with giant cells were seen without worms in 15% of cases. No histologic reaction to worms in the vessels were observed in 12%. Neutrophilic microabscess were rare and seen in less 1% along with epithelioid histiocytes and suppurative central necrosis containing fragments of worm. (See Table 20.2.)

TABLE 20.2 Key Findings in Bancroftian Lymphadenopathy

Follicular hyperplasia and granulomatous endolymphangitis
Presence of variably preserved worm
Lymphatic dilation without inflammation
Exudative abscess
Lymphangitis
Epithelioid granulomas

The most common findings were a mixed pattern with follicular hyperplasia and granulomatous response in 64% of cases. The histopathologic diagnosis of filariasis can often be made even in the absence of identifiable parasites. The histopathology of lymph nodes removed from immigrants is similar to the lymph nodes of patients from endemic zones (Wartman, 1946).

Brugia spp. Lymphadenopathy

The first published report of human infection in the United States with *Brugia spp.* presented with painless swelling of inguinal lymph nodes initially diagnosed as lymphoma. (Rosenblatt, Beaver, and Orihel, 1962). Since then more than 30 cases have been reported, and most are discovered in lymph nodes.

Epidemiology

In the United States, *B. beaveri*, in raccoons, rabbits, and bobcats can be found in Louisiana and Florida.

Morphology

Reactions of the lymph node range from nonspecific lymphoid hyperplasia to granulomatous response and florid monocytoid hyperplasia (Elenitoba-Johnson et al., 1996). The classic description of Baird is summarized for *Brugia spp.* lymphadenitis (Baird et al., 1986).

In *Brugia spp.* lymphadenopathy the lymph vessels containing intact worms are dilated (Baird et al., 1986). Around the degenerated worms the vessel walls may be thickened and inflamed. Necrotizing granuloma with palisading epithelioid cells and foreign body giant cells can be seen along with either follicular hyperplasia or germinal center atrophy. In addition 30% show sinus histiocytosis and dense eosinophils infiltrate. Fibrosed capsules with capsulitis are always seen. A third of cases show necrotizing granulomas on the capsule, possibly as worm tracks. The hilum show dilated vessels, which may be scarred and inflamed.

Differential Diagnosis

Morphologically, *Brugia spp.* worms differ markedly from Dirofilaria and W. bancrofti, both of which have larger transverse girth and longitudinal length. Females are larger than males. Cuticles are smooth with no cuticular or external longitudinal ridges. The diameter of females range from 50 to 120 μm, and the male diameters are generally 35 to 55 μm at mid-body. Reproductive tubes may show eggs or sperms.

Treatment

Complaints and symptoms are result of an inflammatory reaction adjacent to dead or dying worm and may present as a painful or inflamed node. In the absence of systemic symptoms or microfilaremia, treatment is generally not required.

Loa Loa Lymphadenitis

Loa loa is one of the first nematode studied and first described by Mongin in 1770.

Definition

Loa loa is a filarial nematode that infects human and some other primates in West and Central Africa. Loiasis is the disease caused by Loa loa.

Synonyms

Calabar swelling, eyeworm, fugitive swelling, loasis.

Clinical Aspects

"Calabar swelling" is characterized by recurrent swelling of hand, wrist, and forearm caused by migrating worms lasting about 3 days. Eosinophilia or eye involvement is common.

Incidence

The Armed Forces Institute of Pathology/WHO collaborating center had records of 2650 patients, and 168 (6%) of these patients have loiasis (Paleologo, Neafie, and Connor, 1984).

Approach to Diagnosis

The diagnosis of loiasis was established by demonstrating microfilariae of *L. loa* in the blood, tissues, or both, or by finding adult worms in tissue sections in each patients. Of 168 patients with loiasis, there were 13 cases with lymphadenitis, 10 of which had worms visible microscopically. These nodes measured 2 to 5 cm.

Histology

The 10 nodes with distinctive microscopic features were characterized microscopically as follows: sinus histiocytosis with eosinophils and histiocytes and atrophic lymphoid follicles in most of the lymph nodes. There were fibrous thickened capsule and plasma cells with Russell bodies in parenchyma. There were no granulomas, necrosis, or endothelial cell proliferation or eosinophilic abscess identified. Microfilariae of *L. loa* were seen in the nodes of each of the 10 patients. These worms were inside the vessels, and in trabecular, subcapsular, and septal sinuses.

TABLE 20.3 Histopathologic Features of Loa Loa Lymphadenitis

Major features
Distension of subcapsular and medullary sinuses by histiocytes and eosinophils
Atrophy of lymphoid follicles
Microfilaria in tissue
Minor features
Fibrous thickening of capsules/trabeculae
Dilatation of lymphatic vessels of the capsule and medulla
Prominent collections of mast cells, plasma cells, and Russell bodies in lymphoid tissues, capsule, and trabeculae

Source: Paleologo, Neafie, and Connor, (1984).

The microfilariae were quite small when compared with other types of microfilariae: these were 5 μm wide and has a clear cephalic space 5 μm long. (See Table 20.3.)

Tropical (Filarial) Eosinophilia Diagnosed by Tissue Biopsy

Tropical pulmonary eosinophilia is also known as Weingartner's syndrome. It is believed to be a form of "occult filariasis" because these patients do not demonstrate a microfilaremia on blood smear (Webb, Job, and Gault, 1960).

Definition
Weingartner's syndrome is characterized by cough, wheezing, hypereosinophilia, and pulmonary infiltrates. Many patients show impaired lung function with reduction of vital capacity, total lung function, and residual volume.

Pathogenesis
There is an IgE-mediated hypesensitivity to microfilariae in tropical pulmonary eosinophilia. Both IgE and eosinophils may be secondary to secretion of IL-4 and IL-5, respectively, by filaria-specific TH2 helper T cells (Vijayan, 2007)

Diagnosis
A constant and characteristic feature is peripheral blood hypereosinophilia (3000–50,000 cells/mm^3) in the presence of circulating filarial antibodies. A filarial origin can be diagnosed histopathologically when lymph node and other biopsies show trapped microfilariae. The previously described histology of lymph nodes in different types of microfilariae may guide in determining the subtype of filariasis.

Morphology
Lung biopsy specimens show eosinophilic bronchitis and bronchopneumonia, with multiple small granulomas and areas of necrosis (eosinophilic microabscesses). Foreign body giant cells are common, forming tubercle-like nodules. While intact microfilariae are not generally seen, there may be fragments in the granulomata. The eosinophilic debris, in the form of Splendore–Hoeppli material, implicates helminthic infection.

SCHISTOSOMIASIS

After malaria, schistosomiasis is the second most prevalent tropical disease in the world. Despite the high prevalence, it received less attention and is considered a neglected tropical disease.

Synonym
Bilharziasis.

Epidemiology
Recent World Health Organization reports estimated that 500 to 600 million people in 74 tropical and subtropical countries were at risk for schistosomiasis. More than 200 million people in these countries were infected. Of these, 120 million were symptomatic, and 20 million have severe clinical disease. In the United States 400,000 cases were seen exclusively in immigrants (Fenwick, Rollinson, and Southgate, 2006).

Etiology
The main forms of human schistosomiasis are caused by 5 species of flatworm in the genus Schistosoma: *Schistosoma hematobium, Schistosoma mansoni, Schistosoma japonicum, Schistosoma intercalatum, and Schistosoma mekongi*. The worms also are called blood flukes because they live in the vascular system. *S. hematobium* further causes urinary and bladder pathology. *S. mansoni* and *S. japonicum* cause an intestinal form schistosomiasis. The ova differs among species: *S. hematobium* and *intercalatum* have a terminal spine, *S. mansoni* and *mekongi* have a lateral spine, and *S. japonicum* has no spine.

Pathogenesis
The pathology derives from immune response against the schistosome eggs or direct invasion of worms. Skin invasion of cercariae produces hypersensitivity dermatitis. Cercariae are transported through blood or lymphatics and cause fever, cough, and eosinophilia. Antigens released from the eggs

stimulate a granulomatous reaction comprised of T cells, macrophages, and eosinophils that result in clinical disease. A delayed type of hypersensitivity granuloma is the pathogenesis (Doughty et al., 1984).

Katayama fever is a form of schistosomiasis believed to be due to the excessive parasitic antigen stimuli resulting in immune complex formation and a serum sickness-like illness. It occurs 4 to 6 weeks after infection and is usually associated with *S. japonicum or S. mansoni*.

Diagnosis

Characteristic schistosoma eggs could be found in feces, urine, as well as in tissue sections. See Table 20.4 for diagnostic features.

Lymph Node Pathology

Early stages cause sinus histiocytosis and capsular fibrosis. Later on, the ova incites parenchymal

TABLE 20.4 Key Diagnostic Features of Schistosomiasis

Etiology *Schistosoma hematobium, Schistosoma mansoni, Schistosoma japonicum, Schistosoma intercalatum*, and *Schistosoma mekongi*
Regions Worldwide
Transmission Freshwater snail
Population at risk Persons at risk include those who live or travel in areas where schistosomiasis occurs
Organs involved Skin lymph nodes bladder, gastroenteric region
Lymph Node pathology Granulomas, fibrosis, eggs
Differential Diagnosis Leishmaniasis, malaria, typhoid fever, hepatitis
Diagnosis Microscopic appearance of the egg allows diagnostic differentiation of the 5 species identified in urine or stool; also by rectal biopsy or bladder mucosal biopsy
Unsual feature Katayama fever

TABLE 20.5 Causes of Palisading Granulomas

Palisading Granulomatous Pattern
Nontuberculous mycobacteriosis
Cat-scratch disease
Phaeohyphomycosis
Sporotrichosis,
Cryptococcosis
Coccidioidomycosis
Syphilis
Brucellosis
Foreign body granulomatous reactions
Post-surgical necrobiotic granulomas
Churg–strauss granulomatous disease
Wegener's granulomatosis

fibrosis and granulomatous response with histiocytic and eosinophilic collections (Sharaf, Nada, and Eldosoky, 2008). Splendore–Hoeppli phenomenon can be seen around the ova as pink proteinaceous necrotic response. Frank fibrous tissue may surround the ova, which are progressively degenerated in chronic infections (Doenhoff, 1997).

Treatment

Praziquantel is the treatment of choice for all species of schistosomiasis. Combination of artemether and praziquantel show effective results.

LEISHMANIASIS

Leishmaniases can be divided into visceral leishmaniasis (VL) and cutaneous leishmaniasis (CL) (Kolaczinski et al., 2007; Reithinger et al., 2007).

Definition

Kala-azar or visceral leishmaniasis is a chronic systemic disease characterized by fever, splenomegaly, lymphadenopathy, pancytopenia, and with a fatal course if untreated. Cutaneous leishmaniasis is generally nonfatal and is characterized by a relatively benign disease that is limited to the skin and may spontaneously resolve (Reithinger et al., 2007) (see Figure 20.7).

ICD-10 Code B55

Synonyms

Leishmania; Delhi, Baghdad, or Jericho boil; Aleppo boil; Bouton de Cretem; Biytib d'orient; little

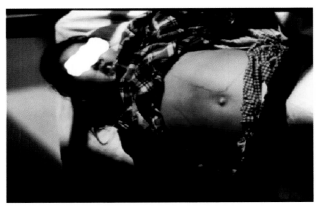

FIGURE 20.7 **Kala-azar in a Nepalese child**. The child's massive hepatosplenomegaly is outlined on abdomen.

sister; Chiclero ulcer, Biskra button; kala-azar; espundia; Dum-Dum fever; Pian bois; Uta; Mucocutaneous Espundia.

Epidemiology

Leishmaniasis occurs worldwide, in tropical and subtropical regions, including the Middle East, India, Africa, China, and central and southern America, altogether described in 88 countries. Leishmaniasis directly affects 1.5 to 2 million patients per year, up to 51,000 deaths, and more than 350 million persons are at risk worldwide (Reithinger, 2008).

About 90% of Kala-azar cases are reported in Bangladesh, Brazil, Ethiopia, India, Nepal, and Sudan, while 90% of cutaneous forms occur in Afghanistan, Algeria, Brazil, Pakistan, Peru, Saudi Arabia, and Syria.

Three distinct reservoir patterns are described: canine, rodent, and human reservoir. In the United States and Europe, Leishmaniasis is an emerging disease found in canines (Petersen 2009a, b; Rosypal et al., 2003). The dog is the primary peridomestic reservoir of the infection and phlebotomine sandflies are the only confirmed vector (Capelli et al., 2004; Gravino, 2004). In Africa, rodents are the reservoir of *L. donovani*. Human-reservoir epidemics caused by *P. argentipes*, a sandfly with predilection for humans are prevalent in India, Bangladesh, and Burma. In addition transmission via needle sharing from patients with human immunodeficiency virus (HIV) is reported as an important cause of human to human nonvector transmission (Magill, 1995). Occupational travel exposure is a recognized risk factor shown in veterans of Desert Storm coming back to their country infected by viscerotropic *L. tropica* during their deployment in endemic areas of the Middle East (Magill et al., 1994).

Etiology

Leishmaniasis is a disease with complex range of presentations from cutaneous to disseminated forms caused by protozoa of genus Leishmania, transmitted largely by sandfly, *Phlebotomus spp*. The phlebotomine sandfly, a tiny 2- to 3-mm long weakly flying insect transmits the protozoa. Several vectors are described: *P. perniciousus* and *ariasi* in western Europe, *P. chinensis* in China, *P. papatasi* in the Middle East (also called *P. infantum* since the disease is most common among very young children).

About 24 Leishmania species are pathogenic for humans. Each species can cause a variety of clinical manifestations, and each form of disease can be caused by equally varied species. Two subgenera

are generally recognized from the genus Leishmania: Leismania sensu stricto and Viannia, restricted to the New World. Genomic identification is by DNA hybridization and phenotypic identification is by isoenzyme electrophoresis called zymodeme pattern. (Lopes et al., 1984).

Pathogenesis

The variability of the diseases is secondary to both the species diversity and the response of the infected host. *L. donovani* and *L. infantum* or *chagasi* can cause fatal disease. These species are more viscerotropic than *L. brazilienses* and *L. panamensis*, which are more dermotropic. However, in patients with immune deficiency, these dermotropic species cause viscerotropism. Localized cutaneous leishmaniasis is characterized by active immune response, an early development of skin test positivity, and a T helper-1 phenotype response (Melby et al., 1994). The diffuse cutaneous form is characterized by a T helper-2 dominant response (Pirmez et al., 1993), and the visceral form, a lack of effective response or anergy. These patients characteristically lack host cell-mediated specific response to Leishmania antigens and a weak T-cell function. The Leishmania skin test is often negative unlike the dermotropic leismaniasis.

Leishmani spp. have a dual life cycle: an amastigote or Leishman–Donovan stage, which are intracellular in the host and the promastigotes cycle. In the sandfly, the parasite contains flagellae, called "promastigotes." The inoculation of promastigotes in the host with vector saliva enhances contagion by vasodilation, immunosuppression, and anticoagulation. The promastigote coat of the lipophosphoglycan contributes to the microorganisms' escape from complement lysis, and hence intact organisms are ingested by macrophages. The amastigote is an oval 2 to 6 μm protozoa with a nucleus and a kinetoplast identifiable by Giemsa stain. Amastigotes divide and multiple inside the parasitophorous vacuoles of macrophages, eventually causing rupture and release. These organisms have high tropism for the mononuclear-phagocytic system, causing diseases found in liver, spleen, bone marrow, and the lymph nodes as well as in extralymphatic areas rich in antigen-presenting cells like the skin.

The outcome of infection depends on the Th1 or Th2 response, where the Th1 cells secretes IFN-gamma and IL-2 interleukins, and the Th2 response cells produce IL-4-5 and IL-10. These two response types are counter-responsive to each other and both are modulated by the microorganisms (Gravino, 2004). Interleukin-12, a Th1 shift promoter, is actively inhibited by the organism (Carrera et al., 1996). Similar Th1 and Th2 yin-yang-like patterns have been described in lymphadenopathy phases secondary to American cutaneous leishmaniasis (Bomfim et al., 2007).

Clinical Aspects

In addition to the two clinical forms a third form is suggested as a localized lymphadenopathic form with or without cutaneous symptoms.

Kala-azar or Visceral Form. The incubation period is generally 2 to 6 months, but earlier and later presentations have been described. Fever heralds the acute infection, which may be intermittent and could also persists in the chronic form. The chronic classic form shows a patient with protruberant abdomen with enlarged spleen and liver and wasting and may be obtunded. The classic clinical triad is: fever, anemia, and splenomegaly (see Figure 20.7).

Lymphadenopathy has been described as about 5% in Iran (Azadeh, 1985) but much higher upward of 90% in Sudan, Kenya, and African patients (Babiker et al., 2007).

Cutaneous Disease. Two types are described: ulcerative and dry type (see Figures 20.8, 20.9). The ulcerative type is the most common, and shows as a volcano-like wet lesion covered with scab. This is the form that has earned several names such as oriental boils and chichero's ulcer. The dry type shows an elevated dry plaque often with satellite or daughter papules. The mucocutaneous form, also called espundia, is caused by *L. braziliensis*. This leads to the involvement of oral, buccal, and the nasal mucosae with a complication of nasal septum perforation.

Localized Leishmania Lymphadenopathy. The pattern is mixed, with histiocytic collections, necrotic macrophages, and epithelioid granulomatas (Azadeh, 1985). Three patterns are seen, in order of frequency:

1. Histiocytic necrotizing granulomas with microorganism in granulomas and subcapsular areas.
2. Follicular hyperplasia and microgranulomatas. Prominent macrophages present as tingible bodies in germinal centers showing clusters of amastigotes as Leishmania–Donovan bodies.
3. Sarcoidal type dry granulomas with no necrosis and no microorganisms.

Cutaneous Leishmania with Lymphadeno-pathy. In South America, cutaneous infections are also associated with a higher frequency of

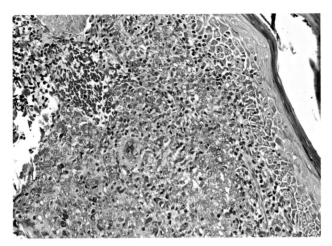

FIGURE 20.8 **Cutaneous leishmania infection**. Giemsa stained with sheets of basophilic histiocytes shows these to be laden with intracellular organisms. (Courtesy of Dr. Wun-Ju Shieh and Dr. Sherif Zaki, Infectious Diseases Pathology Branch, Centers for Disease Control and Prevention.)

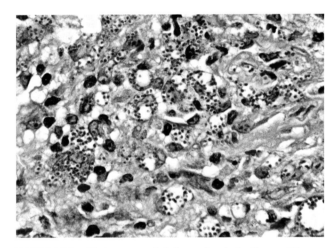

FIGURE 20.9 **Cutaneous leishmania infection**. Giemsa stained with histiocytes show these to be laden with intracellular Giemsa-positive leishmania-donovan bodies. (Courtesy of Dr. Wun-Ju Shieh and Dr. Sherif Zaki, Infectious Diseases Pathology Branch, Centers for Disease Control and Prevention.)

lymphadenopathy. Thirty-six cases of untreated cutaneous form showed 67% lymphadenopathy (Barral et al., 1992). The cultures from excised lymph nodes were positive for promastigotes in 62%, with most of the isolates identified as *L. braziliensis*. Lymphadenopathy presented with either persistently enlarged lymph nodes or transitory lymphadenopathy (Barral et al., 1995).

Approach to Diagnosis

Leishmania disease is classically diagnosed by demonstrating parasites in smears from spleen, bone marrow, lymph nodes, or liver biopsy specimens. Skin biopsy and blood may show organisms sometimes by Giemsa stain in tissue or on a buffy coat. In histologically equivocal cases, a polymerase chain reaction (PCR) for leishmania-specific DNA is useful (Harms et al. 2005).

Lymph Node Morphology. A depletion of small lymphocytes, along with plasmacytosis and histiocytosis, can be seen in the paracortical areas of the lymph nodes. A granulomatous response may be seen, resembling sarcoidosis, along with the presence of epithelioid and multinucleated giant cells. Identification of Leishmania–Donovan bodies provides the most reliable diagnostic approach (Veress et al., 1977; Veress, Malik, and el-Hassan, 1974).

As in the lymph nodes, the spleen and extranodal tissue may show histiocytes with leishmania organisms. Splenic involvement by visceral leishmania causes massive splenomegaly as well as hepatomegaly. Microscopically the red pulp is expanded with numerous macrophages and the white pulp tends to be a atropic. Histiocytes with pink granular cytoplasm filled with intracytoplasmic bodies or Donovan bodies are easily seen. Wright–Giemsa imprints on oil magnification will show the teardrop-shaped microorganisms with a central kinetoplast and a pale blue cytoplasm. These are negative for PAS, Grocott, or GMS stains. Routine H&E stains will show the microorganisms to be basophilic. Both plasmacytic and lymphocytic reactions are prominent, and occasional granulomas may be seen.

In tissue Giemsa stain reveals Leishmania–Donovan bodies better than H&E. In the skin, sheets of basophilic histiocytes in the dermis show Giemsa-positive Leishmania–Donoval bodies as intracellular blue bodies (see Figures 20.8, and 20.9).

A fine needle aspirate for a diagnosis of leishmania was successfully used in Nepal and Iran (Kumar et al., 2001). However, a microscopic demonstration of the parasites proved to be highly specific, and correlated with histopathology (Sah, Prasad, and Raj, 2005), this may be a better diagnostic than bone marrow aspiration (Zijlstra and el-Hassan, 2001).

Differential Diagnosis

In contrast to infections with Toxoplasma, the microorganisms are readily seen and numerous. Unlike Histoplasma, with which they are often confused, these microorganisms are smaller and lack reactivity with most special stains for fungi. The

TABLE 20.6 **Mixed Pattern with Non-necrotizing Granulomas**

Non-necrotizing Granulomatous Pattern
Tuberculoid leprosy
Lepromatous leprosy
Leishmaniasis
Sarcoidal granulomas

granulomatous response raise several differential diagnosis. (See Table 20.6.)

Treatment of Choice and Prognosis. Untreated Kala-azar is fatal in 90% of the cases, but treatment generally leads to a cure. Treatment with antimony-containing drugs and Amphotericin B, or a topical application with an antimony-based ointment, has proved successful. Spontaneous cure albeit with a depressed scar is the rule in cutaneous lesions, but reactivation occurs in about 10% of the cases.

Other Information. *Leishmania tropicana* caused viscerotropic disease in servicemen in the Desert Storm conflict. In the case of imported cutaneous leishmaniasis, Latin America is the common source of infection (Schwartz, Hatz, and Blum, 2006).

MIXED PATTERN WITH GRANULOMAS AND FOAMY MACROPHAGES

Leprosy

Leprosy is primarily a granulomatous disease affecting peripheral nerves, mucosa, skin, and lymph nodes. The disease may take a lepromatous or tuberculoid form.

ICD-10 Code A30

BOX 20.1 **Leprosy: Historical Vignette**

Leprosy

Humanity has been afflicted by leprosy, or Hansen's disease, for over 4000 years. In Old Jerusalem, the earliest human to have leprosy was discovered based on DNA taken from the shrouded remains. Since then, the World Health Organization (WHO), estimated in 1995 that between 2 and 3 million people are still suffering from this infection. Many leper colonies still remain around the world in countries such as India (where there are still more than 1000 leper colonies), China, Romania, Egypt, Nepal, Somalia, Liberia, Vietnam, and Japan. Unlike the reputation in olden times, now we know that the bacteria is not highly infectious after treatment. About 95% of people are naturally immune, and patients are noncommunicable after 2 weeks of treatment. Adversely, about 5% of the world's population is susceptible to the disease. Venezuelan Dr. Jacinto Convit synthesized a vaccine for *Mycobacterium leprae*, a feat that earned him a nomination for the 1988 Nobel prize in medicine.

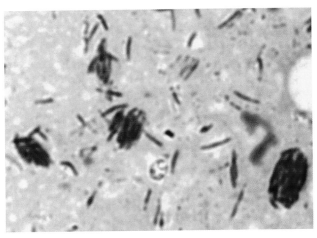

FIGURE 20.10 **Mycobacterium leprae**. The Ziehl–Neelsen staining of skin smears was from a patient with cutaneous leprae showing pink, acid-fast bacilli. (Courtesy of Dr. Rito Zerpa Larrauri, Servicio de Microbiologia, Int Nac de Salud del Ni no, Lima, Peru.)

Definition

The lepromatous form commonly involves lymph nodes, and has a worse prognosis compared to the tuberculoid form.

Synonyms

Hansen's disease, elephantiasis graecorum.

Epidemiology

Hansen's disease is worldwide in distribution. The disease is endemic in 91 countries with a high prevalence in Brazil, India, Nepal, some parts of Africa (Tanzania, Madagascar, Mozambique), and the western Pacific. In some parts of southern India the infection rates for lepromatous leprosy vary up to 55.8 per 1000 a year. (Noordeen & Neelan, 1978) In the United States the Centers for Disease Control and Prevention reported a total of 92 cases in 2002.

Etiology

Mycobacterium leprae and *Mycobacterium lepromatosis* are the causative agents of leprosy. *M. lepromatosis* is a relatively newly identified mycobacterium that was isolated from a fatal case of diffuse lepromatous leprosy in 2008. An intracellular, acid-fast bacterium, *M. leprae* are aerobic, rod-shaped, and posses a cell membrane characteristic of the Mycobacterium species (Figure 20.10).

Pathogenesis

Persons with low immunity are predisposed to infection. A Th1 response characterizes tuberculoid, and a Th2 response are the lepromatous form. The skin and the upper respiratory tract are the most likely portals of entry.

Clinical aspects

The two clinical types show overlapping features. The tuberculoid type rarely involves lymph nodes and manifests in patients with immunity. The lepromatous type shows the common lymph node involvement and is seen in immunocompromised patients. The lepromin test is negative for the lepromatous form.

Morphology. In lepromatous leprosy the lymph nodes show a sinus pattern (see Figure 20.10 and Figure 20.11). In low-power view, there are seen sinus histiocytosis and sheets of foamy histiocytes. The architecture is preserved and there is no necrotizing focus. In the florid disease, the lymph nodes or spleen show mononuclear or multinuclear phagocytic vacuolated histiocytes. Bluish rounded bodies known as Globi are visible, representing clumps of lepromatous organisms. Cells containing these vacuoles or Globi are known as Leprae cells.

Tuberculoid. The nonnecrotizing granulomas resemble sarcoidosis but with discrete epithelioid giant cells without necrosis. The acid-fast bacilli are rarely revealed by cytochemistry, and in suspected cases, a lepromin skin test may be done to confirm diagnosis.

Cytochemistry. Staining with Wade–Fite or the Ziehl–Neelsen technique will show clumps or globi with a large number of acid-fast bacilli (Figure 20.10).

Differential Diagnosis

Silicone lymphadenopathy presents as foamy vacuolated histiocytes and at low power is

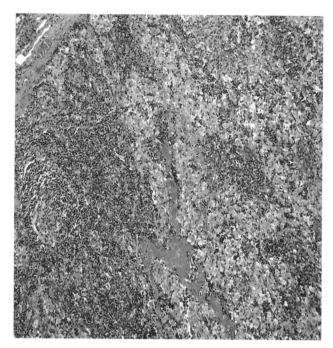

FIGURE 20.11 **Lymph node with sheets of foamy vacuolated to clear histiocytes**. Lepromatous leprosy imparts this sinus pattern in the lymph node.

morphologically similar to leprosy. Staining with Wade–Fite or Ziehl–Neelsen technic should show vacuoles with large number of acid-fast bacilli in leprosy. (See Tables 20.6 and 20.10 for the differential diagnosis.)

Treatment

A multidrug therapy, introduced in the early 1980s, has treated the disease successfully. The treatment consists of rifampicin, dapsone, and clofazimine taken over 12 months.

MIXED PATTERN WITH DEPOSITION OF INTERSTITIAL SUBSTANCE

Pneumocystiis jiroveci Lymphadenitis

Pneumocystis pneumonia (PCP) or pneumocystosis is a form of pneumonia, caused by the yeast-like fungus called *Pneumocystis jirovecii*. This pathogen is specific to humans; it has not been shown to infect other animals, while other species of Pneumocystis that parasitize other animals have not been shown to infect humans. Pneumocystis is commonly found in the lungs of healthy people, but being a source of opportunistic infection it can cause a lung infection in people with a weak immune system. Pneumocystis pneumonia is especially seen in people with cancer and HIV/AIDS, and in people who use medications that affect the immune system.

Definition

Pneumocystis jiroveci lymphadenitis is infection of the lymph nodes characterized by deposition of amorphous interstial substance.

ICD-10 Code B20.6

Synonyms

Pneumocystis jirovecii formerly *Pneumocystis carinii*.

Epidemiology

Pneumocystis jirovecii infection is prevalent in developing countries, specifically in the inner city populations, in malnourished children. Pneumocystis pneumonia occurs in immunosuppressed individuals and in premature and malnourished infants.

Etiology

Pneumocystis jirovecii was previously classified as *Pneumocystis carinii*. It was previously classified as a protozoa. Currently it is considered a fungus based on a nucleic acid and biochemical analysis. It is the most common opportunistic infection associated with AIDS and is the first indication of an HIV infection.

Pathogenesis

The risk of pneumonia due to *Pneumocystis jirovecii* increases when CD4-positive cell levels are less than 200 cells/μl. In immunosuppressed individuals the manifestations of the infection are highly variable. The disease attacks the interstitial, fibrous tissue of the lungs, with marked thickening of the alveolar septa and alveoli, leading to significant hypoxia. This can be fatal if not treated aggressively, since LDH levels increase and gas exchange is compromised. Oxygen is less able to diffuse into the blood, leading to hypoxia. Hypoxia, along with high arterial carbon dioxide (CO_2) levels, stimulates ventilation, thereby causing dyspnea.

Clinical Aspects

Symptoms of PCP include fever, shortness of breath (especially on exertion), weight loss, and night sweats. The fungus can invade other visceral organs, such as the liver, spleen, and kidney, but only in a minority of cases.

Sites of Involvement. In addition to the lungs, the organism affects the lymph nodes, spleen, liver, and bone marrow. The symptoms of Pneumocystis pneumonia (PCP) include dyspnea and nonproductive cough, and fever. The nonproductive cough is due to sputum that is too viscous to become productive. There is usually not a large amount of sputum with PCP unless the patient has an additional bacterial infection. Chest radiography demonstrates bilateral infiltrates. Extrapulmonary lesions occur in a minority of patients, involving most frequently the lymph nodes, spleen, liver, and bone marrow.

Approach to Diagnosis

The diagnosis can be confirmed by the characteristic appearance of the chest X ray which shows widespread pulmonary infiltrates, and an arterial oxygen level (pO$_2$) strikingly lower than would be expected from symptoms. The diagnosis can be definitively confirmed by histological identification of the causative organism in sputum or bronchio-alveolar lavage (lung rinse).

Laboratory Diagnosis

Staining with toluidine blue, silver stain, or periodic-acid-Schiff or immunofluorescence assay, will show characteristic cysts. The cysts resemble crushed ping-pong balls and are present in aggregates of 2 to 8 (not to be confused with Histoplasma or Cryptococcus, which typically do not form aggregates of spores or cells). A lung biopsy would show thickened alveolar septa with fluffy eosinophilic exudate in the alveoli. Both the thickened septa and the fluffy exudate contribute to dysfunctional diffusion capacity, which is characteristic of this pneumonia.

Pneumocystis infection can also be diagnosed by immunofluorescent or histochemical staining of the specimen, and more recently by molecular analysis of polymerase chain reaction products comparing DNA samples. Notably simple molecular detection of *Pneumocystis jirovecii* in lung fluids does not mean that a person has Pneumocystis pneumonia or infection by HIV. The fungus appears to be present in healthy individuals also in the general population.

The specific diagnosis is based on identification of *P. jirovecii* in bronchopulmonary secretions obtained as induced sputum or bronchoalveolar lavage material. In situations where these two techniques cannot be used, transbronchial biopsy or open lung biopsy may prove necessary. Microscopic identification of *P. jiroveci* trophozoites and cysts is performed with stains that demonstrate either the nuclei of trophozoites and intracystic stages (e.g., Giemsa) or the cyst walls (e.g., silver stains). In addition immunofluorescence microscopy using monoclonal antibodies can identify the organisms with higher sensitivity than conventional microscopy.

Lymphadenopathy

Lymph nodes, commonly of the mediastinal and retroperitoneal nodes, are enlarged and show irregular shaped creamy and yellowish necrotic areas. Microscopically, such areas consists of necrotic tissues that are characterized as eosinophilis, periodic-acid-Schiff-positive, fibrinous foamy exudate. Epitheliod cells and multi-nucleated grant cells may be present in some organs as the periphery of necrotic areas. The lymphadenopathy is unusual with large amount of PAS-positive fibrinous foamy exudate forming nodules in between residual lymphocytes and histiocytes.

Differential Diagnosis

The organism affects humans and can be found in individuals with no previous clinical or history of infection. The Pneumocystis organism may be inactive for a long time but turn active as soon as the individual become immunocompromised. Cellular immunity can keep the organism under control or latent. Recent studies show that even healthy individuals can be carriers. (See Table 20.10 for patterns of lymph node reactions.)

Treatment of Choice and Prognosis

Typically, in untreated PCP, increasing pulmonary involvement leads to death. Pneumothorax is a well-known complication of PCP. An acute history of chest pain with breathlessness and diminished breath sounds is typical of pneumothorax.

Antipneumocystic medication is used with concomitant steroids in order to avoid inflammation, which causes an exacerbation of symptoms about 4 days after treatment begins if steroids are not used. The most commonly used medication is co-trimoxazole, but some patients are unable to tolerate this treatment due to allergies. Other medications that are used, alone or in combination, include pentamidine, trimetrexate, dapsone, atovaquone, primaquine, pafuramidine meleate (under investigation), and clindamycin. Treatment is usually for a period of about 21 days. Pentamidine is less often used as its major limitation is the high frequency of side effects. These include acute pancreatitis, renal failure, hepatotoxicity, leukopenia, rash, fever, and hypoglycaemia. In immunocompromised patients, prophylaxis with Bactrim or regular pentamidine inhalations may help prevent PCP.

MIXED PATTERN WITH CASEATION NECROSIS

Mycobacteria tuberculosis, BCG Lymphadenitis, and Systemic Fungal Lymphadenitis

Mycobacterium tuberculosis lymphadenitis is the second leading cause of death from communicable disease worldwide, next to HIV. *M.* tuberculosis was described by Koch in 1882 for which he received the 1905 Nobel Prize in Medicine for this discovery. The other mycobacteria are collectively known as MOTTS (mycobacteria other than tuberculosis) and some can cause opportunistic infections in immunocompromized people and those with AIDS. *M. tuberculosis* is an obligate human pathogen that has a relatively high requirement for oxygen, hence it usually inhabits the lungs.

Definition

Lymph node infection with characteristic caseating granulomatous pattern and presence of the acid-fast bacillus, *Mycobacterium tuberculosis*. (See Table 20.7.)

ICD-10 Code A18.2

Synonyms

Pott's disease, the white plague, Koch's bacillus, tubercle bacillus, consumption.

Epidemiology

It is estimated that about 30% of the world's inhabitants test positive for MTB and about 10% develop the disease. An estimated 13% developed tuberculous lymphadenitis in a Canadian study (Cook, Manfreda, and Hershfield, 2004). The typical background was a young female of western Pacific origin. The incidence of TB has been declining in western Europe and North America, but emigration from high-incidence areas such as sub-Saharan Africa, western Pacific, and Asia has been reversing this trend.

TABLE 20.7 **Mixed Pattern with Caseating Granulomas**

Caseating Necrotizing Granulomatous Pattern
Mycobacteria
Systemic fungal lymphadenitis

Clinical Aspects

Etiology. Most of the etiology of TB lymphadenitis is from the *Mycobacterium tuberculosis* with rare instances of *Mycobacterium bovis*. This pattern is attributed to the pasteurization of milk, but in areas and among ethnic groups where pasteurization of milk is less practiced, the incidence of lymphadenitis from *M. bovis* is high. In addition coinfection with HIV is high in countries with high prevalence of MTB. In cases of coinfection, extrapulmonary MTB is higher in incidence. The most common extrapulmonary site is the lymph node.

Sites of Involvement. Most cases involve a single lymph node site. Most common is a cervical location followed by supraclavicular lymph nodes. In patients with multiple sites, coexistent lung TB only accounted for 8% (Cook, Manfreda, and Hershfield, 2004).

Symptoms. The symptoms of tuberculosis were well known in the eighteenth and nineteenth century when the disease claimed many lives. Bloody sputum, fever, cough, and weight loss were the classic picture of "consumption." Swelling and pain were the most common presenting symptoms of TB lymphadenitis with ulceration and fistulous drainage in a few cases.

Pathophysiology. MTB rapidly invade lung macrophages where they are protected from phagosomal digestion by their mycolic acid coating. They replicate slowly and steadily, forming persistent granulomas that can last for years.

Diagnosis. Chest X rays of patients with active tuberculosis reveal characteristic lucent cavities with opaque nodular or fibrotic areas. Old cases of TB may leave fibrotic scars or calcified nodules usually in the upper lobes. Miliary TB can manifest with many small nodules (1–2 mm) throughout the parenchyma. Pleural effusions may also be seen. Tuberculin skin testing is a simple and common method for detecting old or latent TB infections, although it is not very sensitive. Prior vaccination with BCG can cause a positive reaction. The size of the induration is the clinical determinant considered together with other factors, such as presence of HIV infection, silicosis, immunosuppression, immigration from a high-risk country, contact with known TB patients, or diagnosis of diabetes or cancer.

Laboratory Findings. Examination of stained sputum samples is the usual lab method for MTB diagnosis. The mycobacteria all take up the

Ziehl–Neelsen acid-fast stain, but MTB has a waxy envelope made up of mycolic acid that prevents it from staining with Gram's. MTB stained with Ziehl–Neelsen are red. Several specimens should be examined because the bacteria may be present in low numbers. They may be cultured from sputum, but their slow growth rate makes this a relatively long process. Rapid identification by PCR, however, can give results in 24 hours (Figures 20.12, 20.13).

Morphology. The classic lymph node histopathology is a caseating granuloma with multinucleated Langhans type giant cells (Figure 20.13).

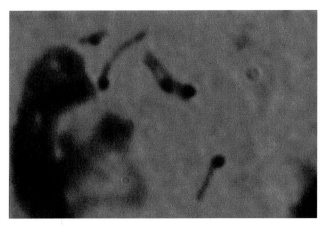

FIGURE 20.12 AFB bacilli in smear stained with Ziehl–Neelsen. (Courtesy of Dr. Rito Zerpa Larrauri, Servicio de Microbiologia, Int Nac de Salud del Ni no, Lima, Peru.)

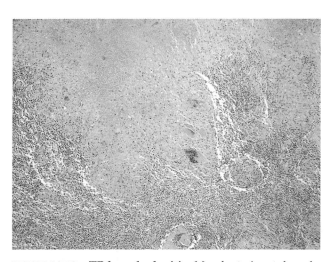

FIGURE 20.13 **TB lymphadenitis**. *Mycobacterium tuberculosis lymphadenitis* shows a classic caseating tubercle with necrosis and multinucleated Langhans-type giant cells. (Courtesy of Drs. Shieh and Zaki.)

Differential Diagnosis

Fungal lymphadenitis could show caseating granulomas and should be considered and appropriate culture and cytochemical studies performed. Specific PCR on sputum samples can reveal the presence of different species of bacteria. (See Tables 20.7 and 20.8 for lists of diseases to consider.) See

TABLE 20.8 Mixed Pattern with Suppurative Granulomas

Cat scratch (*Bartonella henselae*)
Tularemia *Francisella tularensis*
Lymphogranuloma venereum (*Chlamydia trachomatis*)
Chancroid (*H. ducreyi*)
Yersiniosis (*Yersinia enterocolitica/pseudotuberculosis*)
Brucellosis lymphadenitis
Melioidosis(*Burkholderia pseudomallei*)
Typhoid lymphadenitis (*Salmonella typhi*)
Fungal and mycobacterial granulomas

TABLE 20.9 Mixed Pattern with Hemorrhage

Hemorrhagic Pattern
Anthrax
Rocky Mountain spotted fever

TABLE 20.10 Mixed Patterns with Other Changes

Mixed pattern with follicular hyperplasia, granulomas, and histiocytosis
• *Visceral Leishmaniasis,*
Mixed pattern with follicular hyperplasia, microgranulomas, and monocytoid cells
• Toxoplasmosis
Mixed pattern with sinus pattern, foamy histiocytes, and foreign body-type giant cells
• Whipple's disease (*Tropheryma whippelii*)
• Lepromatous Leprosy
Mixed pattern with obscured follicles and diffuse paracortical areas
• Cytomegalovirus
• Epstein–Barr virus
• Measles
Mixed pattern with follicular hyperplasia, plasmacytosis, and vasculitis
• Syphilis

Tables 20.9 and 20.10 for differential diagnosis using other types of mixed histologic patterns.

Treatment and Prognosis

Isoniazid given over a period of 6 to 12 months is the usual regimen for latent tuberculosis. If the infection is active, then rifampin, ethambutol or pyrazinamide may be added. Drug-resistant strains of TB are becoming more common, especially in AIDS patients, and identification of these is critical for an effective treatment regimen. New methods for determining drug resistance employ rapid DNA sequencing of those regions of the bacterial genome responsible for resistance. The presence of specific sequences tells the clinician that a certain drug would not be effective on that strain of TB and allows the clinician to choose a drug that will most likely destroy the bacteria.

MIXED PATTERN ATYPICAL MYCOBACTERIAL INFECTIONS IN AIDS

Immunocompromised, HIV-infected patients are susceptible to a variety of bacterial infections including those from mycobacteria, especially atypical species. The increased incidence of atypical, nontuberculous mycobacterial (NTM) infection stems in part from improvements in detection methods but primarily from the growing population of immunodeficient AIDS patients with low CD4+ T lymphocyte counts.

Definition

Atypical mycobacteria are opportunistic human pathogens that are normally kept in check by the healthy immune system. Immunodeficiency that occurs in HIV-AIDS patients may allow infections by the mycobacterium avium complex, the mycobacterium fortuitum complex, or other nontubercular species.

ICD-10 Code A31—infection with other mycobacteria (excluding leprosy and TB).

Synonyms

Nontuberculous mycobacterial infection, Lady Windermere syndrome, Buruli ulcer.

Epidemiology

Atypical mycobacteria are found in soil and water worldwide, and opportunistic infection is relatively common. The majority of NTM co-infections in AIDS patients are caused by bacteria of the *M. avium-intracellulaire* complex. There have been reports of a number of other mycobacterial species in AIDS patients, such as *M. ulcerans, M. abscessus, M. kansasii, M. xenopi, M. scrofulaceum, M. marinum,* and *M. gordonae.* Appropriate antibiotic treatment may be necessary to prevent such complications.

Defective host immunity is the major factor in mycobacterial infection. NTM infections are quite common in immunodeficient persons, and they range from mild and self-limiting to highly virulent and life threatening.

Mycobacteria are classified according to their growth rate and whether or not they are pigmented. The pigmented varieties such as *M. phlei* and *M. aurum* are rarely associated with human disease. Among the important nonpigmented types, the *M. fortuitum* complex, which includes *M. abscessum,* can cause severe disease in HIV/AIDS patients (Benwill 2010). *M. kansasii* can cause a serious disseminated infection that requires rapid and aggressive treatment. The *M. avium* complex is a commonly found agent in AIDS patients and in persons with other types of immunodeficiency, but improved recognition and aggressive treatment has reduced the morbidity and mortality associated with this infection.

M. ulcerans can cause a chronic skin disease called Buruli ulcer in which the bacteria secrete a compound that inhibits the antibacterial immune response, resulting in a persistent colonization of the tissues erupting as skin ulcers. *M. chelonae, M. kansasii,* and *M. xenopi* have all been associated with mycobacterial disease in immunodeficient individuals. In children, the *M. avium-intracellulaire* complex and *M. scrofulaceum* are typically seen.

Clinical Aspects

It is important to distinguish tuberculous mycobacterial infections from NTM infections because the treatment methods are different. Also early detection and identification of the mycobacterial species infecting an immunocompromised person is critical for initiating an appropriate antibiotic treatment regimen.

Sites of Involvement. NTM infection of immunocompromised persons results in lymphadenitis, but may also involve the lungs or cause skin abscesses. Lymphadenitis involving the nodes of the cervical chain is the usual observation in NTM infection but generalized lymphadenopathy can occur in disseminated disease.

HIV-infected children with low CD4+ T cell counts are especially prone to disseminated NTM infections, and they require quick identification and treatment. In addition to granulomatous lymphadenopathy, fever, diarrhea, leukopenia, and hepatosplenomegaly are also commonly seen. In HIV-infected children, failure to gain weight or thrive and chronic fatigue may be symptoms of NTM infection. Death from NTM infection is relatively rare, and infections can be successfully treated with the appropriate antibiotics when diagnosed early.

Highly aggressive antiretroviral therapy (HAART) can lead to a condition called immune reconstitution inflammatory syndrome, or IRIS, and infection with certain nontuberculous mycobacteria has been linked to IRIS. Testing HIV patients undergoing HAART for mycobacteria and prophylaxis with antibiotics might be effective in limiting IRIS.

Pathophysiology

Host immune defense is the most important factor in the pathophysiology of NTM infections and low CD4+ T cell count and weak IFN-g responsiveness are directly correlated with NTM disease. HIV-AIDS patients are the usual target for NTM infection, but there have been a number of reports of infections in subjects with mutations in the interferon gamma response pathway, suggesting that that IFN-g is a key component of the antimycobacterial defense system.

The route of NTM infection in immunocompromized individuals is commonly through the gut, but bacteria may also gain entry through the respiratory tract or as a result of surgery, injection, or trauma. Catheter-related infections have also been reported.

Lab Workup

Specimens of blood, purulent discharge, or stool may be cultured on selective media to identify NTMs and DNA. Sequence-specific probes can be used for identification by DNA hybridization or PCR amplification.

Morphology. Histology may show the presence of granulomas, and bone marrow aspirates may contain foam cells. The granulomas in NTM of immunocompromized persons are different morphologically from those with competent immunity. Unless undergoing immune reconstitution, the granulomas are vaguely formed, large nodules of a mixed inflammatory process with spindly or nonepithelioid histiocytes, sometimes with vascularized and angiomatoid pattern. In contrast, granulomas of immunocompetent patients tend to be well-formed discrete epithelioid granulomas with or without caseation necrosis (see Figures 20.14, 20.15). (See Tables 20.5, 20.6 and 20.12 for differential diagnosis.)

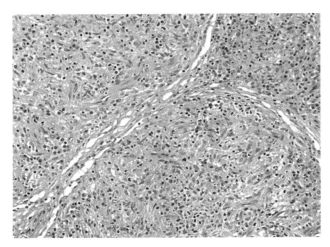

FIGURE 20.14 **Atypical mycobacteria with poorly formed granulomas and increased vascularity.**

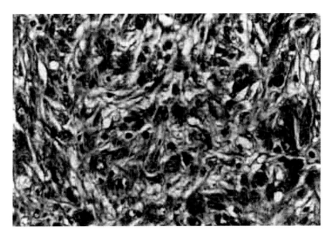

FIGURE 20.15 **Atypical mycobacteria with Ziehl–Neelsen AFB.**

Differential Diagnosis

Suppurative lymphadenitis may result from a number of different types of microbial infection and positive identification of atypical mycobacteria by culturing is still the gold standard for treatment. Malignancies should be ruled out as well as lymphadenitis of fungal origin (see Table 20.8). Non-HIV patients manifesting NTM disease should be tested for immunodeficiencies caused by mutations such as those in genes in the IFN-g response pathway.

Coccidiomycosis Lymphadenitis. The endemic areas include Mexico, the western US region, and parts of South America. This infection is a deep-seated fungal infection *Coccidioides immitis.* Lungs are primarily involved, but dissemination occurs in many other organs including lymph nodes.

Lymph node pathology characteristically results in granulomas, often with a central microcyst, giant cells, and spherules of *C. immitis*. Since the disease causes caseation necrosis, it is likely to be confused with tuberculosis. The spherules, also called "sporangia," are often seen within giant cells. The spherules are surrounded by a thick wall and closing endospores that appear granular (see Figure 20.17). Sometimes the granuloma is surrounded by eosinophilic material with a proteinaceous (concentric to irregular) contour, a phenomenon called

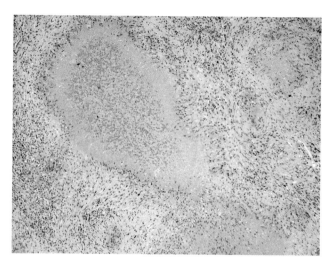

FIGURE 20.16 *Coccidiodis immitis* causing a palisaded caseating granulomatous inflammation (H&E, 50×). (Courtesy of Drs. Shieh and Zaki.)

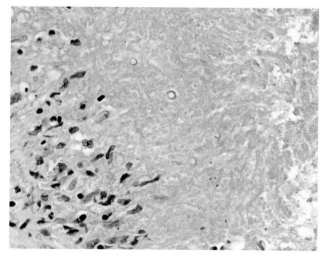

FIGURE 20.17 *Coccidiodis immitis* showing caseating granuloma with yeast forms (H&E, 400×). (Courtesy of Drs. Shieh and Zaki.)

"Splendore hoeppli" (see Figure 20.16). This characteristic is often observed in cases of sporotrichosis by another fungal infection. The surrounding organisms are characteristically a plasmacytic reaction, but neutrophilic response surrounding the granuloma is common in the acute phase. See Tables 20.5 and 20.7 for a differential diagnosis.

Cryptococcal n. Lymphadenitis. *Cryptococcus neoformans* and *Cryptococcus gattii* (formerly known as *C. neoformans* var *gattii*) are yeasts that act as opportunistic human pathogens in immunocompromized and healthy individuals. The fungi can be found in nearly all parts of the body, but the most common manifestation is meningitis or meningoencephalitis. The fungal infection can result in lymphadenitis, but it is usually accompanied by other symptoms. In immunocompetent persons the disease is mild and self-limiting. It may be life threatening, however, in HIV patients with low CD4+ T lymphocyte counts.

The cryptococcal fungi appear to have a worldwide distribution but are most prevalent in the tropics and subtropics. Recent outbreaks in Canada and the Pacific Northwest, however, suggest that their range may be increasing (CDC, 2010). *C. neoformans* is commonly found associated with bird droppings, while *C. gattii* occurs around trees, especially eucalyptus (Levitz, 1991). Inhalation of dust containing the spores may be the usual route for dissemination of the yeasts in the body. The increased incidence of HIV infection in the 1980s caused a spike in cryptococcosis that has since been declining because of better treatments and control of transmission. The prevalence of cryptococcosis among AIDS patients in the United States is 3-6%, while in Africa it is around 12%.

Cryptococcosis is one of the most common and serious opportunistic infections of AIDS patients (Kwon-Chung, 2000). The fungi may colonize any part of the body including the lymph nodes, but the most prevalent forms of cryptococcosis are meningitis or meningoencephalitis. The cryptococcal fungi are naturally occurring in nature associated with certain trees, rotting vegetation, and bird droppings. Inhalation of dust containing the spores can result in a respiratory focus of the disease with dissemination to the thoracic lymph nodes and frequently the nervous system for which *C. neoformans* seems to have a predisposition. The spores can also enter the circulation through a wound. The symptoms of cryptococcosis depend somewhat on the route of entry with respiratory effects such as coughing and chest pain accompanied by fever and fatigue being the most common. Immunocompetent persons may show few symptoms, and person-to-person transmission has not been well documented.

Lymphadenitis, primarily of the mediastinal and cervical nodes is relatively rare but is well documented. Fine needle aspiration cytology of suspected nodes can reveal a cryptococcal infection. A condition called "immune reconstitution inflammatory syndrome" can result in cryptococcal lymphadenitis in AIDS patients undergoing highly active antiretroviral therapy (HAART) (Putignani, 2001). While the antiviral medications reduce HIV titers, a loss of immune responsiveness to other microbial infections can occur, allowing opportunistic pathogens such as cryptococcus to gain a foothold in the body. Lymph node aspirates can be tested for cryptococcus.

Bacillus Calmette–Guarine Lymphadenopathy

Definition

Bacillus Calmette–Guérin (BCG) is a live attenuated vaccine strain of *Mycobacterium bovis* for prevention of human tuberculosis. It has been used against TB since 1921 and is generally safe. Immunotherapy for bladder cancer is another application. A few complications, however, can develop, including innoculation site abscess or keloid formation. BCG lymphadenopathy is a common sequelae seen in infants and young children post-BCG vaccination especially those that received the higher intradermal dose (Guerin and Bregere, 1992). BCG is contraindicated in symptomatic children with AIDS, according to WHO, but not indicated for HIV-positive individuals. Some of the severe cases develop in adults and older children coinfected with human immunodeficiency virus (Waddell et al., 2001).

Synonyms

BCGitis, BCGosis for disseminated disease)

Incidence

The complication occurs in 1.9% of the infants post-BCG vaccination, with severe infection seen in up to 3.4 per 1 million children (Al-Bhlal, 2000). The incidence of lymphadenopathy ranges between 0.73 and 2.2% (Mori, Yamauchi, and Shiozawa, 1996), with frequency of up to 38 per 1000 reported (Aggarwal et al., 1990). Lymphadenopathy occurs within one year of vaccination, with an average of 2.5 months interval from vaccination to adenopathy.

Pathogenesis

Many infants develop mild enlargement of lymph nodes after vaccination. This lymphadenitis is, however, subclinical and regresses spontaneously. Persistent lymphadenopathy or development of tenderness or suppuration heralds clinically worrisome lymphadenitis.

BCG lymphadenitis in an immunocompromised patient can develop into severe systemic dissemination, which is regarded as a result of acquired or congenital immune deficiency (Abramowsky, Gonzalez, and Sorensen, 1993; Al-Bhlal, 2000). Rarely, bone marrow and other organs become involved by fatal disseminated post-BCG systemic form (Kumar et al., 2005).

Clinical Aspects

Enlargement of axillary or cervical lymph nodes are a rare sequela of BCG vaccination (Chaves-Carballo and Sanchez, 1972). Maculopapular skin rash and skin nodules or osteitis may also be seen. Rarely disseminated visceral disease develop in immunosuppressed patients with an estimated frequency of 1 in 1 million vaccination.

Laboratory Tests. Multiplex PCR can differentiate BCG DNA from mycobacterium tuberculosis DNA (Talbot, Williams, and Frothingham, 1997; Waddell et al., 2001a).

Morphology. Two types of granulomatous patterns are seen: a tuberculoid type with suppuration and and a nonsuppurative type that resemble sarcoidosis. Variable numbers of neutrophils to the formation of frank suppurative lymphadenitis are seen (Teo, Smeulders, and Shingadia 2005). The epithelioid histiocytes in both are admixed with variable numbers of Langhans-type giant cells. Also disseminated BCG can show diffuse parenchymal foamy histiocytosis containing numerous acid-fast bacilli.

Skin lesions show dermal epithelioid granulomas, some with central necrosis and Langhans giant cells. The Ziehl–Neelsen stain for acid-fast bacilli typically shows numerous bacilli within the cytoplasm of the histiocytes, and these correspond to the rod-like structures seen on routine stains.

Differential Diagnosis

Unlike de novo tuberculous lymphadenitis, caseous necrosis is not common. Unlike MTB, clusters of intracellular acid-fast bacilli are typical. When a biopsy of the bone marrow and visceral organs reveals foamy histiocytosis in an infant, this finding may raise a concern for histiocytosis of storage disease. Additionally, since the acid-fast bacilli are PAS positive, the picture may be futher confused with certain storage diseases.

Lepromatous leprosy is also a differential diagnosis given the high incidence of skin granulomas and the acid-fast intracytoplasmic organisms that may resemble Hansen's bacilli. Leprae cells contain prominent vacuoles with bluish tingible bodies known as Globi bodies, a feature not seen in BCG lymphadenitis. A morphologic clue also includes finding negative images in the cytoplasm of the bacilli appearing as grayish rods when examined using hematoxylin and eosin stains.

Treatment

The treatment ranges from no therapy for patients with nonsuppurative lymphadenitis to antituberculosis therapy or surgical excision for large suppurative lymph nodes (Nazir and Qazi, 2005). Prognosis is excellent. The lymphadenopathy resolves spontaneously after a few months but complications of dissemination (Kumar et al., 2005), or fistula, may require surgery or antibiotic therapy. The predictor of nonresponse to antituberculous drugs includes large lymph nodes or the disseminated disease (Chaves-Carballo and Sanchez, 1972).

MIXED PATTERN WITH ANGIOMATOID CHANGE

Bartonella bacilliformis Bacillary Angiomatosis

Bartonellosis are infections caused by pathogens in the family Bartonellaceae. In 1909 Alberto Barton, a Peruvian bacteriologist, first described these microorganisms that adhered to RBCs. Since then, other species etiologic for cat-scratch disease and bacillary angiomatosis (*B. henselae*), and trench fever (*B. quintana*), are included under this family. Since these organisms are frequent opportunistic infectious, they are regarded as re-emerging infectious diseases. Historically a case of interest is a Peruvian medical student Daniel Carrión who innoculated himself in 1885 with blood from a lesion of a patient with a Peruvian wart from the Oroya valley to study the relation of skin lesion with the more severe Oroya disease prevalent in the river basin. He developed the classic Oroya infection and died. In his tribute and for his mortal contribution, Oroya fever and the skin lesions called verruga peruana are now considered one disease and collectively called Carrión disease.

Definition

Bartonellosis, of the classic form secondary to *Bartonella bacilliformis*, is a cutaneous and systemic disease with endemicity in distinct South American countries.

ICD-10 Code A44.0

Synonyms

Oroya fever, Carrion's disease for the systemic form, and Peruvian wart or verruga peruana for the eruptive cutaneous form.

Epidemiology

Bartonellosis has occurred only in certain regions of Peru, Ecuador, and Colombia. The endemic sites are waterways basins (quebradas) in the Andes mountains at altitudes between 700 and 3000 meters. About 10 to 15% of the population have underlying infections in these areas. Visitors are at risk, whereas the native population is immune, a difference attributed to the latent infection and resistance shown by the indigenous people. Carrión disease typically affects the young population in Peru and Ecuador.

Etiology

Bartonella bacilliformis is the etiologic agent of Carrion's disease or Oroya fever (acute phase of infection) and Verruga peruana or Peruvian wart (chronic cutaneous phase of infection). Bartonella bacilliformis is a Gram-negative aerobic, motile, facultative intracellular coccobacillary bacterium. The disease is transmitted by the sandflies *Phlebotomus verrucarum* and *P. noguchi*. The vectors are vulnerable to cold and arid conditions, hence the lack of bartonellosis in coastal and at higher elevations. Unlike other Bartonella species, humans are the only reservoir. Infections are common at evening and night, when sandflies are most vigorous.

Pathogenesis

B. bacilliformis, which has flagellum for motility, attaches to erythrocytes. The infection multiplies inside vacuoles and causes deformities and invaginations of the red cell membrane, contributing to red blood cell fragility and hemolysis. In tissue, this species also causes proliferation of both endothelial cells and blood vessels by secreting an endothelial cell stimulating factor. In contrast, *B. henselae* and *B. quintana* do not bind to human red blood cells; however, these organisms adheres to feline red cell membranes, leading to diseases transmitted by cats. Erythrocytes may serve as an infective pool for Bartonella species. Virulence is secondary to the following bacterial factors: the motile flagellum as well as the deformin proteins, and invasion-associated loci A and B (Li et al., 2004).

Clinical Aspects

At about 21 days the sandflies's bite inoculation causes bacteremia, and the infection of human red blood cells results in a severe intravascular hemolytic anemia (Carrion's disease) (Maguiña, 2000). This acute hemolytic phase is associated with anemia, high fever, and transient immune suppression and typically develops in 2 to 4 weeks. During this time thrombocytopenia can occur and can be severe. Neurologic involvement heralds poor prognosis. Complications secondary to immune suppression lead to debilitating co-infections with other bacteria and parasites such as *Pneumocystis spp.* or *Toxoplasma gondii*. If the patient survives this acute phase, chronic infection can supervene. At this phase a chronic eruptive phase called verruga peruana may occur, and this consists of a skin lesions characterized as reddish-purple lumps called angiomatous tumors.

The eruptive phase of bartonellosis may overlap with the anemic phase, but both phases often show a hiatus interval of several months. Sometimes the eruptive form occurs without prior evidence of bartonellosis. In this case the lesions are usually miliary (*forma miliar*), and many small hemangioma-like lesions are seen. Nodular eruptions (*forma nodular*) are bigger but more scattered and may be frequent on the extensor surfaces of the arms and legs. Rarely, a few large ulcerated lesions may appear near articular joints and limit movement. The eruptive phase is often protracted, but ultimately heals.

Sites of Involvement. Besides skin and blood, bartonellosis affects liver, bone marrow, and other visceral organs, and frequently it causes generalized lymphadenopathy and hepatosplenomegaly. Neurologic involvement is rare, but when seen, it often indicates a fatal outcome.

Approach to Diagnosis

Diagnosis could be made by visualizing the coccobacilli in peripheral smears (see Figure 20.18) or cytologic preparations or lymphoid tissue sections. In patients with skin lesions, mucosal involvement is signaled by dysphagia and gastrointestinal bleeding. Clinically the onset is abrupt with fever, skeletal pains, and a severe hemolytic anemia that is often macrocytic. Changes characteristic of acute hemolytic anemia are present with prominent pallor and jaundice. Reticulocytosis is present. The anemia can be severe, and the blood red cell count may fall in a few days from normal to lower than 500,000/μl.

Laboratory Findings. Serology is not practical in immunocompromised patients. For healthy

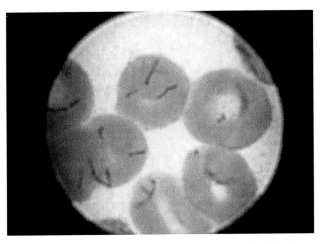

FIGURE 20.18 *Bartonella bacilliformis* **on red cells forming Y- or V-shaped patterns**. Oroya fever and blood cells with adhered microorganisms. (Courtesy of Dr. Rito Zerpa of Peru.)

transient travelers, blood or tissue cultures are diagnostic. PCR for *B. bacilliformis* can be fixed by embedding the tissue in paraffin (Maass, Schreiber, and Knobloch, 1992). In skin biopsies, with the characteristic angiomatoid histology present, Warthin–Starry or Steiner modification silver stain can be used to identify L-shaped or branching bacilli with endothelial cell tropisms (see Figure 20.19).

Morphologic Aspects

Peripheral blood smears should show macrocytosis with many branching clustered cocci or bacilli on erythrocytes. These Giemsa-stained rods or bacilli (2 × 0.5 μm in size) form Y or V patterns end to end and X-shaped forms are not observed (see Figure 20.18). The coccoid forms are smaller. In tissue, because the bacteria secretes an endothelial cell stimulating factor and also because of the by-products of hemolysis, the reticuloendothelial cells proliferate systemically and the sinusoidal vessels are distended with entrapped blood, hemosiderin, and packed bacilli. There is lymphadenopathy with sinusoidal hyperplasia, and also seen are cytophagic macrophages with ingested microorganisms. Splenic necrosis with hemosiderin pigments and thrombosed vessels may be seen, with infarcts and sinusoidal congestion. Hepatic necrosis may also be present. The verruga peruana cutaneous lesions will show an angiomatoid proliferation of high endothelial venules, capillaries, and hemorrhage that is positive for Warthin–Starry pleomorphic bacilliform organisms, the same as the histology of bacillary angiomatosis secondary to *B. henselae* (see Figure 20.19). The lesions are granulomatous,

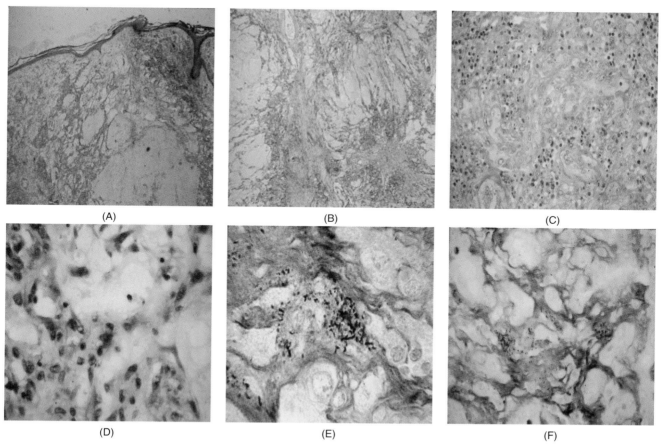

FIGURE 20.19 *Bacillary angiomatosis,* **chest lesion**. **(A)** Dermal loose angiomatoid pattern. **(B)** Solid and edematous areas. **(C)** PAS outlining back-to-back endothelial venules with plump lining and admixed inflammatory plasma cells, neutrophils, and lymphocytes. **(D)** Interdigitating endotheliawith smudgy cytoplasm, suggestive of intracellular bacilli. **(E, F)** Warthin–Starry Steiner stain-pleomorphic branching and coccoid forms of *Bartonella spp.*

with extensive infiltrations of various types of cells along with the proliferation of the endothelial cells, histiocytes, plasma cells, and lymphocytes. The blood vessels are dilated, with plump and swollen endothelial cells. Endothelial cells show a smudgy cytoplasm that may correspond to Rocha–Lima's cytoplasmic inclusions. Under ultrastructure these inclusions show endothelial cells as a phagocytosed labyrinth of channels and vacuoles containing degraded bacteria, extracellular matrix components, or both (Arias-Stella et al. 1986).

Immunohistochemistry/Cytochemistry

Silver stains and PCR can be performed on pus collected from a node via fine needle aspiration, sparing the patient a surgical biopsy. A biopsy of the skin lesion allows the bacterium to be observed using a silver stain such as Warthin–Starry or the Steiner stain. The Warthin–Starry stain better identifies *Bartonella spp.*

Differential Diagnosis

The skin eruptive form must be distinguished from secondary syphilis, Yaws, or Kaposi sarcoma. A single large violaceous hemorrhagic tumor may resemble a vascular neoplasm of skin. The systemic acute form must be separated from acute hemolytic crisis of malaria, typhoid, typhus, and other hemolysis associated acute bacteremic infections. See Tables 20.11 and 20.12 for differenital diagnosis.

Treatment of Choice and Prognosis

Treatment of Oroya hemolytic disease and the dermal eruptions has been reported with chloramphenicol, streptomycin, tetracycline, and penicillin, but therapy has not always worked. The mortality in the eruptive phase is less than 5%. The acute phase of the disease is fatal, characterized by massive red blood cells hemolysis and fever. Where the infection is not treated, the case fatality rate is reported to be on average 40% and rising up to 85% (Maguiña, 2000).

TABLE 20.11 Mixed Pattern with Depletion and Immunoblastic Reaction

Mixed pattern with depletion and immunoblastic reaction
- Dengue hemorrhagic fever
- Ehrlichiosis lymphadenopathy
- Lassa hemorrhagic fever-
- Nipah virus

TABLE 20.12 Mixed Pattern with Angiomatoid changes

Mixed Pattern with Angiomatoid Change	Malignant Simulating Lesions
Bartonellosis bacilliformis verruga peruana	Kaposi sarcoma
Bacillary angiomatosis *B. henselae* in HIV	Angiosarcoma
Atypical mycobacterial Infections In HIV	

MIXED PATTERN WITH SPENT GRANULOMAS AND EXTRACELLULAR ORGANISMS

Histoplasmosis Secondary to *H. Capsulatum*

Histoplasmosis is the most frequent fungal infection in the United States. Most endemic infections are asymptomatic, but some individuals develop disseminated disease with acute pulmonary infection or severe involvement of blood-perfused organs like spleen, liver, and bone marrow. See Chapter 9 for the morphology and microbiology of clinically significant fungi.

Subclinical Histoplasmosis: Fibrotic Granulomas

Subclinical infection with *H. capsulatum* is common in persons residing in disease-endemic areas. The ensuing granulomas are an incidental surgical pathology finding or observed radiographically. Human histoplasmosis is caused by two varieties of Histoplasma, the classic or common *H. capsulatum var capsulatum* and the rarer *H. var. duboisii*, or African histoplasmosis. The incidental fibrotic granulomas, in surgical specimen, are caused by the common *H. capsulatum*.

Definition
Classic or common histoplasmosis is an infection transmitted by airborne spores of a fungus *Histoplasma capsulatum*.

ICD-10 Code B39.4

Synonyms
Cave disease, Darling's disease, Ohio River Valley fever, and reticuloendotheliosis.

Epidemiology
Subclinical histoplasma granulomas are frequently observed in residents of Ohio and Mississippi River valleys. This central part of the United States is an area where histoplasmosis is endemic. Most cases of histoplasmosis are associated with mediastinal lymphadenopathy, which can calcify and may cause asymptomatic or symptomatic disease. Travelers or recreational cave explorers are at risk of exposure to airborne spores. Aerosolized dust can cause unusual outbreaks in residences or hotels with ongoing dust-laden building constructions. Bird or bat droppings, known as guano are a rich source of *H. capsulatum* and pose risk for spelunkers and cave visitors (Morgan et al., 2003).

Etiology
Histoplasmosis is caused by a dimorphic fungus *Histoplasma capsulatum var. capsulatum*. This is also the most common variety worldwide. It has been reported in many HIV -endemic areas and has been an AIDS-defining opportunistic infection in patients who are living in or have traveled to histoplasmosis-endemic areas (see Figures 20.20, 20.21).

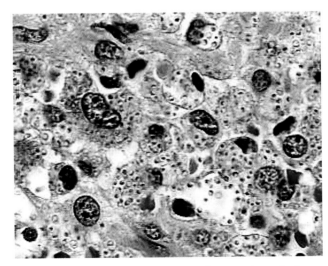

FIGURE 20.20 Histoplasma capsulatum lymphadenopathy in HIV. (Courtesy of Tony Hernandez, MD, Ameripath, FL.)

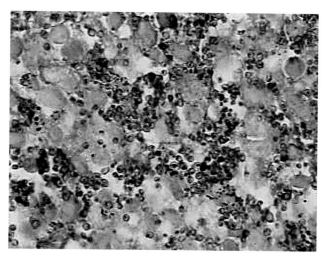

FIGURE 20.21 **Histoplasma capsulatum lymphadenopathy in HIV.** The PAS stain is on an imprint. (Courtesy of Tony Hernandez, MD, Ameripath, FL.)

Pathophysiology

The natural habitat is the soil, especially if enriched with bird and bat excrements. Infection is acquired during aerosol-creating activities around infected areas. Inhalation of *H. capsulatum conidia* from the environment leads to primary lung infection and hematogenous seeding. This leads to visible foci noted in splenectomy or other viscerae both radiologically or in surgical specimen. Sometimes the lymph nodes "crystalize" and commonly seen as calcified nodules in X ray. Histologically, these nodes are fibrotic; later stages may be densely calcified, especially those biopsied from the mediastinum. There is often a central caseation surrounded by inflamed or fibrotic capsule, and histiocytes with encapsulated yeasts (see Figures 20.22, 20.23).

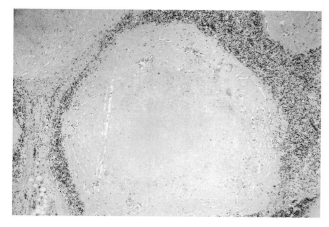

FIGURE 20.22 **Lymph node with multifocal granulomas with central caseation and fibrotic wall (H&E, 50×).** (Courtesy of Dr. Shieh and Zaki.)

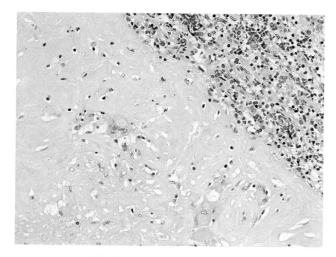

FIGURE 20.23 **Wall of granulomas with fibrosis.** Note the entrapped histiocytes laden with intracellular histoplasma organisms (H&E, 400×). (Courtesy of Dr. Shieh and Zaki.)

Approach to Diagnosis

Most subclinical cases of histoplasmosis are diagnosed serologically. The most widely accepted serologic tests are the immunodiffusion test and/or the complement-fixation test. Positive Histoplasmin skin tests occur in as many as 90% of the people living in endemic areas, but skin tests are seldom used for diagnosis of acute disease.

Morphology

The common histoplamosis, *H. capsulatum var capsulatum*, often are intracellular organisms, averaging in size from 2 to 3 µm. Histologic features of splenic, pulmonary, or hepatic lesions are characteristic. Spent fibrotic granulomas are often an incidental finding in the pathology specimen. Grocott staining on sequential sections are necessary to demonstrate *H. capsulatum* (Grocott, 1955). Lung, lymph nodes, spleen, and liver stained sections yielded 92%, 86%, 73%, and 62% positivity, respectively, on first microscopic evaluation (Okudaira, Straub, and Schwarz, 1961). The changes observed are as described previously by Schwartz (1954) who described "early" and "old" lesions (see also Okudaira, Straub, and Schwarz, 1961). All figures are from Ohio River Valley and Cincinnati specimen in surgical pathology. See Figures 20.24, 20.25, and Table 20.13.

Acute Histoplasmosis

Definition

Acute pulmonary form follows massive exposure to spores, usually seen up to 2 weeks where a history of travel to a cave is typical.

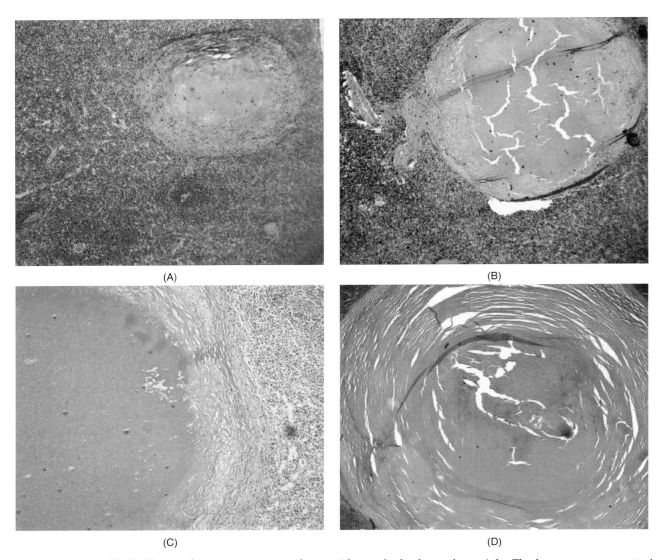

FIGURE 20.24 **(A)** "Early" lesion showing spent granuloma with attached sclerosed arteriole. The hematogenous route is probably embolic, and the intrasplenic trapping at the marginal sinus may account for the associated vessels. **(B)** Early granuloma with tethered arteriole (at top of white pulp marginal zone) showing a central necrosis with no calcification. **(C)** Incidental splenectomy for splenic rupture showing several fibrotic circular granulomas, one with a completely hyalinized nodule with central cores of pink amorphous necrotic material. **(D)** "Old" lesion. The more advanced sclerosis shows calcific basophilic change (left) at the inner half of the capsule, concentrically sclerosed center and clefts. Incomplete decalcification likely caused tissue fragmentation (right).

Risk factors are travel to or residence within the central or eastern United States, and exposure to the droppings of birds and bats. Symptoms of cough, skin rash, and joint pains usually abate without treatment. Rarely, a disseminated disease occurs in about 1 in 2000 patients with acute infection.

Most patients who develop disseminated histoplasmosis are immunosuppressed. In disseminated disease, the infection has spread to other organs from the lungs through the bloodstream. The lymph nodes, liver and spleen are usually enlarged, and the bone marrow is infiltrated. Ulcerations of the mouth or gastrointestinal tract may occur, especially in the chronic indolent form of disseminated histoplasmosis.

Laboratory Test and Approach to Diagnosis

In general, the test used depends on the histoplasmosis type. In the acute or chronic pulmonary type, serology, culture, and chest radiography are useful. In the acute and chronic disseminated type, cuture of bone marrow or the involved tissue, antigen detection by anti-Histoplasma, and histopathology

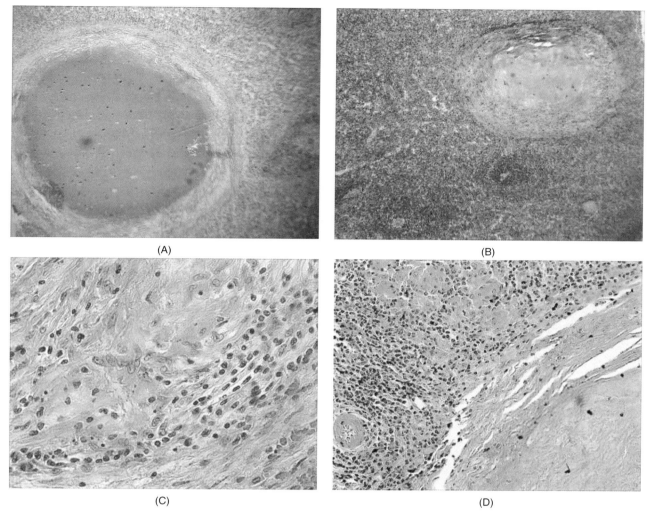

(A) (B) (C) (D)

FIGURE 20.25 **Early lesion in spleen. (A)** PAS (10×) and **(B)** H&E (10×) show adjacent white pulp and arterioles with spent fibrous granulomas. There is a pink accellular necrotic center surrounded by a wall of loose fibrous tissue with no calcification. **(C D)** Loosely organized rim of epithelioid histiocytes, plasma cells, lymphocytes, eosinophils and fibroblasts arrayed with hyaline circumferential fibrous wall. The inflammatory wall is filled with loose granuloma, fibroblasts, lymphocytes, neutrophils and plasma cells with a fibrosing acellular center (H&E).

TABLE 20.13 **Mixed Patterns with Unusual Granulomas**

Mixed pattern with unusual granulomata: extracellular yeast or spent granulomas
• *Histoplasma capsulatum*
• *Histoplasmosis duboisii (African Histoplasmosis)*

are the diagnostic modalities (see Figure 20.26). The histoplasmin test is often negative in acute histoplasmosis. Direct microscopy of the affected organ including bone marrow smears, aspirate, or sputum is useful. Histopathology is helpful.

Morphology

The microorganisms are intracellular, usually packed inside histiocytes, (Figure 20.20) and they can be seen in routine as well as PAS-stained tissue (Figure 20.21). Granulomatous inflammation is seen with the typical fibrosing wall and central caseation necrosis. Up to 5 μm in size, the intracellular organisms are usually uniform in appearance, except in AIDS, where the organisms tend to be variable in size and shape.

Differential Diagnosis

H. capsulatum infection is a common cause of diffuse or nodular pulmonary or splenic calcification;

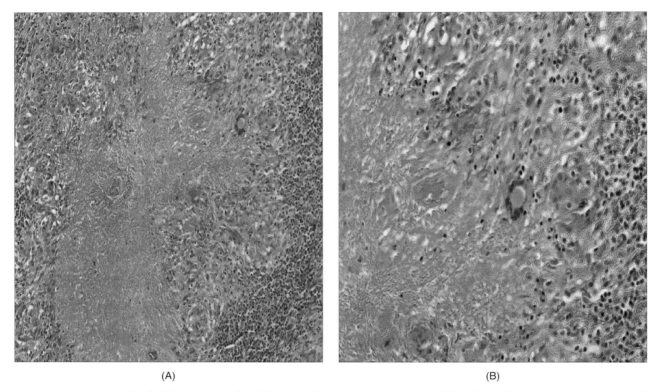

(A)   (B)

FIGURE 20.26   **Acute splenic histoplasmosis with caseating granuloma and multinucleated Langhans-type giant cells resembling mycobacterium TB**.

other considerations include brucellosis and tuberculosis. The differential diagnosis includes *Cryptococcus neoformans*, which can be differentiated by demonstration of positive mucicarmine staining. Cryptococcus, however, unlike both *Histoplasma spp.* rarely involves the lymph nodes and often presents with suppurative foci.

In Southeast Asia (Navarro et al., 1992) organisms such as *Cryptococcus neoformans* and *Peniciiium marneffei* are etiologies of disseminated mycoses. These can resemble *H. capsulatum* in tissues. *P. marneffei* may also appear as a small yeast within the macrophages, although these often appears septate. *P. marneffei* reproduction is by binary fission, in contrast to sporulation, which occurs in Histoplasma. *P. marneffei* is a pathogen of bamboo rats found in Southeast Asia and China and is also commonly seen in AIDS patients. The organisms' mode of entry, course, and dissemination mimic the Histoplasma species, but they are morphologically different. They do not form budding yeasts but show bilobed curved or round yeast separated by septa.

In subSaharan Africa, the large form of Histoplasma (*H. duboissi*) is a differential and description is shown in the following part.

Treatment

The incidental granulomas of Histoplasma require no treatment unless they are part of a disseminated disease. Amphotericin B and itroconazole are the usual therapy in the acute and relapsing chronic forms.

Prognosis

Clinically, disseminated disease is rare except in the AIDS or organ transplant setting, where the prognosis is guarded and multifactorial (Tobon et al., 2005).

AFRICAN HISTOPLAMOSIS SECONDARY TO *H. CAPSULATUM VAR DUBOISII*

African histoplasmosis is caused by *H. capsulatum var duboisii*. Skin and lymph node infections are common.

ICD-10 Code B39.5

Definition

Histoplasma capsulatum var. duboisii is an invasive fungal infection endemic in central and west Africa.

Epidemiology Including Geolocation

This condition occurs only in about 20 countries in the tropical belt of Africa: in the western and central regions of sub-Saharian Africa, the island of Madagascar between the Kalahari and Sahara deserts, with about 50% of the infection detected in Nigeria (Gugnani, 2000). Cases due to *H. capsulatum var. duboisii* or African histoplasmosis are scarce in western countries but are sometimes encountered in travelers or immigrants. The cases described in the United States and Europe were in former residents of the endemic areas in Africa. Skin sensitivity test reveals a prevalence of 3% (Gugnani, Egere, and Larsh 1991).

Etiology

African histoplasmosis caused by *Histoplasma capsulatum var. duboisii* is an invasive fungal infection endemic in central and west Africa. A natural reservoir of this fungus is soil admixed with bat guano usually found in the bat caves (Gugnani and Muotoe-Okafor, 1997). *H. capsulatum var. capsulatum* coexists with another variety, *H. capsulatum var. duboisii*, whose pathogenesis is not as well described.

Pathogenesis

Lymphadenopathy may be the only manifestation or be part of a cutaneous or systemic disease. Abscess is rare, but necrosis with caseation can usually be seen.

Clinical Aspects

Histoplasmosis encompasses a spectrum of clinical forms, with disseminated histoplasmosis being the most severe. Unlike the common Histoplasma, opportunistic and animal infections are rarely seen. Although both pathogens coexist in those regions, reports concerning African histoplasmosis during HIV infection are rare. Endemic histoplasmosis is caused by *Histoplasma spp.*, both the severe and localized clinical forms.

Sites of Involvement. Unlike the common Histoplasma where primary lung infection is seen, *H. duboisii* rarely involves the lungs. Skin, bones, and lymph nodes are the usual organ affected with dissemination to other organs. Rare mucosal involvement in the intestinal tract may appear as a large ulcer mimicking carcinoma. Although the most common location is the skin, lymphadenopathy is often seen in African histoplasmosis. Lymphadenitis may be associated with cutaneous lesion but may be part of a systemic infection. From 45 to 65% of immunocompromised persons present with involvement of lymph nodes, followed by skin at 25% (Loulergue et al., 2007).

The cutaneous lesions are varied and present as papulo-nodules, ulcerated abscess, fistulas, or pigmentary changes. The papules and nodules have a pathognomonic hyperpigmented halo around them (Williams, Lawson, and Lucas, 1971; Gugnani, 2000) Abscess yields the typical yeasts. Fistulas may also result from the inflamed lymph nodes. The bones lesions often resemble multiple myeloma and mainly seen in ribs and long bones (Williams, Lawson, and Lucas, 1971; Gugnani, 2000).

Approach to Diagnosis

The disease presents initially with focal infection but becomes rapidly disseminated. Eventually multiple sites, including the lungs, gastrointestinal tracts, and bones, may be affected. Diagnosis is by tissue or aspirate biopsy and demonstration of large oval yeasts measuring 8 to 14 microns by direct microscopy. Tissue biopsy shows the large yeasts in intracellular and extracellular location, and the culture may be positive. Serology is often not contributory.

Morphologic Aspects

Direct microscopy under a 10% potassium hydroxide solution of skin scrapings or pus aspirate from skin ulcer may reveal yeasts wtih double refractile walls. Histopathologic examination of the involved lymph node may present with a necrotizing or granulomatous lymphadenitis with epithelioid histiocytes but without caseation. Most characteristic besides necrosis are the presence of multinucleated giant cells and extracellular microorganisms. Unlike the smaller *Histoplasma capsulatum, H. duboissi*, are much larger, ranging from 8 to 14 μm and show a double-contoured wall. The organism may sometimes be confused with other deep mycoses that are difficult to see on a routine hematoxylin and eosin (H&E) stain. The African type, however, is easily identified on routine H&E stains as large yeasts with clear refractile walls. Epithelioid granulomas are often present with many organisms outside the macrophages, as are giant cells filled with organisms (see Figure 20.27).

Differential Diagnosis

Between *H. capsulatum* and African histoplasmosis (*H. c. duboissi*), the size difference is key. Whereas

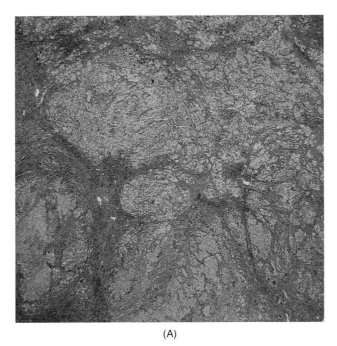

(A)

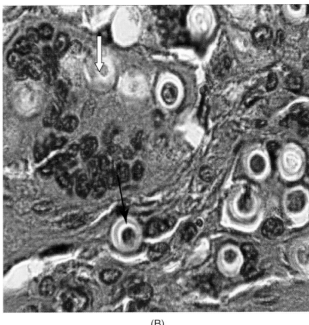

(B)

FIGURE 20.27 African histoplasmosis or *H. duboisii* granulomatous lymphadenitis. (A) Numerous granulomatous foci efface the lymph node with thickened capsule, pale areas of epithelioid granulomas, and few dark foci of residual lymphoid tissue. **(B)** Intracellular and extracellular *H. duboisii* with characteristic refractile double contoured wall (arrow) are seen in routine H&E. Some are inside a multinucleated giant cell (open arrow), but the majority of yeasts are extracellular.

H. capsulatum is 2 to 5 μm, *H. duboisii* is 8 to 14 μm, which is larger than the diameter of the lymphocytes (see Figure 20.27). Leismaniasis shows kinetoplasts, and *Cryptococcus n.* shows carminophilia when stained with mucicarmine. *Blastomycosis dermatitidis* may be in the same endemic belt in Africa and may be confused with African histoplasmosis. Unlike the latter, however, the multiple condensed nuclei of *Blastomyces dermatitidis* can be visualized by silver stains but be difficult to see on H&E stained sections, also unlike *H. duboisii*. Moreover the *B. dermatitdis* granulomas often show abscessed neutrophils, which is uncommon in *H. duboisii*.

Immunohistochemistry/Cytochemistry

Routine H&E stains allow for a microscopic visualization of the organisms. PAS does not stain the walls, and the cytoplasm looks clear.

Treatment of Choice and Prognosis

Amphotericin B, ketoconazole, and itraconazole are the mainstay agents used for therapy.

REFERENCES

Abramowsky C, Gonzalez B, Sorensen RU. 1993. Disseminated bacillus Calmette–Guerin infections in patients with primary immunodeficiencies. Am J Clin Pathol 100:52–6.

Aggarwal NP, Kallan BM, Grover PS, Aggarwal M. 1990. Clinico-excisional study of lymphadenitis following B.C.G. vaccination. Indian J Pediatr 57:585–6.

Al-Bhlal LA 2000. Pathologic findings for bacille Calmette–Guerin infections in immunocompetent and immunocompromised patients. Am J Clin Pathol 113:703–8.

Arias-Stella J, Lieberman PH, Erlandson RA, Rias-Stella J Jr. 1986. Histology, immunohistochemistry, and ultrastructure of the Verruga in Carrion's disease. Am J Surg Pathol 10:595–610.

Azad AF, Radulovic S, Higgins JA. 1997. Flea-borne rickettsioses: ecologic considerations. Emerg Infect Dis 3:319–27.

Azadeh B 1985. "Localized" Leishmania lymphadenitis: a light and electron microscopic study. Am J Trop Med Hyg 34:447–55.

Babiker ZO, Davidson R, Mazinda C, Kipngetich S, Ritmeijer K. 2007. Utility of lymph node aspiration in the diagnosis of visceral leishmaniasis in Sudan. Am J Trop Med Hyg 76:689–93.

Baird JK, Alpert LI, Friedman R, Schraft WC, Connor DH. 1986. North American Brugian filariasis: report of nine infections of humans. Am J Trop Med Hyg 35:1205–9.

Barral A, Barral-Netto M, Almeida R, de Jesus AR, Grimaldi JG, Netto EM, Santos I, Bacellar O, Carvalho EM. 1992. Lymphadenopathy associated with

Leishmania braziliensis cutaneous infection. Am J Trop Med Hyg 47:587–92.

Barral A, Guerreiro J, Bomfim G, Correia D, Barral-Netto M, Carvalho EM. 1995. Lymphadenopathy as the first sign of human cutaneous infection by *Leishmania braziliensis*. Am J Trop Med Hyg 53:256–9.

Bomfim G, Andrade BB, Santos S, Clarencio J, Barral-Netto M, Barral A. 2007. Cellular analysis of cutaneous leishmaniasis lymphadenopathy: insights into the early phases of human disease. Am J Trop Med Hyg 77:854–9.

Capelli G, Baldelli R, Ferroglio E, Genchi C, Gradoni L, Gramiccia M, Maroli M, Mortarino M, Pietrobelli M, Rossi L, Ruggiero M. 2004. [Monitoring of canine leishmaniasis in northern Italy: an update from a scientific network]. Parassitologia 46:193–7. (In Italian)

Carrera L, Gazzinelli RT, Badolato R, Hieny S, Muller W, Kuhn R, Sacks DL. 1996. Leishmania promastigotes selectively inhibit interleukin 12 induction in bone marrow-derived macrophages from susceptible and resistant mice. J Exp Med 183:515–26.

Centers for Disease Control and Prevention (CDC). 2010. Emergence of *Cryptococcus gattii*—Pacific northwest, 2004–2010. MMWR Morb Mortal Wkly Rep 59(28):865–8.

Chaves-Carballo E, Sanchez GA. 1972. Regional lymphadenitis following BCG vaccination (BCGitis): clinical comments based upon 25 instances among 1295 childhood vaccinees. Clin Pediatr (Phila) 11:693–7.

Cook VJ, Manfreda J, Hershfield ES. 2004. Tuberculous lymphadenitis in Manitoba: incidence, clinical characteristics and treatment. Can Respir J 11:279–86.

Cuellar-Rodriguez J, Avery RK, Lard M, Budev M, Gordon SM, Shrestha NK, van Duin D, Oethinger M, Mawhorter SD. 2009. Histoplasmosis in solid organ transplant recipients: 10 years of experience at a large transplant center in an endemic area. Clin Infect Dis 49:710–6.

Cualing H, Sandin R. 2010. Epitrochlear lymphadenitis infection with *Dirofilaria immitis*: morphohistologic findings. Am J Trop Med Hyg 83(5)suppl p. 91.

Doenhoff MJ 1997. A role for granulomatous inflammation in the transmission of infectious disease: schistosomiasis and tuberculosis. Parasitology 115(suppl):S113–25.

Doughty BL, Zodda DM, el KA, Phillips SM. 1984. Delayed type hypersensitivity granuloma formation around schistosoma: Mansoni eggs in vitro. IV. Granuloma formation in human schistosomiasis. Am J Trop Med Hyg 33:1173–7.

Doull JA, Guinto RA, Rodriguez RS, et al. 1942. The incidence of leprosy in Cordova and Talisay, Cebu, Philippines. Int J Leprosy 10:107–31.

Elenitoba-Johnson KSJ, Eberhard ML, Dauphinais RM, Lammie PJ, Khorsand J. 1996. Zoonotic brugian lymphadenitis: an unusual case with florid monocytic B-cell proliferation. Am J Clin Pathol 105:384–7.

Fenwick A, Rollinson D, Southgate V. 2006. Implementation of human schistosomiasis control: challenges and prospects. Adv Parasitol 61:567–622.

Garred P, Larsen F, Seyfarth J, Fujita R, Madsen HO. 2006. Mannose-binding lectin and its genetic variants. Genes Immun 7:85–94.

Gravino AE 2004. [Interpretation of laboratory data during cryptic leishmaniasis in dog]. Parassitologia 46:227–9. (In Italian)

Grocott RG 1955. A stain for fungi in tissue sections and smears using gomori's methenamine-silver nitrate technic. Am J Clin Pathol 25:975–9.

Grove DI, Cabrera BD, Valeza FS, Guinto RS, Ash LR, Warren KS. 1977. Sensitivity and Specificity of skin reactivity to *Brugia malayi* and *Dirofilaria immitis antigens* in Bancroftian and Malayan filariasis in the Philippines. Am J Trop Med Hyg 26:220–9.

Guerin N, Bregere P. 1992. BCG vaccination. Child Trop (196–197):72–76.

Gugnani HC 2000. Histoplasmosis in Africa: a review. Indian J Chest Dis Allied Sci 42:271–7.

Gugnani HC, Egere JU, Larsh H. 1991. Skin sensitivity to capsulatum and *Duboisii histoplasmins* in Nigeria. J Trop Med Hyg 94:24–6.

Gugnani HC, Muotoe-Okafor F. 1997. African histoplasmosis: a review. Rev Iberoam Micol 14:155–9.

Harms G, Fraga F, Batroff B, Oliveira F, Feldmeier H. 2005. Cutaneous leishmaniasis associated with extensive lymphadenopathy during an epidemic in Ceara State, Northeast Brazil. Acta Trop 93:303–10.

Itoh M, Wu W, Sun D, Yao L, Li Z, Islam MZ, Chen R, Zhang K, Wang F, Zhu S, Kimura E. 2007. Confirmation of elimination of lymphatic filariasis by an IgG4 enzyme-linked immunosorbent assay with urine samples in Yongjia, Zhejiang Province and Gaoan, Jiangxi Province, People's Republic of China. Am J Trop Med Hyg 77:330–3.

Jungmann P, Figueredo-Silva J, Dreyer G. 1991. Bancroftian lymphadenopathy: a histopathologic study of fifty-eight cases from northeastern Brazil. Am J Trop Med Hyg 45:325–31.

Kolaczinski JH, Worku DT, Chappuis F, Reithinger R, Kabatereine N, Onapa A, Brooker S. 2007. Kala-Azar control, Uganda. Emerg Infect Dis 13:507–9.

Kramer LH, Kartashev VV, Grandi G, Morchon R, Nagornii SA, Karanis P, Simon F. 2007. Human subcutaneous dirofilariasis, Russia. Emerg Infect Dis 13:150–2.

Kumar PV, Monabati A, Kadivar R, Soleimanpour H. 2005. Peripheral blood and marrow findings in disseminated bacille calmette–guerin infection. J Pediatr Hematol Oncol 27:97–9.

Kumar PV, Moosavi A, Karimi M, Safaei A, Noorani H, Abdollahi B, Bedayat GR. 2001. Subclassification of localized leishmania lymphadenitis in fine needle aspiration smears. Acta Cytol 45:547–54.

Kwon-Chung KJ, Sorrell TC, Dromer F, Fung E, Levitz SM. 2000. Cryptococcosis: clinical and biological aspects. Med Mycol 38(suppl 1):205–13.

Levitz SM. 1991. The ecology of *Cryptococcus neoformans* and the epidemiology of cryptococcosis. Rev Infect Dis 13:1163–9.

Li DM, Yu DZ, Liu QY, Hai R, Guo BH. 2004. [Study on Bartonella infection using molecular biological diagnostic techniques from China]. Zhonghua Liu Xing Bing Xue Za Zhi 25:602–6. (In Chinese)

Lopes UG, Momen H, Grimaldi G Jr., Marzochi MC, Pacheco RS, Morel CM. 1984. Schizodeme and zymodeme characterization of leishmania in the investigation of foci of visceral and cutaneous leishmaniasis. J Parasitol 70:89–98.

Loulergue P, Bastides F, Baudouin V, Chandenier J, Mariani-Kurkdjian P, Dupont B, Viard JP, Dromer F, Lortholary O. 2007. Literature review and case histories of Histoplasma capsulatum var. duboisii infections in HIV-infected patients. Emerg Infect Dis 13:1647–52.

Maass M, Schreiber M, Knobloch J. 1992. Detection of Bartonella bacilliformis in cultures, blood, and formalin preserved skin biopsies by use of the polymerase chain reaction. Trop Med Parasitol 43:191–4.

Magill AJ 1995. Epidemiology of the leishmaniases. Dermatol Clin 13:505–23.

Magill AJ, Grogl M, Johnson SC, Gasser RA Jr. 1994. Visceral infection due to Leishmania tropica in a veteran of operation desert storm who presented 2 years after leaving Saudi Arabia. Clin Infect Dis 19:805–6.

Melby PC, Andrade-Narvaez FJ, Darnell BJ, Valencia-Pacheco G, Tryon VV, Palomo-Cetina A. 1994. Increased expression of proinflammatory cytokines in chronic lesions of human cutaneous leishmaniasis. Infect Immun 62:837–42.

Meyrowitsch DW, Simonsen PE, Garred P, Dalgaard M, Magesa SM, Alifrangis M. 2010. Association between mannose-binding lectin polymorphisms and Wuchereria Bancrofti infection in two communities in northeastern Tanzania. Am J Trop Med Hyg 82:115–20.

Morgan J, Cano MV, Feikin DR, Phelan M, Velazquez MO, Kuri Morales P, Carpenter J, Weltman A, Spitzer PG, Liu HH, Mirza SA, Bronstein DE, Morgan DJ, Kirkman LA, Brandt ME, Iqbal N, Lindsley MD, Warnock DW, Hajjeh RA. 2003. A large outbreak of histoplasmosis among American travelers associated with a hotel in Acapulco, Mexico, spring 2001. Am J Trop Med Hyg 69:663–9.

Mori T, Yamauchi Y, Shiozawa K. 1996. Lymph node swelling due to bacille Calmette–Guerin vaccination with multipuncture method. Tuber Lung Dis 77:269–73.

Navarro EE, Tupasi TE, Verallo VM, Romero RC, Tuazon CU. 1992. Disseminated histoplasmosis with unusual cutaneous lesions in a patient from the Philippines. Am J Trop Med Hyg 46:141–5.

Nazir Z, Qazi SH. 2005. Bacillus Calmette–Guerin (BCG) lymphadenitis—changing trends and management. J Ayub Med Coll Abbottabad 17:16–8.

Noordeen SK, Neelan PN. 1978. Extended studies on chemoprophylaxis against leprosy. Indian J Med Res 67:515–27.

Okudaira M, Straub M, Schwarz J. 1961. The etiology of discrete splenic and hepatic calcifications in an endemic area of histoplasmosis. Am J Pathol 39:599–611.

Orihel TC, Beaver PC. 1989. Zoonotic Brugia infections in North and South America. Am J Trop Med Hyg 40:638–647.

Paleologo FP, Neafie RC, Connor DH. 1984. Lymphadenitis caused by Loa Loa. Am J Trop Med Hyg 33:395–402.

Petersen CA. 2009a. Leishmaniasis, an emerging disease found in companion animals in the United States. Top Companion Anim Med 24:182–8.

Petersen CA. 2009b. New means of canine leishmaniasis transmission in North America: the possibility of transmission to humans still unknown. Interdiscip Perspect Infect Dis 2009:802712. Epub. pp 1–5.

Pirmez C, Yamamura M, Uyemura K, Paes-Oliveira M, Conceicao-Silva F, Modlin RL. 1993. Cytokine patterns in the pathogenesis of human leishmaniasis. J Clin Invest 91:1390–5.

Putignani L, Antonucci G, Paglia MG, Vincenzi L, Festa A, De Mori P, Loiacono L, Visca P. 2008. Cryptococcal lymphadenitis as a manifestation of immune reconstitution inflammatory syndrome in an HIV-positive patient: a case report and review of the literature. Int J Immunopathol Pharmacol 21(3):751–6.

Reithinger R 2008. Leishmaniases' burden of disease: ways forward for getting from speculation to reality. PLoS Negl Trop Dis 2:e285.

Reithinger R, Dujardin JC, Louzir H, Pirmez C, Alexander B, Brooker S. 2007. Cutaneous leishmaniasis. Lancet Infect Dis 7:581–96.

Rosenblatt P, Beaver PC, Orihel TC. 1962. A filarial infection apparently acquired in New York City. Am J Trop Med Hyg 11:641–5.

Rosypal AC, Troy GC, Zajac AM, Duncan RB Jr., Waki K, Chang KP, Lindsay DS. 2003. Emergence of zoonotic canine leishmaniasis in the United States: isolation and immunohistochemical detection of Leishmania infantum from foxhounds from Virginia. J Eukaryot Microbiol 50(suppl):691–3.

Sah SP, Prasad R, Raj GA. 2005. Fine needle aspiration of lymphadenopathy in visceral leishmaniasis. Acta Cytol 49:286–90.

Schwartz E, Hatz C, Blum J. 2006. New world cutaneous leishmaniasis in travellers. Lancet Infect Dis 6:342–9.

Schwartz B 1954. Histoplasmosis of lungs. AMA Arch Intern Med 94:970–94.

Sharaf EO, Nada N, Eldosoky I. 2008. Bilharzial lymphadenitis, a case report. Histopathology 52:655–6.

Sidrim JJ, Costa AK, Cordeiro RA, Brilhante RS, Moura FE, Castelo-Branco DS, Neto MP, Rocha MF. 2010. Molecular methods for the diagnosis and characterization of Cryptococcus: a review. Can J Microbiol 56:445–58.

Srinivasan R, Gupta N, Shifa R, Malhotra P, Rajwanshi A, Chakrabarti A. 2010. Cryptococcal lymphadenitis diagnosed by fine needle aspiration cytology: a review of 15 cases. Acta Cytol 54:1–4.

Talbot EA, Williams DL, Frothingham R. 1997. PCR identification of Mycobacterium bovis BCG. J Clin Microbiol 35:566–9.

Teo SSS, Smeulders N, Shingadia DV. 2005. BCG vaccine-associated suppurative lymphadenitis. Vaccine 23:2676–9.

Tobon AM, Agudelo CA, Rosero DS, Ochoa JE, De Bedout C, Zuluaga A, Arango M, Cano LE, Sampedro J, Restrepo A. 2005. Disseminated histoplasmosis: a comparative study between patients with acquired immunodeficiency syndrome and non-human immunodeficiency virus-infected individuals. Am J Trop Med Hyg 73:576–82.

Veress B, Malik MO, el-Hassan MA. 1974. [Pathological morphology of visceral leishmaniasis (Kala-Azar)]. Morphol Igazsagugyi Orv Sz 14:198–206. (In Hungarian)

Veress B, Omer A, Satir AA, el-Hassan AM. 1977. Morphology of the spleen and lymph nodes in fatal visceral leishmaniasis. Immunology 33:605–10.

Vijayan VK 2007. Tropical pulmonary eosinophilia: pathogenesis, diagnosis and management. Curr Opin Pulm Med 13:428–33.

Waddell RD, Lishimpi K, von Reyn CF, Chintu C, Baboo KS, Kreiswirth B, Talbot EA, Karagas MR. 2001. Bacteremia due to Mycobacterium tuberculosis or M. bovis, Bacille Calmette–Guerin (BCG) among HIV-positive children and adults in Zambia. AIDS 15:55–60.

Wartman WB 1946. Filariasis in American armed forces. Am J Pathol 22:653.

Webb JK, Job CK, Gault EW. 1960. Tropical eosinophilia: demonstration of microfilariae in lung, liver, and lymphnodes. Lancet 1:835–42.

Weil GJ, Lammie PJ, Weiss N. 1997. The ICT filariasis test: a rapid-format antigen test for diagnosis of Bancroftian filariasis. Parasitol Today 13:401–4.

Weil GJ, Ramzy RM. 2007. Diagnostic tools for filariasis elimination programs. Trends Parasitol 23:78–82.

WHO. 2004. WHO Report on the mid-term assessment of microfilaraemia reduction in sentinel sites of 13 countries of the Global Programme to Eliminate Lymphatic Filariasis. Wkly Epidemiol R 79:358.

Williams AO, Lawson EA, Lucas AO. 1971. African histoplasmosis due to Histoplasma duboisii. Arch Pathol 92:306–18.

Zagaria N, Savioli L. 2002. Elimination of lymphatic filariasis: a public-health challenge. Ann Trop Med Parasitol 96(suppl 2):S3–13.

Zijlstra EE, el-Hassan AM. 2001. Leishmaniasis in Sudan: visceral leishmaniasis. Trans R Soc Trop Med Hyg 95(suppl 1):S27–58.

CHAPTER TWENTY-ONE

CYTOPATHOLOGY OF NON-NEOPLASTIC AND INFECTIOUS LYMPHADENOPATHY

Sara E. Monaco, Liron Pantanowitz, and Walid E. Khalbuss

Fine needle aspiration (FNA) biopsies have been used in the evaluation of patients with lymphadenopathy for decades (Thomson et al., 1978; Cardillo, 1989; Sarda et al., 1990). The FNA provides a minimally invasive means to obtain clinical answers that guide treatment decisions. Because it is a rapid, safe, accurate, and cost-effective diagnostic technique, FNA can quickly alleviate patient anxiety in benign scenarios, and this procedure can appropriately triage specimens for infectious or neoplastic conditions in most scenarios (Rimm et al., 1997; Sarda et al., 1990). Nevertheless, FNA remains fairly underutilized in major academic centers and in some resource-poor areas for the evaluation of lymphadenopathy in both children and adults. The under utilization of FNAs may partially be attributed to the lack of expertise available for the performance and interpretation of FNA cytology.

Lymphadenopathy, or persistent enlargement of lymph nodes, is worrisome for the patient, as well as for clinicians, particularly in situations where the lymph nodes are superficial, palpable, and noticed by the patient. In some scenarios, lymphadenopathy may be observed closely to see if the lymph nodes diminish in size, especially following empiric antibiotics. With persistent lymphadenopathy that is unresponsive to

antibiotics, treating clinicians may decide to obtain a tissue diagnosis using an FNA, core biopsy, or excisional biopsy. The drawback of continuing observation is the danger of possibly delaying a diagnosis, and therefore subsequent treatment of a potential malignancy or infection that could have dramatic consequences for the patient. However, performing a surgical excision of enlarged lymph nodes with a low risk for malignancy, and in nonsurgical malignancies (e.g., lymphoma), is associated with morbidity for the patient and requires anesthesia. FNA provides a minimally invasive modality to get quick answers in most cases that can facilitate further management. In addition, FNA is particularly advantageous in nonsurgical diseases, such as infections or lymphomas, and in patients with poor medical status who may not be surgical candidates.

Since FNA is a cost-effective tool, it is particularly beneficial in areas with economic limitations and limited access to imaging techniques or operating rooms, such as developing countries. In these settings, FNA of superficial palpable lymphadenopathy can provide quick answers on an outpatient basis (Sarda et al., 1990; Gupta AK, 1992; Thomas et al., 1999). Furthermore, in many developing countries where infectious etiologies such as tuberculosis

Non-Neoplastic Hematopathology and Infections, First Edition. Edited by Hernani D. Cualing, Parul Bhargava, and Ramon L. Sandin.
© 2012 Wiley-Blackwell. Published 2012 by John Wiley & Sons, Inc.

pose common major health problems, a quick and reliable FNA diagnosis can lead to significant cost-effective management and treatment. For example, in one study looking at an outpatient setting in India with over 1400 FNAs, over 68% of cases were benign, and included 31% cases with reactive hyperplasia and 38% with tuberculous lymphadenitis (Gupta AK et al., 1992). Furthermore, in some areas where facilities for tissue biopsy or excision and high complexity testing (e.g., PCR, microbiology culture) are not readily available, FNA may be the only feasible option. In terms of cost, the reported cost savings per 1000 FNAs as compared to surgical biopsies have been calculated at approximately $250,000 to $750,000 (Rimm et al., 1997). Moreover the use of rapid on-site evaluation (ROSE) has also been shown to increase the diagnostic yield by reducing the number of inadequate specimens to less than 1%, and thereby decreasing the need for additional diagnostic procedures, which are more costly and delay the diagnosis (Nasuti et al., 2002; Egea et al., 2002).

Deep-seated nonpalpable lymphadenopathy is aspirated under image guidance, while superficial lymphadenopathy can be sampled by palpation or image guidance. Having cytologists or pathologists provide ROSE evaluation for lymph node FNAs can be crucial for the appropriate triage. ROSE can also help minimize the number of needle passes required by assessing for adequacy, which can maximize the diagnostic yield and decrease the need for additional procedures. In addition, a pathologist can provide a preliminary diagnosis that can quickly help guide treatment.

An FNA can be done without anesthesia and does not require hospitalization; thus, it is a very quick procedure with a minimal risk to the patient. For this reason, some practitioners have used the pneumonic SAFE (safe, accurate, fast, and economic) to summarize the advantages of FNA in making diagnoses. Moreover, FNA may be the only option to obtain a diagnosis for patients with deep-seated lymphadenopathy or those with an emergent condition (e.g., superior vena cava syndrome or spinal cord compression). The potential complications include a low risk of hemorrhage or hematoma, infection, pneumothorax (in deep-seated chest wall, lung, or supraclavicular FNAs), tissue infarction, reactive changes (Nasuti et al., 2001; Tsang and Chan, 1992), and the possibility of missing the lesion, particularly in small or deep lymph nodes. The complication rate is usually less than 1%, and the majority of complications occur when larger gauge needles are used (Schultenover et al., 1984). The drawbacks of FNA include false-negative diagnoses, which are largely attributed

to sampling error or suboptimal specimens, inability to evaluate for architecture in some cases, and interpretation error due to lack of experience with nongynecologic aspiration cytology. Sampling errors may be attributed to lack of experienced aspirators, partial involvement of a lymph node, small node size, or deep location. In addition, certain disease processes, particularly those that are fibrotic (e.g., nodular sclerosing Hodgkin lymphoma, sclerosing mediastinal lymphadenopathy due to histoplasmosis), necrotic, or cystic (e.g., lymphangiomas) it may be difficult to aspirate sufficient viable cells to make a definitive diagnosis. Last, the distinction between reactive lymphoid hyperplasia and low-grade lymphomas based solely on cytology can be diagnostically difficult, thus material for ancillary studies is crucial (Lioe et al., 1999) (Table 21.1).

In general, FNA of lymph nodes is a very sensitive diagnostic modality, particularly when performed by those with experience in the performance and interpretation of FNA cytology in both children and adults. In children, FNA of lymph nodes has a reported sensitivity of 78 to 100% and specificity of 91 to 100%, with a nondiagnostic rate of 13% or less (Eisenhut et al., 1996; Buchino and Jones, 1994; Silverman et al., 1991; Kardos et al., 1989; Wakely et al., 1988; Wright et al., 2008; Wakely, 2001). The overall diagnostic accuracy for lymph node FNAs, largely in adult populations, has been reported to be approximately 90% (Thomas et al., 1999). The accuracy improves over time, with increasing experience and expertise of the cytopathologist in performing and interpreting FNAs. A way to minimize the unsatisfactory aspirates and maximize diagnostic yield is to have pathologists perform the aspirates on superficial nodes and perform ROSE to guide appropriate specimen triage, which is particularly important in the evaluation of lymph nodes. False-positive diagnoses are rare, with only occasional reports of overcalling Hodgkin lymphoma based on reactive macrophages that were mistaken for Reed–Sternberg cells (Thomas et al., 1999). False-negative cases are more common, and as alluded to above, may be due to inadequate sampling, partial or early involvement of lymph nodes, and unrecognized low-grade lymphomas (Thomas et al., 1999). In one series of lymphomas diagnosed by FNA, 12% of the cytologic diagnoses were falsely negative, largely due to mistaking low-grade lymphomas and Hodgkin lymphomas as benign conditions (Steel et al., 1995; Prasad et al., 1996). However, FNA has a very high sensitivity, so false negatives for metastatic tumors are rare (Prasad et al., 1996).

TABLE 21.1 **Pros and Cons of Lymph Node Fine Needle Aspiration (FNA)**

Advantages	Disadvantages
Confirmation of lymphoid tissue	Need for expertise in performance and interpretation of FNA
Rapid turn around time	Interpretation error: lack of operator expertise
Immediate preliminary diagnosis	Lack of architecture
Minimal complications (hematoma, hemorrhage, infection, scarring)	Need for sufficient material for ancillary studies
No general anesthesia	
Less expensive than surgical excision	
Outpatient or inpatient procedure	
Alleviate anxiety for the patient	
Triage of material for cytomorphology, culture, immunohistochemical stains, flow cytometry, and/or molecular studies	Sampling errors: operator dependent, lack of on-site evaluation, nonrepresentative areas due to fibrosis, necrosis, or cystic change, partial/incomplete involvement of LN, small or difficult to sample lesions

TECHNICAL COMPONENTS

When performing an FNA, there are a variety of technical issues to consider. A clinical history is helpful to obtain pertinent information that allows one to formulate a differential diagnosis. The duration of symptoms and review of systems are also important. For example, the patient may report that their lymphadenopathy waxes and wanes, which would favor a reactive process; however, if the lymphadenopathy persists and enlarges, then it would be more concerning for potential malignancy. A prior history of malignancy is also important information, as they are likely to have greater than a twofold higher risk of having malignancy diagnosed on FNA of a lymph node, compared to those without such a history (Schafernak et al., 2003). Other symptoms may also be important, such as pharyngitis with infectious mononucleosis, and a fever associated with infection or B symptoms of lymphoma. The patient's immune status, travel history, and list of exposures (to cats, other animals, insect bites, or contagious diseases) can be helpful. Furthermore, any recent laboratory data such as Monospot test results, serologies, and microbiology culture results can be helpful. After obtaining a history, a directed physical examination is important. This allows one to determine if lymphadenopathy is localized or generalized, the size of the lymph nodes, and other palpable characteristics such as mobility (mobile or fixed), contour (ill-defined or well-defined), texture (soft, doughy/cystic or firm), and tenderness (usually from rapid enlargement or stretching of the capsule in benign/infectious processes or rapidly proliferating lymphomas).

An FNA can be performed on almost any patient, which is a distinct advantage of the procedure. In some nodal targets, proximity to large blood vessels or bleeding disorders may make the procedure unsafe. However, even patients on heparin and coumadin can have an FNA without risk of significant bleeding, unlike other more invasive procedures. Contraindications to performing an FNA include vascular carotid body tumors or pheochromocytomas, in which sampling may lead to syncope or acute hypertension. However, there are very few other contraindications. Hydatid cysts are usually not aspirated due to the risk of anaphylactic shock from spilled parasitic contents. FNA is typically performed without anesthesia in an outpatient or inpatient setting at the bedside. Local anesthesia, such as topical sprays or creams like EMLA (Eutectic Mixture of Local Anesthetic, which includes lidocaine 2.5% and prilocaine 2.5%) may be particularly helpful in children. In deep (visceral) locations, an injection of lidocaine is frequently used. The skin is cleaned (e.g., with alcohol) prior to puncture for superficial locations, whereas sterile procedures are usually necessary for deeper aspirates.

FNA can be performed with suction or without suction (the Zajdela technique, also called fine needle nonaspiration) (Zajdela et al., 1987). Aspirates without suction (relying largely on capillary action of material moving in the needle) are particularly useful for vascular lesions (e.g., neuroendocrine and thyroid lesions) to minimize peripheral blood dilution and in very small (<1-cm) mobile lesions (e.g., small mobile lymph nodes in children) where fine motor control to joggle (rapidly move) needles is required. Aspirates performed with suction usually yield more material and are helpful in lesions that are cystic in order to drain fluid. Most aspirates preformed with suction

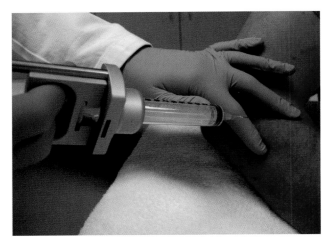

FIGURE 21.1 **FNA technique with aspiration and syringe holder**. Stabilization of the targeted lesion with the pointer finger and middle finger allows the thumb to be free for stabilizing the syringe.

rely on a syringe holder that fits a 10-cc syringe, allowing negative pressure to be applied using one hand while the other hand is free to immobilize the patient's lesion. Careful positioning of one's thumb under the syringe can help stabilize the needle and reduce the likelihood of the aspirator puncturing the user's own skin (Figure 21.1).

About 3 to 5 passes are performed with every FNA, depending on the ability to obtain lesional cells and adequate material. At least three aspirates should be obtained from different areas of an enlarged lymph node in order to ensure good, representative sampling (Ersoz et al., 1998). If needed, subsequent passes should be performed in slightly different areas to sample the lymph node better and to avoid blood dilution. With each pass, approximately 15 to 20 excursions are taken with a cutting motion to obtain cells from the lymph node. Occasionally separate dedicated passes can be performed for ancillary studies if the aspirates appear hypocellular; however, expelling a little material from each pass on a glass slide allows one to determine whether the lesion has been sampled and how cellular or representative the sample is of the target. With each pass, smears can be air dried or fixed in 95% alcohol. Air dried smears are usually stained with a Romanowsky stain such as Diff-Quik, but unstained air-dried smears can also be saved for potential ancillary studies (e.g., FISH) (Monaco et al., 2009). The Diff-Quik stain is a particularly helpful stain for the evaluation of lymphoid cells because lymphoglandular bodies can be easily identified. It also provides similar staining of cells to that seen in peripheral blood and bone marrow aspirate samples.

APPROACH TO CYTOMORPHOLOGIC EVALUATION OF LYMPH NODES

In lymph node FNA the first goal is to confirm that you have aspirated lymphoid tissue, which includes a discohesive population of cells with lymphoglandular bodies (fragments of lymphocyte cytoplasm) in the background, which is best appreciated on a Romanowsky stain such as Diff-Quik. In many cases, aspirates tend to be cellular with a predominance of small mature lymphocytes with round nuclei, dark chromatin, and scant cytoplasm. At low power, it is important to look for cell clustering, which may be due to technical components causing benign lymphocytes to cluster (e.g., thick smear, suboptimal spreading technique, or trapping within blood clot), granulomas, or metastatic carcinoma. Aggregates of lymphocytes adherent to follicular dendritic cells can also occur in follicular hyperplasia (O'Dowd et al., 1985). Low-power examination helps in evaluating background material, such as necrosis, inflammatory debris, and cyst contents. After establishing that one has a lymphoid population, the next goal is to evaluate the types of cells present, uniformity of these cells, their cell size, and associated background to further classify the lesion. Aspirates raising concern for a lymphoproliferative process tend to have monomorphic cell populations, larger cells, and an absence of macrophages. Benign/reactive processes tend to be more polymorphous, have a predominance of small cells, and a conspicuous presence of macrophages (Tables 21.2, 21.3; Figures 21.2, 21.3). One clue for evaluating the uniformity of lymphoid cells is to use the "string-of-pearls" technique, whereby if you can find a population of atypical or immature lymphocytes and connect them at high-power from one side

TABLE 21.2 **Key Cytomorphologic Features Used to Examine Lymph Node FNA Biopsies**

Adequacy (unsatisfactory, limited for evaluation, satisfactory)
Cellularity
Pattern of arrangement: cohesive, discohesive
Major cell type: lymphocytes (small, intermediate, or large), neutrophils, eosinophils, histiocytes
Cellular homogeneity or heterogeneity
Presence/absence of tingible body macrophages
Background: lymphoglandular bodies, necrosis, organisms
Granulomatous inflammation (present/absent and necrotizing/non-necrotizing)

TABLE 21.3 Cytomorphologic Differences between RLH and Non-Hodgkin B-Cell Lymphoma

Cytomorphologic Features	RLH	B-Cell Lymphoma
Cell population	Heterogeneous	Homogeneous
Cell types	T cells > B cells	B cells > T cells
Tingible-body macrophages	Present	Absent/rare
Lymphocyte nuclear features	Absence of cleaved nuclei or nucleoli	Cleaved nuclei or immature chromatin
Immunoglobulin light chain	Polyclonal	Monoclonal
CD10	Positive in germinal center only	Positive, diffuse for germinal center type
Bcl-2	Negative in germinal center	Positive in GC for germinal center type lymphoma
Mitoses	Frequent	Less frequent, unless high grade

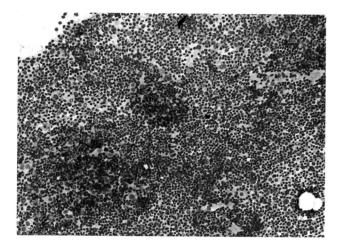

FIGURE 21.2 **Reactive lymphoid hyperplasia (low power, DQ stain).** At low power, a follicular architecture is apparent with scattered dense aggregates of dendritic cells, lymphocytes, and tingible body macrophages.

of the field to the other, then it is a homogeneous or monotonous population in which lymphoma should be excluded. An algorithmic approach on how to evaluate benign lymph nodes is shown in Figure 21.4.

FNA REPORTING TERMINOLOGY

In general, FNA results for nongynecologic specimens such as lymph nodes are reported with an adequacy determination (adequate, less than optimal, unsatisfactory) and a general interpretation (nondiagnostic, negative for malignant cells, atypical cells present, suspicious for malignant cells, positive for malignant cells). The frequency of nondiagnostic/unsatisfactory specimens is variable, but ranges from about 5 to 15%, with more nondiagnostic cases arising in small lymph

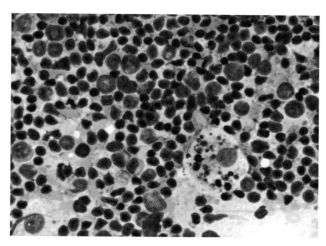

FIGURE 21.3 **Reactive lymphoid hyperplasia (high power, DQ stain).** The predominant cell type is the small mature lymphocyte, in addition to the follicle center cell, including centrocytes, centroblasts, and immunoblasts. Scattered tingible-body macrophages and plasmacytoid cells can also be seen.

nodes or those that are difficult to access (Lioe et al., 1999; Nasuti et al., 2000; Prasad et al., 1996; Steel et al., 1995). Unsatisfactory aspirates include those cases with insufficient cellularity or bloody aspirates, and cases where the material is obscured or uninterpretable (Thomas et al., 1999). A free text diagnosis can also be added to describe the lesion, to highlight the presence of organisms, or communicate another diagnoses to the clinician. A comment can be added to further describe findings in more detail and/or to report the findings from ancillary studies that support your diagnosis. A negative result does not necessarily exclude the possibility of malignancy. Thus, all FNA diagnoses really require correlation with clinical findings, other laboratory tests (e.g., microbiology studies), and available imaging results.

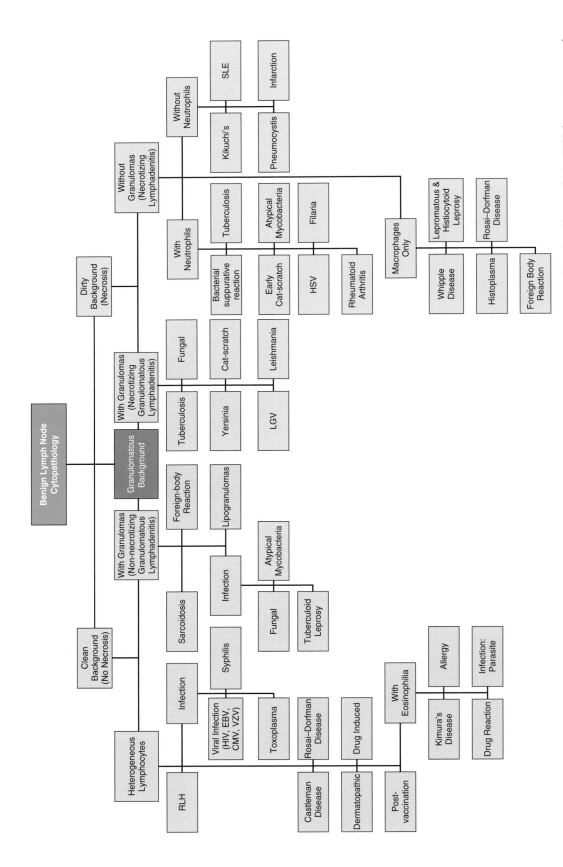

FIGURE 21.4 **Practical approach to the cytomorphologic evaluation of benign lymphadenopathy.** RLH, reactive lymphoid hyperplasia; HIV, human immunodeficiency virus; EBV, Epstein–Barr virus; CMV, cytomegalovirus; VZV, varicella zoster virus; HSV, herpes simplex virus; LGV, lymphogranuloma venereum; SLE, systemic lupus erythematosus.

INTRAOPERATIVE TOUCH PREPARATION

Intraoperative cytologic preparations, including touch imprint or scrapes, can be very helpful in the intraoperative evaluation of lymphoid lesions. They provide greater cytologic detail, particularly if air-dried Romanowsky stained material is available. Touch preps nicely complement or enhance the findings seen on frozen section, which can have many artifacts causing distortion. In some scenarios, such as lesions that are entirely necrotic, comprised predominantly of adipose tissue or calcified, a frozen section may not be possible, and thus cytology preparations may be the only option (Wilkerson, 1985). In addition, by using cytology preparations intraoperatively, more of the specimen can be preserved for final histology and ancillary studies.

REACTIVE LYMPHOID HYPERPLASIA

Definition

Reactive lymphoid hyperplasia (RLH) is one of the most common reasons for lymphadenopathy and involves chronic lymph node enlargement due to a reactive process. Nodal enlargement may be due to follicular or paracortical hyperplasia, as well as sinus histiocytosis.

ICD-9-CM Code 785.6

Synonyms

Chronic lymphadenitis, reactive lymphadenopathy, and follicular hyperplasia.

Clinical Aspects

RLH is the most common cause of lymphadenopathy, particularly in children. RLH can account for 50% or more of pediatric lymphadenopathy cases due to the repeated antigenic stimulation encountered in the early years of life (Anne et al., 2008). RLH is also relatively common in adults, comprising approximately 30% of cases of lymphadenopathy. However, in the adult population the possibility of lymphoma or metastatic carcinoma is markedly increased compared to children (Tatomirovic et al., 2009). Most cases involve the cervical, axillary, and inguinal lymph nodes. In general, involved nodes tend to be less than 3 cm in the greatest dimension. Patients with RLH can be followed clinically. Typically lymphadenopathy spontaneously resolves over a period of time, which may be variable. If the lymphadenopathy does not subside in 3 to 6 months or if the findings do not match the clinical suspicion, then a repeat biopsy should be recommended (Thomas et al., 1999).

Cytomorphology

The lymphoid population in RLH is polymorphous with a predominance of small mature lymphocytes that have round nuclei with condensed dark chromatin. The aspirates are usually cellular due to the lack of stroma to trap cells. There are also scattered plasmacytoid cells (which have moderate amounts of cytoplasm and an eccentrically placed nucleus) and immunoblasts (larger lymphoid cells with nucleoli and dark basophilic cytoplasm). Tingible body macrophages that contain apoptotic debris within their cytoplasm, and lymphohistiocytic aggregates or follicular center fragments are also usually seen. Mitotic figures are common. Occasional neutrophils, eosinophils, and mast cells may also be present. Moreover dendritic cells with pale oval nuclei (some bi/multinucleated), indistinct nucleoli, and long cytoplasmic processes can be identified (Figures 21.2, 21.3).

Differential Diagnosis

The diagnostic possibilities for a heterogeneous lymphoid population, as seen in RLH, include Hodgkin lymphoma (usually has more conspicuous eosinophils and Reed–Sternberg cells), partial lymph node involvement by a malignancy, post-transplant lymphoproliferative disorder, T-cell lymphomas, and some non-Hodgkin lymphomas (e.g., marginal zone lymphoma, low grade follicular lymphoma, T-cell-rich large B-cell lymphoma). In many of these mimics, the range of heterogeneity is limited, and a careful search for atypical cells can usually help raise the suspicion for a neoplastic process. In addition, although tingible body macrophages are frequently associated with RLH, these cells can also be a feature of high-grade lymphomas (including Burkitt lymphoma and plasmablastic lymphoma with a "starry sky" appearance). Early stages of infection, such as cat-scratch disease and tuberculosis, may also have a paucity of granulomas and inflammation, thereby mimicking RLH. Granulomas can sometimes be confused with lymphohistiocytic aggregates; however, the epithelioid histiocytes in granulomas have a characteristic nuclear morphology (kidney bean or boomerang shaped elongated nuclei and prominent nucleoli) that can help in recognizing them. Also included in the differential diagnosis are progressive transformation of germinal centers, Castleman disease, other causes of inflammatory lymphadenitis, chronic infection (e.g., HIV or syphilitic lymphadenitis), vaccinia (post-vaccination) lymphadenitis, and Kimura disease.

INFLAMMATORY AND INFECTIOUS CAUSES OF LYMPHADENOPATHY

Acute Suppurative Lymphadenitis

Definition
Lymph nodes with a predominance of acute neutrophilic inflammation.

ICD-9-CM Code 683

Synonyms
Acute lymphadenitis and ordinary bacterial lymphadenitis.

Clinical Aspects
Acute suppurative lymphadenitis is typically caused by bacterial organisms (e.g., *Staphylococcus* or *Streptococcus spp*, Gram-negative bacilli), and can give rise to tender, enlarged lymph nodes. Less likely causes include actinomycetes and some fungi.

Cytomorphology
The first key to this diagnosis is the finding of pus or purulent material (yellow, viscous material) upon aspiration. Specimens will have a large population of neutrophils admixed with inflammatory debris, lymphocytes, and tingible body macrophages (Figure 21.5). Careful examination is required to look for intracellular and extracellular organisms (fungus, bacteria, mycobacteria). Special stains should be performed including a Gram stain, GMS/Grocott stain, and AFB stain on available material to look for microorganisms. A portion of the specimen should be sent for microbial cultures in a sterile container, to help assist in subclassification of organisms if present, and provide information regarding antibiotic effectiveness (antibiotic sensitivity/resistance). The microbiologic culture yield (30%) from lymph node FNA is comparable with open biopsy (Layfield et al., 1985). With prior antibiotic therapy, microorganisms may not be detected.

Differential Diagnosis
The diagnostic possibilities for acute lymphadenitis primarily include bacterial etiologies

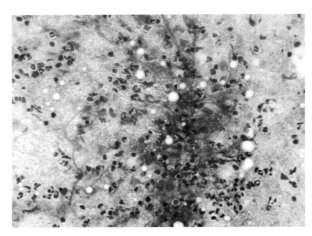

FIGURE 21.5   Acute suppurative lymphadenitis (medium power, DQ stain). Acute suppurative lymphadenitis yields numerous neutrophils in a background of granular inflammatory debris.

(Table 21.4). Fungus or mycobacteria may also occur in the absence of a granulomatous response, particularly in immunocompromised patients (e.g., AIDS patients). Cat-scratch disease, tularemia, and lymphogranuloma venereum may all cause a suppurative lymphadenitis with or without granulomas. The differential diagnosis includes the possibility of an abscess or developmental cyst of the neck with cystic and inflammatory changes. Kikuchi's lymphadenitis or other causes of necrotizing lymphadenitis may be considered if the background debris is predominant. However, in Kikuchi's lymphadenitis, while there is an absence of neutrophils, karyorrhectic debris present may mimic neutrophils.

Lymphoma is infrequently associated with abscess-type material. However, some malignancies, particularly keratinizing squamous cell carcinomas, can be associated with a prominent inflammatory component, and thus can give rise to a potential false-negative diagnosis if the inflammatory component obscures the malignant cells (Silverman and Kardos, 1991).

TABLE 21.4   Causes of Acute Suppurative Lymphadenitis

Infection: bacteria, cat-scratch disease, tuberculosis, fungal, HSV, other
Immunodeficiency: CGD, other
Infarction of lymph node
Mimics: Kikuchi's lymphadenitis, autoimmune-related lymphadenopathy

Cat-Scratch Lymphadenitis

Definition
Infection by the gram-negative bacillus *Bartonella henselae* causing an acute self-limited necrotizing granulomatous lymphadenitis.

ICD-9-CM Code 683

Synonyms
Cat-scratch disease, CSD.

Clinical Aspects
CSD is a form of lymphadenopathy that is relatively common among children and young adults. The major etiologic agent is *Bartonella henselae*, which enters via the skin at the time of a cat scratch or bite and causes regional (localized) lymphadenopathy 1 to 3 weeks later, usually in the axilla or head and neck region. The skin lesion (papule/vesicle) is usually present at the time of lymphadenopathy. Serologic studies have a low sensitivity and specificity because some patients never have a detectable antibody response. Patients may have a fever, headache, and body aches. Histologically, one of the hallmark findings are stellate microabscesses within lymph nodes. *B. henselae* has also been known to cause clinical manifestations, such as oculoglandular syndrome, bacillary angiomatosis, pelosis hepatica, bacteremia, endocarditis, and aseptic meningitis. In patients with AIDS, CSD can cause fatal systemic illness.

Cytomorphology
Cytology specimens can show three patterns: the initial phase will usually show florid reactive lymphoid hyperplasia, the second phase involves loose granulomas and single histiocytes, and the final phase is the most characteristic with an acute suppurative and granulomatous lymphadenitis containing neutrophils admixed with granulomas (cohesive groups of epithelioid macrophages) and sometimes necrotic/inflammatory debris and multinucleated giant cells (Table 21.4; Figure 21.6). The diagnosis can be confirmed with PCR or stains to detect *B. henselae*. Since this bacteria does not stain well with a Gram stain, silver impregnation stains such as a modified silver stain (modified Steiner stain) or Warthin–Starry stain have been used to identify organisms, which appear as pleomorphic aggregates of bacilli or single organisms. A modified silver stain is reportedly positive in 69% cases (Donnelly et al., 1995). However, given the difficulty interpreting silver stains due to the background nonspecific staining seen with necrotic debris and macrophages,

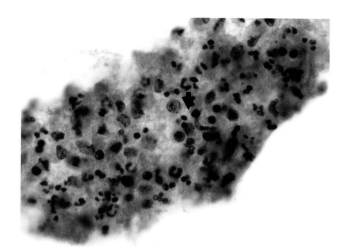

FIGURE 21.6 **Cat-scratch disease (high power, Pap stain).** A cluster of epithelioid histiocytes intermixed with neutrophils with a rare probable bacillus (arrowhead) is seen in a patient with cat-scratch disease.

an immunohistochemical stain using *B. henselae* monoclonal antibody is now available but will only detect *B. henselae* (Caponetti et al., 2009). Serologic studies for Bartonella are also available. Molecular testing with PCR is the most sensitive way to detect the organism, but immunostaining is a more cost effective, widely available, and rapid test.

Differential Diagnosis
The differential diagnosis includes abscess and an acute suppurative lymphadenitis due to other causes, such as tuberculosis, fungal or bacterial organisms (Table 21.4). Kikuchi necrotizing lymphadenitis may cause patchy necrosis with debris but lacks granulomatous inflammation and neutrophils. In some cases, the features may also resemble a lymphoproliferative disorder.

Granulomatous Lymphadenitis

Definition
Inflammation within a lymph node composed of epithelioid macrophages (granulomas).

ICD-9-CM Code 289.1

Synonyms
Necrotizing/non-necrotizing lymphadenitis, and caseating/noncaseating lymphadenitis

Clinical Aspects
Granulomatous lymphadenitis can be seen in the setting of infectious processes, in addition to noninfectious processes such as sarcoidosis, foreign body

reactions, and malignancies. Patients usually present with regional or multiple enlarged lymph nodes, such as in the mediastinal or head and neck region.

Cytomorphology

At low power, granulomatous lymphadenitis will show clusters of epithelioid histiocytes intermixed with lymphocytes and occasionally multinucleated giant cells (Figures 21.7, 21.8). In addition there may be a necrotic background in cases of necrotizing (or caseous) granulomas. The macrophages are typically epithelioid and contain elongated, kidney bean, or boomerang shaped nuclei with nucleoli and a moderate amount of cytoplasm. Macrophages may sometimes radiate around the edges of cell clusters in a starburst configuration or be scattered as single epithelioid cells. On occasion, macrophages may form bundles of elongated spindle cells. Suppurative granulomatous inflammation has a prominent neutrophilic infiltrate admixed with granulomas and necrotic/inflammatory debris. The three main patterns encountered are listed below with tables showing the differential diagnosis for each type:

1. Suppurative/acute granulomatous inflammation (Table 21.4; Figure 21.6)
2. Necrotizing granulomatous inflammation (Table 21.5; Figure 21.7)
3. Non-necrotizing granulomatous inflammation (Table 21.5; Figure 21.8)

Foreign material may be encountered, and this may require polarization of procured nodal material. Special stains for mycobacteria and fungi should be routinely performed to exclude an infectious etiology. Immunocytochemistry using markers such as S-100 and CD68 (KP1) can be used to confirm the presence of macrophages.

TABLE 21.5 Causes of Granulomatous Inflammation in Lymph Node

Non-necrotizing	Necrotizing
Infection: atypical mycobacteria, schistosomiasis	Infection: tuberculosis, fungal, cat scratch
Sarcoidosis	Kikuchi's lymphadenitis
Foreign-body reaction (silicosis, berylliosis)	Lymph node infarction
Other: malignancies (Lymphoma, Seminoma, squamous cell carcinoma)	Immunodeficiency: Chronic granulomatous disease, other

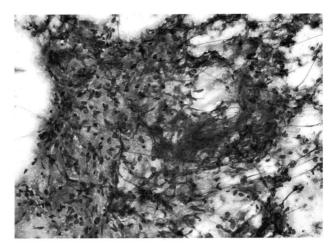

FIGURE 21.7 **Necrotizing lymphadenitis due to histoplasmosis (medium power, DQ stain)**, Ill-defined clusters of epithelioid histiocytes are intermixed with dense granular debris and lymphocytes in an FNA from a patient with histoplasmosis.

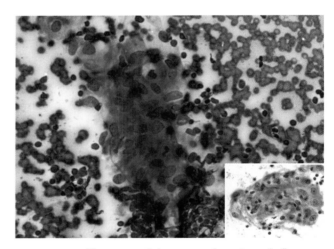

FIGURE 21.8 **Non-necrotizing granulomatous inflammation in a patient with sarcoidosis (high power, DQ stain; inset: high power, Pap stain)**. Well-defined rounded aggregates of epithelioid histiocytes with small lymphocytes are observed in a clean background from an FNA of a lymph node in a patient clinically diagnosed with sarcoidosis.

Differential Diagnosis

Granulomas can mimic malignancies like metastatic carcinomas, particularly in the setting of a necrotic background. Some malignancies including lymphoma (e.g., Hodgkin lymphoma), squamous cell carcinoma, and seminoma can be associated with granulomatous inflammation. Therefore it is crucial to exclude the presence of malignant cells in the setting of granulomatous inflammation (Monaco et al., 2010; Zardawi et al., 2005). Granulomas

TABLE 21.6 Neoplastic Processes that Mimic Benign Lymph Node Conditions

Low-grade small-cell lymphoma (mimic of reactive lymphoid hyperplasia)

Metastatic bland malignancies (mimic of granulomatous inflammation)

Hodgkin lymphoma (mimic of reactive lymphoid hyperplasia)

Tumors associated with granulomas (mistaken for granulomatous inflammation)

T-cell lymphomas (mimic of RLH because mostly T cells, clonality not established easily, heterogeneous)

can also mimic lymphohistiocytic aggregates in RLH, sinus histiocytosis, dendritic reticulum cells, low-grade neoplasms, and occasionally spindle cell lesions/tumors or fibroblasts; however, the characteristic morphology of the nucleus of epithelioid macrophages is key to making this distinction (Table 21.6). Other entities to consider are lipogranulomatous reactions and allergic granulomatosis in lymph nodes. Moreover, in the appropriate setting (e.g., young patients with recurrent lymphadenitis, hepatosplenomegaly, skin rash, and pulmonary edema), congenital enzymatic defects of NADPH oxidase in granulocytes and monocytes should be considered, as seen in chronic granulomatous disease.

Mycobacterial Lymphadenitis

Definition

Lymphadenitis due to infection by mycobacteria, either *Mycobacterium tuberculosus* (Tuberculosis, TB) or non-tuberculous (atypical) mycobacteria, such as *Mycobacterium avium-intracellulare*.

ICD-9-CM Code 031.8, 017.2 (tuberculous)

Synonyms

Tuberculous or nontuberculous lymphadenitis.

Clinical Aspects

TB is the most common form of mycobacterial lymphadenitis in the world and the most common extrapulmonary manifestation of TB, predominantly in less developed countries (Wright et al., 2008). Patients may have a known history of tuberculosis or a positive tuberculin test, and often have multiple nodes involved. Lymphadenitis due to mycobacteria is most frequent in the head and neck lymph nodes, followed by the axilla (Sharma et al., 2007; Gupta AK et al., 1992). The individuals most at risk for

mycobacterial infection are young children, elderly adults, and immunocompromised or immunosuppressed patients such as HIV-positive patients. Disseminated *M. bovis* infection following BCG therapy may rarely involve lymph nodes. The sensitivity for the detection of mycobacteria, in particular *M. tuberculosis*, by FNA cytology ranges from about 25% (Ellison et al., 1999) to a high of about 70% (Aljafari et al., 2004; Thomas et al., 1999; Wright et al., 2008). In general, FNA detects around half the cases of mycobacterial lymphadenitis and has a high specificity and positive predictive value (Ellison et al., Gupta AK et al., 1992; Jain et al., 2005; Ersöz et al., 1998). However, there is a high false-negative rate due to the absence of granulomas and/or necrosis in cases of early tuberculous lymphadenitis. FNA supplemented with mycobacterial cultures increases the sensitivity of diagnosing TB lymphadenitis. Rare cases may be positive by cytology but have false-negative culture results due to the inhibitory effect of prior treatment or inadequacy of the material sent. Nevertheless, culture should always be done in each case for characterization and determination of drug sensitivity if the growth for mycobacteria turns positive (Kishore et al., 2008; Gupta SK et al., 1993). If available, PCR may be helpful in cases with a strong suspicion, equivocal tests (e.g., ELISA), and in the early diagnosis of TB when other, less sensitive tests may be negative (Goel et al., 2001). Overall, PCR detects approximately 83% of cases, FNA detects about 50%, and staining for acid fast bacilli (AFB) detects about 33% of cases (Jain et al., 2005) Thus, a combination of these modalities can optimize sensitivity and specificity.

Cytomorphology

At the time of aspiration, many of these cases will demonstrate cheesy (caseous) or purulent material on gross examination, similar to acute suppurative lymphadenitis. This can be a helpful clue to save material for culture and other ancillary studies. On microscopic examination, aspirates often have a dirty or granular background with macrophages, including multinucleated Langhans giant cells, epithelioid histiocytes, and aggregates of macrophages forming granulomas. Extensive necrosis and suppuration occurs more frequently in atypical mycobacterial lymphadenitis. The four different cytomorphological patterns of TB include granulomas with necrosis (50%), granulomas without necrosis (32%), necrosis/pus without granulomas or giant cells (15%), and epithelioid macrophages without necrosis or giant cells (3%) (Gupta AK et al., 1992). Markedly foamy macrophages may be encountered, especially with atypical mycobacterial infections where the

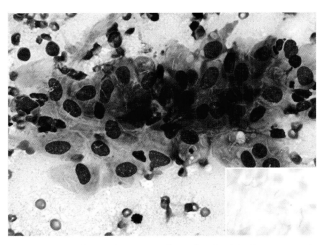

FIGURE 21.9 **Granulomatous lymphadenitis due to atypical mycobacteria (high power, DQ stain; inset: high power, AFB stain).** A cluster of epithelioid histiocytes with the negative image of long, beaded mycobacterial organisms is seen on DQ stain, and highlighted with the AFB stain (inset).

macrophages are loaded with microorganisms. If numerous, bacilli may sometimes be seen as a negative image (i.e., clear area in the shape of a rod that fails to stain) in air-dried Romanowsky stained smears (Stanley et al., 1990) (Figure 21.9). Bacilli can also be visualized by acid-fast stains (Ziehl-Neelsen, Kinyoun, Fite) and/or immunostains. In *M. tuberculosis*, bacilli may be hard to find and appear as slightly curved, slender rods measuring 2 to 4 μm in length. With atypical mycobacteria there are usually more abundant acid-fast bacilli, and the rods appear more beaded. An AFB stain is most often positive in those cases where abundant pus or necrosis is aspirated. There appears to be an inverse relationship between the presence of granulomas and the chance of identifying AFB-positive mycobacteria (i.e., the greatest chance of finding AFB is in patients with an abscess and no granulomas) (Prasoon, 2000). Negative staining results do not entirely exclude an infectious origin. A definitive diagnosis may depend on the microbiology results.

Differential Diagnosis

In the early stages of mycobacterial lymphadenitis the findings may mimic an acute suppurative lymphadenitis or necrotizing lymphadenitis. Later, with the formation of granulomas, the differential diagnosis would include the multitude of inciting agents for granulomatous lymphadenitis (Table 21.5). In the setting of atypical mycobacterial infection with foamy histiocytes, one needs to consider metabolic storage diseases (e.g., Gaucher's disease with Gaucher

cells) or lepromatous leprosy with vacuolated histiocytes containing lepra bacilli (Gupta SK et al., 1981). In the setting of a necrotic background, one should consider malignancy and the variety of other possibilities (Figure 21.4).

Fungal Lymphadenitis

Definition

Lymph node enlargement due to infection by fungal organisms.

ICD-9-CM Code 683, 117.5 (Cryptococcus), 115.90 (Histoplasmosis)

Synonyms

Lymphadenitis due to a specific fungal infection (cryptococcal lymphadenitis, histoplasma lymphadenitis, etc.).

Clinical Aspects

Fungal infections most often detected as causative agents in lymphadenitis include *Histoplasma capsulatum* (dimorphic fungus), *Coccidioides immitis* (dimorphic fungus), and *Cryptococcus neoformans* (monomorphic fungus). There is a relatively high incidence in AIDS patients from endemic areas. Pneumocystis lymphadenitis is rare, and also usually arises in the setting of underlying HIV infection. Histoplasmosis is endemic in the central United States (Ohio River Valley). There are only rare reports of histoplasmosis involving lymph nodes, particularly in HIV-positive patients with widespread disease (Neumann et al., 1992).

Coccidioidomycosis is endemic in the southwestern United States and has rarely been reported to cause lymphadenopathy (Stephany et al., 2005). Cryptococcus occurs most commonly (about 67% of the time) as an opportunistic infection in the immunocompromised host. Cryptococcus (mainly *C. neoformans*) can cause lymphadenitis, but usually infection with this fungus results in a systemic disease that can also involve the respiratory system, CNS, skin, and other organs. Since Cryptococcus can disseminate and become life-threatening, a rapid diagnosis is important (Garbyal et al., 2005; Gustafson et al., 2007; Srinivasan et al., 2010).

Cytomorphology

The aspirates in fungal lymphadenitis usually show necrotic and/or inflammatory debris with acute inflammation and/or chronic granulomatous inflammation. Fungal histochemical stains including Grocott or Gomori methenamine silver (GMS), Periodic acid-Schiff (PAS) or mucicarmine stains performed

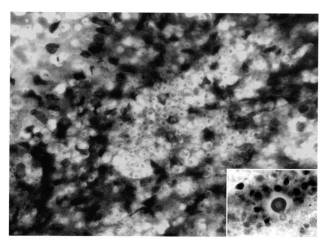

FIGURE 21.10 Fungal lymphadenitis due to *Cryptococcus neoformans* (high power, DQ stain; inset: high power, Pap stain). Yeast forms with narrow-based, teardrop-shaped budding and a thick capsule are identified on the DQ stain and Pap stain (inset), which are morphologically consistent with *Cryptococcus neoformans*.

on cytology material can help identify organisms and aid in their subclassification. Cryptococcus appears as encapsulated yeast forms, 5 to 15 μm in diameter with narrow-based budding (teardrop shape), and a thick mucopolysaccharide capsule that appears as a clear halo on a DQ stain and stains positive with muci-carmine, Alcian blue, and PAS stains (Figure 21.10). A Fontana–Masson stain can be helpful to identify capsule-deficient Cryptococcus (Lazcano et al., 1993). Histoplasmosis will show small round to oval, intra-cytoplasmic, narrow-based budding yeast forms that measure 2 to 4 μm. Macrophages in these cases are usually laden with yeast. Histoplasma stains best with GMS, and may fail to stain with hematoxylin and eosin (H&E), PAS, and mucicarmine stains. *C. immitis* forms mature, thick-walled spherules (cysts) that are 20 to 150 μm in size, containing 3 to 5 μm endospores. Endospores may sometimes form long, thin, branching septate hyphae. These fungal organisms should stain well with GMS and PAS stains. The findings in any case of fungal lymphadenitis should be correlated with culture results. Some cases of fungal infection may be associated with eosinophilia, which can also be seen with a variety of other lesions in lymph nodes (Table 21.7).

Differential Diagnosis

The cytomorphology of fungal lymphadenitis can mimic that seen in tuberculosis, granulomatous disease, and acute suppurative lymphadenitis. Blas-tomycosis can look very similar to Cryptococcus but is

TABLE 21.7 Differential Diagnosis of Increased Eosinophils within a Lymph Node

Infection: parasite, fungal
Drug and allergic reaction
Kimura disease
Langerhan cell histiocytosis
Hodgkin lymphoma
T-cell lymphoma
Other: hypereosinophilic syndrome

not a common cause of lymphadenitis. Usually blas-tomycosis shows larger organisms with broad-based budding, and does not have a mucoid capsule.

Sarcoidosis

Definition

Sarcoidosis is a multisystem granulomatous dis-ease that is due to an unknown inciting factor or antigen, and is characterized by a non-necrotizing granulomatous inflammation.

ICD-9-CM Code 289.1, 135 (sarcoidosis)

Synonyms

Besnier-Boeck disease.

Clinical Aspects

Sarcoidosis occurs worldwide and typically affects young adult females, especially in African-Americans. It is a granulomatous disease that can involve a variety of organs. Although there is frequently involvement of bilateral hilar and mediastinal lymph nodes, any lymph node can be affected. The onset is gradual and patients may be asymptomatic or present with a chronic illness. Clini-cal clues may include erythema nodosum, chest X-ray findings (e.g., pulmonary infiltrates), and elevated angiotensin-converting enzyme (ACE) blood levels.

Cytomorphology

The predominant pattern is granulomatous inflammation with a clean background. Clusters of macrophages usually make well-formed discrete granulomas with fewer multinucleated giant cells compared to cases of tuberculosis (Figure 12.8) The macrophages may show asteroid bodies (star-shaped), Hamazaki–Wesenberg inclusions (PAS+, yellow-brown inclusions), or Schaumann bodies (concentrically laminated spherical structures made of calcium and iron). In long-standing cases there can be extensive fibrosis and hyalinization of the granulomas as well as the entire lymph node, giving rise to scant aspirates and inadequate material for a cytology diagnosis. The diagnosis of sarcoidosis is essentially a diagnosis of exclusion, which requires the exclusion of other causes of granulomatous inflammation, particularly infectious etiologies. Thus special stains (e.g., AFB, GMS) and culture are usually performed on these specimens.

Differential Diagnosis

The differential diagnosis includes the variety of etiologies of granulomatous inflammation. Given that some patients with severe sarcoidosis are treated with immunosuppression, it is important to exclude the possibility of concurrent infection. The three types of inclusions seen in sarcoidosis (asteroid bodies, Hamazaki–Wesenberg bodies, or Schaumann bodies) may also be mistaken for fungus but should not stain with GMS. In addition, the possibility of an associated lymphoma or metastatic carcinoma should always be considered in these patients.

Toxoplasma Lymphadenitis

Definition

The lymph node infection is caused by the protozoan *Toxoplasma gondii*.

ICD-9-CM Code 130.7

Synonyms

Toxoplasmosis, Piringer-Kuchinka Lymphadenopathy.

Clinical Aspects

Toxoplasma is a parasitic infection in which the definitive host is the cat. Infections can be congenital and severe (fetal toxoplasmosis), or acquired where it usually remains latent and only causes tissue damage if the host is immunocompromised. Toxoplasmosis lymphadenitis has been reported and tends to be localized (e.g., mainly posterior cervical nodes) in normal hosts (Pathan et al., 2003). Systemic toxoplasmosis is seen mainly in immunodeficient patients. Acute disease can be similar in presentation to infectious mononucleosis (EBV) or other viral infections manifesting with chills, fever, fatigue, and lymphadenitis.

Cytomorphology

The key findings include cellular specimens with a polymorphous lymphoid population arising from reactive germinal centers, epithelioid cell clusters (epithelioid microgranulomas), and aggregates of monocytoid B cells with or without a necrotic background (Shimizu et al., 2001). Plasma cells may be seen, but neutrophils are not. Cysts with many

bradyzoites ("bag of parasites") of *T. gondii* are rarely found in aspirates but have been reported (Pathan et al., 2003). Free extracellular tachyzoites can rarely be seen and may be missed with a routine Pap stain. Toxoplasma organisms are best stained with a Wright–Giemsa stain or specific immunohistochemical stain (Zaharopoulos, 2000). PCR using primers designed for the ribosomal DNA of *T. gondii* can also be performed on blood or cytology material. Serologic testing (high titers of IgG- and IgM-specific antibodies to *T. gondii*) is usually necessary for the diagnosis, and the IgM is usually positive within three months of infection.

Differential Diagnosis

Several different causes of lymphadenitis with granulomas or monocytoid cells are included in the differential. This includes sarcoidosis, which usually has more well-defined granulomas and multinucleated giant cells. Leishmaniasis lymphadenitis and Brucella infection (undulant fever) can be very similar to toxoplasmosis, and may require electron microscopy or culture to make the distinction. Acute suppurative lymphadenitis or granulomatous lymphadenitis, as seen with cat-scratch disease or tuberculosis, can be considered and excluded with special stains and culture. The differential diagnosis also includes infectious mononucleosis lymphadenitis, given the presence of monocytoid cells without distinct granulomas, and dermatopathic lymphadenopathy.

Herpes Simplex Virus Lymphadenitis

Definition

The lymph node infection and enlargement is due to infection by the Herpes simplex virus (HSV).

ICD-9-CM Code 054.9

Synonyms

HSV lymphadenitis.

Clinical Aspects

Lymphadenitis due to HSV is rare, but has been reported in inguinal lymph nodes, particularly in patients with hematological malignancies (Gaffey et al., 1991). Apart from manifesting with localized lymphadenopathy, patients may have disseminated infection with a herpetic rash, particularly individuals who are immunosuppressed.

Cytomorphology

HSV may cause a necrotizing lymphadenitis in lymph nodes that lacks granulomas but has abundant necrotic debris with scattered neutrophils and a mixed lymphoplasmacytic infiltrate. Intranuclear inclusions characteristic of herpes with margination of the chromatin, multinucleation, and molding can help, if present, and have been reported to occur in stromal cells, not lymphoid cells (Gaffey et al., 1991). Ancillary studies that can be ordered include an immunohistochemical or in-situ hybridization stain for HSV1/2 ("cocktail"), viral culture, and molecular methods (to prove whether the infection is due to HSV1 or HSV2).

Differential Diagnosis

The suppurative nature of the reaction may mimic cat-scratch disease. However, the lymph nodes involved in HSV infection are not associated with granulomatous inflammation. Necrotic lymph nodes with neutrophils can also be attributed to bacterial infection, infarction from vascular compromise or vasculitis, and Kikuchi disease (Table 21.4). Varicella-Herpes Zoster lymphadenitis exhibits different intranuclear viral inclusions and does not characteristically have associated acute inflammation. Measles lymphadenitis has Warthin–Finkeldey giant cells. Furthermore, given that HSV lymphadenitis typically occurs in patients with a history of a hematological malignancy, one of the possibilities in the differential is a Richter transformation to a non-Hodgkin lymphoma or Hodgkin lymphoma given the presence of large cells with bi- and multi-nucleation.

Infectious Mononucleosis Lymphadenitis

Definition

Lymphadenopathy due to infection by Epstein–Barr virus (EBV) that is part of the clinical syndrome is called infectious mononucleosis, which includes a constellation of symptoms such as fatigue, fever, pharyngitis, lymphadenopathy, splenomegaly, and sometimes hepatomegaly.

ICD-9-CM Code 075

Synonyms
EBV-related lymphadenopathy.

Clinical Aspects
EBV is a DNA virus that is part of the Herpesviridae family. The manifestations of the infection are variable. Young children and toddlers typically have asymptomatic self-limiting infections, whereas teenagers may have a more serious illness. The condition is highly contagious. EBV-infected patients may have a leukocytosis and atypical lymphocytes

(Downey cells) reported in their peripheral blood smears. Heterophil antibody testing (Paul–Bunnell test), the MonoSpot test (more sensitive assay), and EBV-specific serology studies can be helpful and should be performed when infection is clinically suspected. Given that the incubation for the virus is 40 to 60 days, serology is usually positive at presentation. Some cases that have an infectious mononucleosis-like syndrome may be caused by other viruses such as CMV or HIV (Rinaldo et al., 1980). Lymph node biopsies are usually performed when the clinical presentation is atypical, lymphadenopathy is in unusual sites (axilla or groin), or a neoplastic process is suspected.

Cytomorphology

The diagnosis usually relies on a combination of clinical and serologic findings, in addition to the morphologic features when lymph nodes are aspirated. FNAs will show a polymorphous population of lymphocytes admixed with tingible-body macrophages, as well as plasmacytoid lymphocytes and many immunoblasts. An intermediate- to large-size polymorphic immunoblast proliferation should be a clue to making this diagnosis (Stanley, et al., 1990) (Figure 21.11). Occasionally pleomorphic atypical immunoblasts with binucleation, mimicking Reed–Sternberg cells, or mitoses will be seen. No viral inclusions are present.

Differential Diagnosis

The aspirates in this condition can look very concerning for malignancy, including a large cell lymphoma, given the prominent atypical immunoblastic proliferation. (Tables 21.8 and 21.9). The key features that help distinguish EBV lymphadenopathy from lymphoma are the range (polymorphous appearance) of lymphoid cells present. Flow cytometry in infectious mononucleosis cases will show predominantly heterogeneous T cells with polyclonal B cells, and this should be performed in those cases with an exuberant immunoblastic reaction that mimics lymphoma. In cases that are not supported by positive

TABLE 21.8 Differential Diagnosis of Prominent Immunoblast Proliferation

Viral infection: Epstein-Barr virus
Autoimmune disease: Systemic lupus erythematosus, rheumatoid arthritis
Drug-related lymphadenopathy: Dilantin
Hematolymphoid malignancy: immunoblastic diffuse large B-cell lymphoma acute prolymphocytic leukemia/lymphoma, others
Mimics: plasmablasts, Reed–Sternberg cells in Hodgkin lymphoma, non-lymphoid cells

TABLE 21.9 Non-neoplastic Processes That Mimic Malignancy in Lymph Nodes

EBV-related lymphadenopathy that mimics lymphoma

Atypical reactive lymphoid hyperplasia that mimics lymphoma

Extramedullary hematopoiesis with megakaryocytes that mimic malignant cells

Eosinophilic infiltrates that mimic Hodgkin lymphoma

Cellular granulomas that mimic metastatic carcinoma

Benign nodal reactions (e.g., decidual reaction) that mimic metastases

Benign lymph node inclusions that mimic metastases

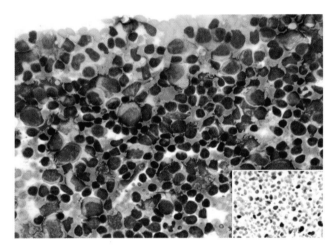

FIGURE 21.11 **Infectious mononucleosis (high power, DQ stain; inset: high power, EBER in-situ hybridization).** A polymorphous population of lymphoid cells is seen with a prominent immunoblastic population and plasmacytoid cells, in this case of EBV-related infectious mononucleosis in an 8-year-old boy. Flow cytometry confirmed the absence of a monoclonal population.

serologic studies and in which lymphadenopathy persists, a lymph node biopsy or excision should be performed to exclude a lymphoproliferative disorder (Stanley et al., 1990). Unlike classical type Hodgkin lymphoma, the Reed–Sternberg-like cells that may be seen in cases of infectious mononucleosis are positive for pan-B-cell markers (CD20) and negative for CD15 and CD30. The cytomorphology may resemble that seen in other reactive viral lymphadenitides, as well as toxoplasma lymphadenitis.

HIV-Associated Lymphadenopathy

Definition

Lymphadenopathy arises in association with a patient that has human immunodeficiency virus (HIV) infection.

ICD-9-CM Code 042

Synonyms

HIV lymphadenitis and persistent generalized lymphadenopathy, PGL.

Clinical Aspects

Lymphadenopathy in HIV-positive persons may be due to the HIV infection and/or be secondary to coinfection (e.g., tuberculosis), an inflammatory process (e.g., Castleman disease or immune reconstitution inflammatory syndrome), or malignancy (e.g., lymphoma, Kaposi sarcoma, metastases). Lymph node FNA and/or biopsy is usually performed if any of these conditions are suspected (Lowe et al., 2008; Martin-Bates et al., 1993). Acute HIV infection in children can create a mononucleosis-like syndrome with lymphadenopathy, pharyngitis, rash, and malaise. Chronic HIV-related lymphadenopathy tends to be progressive and generalized (i.e., PGL), with relatively small-sized lymph nodes. However, in some patients, localized lymphadenopathy (e.g., intraparotid lymph node enlargement) may occur. Lymph node architecture changes with HIV chronicity and declining immunodeficiency (diminishing CD4 cell count); progressing initially from hyperplastic geographic reactive follicles (pattern A), to follicle regression (pattern B), and ultimately a "burnt-out" fibrotic node (pattern C). In one series of lymph node FNAs in HIV patients, reactive hyperplasia was the most common FNA diagnosis (52%), followed by necrotizing granulomatous lymphadenitis (20%) (Sarma et al., 2010). Nodal morphology may also be altered by highly active antiretroviral therapy (HAART).

Cytomorphology

The three patterns (phases) of HIV lymphadenitis may not be easy to recognize by FNA alone. Nevertheless, with pattern A (early HIV infection) and B (chronic HIV infection) in which nodes contain prominent or involuting follicular hyperplasia, aspirates are likely to contain lymphoid elements representative of reactive follicles such as tingible-body macrophages and follicular dendritic cells. Giant cells produced by the syncytial aggregate of HIV-infected macrophages or cells resembling Warthin–Finkeldey giant cells (hyperchromatic overlapping nuclei and scant cytoplasm) may rarely be seen. Cytology samples usually always have admixed plasma cells. Late phase lymphadenopathy today is uncommon but, if aspirated, will demonstrate lymphocytic depletion with follicular dendritic cells. If HIV is suspected, a p24 immunohistochemical stain can be performed, with positive staining best localized to dendritic cells. Coexistent pathology should always be excluded, including stains for mycobacteria and fungal infection. Mycobacteria are particularly likely to be encountered in necrotic aspirates with or without granulomas (Sarma et al., 2010; Gupta SK et al., 1993).

Differential Diagnosis

The differential diagnosis includes a variety of causes of reactive hyperplasia, infectious etiologies, and Castleman disease. In this setting there is also a need to carefully exclude the possibility of lymphoma, since these patients have an increased risk for high-grade lymphomas (Sarma et al., 2010).

Leishmania Lymphadenitis

Definition

Lymphadenitis due to Leishmania infection.

ICD-9-CM Code 085.9

Synonyms

Leishmaniasis.

Clinical Aspects

Leishmania lymphadenitis is an uncommon cause of lymphadenopathy, caused by infection with the protozoan Leishmania transmitted by sandflies. The disease is usually self-limited and requires no treatment. Lymphadenitis may be due to localized nodal infection, or may be associated with cutaneous or visceral forms of the disease.

Cytomorphology

The FNA findings in leishmaniasis include a polymorphic background population of cells composed of lymphocytes, histiocytes, epithelioid cells, plasma cells, tingible-body macrophages, and macrophages infiltrated with Leishmania amastigotes (Beljan et al., 2010). Amastigotes are round to oval in shape and range in size from 1 to 3 μm. Multinucleated giant cells and small granulomas may also be seen. Histiocytes with cytoplasmic Leishmania organisms that have a nucleus and small rod-shaped paranucleus (kinetoplast), which are called Leishman–Donovan (LD) bodies, are usually seen intracellularly and extracellularly, and are characteristic of this condition (Sah et al., 2005; Vera-Alvarez et al., 1999; Tallada et al., 1993; Kumar et al., 2001). LD bodies are negative for PAS and do not stain with silver stains. LD bodies are more commonly found in cases with more acute inflammation and less often in cases with granulomas or numerous plasma cells. An immunostain is available if needed.

Differential Diagnosis

The differential diagnosis depends on the predominant cytomorphologic findings. In cases with prominent granulomas, tuberculosis, fungal granulomas, and cat-scratch disease are diagnostic considerations (Table 21.5) In cases with prominent eosinophils, the possibility of Hodgkin lymphoma or other possibilities may arise (Table 21.7). Toxoplasma lymphadenitis and other rare infections are also in the differential including filariasis in lymph node FNAs (Dey et al., 1993). Histoplasma yeasts that may mimic amastigotes can be differentiated using a GMS stain, which will not stain Leishmania organisms.

OTHER CAUSES OF LYMPHADENOPATHY

Histiocytic Necrotizing Lymphadenitis

Definition

Necrotizing lymphadenopathy of unknown origin arise typically in young Asian females with associated fever.

ICD-9-CM Code 289.3

Synonyms

Kikuchi–Fujimoto disease and Kikuchi disease.

Clinical Aspects

This is a benign, self-limited condition, seen most frequently in young Asian women with painless cervical lymphadenopathy, fever and night sweats. Cellular debris from patchy necrosis in lymph nodes is actively phagocytosed by abundant macrophages. The etiology is unknown, but a viral or autoimmune pathogenesis is suspected. The diagnosis can be difficult based on cytomorphology alone, with some reporting an overall accuracy of 56%, with around 38% false-positive cases and 50% false-negatives. Typically the condition resolves spontaneously, and usually within six months of diagnosis (Tong et al., 2001; Schinstine 2009; Kishimoto et al., 2010).

Cytomorphology

The key findings include increased tingible-body macrophages, prominent karyorrhectic debris, and an absence of neutrophils in the background (Figure 21.12). There are two characteristic cell types present: macrophages with crescent-shaped nuclei and monocytes with eccentric nuclei and perinuclear clearing, imparting a plasmacytoid appearance

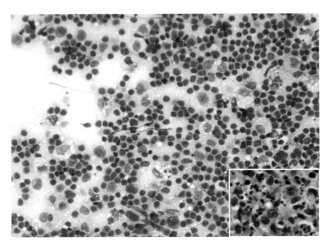

FIGURE 21.12 Histiocytic necrotizing lymphadenitis (medium power, DQ stain; inset: high power, H&E stain of lymph node excision). Histiocytes are seen with karyorrhectic debris and necrosis. No neutrophils are identified, but the karyorrhectic debris can mimic polymorphonuclear neutrophils in some cases. The lymph node excision confirmed the diagnosis (inset).

(Viguer et al., 2001). The macrophages are positive for CD68. In addition a myeloperoxidase (MPO) special stain may be positive in macrophages, which is a unique finding compared to other histiocytic conditions. Although the finding of macrophages with crescentic nuclei are helpful, they have been reported in other reactive lymph node conditions as well as lymphoma (Tong et al., 2001). Background lymphocytes show a predominance of CD8+ T cells.

Differential Diagnosis

The differential diagnosis includes an acute suppurative lymphadenitis due to the karyorrhectic debris, which can mimic the multilobulated nuclei of neutrophils. However, at high-power magnification, cytology specimens of Kikuchi lymphadenitis should be noted to lack neutrophils, which will be abundant in acute suppurative lymphadenitis. The findings in Kikuchi lymphadenitis also overlap significantly with the changes seen in autoimmune conditions, like systemic lupus erythematosus (SLE) lymphadenitis, which contains areas of fibrinoid necrosis. The presence of hematoxyphilic bodies favors lupus lymphadenopathy. Necrotizing granulomatous conditions should be considered, like tuberculous lymphadenitis (Tong et al., 2001). A less likely diagnostic consideration in some cases is malignant lymphoma, which can be excluded with appropriate triage for ancillary studies. Finally, any entity that may have necrosis (e.g., lymph node infarction, tumor necrosis) can mimic Kikuchi lymphadenopathy.

Kimura Disease

Definition

This is a chronic inflammatory disorder characterized by angiolymphoid hyperplasia and eosinophilia involving lymph nodes and subcutaneous tissue that may represent an abnormal immune response to an unknown stimulus.

ICD-9-CM Code 289.3

Synonyms

Angiolymphoid hyperplasia with eosinophilia (now a distinct entity).

Clinical Aspects

This disease typically affects Asians, like Kikuchi lymphadenitis, but unlike Kikuchi's, which occurs in women, lymphadenopathy in Kimura's disease is more often seen in men. The symptoms include painless lymphadenopathy mainly in the head and neck region, with associated lymphoid infiltrates in the skin. There is usually an elevation in the serum IgE level and peripheral blood eosinophilia. This is a benign condition, but recurrence is common.

Cytomorphology

The involved lymph nodes show reactive lymphoid hyperplasia with Warthin–Finkeldey-type multinucleated giant cells and a background of numerous eosinophils. Occasionally one may encounter Charcot–Leyden crystals. The background may also contain a few plasma cells and mast cells.

Differential Diagnosis

The other diagnostic possibilities include all conditions that are associated with reactive lymphoid hyperplasia. The prominence of eosinophils in the background may lead one to think about drug reactions, parasitic lymphadenitis, Hodgkin lymphoma, and T-cell lymphomas (Table 21.7).

Sinus Histiocytosis with Massive Lymphadenopathy

Definition

The histiocytic condition is characterized by massive, painless lymphadenopathy of unknown origin characterized by a proliferation of histiocytes with engulfed lymphocytes (emperipolesis).

ICD-9-CM Code 785.6

Synonyms

SHML and Rosai–Dorfman disease.

Clinical Aspects

SHML is a benign, self-limited condition that usually presents in young patients with bilateral cervical lymphadenopathy (Deshpande et al., 1998). Patients may also develop extranodal pseudotumors. The characteristic finding is the presence of emperipolesis, or engulfment of hematopoietic cells by macrophages, which may be due to M-CSF stimulating macrophages to phagocytose other cells (Jadus et al., 1995).

Cytomorphology

The key finding is emperipolesis, whereby histiocytes engulf other viable cells, including lymphocytes, and occasionally other hematopoietic cells. These large histiocytes are easily identified at low-power magnification. The engulfed cells usually have a narrow halo or vacuole around them within the histiocytic cytoplasm, which can help distinguish these characteristic histiocytes from tingible-body macrophages, or just cells overlapping macrophages in a smear (Figure 21.13) The histiocytes can also have fine cytoplasmic vacuoles, and characteristically stain positive for CD68 and S100, but are negative for CD1a. The background contains lymphocytes and plasma cells (Deshpande et al., 1998).

Differential Diagnosis

The differential diagnosis includes Langerhan cell histiocytosis (LCH), where the histiocytes are positive for the immunomarkers CD1a, fascin, and Langerin, but usually negative for S100. In addition the histiocytes in LCH have an irregular nucleus with nuclear grooves. Emperipolesis has only rarely been reported in LCH (Kakkar et al., 2001). Phagocytosis of viable lymphocytes distinguishes the histiocytes from tingible-body macrophages with apoptotic debris and other benign histiocytes in RLH, which are also S100 negative. In rare cases SHML may mimic Hodgkin lymphoma due to the presence of binucleated histiocytes resembling Reed–Sternberg cells in the heterogeneous background (Deshpande et al., 1998). Other diagnoses to consider are granulomatous lesions and hemophagocytosis (viral associated, familial, or related to neoplasms). SHML may rarely coexist with lymphoma in same node.

Dermatopathic Lymphadenitis

Definition

Lymph node enlargement occurs in response to an exfoliative dermatitis with pigment-containing macrophages.

ICD-9-CM Code 695.89

Synonyms

Lipomelanosis reticularis of Pautrier.

Clinical Aspects

Lymphadenopathy is typically due to a chronic dermatitis that is pruritic. Usually patients present with isolated lymphadenopathy (axillary or inguinal) without a known skin disorder (Iyer et al., 1998; Sudilovsky, 1998).

Cytomorphology

The cytology specimens tend to be cellular with numerous melanin-laden macrophages and histiocytoid cells that exhibit nuclear grooves and S100 immunopositivity. There are prominent proliferative postcapillary venules present as well as occasional plasma cells and eosinophils. Melanin pigment will stain with Fontana–Masson stains, and unlike hemosiderin pigment containing iron, will not stain with Prussian blue.

Differential Diagnosis

The differential diagnosis includes reactive lymphoid hyperplasias and other conditions associated with pigment within lymph nodes such as a tattoo, nodal nevi inclusions, and metastatic melanoma. In addition the possibility of Hodgkin lymphoma or mycosis fungoides may also be in the differential diagnosis.

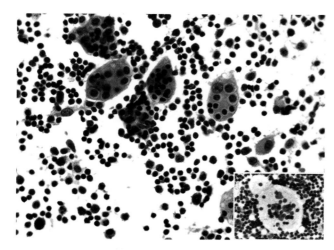

FIGURE 21.13 **Sinus histiocytosis with massive lymphadenopathy (high power, H&E stain; inset: high power, DQ stain)**. Prominent emperipolesis is seen in this case of Rosai–Dorfman disease with phagocytosed hematopoietic cells within histiocytes. A prominent halo is seen around the engulfed cells on the H&E stained slide.

Castleman Disease

Definition

This is a reactive condition that presents with findings of a mediastinal mass or lymphadenopathy.

ICD-9-CM Code 785.6

Synonyms

CD, Castleman lymphadenopathy, and giant lymph node or angiofollicular lymph node hyperplasia.

Clinical Aspects

The pathologic lesions of Castleman's disease (CD) include lymphadenopathy and/or localized extranodal lymphoid tumors. CD has several morphologic subtypes: hyaline-vascular variant, plasma cell variant, mixed variant, and plasmablastic variant (Cronin et al., 2009). Hyaline-vascular lesions tend to be localized (unicentric), often as lymphadenopathy confined to the mediastinum or abdomen. Plasma cell type CD tends to be multicentric, and may involve several lymph nodes, form extranodal masses such as mesenteric or retroperitoneal tumors, and/or result in hepatosplenomegaly. Castleman-like changes within lymph nodes may also be nonspecific and have been associated with various disorders. The hyaline-vascular pattern has been described in autoimmune disease, primary immune deficiency, and chronic HIV infection. The plasma cell pattern has been associated with rheumatoid arthritis, syphilis, and POEMS (polyneuropathy, organomegaly, endocrinopathy, monoclonal gammopathy, skin changes) syndrome. Patients with CD can be very ill and have systemic symptoms like fever and hypergammaglobulinemia. In HIV-affected patients, CD is associated with human herpesvirus 8 (HHV-8) infection. Occasional cases may be complicated by the development of non-Hodgkin lymphoma or follicular dendritic cell sarcoma. In lymph nodes from HIV+ patients there may be coexistent Kaposi's sarcoma in up to 40% of cases (Oksendhendler et al., 1996).

Cytomorphology

Although challenging (Cangiarella et al., 1997), FNA biopsy of CD lesions may be diagnostically helpful (Meyer et al., 1999; Taylor et al., 2000). The cytopathology appears similar to that seen in RLH. The vascular patterns and hyalinized germinal centers are not often seen in aspirates. There can be large tissue fragments with clusters of atypical follicular dendritic cells, traversing capillaries, increased plasma cells, and hyalinized material. The amount of tingible-body macrophages and small cleaved cells are fewer than that seen in RLH (Bachowski et al., 2000). Aspirates from cases of multicentric CD tend to have a polymorphous lymphoid population with a higher than normal number of plasma cells (Caraway et al., 1996). The plasmablastic variant of CD is characterized by increased numbers of plasmablasts that morphologically resemble immunoblasts. Plasmablasts are approximately twice the size of lymphocytes, have a moderate amount of amphophilic cytoplasm, and a large vesicular nucleus with 1 to 2 prominent nucleoli. Immunohistochemistry can be performed to demonstrate follicular dendritic cells, which are S100+, CD21+, CD23+, and CD35+. These specimens should be carefully examined and triaged (e.g., flow cytometry) to exclude lymphoma. Lymphocytes in the vast majority of cases are polyclonal, typically showing a mixed B-cell population. The use of LNA-1 immunohistochemistry to demonstrate HHV8 in dendritic cells, immunoblasts, and/or plasmablasts is helpful in the setting of HIV-positive patients.

Differential Diagnosis

The differential diagnosis includes Hodgkin lymphoma, given the location of these masses in the mediastinum and the occurrence of large atypical cells that can be bi-nucleated. Non-Hodgkin lymphoma should also be excluded. In the plasmablastic variant of CD, plasmablasts can coalesce to form "microlymphomas" or develop into frank lymphoma. Plasmablasts in such microlymphomas show lambda light chain restriction (Dupin et al., 1999). Despite this monotypic appearance, immunoglobulin gene rearrangement studies performed on these plasmablasts has shown them to be polyclonal (Du et al., 2001). However, frank plasmablastic lymphomas arising in this setting are monoclonal.

Extramedullary Hematopoiesis

Definition

This disease is characterized by a proliferation of marrow elements (myeloid, erythroid, megakaryocytic) outside the environment of the bone marrow.

ICD-9-CM Code 288.02

Synonyms

EMH or myeloid proliferation.

Clinical Aspects

Extramedullary hematopoiesis may occur in patients with hyposplenism, compromised marrow space (e.g., myelofibrosis), chronic anemia states, or after the administration of hematopoietic growth factors like granulocyte colony-stimulating factor (G-CSF) (O'Malley, 2007). EMH has also been reported in axillary sentinel nodes of breast cancer patients following neoadjuvant therapy (Millar et al., 2009). Abnormal hematopoietic tissue usually develops in sites involved in hematopoiesis during fetal development such as the spleen, liver, and kidneys. However, other locations such as lymph nodes may also be involved.

Cytomorphology

In nodal EMH, one may identify varying amounts of marrow elements including myeloid precursors, erythroid cells, and/or megakaryocytes (Figure 21.14). This finding is an indication to search for an underlying hematological condition (e.g., bone marrow neoplasm or anemia). Immunohistochemical stains may help confirm immature myeloid cells (myeloperoxidase, CD117, CD34), erythroid cells (hemoglobin or glycophorin), and megakaryocytic elements (factor VIII antigen, CD61).

Differential Diagnosis

The differential diagnosis includes benign entities such as myelolipoma as well as proliferations of neoplastic hematopoietic elements as occurs in leukemia and myeloid sarcoma. Megakaryocytes can be differentiated from multinucleated histiocytes, which tend to be larger, have more cytoplasm, have vesicular nuclei that are not multilobated, and be CD68

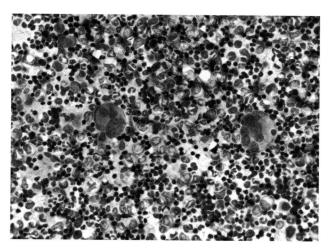

FIGURE 21.14 **Extramedullary hematopoiesis (medium power, DQ stain).** The megakaryocytes in nodal extramedullary hematopoiesis are the first clue to the diagnosis due to their large size and multilobulated nuclei, which may mimic a neoplastic process. The background shows immature myeloid and erythroid cells.

positive. Immature hematopoietic cells may also be mistaken for metastatic carcinoma to a lymph node (Hoda et al., 2002). Immature cells may also resemble a decidual reaction (ectopic decidua) within lymph nodes.

Foreign Body or Iatrogenic Related Changes in Lymph Nodes

Definition

The migration or drainage of small foreign material fragments to regional lymph nodes that evoke a variable foreign body reaction.

ICD-9-CM Code 785.6

Synonyms

Foreign body lymphadenopathy.

Clinical Aspects

Lymph nodes can develop reactive changes and create mass lesions or pronounced lymphadenopathy in response to foreign material, such as metal particles after hip replacement with cobalt-chromium or titanium prostheses (Munichor et al., 2003), radiocontrast material, talc from intravenous drug abuse (Housini et al., 1990), and silicone (silicone lymphadenopathy) after breast augmentation/reconstruction (Tabatowski et al., 1990; Santos-Briz et al., 1999). Lipogranulomatous reactions (lipid lymphadenopathy) can be seen in response to endogenous or exogenous lipids. Lymphadenopathy can also develop in regional lymph nodes as a result of oil droplets from lymphangiography (lymphangiogram effect). Anthracosis is common in thoracic and mediastinal lymph nodes.

Cytomorphology

The key finding includes numerous macrophages with foamy cytoplasm that corresponds to the prominent sinus histiocytosis seen on histologic evaluation. Foreign body multinucleated giant cells may be a frequent finding. On close examination, one may see small intracytoplasmic particles within macrophages that may be refractile or birefringent. In silicone lymphadenopathy, multivacuolated histiocytes become distorted by rigid large globules of refractive, faint yellow, homogeneous material that is not birefringent (Tabatowski et al., 1990). In lymphadenopathy after lymphangiograms, lymph nodes may show a histiocytic response with ingested lipid droplets of contrast material. In any case suspected of having foreign material, microscopy with polarization should be employed to help identify polarizable foreign

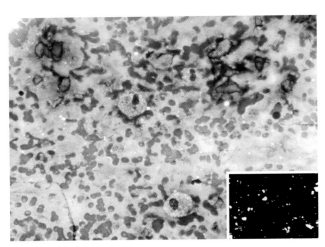

FIGURE 21.15 **Foreign body lymphadenopathy (high power, DQ stain; inset: low power, polarization).** Abundant refractile material is seen in the background of this aspirate with scattered multivacuolated histiocytes. Using microscopy with polarization, the refractile material is highlighted.

material easily (Figure 21.15). Ultrastructural evaluation by electron microscopy or energy dispersive X-ray microanalysis has been reported to further help identify and characterize potential foreign material (Munichor et al., 2003).

Differential Diagnosis

Xanthogranulomatous inflammation can mimic the changes produced by foreign body reactions. In addition histiocytic proliferations due to organisms, such as atypical mycobacterial infections and Whipple disease, or metabolic storage diseases, such as Gaucher disease, are included in the differential diagnosis. In thoracic and mediastinal lymph nodes, metal pigment may be difficult or impossible to distinguish from carbon and anthracotic pigment commonly seen in this location.

Non-neoplastic Inclusions in Lymph Node

Definition

Incidental finding of squamous, glandular, or nevus inclusions are seen within lymph nodes due to developmental heterotopia.

ICD-9-CM Code 785.6

Synonyms

Lymph node inclusions.

Clinical Aspects

Non-neoplastic lymph node inclusions in capsule or cortical sites are an incidental finding. Benign

epithelial inclusions include salivary glands in upper cervical nodes, thyroid follicles in lower cervical nodes, mammary glands in axillary nodes, mesothelial inclusions in mediastinal nodes, and endosalpingiosis within pelvic nodes. (Pantanowitz et al., 2003). Rare reports of benign epithelial inclusions in lymph nodes have been detected by FNA cytology (Paull et al., 2003; Kloboves-Prevodnik et al., 2007). Aggregates of nevus cells (nevus cell inclusions) are seen most frequently in axillary lymph nodes. Such nodal nevi have been detected by FNA (Zaharopoulos et al., 2004).

Cytomorphology

Epithelial inclusions have a benign appearance. Mesothelial inclusions, in particular, resemble typical mesothelial cell clusters present in a background of lymphocytes. Nodal nevi show uniform cells with round nuclei and faint, dusty melanin pigment (Zaharopoulos et al., 2004). If required, the type of inclusion can be confirmed using immunostains (e.g., nevus cells are positive for S100, MART1, and tyrosinase, but rarely HMB45).

Differential Diagnosis

The main differential diagnosis is that of metastases. Benign epithelial inclusions can be differentiated from metastatic carcinoma because the benign inclusions lack nuclear pleomorphism and mitoses. Similarly, excluding the possibility of metastatic melanoma is important for nodal nevi. Endometriosis should be considered if one finds benign endometrial type glands associated with endometrial-type stromal elements.

Autoimmune Lymphoproliferative Syndrome

Definition

Autoimmune lymphoproliferative syndrome (ALPS) is an inherited disorder due to genetic and immunological abnormalities (defects in Fas/CD95/Apo-1 mediated apoptosis) that causes generalized benign lymphadenopathy, hypergammaglobulinemia, lymphocytosis, splenomegaly, and autoimmune phenomena.

ICD-9-CM Code 279.4

Synonyms

Canale-Smith syndrome.

Clinical Aspects

In afflicted patients with ALPS, there is childhood onset of lymphadenopathy, hepatosplenomegaly, hypergammaglobulinemia, cytopenias, and autoimmunity. The distinct feature of ALPS is the presence of increased double negative (CD4- CD8-) T-cell receptor (TCR)-alpha beta T cells in circulation and lymphoid tissues. Recently these patients were also found to have functional CD95 (Fas/Apo1) mutations, which impair apoptosis of normal and autoreactive lymphocytes, which lead to their accumulation (Lim et al., 1998). These patients are at increased risk of developing lymphoma.

Cytomorphology

Cytology specimens appear similar to that seen in RLH. There may be a conspicuous absence of macrophages with apoptotic debris, which is usually seen in cases of RLH. Other features of ALPS include follicular hyperplasia, prominent vascularity of interfollicular areas, and florid polyclonal plasmacytosis. Flow cytometry of the lymph nodes in ALPS patients shows an increase in double-negative T cells ranging from 27 to 54% of mononuclear cells, and representing 51 to 78% of alpha beta T cells (Lim et al., 1998).

Differential Diagnosis

The differential diagnosis includes many other causes of reactive lymphoid hyperplasia, sinus histiocytosis with massive lymphadenopathy, dermatopathic lymphadenitis, and lymphoma.

Lymphadenopathy in Autoimmune Diseases

Definition

Autoimmune diseases include a variety of different disorders causing patterns of systemic inflammation. Two of the most common conditions associated with lymphadenopathy include systemic lupus erythematosus (SLE) and rheumatoid arthritis (RA).

ICD-9-CM Code 279.4, 785.6, 710.1 (systemic lupus erythematosus)

Synonyms

Acute lupus lymphadenitis, systemic lupus erythematosus or SLE, as well as rheumatoid arthritis or RA.

Clinical Aspects

SLE is an autoimmune disease of unknown etiology, characterized by the presence of antinuclear antibodies in the blood. Many patients with SLE are young woman that manifest with nonspecific autoimmune-related symptoms and varying lymphadenopathy. Lymphadenopathy in

SLE is common and occurs in about 26 to 65% patients. When SLE lymphadenopathy occurs as the primary symptom (usually cervical), it may lead to a clinical suspicion for lymphoma. The histologic findings in nodal SLE include prominent lymphoid hyperplasia, fibrinoid necrosis, and vasculitis with possible florid necrotizing lymphadenitis and infarction. In RA, around 82% of individuals may have associated lymphadenopathy (usually axillary and supraclavicular). These enlarged lymph nodes usually disappear during RA disease remission. RA lymphadenopathy is associated with florid reactive hyperplasia, marked plasmacytosis, and focal necrosis. Lymphadenopathy with similar features may also occur in other autoimmune diseases like Still disease, Sjögren syndrome, Hashimoto thyroiditis, dermatomyositis, scleroderma, and polyarteritis nodosa. Lymphadenopathy may also be associated with methotrexate therapy.

Cytomorphology

The cytomorphology of these autoimmune diseases is rarely described, but comprises features showing reactive lymphoid hyperplasia. In RA, there is a prominence of plasma cells with eosinophilic, cytoplasmic inclusions (Russell bodies) in a polymorphous, reactive background of lymphocytes. In SLE, there is typically a necrotic/apoptotic background (i.e., necrotizing lymphadenitis), absence of neutrophils, and dispersed karyorrhectic nuclear debris or basophilic bodies (hematoxylin bodies) (Ko et al., 1992). These basophilic or hematoxylin bodies are variable in size (measuring approximately 1–10 μm), stain blue on Pap stain and a deep violet color with H&E, and are crucial to making the diagnosis of SLE based on cytology. They are thought to consist of depolymerized DNA, protein, and carbohydrates. Other features of SLE that may be seen in a lymph node FNA include the presence of a prominent atypical immunoblastic population and occasional Reed–Sternberg-like cells (Pai et al., 2000). Granulomas are unusual, but may be seen in occasional RA cases or if there is a coexistent infection. In some cases (e.g., RA, systemic sclerosis), amorphous hyaline-like extracellular material may be seen that is PAS positive but congo red negative (McCluggage et al., 1994).

Differential Diagnosis

In cases of RA-associated lymphadenopathy, the main differential diagnosis includes reactive lymphoid hyperplasia, plasma cell variant of Castleman's disease, or a low-grade lymphoma with plasma cells, such as a marginal zone lymphoma. The differential diagnosis of necrotizing lymphadenopathy in SLE includes Kikuchi lymphadenitis. Other causes of nodal necrosis that need to be included are infarction, high-grade lymphomas, tuberculosis, cat-scratch lymphadenitis, lymphogranuloma venereum, and Yersinia infection. The presence of a prominent infiltrate of neutrophils favors infarction or acute suppurative lymphadenitis over lupus lymphadenopathy. In addition careful examination of the lymphoid cells for cytological atypia should be done to exclude the possibility of lymphoma. The prominent immunoblastic proliferation seen in some autoimmune cases can mimic Hodgkin lymphoma, infectious mononucleosis, and dilantin lymphadenopathy (Table 21.8). Another important diagnostic consideration is that a given patient with SLE or RA may be on immunosuppressant medications, such as corticosteroids, which can increase the risk of reactivated or new infections. Proteinaceous (nonamyloid) or amyloid lymphadenopathy should be considered if one finds abundant acellular, amorphous eosinophilic material.

LYMPHADENOPATHY IN THE PEDIATRIC PATIENT

In the pediatric patient, FNA cytology is particularly advantageous because the likelihood of a reactive or infectious process is much higher than a neoplastic process, compared to adults where metastases and hematolymphoid malignancies are much more of a diagnostic consideration (Handa et al., 2003), In addition, where infections such as tuberculosis are a major cause of morbidity and mortality, rapid diagnosis and treatment are crucial. When a childhood malignancy is suspected (e.g., small round blue cell tumor), adequate material can also be acquired by FNA for diagnosis and ancillary studies, including flow cytometry, FISH studies, and immunohistochemical stains (Wakely, 2001).

When a child is the patient, time is often spent talking with the parents and family about the procedure and to obtain consent. Although informed consent is obtained from the parent or legal guardian in these cases, when old enough, assent is obtained from the pediatric patient as well. In addition an extensive review of systems with emphasis on recent exposures (animals, infections, etc.), birth history, and developmental/growth history can be helpful. If the FNA is being performed on children without anesthesia, EMLA cream can be applied to the skin prior to the procedure. A child can also be swaddled in a "papoose" fashion to minimize movement, particularly in areas difficult to biopsy, like the head and neck region. When performing the FNA, usually the target is a small, mobile lymph node that is difficult to immobilize. In these scenarios, performing the FNA without suction, allows one to avoid scaring an awake child, and allows the aspirator to have better fine motor control. If needed, one can try aspiration with a syringe if the lesion is larger, the patient is under anesthesia, or there is insufficient material aspirated with the needle-only technique.

USE OF ANCILLARY STUDIES

Recent advances in molecular diagnostics and immunologic methods have resulted in a multitude of ancillary studies available to obtain accurate and reliable diagnoses and prognostic information using FNA (Clark et al., 2009). In addition it has been shown that ancillary studies preformed on aspirate material provides critical diagnostic information in about 86% cases that is important for patient management (Nasuti et al., 2001).

Flow Cytometry

If there are adequate numbers of viable cells present, flow cytometry can help determine the immunophenotype of cells, and if needed, can document light chain restriction or clonality in a B-cell lymphoma. A predominant clonal B-cell population is rare in reactive lymphadenopathy, but given that subpopulations of cells can be clonal, correlation with morphology is essential (Kussick et al., 2004). The advantages of flow cytometry include rapid turn around time, quantitative analysis, and good sensitivity. The disadvantages include need for sufficient viable cells; inability to perform testing on fixed cells, archived material, or low viability specimens; and inability to look at clonality in surface immunoglobulin negative cells (Monaco et al., 2009).

Microbiology Culture

Although culture specimens are usually sent in cases suspected of infection, alone it has a low diagnostic sensitivity. However, a microbiology culture can be very helpful in determining sensitivity to different antimicrobial drugs. Culture positivity in TB only ranges from 8 to 50%, causing some to doubt its usefulness as a diagnostic modality (Radhika et al., 1989; Jain et al., 2005; Gupta SK et al., 1993; Lau et al., 1990). Also, appropriate facilities are required to perform cultures, and results can take several days.

Immunohistochemistry and Special Stains

Special stains and immunocytochemical stains can be readily utilized on cytology material. In general, these tests are relatively cheap in comparison to complex molecular studies. Furthermore, they can help identify organisms (AFB, GMS, Mucicarmine, and PAS stains) and subtype cells based on their immunoprofile, and help evaluate a lymphoid population for abnormalities. Special stains, such as the AFB stain and Grocott stain, are routinely done on cases with granulomatous inflammation to look for acid fast bacilli and fungal organisms, respectively (Figures 21.16, 21.17). Although special stains are one of the least expensive studies, they tend to lack sensitivity (Jain et al., 2005). Thus, pathologists are looking more to using specific immunohistochemical stains for different organisms (e.g., LMP for EBV and LNA-1 for HHV8 infection). Immunostains and special stains can be performed on a variety of different types of cytology material, including smears, cytospins, liquid-based preparations, and cell blocks. However, results may differ based on the type of fixative used (alcohol based vs. formalin), cellularity, and the amount of background artifact or nonspecific staining. In general, when using these stains, appropriate positive and negative controls are crucial, and each stain should be validated prior to diagnostic use in each individual laboratory. Often cytology samples contain limited material and may not include an internal tissue control for evaluation.

Microorganisms

A variety of special histochemical stains (acid-fast stains, Gram, GMS/Grocott, PAS, Mucicarmine,

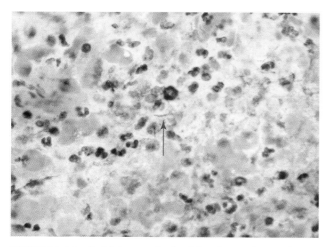

FIGURE 21.16 Acid-fast stain in *Mycobacterium tuberculosis* **(high power, AFB stain).** Long beaded bacilli appear as a dark pink or red color (arrow) on the AFB stain in this case of *Mycobacterium tuberculosis*.

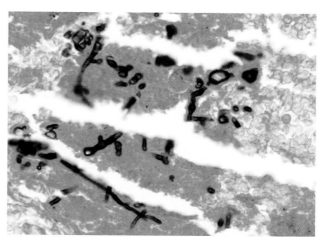

FIGURE 21.17 Grocott stain in *Aspergillus* **infection (high power, Grocott stain).** Narrow angle branching hyphae with septae are visualized well on this cell block section stained with the Grocott stain.

Steiner, Giemsa, etc.) and immunostains (HSV, HPV, EBV-LMP, Toxoplasmosis, Aspergillus, Bartonella, LNA-1, p24, etc.) are available to help characterize microorganisms within lymph node specimens. Special stains like AFB are generally regarded as being insensitive for the detection of organisms, with some reporting positivity in only about 20% cases with known culture positivity, which may be due to problems with the stain itself, interpretation of the stain, or a low bacterial load. While some authors have reported sensitivities of up to 62% to detect mycobacteria using special stains (Wright et al., 2008), others have reported a low positivity rate of only 33% for acid-fast-stained mycobacteria, even in cases with identifiable necrosis and granulomas (Radhika et al., 1989). Silver stains (e.g., Steiner stain) sometimes used for cat-scratch disease to detect bacteria are reported to be positive in about 69% of cases (Donnelly et al., 1995). Because there is often much nonspecific silver impregnation related to background necrosis and intracellular debris within macrophages, these stains are difficult to interpret. An immunohistochemical stain with monoclonal antibodies to *B.henselae* may therefore be more helpful (Caponetti et al., 2009).

Lymphocytes

Immunocytochemistry is frequently relied on to help distinguish reactive from clonal nodal processes. IHC can also help to determine the immunophenotype of cells, like FC. Unlike FC, morphology is preserved and it can be performed on fewer cells. In addition some neoplastic lymphoid populations, like Hodgkin lymphoma (CD30 and CD15) and mantle cell lymphoma (cyclin D1), require immunostains.

Also Ki67, along with morphology, has been shown to be helpful in grading of lymphomas (Ali et al., 2010). The disadvantage is that the analysis is subjective and qualitative, and each antibody must be performed on an individual slide, making it difficult to definitively establish an immunophenotype of a population.

In-situ Hybridization

Occasionally in-situ hybridization (ISH) techniques may prove useful in evaluating cytology material. EBER (EBV-encoded RNA) detected by ISH can help demonstrate EBV infection. EBERs are the most abundant EBV RNAs present in latently infected B cells, and can be seen in cases of infectious mononucleosis.

Fluorescence Microscopy

The use of fluorescence microscopy to detect autofluorescence is a rapid, simple, and sensitive modality, but not widely utilized due to the expensive equipment and expertise required. It can only be performed on alcohol-fixed, Papanicolaou-stained material, not cell block material. In addition, false-positive results have been reported with fluorescence given that bacterial forms other than tuberculosis can exhibit autofluorescence. Moreover, red blood cells and amorphous bodies in the background can also cause green fluorescence, and the staining patterns can be variable (Wright et al., 2004; Mathai et al., 2008). Although usually used for mycobacteria, autofluorescence of other organisms, including cryptococcus (Mathai et al., 2008), has been reported (Figure 21.18).

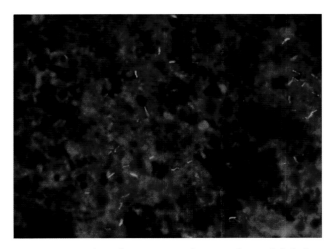

FIGURE 21.18 Autofluorescence in mycobacterial infection (high power, Pap stain). The long beaded mycobacterial organisms stand out with a yellow-green color due to autofluorescence.

MOLECULAR STUDIES

FISH

This test involves DNA probes targeting specific chromosomal regions of interest are labelled with fluorochrome, and hybridized with intact nuclei. This is useful for the detection of gene rearrangements, translocations, deletions, and gene amplifications. Such studies are helpful in cytology specimens where lymphoma is a diagnostic consideration (Monaco et al., 2009).

PCR

PCR can amplify small regions of DNA through repeated cycles of denaturation and DNA synthesis, resulting in superior sensitivity in comparison to other aforementioned tests (i.e., special stains and culture). However, false positives can occur, especially if there has been contamination of the specimen. PCR testing can be done on formalin-fixed cell block material or dedicated samples submitted in the correct media. PCR is expensive and requires expertise to perform and interpret results. However, if available, the remarkable sensitivity of PCR to detect and subtype microbial agents, like tuberculosis, can be crucial (Ersoz et al., 1998).

REFERENCES

ALI AE, MORGEN EK, GEDDIE WR, BOERNER SL, MASSEY C, BAILEY DJ, DA CUNHA SANTOS G. 2010. Aspirates. Cancer Cytopathol 118:166–72.

ALJAFARI AS, KHALIL EAG, ELSIDDIG KE, EL HAG IA, IBRAHIM ME, ELSAFI MEMO, HUSSEIN AM, ELKHIDIR IM, SULAIMAN GS, ELHASSAN AM. 2004. Diagnosis of tuberculous lymphadenitis by FNAC, microbiological methods and PCR: a comparative study. Cytopathology 15:44–8.

ANNE S, TEOT LA, MANDELL DL. 2008. Fine needle aspiration biopsy: role in diagnosis of pediatric head and neck masses. J Ped Otorhinolaryngology 72:1547–53.

BACHOWSKI G, GEISS M, LUNDEEN S, PAMBUCCIAN S. 2000. Fine needle aspiration findings of cervical Castleman's disease. Acta Cytol 44:896–7.

BELJAN R, SUNDOV D, LUKSIĆ B, SOLJIĆ V, BURAZER MP. 2010. Diagnosis of visceral leishmaniasis by fine needle aspiration cytology of an isolated cervical lymph node: case report. Coll Antropol 34:237–9.

BUCHINO JJ, JONES VF. 1994. Fine needle aspiration in the evaluation of children with lymphadenopathy. Arch Pediatr Adolesc Med 148:1327–30.

CANGIARELLA J, GALLO L, WINKLER B. 1997. Potential pitfalls in the diagnosis of Castleman's disease of the mediastinum on fine needle aspiration biopsy. Acta Cytol 41:951–2.

CAPONETTI GC, PANTANOWITZ L, MARCONI S, HAVENS JM, LAMPS LW, OTIS CN. 2009. Evaluation of immuno-histochemistry in identifying Bartonella henselae in cat-scratch disease. Am J Clin Pathol 131:250–6.

CARAWAY NP, KATZ RL. 2006. Lymph nodes. In: Koss LG, Melamed MR, ed., Koss' Diagnostic Cytology and Its Histopathologic Bases, 5th ed. Lippincott Williams and Wilkins, Philadelphia, 1190–1227.

CARDILLO MR. 1989. Fine-needle aspiration cytology of superficial lymph nodes. Diagn Cytopathol 5:166–73.

CLARK DP. 2009. Seize the opportunity: underutilization of fine-needle aspiration biopsy to inform targeted cancer therapy decisions. Cancer Cytopathol 117:289–97.

CRONIN DM, WARNKE RA. 2009. Castleman disease: an update on classification and the spectrum of associated lesions. Adv Anat Pathol 16:236–46.

DESHPANDE V, VERMA K. 1998. Fine needle aspiration (FNA) cytology of Rosai–Dorfman disease. Cytopathology 9:329–35.

DEY P, RADHIKA S, JAIN A. 1993. Microfilariae of Wuchereria bancrofti in a lymph node aspirate: a case report. Acta Cytol 37:745–6.

DONNELLY A, HENDRICKS G, MARTENS S, STROVERS C, WIEMERSLAGE S, THOMAS PA. 1995. Cytologic diagnosis of cat scratch disease (CSD) by fine-needle aspiration. Diagn Cytopathol 13:103–6.

DU MQ, LIU H, DISS TC, YE H, HAMOUDI RA, DUPIN N, MEIGNIN V, OKSENHENDLER E, BOSHOFF C, ISAACSON PG. 2001. Kaposi sarcoma-associated herpesvirus infects monotypic (IgM lambda) but polyclonal naive B cells in Castleman disease and associated lymphoproliferative disorders. Blood 97:2130–6.

DUPIN N, FISHER C, KELLAM P, ARIAD S, TULLIEZ M, FRANCK N, van MARCK E, SALMON D, GORIN I, ESCANDE JP, WEISS RA, ALITALO K, BOSHOFF C. 1999. Distribution of human herpesvirus-8 latently infected cells in Kaposi's sarcoma, multicentric Castleman's disease, and primary effusion lymphoma. Proc Nat Acad Sci USA 96:4546–51.

EGEA AS, MARTINEZ-GONZALEZ MA, BARRIOS AP, MASGRAU NA, de AGUSTIN P. 2002. Usefulness of light microscopy in lymph node fine needle aspiration biopsy. Acta Cytol 46:364–8.

EISENHUT CC, KING DE, NELSON WA, OLSON LC, WALL RW, GLANT MD. 1996. Fine-needle biopsy of pediatric lesions: a three-year study in an outpatient biopsy clinic. Diag Cytopathol 14:43–50.

ELLISON E, LAPUERTA P, MARTIN SE. 1999. Fine needle aspiration diagnosis of mycobacterial lymphadenitis. Sensitivity and predictive value in the United States. Acta Cytol 43:153–7.

ERSÖZ C, POLAT A, SERIN MS, SOYLU L, DEMIRCAN O. 1998. Fine needle aspiration (FNA) cytology in tuberculous lymphadenitis. Cytopathology 9:201–7.

GAFFEY MJ, BEN-EZRA JM, WEISS LM. 1996 Herpes simplex lymphadenitis. Am J Clin Pathol 95:709–14.

GARBYAL R, BASU D, ROY S, KUMAR P. 2005. Cryptococcal lymphadenitis: report of a case with fine needle aspiration cytology. Acta Cytol 49:58–60.

GOEL MM, RANJAN V, DHOLE TN, SRIVASTAVA AN, MEHROTRA A, KUSHWAHA MRS, JAIN A. 2001. Polymerase chain reaction vs. conventional diagnosis in fine needle aspirates of tuberculous lymph nodes. Acta Cytol 45:333–40.

GUPTA SK, KUMAR B, KAUR S. 1981. Aspiration cytology of lymph nodes in leprosy. Int J Lepr Other Mycobact Dis 49:9–15.

GUPTA SK, CHUGH TD, SHEIKH ZA, al-RUBAH NA. 1993. Cytodiagnosis of tuberculosis lymphadenitis: A correlative study with microbiologic examination. Acta Cytol 37:329–32.

GUPTA AK, NAYAR M, CHANDRA M. 1992. Critical appraisal of fine needle aspiration cytology in tuberculous lymphadenitis. Acta Cytol. 36:391–4.

GUSTAFSON KS, FELDMAN L. 2007. Cryptococcal lymphadenitis diagnosed by fine-needle aspiration biopsy. Diagn Cytopathol 35:103–4.

HANDA U, MOHAN H, BAL A. 2003. Role of fine needle aspiration cytology in evaluation of pediatric lymphadenopathy. Cytopathology 14:66–9.

HODA SA, RESETKOVA E, YUSUF Y, CAHAN A, ROSEN PP. 2002. Megakaryocytes mimicking metastatic breast carcinoma. Arch Pathol Lab Med 126:618–20.

HOUSINI I, DABBS DJ, COYNE L. 1990. Fine needle aspiration cytology of talc granulomatosis in a peripheral lymph node in a case of suspected intravenous drug abuse. Acta Cytol 34:342–4.

IYER VK, KAPILA K, VERMA K. 1998. Fine-needle aspiration cytology of dermatopathic lymphadenitis. Acta Cytol 42:1347–51.

JADUS MR, SEKHON S, BARTON BE, WEPSIC HT. 1995. Macrophage colony stimulating factor-activating bone marrow macrophages suppress lymphocytic responses through phagocytosis: a tentative in vitro model of Rosai–Dorfman disease. J Leukoc Biol 57:936–42.

JAIN A, VERMA RK, TIWARI V, GOEL MM. 2005. Dot-ELISA vs. PCR of fine needle aspirates of tuberculous lymphadenitis: a prospective study in India. Acta Cytol 49:17–21.

KARDOS TF, MAYGARDEN SJ, BLUMBERG AK, WAKELY PE JR, FRABLE WJ. 1989. Fine needle aspiration biopsy in the management of children and young adults with peripheral lymphadenopathy. Cancer 63:703–7.

KAKKAR S, KAPILA K, VERMA K. 2001. Langerhans cell histiocytosis in lymph nodes: cytomorphologic diagnosis and pitfalls. Acta Cytol 45:327–32.

KISHIMOTO K, TATE G, KITAMURA T, KOJIMA M, MITSUYA T. 2010. Cytologic features and frequency of plasmacytoid dendritic cells in the lymph nodes of patients with histiocytic necrotizing lymphadenitis (Kikuchi–Fujimoto disease). Diagn Cytopathol 38:521–6.

KISHORE REDDY VC, APARNA S, PRASAD CE, SRINIVAS A, TRIVENI B, GOKHALE S, KRISHNA MOORTHY KV. 2008. Mycobacterial culture of fine needle aspirate—a useful tool in diagnosing tuberculous lymphadenitis. Indian J of Med Microbiol 26:259–61.

KLOBOVES-PREVODNIK V, REPSE-FOKTER A, BRACKO M. 2007. Cytological features of benign mesothelial inclusions in lymph node: a case report of a patient presenting with cervical lymphadenopathy after in vitro fertilization. Cytopathology 18:56–8.

Ko YH, Lee JD. 1992. Fine needle aspiration cytology in lupus lymphadenopathy: a case report. Acta Cytol 36:748–51.

Kumar PV, Moosavi A, Karimi M, Safaei A, Noorani H, Abdollahi B, Bedayat GR. 2001. Subclassification of localized leishmania lymphadenitis in fine needle aspiration smears. Acta Cytol 45:547–54.

Lau SK, Wet WI, Hsu C, Engzell UCG. 1990. Efficacy of fine needle aspiration cytology in the diagnosis of tuberculous cervical lymphadenopathy. J Laryngol Otol 104:24–27.

Layfield LJ, Glasgow BJ, DuPuis MH. 1985. Fine-needle aspiration of lymphadenopathy of suspected infectious etiology. Arch Pathol Lab Med 109:810–2.

Lazcano O, Speights VO Jr, Strickler JG, Bilbao JE, Becker J, Diaz J. 1993. Combined histochemical stains in the differential diagnosis of *Cryptococcus neoformans*. Mod Pathol 6:80–4.

Lioe TF, Elliott H, Allen DC, Spence RAJ. 1999. The role of fine needle aspiration cytology (FNAC) in the investigation of superficial lymphadenopathy: uses and limitations of the technique. Cytopathology 10:291–7.

Lim MS, Straus SE, Dale JK, Fleisher TA, Stetler-Stevenson M, Strober W, Sneller MC, Puck JM, Lenardo MJ, Elenitoba-Johnson KSJ, Lin AY, Raffeld M, Jaffe ES. 1998. Pathological findings in human autoimmune lymphoproliferative syndrome. Am J Pathol 153:1541–50.

Lioe TF, Elliott H, Allen DC, Spence RAJ. 1999. The role of fine needle aspiration cytology (FNAC) in the investigation of superficial lymphadenopathy; uses and limitations of the technique. Cytopathology 10:291–7.

Lowe SM, Kocjan GI, Edwards SG, Miller RF. 2008. Diagnostic yield of fine-needle aspiration cytology in HIV-infected patients with lymphadenopathy in the era of highly active antiretroviral therapy. Int J STD AIDS 19:553–6.

Martin-Bates E, Tanner A, Suvarna SK, Glazer G, Coleman DV. 1993. Use of fine needle aspiration cytology for investigating lymphadenopathy in HIV positive patients. J Clin Pathol 46:564–6.

Mathai AM, Rau AR, Kini H. 2008. Cryptococcal autofluorescence on fine needle aspiration cytology of lymph node. Diagn Cytopathol 36:689–90.

McCluggage WG, Bharucha H. 1994. Lymph node hyalinisation in rheumatoid arthritis and systemic sclerosis. J Clin Pathol 47:138–42.

Meyer L, Gibbons D, Ashfaq R, Vuitch F, Saboorian MH. 1999. Fine-needle aspiration findings in Castleman's disease. Diagn Cytopathol 21:57–60.

Millar EK, Inder S, Lynch J. 2009. Extramedullary haematopoiesis in axillary lymph nodes following neoadjuvant chemotherapy for locally advanced breast cancer—a potential diagnostic pitfall. Histopathology 54:622–3.

Monaco SE, Teot LA, Felgar RE, Surti U, Cai G. 2009. Fluorescence in situ hybridization studies on direct smears: an approach to enhance the fine-needle aspiration biopsy diagnosis of B-cell non-Hodgkin lymphomas. Cancer Cytopathol 117:338–48.

Monaco SE, Schuchert MJ, Khalbuss WE. 2010. Diagnostic difficulties and pitfalls in rapid on-site evaluation of endobronchial ultrasound guided fine needle aspiration. Cytojournal 7:9.

Munichor M, Cohen H, Volpin G, Kerner H, Iancu TC. 2003. Chromium-induced lymph node histiocytic proliferation after hip replacement: a case report. Acta Cytol 47:270–4.

Nasuti JF, Yu G, Boudousquie A, Gupta P. 2000. Diagnostic value of lymph node fine needle aspiration cytology: An institutional experience of 387 cases observed over a 5 year period. Cytopathology 11:18–31.

Nasuti JF, Gupta PK, Baloch ZW. 2002. Diagnostic value and cost-effectiveness of on-site evaluation of fine-needle aspiration specimens: review of 5,688 cases. Diagn Cytopathol 27:1–4.

Nasuti JF, Gupta PK, Baloch ZW. 2001. Clinical implications and value of immunohistochemical staining in the evaluation of lymph node infarction after fine-needle aspiration. Diagn Cytopathol 25:104–7.

Nasuti JF, Mehrotra R, Gupta PK. 2001. Diagnostic value of fine-needle aspiration in supraclavicular lymphadenopathy: a study of 106 patients and review of the literature. Diagn Cytopathol 25:351–5.

Neumann MP, Eng MH, Rholl KS, Swedo GJ, Meranze SG. 1992. Disseminated histoplasmosis diagnosed by percutaneous needle biopsy of a retroperitoneal lymph node: a case report. Acta Cytol 36:527–8.

O'Dowd GJ, Frable WJ, Behm FG. 1985. Fine needle aspiration cytology of benign lymph node hyperplasia: Diagnostic significance of lymphohistiocytic aggregates. Acta Cytol 29:554–8.

Oksenhendler E, Duarte M, Soulier J, Cacoub P, Welker Y, Cadranel J, Cazals-Hatem D, Autran B, Clauvel JP, Raphael M. 1996. Multicentric Castleman's disease in HIV infection: a clinical and pathological study of 20 patients. AIDS 10:61–7.

O'Malley DP. 2007. Benign extramedullary myeloid proliferations. Mod Pathol 20:405–15.

Pai MR, Adhikari P, Coimbatore RV, Ahmed S. 2000. Fine needle aspiration cytology in systemic lupus erythematosus lymphadenopathy. A case report. Acta Cytol 44:67–9.

Pantanowitz L, Upton MP. 2003. Benign axillary lymph node inclusions. Breast J 9:56–7.

Pathan SK, Francis IM, Das DK, Mallik MK, Sheikh ZA, Hira PR. 2003. Fine needle aspiration cytologic diagnosis of toxoplasma lymphadenitis: a case report with detection of toxoplasma bradycyst in papanicolaou-stained smear. Acta Cytol 47:299–303.

Paull G, Mosunjac M. 2003. Fine-needle aspiration biopsy and intraoperative cytologic smear findings in a case of benign mesothelial-cell inclusions involving a lymph node: case report and review of the literature. Diagn Cytopathol 29:163–6.

Prasad RR, Narasimhan R, Sankaran V, Veliath AJ. 1996. Fine-needle aspiration cytology in the diagnosis of superficial lymphadenopathy: an analysis of 2,418 cases. Diagn Cytopathol 15:382–6.

Prasoon D. 2000. Acid-fast bacilli in fine needle aspiration smears from tuberculous lymph nodes: where to look for them. Acta Cytolog 44:297–300.

Radhika S, Gupta SK, Chakrabarti A, Rajwanshi A, Joshi K. 1989. Role of culture for mycobacteria in fine-needle aspiration diagnosis of tuberculous lymphadenitis. Diagn Cytopathol 5:260–2.

Rimm DL, Stastny JF, Rimm EB, Ayer S, Frable WJ. 1997. Comparison of the costs of fine needle aspiration and open surgical biopsy as methods for obtaining a pathologic diagnosis. Cancer 81:51–56.

Rinaldo CR, Carney WP, Richter BS, Black PH, Hirsch MS. 1980. Mechanisms of immunosuppression in cytomegaloviral mononucleosis. J Infect Dis 141:488.

Sah SP, Prasad R, Raj GA. 2005. Fine needle aspiration of lymphadenopathy in visceral leishmaniasis. Acta Cytol 49:286–90.

Santos-Briz A Jr, Lopez-Rios F, Santos-Briz A, De Agustin PP. 1999. Granulomatous reaction to silicone in axillary lymph nodes: a case report with cytologic findings. Acta Cytol 43:1163–5.

Sarda AK, Bal S, Singh MK, Kapur MM. 1990. Fine needle aspiration cytology as a preliminary diagnostic procedure for asymptomatic cervical lymphadenopathy. J Assoc Phys India 38:203–5.

Sarma PK, Chowhan AK, Agrawal V, Agarwal V. 2010. Fine needle aspiration cytology in HIV-related lymphadenopathy: experience at a single centre in north India. Cytopathology 21:234–9.

Schafernak KT, Kluskens LF, Ariga R, Reddy VB, Gattuso P. 2003. Fine-needle aspiration of superficial and deeply seated lymph nodes on patients with and without a history of malignancy: review of 439 cases. Diagn Cytopathol 29:315–9.

Schinstine M. 2009. Kikuchi's lymphadenitis. Diagn Cytopathol 38:190.

Schultenover SJ, Ramzy I, Page CP, LeFebre SM, Cruz AB Jr. 1984. Needle aspiration biopsy: role and limitations in surgical decision making. Am J Clin Pathol 82:405–10.

Sharma M, Agarwal S, Wadhwa N, Mishra K, Gadre DJ. 2007. Spectrum of cytomorphology of tuberculous lymphadenitis and changes during anti-tubercular treatment. Cytopathology 18:180–3.

Shimizu K, Ito I, Sasaki H, Takada E, Sunagawa M, Masawa N. 2001. Fine-needle aspiration of Toxoplasmic lymphadenitis in an intramammary lymph node: a case report. Acta Cytol 45:259–62.

Silverman JF, Gurley AM, Holbrook CT, Joshi VV. 1991. Pediatric fine-needle aspiration biopsy. Am J Clin Pathol 95:653–9.

Silverman JF and Kardos TF. 1991. Cytomorphologic patterns of inflammatory aspirates. In: Silverman JF, ed., Guides to Clinical Aspiration Biopsy: Infectious and Inflammatory Diseases and Other Nonneoplastic Disorders. Igaku-Shoin, New York, 85–104.

Srinivasan R, Gupta N, Shifa R, Malhotra P, Rajwanshi A, Chakrabarti A. 2010. Cryptococcal lymphadenitis diagnosed by fine needle aspiration cytology: a review of 15 cases. Acta Cytologica 54:1–4.

Stanley MW, Steeper TA, Horwitz CA, Burton LG, Strickler JG, Borken S. 1990. Fine-needle aspiration of lymph nodes in patients with acute infectious mononucleosis. Diagn Cytopathol 6:323–9.

Stanley MW, Horwitz CA, Burton LG, Weisser JA. 1990. Negative images of bacilli and mycobacterial infection: a study of fine needle aspiration smears from lymph nodes in patients with AIDS. Diagn Cytopathol 6:118–21.

Steel BL, Schwartz MR, Ramzy I. 1995. Fine needle aspiration biopsy in the diagnosis of lymphadenopathy in 1103 patients: role, limitations, and analysis of diagnostic pitfalls. Acta Cytol 39:76–81.

Stephany JD, Lucero S, Walsh AF. 2005. Mediastinal mass in a 27-year-old man: extrapulmonary *Coccidioides immitis*. Arch Pathol Lab Med 129:699–700.

Sudilovsky D, Cha I. 1998. Fine needle aspiration cytology of dermatopathic lymphadenitis. Acta Cytol 42:1341–7.

Tabatowski K, Elson CE, Johnston WW. 1990. Silicone lymphadenopathy in a patient with a mammary prosthesis: fine needle aspiration cytology, histology, and analytical electron microscopy. Acta Cytolog 34:10–14.

Tallada N, Raventós A, Martinez S, Compañó C, Almirante B. 1993. Leishmania lymphadenitis diagnosed by fine-needle aspiration biopsy. Diagn Cytopathol 9:673–6.

Tatomirovic Z, Skuletic V, Bokun R, Trimcev J, Radic O, Cerovic S, Strbac M, Zolotarevski L, Tukic Lj, Stamatovic D, Tarabar O. 2009. Fine needle aspiration cytology in the diagnosis of head and neck masses: accuracy and diagnostic problems. J BUON 14:653–9.

Taylor GB, Smeeton IW. 2000. Cytologic demonstration of "dysplastic" follicular dendritic cells in a case of hyaline-vascular Castleman's disease. Diagn Cytopathol 22:230–4.

Thomas JO, Adeyi D, Amanguno H. 1999. Fine-needle aspiration in the management of peripheral lymphadenopathy in a developing country. Diagn Cytopathol 21:159–62.

Thomson KR, House AJ, Göthlin JH, Dolin TE. 1978. Percutaneous lymph node aspiration biopsy: experience with a new technique. Clin Radiol 29:329–32.

Tong TRS, Chan OW, Lee K. 2001. Diagnosing Kikuchi disease on fine needle aspiration biopsy: a Retrospective study of 44 cases diagnosed by cytology and 8 by histopathology. Acta Cytol 45:953–7.

Tsang WYW, Chan JKC. 1992. Spectrum of morphologic changes attributable to fine-needle aspiration. Hum Pathol 23:562–5.

Vera-Alvarez J, Marigil-Gomez M, Abascal-Agorreta M, Lacasa-Laliena M. 1999. Diagnosis of localized Leishmania lymphadenitis by fine needle aspiration cytology. Acta Cytol 43:529–30.

Viguer JM, Jiménez-Heffernan JA, Pérez P, López-Ferrer P, Gónzalez-Peramato P, Vicandi B. 2001.

Fine-needle aspiration cytology of Kikuchi's lymphadenitis: a report of ten cases. Diagn Cytopathol 25:220–4.

WAKELY PE JR, KARDOS TF, FRABLE WJ. 1988. Application of fine needle aspiration biopsy to pediatrics. Hum Pathol 19:1383–6.

WAKELY PE JR. 2001. Lymph node aspiration cytopathology. In: Collins RD, Swerdlow SH, ed., Pediatric Hematopathology. Churchill Livingstone, New York, 12–19.

WILKERSON JA. 1985. Intraoperative cytology of lymph nodes and lymphoid lesions. Diag Cytopathol 1:46–52.

WRIGHT CA, VAN ZYL Y, BURGESS SM, BLUMBERG L, LEIMAN G. 2004. Mycobacterial autofluorescence in Papanicolaou-stained lymph node aspirates: a glimmer in the dark? Diagn Cytopathol 30:257–60.

WRIGHT CA, VAN DER BURG M, GEIGER D, NOORDZIJ JG, BURGESS SM, MARAIS BJ. 2008. Diagnosing mycobacterial lymphadenitis in children using fine needle aspiration biopsy: cytomorphology, ZN staining, and autofluorescence-making more of less. Diagn Cytopathol 36:245–51.

ZAHAROPOULOS P, HUDNALL SD. 2004. Nevus-cell aggregates in lymph nodes: fine-needle aspiration cytologic findings and resulting diagnostic difficulties. Diagn Cytopathol 31:180–4.

ZAHAROPOULOS P. 2000. Demonstration of parasites in toxoplasma lymphadenitis by fine-needle aspiration cytology: report of two cases. Diagn Cytopathol 22:11–5.

ZAJDELA A, ZILLHARDT P, VOILLEMOT N. 1987. Cytological diagnosis by fine needle sampling without aspiration. Cancer 59:1201–5.

ZARDAWI IM, BARKER BJ, SIMONS DP. 2005. Hodgkin's disease masquerading as granulomatous lymphadenitis on fine needle aspiration cytology. Acta Cytol 49:224–6.

CHAPTER TWENTY-TWO

MIXED PATTERNS IN LYMPH NODE: TROPICAL INFECTIOUS LYMPHADENOPATHY AND HEMATOPATHOLOGY, NOT OTHERWISE CHARACTERIZED

Hernani D. Cualing

INTRODUCTION

In many tropical infections lymphadenopathy is a prominent sign, owing to the strategic location of the lymph nodes and the role that they and the immune system play in response to infections. A number of infections that cause lymphadenopathy are included in this chapter not because they are tropical in endemicity but because of their potential biothreat importance in the West. Many tropical and biothreat infections have a zoonotic mode of transmission.

Zoonoses are animal diseases that can be transmitted to humans by contact with infected animals. Hunters, farmers, abattoir workers, and wildlife tourists are at greatest risk for zoonoses but the diseases can occur in anyone and are astonishingly widespread. Of the 1415 known human infectious pathogens, 62% are of zoonotic origin (Taylor, Latham, and Woolhouse, 2001). Prominent among

the list are vector-transmitted and arthropod-borne illnesses.

Many of the infections show prominent hematopathology in lymph nodes and spleen, but a number are characterized by lymphadenopathy features with only provisional findings (see Table 22.1 and 22.2). The patterns described herein for the known diseases are characteristic and unequivocal, but for others the features have been less well studied. Therefore, in those cases, the features described are labeled as not otherwise characterized or provisional (see Box 22.4 and Box 22.6).

HEMORRHAGIC LYMPHADENOPATHY

Anthrax

Although rare in the United States, anthrax as a potential bioterrorism agent during the Middle East

Non-Neoplastic Hematopathology and Infections, First Edition. Edited by Hernani D. Cualing, Parul Bhargava, and Ramon L. Sandin.
© 2012 Wiley-Blackwell. Published 2012 by John Wiley & Sons, Inc.

TABLE 22.1 Emergent/Tropical Infections with Lymphadenopathy (Not Otherwise Characterized)

Hemorrhagic lymphadenopathy

- *Bacillus anthracis* (anthrax) lymphadenopathy: hemorrhage, necrosis
- RMSF-hemorrhage, necrosis, edema, vasculitis, lymphohistiocytosis, endothelial necrosis

Sinus pattern

- *Yersinia pestis* (bubonic plaque) lymphadenopathy: histiocytosis, necrosis, edema, congestion, vascularity, sinus proliferation
- *Leptospira interogans* lymphadenopathy: sinus pattern, hemophagocytosis
- Scrub typhus lymphadenopathy: sinus hemophagocytosis, vasculitis, necrosis

Diffuse pattern with depletion and atypical immunoblastic reaction

- Dengue hemorrhagic fever lymphadenopathy: depletion, congestion, paracortical immunoblasts
- Ehrlichiosis lymphadenopathy: immunoblastic, lymphoplasmacytosis, histiocytosis, morulae
- Lassa hemorrhagic fever: atypical immunoblasts, necrosis, apoptosis, depletion
- Nipah virus: atypical immunoblasts, endothelial cell multinucleation

Unusual granulomas

- Q fever

TABLE 22.2 Tropical/Emergent Diseases with Prominent Hematopathology

Anthrax
Bartonellosis
Brucellosis
Bubonic plaque
Chaga's disease
Dengue
Ehrlichiosis
Filariasis
Lassaviruses
Leismaniasis
Leprosy
Leptospirosis
Melioidiosis
Nipah virus
Rocky Mountain spotted fever
Schistosomiasis
Scrub typhus
Syphilis, secondary
TIBOLA (Tick Borne Lymphadenopathy)
Trypanosomiasis, African
Tuberculosis
Tularemia

TABLE 22.3 Hemorrhagic Lymphadenopathy Findings

Bacillus anthracis (anthrax) lymphadenopathy: hemorrhage, necrosis
Rocky Mountain spotted fever lymphadenopathy: hemorrhage, necrosis, edema, vasculitis, lymphohistiocytic, endothelial necrosis

and post-911 conflicts raised the attention of the public and healthcare workers to a level normally accorded to diseases like smallpox, tularemia, plague, and botulism (see Table 22.2).

Definition

Anthrax is an acute disease caused by the bacterium *Bacillus anthracis*, which in less virulent forms and if treated early responds well to antibiotics. The spectre of *B. anthracis* being used in biowarfare has stimulated interest in the development of more effective vaccines.

ICD-10 Code A22

Synonyms

Malignant pustule, malignant edema, woolsorter's disease, ragpicker's disease.

Epidemiology

Anthrax occurs globally. The disease is an occupational risk of veterinarians and workers who process hides, goat hair, or sheep's wool. Bioterrorist groups

may develop "weaponized" versions of the bacterium such as those reported after the World Trade Center attack that involved a number of mail handlers (Guarner et al., 2003). These highly virulent, inhalable preparations could result in serious exposure to large numbers of people.

Pathogenesis

In addition to being able to evade immune effector cells with an antiphagocytic capsule, *B. anthracis* secretes three virulence proteins, a protective antigen, a lethal factor, and an edema factor that generate exotoxins (Mikesell et al., 1983; Farrar, 1994; Duesbery et al., 1998). The toxins cause edema with perivascular and intravascular hemorrhage of mediastinal lymph nodes. The lymphadenopathy leads to lymphatic blockage that, with the extensive inflammatory reaction to the bacilli, contributes to the hemorrhagic pleural effusion. Septicemia supervenes upon entry of bacilli into the blood stream and death is the usual outcome. Published findings about inhalation anthrax observed in Sverdlovsk, Russia (Abramova and Grinberg, 1993) showed prominent vessel necrosis, capillaritis, and vasculitis resulting in blood dissemination and hemorrhagic pathology. These cases in addition showed hematogenous involvement of intestinal mucosa and mesenteric lymph nodes.

Clinical Aspects

Etiology. The anthrax bacillus is a Gram-positive, aerobic, spore-forming microorganism. *B. anthracis* spores remain infective in the soil for many years and are inert reservoirs of infection for herbivorous animals.

Sites of Involvement. The spores may cause infection through skin contact, ingestion, or inhalation leading to cutaneous, oropharyngeal-intestinal, or pulmonary forms of anthrax, respectively.

Cutaneous anthrax, commonly affects the head, forearms or hands. Infection is characterized by itching followed by papular-vesicular lesions in 2 to 6 days that become indented black eschars, with edema and formation of more vesicles. Pain is unusual and the cutaneous appearance has been confused with human Orf virus and other skin lesions (Table 22.4) (Brachman, 1965).

TABLE 22.4 Differential Diagnosis of Anthrax

Type	Etiology
Cutaneous anthrax	• Spider bite of brown recluse, *Loxosceles*: painful red, white, blue sign (hemorrhage then, blue central necrosis then depressed white skin) • Tick bite: no edema, no pain, no necrosis, *tache noir* sign • Cat-scratch disease: slower course than anthrax • *Staphylococcus aureus* furuncle: lesion emits pus and is painful • Ecthyma gangrenosum: *Pseudomonas* bacteraemia seen in neutropenic patients • Cutaneous leishmaniasis: lesion resembles the eschar but develops slowly
Inhalation and GI anthrax	• Pneumonia, influenza, viral syndrome, septicemia, bronchitis, central nervous system infection, and gastroenteritis

> **BOX 22.1 Inhaled Anthrax as a Cause of Lymphadenopathy and Mediastinal Hemorrhage**
>
> Mediastinal hemorrhage with lymphadenopathy, in an acutely ill patient with no history of trauma should raise concern for inhalational anthrax infection.

Intestinal and oropharyngeal anthrax may arise from ingestion of undercooked infected meat, but there is no evidence that milk from infected animals can cause anthrax. Presentations include fever, dysphagia, sore throat, and regional lymphadenopathy. Acute inflammation of the bowel is accompanied by nausea, vomiting, fever, loss of appetite, and abdominal pain and sometimes hematemesis or hematochezia (Tekin, Bulut, and Unal, 1997; Jena, 1980). Primary intestinal anthrax is usually localized in the terminal ileum unlike the diffuse intestinal distribution of hematogenous anthrax (Kanafani et al., 2003).

Inhalation of aerosolized spores leads to pulmonary anthrax (see Box 22.1). This is a lethal form of the disease often with complicating pleural effusion, pneumonia, and mediastinal lymphadenopathy (Van Ness, 1971).

The inhaled spores are trapped in the upper airways and ingested by macrophages, which migrate to the perihilar and mediastinal lymph nodes. There the bacilli become vegetative again, and multiply causing hemorrhagic lymphadenitis. The enlarged mediastinal masses become visible on X-ray images (Frazier, Franks, and Galvin, 2006; Brachman, 1980) and in postmortem examinations (Guarner et al., 2003). There may be hemorrhagic pericardial effusion and lung edema. (Barakat et al., 2002; Guarner et al., 2003). There is often no associated meningitis, splenomegaly, or mesenteric lymphadenopathy. Despite mediastinal and lung involvement, there is often no bronchopneumonia. The rapid macrophage shuttling of bacilli from alveoli to the pleura and lymph nodes is believed to account for the scant pulmonary lesions. There are no hemorrhagic lesions of the liver or kidney. The most common gross autopsy findings include serosanguinous pleural effusion and hemorrhages of mediastinal lymph nodes and adjacent soft tissues (Guarner et al., 2003).

Approach to Diagnosis

The diagnosis of anthrax is best approached clinically because of the urgent need to treat early, keeping in mind all three clinical presentations. A severely ill, febrile patient with a widened mediastinum should prompt an empirical diagnosis of inhalation anthrax.

Drawing blood or cerebral spinal fluid to isolate *B. anthracis* is the definitive diagnostic step. Cutaneous anthrax is suspected in a patient that presents with a painless, pruritic, papular lesion that ends in vesicles and a "black eschar." Fluid within the vesicles may contain numerous, large Gram-positive bacilli with characteristic Gram-negative segments, and this fluid may be submitted for rapid microbiology stain or culture. Intestinal anthrax is characterized by acute abdominal distress associated with severe gastrointestinal symptoms that mimics a "surgical abdomen," along with ascites, perforation and mesenteric lymphadenitis (Kanafani et al., 2003). In all instances, regional lymphadenopathy is common. Gram-positive bacilli in chains and bacterial cultures from excised lymph nodes is diagnostic for *Bacillus anthracis*.

Laboratory Findings. Laboratory workups of blood, tissue, and skin lesions or discharges can demonstrate the organism directly in polychrome methylene blue (M'Fadyean)-stained smears or by culture. Immunodiagnostic testing, ELISA and PCR may be available in some reference laboratories.

Morphology. Postmortem mediastinal lymph node specimens show florid hemorrhagic mediastinitis (see Figure 22.1). Hilar and peribronchial lymph nodes are enlarged, hemorrhagic and necrotic, and appear replaced by hematoma. Lymph nodes show a mixed pattern with effacement of the normal architecture replaced by florid hemorrhages, a condition called hemorrhagic lymphadenitis (see Figure 22.2) *B. anthracis* is sometimes seen in routine tissue stains but is more clearly seen by using Steiner silver stains or immunohistochemistry (available at CDC pathology). If antibiotics were given for more than 3 days, ghostly, distorted, and knobbed bacillary fragments may be seen. Granular cytoplasmic antigens are a characteristic immunostaining feature.

The most common lymph node findings (Guarner et al., 2003) include necrosis, hemorrhage, paucicellular presence of immunoblasts, neutrophils, and apoptotic and necrotic debris. The spleen may exhibit one or more of the following changes: congestion, immunoblastosis, neutrophilic infiltration or necrosis similar to that seen in experimental animals. [Fritz et al. 1995].

In lungs, hematoxylinophilic bacilli completely filling the perivascular lymphatic space with pigmented macrophages may be seen. Hemorrhages secondary to erosion or break in the lumen of the pulmonary vessels may be noted (see Box 22.2) There are often few neutrophils despite the presence of

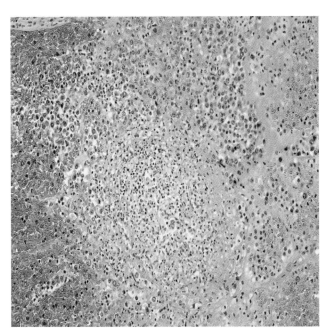

FIGURE 22.1 **Anthrax: mediastinal lymph node with effaced architecture and hemorrhagic necrotizing lymphadenitis (100×, H&E).** (Courtesy Dr. Wun-Ju Shieh and Dr. Sherif Zaki, Infectious Diseases Pathology Branch, Centers for Disease Control and Prevention.)

many microorganisms. Clusters of bacilli end to end, typically with square-ended "box car" morphology may be observed. Pleural fluid cell blocks often show bacilli by immunohistochemisty.

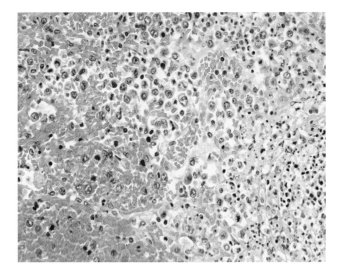

FIGURE 22.2 **Anthrax: mediastinal lymph node with hemorrhagic necrotizing lymphadenitis with interstitial convoluted hemorrhages, necrotic nuclear debris, and nucleolated large cells (200×, H&E).** (Courtesy Dr. Wun-Ju Shieh and Dr. Sherif Zaki, Infectious Diseases Pathology Branch, Centers for Disease Control and Prevention.)

Stained skin biopsies from suspected cases of cutaneous anthrax infection may show the bacilli, but if the numbers are small, they are best seen by immunohistochemical staining for the *B. anthracis* cell wall antigen (Tatti et al., 2006; Guarner et al., 2003).

Immunohistochemistry/Cytochemistry. Touch Preps Diff-Quick cytology should reveal intracellular and free bacilli. The Gram stain shows Gram-positive (dark blue) areas due to cell wall staining along with Gram-negative regions (red) where the bacilli appear less thick.

Differential Diagnosis

Because of the rare occurrence of inhalation, cuta-neous, and intestinal anthrax, a high level of suspicion on the most common illness seen by primary care practitioners is essential for an earlier diagnosis and treatment. The nonfatal cases may have been seen and diagnosed earlier than the fatal cases. In a pri-mary care setting, pneumonia, influenza, bronchitis, and viral syndrome accounted for 80% of nonfatal anthrax diagnoses while pneumonia, septicemia, CNS infection, bronchitis, and gastroenteritis accounted for 70.1% of fatal anthrax cases (Temte and Zinkel, 2004). In cutaneous form, the black eschar can clini-cally mimic a spider bite, or Orf's virus skin lesions. A *tache noir* skin lesion resembling the eschar may be seen in patients living in areas where tick bites are common. The intestinal form resembles an acute sur-gical abdomen and may mimic an acute appendicitis when localized in the ileo-cecal area (see Table 22.4).

Treatment of Choice. Ciprofloxacin or doxycy-cline administered for 60 days are the most effective antibiotics. Ciprofloxacin should be given to adults (including pregnant women and immunocompro-mised persons) and doxycycline to children.

Prognosis. Case fatality rates for inhalational anthrax are high (estimated at 75%; http://www.bt.cdc.gov/agent/anthrax/faq/signs.asp) despite administration of antibiotics and intensive care. The mortality rate for cutaneous anthrax is lower than for the inhaled form: 20% without, and <1% with antibiotic treatment. The fatality rate for the intestinal form is 25 to 60%, but the effect of early antibiotic treatment on mortality has not been established.

Rocky Mountain Spotted Fever

Rocky Mountain spotted fever (RMSF) is the most lethal and commonly reported rickettsial illness in the United States (see Box 22.3).

ICD-10 Code A77

Synonyms

"Black measles," "tick typhus," "Tobia fever" (Colombia), "São Paulo fever" or "febre maculosa" (Brazil), and "fiebre manchada" (Mexico).

Epidemiolology

It is now known that the name is a misnomer and that this disease is widely found throughout the United States as well as in the Americas. The disease was reported from every US state except Hawaii, Vermont, Maine, and Alaska. Most cases, however, are found in eastern United States and more recently in Arizona. About 250 to 1200 cases are reported each year. RMSF occurs as far as Canada and as far as Central America and parts of South America. *R. rickettsii* spread to humans by bite of *Dermacentor variabilis* (dog tick) or *D. andersoni* (Rocky Mountain wood tick). In Arizona, where most cases are reported, *Rhipicephalus sanguineaus* (brown dog tick) transmits the disease.

Pathogenesis

Endothelial cells are the organism's target leading to vascular injury. A vigorous Th1 response is seen. Interferon (IFN)gamma and tumor necrosis factor (TNF) alpha activated by obligate intracellular rickettsia activate macrophages. These injuries lead to increased vascular permeability, leakage of blood fluids, then to hypovolemia and hypoperfusion of some organs such as the kidneys (Walker, Valbuena, and Olano, 2003).

Clinical Aspects

Etiology. The *R. rickettsii* bacteria is a Gram-negative intracellular bacilli that invades and injure endothelial cells.

Sites of Involvement. Skin rash is the most visible manifestation. The rash are characteristically red, flat, and macular, spreading from wrists or ankles to the chest, back and abdomen. Most of the infection occur in children and the vast majority happens between late spring to early fall.

The initial presentation is a nonspecific flu-like illness. Later on, a triad of fever, rash, and headache coupled with a history of previous tick bite point to the disease. The illness could be severe, with abdominal and joint pains associated with diarrhea, causing the majority of patients to be hospitalized. Dyspnea, heart rhythm disturbance, renal insufficiency, and encephalitis are severe manifestations (see Table 22.5).

Approach to Diagnosis

The characteristic symptoms, history of tick bite, and exposure to a location known to have ticks are the basis of clinical diagnosis. Since only a few laboratories perform specialized time-consuming diagnostic tests, diagnosis is rendered empirically to avoid fatalities. In specialized laboratories, the biopsy of a skin rash may be diagnostic.

Laboratory Findings. *R. rickettsii* is not visible in blood smears, and these bacteria fail to stain with the majority of conventional stains. A CBC, metabolic panel, and peripheral blood smear examination are helpful in developing a differential diagnosis. The total white blood cell (WBC) count is typically normal, but WBC that show a left shift with increased bands, coupled with thrombocytopenia, are hematology findings in patients with RMSF (Walker, 1995).

Morphology. Because of injury to endothelial lining cels, the lymph node pathology is characterized by endothelial lining necrosis, vasculitis, and subsequent diffuse hemorrhagic lymphadenopathy

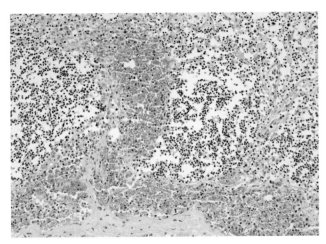

FIGURE 22.3 **RMSF: subcapsular hemorrhage and effaced architecture (H&E, 100×).** (Courtesy Dr. Wun-Ju Shieh and Dr. Sherif Zaki, Infectious Diseases Pathology Branch, Centers for Disease Control and Prevention.)

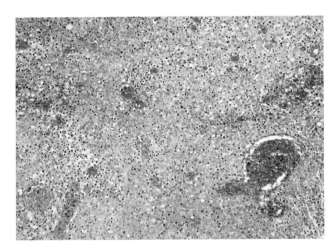

FIGURE 22.4 **RMSF: hemorrhagic lymphadenopathy with hypocellularity, hemorrhagic necrosis, congestion, and edema (H&E, 100×).** (Courtesy Dr. Wun-Ju Shieh and Dr. Sherif Zaki, Infectious Diseases Pathology Branch, Centers for Disease Control and Prevention.)

(See Figures 22.3–22.5). Sometimes the hemorrhages include capsular and subcapsular areas associated with edema and congestion. Scattered immunoblasts are seen and at time numerous, imparting a diffuse immunoblastic pattern. Skin biopsy findings include predominantly perivascular lymphohistiocytic vasculitis with edema and extravasation of erythrocytes (Kao et al., 1997).

Immunohistochemistry/Cytochemistry. For patients with a rash, immunostaining of skin biopsy specimens has been reported to be 100% specific and

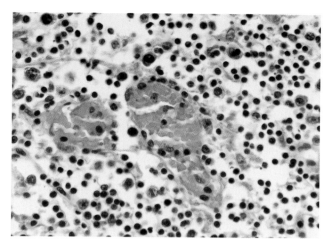

FIGURE 22.5 **RMSF: endothelial cell necrosis, vasculitis, immunoblastic proliferation (H&E, 400×).** (Courtesy Dr. Wun-Ju Shieh and Dr. Sherif Zaki, Infectious Diseases Pathology Branch, Centers for Disease Control and Prevention.)

70% sensitive in diagnosing RMSF (Walker, 1989, 1995).

Differential Diagnosis

The differential diagnosis is wide in a young patient with fever and rash. These include viral exanthems, drug reactions, Fifth disease, as well as other tick-borne diseases like anaplasmosis and ehrlichiosis (Chapman et al., 2006). Microscopic examination of Wright–Giemsa stained blood smears may show morulae in the cytoplasm of infected circulating leukocytes (1–20%) of patients with and 20 to 80% of patients with granulocytic anaplasmosis. (Dumler et al., 2007; Paddock and Childs, 2003). (See Chapter 8 for blood smear findings in ehrlichiosis and anaplasmosis.)

Treatment and Prognosis

Untreated cases have up to 25% mortality and 4% mortality after antibiotic treatment. Tetracycline

TABLE 22.5 Key Diagnostic Features of Rocky Mountain Spotted Fever

Etiology: *Rickettsia rickettsii*
Regions: widespread in US
Transmission: ticks
Population at risk: travelers, campers, naturalists
Organs involved: skin lymph nodes
Lymph node pathology: vasculitis, pulp and capsular hemorrhages, prominent edema
Differential diagnosis: human monocytic ehrlichiosis
Diagnosis: immunohistochemistry using polyclonal antibody to *R. rickettsii* with 100% sensitivity
Unusual feature: hemorrhages, vasculitis

or doxycyline is the treatment of choice. Standard duration of treatment is 5 to 10 days and best initiated based on clinical epidemiological information because laboratory confirmation may not be available during the acute illness.

SINUS PATTERN

Bubonic Plaque

Bubonic plague, caused by *Yersinia pestis*, a flea-borne zoonotic, is the cause of three pandemics that are unmatched in history. The bubonic plague was responsible for killing about 200 million people and destabilizing civilized world's economy, social fabric, and course of history (Sherman, 2006). It is worldwide in scope with Asia, Africa, and the Americas as the main endemic areas. From its origin in China, carried via the ancient shipping lanes, *Y. pestis* spread to the United States in 1900 (Perry, 1997; Khan, 2004, Achtman et al., 1999), with outbreaks that started and spread eastward from the Pacific coast, from populous cities like San Francisco (Link, 1955). This spread continued and has since then stopped expanding on the plaque line, at the 103 meridian, located on the western Great Plains (Antolin, Biggins, and Gober, 2010). Case fatality rate is high if not detected early or if there is inappropriate or inadequate antibiotic therapy, so early detection is crucial for a life-saving outcome (see Box 22.5).

BOX 22.4 Sinus Pattern with Salient Findings

Yersinia pestis **(bubonic plaque) lymphadenopathy:** histiocytosis, necrosis, edema, congestion, vascularity, sinus proliferation

Leptospira interogans **lymphadenopathy:** sinus pattern, hemophagocytosis

Scrub typhus *O. tsutsugamushi* lymphadenopathy: sinus pattern, hemophagocytosis, vasculitis, necrosis

---

BOX 22.5 Historical Vignette: Plaque

A possible epidemic of bubonic plague was described in the Old Testament, in the First Book of Samuel. The so-called "Black Death" emerged in the fourteenth century and caused vast losses throughout Asia, Africa, and Europe. The epidemic, which originated in the Far East, killed approximately one-third of Europe's population. However, bubonic plague still occurs in Asia, Africa, and the Americas, and the World Health Organization annually reports 1000 to 3000 cases. In the western United States, acquisition of plague in humans in linked to companion animals infested with *Yersinia pestis*–carrying fleas in areas of endemic sylvatic disease (Perry and Fetherston, 1997).

Definition

A zoonotic disease, transmitted from a bite of an infected rat flea carrying *Yersinia pestis* leading to painful swollen nodes, called buboes, and death.

ICD-10 Code A200

Synonyms

Black death, third pandemic, plague of Justinian, the plaque.

Epidemiology

Historically, over the course of the past five centuries, rat and flea-borne bubonic plague caused by *Yersinia pestis* developed into pandemics that claimed more than 200 million lives and killed about a third of the population of Europe. However, bubonic plague still occurs in Asia, Africa, and the Americas, and the World Health Organization annually reports 1000 to 3000 cases. In the United States, New Mexico and adjacent states have the highest CDC reported cases. The incidence was linked to companion animals infested with *Y. pestis*–carrying fleas (Perry and Fetherston, 1997). An average of 8 cases (1–40) per year have been reported during 1950 to 2008 in the United States. During this time, more than 80% of all US cases were reported from New Mexico, with the remainder in Arizona, Colorado, or Utah (Brown et al., 2010).

From its origin in rats, *Y. pestis* subsequently became established in wild rodent populations in several western states with wood rats, squirrels, rabbits, chipmunks, deer mice, ground squirrel, and prairie dogs as reservoirs (Ingelsby et al., 2000).

Worldwide, and in the recent past, the incidence is much higher, with more than 200 different rodents and species that can serve as hosts. From 1987 to 2001, the World Health Organization has reported an annual average of 38,876 cases of the plague with 2847 deaths. Most cases occur in the developing countries of Africa and Asia and the more recent outbreaks have occurred in India, northeast Congo, Algeria, Vietnam, and Madagascar. During 2000 to 2001, 95% of the world's cases occurred in Africa.

Pathogenesis

The bacillus exerts a wide ranging effect from its innate virulence factors and by interfering with hosts cellular mechanisms. The effect starts in the flea, where the bacilli clogs its esophagus and to overcome hunger starts its parasitical bites. With this blood-sucking flurry, *Y. pestis* bacillus gets deposited in the skin. The vast majority of virulence factors in *Y. pestis* are encoded by 70 Kb plasmids producing a host of Yersinia outer proteins (Yops) (Huang, Nikolich, and Lindler, 2006). Direct contact between Yersiniae and phagocytic cells induces secretion of bacterial Yop proteins into the cytophagic cell cytoplasm, which (1) block phagocytosis, (2) induce apoptosis, and, (3) modulate cytokine networks to inhibit the inflammatory response (Cornelis et al., 1998; Ruckdeschel et al., 1997, Monack et al., 1997). Unlike the more suppurative cellular host response caused by other Yersinia species, neutrophils and macrophage reaction are decreased as disease advanced and may partly explain the depleted lymph node morphology. In addition other factors associated with virulence exploit Toll-like recognition molecules and defense mechanisms using virulence V-antigen to evade the host immune response (Sing et al., 2002).

Clinical Aspects

Etiology. The agent of the plaque, *Y. pestis*, is a facultative anaerobic, intracellular, Gram-negative bacillus with vector as well as passive material modes of propagation. The vector is usually the rat flea, *Xenopsylla cheopis*, with 30 different species identified worldwide. Rare carriers include ticks and human lice. Also virulent plague bacteria can survive dormant in grain, dried sputum, flea feces, soil, and buried carcasses. *Y. pestis* can be transmitted via close contact with infected tissue or body fluids, and via direct inhalation of aerosolized bacteria. The most common form of transmission is from the bite of an infected flea. In the United States the most common form of exposure is through flea bites, primarily those of ground squirrel fleas (*Oropsylla montana*), which are believed to serve as the primary bridging vector to humans (Eisen et al., 2006). Bubonic, pneumonic, and septicemic plagues are the three forms commonly seen.

Sites of Involvement. In bubonic plague the bacilli spread from the flea bite abscess to lymph nodes, followed by septicemia and pneumonia. Two to 8 days after the bite, bubonic plague begins with painful draining lymph ''buboes,'' fever, chills, and prostration. The most virulent form, pneumonic plague, results from inhalation due to direct animal contact or from bioterrorist aerosolized bacteria. In systemic plague the bacteria are primarily inoculated directly into the blood and do not produce a bubo. The bacillus may seed each organ, including the spleen, kidneys, liver, lungs, and rarely the meninges.

The bubonic form makes up approximately 80 to 95% of cases. The bacillus invades nearby lymphoid tissue, and distributed along the lymphatic vessels, with eventual vascular seeding with ensuing bacteremia and septicemia. Lymphadenitis ensues with inflamed, hemorrhagic, and necrotic lymph nodes.

In primary pneumonic plague, cough, dyspnea, and high fever show after 2 to 3 days. A severe bronchopneumonia follows with subsequent bacteremia.

Chest Radiography. Pneumonic plague shows alveolar infiltrates with or without hilar lymphadenopathy. No chest radiograph pattern is characteristic of plague, but bilateral interstitial infiltrates are most commonly seen. This finding contrast with anthrax where pneumonia is seldom seen and mediastinal masses are frequent.

The third type of plague is a primary septicemic plague. Rapid spread occurs. Bites typically occur in the highly vascularized areas of the oro-pharynx which are also adjacent to the thoracic duct drainage.

Approach to Diagnosis

Diagnosis depends on clinical appearance, history of animal contact, and results of culture on blood agar. Colonies are small, nonhemolytic, and iridescent. The organisms are identified by biochemical and serologic methods. *Y. pestis* fluorescent antibody titer, acute and convalescent passive hemagglutination (PHA) titers, should be taken 10 days apart. A fourfold difference or a single convalescent PHA titer of 1:16 is evidence of infection.

In general, after an incubation period of 1 to 6 days, the history suggests a severe and rapidly progressive sepsis. Several key clinical findings are important: Recent travel to endemic areas is important, even though less than 10% of patients recall a flea bite, and should raise suspicion for the plague. Close contact with ground squirrel or domestic cat is another. Sudden severe pneumonia in a group of previously healthy individuals should raise concern for pneumonic plague possibly deployed as a bioterrorism weapon. A painful bubo of the femoral lymph node, the most common site, should make one suspect a plague victim. The other lymph node regions involved are the inguinal, axillary, and cervical areas. Black-blue necrosis of nose, lips, fingers, and toes and residual ecchymoses are helpful signs.

Laboratory Findings. The diagnosis is made by blood culture and smears of aspirate from buboes, cerebrospinal fluid, sputum, and intratracheal aspirates. Blood culture results are positive in 85 to 96% of patients. Bubo aspirate culture results are positive in 80 to 85% of patients. WBC count may be markedly elevated to levels of $20,000/\mu l$ or greater, unless there is septicemic shock. Urinalysis may show hematuria, RBC casts, and/or proteinuria.

A rapid diagnostic test using monoclonal antibodies to F1 antigen is available at CDC. This may be used in the early detection of the plague. *Y. pestis* fluorescent antibody stain may be performed on blood, sputum, or bubo aspirate samples. Sputum may show large numbers of small bacilli when stained with fluorescent antibody (CDC, Plague Branch, PO Box 2087, Fort Collins, CO 80522). Rapid urine dipstick tests have been developed to screen for *Y. pestis* antigen and can be used in the field for rapid identification during outbreak situations.

Morphology

Aspiration of lymph node may be attempted. If hard, bloody, or nondiagnostic, histologic examination of an excisional biopsy may be diagnostic (see Figures 22.6, 22.7).

Two patterns are seen: Mixed pattern with acute lymphadenitis and mixed pattern with lymphoid depletion. Acute lymphadenitis shows a mixed pattern with focal hemorrhage, necrosis, edema, and vessels with small thrombi can be seen in bubonic and septicemic plague (Sebbane et al., 2006). The bacterial clumps appear on routine stains as finely

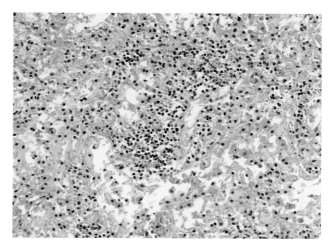

FIGURE 22.6 **Plaque with sinus histiocytic necrosis, lymphoid depletion and foamy histiocytosis with tingible bodies 100×, H&E).** (Courtesy Dr. Wun-Ju Shieh and Dr. Sherif Zaki, Infectious Diseases Pathology Branch, Centers for Disease Control and Prevention.)

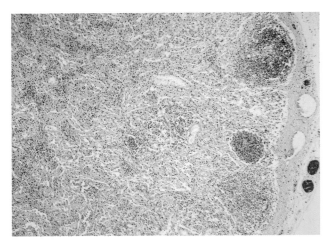

FIGURE 22.7 **Plaque with lymphocyte depletion imparting a sinus or interfollicular pattern**. There is increased vascularity, edema, and widespread necrosis of interfollicular areas. Congestion and preserved architecture with residual follicles are present (50×, H&E). (Courtesy Dr. Wun-Ju Shieh and Dr. Sherif Zaki, Infectious Diseases Pathology Branch, Centers for Disease Control and Prevention.)

granular material. The architecture is generally preserved despite hemorrhages or necrosis. The bacteria are seen within hemorrhagic foci and within necrotic blood vessels. In a more chronic but fatal form, there is lymphoid depletion, foamy macrophages in sinusoids, and tissue abscess. Splenic hyperplasia and thrombosed perisplenic blood vessels contain fibrin mixed with bacilli. Multifocal hemorrhage is present in the capsular and perisplenic tissue (Guarner et al., 2002; Guarner and Zaki, 2006).

Cytochemistry. Y. pestis coccobacillus is identified by microbial stains in peripheral smears in up to 20% of patients. When stained with Wright–Giemsa, a bipolar safety pin structure may be identified. Gram stain may identify the Gram-negative, pleomorphic coccobacillus. Gram stain can be performed on bubo aspirate, sputum, and blood. In 70% of patients, the Gram-negative bipolar-stained coccobacillus is visualized if present.

Immunohistochemistry. Mouse monoclonal antibody against F1 antigen (CDC and Naval Research "Institute", Bethesda, MD) can detect the organisms in tissue. In lymph nodes with lymphoid depletion, bacteria were found in blood vessels only, but in those with other mixed patterns, granular stained bacteria are seen inside macrophages and abundant extracellular bacilli in subcapsular sinuses (Guarner et al., 2002).

Differential Diagnoses

Clinical considerations include pneumonia, acute respiratory distress syndrome, tick-borne diseases, and any acute lymphadenitis with a rapidly progressive systemic illness. Because of the focal nodal hemorrhage, anthrax is also a consideration, but the presence of pneumonia constrasts with absence of pneumonic lesions in inhalation anthrax.

Treatment of Choice. Tetracycline, sulfadiazine, and streptomycin are effective if started early, and chloramphenicol is used for patients with meningitis.

Prognosis. In about 48 hours, respiratory failure, bacteremic shock, and coagulopathy herald death. Septicemic plague (whether primary or secondary) has a 40% mortality rate when treated and 100% mortality rate untreated. Pneumonic plague (whether primary or secondary) has 100% mortality rate untreated within the first 24 hours of infection. Bubonic plaque, without septicemia, has a 1 to 15% mortality rate in treated cases and a 40 to 60% mortality rate in untreated cases.

Additional Information

Prevention recommendations focus on animal vectors or use of vaccination. These include avoiding handling sick or dead animals, reducing rodent food, and not allowing pets to roam and hunt, and eliminating fleas from pets. Control of rats and rat fleas is crucial. Several vaccines are available for animal use, but their effectiveness is controversial. Laboratory personnel should be vaccinated. Y. pestis is a grave hazard for nursing and laboratory personnel in close contact with the infection. Noncommercial vaccines in addition to administration of prophylactic antibiotics are available for humans at high risk.

Leptospirosis

Leptospirosis is the most common zoonotic disease found in tropical countries. In temperate regions, leptospirosis occurs sporadically during summer and fall months.

Definition

Leptospirosis is a systemic illness caused by the spirochete *Leptospira interrogans* and other *Leptospira spp.* and is considered the most common zooosis worldwide.

ICD-10 Code A27

Synonyms

Seven-day fever, Autumn fever or Akiyami, cane field fever, Canicola fever, cave fever flu, Fort Bragg fever, hemorrhagic jaundice, infectious jaundice, mud fever, Nanukayami fever, pretibial fever, rat catcher's yellows, redwater of calves, ricefield fever, spirochetal jaundice, Stuttgart disease, swamp fever, swineherd's disease, swamp or mud fever, Sewerman's flu, Weil's disease, Weil's syndrome.

Epidemiology

The worldwide incidence of leptospirosis is alarming and, if unabated, threatens to be an emergent epidemic (see Table 22.6). Exacerbating factors may include the flood-related effects of global warming, long-lasting popularity of water recreation activities, and occupational hazards, which when combined may hasten the resurgence of leptospirosis. The onslaught of changing climactic conditions is associated with reports of increasing case to fatality ratios that ranges from 5% up to 30%. Urban populations are at increased risk because of deteriorating housing and poor health conditions. Seasonal outbreaks are most common during rainy season (Bharti et al., 2003), highlighted by the 2009 flooding in the Philippines in which 2000 cases are reported with more than 100 people dead. In endemic areas, seroprevalence rate increased from 0.7 to 28% in flooded areas. In Hawaii since the 1970s, most cases followed recreational exposures involving water sports like swimming in canals and white water rafting (Kaufmann, 1976, Martone and Kaufmann, 1979). Similarly, in 2004, tainted floodwaters at the University of Hawaii campus infected the cleanup workers. In 2000, during a sporting competition in

TABLE 22.6 Key Diagnostic Features of Leptospirosis

Etiology: *Leptospira interrogans*
Regions: worldwide
Transmission: rodents and rats as reservoir
Population at risk: recreational and occupational disease affecting farmers, veterinarians, abattoir workers, rodent-control workers, military troops
Organs involved: blood, and in Weil's syndrome: renal, liver, pulmonary
Lymph node pathology: sinusoidal hyperplasia with erythrophagocytosis
Differential diagnosis: tuberculous lymphadenitis; for systemic presentation: influenza, dengue, viral hepatitis
Diagnosis: serology, ELIZA or Leptodiptick for serum or urine
Unusual feature: Immune phase heralds severe symptoms

Malaysia, an infection outbreak occurred in athletes playing water sports. From Springfield, Illinois, in 1998, 100 leptospirosis cases developed from the 700 exposed during a triathlon competition. "Swamp fever" appeared in water-rafting visitors to Costa Rica in 1997. The estimated incidence of leptospira cases in the United States is about 100 annually, which may be below the real frequency. Recent fall 2011 outbreak of illnesses from Leptospira contaminated cantaloupes caused many fatalities in US traced to produce that were stored in waterlogged floors.

Spread of the disease, however, remains related mainly to occupational involvement. Groups at risk include farm and agricultural workers, veterinarians, pet and pet shop owners, those working in abattoirs and slaughterhouses, including meat handlers. Historically, military troops, veterinarians, and rodent-control workers are most commonly infected (Levett, 2001). A rodent, especially rats, is considered the most important reservoir or maintenance hosts but has also been reported in ducks, livestock, foxes, and skunks. Several leptospirosis serovars and serogroups are present in rats, a common source of leptospirosis in the Philippines (Villanueva et al., 2010).

Pathogenesis

Leptospirosis is a two-phased illness involving blood and tissue. The first or septicemic phase is characterized by nonspecific flu-like symptoms, which include fever, chills, muscle aches, myalgia, and photophobia. Muscle tenderness is present with the myositis of early infection; most often found in the paraspinal and calf muscles but can involve any muscle. This phase is followed by a brief afebrile period, as symptoms seem to disappear by the fifth to the ninth day. The second or immune phase triggers the onset of Weil's disease. It begins after a few days of feeling well then recurring with fever, muscle ache, and stiffness of the neck.

Virulence factors may include the spiral motility of the hooked ends and hyaluronidase that could enable penetration of intact mucosa and blood vessels. The outer membrane contains a variety of lipoproteins, which may be important for adhesion of *Leptospira spp.* to host tissues. The outer membrane of Leptospira, like those of most other Gram-negative bacteria, contains lipopolysaccharide (LPS), a highly immunogenic structure that accounts for the numerous serovars of Leptospira.

Clinical Aspects
Sites of Involvement. Blood dissemination and pathologic immune response lead to Weil's disease.

Almost all patients present with jaundice. These patients develop renal, pulmonary, and multi-organ dysfunction. Skin, eyes, muscle, lymph nodes, and viscera are involved in varying degree and severity. Redness of the eyes occurs, with rash, cough, anorexia, vomiting, and lymphadenopathy. Alveolar hemorrhage manifesting as dyspnea and hemoptysis are the main pulmonary aspects. Some patients develop meningitis. Pulmonary involvement has emerged as a serious cause of mortality in some countries. Hypotension, oliguria, and abnormal chest auscultation are grave signs of severe disease.

Etiology. *Leptospira interrogans* are spiral bacteria 0.6 μm in diameter and 6 to 20 μm in length terminating with hooked ends and move in a spin. *Leptospira interrogans* and the serovar, *L. interrogans icterohemorrhagiae*, cause Weil's disease (Herrmann-Storck et al., 2010).

Approach to Diagnosis

A combination of clinical data, epidemiologic factors, and lab findings is an optimal approach to diagnosis (Table 22.6). (Chappel et al., 1998; Vijayachari and Sehgal, 2006). Isolation of leptospira is considered the gold standard in diagnosis. However, because isolation of leptospira is usually difficult, microscopic agglutination testing (MAT) and ELISA may be helpful in detecting elevated antibody titers. Enzyme-linked immunosorbent assay (ELISA) uses a broadly reactive antigen, from the patient's blood or urine and detects IgM. It may be useful for diagnosis within 3 to 5 days. ELISA tests are available as color-changing dipsticks. Polymerase chain reaction, ribotyping, and pulse field gel electrophoresis are molecular tests that can be used if available (Villanueva et al., 2010).

Laboratory Findings. The results vary with increasing severity of disease. In patients with mild disease, elevated erythrocyte sedimentation rates and peripheral leukocytosis with a left shift are noted. Cerebral spinal fluid cells may reveal polymorphonuclear leukocytes early on followed by monocytes later. In Weil's disease, about half the patients show mild thrombocytopenia, often accompanied by renal failure. Marked leukocytosis and elevated creatine phosphokinase (CPK) and prothrombin times are seen at this stage.

Morphology. Lymphadenopathy is one of the features of Weil's disease and is commonly seen in fatal cases. Enlarged lymph nodes were clinically seen in 10%, but fatal cases showed generalized

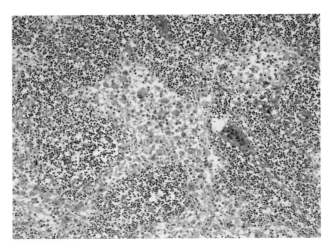

FIGURE 22.8 **Leptospirosis: sinus pattern with congestion, histiocytosis, and focal hemorrhages.** (Courtesy Dr. Wun-Ju Shieh and Dr. Sherif Zaki, Infectious Diseases Pathology Branch, Centers for Disease Control and Prevention.)

lymphadenopathy in 66% of autopsy cases (Arean, 1962). The lymph nodes were soft, with reddish hemorrhagic cut surfaces. More common were the marked sinus histiocytosis (see Figure 22.8) and histiocytic erythrophagocytosis (see Figure 22.9). The spleen was mostly normal in size but histologically showed zones of hemorrhage disrupting the normal architecture. The bone marrow showed granulocytic hyperplasia with left shift and normal or slightly reduced erythropoietic activity. Megakaryocytes were normal in number and appearance. Foci of hemorrhage, erythrophagocytosis, and increased numbers of plasma cells or lymphocytes were also noted. In autopsy cases, the mucosa of the gastrointestinal tract contained hemorrhages. Peyer's patches showed lymphoid hyperplasia with erythrophagocytosis, and scattered hemorrhages. Liver showed hepatic degeneration, Kupffer cell hyperplasia, and erythrophagocytosis. Pulmonary hemorrhage was a very prominent histopathology finding in fatal cases of leptospirosis (Arean, 1962).

Differential Diagnosis

Leptospirosis in the early stages of acute infection can be mistaken for many other infections. The following diseases should be considered in the differential diagnosis of leptospirosis. Clinically, influenza, dengue hemorrhagic fever, hantavirus infection, yellow fever, and other viral hemorrhagic fevers, rickettsiosis, borreliosis, brucellosis, malaria, typhoid fever, and other enteric fevers, are only a short list of many other considerations.

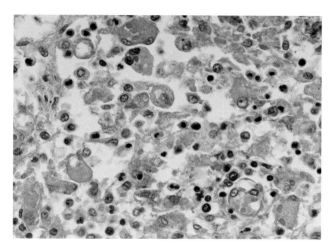

FIGURE 22.9 **Leptospirosis: Hemophagocytic histiocytosis in Leptospiral lymphadenopathy.** (Courtesy Dr. Wun-Ju Shieh and Dr. Sherif Zaki Infectious Diseases Pathology Branch, Centers for Disease Control and Prevention.)

Treatment of Choice

Oral doxycycline, ampicillin, streptomycin, and amoxicillin are commonly used for some of the milder cases. For the more severe cases, intravenous penicillin G is used, and alternatives include ampicillin, amoxicillin, and erythromycin. Currently, no human vaccine against leptospirosis is available.

Prognosis

Most patients with leptospirosis recover. The highest mortality rates are in elderly patients and in those with Weil's syndrome. Mortality rate ranges from five to 14% in diagnosed cases.

Newer diagnostic modalities have proved useful in developed and developing countries: Leptospira DipS-Ticks® (PanBio InDx Inc., Baltimore, MD). Screening with Leptospira Dip-S-Ticks had poor sensitivity but 100% specificity when compared with the Leptospira IgM ELISA (Myint et al., 2007).

Scrub Typhus

Scrub typhus needs to be differentiated from other rickettsiosis and other causes of febrile rash because of its high mortality rate if untreated.

ICD-10 Code A75.3

Synonym

Tsutsugamushi. Rickettsia *tsutsugamushi*.

Definition

Scrub typhus is an acute febrile illness characterized by the presence of a vasculitis and organomegaly caused by *Orientia tsutsugamushi*.

Epidemiology

Endemic in the "tsutsugamushi triangle," which extends from Japan and eastern Russia in the north, to northern Australia in the south, and to Pakistan and Afghanistan in the west. Scrub typhus is a chigger-borne zoonosis that is endemic in tropical Asia and the islands of the western Pacific Ocean and of grave public concern (Brown, 1978).

Pathogenesis

Disseminated vasculitis with perivasculitis is the foremost pathology. Multiorgan involvement with hemorrhages of the brain and lungs are associated with fatal outcome. Vascular damage from disseminated endothelial infection is the key pathogenesis for tsutsugamushi disease, with immune and inflammatory factors playing a role (see Table 22.7) (Moron et al., 2001).

Clinical Aspects

Etiology. *Orientia* (formerly Rickettsia) *tsutsugamushi* (Tamura et al., 1995), the etiologic agent of scrub typhus, is transmitted to humans by the larval mite (chigger) during feeding (Brown et al., 1976).

Sites of Involvement. Typical physical findings are eschars and maculopapular skin rashes, which develop over the trunk and limbs and lymphadenopathy. Lee et al., studied 92 cases from Hong Kong, and lymphadenopathy was present in 22.8% of the cases, with hepatosplenomegaly in up to 15% (Lee et al., 2008). A study of 140 cases in Taiwan detected 8% lymphadenopathy along with the most common presentation of fever, chills, cough, myalgia, and bradycardia. Hematologic findings include thrombocytopenia in most cases and leukocytosis or lymphopenia is a minority. Hepatosplenomegaly were

TABLE 22.7 **Key Diagnostic Features of Scrub Typhus**

Etiology: *Orientia tsutsugamushi*
Regions: Asia and Pacific Islands
Transmission: mites or "chiggers"
Population at risk: travelers, indigenous people
Organs involved: blood, lymph nodes, liver, spleen
Lymph node pathology: eschar at the site of chigger feeding, and a maculopapular rash.
Regional lymphadenopathy: sinus histiocytosis with hemophagocytosis, vasculitis, and monocytoid lymphoid hyperplasia.
Differential diagnosis: dengue fever, leptospirosis, other rickettsiosis
Diagnosis: Giemsa or Gimenez stain or immunohistochemistry
Unusual feature: high mortality of up to 35%

present in 20% and elevated liver enzyme in majority of the cases (Lai et al., 2008).

Approach to Diagnosis

When flu-like symptoms and thrombocytopenia present in a patient with generalized lymphadenopathy, scrub typhus or other rickettsiosis should be considered in the differential diagnosis, especially if the patient lives in, or has a history of travel to, scrub typhus-endemic areas.

Laboratory Findings. Initial misdiagnosis were common in 90% with false-negative serologic tests including IFA or Weil–Felix test probabaly due to delayed antibody response or blunted response post-treatment. The gold standard is indirect immunofluorescence. The diagnosis may be by ELISA, immunofluorescence, molecular detection polymerase chain reaction (PCR), and real-time PCR. Histology and immunohistochemistry may be helpful in serology negative cases (see Table 22.7).

Morphology. Forty-seven lymph nodes and 68 splenic autopsy pathology were described early on by Allen and Spitz (1945). Sinus expansion with hemophagocytosis are the characteristic findings (see Figure 22.10). Erythrophagocytic histiocytes are seen expanding the sinuses (see Figure 22.11). Infarction of the lymph node or focal necrosis of the nodes with karyorrhexis, hemorrhage, and deposits of fibrin within germinal centers or sinuses are less common findings. Some degree of monocytoid, lymphocytic, and immunoblastic proliferation are seen. These immunoblast cells were called basophilic macrophages, Turk cells, large lymphocytes, in the pre-modern description of Allen. Also vasculitis and endothelial necrosis may be present (see Figure 22.12).

Cutaneous pathology was described in one case of scrub typhus eschar and showed leucoclastic vasculitis and atypical CD30+ lymphocytes (Lee et al., 2009). Atypical multilobated lymphocytes have also been described in skin lesions (Iwasaki et al., 1991). Spleen similarly showed erythrophagocytosis in all cases and rarely thrombophlebitis and necrotic infarcts. Bone marrow was hyperplastic with hemophagocytic histiocytes (Allen and Spitz, 1945).

Immunohistochemistry/Histochemistry. Rickettsiae can been detected occasionally in tissue specimens by various histochemical stains, including Giemsa or Gimenez stains. Immunohistochemical methods provide visualization of rickettsiae when applied to formalin-fixed, paraffin-embedded tissue specimens obtained at autopsy or cutaneous

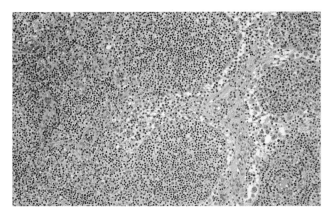

FIGURE 22.10 **Scub typhus with nodules of primary follicles, a degree of sinus expansion with histiocytosis, and interfollicular congestion (5×, H&E).** (Courtesy Dr. Wun-Ju Shieh and Dr. Sherif Zaki, Infectious Diseases Pathology Branch, Centers for Disease Control and Prevention.)

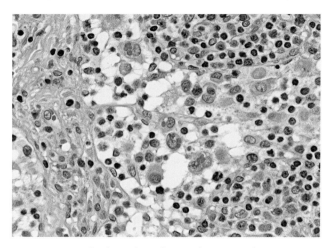

FIGURE 22.11 Scub typhus: hemophagocytic histiocytosis. (40×, H&E). (Courtesy Dr. Wun-Ju Shieh and Dr. Sherif Zaki, Infectious Diseases Pathology Branch, Centers for Disease Control and Prevention.)

biopsy (particularly eschars). Immunofluorescence or immunoperoxidase assay is the gold standard for the diagnosis of scrub typhus (Kim et al., 2007; Tseng et al., 2008; Moron et al., 2001).

Differential Diagnosis

There are many species of Rickettsia that cause illnesses, so scrub typhus can be easily confused with other viral, bacterial, and parasitic diseases because of the similarity in their clinical manifestations. Leptospirosis and dengue fever come into the differential in the right epidemiologic settings.

Treatment of Choice and Prognosis

Among the causes of mortality are leucocytosis and pulmonary complications, and also failure to

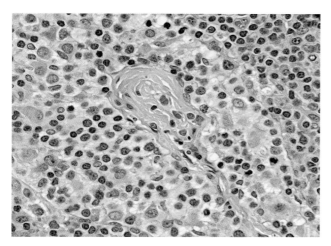

FIGURE 22.12 **Scub typhus: vascular sclerosis and vasculitis with surrounding monocytoid hyperplasia (40×, H&E)**. (Courtesy Dr. Wun-Ju Shieh and Dr. Sherif Zaki, Infectious Diseases Pathology Branch, Centers for Disease Control and Prevention.)

BOX 22.6 **Diffuse Pattern with Depletion and Atypical Immunoblastic Reaction**

Dengue hemorrhagic fever lymphadenopathy: depletion, lymphoplasmacytosis, HEV hyperplasia, congestion, hemolysis, hemosiderin pigments

Ehrlichiosis lymphadenopathy: atypical immunoblastic lymphoplasmacytosis, histiocytosis, morulae

Lassa hemorrhagic fever: atypical immunoblasts, necrosis, apoptosis, depletion

Nipah virus: atypical immunoblasts, endothelial cell multinucleation and syncitia formation

---

initiate doxycyline therapy with in the first three days. Without treatment, the disease is highly fatal. Unlike other rickettsiae cases scrub typhus without treatment has as high as 35 to 37% death rate (Lee et al., 2008). Ever since the use of antibiotics, case fatalities have decreased from a high of 37% to less than 2% (Box 22.6).

DIFFUSE PATTERN WITH DEPLETION AND ATYPICAL IMMUNOBLASTIC REACTION

Dengue

Dengue, a mosquito-borne infection, is a leading cause of illness and death in the tropics and subtropics, and incidence of dengue has increased globally in the last decades. Dengue haemorrhagic fever (DHF), a potentially deadly complication, was first recognized in the 1950s during dengue epidemics in the Philippines (Fresh et al., 1969) and Thailand. Dengue is a principal travel diagnosis and along with Chikungunya and African tick-bite fever, a leading cause of tourist febrile rash (Hochedez et al., 2008a). Although dengue rarely occurs in the continental United States, it is endemic in many popular tourist destinations in Latin America and Southeast Asia, and unlike malaria, dengue is just as prevalent in cities as well as in rural spots. A dengue fever vaccine, developed by France's Sanofi Pasteur, is the first to undergo Phase III trial in 2011 for 2000 children who are at risk in the Philippines.

Definition
Dengue is a mosquito-borne viral infection that presents as an acute flu-like illness, and sometimes a potentially fatal development called dengue haemorrhagic fever (DHF).

ICD-10 Code A90

Synonyms
Break-bone fever, Dengue fever.

Epidemiology
Dengue fever occurs in similar insect habitats of tropical areas in the Pacific and the Americas and is estimated to infect 120 million people worldwide. Infected humans are the main transporters and reservoirs of the virus, with monkeys likely as secondary carriers. Dengue infection occurs in more than 100 countries in the Asia–Pacific region, the Americas, the Middle East, Africa, and cases continue to rise worldwide (Guzman and Khouri, 2006; Periago, 2007). Some 2.5 billion people—two-fifths of the world's population—are now at risk from dengue. In 2007 alone there were more than 890,000 reported cases of dengue in the Americas, of which 26,000 were DHF (WHO, 1999). Over the last three decades, about a fivefold increase in reported cases was observed in the Americas.

The United States is not spared as recent events of dengue outbreaks were reported in Key West, Florida, in 2010, mostly contacted by tourists coming from the Caribbean islands. In the continental United States, *Aedes aegypti* vector is seasonally abundant, and since 1985, a vector mosquito from Asia, *Aedes albopictus*, along with *A. aegypti*, is now found in most states in the southeastern part of the United States.

Pathogenesis

For about 7 days, viremia and fever occur together. After inoculation, the virus replicates and spread in the blood, skin, and lymphatic tissue. Immune cross-reactivity is understood to be the core pathogenesis, since antibodies directed against nonstructural protein 1 (NS1) showed cross-reactivity with human platelets, and mononuclear and endothelial cells. Dengue infection causes platelet and endothelial cell damage, which activates inflammatory (Lin et al., 2006) as well as direct endothelial damage (Luplertlop et al., 2006). Infected dendritic cells produce matrix metalloproteinases that enhance endothelial permeability. Target cells may include dendritic cells, monocytes, and lymphocytes. A viral replication appears to occur in the dendritic cells and monocytes. Immune-mediated and cross-reacting antibodies and cytokines released by these cells trigger cytotoxicity and immune suppression (Leong et al., 2007). In patients with DHF and re-infection, there is T-cell depletion. Anti-NS1 antibodies cross-reacted with human platelets, fibrinogen, and human clotting factors (Falconar, 1997). Hence the pathogenesis is considered multifactorial (Pang, Wong, and Pathmanathan, 1982).

Serotypes may have different virulences. Type DENV-2 may be the most severe in the Thailand cases, with high viremia titer contributing to severe disease (Vaughn et al., 2000). In the Philippines, DENV-3 infections cover a wide spectrum of disease severity, ranging from inapparent infection to dengue hemorrhagic fever (DHF) (Capeding et al., 2010).

Clinical Aspects

Etiology. Dengue belongs to single-strand RNA viruses. These viruses have been grouped into antigenically distinct serotypes (DENV-1 through DENV-4) belonging to the genus Flavivirus (family Flaviviridae) (Chang, 1997). *Aedes aegypti* is the principal mosquito vector, but *Aedes albopictus* can also cause dengue virus transmission.

Sites of Involvement. Lymphadenopathy can range from 16% (Agarwal et al., 1999; Butt et al., 2008b) to 50% of the cases (Nimmannitya, 1997). Conjunctival infection is present in 89.4%, hepatomegaly 56.7%, and splenomegaly in 12.5% (Butt et al., 2008b). Cutaneous dengue exanthems, usually beginning at lower limbs and the chest, show as morbilliform rash associated with petechial hemorrhages.

Dengue fever is a severe, flu-like illness that affects infants, young children, and adults but seldom causes death. DHF, a disease of children, is characterized by a rapid vascular leakage, hemoconcentration, coagulopathy, and hypovolemic shock (Wills et al., 2004). Generalized lymphadenopathy is often associated with leucopenia and neutropenia.Febrile seizures, petechiae, rashes, and thrombocytopenia among infants is a constellation of signs indicating a Dengue infection. [Capeding et al., 2010] The clinical spectrum of disease range from asymptomatic infection to mild dengue fever (DF) to dengue hemorrhagic fever (DHF), or dengue shock syndrome. The latter is frequently fatal. [Nimmannitya S, 1997].

Approach to Diagnosis

The diagnosis of dengue is usually made clinically. Fever, rash, thrombocytopenia, and leukopenia are the classic findings (Lin et al., 1989).

Laboratory Findings. Hematologic findings are found in 90% of cases (Hochedez et al., 2008b). Thrombocytopenia of less than 100,000 is reported in more than 50% of cases. Although there is activation of complements, there is no disseminated intravascular coagulation To diagnose dengue, the laboratory requires a blood sample taken during the acute period and a second sample taken from day 6 after the onset of symptoms. A seroconversion from negative to positive IgM antibody to dengue or demonstration of a fourfold or greater increase in IgG antibody titers in paired (acute and convalescent) serum specimens indicates infection. IgM antibodies for dengue remain elevated for 2 to 3 months after the illness. Acute infection with dengue virus is confirmed when the virus is isolated from serum or autopsy tissue specimens, or the specific dengue virus genome is identified by reverse transcription-polymerase chain reaction (RT-PCR). RT-PCR is a more sensitive technique for detecting dengue virus or its components in human tissue (Rosen, Drouet, and Deubel, 1999).

Morphology. Lymphoid depletion and congestion is present in lymph nodes, thymus,spleen, and bone marrow (see Figure 22.13). The cellularity is composed of lymphocytes, plasma cells, and scattered immunoblasts (see Figure 22.14). There is depletion of the paracortical areas of the lymph nodes (ung-Khin, Ma-Ma, and Thant, 1975). There is acute atrophy of the thymus and depletion of cuffs of cells in the periarterial lymphatic sheaths (PALS) of the spleen. Bone marrow histologic findings suggest myelosuppression. There may be also a virus-induced repression of myeloid progenitor cells.There is hypocellularity in the early infection, and normal cellularity in the recovery stage usually after 1 week. Megakaryocytes are increased. Nuclear vacuolization of megakaryocytes could also be found (La and Innis, 1995). Thrombocytopenia may result

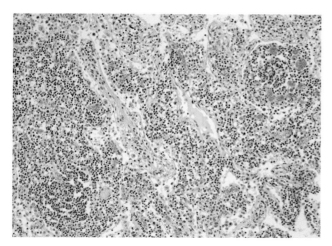

FIGURE 22.13 Dengue lymphadenitis: lymphoid depletion of the paracortex and congestion (100×, H&E). (Courtesy Dr. Wun-Ju Shieh and Dr. Sherif Zaki, Infectious Diseases Pathology Branch, Centers for Disease Control and Prevention.)

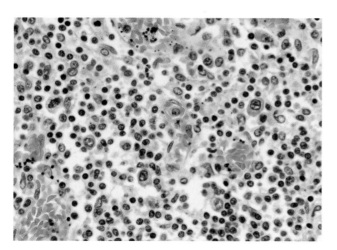

FIGURE 22.14 Dengue lymphadenitis dengue scattered atypical lymphocytes, plasma cells, and immunoblasts (400×, H&E). (Courtesy Dr. Wun-Ju Shieh and Dr. Sherif Zaki, Infectious Diseases Pathology Branch, Centers for Disease Control and Prevention.)

from peripheral immune destruction of platelet or cytopathic effect on megakaryocytes by viruses (Bhamarapravati, Tuchinda, and Boonyapaknavik, 1967). The skin pathology includes mononuclear, perivascular lymphoplasmacytic infiltrate, edema, and endothelial cell hyperplasia.

In patients dying of dengue hemorrhagic fever, germinal center hyperplasia can occasionally be seen, but this is not a consistent finding in dengue fever. Hemorrhage in lymph node is rarely seen, even in those fatal DHF cases that may show nonspecific changes.

Immunohistochemistry/Cytochemistry. The virus can be detected by immunohistochemistry. Acute infections can be confirmed by identification of dengue viral antigen or RNA in autopsy tissue specimens by immunofluorescence or immunohistochemical analysis.

Differential Diagnosis

Dengue should be considered in a dengue-endemic area. Clinical symptoms may mimic leptospirosis, enterovirus, influenza, rubella, or measles infection.

Treatment of Choice and Prognosis

The overall mortality was 2.8% without proper treatment (Butt et al., 2008a). Treatment comprises of supportive care, maintenance of blood volume, and platelets transfusions to prevent bleeding. DHF fatality rates exceed 20%. Access to medical care and to knowledgeable medical workers reduce death rates to less than 1%.

Additional Information

If a dengue-like illness is observed in a person who has recently traveled to a tropical area, acute and convalescent blood specimens, associated clinical information, and a brief travel history should be sent to the state public health laboratory or sent to CDC's Dengue Branch. The blood sample is taken in a red-top tube or a green-top tube, and serum must be maintained on dry ice or in a refrigerator until it is delivered to the CDC's Dengue Branch.

Newer vaccine trials are needed in developed and developing countries. Vaccine research is ongoing, and one based on recombinant live attenuated vaccine on the backbone of yellow fever vaccine (YF 17D) is being tested in the Philippines and Mexico, but the current method of controlling or preventing dengue virus transmission is to combat the vector mosquitoes.

Human Monocytic Ehrlichiosis Lymphadenopathy

Definition

Ehrlichiosis is a disease caused by bacteria *Ehrlichia chaffeensis* and *Ehrlichia ewingii*.

Synonym

Human monocytic ehrlichiosis.

ICD-10 Code A79.8

Epidemiology

Humans acquire *Ehrlichia chaffeensis* through the bite of a tick, most often the Lone Star tick. Lone Star ticks are common in Texas and the southeastern and mid-Atlantic United States. The name actually comes from the white spot on the tick's back. Several other ticks transmit *Ehrlichia chaffeensis*, including the dog tick, the deer tick, and possibly the Gulf Coast tick. A large number of reservoir animals carry *Ehrlichia chaffeensis*, namely white-tailed deer, goats, domestic dogs, red foxes, and some birds.

Pathogenesis

The mechanism of disease is twofold: direct cytologic injury and cytokine dysregulation. Monocytic Ehrlichia attaches and invades lymphocytes, monocytes, and macrophages. Once the bacteria are inside white blood cells, they reproduce by dividing into two microorganisms and multiply continuously. They form inside the cytoplasmic vacuoles large dark-stained cytoplasmic aggregates called morulae. The multiplying organisms eventually lead to white blood cell death and contribute to the development of leukopenia. Cytokine dysregulation is linked to the production of dysfunctional TNF alpha by CD8, aberrant macrophage function, and stimulation of natural killer cells to produce IFN gamma. Excessive cytokine production induced by Ehrlichia infection lead to edema, septic shock-like presentation. Th1-mediated reaction with increased CD8 response is seen.

Clinical Aspects

The triad of findings include fever, myalgias, and pancytopenia. Symptoms of ehrlichiosis resemble those of influenza, namely chills, cough, fever, headache, and muscle pains. Nausea, abdominal pain, and lack of appetite are observed. Unlike other tick-borne illnesses, skin rash is not common in monocytic ehrlichiosis, about 30% of the time.

Etiology. Ehrlichia are Gram-negative bacteria that infect mononuclear cells and granulocytes. Ehrlichia, are obligate intracytoplasmic organisms that resemble Rickettsia.

Approach to Diagnosis. A constellation of clinical and laboratory findings needs to be correlated to suspect the disease. The diagnosis of ehrlichiosis is usually based on symptoms and a history of exposure to ticks and corresponding laboratory findings (see Table 22.8).

Laboratory Findings. A complete blood count is useful and the following findings suggest HME infection: low white blood cell count, low platelet count, and elevated liver enzymes or serum transaminases. Serology is not useful in acute infection and

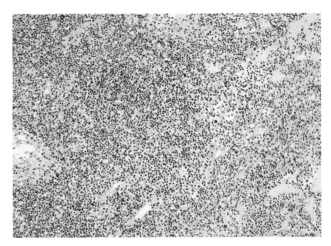

FIGURE 22.15 **Human monocytic ehrlichiosis lymphadenopathy: mild lymphoid depletion, with monocytois and absence of lymphoid follicles (10×).** (Courtesy Dr. Wun-Ju Shieh and Dr. Sherif Zaki, Infectious Diseases Pathology Branch, Centers for Disease Control and Prevention.)

the organism does not grow on standard blood culture media. In equipped laboratories, acute infection is best diagnosed with molecular detection by PCR (Prince et al., 2007).

Morphology. Peripheral blood smears could be diagnostic of HME by finding the characteristic morulae in leukocytes (see Chapter 8). Morulae are intracytoplasmic punctate, bluish-gray coccobacilli arranged in spheres. Examination of at least 500 leukocytes is recommended (Hamilton, Standaert, and Kinney, 2004). Toxic granulation and large granular lymphocytes may be seen.

Lymph nodes show lymphoid depletion, erythrophagocytosis, and infiltrate of foamy macrophages. There is absence of follicles and diffuse monocytosis (see Figure 22.15). Along with paucicellularity is the presence of atypical immunoblastic and monocytic reaction (see Figure 22.16). Intracytoplasmic morulae could seen under high power inside monocyte. The spleen shows depletion, increased apoptotic bodies, and erythrophagocytosis (Lepidi et al., 2000b). Bone marrow is hypercellular or rarely normocellular, with some macrophages showing morulae (Dumler, Dawson, and Walker, 1993).

Differential Diagnosis

The most common differential diagnosis is Rocky Mountain spotted fever which clinically presents with characteristic rash compared to HME.

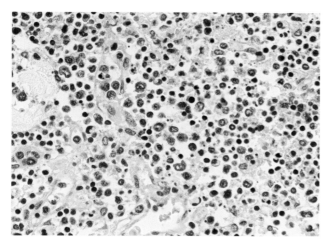

FIGURE 22.16 **Ehrlichia monocytic and immunoblastic reaction with paucicelllularity (40×).** (Courtesy Dr. Wun-Ju Shieh and Dr. Sherif Zaki, Infectious Diseases Pathology Branch, Centers for Disease Control and Prevention.)

TABLE 22.8 **Key Diagnostic Features of Human Monocytic Ehrlichiosis Lymphadenopathy**

Etiology: *Ehrlichia chaffeensis*
Regions: widespread in US
Transmission: Lone Star tick *Amblyoma americanum*
Population at risk: travelers, campers
Organs involved: monocytes and macrophages and organs rich in these such as lymphoid reticuloendothelial system.
Lymph node pathology: Lymphoid depletion, immunoblastic and histiocytic reaction with intracellular morulae organisms
Differential diagnosis: Rocky mountain spotted fever,
Diagnosis: immunohistochemistry monoclonal antibody to *E. chaffeensis* sensitivity of 67%
Unusual feature: Cytophagocytosis, CD8 predominant reaction

Treatment

Antibiotics (tetracycline or doxycycline) are used to treat the disease.

Human Granulocytotropic (or Granulocytic) Anaplasmosis

Definition

Anaplasma phagocytophilum (formerly *Ehrlichia phagocytophilum*) is responsible for anaplasmosis.

ICD-9 Code 082.4

Synonym

Ehrlichia phagocytophilum, anasplasmosis, HGA.

Epidemiology

Various types of Ixodes ticks are vectors for anaplasma. In the United States, the deer tick, western black-legged tick or bear tick, and *Ixodes spinipalpis* most often transmit the bacteria. The reservoir animals for these bacteria are mainly mice, rabbits, lizards, and deer. The life cycle of anaplasma is similar to that of *Borrelia burgdorferi* and *Babesia microti*.

Pathogenesis

After entering the dermis via tick bite inoculation and spread, presumably via lymphatics or blood, ehrlichiae invade target cells of the hematopoietic and lymphoreticular systems. The major infected target cells during the *E. phagocytophila*-group infections are granulocytic leukocytes, mostly neutrophils. Anaplasma also favors basophils and eosinophils.

Clinical Aspects

Symptoms of anasplamosis resemble those of ehrlichiosis and influenza, namely chills, cough, fever, headache, and muscle pains. Rash is rare in anaplasmosis.

Etiology. The bacterium is an obligate intracellular pathogen of neutrophils (Dumler and Brouqui, 2004).

Approach to Diagnosis. Early diagnosis is best achieved by amplification of nucleic acids from the blood (see Table 22.9) (Dumler and Brouqui, 2004).

Laboratory Findings. Microscopic examination of Wright-stained peripheral blood smears may be helpful for the presence of neutrophilic morulae. Polymerase chain reaction (PCR) analysis of blood samples for the *E. phagocytophila*-group DNA, and evaluation of serologic responses by indirect immunofluorescent antibody assay have been used for diagnosis.

Morphology. Lymph nodes show lymphoid depletion but initially may show neutrophil infiltrates and macrophage aggregates or paracortical hyperplasia with erythrophagocytosis (Lepidi et al., 2000a). The splenic pathology also shows lymphoid depletion with variable degrees of macrophage infiltrates and erythrophagocytosis and leukophagocytosis.

Treatment

Doxycycline therapy (100 mg twice daily) until the patient is afebrile for at least 3 days are effective as well as other tetracycline drugs.

TABLE 22.9 Key Diagnostic Features of Human Granulocytic Lymphadenopathy

Etiology: *Anaplasma phagocytophila* group
Regions: widespread in US
Transmission: ticks are the vectors, small mammals and deer are the likely reservoirs.
Population at risk: travelers, campers
Organs involved: blood neutrophils and reticuloendothelial system including liver, spleen, lymph nodes
Lymph node pathology: lymphoid depletion, interfollicular and paracortical hyperplasia, histiocytosis with hemophagocytosis
Differential diagnosis: Rocky Mountain spotted fever
Diagnosis: tissue detection by polyclonal antibody *to E. phagocytophila*. Microscopic examination of Wright-stained peripheral blood smears for presence of neutrophilic morulae, polymerase chain reaction (PCR) analysis of blood samples for the *E. phagocytophila*-group DNA, and evaluation of serologic responses by indirect immunofluorescent antibody assay
Unusual feature: ehrlichiae differ from rickettsiae because they replicate within vacuoles of the host cell, whereas vasculotropic rickettsiae grow freely within the cytoplasm

Lassa Hemorrhagic Fever

Lassa acute viral hemorrhagic fever was first described in the town of Lassa, Nigeria, in 1969 but may be endemic in other countries of West Africa.

ICD-10 Code A96.2

Definition

Lassa fever is an endemic acute zoonotic viral illness transmitted by rodent and causes human to human spread.

Epidemiology

In West Africa, about 100,000 to 300,000 are affected with an estimated 5000 deaths. In some areas of high endemicity, approximately 10 to 16% of hospitals admissions have Lassa fever. The known reservoir of Lassa virus is a rodent called "multi-mammate rat" of the genus Mastomys. Mastomys are common cohabitants of human homes and thus directly contribute to transmission of Lassa virus. Like other hemorrhagic fevers, it can be contracted by an airborne route or with direct contact with infected blood or urine. Transmission through breast milk or sexual contact has also been reported. During illness, the virus is excreted in urine for three to nine weeks and in semen for three months.

Pathogenesis

Lassa virus will infect almost every tissue in the human body, including the reticulo-endothelial system. It starts with the mucosa, intestine, lungs, and urinary system, and then progresses to the vascular and systemic-lymphatic system. In the lymph nodes Lassa virus, including other viral hemorrhagic fever viruses like Ebola virus, targets the fibroblastic reticulum cell framework inducing lymphoid dysregulation and fibrinoid necrosis (Steele, Anderson, and Mohamadzadeh, 2009).

Clinical Aspects

Illness manifests one to three weeks after the patient comes into contact with the virus. About 80% of human infections are subclinical, but the remaining cases may have severe multi-organ disease.

Etiology. The virus, a member of the virus family Arenaviridae, is a single-stranded RNA virus.

Approach to Diagnosis. The best clinical predictor of Lassa fever includes fever, pharyngitis, retrosternal pain, and proteinuria. Lassa fever is most often diagnosed by using enzyme-linked immunosorbent serologic assays (ELISA), which detect IgM and IgG antibodies as well as Lassa antigen. The virus itself may be cultured in 7 to 10 days. Immunohistochemistry performed on tissue specimens can be used to make a tissue ante- or postmortem diagnosis.

Morphology. Lassa fever lymphadenopathy shows enlargement grossly, but microscopically there is follicle depletion, sinusoidal fibrinoid necrosis, and scattered cytophagic histiocytes (see Figures 22.17, 22.18). Spleen shows white pulp atrophy and circumferential deposits of amorphous eosinophilic material in the white pulp were seen in most cases (Winn, Jr., and Walker, 1975). These represent fibrinoid necrosis of splenic marginal zone is seen frequently as presence of lymphocytic intimal deposits of splenic venules (Walker et al., 1982).

Immunohistochemistry. Usually a large amount of viral antigens is seen in the mononuclear cell, endothelial cells, and fibroblastic cells.

Differential Diagnosis

Clinically, Lassa fever infections are difficult to differentiate from other viral hemorrhagic fevers, including dengue and Kyasanur forest disease. The lymphoid depletion with focal necrosis can be seen in lymph node and spleen in Lassa fever infection. These are nonspecific features that can also be observed in

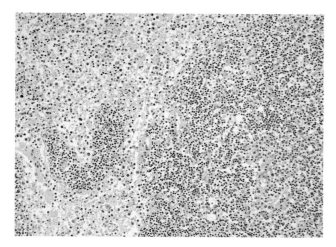

FIGURE 22.17 **Lassa viral hemorrhagic fever lymphadenopathy**. There is lymphoid depletion, sinusoidal histiocytic fibrinous necrosis and scattered cytophagic histiocytes (**100×, H&E**). (Courtesy Dr. Wun-Ju Shieh and Dr. Sherif Zaki, Infectious Diseases Pathology Branch, Centers for Disease Control and Prevention.)

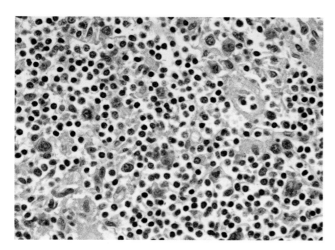

FIGURE 22.18 **Lassa viral lymphadenopathy: atypical lymphocytes, lymphoplasmacytes, and immunoblasts** (**400×, H&E**). (Courtesy Dr. Wun-Ju Shieh and Dr. Sherif Zaki, Infectious Diseases Pathology Branch, Centers for Disease Control and Prevention.)

other viral hemorrhagic fevers, such as ebola, Marburg, and CCHF.

Treatment

Ribavirin, an antiviral drug, has been used sucessfully in these patients.

Prognosis

Only about 1% of infections with Lassa virus result in death. Women in the third trimester of pregnancy are particularly affected. About 95% of fetuses die in the uterus of infected pregnant mothers.

Prevention

The primary transmission of the Lassa virus from its host to humans can be prevented by avoiding contact with Mastomys rodents, especially in the geographic regions where outbreaks occur.

Additional Information

On rare occasions, travelers from endemic areas export the disease to other countries. In addition to the more common etiologies such as malaria, typhoid fever, and other tropical infections, the diagnosis of Lassa fever should be entertained in febrile patients returning from West Africa, especially if they have had visits in areas or hospitals in countries where Lassa fever is endemic.

Nipah Virus

Definition

Nipah virus (NiV) fever is one of the emergent zoonotic viral illness that causes flu-like symptoms and encephalitis.

Etiology

New genus of Henipavirus in the subfamily Paramyxovirinae.

Epidemiology

Nipah is named after the Malaysian village where it was first discovered. It is prevalent in Southeast Asia with identified transmission from carrier fruit bats and sick pigs. Most of the infection has occurred in pig farmers. The case fatality rate is high, and Nipah virus is classified internationally as a biosecurity level (BSL) 4 agent. Diagnosis of the Nipah virus includes serology, histopathology, PCR, and virus isolation.

Histopathology shows characteristic endothelial cell multinucleation (similar to polykaryotes) (see Figure 22.19) along with immunoblastic and lymphoplasmacytic cellularity (see Figure 22.20). At times, the sinus lining cells show multinucleation—likely a viral cytopathic effect of Nipah virus.

UNUSUAL GRANULOMAS Q FEVER

Definition

Q fever is a zoonotic infection caused by *Coxiella burnetii*.

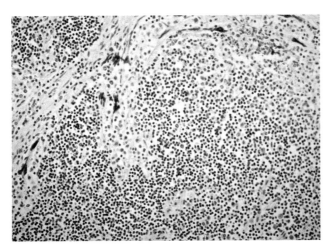

FIGURE 22.19 **Nipah virus: diffuse immunoblastic and lymphoplasmacytic paracortical pattern with polykaryotes-like endothelial cell multinucleation (10×, H&E).** (Courtesy Dr. Wun-Ju Shieh and Dr. Sherif Zaki, Infectious Diseases Pathology Branch, Centers for Disease Control and Prevention.)

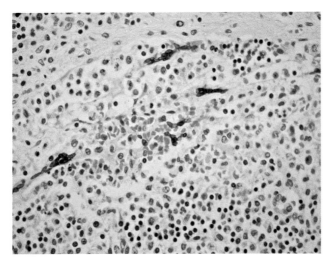

FIGURE 22.20 **Nipah virus multinucleated sinus lining cells.** Diffuse immunoblastic and lymphoplasmacytic paracortical cellularity (**20×, H&E**). (Courtesy Dr. Wun-Ju Shieh and Dr. Sherif Zaki, Infectious Diseases Pathology Branch, Centers for Disease Control and Prevention.)

Etiology

Coxsiella burnetti is an obligate, intracellular, Gram-negative microorganism.

Epidemiology

The disease is endemic in southwest United States, Canada (Ontario), France, and Australia. Exposure of humans with ruminant animals in endemic areas and exposure of veteran troops that served foreign wars are risk factors (Gleeson et al., 2007).

The disease is more common in male adults. Goats, sheep, and cattles (Hatchette et al., 2003) shed large number of infective organism in feces, urine, milk, and products of conception (Hartzell et al., 2008).

Clinical Aspect

The classic presentation is a flu-like illness manifested by fevers, myalgias, arthralgias and comes with a high incidence of pneumonia and hepatitis, at times with hepatosplenomegaly. Acute flu-like syndrome without rash distinguish Q fever from other Rickettsiae. Chronic disease manifests mainly as endocarditis. Endocarditis, the most common form of chronic Q fever, is seen in more than two-thirds of the cases.

Approach to Diagnosis

Morphology. The presence of fibrin rings granulomas in liver or bone marrow histopathology specimens is the classic morphologic finding associated with Q fever but is not specific for the disease (see Table 22.10). Central fat droplets inside a rim of histiocytes and fibrin ring characterize this lesion (see Figure 22.21).

Lab diagnosis is by complement fixing antibody to phase II *C. burnetii* antigen. A titer of 200 or greater for IgG and 50 or greater for IgM against phase II antibodies indicates a recent Q fever infection; an IgG titer of 800 or greater against phase I antibodies suggests chronic infection.

Treatment

The treatment of choice is 100 mg of oral doxycycline every 12 hours for 14 days. The current recommendation for treatment of Q fever endocarditis

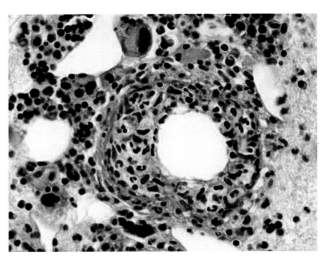

FIGURE 22.21 **Q fever: bone marrow fibrin ring granuloma.** (Courtesy of Dr. Tony. Hernandes, Ameripath, Orlando FL.)

TABLE 22.10 **Causes of Ring Granulomas**

Granulomas with Fibrin Ring
Q fever
CMV
EBV
Mycobacterium avium (MAI)
Hepatitis A
Infectious mononucleosis
Visceral leishmaniasis
Lyme disease
Boutonneuse fever
Toxoplasmosis
Hodgkin disease
Non-Hodgkin lymphomas
Drug reactions

is oral doxycycline (100 mg twice daily) plus hydroxychloroquine (200 mg 3 times daily), 1 for at least 18 months.

REFERENCES

ABRAMOVA AA, GRINBERG LM. 1993. [Pathology of anthrax sepsis according to materials of the infectious outbreak in 1979 in Sverdlovsk (microscopic changes)]. Arkh Patol 55:18–23. (In Russian)

AGARWAL R, KAPOOR S, NAGAR R, MISRA A, TANDON R, MATHUR A, MISRA AK, SRIVASTAVA KL, CHATURVEDI UC. 1999. A clinical study of the patients with dengue hemorrhagic fever during the epidemic of 1996 at Lucknow, India. Southeast Asian J Trop Med Public Health 30:735–40.

ALLEN AC, SPITZ S. 1945. A comparative study of the pathology of scrub typhus (Tsutsugamushi disease) and other rickettsial diseases. Am J Pathol 21:603–81.

ANTOLIN MF, BIGGINS DE, GOBER P. 2010. Symposium on the ecology of plague and its Effects on wildlife: a model for translational research. Vector Borne Zoonotic Dis 10:3–5.

AREAN VM 1962. The pathologic anatomy and pathogenesis of fatal human leptospirosis (Weil's disease). Am J Pathol 40:393–423.

BARAKAT LA, QUENTZEL HL, JERNIGAN JA, KIRSCHKE DL, GRIFFITH K, SPEAR SM, KELLEY K, BARDEN D, MAYO D, STEPHENS DS, POPOVIC T, MARSTON C, ZAKI SR, GUARNER J, SHIEH WJ, CARVER HW, MEYER RF, SWERDLOW DL, MAST EE, HADLER JL. 2002. Fatal inhalational anthrax in a 94-year-old Connecticut woman. JAMA 287:863–8.

BHAMARAPRAVATI N, TUCHINDA P, BOONYAPAKNAVIK V. 1967. Pathology of Thailand haemorrhagic fever: a study of 100 autopsy cases. An Trop Med Parasitol 61:500–10.

BHARTI AR, NALLY JE, RICALDI JN, MATTHIAS MA, DIAZ MM, LOVETT MA, LEVETT PN, GILMAN RH, WILLIG MR, GOTUZZO E, VINETZ JM. 2003. Leptospirosis: a zoonotic disease of global importance. Lancet Infect Dis 3:757–71.

BRACHMAN PS 1965. Human anthrax in the United States. Antimicrob Agents Chemother (Bethesda) 5:111–4.

BRACHMAN PS 1980. Inhalation anthrax. An NY Acad Sci 353:83–93.

BROWN GW 1978. Recent studies in scrub typhus: a review. J R Soc Med 71:507–10.

BROWN GW, ROBINSON DM, HUXSOLL DL, NG TS, LIM KJ. 1976. Scrub typhus: a common cause of illness in indigenous populations. Trans R Soc Trop Med Hyg 70:444–8.

BROWN HE, ETTESTAD P, REYNOLDS PJ, BROWN TL, HATTON ES, HOLMES JL, GLASS GE, GAGE KL, EISEN RJ. 2010. Climatic predictors of the intra- and inter-annual distributions of plague cases in New Mexico based on 29 years of animal-based surveillance data. Am J Trop Med Hyg 82:95–102.

BUTT N, ABBASSI A, MUNIR SM, AHMAD SM, SHEIKH QH. 2008b. Haematological and biochemical indicators for the early diagnosis of dengue viral infection. J Coll Physicians Surg Pak 18:282–5.

CAPEDING RZ, BRION JD, CAPONPON MM, GIBBONS RV, JARMAN RG, YOON IK, LIBRATY DH. 2010. The incidence, characteristics, and presentation of dengue virus infections during infancy. Am J Trop Med Hyg 82:330–6.

CHAPMAN AS, BAKKEN JS, FOLK SM, PADDOCK CD, BLOCH KC, KRUSELL A, SEXTON DJ, BUCKINGHAM SC, MARSHALL GS, STORCH GA, DASCH GA, MCQUISTON JH, SWERDLOW DL, DUMLER SJ, NICHOLSON WL, WALKER DH, EREMEEVA ME, OHL CA. 2006. Diagnosis and management of tickborne rickettsial diseases: Rocky Mountain spotted fever, ehrlichioses, and anaplasmosis—United States. A practical guide for physicians and other healthcare and public health professionals. MMWR Recomm Rep 55:1–27.

CHAPPEL RJ, KHALIK DA, ADLER B, BULACH DM, FAINE S, PEROLAT P, VALLANCE V. 1998. Serological titres to Leptospira Fainei Serovar Hurstbridge in human sera in Australia. Epidemiol Infect 121:473–5.

CORNELIS GR, BOLAND A, BOYD AP, GEUIJEN C, IRIARTE M, NEYT C, SORY MP, STAINIER I. 1998. The virulence plasmid of yersinia, an antihost genome. Microbiol Mol Biol Rev 62:1315–52.

DUESBERY NS, WEBB CP, LEPPLA SH, GORDON VM, KLIMPEL KR, COPELAND TD, AHN NG, OSKARSSON MK, FUKASAWA K, PAULL KD, VANDE WOUDE GF. 1998. Proteolytic inactivation of MAP-kinase-kinase by anthrax lethal factor. Science 280:734–7.

DUMLER JS, BROUQUI P. 2004. Molecular diagnosis of human granulocytic anaplasmosis. Expert Rev Mol Diagn 4:559–69.

DUMLER JS, DAWSON JE, WALKER DH. 1993. Human ehrlichiosis: hematopathology and immunohistologic detection of ehrlichia chaffeensis. Hum Pathol 24:391–6.

DUMLER JS, MADIGAN JE, PUSTERLA N, BAKKEN JS. 2007. Ehrlichioses in humans: epidemiology, clinical presentation, diagnosis, and treatment. Clin Infect Dis 45 (suppl 1): S45–51.

EISEN RJ, BEARDEN SW, WILDER AP, MONTENIERI JA, ANTOLIN MF, GAGE KL. 2006. Early-phase transmission of *Yersinia pestis* by unblocked fleas as a mechanism explaining rapidly spreading plague epizootics. Proc Nat Acad Sci USA 103:15380–5.

FALCONAR AK 1997. The dengue virus nonstructural-1 protein (NS1) generates antibodies to common epitopes on human blood clotting, integrin/adhesin proteins and binds to human endothelial cells: potential implications in haemorrhagic fever pathogenesis. Arch Virol 142:897–916.

FARRAR WE 1994. Anthrax: virulence and vaccines. Ann Intern Med 121:379–80.

FRAZIER AA, FRANKS TJ, GALVIN JR. 2006. Inhalational anthrax. J Thorac Imaging 21:252–58.

FRESH JW, REYES V, CLARKE EJ, UYLANGCO CV. 1969. Philippine hemorrhagic fever: a clinical, laboratory, and necropsy study. J Lab Clin Med 73:451–8.

FRITZ DL, JAAX NK, LAWRENCE WB, DAVIS KJ, PITT ML, EZZELL JW, FRIEDLANDER AM. 1995. Pathology of experimental inhalation anthrax in the rhesus monkey. Lab Invest 73:691–702.

GLEESON TD, DECKER CF, JOHNSON MD, HARTZELL JD, MASCOLA JR. 2007. Q fever in US military returning from Iraq. Am J Med 120:e11–2.

GUARNER J, JERNIGAN JA, SHIEH WJ, TATTI K, FLANNAGAN LM, STEPHENS DS, POPOVIC T, ASHFORD DA, PERKINS BA, ZAKI SR. 2003. Pathology and pathogenesis of bioterrorism-related inhalational anthrax. Am J Pathol 163:701–9.

GUARNER J, SHIEH WJ, GREER PW, GABASTOU JM, CHU M, HAYES E, NOLTE KB, ZAKI SR. 2002. Immunohistochemical detection of *Yersinia pestis* in formalin-fixed, paraffin-embedded tissue. Am J Clin Pathol 117:205–9.

GUARNER J, ZAKI SR. 2006. Histopathology and immunohistochemistry in the diagnosis of bioterrorism agents. J Histochem Cytochem 54:3–11.

HAMILTON KS, STANDAERT SM, KINNEY MC. 2004. Characteristic peripheral blood findings in human ehrlichiosis. Mod Pathol 17:512–7.

HARTZELL JD, WOOD-MORRIS RN, MARTINEZ LJ, TROTTA RF. 2008. Q fever: epidemiology, diagnosis, and treatment. Mayo Clin Proc 83:574–9.

HATCHETTE T, CAMPBELL N, HUDSON R, RAOULT D, MARRIE TJ. 2003. Natural history of Q fever in goats. Vector Borne Zoonotic Dis 3:11–5.

HERRMANN-STORCK C, SAINT-LOUIS M, FOUCAND T, LAMAURY I, DELOUMEAUX J, BARANTON G, SIMONETTI M, SERTOUR N, NICOLAS M, SALIN J, CORNET M. 2010. Severe leptospirosis in hospitalized patients, Guadeloupe. Emerg Infect Dis 16:331–4.

HOCHEDEZ P, CANESTRI A, GUIHOT A, BRICHLER S, BRICAIRE F, CAUMES E. 2008a. Management of travelers with fever and exanthema, notably dengue and Chikungunya infections. Am J Trop Med Hyg 78:710–3.

HOCHEDEZ P, THOMAS L, PIERRE-FRANCOIS S, CESAIRE R, CABIE A. 2008b. [Contributions of the 2005 dengue epidemic in Martinique to the understanding of physiopathology]. Med Mal Infect 38 (suppl 2): S92–3. (In French)

HUANG XZ, NIKOLICH MP, LINDLER LE. 2006. Current trends in plague research: from genomics to virulence. Clin Med Res 4:189–9.

IWASAKI H, UEDA T, UCHIDA M, NAKAMURA T, TAKADA N, MAHARA F. 1991. A typical lymphocytes with a multilobated nucleus from a patient with Tsutsugamushi disease (scrub typhus) in Japan. Am J Hematol 36:150–1.

JENA GP 1980. Intestinal anthrax in man: a case report. Cent Afr J Med 26:253–4.

KANAFANI ZA, GHOSSAIN A, SHARARA AI, HATEM JM, KANJ SS. 2003. Endemic gastrointestinal anthrax in 1960s Lebanon: clinical manifestations and surgical findings. Emerg Infect Dis 9:520–5.

KAO GF, EVANCHO CD, IOFFE O, LOWITT MH, DUMLER JS. 1997. Cutaneous histopathology of Rocky Mountain spotted fever. J Cutan Pathol 24:604–10.

KIM DM, LIM SC, WON KJ, CHOI YJ, PARK KH, JANG WJ. 2007. Severe scrub typhus confirmed early via immunohistochemical staining. Am J Trop Med Hyg 77:719–22.

LA RV, INNIS BL. 1995. Mechanisms of dengue virus-induced bone marrow suppression. Baillieres Clin Haematol 8:249–70.

LAI CH, HUANG CK, WENG HC, CHUNG HC, LIANG SH, LIN JN, LIN CW, HSU CY, LIN HH. 2008. Clinical characteristics of acute Q fever, scrub typhus, and murine typhus with delayed defervescence despite doxycycline treatment. Am J Trop Med Hyg 79:441–6.

LEE JS, PARK MY, KIM YJ, KIL HI, CHOI YH, KIM YC. 2009. Histopathological features in both the eschar and erythematous lesions of Tsutsugamushi disease: identification of CD30+ cell infiltration in Tsutsugamushi disease. Am J Dermatopathol 31:551–6.

LEE N, IP M, WONG B, LUI G, TSANG OT, LAI JY, CHOI KW, LAM R, NG TK, HO J, CHAN YY, COCKRAM CS, LAI ST. 2008. Risk factors associated with life-threatening rickettsial infections. Am J Trop Med Hyg 78:973–8.

LEONG AS, WONG KT, LEONG TY, TAN PH, WANNAKRAIROT P. 2007. The pathology of dengue hemorrhagic fever. Semin Diagn Pathol 24:227–36.

LEPIDI H, BUNNELL JE, MARTIN ME, MADIGAN JE, STUEN S, DUMLER JS. 2000b. Comparative pathology, and immunohistology associated with clinical illness after ehrlichia phagocytophila-group infections. Am J Trop Med Hyg 62:29–37.

LEVETT PN 2001. Leptospirosis. Clin Microbiol Rev 14:296–326.

LIN CF, WAN SW, CHENG HJ, LEI HY, LIN YS. 2006. Autoimmune pathogenesis in dengue virus infection. Viral Immunol 19:127–32.

LIN SF, LIU HW, CHANG CS, YEN JH, CHEN TP. 1989. [Hematological aspects of dengue fever]. Gaoxiong Yi Xue Ke Xue Za Zhi 5:12–16. (In Chinese)

Luplertlop N, Misse D, Bray D, Deleuze V, Gonzalez JP, Leardkamolkarn V, Yssel H, Veas F. 2006. Dengue-virus-infected dendritic cells trigger vascular leakage through metalloproteinase overproduction. EMBO Rep 7:1176–81.

Martone WJ, Kaufmann AF. 1979. Leptospirosis in humans in the United States, 1974–1978. J Infect Dis 140:1020–22.

Mikesell P, Ivins BE, Ristroph JD, Dreier TM. 1983. Evidence for plasmid-mediated toxin production in bacillus anthracis. Infect Immun 39:371–6.

Moron CG, Popov VL, Feng HM, Wear D, Walker DH. 2001. Identification of the target cells of Orientia Tsutsugamushi in human cases of scrub typhus. Mod Pathol 14:752–9.

Myint KS, Gibbons RV, Murray CK, Rungsimanphaiboon K, Supornpun W, Sithiprasasna R, Gray MR, Pimgate C, Mammen MP Jr., Hospenthal DR. 2007. Leptospirosis in Kamphaeng Phet, Thailand. Am J Trop Med Hyg 76:135–8.

Paddock CD, Childs JE. 2003. Ehrlichia Chaffeensis: a prototypical emerging pathogen. Clin Microbiol Rev 16:37–64.

Pang T, Wong PY, Pathmanathan R. 1982. Induction and characterization of delayed-type hypersensitivity to dengue virus in mice. J Infect Dis 146:235–42.

Perry RD, Fetherston JD. 1997. Yersinia pestis—etiologic agent of plague. Clin Microbiol Rev 10:35–66.

Prince LK, Shah AA, Martinez LJ, Moran KA. 2007. Ehrlichiosis: making the diagnosis in the acute setting. South Med J 100:825–8.

Rosen L, Drouet MT, Deubel V. 1999. Detection of dengue virus RNA by reverse transcription-polymerase chain reaction in the liver and lymphoid Organs but not in the brain in fatal human infection. Am J Trop Med Hyg 61:720–4.

Ruckdeschel K, Roggenkamp A, Lafont V, Mangeat P, Heesemann J, Rouot B. 1997. Interaction of Yersinia enterocolitica with macrophages leads to macrophage cell death through apoptosis. Infect Immun 65:4813–21.

Sebbane F, Lemaitre N, Sturdevant DE, Rebeil R, Virtaneva K, Porcella SF, Hinnebusch BJ. 2006. Adaptive response of Yersinia pestis to extracellular effectors of innate immunity during bubonic plague. Proc Natl Acad Sci USA 103:11766–71.

Sing A, Rost D, Tvardovskaia N, Roggenkamp A, Wiedemann A, Kirschning CJ, Aepfelbacher M, Heesemann J. 2002. Yersinia V-antigen exploits toll-like receptor 2 and CD14 for interleukin 10-mediated immunosuppression. J Exp Med 196:1017–24.

Steele KE, Anderson AO, Mohamadzadeh M. 2009. Fibroblastic reticular cell infection by hemorrhagic fever viruses. Immunotherapy 1:187–97.

Tamura A, Ohashi N, Urakami H, Miyamura S. 1995. Classification of rickettsia Tsutsugamushi in a new genus, Orientia Gen. Nov., as Orientia Tsutsugamushi Comb. Nov. Int J Syst Bacteriol 45:589–91.

Tatti KM, Greer P, White E, Shieh WJ, Guarner J, Ferebee-Harris T, Bartlett J, Ashford D, Hoffmaster A, Gallucci G, Vafai A, Popovic T, Zaki Sr. 2006. Morphologic, immunologic, and molecular methods to detect Bacillus anthracis in formalin-fixed tissues. Appl Immunohistochem Mol Morphol 14:234–43.

Taylor LH, Latham SM, Woolhouse ME. 2001. Risk factors for human disease emergence. Philos Trans R Soc Lond B Biol Sci 356:983–9.

Tekin A, Bulut N, Unal T. 1997. Acute abdomen due to anthrax. Br J Surg 84:813.

Temte JL, Zinkel AR. 2004. The primary care differential diagnosis of inhalational anthrax. An Fam Med 2:438–44.

Tseng BY, Yang HH, Liou JH, Chen LK, Hsu YH. 2008. Immunohistochemical study of scrub typhus: a report of two cases. Kaohsiung J Med Sci 24:92–8.

ung-Khin M, Ma-Ma K, Thant Z. 1975. Changes in the tissues of the immune system in dengue haemorrhagic fever. J Trop Med Hyg 78:256–61.

Van Ness GB 1971. Ecology of anthrax. Science 172:1303–7.

Vaughn DW, Green S, Kalayanarooj S, Innis BL, Nimmannitya S, Suntayakorn S, Endy TP, Raengsakulrach B, Rothman AL, Ennis FA, Nisalak A. 2000. Dengue viremia titer, antibody response pattern, and virus serotype correlate with disease severity. J Infect Dis 181:2–9.

Vijayachari P, Sehgal SC. 2006. Recent advances in the laboratory diagnosis of leptospirosis and characterisation of leptospires. Indian J Med Microbiol 24:320–2.

Villanueva SYAM, Ezoe H, Baterna RA, Yanagihara Y, Muto M, Koizumi N, Fukui T, Okamoto Y, Masuzawa T, Cavinta LL, Gloriani NG, Yoshida Si. 2010. Serologic and molecular studies of leptospira and leptospirosis among rats in the Philippines. Am J Trop Med Hyg 82:889–98.

Walker DH 1989. Rickettsioses of the spotted fever group around the world. J Dermatol 16:169–77.

Walker DH 1995. Rocky Mountain spotted fever: a seasonal alert. Clin Infect Dis 20:1111–7.

Walker DH, McCormick JB, Johnson KM, Webb PA, Komba-Kono G, Elliott LH, Gardner JJ. 1982. Pathologic and virologic study of fatal lassa fever in man. Am J Pathol 107:349–56.

Walker DH, Valbuena GA, Olano JP. 2003. Pathogenic mechanisms of diseases caused by rickettsia. An NY Acad Sci 990:1–11.

Wills BA, Oragui EE, Dung NM, Loan HT, Chau NV, Farrar JJ, Levin M. 2004. Size and charge characteristics of the protein leak in dengue shock syndrome. J Infect Dis 190:810–8.

Winn WC Jr., Walker DH. 1975. The pathology of human lassa fever. Bull WHO 52:535–45.

PART IV

NON-NEOPLASTIC FINDINGS IN BONE MARROW TRANSPLANTATION

CHAPTER TWENTY-THREE

NON-NEOPLASTIC HEMATOPATHOLOGY OF BONE MARROW TRANSPLANT AND INFECTIONS

Taiga Nishihori and Ernesto Ayala

INTRODUCTION

Hematopoietic cell transplantation (HCT) has the potential to cure a variety of benign and hematologic diseases that are incurable with conventional therapy (Fischer et al., 1994; Gooley et al., 2010; Appelbaum, 2003). Among these are acute leukemia, myelodsyplastic syndrome, multiple myeloma, malignant lymphomas, myelofibrosis, aplastic anemia, hemoglobinopathies, congenital immunodeficiencies, and certain solid tumors (Table 23.1). Although some of these conditions can be controlled or even cured with novel chemotherapeutic agents or molecularly targeted therapy, in patients with high-risk diseases or relapsed/refractory disease, an HCT will significantly improve the chances of survival. Dynamic and dramatic changes in the hematologic and immunologic systems during HCT occur and are commonly appreciated in the morphologic review of the bone marrow biopsy.

In this chapter we review the basic principles of HCT, histopathological features seen in the bone marrow during HCT at different stages, including regeneration of hematopoiesis, and associated infectious complications. It is important for pathologists involved in interpretation of post-transplantation bone marrow biopsies to be familiar with normal or abnormal post-transplant hematologic reconstitution processes.

FUNDAMENTAL PRINCIPLES OF HEMATOPOIETIC CELL TRANSPLANTATION (HCT)

In its broadest form, HCT consists of three parts: a conditioning phase, stem cell infusion, and engraftment. HCT can be performed using autologous (patient's own stem cells), syngeneic (from a human leukocyte antigen (HLA)-identical twin), or allogeneic stem cells (from an HLA-identical sibling or matched unrelated donor) (Barker and Wagner, 2002; Grewal et al., 2003). The sources of stem cells include bone marrow, peripheral blood, and umbilical cord blood. Either the patient or the donor is pretreated with cytokines

Non-Neoplastic Hematopathology and Infections, First Edition. Edited by Hernani D. Cualing, Parul Bhargava, and Ramon L. Sandin.
© 2012 Wiley-Blackwell. Published 2012 by John Wiley & Sons, Inc.

TABLE 23.1 **General Indications for Hematopoietic Cell Transplantation (HCT)**

Type of Conditions	Diseases
Bone marrow failure	Aplastic anemia
	Amegakaryocytic/congenital thrombocytopenia
	Fanconi anemia
	Paroxysmal nocturnal hemoglobinuria (PNH)
Hematologic malignancy	Acute leukemias
	Chronic leukemias
	Myelodysplastic syndromes
	Meyloproliferative disorders
	Non-Hodgkin lymphomas
	Plasma cell dyscrasias
	Histiocytic disorders
Solid tumors	Breast cancer (historic)
	Renal cell carcinoma
	Neuroblastoma
	Ewing sarcoma
	Testicular cancers
Congenital immunodeficiency	Severe combined immunodeficiency (SCID)
	Chronic granulomatous disease
Hemoglobinopathies	Beta-thalassemia major
	Sickle cell disease
Inherited metabolic disorders	Mucopolysaccharidoses
	Hurler's syndrome
	Hunter's syndrome
	Niemann–Pick disease
	Mucolipidosis II
Other inherited disorders	Osteopetrosis
	Glanzmann thromboasthenia
	Lesch–Nyhan syndrome
	Cartilage-hair hypoplasia

Source: Riley et al., (2005).

including granulocyte-colony stimulating factor (G-CSF) for stem cell mobilization to increase the amount of stem cells. Stem cells are collected either from peripheral blood or bone marrow of a suitable donor. For autologous or allogeneic peripheral blood stem cell collection, a leukapheresis machine is used to collect the stem cells. The hematopoietic stem cell can be frozen and stored for a long time before its use. Potential graft manipulation procedures include ex vivo purging to decrease tumor burden (negative selection), CD34 positive selection, and T-cell depletion (TCD). TCD of the allograft reduces the risks of graft-versus-host disease (GVHD) significantly; however, it may be hampered by the increased incidence of graft failure and disease relapse.

Recently peripheral blood stem cells have been used more frequently, although marrow harvesting is still being performed (Figure 23.1A, B). Bone marrow harvesting is performed by multiple aspirations from the posterior iliac crest over approximately 1 hour while the donor is under general or spinal anesthesia. Approximately 10 to 40×10^9 nucleated cells (2×10^8/kg of recipient body weight), up to a maximum of 20 mL/kg of donor body weight, are obtained during this procedure. The marrow aspirate primarily consists of stromal cells and erythroid, myloid, monocytic, megakaryocytic, and lymphoid cell lines in various stages of development. However, undifferentiated stem cells are essential for long-term hematopoiesis for the recipient, while the early committed progenitors provide the earliest peripheral blood cells after engraftment in the allogeneic setting. Particulate material in the marrow will be removed by filtration.

During the conditioning phase, the patient is given intensive chemotherapy and/or total body irradiation to eliminate residual malignancy and suppress the patient's immune system to prevent graft rejection. In autologous transplantation, the curative potential of this therapy comes from the high intensity of the conditioning regimen. In allogeneic transplantation, conditioning regimens can vary considerably in intensity, ranging from high-dose (i.e., myeloablative) regimens that result in complete ablation of the patient's bone marrow to reduced intensity conditioning (RIC) regimens that cause only mild myelosuppression. With the advent of RIC regimens, HCT has been expanded in elderly populations with manageable toxicity (Devine et al., 2002; Ditschkowski et al., 2004; Hessling et al., 2002; Rondelli et al., 2005; McClune et al., 2010). Even though RIC regimens have lesser intensity, they exert a significant impact on hematopoietic cells, bone marrow stromal cells, and the extent of chimerism post-transplant (Elmaagacli et al., 2001). On day 0 (zero), the stem cells are infused into the venous system of the patient to replace patient's hematopoietic and immune system (Figure 23.2).

In the case of allogeneic HCT for hematologic malignancies, the primary goals is to allow engraftment and the subsequent development of a donor-derived immune system, which can effect an immunologic attack against the recipient's lymphohematopoietic system, and in particular against tumor cells. This graft-versus-tumor (GVT) effect is a fundamental and unique aspect of allogeneic HCT. However, because the transplant is performed crossing immunologic barriers, allogeneic transplantation can result in significantly higher transplant-related morbidity and mortality, primarily due to GVHD and infections, compared with

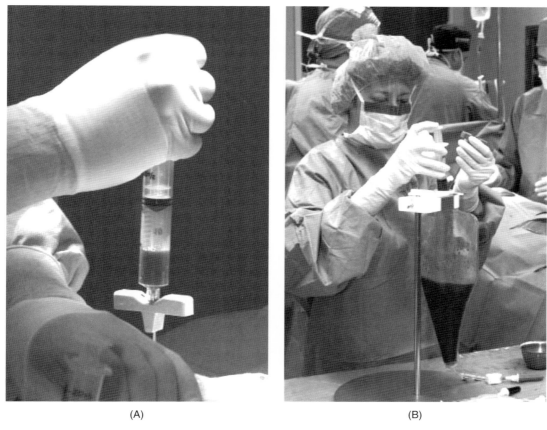

(A)   (B)

FIGURE 23.1   Bone marrow harvest procedure. (**A**) Bone marrow aspiration from the posterior superior iliac spine with a 30 ml syringe. (**B**) Freshly isolated bone marrow will be filtered to remove particulate matter. (Riley et al., 2005)

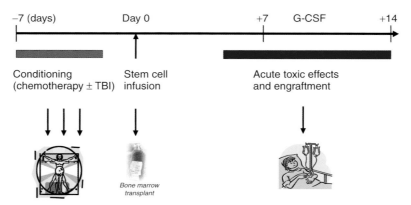

FIGURE 23.2   Schema of HCT conditioning and stem cell Infusion. Abbreviations: HCT: Hematopoietic cell transplantation; G-CSF: Granulocyte-colony stimulating factor (*optional); TBI: Total body irradiation.

autologous or syngeneic transplantation (Gooley et al., 2010). GVHD prophylaxis can be achieved through immunosuppressive medications or graft manipulation (in particular T-cell depletion). The choice of conditioning regimen, stem cell source, and GVHD prophylaxis regimens varies on the basis of

patient and disease characteristics as well as donor availability.

Neutrophil engraftment is defined as the first day the absolute neutrophils count (ANC) is greater than or equal to $500/\mu l$ for 3 consecutive days after transplant. Platelet engraftment is defined as the first day the platelet count is greater than or equal to 20,000/μl for 7 consecutive days independent of transfusions after transplant. Engraftment is usually considered successful (not delayed) if the time to recovery of either neutrophil or platelet achieves the pre-defined time period. For example, if ANC $\geq$ 500/μl is achieved at or prior to 14 days post transplant, then the neutrophil engraftment is successful in the case of autologous HCT.

During the engraftment phase, HCT recipients are profoundly immunocompromised and pancytopenic. Recent significant improvement in the survival of HCT procedures with decreased transplant-related mortality have primarily resulted from advances in supportive care during this period (Gooley et al., 2010). Patients may require red blood cells and platelet transfusion support, together with a protective environment, nutritional support, and prophylactic antimicrobials for bacterial, viral, and fungal infections. To prevent transfusion-acquired GVHD and viral infection, blood products are irradiated and leuko-depleted prior to transfusion. Recipients of allogeneic HCT may have a poor immune function for months to years due to delayed immune reconstitution and GVHD. Monitoring of cytomegalovirus (CMV) and Epstein–Barr virus (EBV) reactivation is performed routinely.

CHARACTERISTICS OF PRETRANSPLANT BONE MARROW

Extensive prior treatments before transplant induce numerous changes in the bone marrow involving hematopoiesis, stromal cells, and interstitial fibrous matrix. These changes are closely related to the underlying lymphoid or myeloid malignancy and a number of other conditions (Rousselet et al., 1996; van den Berg et al., 1990).

A significant reduction of the hematopoiesis is often encountered before the transplant. If it is accompanied by fibrosis, this may indicate an advanced stage of the primary disease. This change may herald impairment in engraftment after transplantation resulting in an unfavorable recovery (i.e., possible prolonged transfusion dependency), especially in patients with underlying myeloproliferative disorders (Thiele et al., 2001(b, c)). Diseases most commonly associated with bone marrow fibrosis include myelodysplastic syndromes, myelofibrosis, chronic myelogenous leukemia (CML), and some acute leukemias. Increased mast cells in the pretransplant marrow have been reported to be associated

with an increased risk of graft failure in patients with aplastic anemia.

Presence of normal cellularity, with normal hematopoietic cell lineage maturations, except slight dysmegakryopoiesis and a reticulin fiber density not exceeding grade II, usually indicates normal engraftment post-transplantation even in patients with preceding idiopathic myelofibrosis (Thiele et al., 2001c; Ni et al., 2005; Daly et al., 2003; Deeg et al., 2003).

In patients with delayed engraftment after transplantation, the pretransplant bone marrow may show little to marked fibrosis, even with reticulin fibrosis grade III/IV and hypocellularity with a patchy aplastic bone marrow, accompanied by dysmegakaryopoiesis and dyserythropoiesis. Therefore an acellular or hypocellular bone marrow and a high degree of reticulin-collagen fibrosis are risks factors for delayed engraftment or graft failure after transplantation (Rousselet et al., 1996; van den Berg et al., 1990; Thiele et al., 2001c; Rajantie et al., 1986; Annaloro et al., 2000; Thiele et al., 2000a).

HEMATOPOIETIC REGENERATION

The speed and quality of post-transplantation hematopoietic regeneration may be variable and generally depend on the underlying marrow disorder, the type of conditioning regimen, and the graft source. In general, bone marrow reconstitution is faster when a nonmyeloablative, or RIC regimen is applied compared to myeloablative strategies, where severe immunosuppression, slower hematopoietic recovery, and long-lasting pancytopenia are seen. If peripheral blood stem cells are used as a graft source, this results in faster hematopoietic recovery than bone marrow grafts (Trenschel et al., 1998; Ottinger et al., 1996). Age also plays an important role. Younger recipients tend to have a faster recovery than older patients or patients with long-standing and advanced stages of disease (Tabata et al., 2005; Eapen et al., 2004; Berkahn and Keating, 2004; Schmitz et al., 2002).

The regenerative capacity of the marrow post-transplantation does not appear to be related to the donor–recipient relationship, degree of HLA matching, or GVHD prophylaxis (Domenech et al., 1997; Chilton et al., 2001; Appleman et al., 2002; Quesenberry et al., 2001). The number of pluripotent stem cells in the graft remains the most important factor in the engraftment kinetics and hematopoietic recovery (Messner, 1998; Quesenberry et al., 2003). A subtype of pluripotent stem cell population, $CD34^+$ progenitor cells, is not only a precursor of hematopoiesis but also appears to be important in producing endothelial cells (Asahara et al., 1997; Gehling et al., 2000; Shi et al., 1998; Choi et al.; 1998; Kvasnicka et al., 2003).

Fat cell regeneration provides the first morphologic evidence of bone marrow regeneration, followed by minute clusters of immature, monotypic hematopoietic cells that gradually mature and enlarge. These colonies are comprised of cells of a single hematopoietic lineage, usually myeloid or erythroid, that presumably arise from committed progenitor cells in the HCT recipients (van den Berg et al., 1990). The regenerating colonies tend to be paratrabecular in patients receiving myeloablative therapy only and interstitial following HCT. Very early erythropoietic hematopoiesis is usually polyclonal but may be monoclonal. Early erythropoietic islands are usually dominated by large basophilic normoblasts that may exhibit dyserythropoietic features. As hematopoietic reconstitution continues, the myeloid precursors are abnormally localized in the intratrabecular areas and erythroid precursors occur near the endosteum (van den Berg et al., 1990). Megakaryocytes are normally the last to engraft. They are usually localized in the central part of the intertrabecular areas, and may appear in clusters, rather than in their normal scattered distribution.

CHIMERISM

Chimerism refers to the presence of donor lymphohematopoietic cells in a transplant recipient. After myeloablative conditioning, a full donor chimerism is commonly achieved early on (within the first 4 to 6 weeks) where all hematopoietic cells in the recipient are derived from the donor. Mixed chimerism is defined as the coexistence of both donor and recipient cells within a given cellular compartment. After an RIC regimen, a mixed donor chimerism is commonly seen, and it takes longer to convert to full donor chimerism. When a mixed donor chimerism is found after full donor chimerism is achieved, it may herald graft loss or disease relapse, which may result in reversion to autologous hematopoiesis (Kvasnicka et al., 2003; Román et al., 1998; Serrano et al., 2000; Tamura et al., 2000; Thiele et al., 2002b,c).

The sensitivity and accuracy of the techniques used to detect chimerism exert an important influence on interpretations of its clinical significance after HCT (Thiele et al., 2003b). Several methods have been reported for this purpose, including cytogenetic,

phenotypic, and molecular techniques (Elmaagacli et al., 2001; Quesenberry et al., 2001; Quesenberry et al., 2003; Ferrand et al., 2003; Antin et al., 2001). However, PCR-based methods are usually preferred because they are independent of gender mismatch, highly sensitive and require only minute amounts of biologic material. Post-transplantation donor/recipient chimerism is determined by the ratio of donor to recipient cells in a variety of subpopulation including bone marrow mononuclear cells, $CD33^+$ sorted and $CD3^+$ sorted peripheral blood mononuclear cells. Based on the guidelines published by the National Marrow Donor Program and the International Bone Marrow Transplant Registry, chimerism analysis should be undertaken using a sensitive technique (<1%) with short tandem repeat (STR) or variable number of tandem repeat (VNTR) analysis being the approach most likely to give reproducible data. Peripheral blood cells are generally more useful than bone marrow cells for chimerism analysis. Lineage-specific chimerism should be considered the assay of choice in the setting of myeloablative and reduced-intensity conditioning. In nonmyeloablative, T-cell depleted transplants, and novel graft-versus-host disease prophylactic regimens, chimerism analysis should be performed at 1, 3, 6, and 12 months because therapeutic interventions may depend on chimerism status. In nonmalignant disorders, chimerism testing should be performed at 1, 2, and 3 months as early patterns of chimerism may determine the need for more frequent testing and therapeutic intervention.

POST-TRANSPLANTATION MARROW

Rapid recovery of bone marrow microenvironment containing an intact stem cell niche is prerequisite for an undisturbed engraftment and regeneration of normal hematopoiesis following HCT. The following phases of hematopoietic reconstitution during the early and last post-transplantation period have been recognized and are described in chronological order (Table 23.2).

First Week after Transplant

In the first few days after HCT, bone marrow biopsies or sampling are almost never performed unless used in a research setting or autopsy. There is a relative lack of knowledge of morphologic examination of early hematopoiesis from a systematic clinical research perspective. However, several reports

TABLE 23.2 Histopathologic Features of Hematopoietic Cell Transplantation (HCT)

Time Period	Histopathologic Features
First week	Cell death and necrosis
	Fibrinoid necrosis with homogenous, PAS+ proteinaceous transudate
	Hemosiderin-laden macrophages
	Edema and focal hemorrhage
	Vascular congestion and sinus ectasia
	Transient reticulin fibrosis
	Small noncaseating granulomas
	Osteocyte necrosis
	Adipocyte proliferation
Second week	Small foci of immature hematopoietic cells
	Frequent hemosiderin-laden macrophages
Third week–first month	Expansion of hematopoietic islands with myeloid and erythroid maturation
	Improvement of fibrosis and fibrinoid necrosis
	Megakaryocyte regeneration

Source: Riley et al. (2005).
Abbreviation: PAS: Periodic acid Schiff.

indicate conspicuous decreases in cellularity, with extensive cell necrosis associated with marked edema and expansion of the adipose tissue or even so-called scleroedema, creating a morphologic condition that is very difficult for microscopic examination of cellular elements and resembling features commonly encountered in radiation and/or drug-induced aplasia (severe toxic myelopathy) (Thiele et al., 2003a). Initially, a slight decrease in reticulin fibrosis may be observed (Thiele et al., 2005; Ni et al., 2005). Adhesion of engraftable hematopoietic CD34$^+$ progenitors to stromal cells within 1 hour of contact has been demonstrated in in vitro studies; however, the timing of cell infusion after appropriate conditioning regimen is of paramount importance (Frimberger et al., 2001; Xu et al., 2004; Madhusudhan et al., 2003; Hardy and Megason, 1996; Whetton and Graham, 1999).

Angiogenesis remains one of the most important factors for the reconstitution of normal hematopoiesis. Survival of a considerable number of recipient endothelial cells even after myeloablative conditioning suggests a persistence of host-derived stromal vascularization, followed by significant disturbances of vascular architecture (Kvasnicka and Thiele, 2004). The differentiation of endothelial cells from hemangioblasts is also implied, resulting in a formation of vascular plexus. Furthermore the engrafted CD34$^+$ progenitors appear to act as precursors for both hematopoietic and endothelial cells, generating a mixed chimeric state after transplantation (Schuh et al., 1999; Shalaby et al., 1995; Lacaud et al., 2001; Asahara et al., 1997). A close functional association is detectable between endothelial and progenitor cells with regard to cell trafficking, expansion, and homing (Möhle et al., 1997, 1999; Rafii et al., 1995).

The distribution of engrafted cells does not occur at random. In the first few hours of engraftment, the donor progenitor cells are evenly distributed in the highly vascularized central regions of the bone marrow and are located adjacent to the endosteal (paratrabecular) borders. In the subsequent hours, the number of donor progenitor cells in the endosteal region decreases and the proportion of cells located in the central regions increases (Nilsson et al., 2001; Thiele et al., 2000a). The distribution of these progenitor cells can be visualized by CD34 immunostaining, and they can be differentiated from endothelial cells by the histologic characteristics (histotopography) (Soligo et al., 1991; Thiele et al., 2002a).

Toward the end of the first week, the bone marrow changes become more evident. A proteinaceous interstitial or stromal edema will be seen. Stroma may contain a homogeneous, periodic acid-Schiff (PAS)-positive proteinaceous transudate resembling fibrinoid necrosis. Small erythroid precursor islands with centrally located macrophages are seen between the stromal edema and fatty tissue (Rousselet et al., 1996; van den Berg et al., 1990). There is a significant correlation between the number of erythroid precursors and the number of macrophages containing cell debris and iron (Thiele et al., 2000b, c).

Macrophages constitute an integral part of the bone marrow microenvironment, responding to fat cell necrosis and playing a major role in the regulation and differentiation of progenitor cells (Rich, 1986; Hanspal, 1997; Wang et al., 1992; Vogt et al., 1989). The CD68$^+$ macrophages also contribute to the generation of erythroblastic islets and mediate the complex mechanism of erythrocyte maturation (Thiele et al., 2000b, c). Regeneration of erythropoiesis in the first several days of transplant may present with marked megaloblastic features accompanied by nuclear abnormalities signaling a maturation arrest, due in part to the toxicity of chemotherapy on DNA synthesis, and can be detected with glycophorin C immunostaining (Gatter et al., 1988). Regenerating erythropoietic islets are located mainly between the fat cells, which provide the microenvironment for erythroid recovery. Isolated megakaryocytes with dysplastic features, granular eosinophilic exudate, and multiloculated fat cells can all be seen during this period.

Second Week after Transplant

Along with the continuous recovery of erythropoietic islets and frequent transfusions required in the transplant, hemoglobin and hematocrit values usually improve over time after transplant. Megaloblastic features on regenerating erythroid precursors are commonly seen. These changes can be accompanied by nuclear contour abnormalities. Regeneration of megakaryopoiesis also ensues (Thiele et al., 2001b). At the beginning of the second week from the transplant, a few colonies of myeloid precursors can be observed around the bony trabeculae (Figure 23.3). There will be an approximately 40 to 50% decrease in the numbers of macrophages found after the second week from the transplant. This change is presumably associated with the degradation of cells and debris after conditioning therapy (scavenger function). Bone marrow in patients with delayed engraftment may demonstrate clusters of large macrophages (Thiele et al., 2000c). A slight increase in inflammatory infiltrates consisting of lymphocytes, mast cells, and plasma cells with perivascular localization can be seen as a reactive change or toxic myelopathy from chemotherapy (Krech and Thiele, 1985; Frisch et al., 1986; Rigolin et al., 1998). The integrity of the stromal cells plays a key role in providing functional microenvironment for marrow regeneration or engraftment. After initial decline, a mild transient increase in the reticulin fibers is seen and is thought to represent a normal recovery of damaged marrow microenvironment, providing adhesion properties that are essential for stem cell homing (Simmons et al., 1992; Liesveld et al., 1991).

Third Week after Transplant

From the third week on, mixed erythroid and myeloid colonies are seen. The amount of lymphoid cells is still low. There is clear rise in the reticulin fibrosis in nearly all patients with preexistent marrow fibrosis as well as in some patients without underlying fibrosis. This transient phenomenon is in contrast to the significant improvement and resolution of fibronecrosis observed at a later time in responding patients with idiopathic myelofibrosis after transplantation (Deeg et al., 2003; Daly et al., 2003; Thiele et al., 2005).

Interestingly there is a correlation between the development of acute GVHD and the number of CD45RO[+] lymphocytes in the bone marrow (Thiele et al., 2001d). In chronic myeloid leukemia, severe

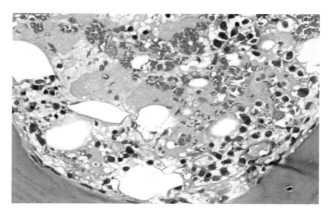

FIGURE 23.3 **Second week after transplant.** A bone marrow biopsy 14 days after hematopoietic cell transplantation clearly depicts sparse regenerating myeloid precursors in paratrabecular location with overall decreased cellularity. (Courtesy of Hernani Cualing, MD, Hematopathologist, USF)

acute GVHD also correlates with increased reticulin fibrosis in the early posttransplant period as well as a delay in achieving transfusion independence (Thiele et al., 2000a). Scattered megakaryocytic regeneration occurs with some dysplastic changes (Thiele et al., 2001b). Normalization of megakaryocyte size and histologic appearance are the hallmarks of successful engraftment. CD61 immunostaining helps identify smaller counterparts of megakaryocytes, including precursor cells (Gatter et al., 1988). The reconstitution of lymphoid cells, especially T cells, begins. Although the absolute lymphocyte counts in the peripheral blood remains low, there has been no significant correlation with the total marrow lymphocyte content. The total lymphocyte numbers in the marrow is estimated to be between 5 and 20 cells per mm^2 (Horny et al., 1993; Thaler et al., 1989).

First Month after Transplant

The time course of the progression from early hematopoiesis to normal marrow cellularity for recipient age is extremely variable; some patients may achieve normal cellularity in as early as 14 days (van den Berg et al., 1990). In peripheral blood transplant, many bone marrow samples may show at least 50% of pretransplant cellularity with conspicuous regeneration of erythropoiesis and neutrophil granulopoiesis occasionally forming loose clusters and sheets approximately 3 weeks after transplantation (Figure 23.4). After the first month of transplant, the number of lymphoid cells may start to increase, depending on the conditioning and GVHD prophylaxis regimens. When GVHD occurs,

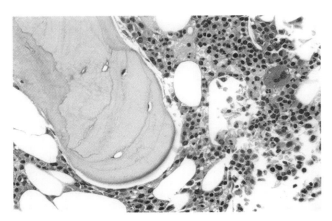

FIGURE 23.4 **One month after transplant**. A bone marrow biopsy performed at day 28 post-transplant shows cellular marrow with abundant regenerating erythroid and myeloid precursors. (Courtesy of Hernani Cualing, MD, Hematopathologist, USF)

subsets of lymphocytes may be increased, especially of CD45RO$^+$ subtype, however, the number of regulatory T cells may be lower (Thiele et al., 2001d).

The kinetics of engraftment depend on the source of donor cell, the dose of infused CD34$^+$ cells, the type and dose of exogenous hematopoietic growth factors, and HLA cross-matching (Keever-Taylor et al., 2001). The rate of marrow recovery is affected by the homing efficiency and clonogenic potential of the transplanted cells. The hematopoietic regeneration may be slower in patients receiving bone marrow grafts and especially umbilical cord blood grafts. In patients receiving double umbilical cord blood transplantations, examination of bone marrow cellularity and chimerism analysis are performed on day +21 and depending on the absolute neutrophil counts and cellularity, the dose of growth factor (e.g., G-CSF) may be increased to facilitate the engraftment. In peripheral blood graft, bone marrow assessment including chimerism analysis is usually performed on day +30.

The effects of hematopoietic growth factors are particularly evident in reconstituting bone marrow and peripheral blood and must be differentiated from other causes. In the peripheral blood, these agents cause an increase in the total white blood cell count and the absolute number of neutrophils, monocytes, and eosinophils. Their effects on the bone marrow include eosinophilic hyperplasia and increases in cellularity and the myeloid:erythroid (M:E) ratio. In addition prominently granulated and/or vacuolated neutrophils and neutrophilic precursors may appear in both the peripheral blood and bone marrow (Ryder et al., 1992).

Second Month after Transplant

In uncomplicated cases, bone marrow cellularity may be close to normal after more than a month from the transplant (Thiele et al., 2001a) (Figure 23.5). The quantity of lymphocytes is likely comparable to that of a normal bone marrow, in contrast to the depression of the amount of lymphocytes in the peripheral blood (Thiele et al., 2001d). Focal necrosis of the bone associated with reactive bone formation may be seen; the newly formed bone will usually disappear within a few months. Particularly in children with acute lymphoblastic leukemia, a vascular type osteonecrosis has been described (Enright et al., 1990).

Beyond Third Month after Transplant

After 3 months from the time of transplant, normal numbers of T and B lymphocytes may be seen in the bone marrow and peripheral blood. However, the qualitative and functional recovery of lymphocytes still remains suboptimal due to various factors including ongoing immunosuppressive therapy, resulting in impaired immune reconstitution (Verma and Mazumder, 1993). There appears to be no clear association between the lymphocyte repopulation in the peripheral blood and the engraftment status in the bone marrow. In patients with underlying myelofibrosis and gross fibro-osteosclerotic changes, a total regression and normalization of the pretransplant increased reticulin fibrosis was seen after approximately 6 months based on the serial bone marrow biopsy examinations (Rondelli et al., 2005; Thiele et al., 2000c; Deeg et al., 2003). The number of endothelial

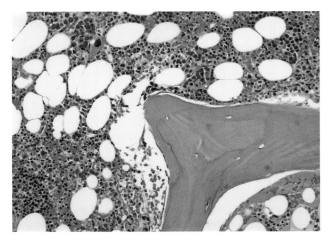

FIGURE 23.5 **Second month after transplant**. A bone marrow biopsy obtained on day 35 after transplant demonstrates close to normal cellular marrow indicating an uncomplicated recovery process of the marrow. (Courtesy of Hernani Cualing, MD, Hematopathologist, USF)

cells may play an important role as evidenced by decreased microvessel density in the bone marrow after transplantation. The CD34$^+$ endothelial cells in the bone marrow could have both a recipient and donor origin; they show mixed chimerism even after the third month after transplantation, with donor-derived elements comprising 18 to 25%. When the disease recurs, there will be almost complete reversal of the endothelial cell chimerism to a recipient (i.e., host) type, indicating a CD34$^+$ progenitor cell origin of the endothelial cells (Kvasnicka et al., 2003; Thiele et al., 2002b).

COMPLICATIONS OF HEMATOPOIETIC REGENERATION

There are a variety of complications known to occur in the post-transplantation bone marrow, and we will describe salient features of these characteristic bone marrow histopathology.

Dyshematopoiesis

Significant disordered hematopoiesis, particularly dysmegakaryopoiesis, can be seen in the first few months after transplantation. These cells show conspicuous cytoplasmic and nuclear abnormalities primarily due to the effect on DNA synthesis from conditioning regimen. One should be cautious in making a new diagnosis of myelodsyplasia in the early post-transplant period, however, therapy-related myelodysplasia and acute leukemia is a form of secondary leukemia following high-dose chemotherapy and should be recognized as a long-term complication of autologous HCT.

Hypocellular or Acellular Marrow

A hypocellular or even acellular marrow can be observed with conspicuous scleroedema and adipocytes in cases where engraftment failure is a diagnostic consideration. Many factors may cause either primary or secondary engraftment failure. Primary engraftment failure is due generally to genetic differences between the donor and recipient, damaged stem cells or an insufficient numbers of stem cells, inadequate immunosuppression or pretreatment conditioning, alloimmunization due to previous multiple blood transfusions, excessive T-cell depletion of the graft, an abnormal recipient bone marrow microenvironment, an abnormal donor graft, drug toxicity, or viral infections (Anasetti et al., 1989). Failure of the graft after initial engraftment,

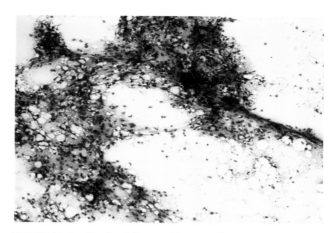

FIGURE 23.6 **Graft failure.** Biopsy shows a markedly hypocellular bone marrow aspirate with few hematopoietic cells. (From ASH Image Bank)

that is, secondary engraftment failure, occurs as a result of drug toxicity, infections, fibrosis, or cell-mediated immune reactions.

Morphologically, bone marrow aspirate smears from patients with engraftment failure are typically markedly hypocellular (Figure 23.6), with a predominance of stromal cells, while core biopsies and clot sections often show diffuse histiocytic proliferation (Rosenthal and Farhi, 1994). Of note, this may not be the case in patients treated for nonmalignant conditions such as thalassemia, sickle cell disease, or immunodeficiency. In those patients engraftment failure is diagnosed by reappearance of the primary disease morphology and loss of donor chimerism markers. In patients who received suboptimal quantity and quality of progenitor cells, hypocellular bone marrow may be seen in the post-transplant period.

Pure Red Cell Aplasia

Currently allogeneic transplantation can be safely performed overcoming the previously perceived barriers of ABO blood type incompatibility. ABO incompatibility is defined as major when the recipient plasma contains isohemagglutinis against donor red blood cell (RBC) antigens, it is an ABO minor mismatch if the donor has isohemagglutinins directed against recipient RBC antigens, and it is bidirectional if both features are present. The time of onset and duration of hemolysis are affected by the titer of iso-hemagglutinin and its rate of clearance, as well as the quantity of target antigen available. In a proportion of major ABO-incompatible HCT, the isohemagglutinin targets not just circulating RBCs but also early marrow precursors expressing the antigen at the level of the colony forming unit-erythroid, leading to pure red cell aplasia (PRCA) (Blacklock et al., 1984; Benjamin et al., 1998; Lee et al., 2000; Barge et al., 1989). The development of RIC regimens to transplant older patients or patients with comorbidities creates an environment of mixed donor and recipient hematopoiesis that persists for protracted periods of time; this has led to concerns for the possibility of higher rates of chronic hemolysis and PRCA (Slavin et al., 1998; McSweeney et al., 2001; Giralt et al., 1997). The reported incidence of PRCA following RIC regimens has varied widely from 6 to 50%, compared with rates of 5 to 16% post high-dose conditioning (Bolan et al., 2001). A study has suggested that recipient plasma cells which lasted longer than B cells were the source of the isohemagglutinin production (Griffith et al., 2005).

Following HCT, patients with ABO incompatibility should be monitored for the emergence of donor-derived erythrocytes, persistence of recipient isohemagglutinins, and evidence of hemolysis using lactate dehydrogenase, reticulocyte counts, and the direct agglutinin test. Patients with major ABO mismatches and high isohemagglunitin titer pre-HCT are particularly at risk for delay of RBC engraftment, hemolysis, and PRCA. Isohemagglutinin titers in recipients with major ABO mismatches should be monitored at least twice monthly until their disappearance. Patients with rising titers and increasing transfusion requirements merit marrow evaluation to exclude PRCA. Of note, iron overload is a potential deleterious condition for those patients who develop PRCA. In the majority of cases of PRCA, tapering of immunosuppression permits a "graft-versus-plasma or B-cell" effect that shuts off isohemagglutinin production by either memory B cells or plasma cells. Other strategies have employed pharmacologic doses of erythropoietin alone or combined with steroids (Taniguchi et al., 1993; Paltiel et al., 1993; Santamaría et al., 1997). In more refractory cases, plasma exchange or the use of rituximab has been successful; rarely, donor lymphocyte infusion has been used to promote full donor chimerism and to ablate isohemagglutinin production (Bavaro et al., 1999; Sorà et al., 2005; Verholen et al., 2004; Selleri et al., 1998). In situations where PRCA develops outside the setting of major ABO incompatibility, a change in calcineurin inhibitor from tacrolimus to cyclosporine, or discontinuation of mycophenolate mofetil, may produce red cell recovery.

Residual Neoplastic Marrow

The presence of the underlying malignant hematologic condition in the marrow may hinder the interpretation of post-transplantation marrow. Some patients may undergo transplantation with either active or minimal residual disease. In reduced-intensity, or nonmyeloablative transplant where graft-versus-tumor effect is the mainstay of anti-tumor activity rather than ablative conditioning therapy, persistence of neoplastic condition in the marrow after transplant is not an uncommon phenomenon. Particular caution should be exercised when recognizable tumor cells are seen in a biopsy specimen before raising the question of recurrent disease in the context of RIC condition regimen. The presence of tumor cells in the marrow during the first few weeks of transplantation can be regarded as residual, in general, unless the disease burden appears to be either similar or decreased in comparison to pretransplant marrow. Substantial residual infiltrate may be detected by morphologic assessment, immunohistochemistry, or flow cytometry. The common dilemma lies in the differentiation of leukemic blasts from normal regenerating myeloblasts, which is usually based on morphologic or characteristic flow cytometric assessment rather than immunohistochemistry where the burden of leukemic blasts may be overestimated. In cases where distinct genetic alterations specific for malignancy are clearly characterized, polymerase chain reaction or short tandem repeat microsatellite markers may be utilized to look for lineage-specific chimerism and minimal residual disease. With these techniques the reappearance or worsening of the known distinct genetic alterations heralds the disease relapse (Serrano et al., 2000; de Weger et al., 2000; Radich et al., 1995; Fehse et al., 2001; Sawyers et al., 1990; Lawler et al., 1991; Alizadeh et al., 2002; van Leeuwen et al., 1991).

Recurrent Disease

Residual disease in the marrow could be encountered in the early phase after transplant. For example, multiple myeloma cells could persist in the marrow for a considerable time before they start to disappear after transplantation. However, in general, an increase in the cells suggestive of the underlying disease is almost always associated with disease relapse. Of note, there is no significant association between delayed engraftment and disease recurrence.

Those residual and clonally transformed CD34+ endothelial cells and myeloblasts may be able to survive myeloablative conditioning and thus could be the potential source for a later relapse. Conversion of lineage-specific mixed chimerism in megakaryocytes might be due to the polyploidy status of these cells; however, abrupt changes from the donor to host type chimerisms in erythroid precursors, megakaryocytes, or CD34$^+$ progenitor cells may herald the recurrent disease. The changes from the donor to host origin in the mature endothelial cells are also seen in patients with evolution to recurrent hematologic malignancies. In the bone marrow macrophage population, leukemia relapse is associated with a lesser degree of host retrieval (Wickenhauser et al., 2002).

Graft-versus-Host Disease (GVHD)

There are no pathognomonic morphologic features of GVHD in the marrow. However, the proliferation of CD68$^+$ macrophages has accompanied acute and chronic GVHD, while bone marrow hypoplasia and myelofibrosis has been reported in chronic GVHD (Kazama et al., 1996; Atkinson et al., 1987). Long-term marrow cultures in patients with GVHD have shown decreased numbers of myeloid, erythroid, and multipotent progenitor cells, as well as reduced numbers of fibroblast colony-forming cells and adherent stromal cells, with the most severe deficiencies in patients with acute GVHD (Martínez-Jaramillo et al., 2001). B-cell precursors are also decreased in patients with chronic GVHD (Storek et al., 1996).

Granulomas and Infectious Disease in the Marrow

It may not be uncommon to encounter intercurrent disease in the bone marrow after HCT. The presence of granulomas in the early post-transplant marrow is one of the most commonly seen marrow conditions. Isolated granulomas could be considered to be therapy or transplant related and may persist for a longer period of time. If granuloma formation is extensive, granulomatous infectious diseases have to be considered as differential diagnoses. These interpretations should be cautiously made in the context of right clinical scenarios. In addition focal necrosis of the bone associated with reactive bone formation may be seen. The newly formed bones usually disappear within a few months. Aside from childhood acute lymphoblastic leukemia where osteonecrosis has been well described, bone changes do not seem to have significant clinical implications (Schulte and Beelen, 2005).

Even with effective prophylaxis and preemptive therapy, some patients may develop infectious diseases in the marrow due to extensive immunosuppressive therapies. Cultured stromal cells infected with Epstein–Barr virus failed to support hematopoiesis and cytomegalovirus (CMV) infection and can also affect stromal cells (Michelson et al., 2001; Mundle et al., 2001). The changes in the bone marrow seen during these viral infections are generally nonspecific and may be accompanied by

an increase in lymphoid cells or macrophages. When erythrophagocytosis is seen, one has to consider CMV infection or toxoplasmosis as a differential diagnosis (Saavedra et al., 2002).

Cytomegalovirus (CMV) Infection

Cytomegalovirus (CMV) infection has been a problem that has limited the success of allogeneic transplant since the era when HCT began (Meyers et al., 1982). The epidemiology of CMV infection in the HCT population is well described and has established that CMV infection can originate from both endogeneous and exogenous sources (Meyers, 1989). The curtailment of blood-borne CMV exposure, by cessation of routine granulocyte transfusion therapy after HCT and by the use of filtered blood product support, demonstrated that CMV can be transmitted in transfused blood cells to a susceptible recipient. However, the major effect on CMV epidemiology was the introduction of effective antiviral agents during the 1980s. The incidence of unmodified CMV infection and disease is best described by the control groups from the blinded studies that attempted to alter the occurrence of CMV complications after HCT. Thus the incidence of CMV infection in both CMV-seronegative donor (−) and CMV-seronegative recipient (−) HCT dropped from approximately 20% to nearly zero % with the introduction of CMV-seronegative blood support (Bowden et al., 1991). Pre-emptive antiviral treatment strategies dramatically reduced the early occurrence of CMV disease but moved disease onset to late times after HCT and altered the natural history of infection, leading to the development of late-onset disease (Boeckh et al., 2003).

Studies have demonstrated the ability to isolate infectious virus from peripheral blood mononuclear cells that were placed in long-term culture with allogeneic stimulation (Söderberg-Nauclér et al., 1997). The actual activation of the virus within the transplanted cells appear to be dependent on cellular activation signals (Söderberg-Nauclér et al., 1997), and such cellular activation might explain the peak period of CMV infection as the new graft becomes established 4 to 8 weeks post-HCT. It is possible that other cells of the blood can serve as a vehicle for transmission of CMV with transfusions, and CMV has been demonstrated in circulating endothelial cells after HCT (Salzberger et al., 1997).

CMV infection per se in HCT recipients is usually defined as the isolation of CMV in tissue culture or the identification of markers of CMV in tissue specimens or blood by histologic and histochemical means, by specific antigen staining, by direct CMV DNA/RNA or CMV antigen detection, or by a fourfold or higher rise in CMV antibody titer (Ljungman et al., 2002). Common CMV disease presentations include CMV-associated interstitial pneumonia, CMV enteritis, and CMV retinitis. Other CMV-associated organ-related syndromes, such as hepatitis and encephalitis, are defined as syndromes with specific organ dysfunction and the concomitant presence of active CMV infection. With the exception of CMV retinitis, the diagnosis of CMV disease cannot be made with confidence without histologic evidence of CMV infection in the involved organ.

Since at least two-thirds of all at-risk transplant recipients develop CMV infection, the accurate association of other syndromes with this infection can be difficult. Nevertheless, in addition to mononucleosis-like syndrome with fever, arthralgia, and malaise, both hepatitis and suppressed marrow function, including neutropenia and thrombocytopenia, have been associated with acute CMV infection (Boeckh et al., 1998). The course of asymptomatic CMV infection is not well described in the allogeneic HCT recipient, but it appears that febrile episodes are a significant part of the CMV infection. In order to understand the clinical effects of asymptomatic CMV infection, a series of consecutive patients with CMV infection during HCT were evaluated and found a significant association of fever between days 42 and 56 in those with otherwise asymptomatic infection (Zaia, 1990). There was no increased rate of neutropenia in this group. However, neutropenia is associated with CMV infection during the same time period (Meyers and Thomas, 1981). There has been a case of CMV-associated marrow suppression with response to therapy using a growth factor and an antiviral agent described (Boeckh et al., 1998). Of note, treatment of CMV infection can cause significant marrow toxicity. The major complications associated with ganciclovir treatment are neutropenia and creatinine elevation. Neutropenia occurs in approximately 30% of patients, and it lasts for a median of 12 days with an upper range of 74 days based on the published experience (Goodrich et al., 1993). The availability of antiviral agents has greatly altered the incidence and management of CMV disease after allogeneic HCT, and yet the control of CMV remains less than optimal because of the toxicity of available agents. Although becoming infrequent, careful evaluation of bone marrow with appropriate histologic examination for CMV is warranted in cases where CMV disease is suspected due to unexplained marrow suppression.

Epstein–Barr Virus (EBV) Infection

Although Epstein–Barr virus (EBV) infection is ubiquitous in all adult human populations (Rickinson and Kieff, 2007; Ambinder and Cesarman, 2007; Cohen, 2000), EBV-associated lymphoproliferative disorder (EBV-LPD) is an occasionally fatal complication of HCT. Its incidence is highly dependent on the specific approach to HCT. In some settings including T-cell depletion, the risk rises to over 25%. EBV infects B cells, establishes latency, and drives these cells to proliferate. The proliferation of latently infected B cells leads to expansion of the pool of latently infected cells. Although antigens are cleared with cellular immune response, viral DNA persists in a tiny percentage of resting memory B cells. EBV is consistently associated with endemic Burkitt's lymphoma, nasopharyngeal carcinoma, nasal-type NK/T-cell lymphoma, AIDS-related lymphoma, primary central nervous system lymphoma, and LPD in transplant recipients (Ambinder and Cesarman, 2007). There is also an association with Hodgkin lymphoma, with 30 to 50% of Hodgkin lymphoma in North America and western Europe harboring the virus.

LPD most commonly presents early after transplantation and as disseminated disease potentially involving bone marrow (Curtis et al., 1999). Fever, generalized lymphadenopathy, respiratory compromise, and rising liver transaminase levels are typical and have usually been associated with a rapidly progressive multiorgan failure and death. Lesions could be nodal and extranodal, frequently involving Waldeyer's ring, the gastrointestinal tract, the liver, and the central nervous system. Tumors that arise later after transplantation (>1 year) are more commonly localized and often have an indolent course. The definitive diagnosis of EBV-LPD requires biopsy with in situ hybridization or immunohistochemistry to define the viral association or flow cytometry (Ambinder and Cesarman, 2007). EBV-encoded RNA in situ hybridization is the most sensitive tool for detecting virus in tumor insofar as these small viral RNAs, which do not code for protein, are expressed in all EBV-associated tumors.

Four categories of post-transplant LPD are recognized in the World Health Organization classification: early lesions, polymorphic lesions, monomorphic lesions, and Hodgkin lymphoma. Early lesions are those of plasmacytic hyperplasia, which resembles infectious mononucleosis. Architecture is preserved and there is little or no cytologic atypia. Polymorphic lesions show loss of architecture (Figure 23.7). These lesions are heterogeneous in their cell population. Cells may or may not show plasmacytic differentiation. There is a spectrum of cytologic atypia. Detailed histologic description of these monomorphic LPDs (e.g., diffuse large B-cell lymphoma, Burkitt or

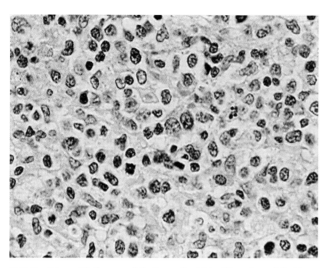

FIGURE 23.7 **Polymorphic lymphoid infiltration**. Medium magnification demonstrates polymorphic lymphoid infiltration of Epstein–Barr virus lymphoproliferative disease (EBV-LPD). (From ASH Image Bank)

Burkitt-like lymphoma, plasma cell myeloma, plasmacytoma, and some peripheral T-cell lymphoma) are beyond the scope of this chapter; however, it is suffice to say that the histologic characteristics of these monomorphic lesions are those seen in immunocompetent individuals. Whereas in solid-organ transplant recipients, EBV-LPD most commonly arises in host B cells, in allogeneic HCT recipient EBV-LPD usually arises in donor B lymphocytes.

A variety of treatments for LPD have been explored (Wagner et al., 2002). Recommended treatment for early EBV-LPD include rituximab, donor lymphocyte infusion or adaptive T-cell transfer of EBV-specific cytotoxic T cells from donor (if available), other sources of EBV-specific T cells, and standard lymphoma chemotherapy. Discontinuation of immunosuppression is sometimes associated with regression of EBV-LPD in solid-organ transplant recipients; however, it is very rarely effective in allogeneic HCT recipients. The use of antivirals, such as acyclovir, ganciclovir, and their congeners, has been advocated; however, there is little evidence to suggest therapeutic efficacy against EBV-LPD in those settings. These agents do not inhibit the proliferation of lymphocytes latently infected by EBV either in vitro or in vivo. The ready availability of rituximab and its lack of toxicity suggest that it should be considered appropriate as first-line therapy, or as a part of first-line regimen, in most instances of EBV-related B-cell LPD. It may also have a role as pre-emptive treatment in high-risk patients (Wagner et al., 2004; van Esser et al., 2002; Comoli et al., 2007).

Parvovirus B19 Infection

Parvoviruses are made of small, naked, single-stranded DNA. Approximately 60% of young adults demonstrate the evidence of past infection. It is most likely spread by respiratory transmission or by blood. Parvovirus B19 can infect erythroid progenitor cells. Parvovirus B19 is commonly associated with aplastic crisis in patients with hemolytic anemia. Immunity to parvovirus B19 is thought to be primarily humoral; neutralizing antibodies to capsid protein have a major role in host defense. IgM antibody detection may be useful in the diagnosis of acute infection in immunocompetent individuals. The reliability of serologic testing in HCT recipients is questionable.

Aplasia in conjunction with parvovirus 19 infection in both HCT and solid-organ transplantation has been reported (Geetha et al., 2000). In addition to transient marrow failure, parvovirus B19 can cause chronic anemia and, rarely, pancytopenia in HCT recipients (Azzi et al., 1993; Schleuning et al., 1999; Florea et al., 2007). Blood PCR is useful as a diagnostic tool (Schleuning et al., 1999). Intravenous immunoglobulin is effective in treating parvovirus B19 symptomatic infection (Kurtzman et al., 1989). Prophylactic intravenous immunoglobulin seems to have a protective effect against parvovirus B19, although this has not been established in a randomized study.

CONCLUSION

More than 25,000 allogeneic HCT procedures are currently performed annually. The number of HCTs is expected to increase due to the increasing use of HCTs in the elderly population, unrelated and mismatched donors, and peripheral blood stem cell and donor lymphocyte infusions. The indication of HCT has been also expanded to nonmalignant conditions and also to autoimmune disorders. Bone marrow examinations are usually scheduled at certain points after transplant; however, many bone marrow biopsies will be performed additionally if there are clinical signs of graft failure or disease relapse. These biopsies remain the most important tool for clinicians to obtain information regarding the hematopoietic status after HCT. Mixed chimerism is dynamic and striking phenomenon of reconstituting hematopoiesis after HCT and has been used in all cell lineages derived from the CD34$^+$ progenitor cells. There is a variety of bone marrow pathology described in the post HCT marrow, including complications from the transplant itself. In-depth knowledge regarding the underlying disease condition as well as characteristics of regenerating marrow are the prerequisite for informative reporting of bone marrow biopsies to help patients undergoing HCT and the challenging task for the pathologist.

REFERENCES

ALIZADEH M, BERNARD M, DANIC B, DAURIAC C, BIREBENT B, LAPART C, LAMY T, LE PRISÉ PY, BEAUPLET A, BORIES D, SEMANA G, QUELVENNEC E. 2002. Quantitative assessment of hematopoietic chimerism after bone marrow transplantation by real-time quantitative polymerase chain reaction. Blood, 99:4618–25.

AMBINDER R, CESARMAN E. 2007. Clinical and Pathological Aspects of EBV and KSHV Infection. Cambridge University Press, New York.

ANASETTI C, AMOS D, BEATTY PG, APPELBAUM FR, BENSINGER W, BUCKNER CD, CLIFT R, DONEY K, MARTIN PJ, MICKELSON E. 1989. Effect of HLA compatibility on engraftment of bone marrow transplants in patients with leukemia or lymphoma. N Engl J Med 320:197–204.

ANNALORO C, ORIANI A, POZZOLI E, DELILIERS DL, BERTOLLI VG, VOLPE AD, SOLIGO D, DELILIERS GL. 2000. Histological alterations in bone marrow in patients with late engraftment after autologous bone marrow transplantation. Bone Marrow Transplant, 25:837–41.

ANTIN JH, CHILDS R, FILIPOVICH AH, GIRALT S, MACKINNON S, SPITZER T, WEISDORF D. 2001. Establishment of complete and mixed donor chimerism after allogeneic lymphohematopoietic transplantation: recommendations from a workshop at the 2001 Tandem Meetings of the International Bone Marrow Transplant Registry and the American Society of Blood and Marrow Transplantation. Biol Blood Marrow Transplant 7:473–85.

APPELBAUM FR. 2003. The current status of hematopoietic cell transplantation. An Rev Med 54:491–512.

APPLEMAN LJ, TZACHANIS D, GRADER-BECK T, VAN PUIJENBROEK AA, BOUSSIOTIS VA. 2002. Induction of immunologic tolerance for allogeneic hematopoietic cell transplantation. Leuk Lymphoma 43:1159–67.

ASAHARA T, MUROHARA T, SULLIVAN A, SILVER M, VAN DER ZEE R, LI T, WITZENBICHLER B, SCHATTEMAN G, ISNER JM. 1997. Isolation of putative progenitor endothelial cells for angiogenesis. Science 275:964–7.

ATKINSON K, DODDS A, CONCANNON A, BIGGS J. 1987. Late onset transfusion-dependent anaemia with thrombocytopenia secondary to marrow fibrosis and hypoplasia associated with chronic graft-versus-host disease. Bone Marrow Transplant 2:445–9.

AZZI A, FANCI R, CIAPPI S, ZAKRZEWSKA K, BOSI A. 1993. Human parvovirus B19 infection in bone marrow transplantation patients. Am J Hematol 44:207–9.

BARGE AJ, JOHNSON G, WITHERSPOON R, TOROK-STORB B. 1989. Antibody-mediated marrow failure after allogeneic bone marrow transplantation. Blood, 74:1477–80.

BARKER JN, WAGNER JE. 2002. Umbilical cord blood transplantation: current state of the art. Curr Opin Oncol 14:160–4.

BAVARO P, DI GIROLAMO G, OLIOSO P, PAPALINETTI G, IACONE A, ACCORSI P, DI BARTOLOMEO P. 1999. Donor lymphocyte infusion as therapy for pure red cell aplasia following bone marrow transplantation. Br J Haematol 104:930–1.

BENJAMIN RJ, CONNORS JM, MCGURK S, CHURCHILL WH, ANTIN JH. 1998. Prolonged erythroid aplasia after major ABO-mismatched transplantation for chronic myelogenous leukemia. Biol Blood Marrow Transplant 4:151–6.

BERKAHN L, KEATING A. 2004. Hematopoiesis in the elderly. Hematology 9:159–63.

BLACKLOCK HA, KATZ F, MICHALEVICZ R, HAZLEHURST GR, DAVIES L, PRENTICE HG, HOFFBRAND AV. 1984. A and B blood group antigen expression on mixed colony cells and erythroid precursors: relevance for human allogeneic bone marrow transplantation. Br J Haematol 58:267–76.

BOECKH M, HOY C, TOROK-STORB B. 1998. Occult cytomegalovirus infection of marrow stroma. Clin Infect Dis 26:209–10.

BOECKH M, LEISENRING W, RIDDELL SR, BOWDEN RA, HUANG ML, MYERSON D, STEVENS-AYERS T, FLOWERS ME, CUNNINGHAM T, COREY L. 2003. Late cytomegalovirus disease and mortality in recipients of allogeneic hematopoietic stem cell transplants: importance of viral load and T-cell immunity. Blood 101:407–14.

BOLAN CD, LEITMAN SF, GRIFFITH LM, WESLEY RA, PROCTER JL, STRONCEK DF, BARRETT AJ, CHILDS RW. 2001. Delayed donor red cell chimerism and pure red cell aplasia following major ABO-incompatible nonmyeloablative hematopoietic stem cell transplantation. Blood 98:1687–94.

BOWDEN RA, SLICHTER SJ, SAYERS MH, MORI M, CAYS MJ, MEYERS J D. 1991. Use of leukocyte-depleted platelets and cytomegalovirus-seronegative red blood cells for prevention of primary cytomegalovirus infection after marrow transplant. Blood 78:246–50.

CHILTON PM, HUANG Y, ILDSTAD ST. 2001. Bone marrow cell graft engineering: from bench to bedside. Leuk Lymphoma 41:19–34.

CHOI K, KENNEDY M, KAZAROV A, PAPADIMITRIOU JC, KELLER G. 1998. A common precursor for hematopoietic and endothelial cells. Development 125:725–32.

COHEN JI. 2000. Epstein–Barr virus infection. N Engl J Med 343:481–92.

COMOLI P, BASSO S, ZECCA M, PAGLIARA D, BALDANTI F, BERNARDO ME, BARBERI W, MORETTA A, LABIRIO M, PAULLI M, FURIONE M, MACCARIO R, LOCATELLI F. 2007. Preemptive therapy of EBV-related lymphoproliferative disease after pediatric haploidentical stem cell transplantation. Am J Transplant 7:1648–55.

CURTIS RE, TRAVIS LB, ROWLINGS PA, SOCIÉ G, KINGMA DW, BANKS PM, JAFFE ES, SALE GE, HOROWITZ MM, WITHERSPOON RP, SHRINER DA, WEISDORF DJ, KOLB HJ, SULLIVAN KM, SOBOCINSKI KA, GALE RP, HOOVER RN,

FRAUMENI JF, DEEG HJ. 1999. Risk of lymphoproliferative disorders after bone marrow transplantation: a multiinstitutional study. Blood 94:2208–16.

DALY A, SONG K, NEVILL T, NANTEL S, TOZE C, HOGGE D, FORREST D, LAVOIE J, SUTHERLAND H, SHEPHERD J, HASEGAWA W, LIPTON J, MESSNER H, KISS T. 2003. Stem cell transplantation for myelofibrosis: a report from two Canadian centers. Bone Marrow Transplant 32:35–40.

DE WEGER RA, TILANUS MG, SCHEIDEL KC, VAN DEN TWEEL JG, VERDONCK LF. 2000. Monitoring of residual disease and guided donor leucocyte infusion after allogeneic bone marrow transplantation by chimaerism analysis with short tandem repeats. Br J Haematol 110:647–53.

DEEG H, GOOLEY T, FLOWERS M, SALE G, SLATTERY J, ANASETTI C, CHAUNCEY T, DONEY K, GEORGES G, KIEM H, MARTIN P, PETERSDORF E, RADICH J, SANDERS J, SANDMAIER B, WARREN E, WITHERSPOON R, STORB R, APPELBAUM F. 2003. Allogeneic hematopoietic stem cell transplantation for myelofibrosis. Blood 102:3912–8.

DEVINE S, HOFFMAN R, VERMA A, SHAH R, BRADLOW B, STOCK W, MAYNARD V, JESSOP E, PEACE D, HUML M, THOMASON D, CHEN Y, VAN BESIEN K. 2002. Allogeneic blood cell transplantation following reduced-intensity conditioning is effective therapy for older patients with myelofibrosis with myeloid metaplasia. Blood 99:2255–8.

DITSCHKOWSKI M, BEELEN D, TRENSCHEL R, KOLDEHOFF M, ELMAAGACLI A. 2004. Outcome of allogeneic stem cell transplantation in patients with myelofibrosis. Bone Marrow Transplant 34:807–13.

DOMENECH J, ROINGEARD F, BINET C. 1997. The mechanisms involved in the impairment of hematopoiesis after autologous bone marrow transplantation. Leuk Lymphoma 24:239–56.

EAPEN M, HOROWITZ MM, KLEIN JP, CHAMPLIN RE, LOBERIZA FR, RINGDÉN, O, WAGNER JE. 2004. Higher mortality after allogeneic peripheral-blood transplantation compared with bone marrow in children and adolescents: the Histocompatibility and Alternate Stem Cell Source Working Committee of the International Bone Marrow Transplant Registry. J Clin Oncol 22:4872–80.

ELMAAGACLI AH, RUNKEL K, STECKEL N, OPALKA B, TRENSCHEL R, SEEBER S, SCHAEFER UW, BEELEN DW. 2001. A comparison of chimerism and minimal residual disease between four different allogeneic transplantation methods in patients with chronic myelogenous leukemia in first chronic phase. Bone Marrow Transplant 27:809–15.

ENRIGHT H, HAAKE R, WEISDORF D. 1990. Avascular necrosis of bone: a common serious complication of allogeneic bone marrow transplantation. Am J Med 89:733–8.

FEHSE B, CHUKHLOVIN A, KÜHLCKE, K., MARINETZ O, VORWIG O, RENGES H, KRÜGER W, ZABELINA T, DUDINA O, FINCKENSTEIN FG, KRÖGER N, KABISCH H, HOCHHAUS A, ZANDER AR. 2001. Real-time quantitative Y chromosome-specific PCR (QYCS-PCR) for monitoring hematopoietic chimerism after sex-mismatched allogeneic stem cell transplantation. J Hematother Stem Cell Res 10:419–25.

FERRAND C, PERRUCHE S, ROBINET E, MARTENS A, TIBERGHIEN P, SAAS P. 2003. How should chimerism be decoded? Transplantation 75:50S–54S.

FISCHER A, LANDAIS P, FRIEDRICH W, GERRITSEN B, FASTH A, PORTA F, VELLODI A, BENKERROU M, JAIS JP, CAVAZZANA-CALVO M. 1994. Bone marrow transplantation (BMT) in Europe for primary immunodeficiencies other than severe combined immunodeficiency: a report from the European Group for BMT and the European Group for Immunodeficiency. Blood 83:1149–54.

FLOREA AV, IONESCU DN, MELHEM MF. 2007. Parvovirus B19 infection in the immunocompromised host. Arch Pathol Lab Med 131:799–804.

FRIMBERGER AE, STERING AI, QUESENBERRY PJ. 2001. An in vitro model of hematopoietic stem cell homing demonstrates rapid homing and maintenance of engraftable stem cells. Blood 98:1012–8.

FRISCH B, BARTL R: CHAICHIK S. 1986. Therapy-induced myelodysplasia and secondary leukaemia. Scand J Haematol (Suppl 45): 38–47.

GATTER KC, CORDELL JL, TURLEY H, HERYET A, KIEFFER N, ANSTEE DJ, MASON DY. 1988. The immunohistological detection of platelets, megakaryocytes and thrombi in routinely processed specimens. Histopathology 13:257–67.

GEETHA D, ZACHARY JB, BALDADO HM, KRONZ JD, KRAUS ES. 2000. Pure red cell aplasia caused by Parvovirus B19 infection in solid organ transplant recipients: a case report and review of literature. Clin Transplant 14:586–91.

GEHLING UM, ERGÜN, S., SCHUMACHER U, WAGENER C, PANTEL K, OTTE M, SCHUCH G, SCHAFHAUSEN P, MENDE T, KILIC N, KLUGE K, SCHÄFER, B., HOSSFELD DK, FIEDLER W. 2000. In vitro differentiation of endothelial cells from AC133-positive progenitor cells. Blood 95:3106–12.

GIRALT S, ESTEY E, ALBITAR M, VAN BESIEN K, RONDÓN, G., ANDERLINI P, O'BRIEN S, KHOURI I, GAJEWSKI J, MEHRA R, CLAXTON D, ANDERSSON B, BERAN M, PRZEPIORKA D, KOLLER C, KORNBLAU S, KØRBLING M, KEATING M, KANTARJIAN H, CHAMPLIN R. 1997. Engraftment of allogeneic hematopoietic progenitor cells with purine analog-containing chemotherapy: harnessing graft-versus-leukemia without myeloablative therapy. Blood 89:4531–6.

GOODRICH JM, BOWDEN RA, FISHER L, KELLER C, SCHOCH G, MEYERS JD. 1993. Ganciclovir prophylaxis to prevent cytomegalovirus disease after allogeneic marrow transplant. An Intern Med 118:173–8.

GOOLEY TA, CHIEN JW, PERGAM SA, HINGORANI S, SORROR ML, BOECKH M, MARTIN PJ, SANDMAIER BM, MARR KA, APPELBAUM FR, STORB R, MCDONALD GB. 2010. Reduced mortality after allogeneic hematopoietic-cell transplantation. N Engl J Med 363:2091–101.

GREWAL SS, BARKER JN, DAVIES SM, WAGNER JE. 2003. Unrelated donor hematopoietic cell transplantation: marrow or umbilical cord blood? Blood 101:4233–44.

GRIFFITH LM, MCCOY JP, BOLAN CD, STRONCEK DF, PICKETT AC, LINTON GF, LUNDQVIST A, SRINIVASAN R,

LEITMAN SF, CHILDS RW. 2005. Persistence of recipient plasma cells and anti-donor isohaemagglutinins in patients with delayed donor erythropoiesis after major ABO incompatible non-myeloablative haematopoietic cell transplantation. Br J Haematol 128:668–75.

HANSPAL M. 1997. Importance of cell-cell interactions in regulation of erythropoiesis. Curr Opin Hematol 4:142–7.

HARDY CL, MEGASON GC. 1996. Specificity of hematopoietic stem cell homing. Hematol Oncol 14:17–27.

HESSLING J, KRÖGER, N., WERNER M, ZABELINA T, HANSEN A, KORDES U, AYUK F, RENGES H, PANSE J, ERTTMANN R, ZANDER A. 2002. Dose-reduced conditioning regimen followed by allogeneic stem cell transplantation in patients with myelofibrosis with myeloid metaplasia. Br J Haematol 119:769–72.

HORNY HP, WEHRMANN M, GRIESSER H, TIEMANN M, BÜLTMANN, B, KAISERLING E. 1993. Investigation of bone marrow lymphocyte subsets in normal, reactive, and neoplastic states using paraffin-embedded biopsy specimens. Am J Clin Pathol 99:142–9.

KAZAMA T, MIYAZAWA M, TSUCHIYA S, HORII A. 1996. Proliferation of macrophage-lineage cells in the bone marrow, severe thymic atrophy, and extramedullary hematopoiesis of possible donor origin in an autopsy case of post-transplantation graft-versus-host disease. Bone Marrow Transplant 18:437–41.

KEEVER-TAYLOR CA, KLEIN JP, EASTWOOD D, BREDESON C, MARGOLIS DA, BURNS WH, VESOLE DH. 2001. Factors affecting neutrophil and platelet reconstitution following T cell-depleted bone marrow transplantation: differential effects of growth factor type and role of CD34(+) cell dose. Bone Marrow Transplant 27:791–800.

KRECH R, THIELE J. 1985. Histopathology of the bone marrow in toxic myelopathy. A study of drug induced lesions in 57 patients. Virchows Arch A Pathol Anat Histopathol 405:225–35.

KURTZMAN G, FRICKHOFEN N, KIMBALL J, JENKINS DW, NIENHUIS AW, YOUNG NS. 1989. Pure red-cell aplasia of 10 years' duration due to persistent parvovirus B19 infection and its cure with immunoglobulin therapy. N Engl J Med 321:519–23.

KVASNICKA HM, THIELE J. 2004. Bone marrow angiogenesis: methods of quantification and changes evolving in chronic myeloproliferative disorders. Histol Histopathol 19:1245–60.

KVASNICKA HM, WICKENHAUSER C, THIELE J, VARUS E, HAMM K, BEELEN DW, SCHAEFER UW. 2003. Mixed chimerism of bone marrow vessels (endothelial cells, myofibroblasts) following allogeneic transplantation for chronic myelogenous leukemia. Leuk Lymphoma 44:321–8.

LACAUD G, ROBERTSON S, PALIS J, KENNEDY M, KELLER G. 2001. Regulation of hemangioblast development. An NY Acad Sci 938:96–107; discussion 108.

LAWLER M, HUMPHRIES P, MCCANN SR. 1991. Evaluation of mixed chimerism by in vitro amplification of dinucleotide repeat sequences using the polymerase chain reaction. Blood 77:2504–14.

LEE JH, LEE KH, KIM S, LEE JS, KIM SH, KWON SW, KIM WK. 2000. Anti-A isoagglutinin as a risk factor for the development of pure red cell aplasia after major ABO-incompatible allogeneic bone marrow transplantation. Bone Marrow Transplant 25:179–84.

LIESVELD JL, WINSLOW JM, KEMPSKI MC, RYAN DH, BRENNAN JK, ABBOUD CN. 1991. Adhesive interactions of normal and leukemic human CD34+ myeloid progenitors: role of marrow stromal, fibroblast, and cytomatrix components. Exp Hematol 19:63–70.

LJUNGMAN P, GRIFFITHS P, PAYA C. 2002. Definitions of cytomegalovirus infection and disease in transplant recipients. Clin Infect Dis 34:1094–7.

MADHUSUDHAN T, RICHHARIYA A, MAJUMDAR SS, MUKHOPADHYAY A. 2003. An in vitro model for grafting of hematopoietic stem cells predicts bone marrow reconstitution of myeloablative mice. J Hematother Stem Cell Res 12:243–52.

MARTINEZ-JARAMILLO G, GÓMEZ-MORALES E, SÁNCHEZ-VALLE E, MAYANI H. 2001. Severe hematopoietic alterations in vitro, in bone marrow transplant recipients who develop graft-versus-host disease. J Hematother Stem Cell Res 10:347–54.

MCCLUNE BL, WEISDORF DJ, PEDERSEN TL, TUNES DA SILVA G, TALLMAN MS, SIERRA J, DIPERSIO J, KEATING A, GALE RP, GEORGE B, GUPTA V, HAHN T, ISOLA L, JAGASIA M, LAZARUS H, MARKS D, MAZIARZ R, WALLER EK, BREDESON C, GIRALT S. 2010. Effect of age on outcome of reduced-intensity hematopoietic cell transplantation for older patients with acute myeloid leukemia in first complete remission or with myelodysplastic syndrome. J Clin Oncol 28:1878–87.

MCSWEENEY PA, NIEDERWIESER D, SHIZURU JA, SANDMAIER BM, MOLINA AJ, MALONEY DG, CHAUNCEY TR, GOOLEY TA, HEGENBART U, NASH RA, RADICH J, WAGNER JL, MINOR S, APPELBAUM FR, BENSINGER WI, BRYANT E, FLOWERS ME, GEORGES GE, GRUMET FC, KIEM HP, TOROK-STORB B, YU C, BLUME KG, STORB RF. 2001. Hematopoietic cell transplantation in older patients with hematologic malignancies: replacing high-dose cytotoxic therapy with graft-versus-tumor effects. Blood 97:3390–400.

MESSNER HA. 1998. Human hematopoietic progenitor in bone marrow and peripheral blood. Stem Cells 16 Suppl 1: 93–6.

MEYERS J, THOMAS E. 1981. *Infection Complicating Bone Marrow Transplantation*. Plenum: New York.

MEYERS JD. 1989. Prevention of cytomegalovirus infection after marrow transplantation. Rev Infect Dis 11 Suppl 7:S1691–705.

MEYERS JD, FLOURNOY N, THOMAS ED. 1982. Nonbacterial pneumonia after allogeneic marrow transplantation: a review of ten years' experience. Rev Infect Dis 4:1119–32.

MICHELSON S, ROHRLICH P, BEISSER P, LAURENT L, PERRET E, PRÉVOST MC, MONCHATRE E, DUVAL M, MAROLLEAU JP, CHARBORD P. 2001. Human cytomegalovirus infection of bone marrow myofibroblasts enhances myeloid progenitor adhesion and elicits viral transmission. Microbes Infect 3:1005–13.

Mundle S, Allampallam K, Aftab Rashid K, Danger-field B, Cartlidge J, Zeitler D, Afenya E, Alvi S, Shetty V, Venugopal P, Raza A. 2001. Presence of activation-related m-RNA for EBV and CMV in the bone marrow of patients with myelodysplastic syndromes. Cancer Lett 164:197–205.

Möhle, R., Bautz F, Rafii S, Moore MA, Brugger W, Kanz L. 1999. Regulation of transendothelial migration of hematopoietic progenitor cells. An NY Acad Sci 872:176–85; discussion 185–6.

Möhle, R., Moore MA, Nachman RL, Rafii S. 1997. Transendothelial migration of CD34+ and mature hematopoietic cells: an in vitro study using a human bone marrow endothelial cell line. Blood 89:72–80.

Ni H, Barosi G, Rondelli D, Hoffman R. 2005. Studies of the site and distribution of CD34+ cells in idiopathic myelofibrosis. Am J Clin Pathol 123:833–9.

Nilsson SK, Johnston HM, Coverdale JA. 2001. Spatial localization of transplanted hemopoietic stem cells: inferences for the localization of stem cell niches. Blood 97:2293–9.

Ottinger HD, Beelen DW, Scheulen B, Schaefer UW, Grosse-Wilde H. 1996. Improved immune reconstitution after allotransplantation of peripheral blood stem cells instead of bone marrow. Blood 88:2775–9.

Paltiel O, Cournoyer D, Rybka W. 1993. Pure red cell aplasia following ABO-incompatible bone marrow transplantation: response to erythropoietin. Transfusion 33:418–21.

Quesenberry PJ, Colvin GA, Abedi M, Lambert JF, Moore B, Demers D, Greer D, Mcauliffe C, Dooner M, Lum LG, Badiavas E, Falanga V. 2003. The marrow stem cell: the continuum. Bone Marrow Transplant 32 (suppl 1): S19–22.

Quesenberry PJ, Stewart FM, Becker P, D'Hondt L, Frimberger A, Lambert JF, Colvin GA, Miller C, Heyes C, Abedi M, Dooner M, Carlson J, Reilly J, Mcauliffe C, Stencel K, Ballen K, Emmons R, Doyle P, Zhong S, Wang H, Habibian H. 2001. Stem cell engraftment strategies. An NY Acad Sci 938:54–61; discussion 61–2.

Radich JP, Gehly G, Gooley T, Bryant E, Clift RA, Collins S, Edmands S, Kirk J, Lee A, Kessler P. 1995. Polymerase chain reaction detection of the BCR-ABL fusion transcript after allogeneic marrow transplantation for chronic myeloid leukemia: results and implications in 346 patients. Blood 85:2632–8.

Rafii S, Shapiro F, Pettengell R, Ferris B, Nachman RL, Moore MA, Asch AS. 1995. Human bone marrow microvascular endothelial cells support long-term proliferation and differentiation of myeloid and megakaryocytic progenitors. Blood 86:3353–63.

Rajantie J, Sale GE, Deeg HJ, Amos D, Appelbaum F, Storb R, Clift RA, Buckner CD. 1986. Adverse effect of severe marrow fibrosis on hematologic recovery after chemoradiotherapy and allogeneic marrow transplantation. Blood 67:1693–7.

Rich IN. 1986. A role for the macrophage in normal hemopoiesis. II. Effect of varying physiological oxygen tensions on the release of hemopoietic growth factors from bone-marrow-derived macrophages in vitro. Exp Hematol 14:746–51.

Rickinson A, Kieff E. 2007. Epstein–Barr Virus. Lippincott Williams and Wilkins, Philadelphia.

Rigolin GM, Cuneo A, Roberti MG, Bardi A, Bigoni R, Piva N, Minotto C, Agostini P, De Angeli C, Del Senno L, Spanedda R, Castoldi G. 1998. Exposure to myelotoxic agents and myelodysplasia: case-control study and correlation with clinicobiological findings. Br J Haematol 103:189–97.

Riley R, Idowu M, Chesney A, Zhao S, Mccarty J, Lamb L, Ben-Ezra J. 2005. Hematologic aspects of myeloablative therapy and bone marrow transplantation. J Clin Lab Anal 19:47–79.

Román, J., Martin, c., Torres A, Garcia, a., Andrés, p., Garcia, m. J, Baiget M. 1998. Importance of mixed chimerism to predict relapse in persistently BCR/ABL positive long survivors after allogeneic bone marrow transplantation for chronic myeloid leukemia. Leuk Lymphoma 28:541–50.

Rondelli D, Barosi G, Bacigalupo A, Prchal J, Popat U, Alessandrino E, Spivak J, Smith B, Klingemann H, Fruchtman S, Hoffman R. 2005. Allogeneic hematopoietic stem-cell transplantation with reduced-intensity conditioning in intermediate- or high-risk patients with myelofibrosis with myeloid metaplasia. Blood 105:4115–9.

Rosenthal NS, Farhi DC. 1994. Failure to engraft after bone marrow transplantation: bone marrow morphologic findings. Am J Clin Pathol 102:821–4.

Rousselet MC, Kerjean A, Guyétant S, François S, Saint-André JP, Ifrah N. 1996. Histopathology of bone marrow after allogeneic bone marrow transplantation for chronic myeloid leukaemia. Pathol Res Pract 192:790–5.

Ryder JW, Lazarus HM, Farhi DC. 1992. Bone marrow and blood findings after marrow transplantation and rhGM-CSF therapy. Am J Clin Pathol 97:631–7.

Saavedra S, Jarque I, Sanz GF, Moscardó F, Jiménez C, Martín, g., Plumé G, Regadera A, Martínez J, De la Rubia J, Acosta B, Pemán, j., Pérez-bellés, c., Gobernado M, Sanz MA. 2002. Infectious complications in patients undergoing unrelated donor bone marrow transplantation: experience from a single institution. Clin Microbiol Infect 8:725–33.

Salzberger B, Myerson D, Boeckh M. 1997. Circulating cytomegalovirus (CMV)-infected endothelial cells in marrow transplant patients with CMV disease and CMV infection. J Infect Dis 176:778–81.

Santamaria, A, Sureda A, Martino R, Domingo-Albós, A, Muñiz-Diaz E, Brunet S. 1997. Successful treatment of pure red cell aplasia after major ABO-incompatible T cell-depleted bone marrow transplantation with erythropoietin. Bone Marrow Transplant 20:1105–7.

Sawyers CL, Timson L, Kawasaki ES, Clark SS, Witte ON, Champlin R. 1990. Molecular relapse in chronic myelogenous leukemia patients after bone marrow transplantation detected by polymerase chain reaction. Proc Natl Acad Sci U S A 87:563–7.

SCHLEUNING M, JÄGER, G., HOLLER E, HILL W, THOMSSEN C, DENZLINGER C, LORENZ T, LEDDEROSE G, WILMANNS W, KOLB HJ. 1999. Human parvovirus B19-associated disease in bone marrow transplantation. Infection 27:114–7.

SCHMITZ N, BEKSAC M, HASENCLEVER D, BACIGALUPO A, RUUTU T, NAGLER A, GLUCKMAN E, RUSSELL N, APPERLEY JF, GORIN NC, SZER J, BRADSTOCK K, BUZYN A, CLARK P, BORKETT K, GRATWOHL A, TRANSPLANTATION EGFBAM 2002. Transplantation of mobilized peripheral blood cells to HLA-identical siblings with standard-risk leukemia. Blood 100:761–7.

SCHUH AC, FALOON P, HU QL, BHIMANI M, CHOI K. 1999. In vitro hematopoietic and endothelial potential of flk-1(-/-) embryonic stem cells and embryos. Proc Natl Acad Sci U S A 96:2159–64.

SCHULTE CM, BEELEN DW. 2005. Low pretransplant bone-mineral density and rapid bone loss do not increase risk for avascular osteonecrosis after allogeneic hematopoietic stem cell transplantation. Transplantation 79:1748–55.

SELLERI C, RAIOLA A, DE ROSA G, LUCIANO L, PEZZULLO L, PICARDI M, ROTOLI B. 1998. CD34+-enriched donor lymphocyte infusions in a case of pure red cell aplasia and late graft failure after major ABO-incompatible bone marrow transplantation. Bone Marrow Transplant 22:605–7.

SERRANO J, ROMAN J, SANCHEZ J, JIMENEZ A, CASTILLEJO JA, HERRERA C, GONZALEZ MG, REINA L, RODRIGUEZ MC, ALVAREZ MA, MALDONADO J, TORRES A. 2000. Molecular analysis of lineage-specific chimerism and minimal residual disease by RT-PCR of p210(BCR-ABL) and p190(BCR-ABL) after allogeneic bone marrow transplantation for chronic myeloid leukemia: increasing mixed myeloid chimerism and p190(BCR-ABL) detection precede cytogenetic relapse. Blood 95:2659–65.

SHALABY F, ROSSANT J, YAMAGUCHI TP, GERTSENSTEIN M, WU XF, BREITMAN ML, SCHUH AC. 1995. Failure of blood-island formation and vasculogenesis in Flk-1-deficient mice. Nature 376:62–6.

SHI Q, RAFII S, WU MH, WIJELATH ES, YU C, ISHIDA A, FUJITA Y, KOTHARI S, MOHLE R, SAUVAGE LR, MOORE MA, STORB RF, HAMMOND WP. 1998. Evidence for circulating bone marrow-derived endothelial cells. Blood 92:362–7.

SIMMONS PJ, MASINOVSKY B, LONGENECKER BM, BERENSON R, TOROK-STORB B, GALLATIN WM. 1992. Vascular cell adhesion molecule-1 expressed by bone marrow stromal cells mediates the binding of hematopoietic progenitor cells. Blood 80:388–95.

SLAVIN S, NAGLER A, NAPARSTEK E, KAPELUSHNIK Y, AKER M, CIVIDALLI G, VARADI G, KIRSCHBAUM M, ACKERSTEIN A, SAMUEL S, AMAR A, BRAUTBAR C, BEN-TAL O, ELDOR A, OR R. 1998. Nonmyeloablative stem cell transplantation and cell therapy as an alternative to conventional bone marrow transplantation with lethal cytoreduction for the treatment of malignant and nonmalignant hematologic diseases. Blood 91:756–63.

SOLIGO D, DELIA D, ORIANI A, CATTORETTI G, ORAZI A, BERTOLLI V, QUIRICI N, DELILIERS GL. 1991. Identification of CD34+ cells in normal and pathological bone marrow biopsies by QBEND10 monoclonal antibody. Leukemia 5:1026–30.

SORÀ F, DE MATTEIS S, PICCIRILLO N, CHIUSOLO P, LAURENTI L, PUTZULU R, LEONE G, SICA S. 2005. Rituximab for pure red cell aplasia after ABO-mismatched allogeneic peripheral blood progenitor cell transplantation. Transfusion 45:643–5.

STOREK J, WITHERSPOON RP, WEBB D, STORB R. 1996. Lack of B cells precursors in marrow transplant recipients with chronic graft-versus-host disease. Am J Hematol 52:82–9.

SÖDERBERG-NAUCLÉR, C., FISH KN, NELSON JA. 1997. Reactivation of latent human cytomegalovirus by allogeneic stimulation of blood cells from healthy donors. Cell 91:119–26.

TABATA M, KAI S, SATAKE A, WAKAE T, TODA A, CHIN M, NISHIOKA K, TANAKA H, ITSUKUMA T, YAMAGUCHI M, OKADA M, TAKATSUKA H, MISAWA M, HARA H. 2005. Relationships between hematological recovery and overall survival in older adults undergoing allogeneic bone marrow transplantation. Intern Med 44:35–40.

TAMURA S, SAHEKI K, TAKATSUKA H, WADA H, FUJIMORI Y, OKAMOTO T, TAKEMOTO Y, HASHIMOTO-TAMAOKI T, FURUYAMA J, KAKISHITA E. 2000. Early detection of relapse and evaluation of treatment for mixed chimerism using fluorescence in situ hybridization following allogeneic hematopoietic cell transplant for hematological malignancies. An Hematol 79:622–6.

TANIGUCHI S, YAMASAKI K, SHIBUYA T, ASAYAMA R, HARADA M, NIHO Y. 1993. Recombinant human erythropoietin for long-term persistent anemia after major ABO-incompatible bone marrow transplantation. Bone Marrow Transplant 12:423.

THALER J, GREIL R, DIETZE O, HUBER H. 1989. Immunohistology for quantification of normal bone marrow lymphocyte subsets. Br J Haematol 73:576–7.

THIELE J, KVASNICKA H, BEELEN D, LEDER L, SCHAEFER U. 2001a. Bone marrow engraftment: histopathology of hematopoietic reconstitution following allogeneic transplantation in CML patients. Histol Histopathol 16:213–26.

THIELE J, KVASNICKA H, BEELEN D, ZIRBES T, JUNG F, RESKE D, LEDER L, SCHAEFER U. 2000a. Relevance and dynamics of myelofibrosis regarding hematopoietic reconstitution after allogeneic bone marrow transplantation in chronic myelogenous leukemia–a single center experience on 160 patients. Bone Marrow Transplant 26:275–81.

THIELE J, KVASNICKA H, DIETRICH H, STEIN G, HANN M, KAMINSKI A, RATHJEN N, METZ K, BEELEN D, DITSCHKOWSKI M, ZANDER, A, KROEGER N. 2005. Dynamics of bone marrow changes in patients with chronic idiopathic myelofibrosis following allogeneic stem cell transplantation. Histol Histopathol 20:879–89.

THIELE J, KVASNICKA HM, BEELEN DW, FLUCKE U, SPOER C, PAPERNO S, LEDER LD, SCHAEFER UW. 2001b. Megakaryopoiesis and myelofibrosis in chronic myeloid leukemia after allogeneic bone marrow transplantation: an immunohistochemical study of 127 patients. Mod Pathol 14:129–38.

THIELE J, KVASNICKA HM, BEELEN DW, LEDER LD, SCHAEFER UW. 2001c. Bone marrow engraftment: histopathology of hematopoietic reconstitution following allogeneic transplantation in CML patients. Histol Histopathol 16:213–26.

THIELE J, KVASNICKA HM, BEELEN DW, PILGRAM B, ROSE A, LEDER LD, SCHAEFER UW. 2000b. Erythropoietic reconstitution, macrophages and reticulin fibrosis in bone marrow specimens of CML patients following allogeneic transplantation. Leukemia 14:1378–85.

THIELE J, KVASNICKA HM, BEELEN DW, WELTER A, SCHNEIDER S, LEDER LD, SCHAEFER UW. 2001d. Reconstitution of the CD45RO(+) and CD20(+) lymphoid marrow population following allogeneic bone marrow transplantation for Ph(+) CML. Bone Marrow Transplant 27:425–31.

THIELE J, KVASNICKA HM, BEELEN DW, WENZEL P, KOEPKE ML, LEDER LD, SCHAEFER UW. 2000c. Macrophages and their subpopulations following allogenic bone marrow transplantation for chronic myeloid leukaemia. Virchows Arch 437:160–6.

THIELE J, KVASNICKA HM, CZIESLICK C. 2002a. CD34+ progenitor cells in idiopathic (primary) myelofibrosis: a comparative quantification between spleen and bone marrow tissue. An Hematol 81:86–9.

THIELE J, KVASNICKA HM, SCHMITT-GRAEFF A, DIEHL V. 2003a. Bone marrow histopathology following cytoreductive therapy in chronic idiopathic myelofibrosis. Histopathology 43:470–9.

THIELE J, WICKENHAUSER C, KVASNICKA HM, VARUS E, BEELEN DW, SCHAEFER UW. 2003b. Dynamics of lineage-restricted mixed chimerism following sex-mismatched allogeneic bone marrow transplantation. Histol Histopathol 18:557–74.

THIELE J, WICKENHAUSER C, KVASNICKA HM, VARUS E, KLEPPE S, BEELEN DW, SCHAEFER UW. 2002b. Mixed chimerism of bone marrow CD34+ progenitor cells (genotyping, bcr/abl analysis) after allogeneic transplantation for chronic myelogenous leukemia. Transplantation 74:982–6.

THIELE J, WICKENHAUSER C, KVASNICKA HM, VARUS E, SCHNEIDER C, MÜLLER H, BEELEN DW. 2003c. Mixed chimerism of erythro- and megakaryopoiesis following allogeneic bone marrow transplantation. Acta Haematol 109:176–83.

TRENSCHEL R, BERNIER M, DELFORGE A, MASSY M, LEBEAU DE, HEMRICOURT E, MAEREVOET M, BADJOU R, STRYCKMANS P, BRON D. 1998. Myeloid and lymphoid recovery following allogeneic bone marrow transplantation: a comparative study between related, unrelated bone marrow and allogeneic peripheral stem cell transplantation. Leuk Lymphoma 30:325–52.

VAN DEN BERG H, KLUIN PM, VOSSEN JM. 1990. Early reconstitution of haematopoiesis after allogeneic bone marrow transplantation: a prospective histopathological study of bone marrow biopsy specimens. J Clin Pathol 43:365–9.

VAN ESSER JW, NIESTERS HG, VAN DER HOLT B, MEIJER E, OSTERHAUS AD, GRATAMA JW, VERDONCK LF, LÖWENBERG, B, CORNELISSEN JJ. 2002. Prevention of Epstein-Barr virus-lymphoproliferative disease by molecular monitoring and preemptive rituximab in high-risk patients after allogeneic stem cell transplantation. Blood 99:4364–9.

VAN LEEUWEN JE, VAN TOL MJ, BODZINGA BG, WIJNEN JT, VAN DER KEUR M, JOOSTEN AM, TANKE HJ, VOSSEN JM, KHAN PM. 1991. Detection of mixed chimaerism in flow-sorted cell subpopulations by PCR-amplified VNTR markers after allogeneic bone marrow transplantation. Br J Haematol 79:218–25.

VERHOLEN F, STALDER M, HELG C, CHALANDON Y. 2004. Resistant pure red cell aplasia after allogeneic stem cell transplantation with major ABO mismatch treated by escalating dose donor leukocyte infusion. Eur J Haematol 73:441–6.

VERMA UN, MAZUMDER A. 1993. Immune reconstitution following bone marrow transplantation. Cancer Immunol Immunother 37:351–60.

VOGT C, PENTZ S, RICH IN. 1989. A role for the macrophage in normal hemopoiesis: III. In vitro and in vivo erythropoietin gene expression in macrophages detected by in situ hybridization. Exp Hematol 17:391–7.

WAGNER HJ, CHENG YC, HULS MH, GEE AP, KUEHNLE I, KRANCE RA, BRENNER MK, ROONEY CM, HESLOP HE. 2004. Prompt versus preemptive intervention for EBV lymphoproliferative disease. Blood 103:3979–81.

WAGNER HJ, ROONEY CM, HESLOP HE. 2002. Diagnosis and treatment of posttransplantation lymphoproliferative disease after hematopoietic stem cell transplantation. Biol Blood Marrow Transplant 8:1–8.

WANG CQ, UDUPA KB, LIPSCHITZ DA. 1992. The role of macrophages in the regulation of erythroid colony growth in vitro. Blood 80:1702–9.

WHETTON AD, GRAHAM GJ. 1999. Homing and mobilization in the stem cell niche. Trends Cell Biol 9:233–8.

WICKENHAUSER C, THIELE J, PÉREZ F, VARUS E, STOFFEL MS, KVASNICKA HM, BEELEN DW, SCHAEFER UW. 2002. Mixed chimerism of the resident macrophage population after allogeneic bone marrow transplantation for chronic myeloid leukemia. Transplantation 73:104–11.

XU H, EXNER BG, CHILTON PM, TANNER MK, MUELLER YM, REZZOUG F, ILDSTAD ST. 2004. A delay in bone marrow transplantation after partial conditioning improves engraftment. Transplantation 77:819–26.

ZAIA J. 1990. Understanding Human Cytomegalovirus Infection. Wiley-Liss, New York.

Index

Non-Neoplastic Hematopathology and Infections, First Edition. Edited by Hernani D. Cualing, Parul Bhargava, and Ramon L. Sandin.
© 2012 Wiley-Blackwell. Published 2012 by John Wiley & Sons, Inc.